Illustrated Surgery

A Basic Road Map for the Postgraduates

Illustrated Surgery
A Basic Road Map for the Postgraduates

Second Edition

Nilay Mandal
MS (General Surgery)
Professor
Department of Surgery
Calcutta National Medical College and Hospital
Kolkata, West Bengal, India

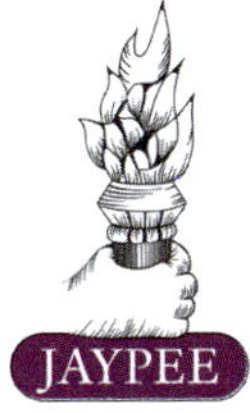

JAYPEE BROTHERS MEDICAL PUBLISHERS
The Health Sciences Publisher
New Delhi | London

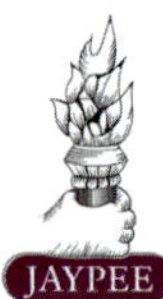

Jaypee Brothers Medical Publishers (P) Ltd

Headquarters
Jaypee Brothers Medical Publishers (P) Ltd
EMCA House, 23/23-B
Ansari Road, Daryaganj
New Delhi 110 002, India
Landline: +91-11-23272143, +91-11-23272703
+91-11-23282021, +91-11-23245672
Email: jaypee@jaypeebrothers.com

Corporate Office
Jaypee Brothers Medical Publishers (P) Ltd
4838/24, Ansari Road, Daryaganj
New Delhi 110 002, India
Phone: +91-11-43574357
Fax: +91-11-43574314
Email: jaypee@jaypeebrothers.com

Overseas Office
JP Medical Ltd.
83, Victoria Street, London
SW1H 0HW (UK)
Phone: +44 20 3170 8910
Fax: +44 (0)20 3008 6180
Email: info@jpmedpub.com

Website: www.jaypeebrothers.com
Website: www.jaypeedigital.com

Inquiries for bulk sales may be solicited at: jaypee@jaypeebrothers.com

Illustrated Surgery: A Basic Road Map for the Postgraduates

First Edition: 2016
Second Edition: **2024**

ISBN: 978-93-5696-705-2

Printed at: Sterling Graphics Pvt. Ltd. India.

Dedicated to

My teachers, students, spouse Dr Tapati, and daughter Tannistha
for their love and support

Preface to the Second Edition

"Both reading and writing are experiences—lifelong—in the course of which we who encounter words used in certain ways are persuaded by them to be brought mind and heart within the presence, the power, of the imagination."

I strongly believe that in the complexity of vast medical knowledge, every medical student needs a mentor, which may be a book or may be his/her teacher. In my short teaching experience, I have experienced that understanding of medical science in students, particularly in undergraduate students, is really lacking. They only remember the theoretical knowledge related to examination purposes, without understanding the basic sciences and pathophysiology of a disease process. In this book, I have attempted to describe the surgical diseases in such an illustrative manner so that any student can understand and remember the underlying pathophysiology of a disease process in a more lucid manner. In this edition, some of the illustrations are removed and texts are added based on the current guidelines and up-to-date informations from reliable resources. Two chapters are also added containing the do's and don'ts in surgery, important facts, classifications, etc.

UG students can also follow this book as reference towards building their concept. I hope that the book will be more of a guidebook for facing examinations as well as real clinical scenarios in everyday practice.

Wish you a happy journey.

Nilay Mandal

Preface to the First Edition

Books are the compass, telescopes, sextants, and charts which other men have prepared to help us navigate the dangerous seas of human life.

I strongly believe that in the seas of life, we all need some help at any moment from others. I also believe that in midst of seas of medical science, all medical personnel, particularly the medical students need a GPS and a philosopher. That GPS can come into his or her life in the form of a teacher or a good book or both.

In my short period of teaching, I have experienced that most of the students can remember the diseases and their management as a whole but without understanding the disease process, its pathophysiology or the principles of treatment. From my understanding, the reason is so many subjects in a too short period.

In this book, I have attempted to describe the diseases in such an illustrative manner so that the students can understand as well as recover his or her memories from the illustrations. Better understanding, not a better memory makes an average medical student to a good doctor.

As the book is based on illustrations, most of the diseases are described in an illustrative manner, less text more illustrations.

I hope that the book will be more of a guidebook for traveling in seas and mountains of medical science than a reference book. Your safe journey can only make me happy.

Wish you a happy journey.

Nilay Mandal

Acknowledgments

I am grateful to my teachers, students, and friends whose encouragement and emotional support made me courageous to do this task.

I am also indebted to my colleagues and residents in the Department of Surgery of Calcutta National Medical College, Kolkata, West Bengal, India, for their emotional and professional support.

I am also obliged to many of my students and residents, who currently occupy faculty positions in different prestigious institutions all over India.

I am also grateful to Shri Jitendar P Vij (Group Chairman), Mr Ankit Vij (Managing Director), Mr MS Mani (Group President), Ms Chetna Malhotra (Senior Director—Professional Publishing, Marketing, and Business Development), and the team of M/s Jaypee Brothers Medical Publishers (P) Ltd, New Delhi, India. I would also like to thank Mrs Pallavi Mehrotra (Development Editor) for her constant support and cooperation to complete this book.

Lastly, I am grateful to my wife Dr Tapati and my daughter Miss Tannistha for bearing with me for years during this work.

Nilay Mandal

Contents

CHAPTER 1 Wound Healing 1

CHAPTER 2 Disorders of Fluid, Electrolyte, and Acid-base Balance 16

CHAPTER 3 Hemostasis–Coagulation–Hemorrhage 30

CHAPTER 4 Gallbladder and Extrahepatic Biliary System 40

CHAPTER 5 Diseases of the Liver 107

CHAPTER 6 Diseases of Pancreas 160

CHAPTER 7 Spleen 205

CHAPTER 8 Abdominal Wall, Peritoneum, Mesentery, and Retroperitoneum 218

CHAPTER 9 Diseases of the Stomach 239

CHAPTER 10 Intestine 292

CHAPTER 11 Appendix 374

CHAPTER 12 Diseases of Rectum and Anal Canal 390

CHAPTER 13 Breast 436

CHAPTER 14 Disorders of Thyroid 487

CHAPTER 15 Parathyroid, Adrenal, Endocrine Pancreas, and MEN 532

CHAPTER 16 Trauma 570

CHAPTER 17 Burn 649

CHAPTER 18 Arterial, Venous, and Lymphatic Diseases 665

CHAPTER 19 Hernia 711

CHAPTER 20 Diseases of Testes, Scrotum, and Penis 752

CHAPTER 21 Diseases of the Esophagus 771

CHAPTER 22 Diseases of the Salivary Gland 801

CHAPTER 23 Diseases of Skin and Adnexa 816

CHAPTER 24 Ulcer, Sinus, and Fistula 841

CHAPTER 25 Urology 856

CHAPTER 26 **Minimally Invasive Surgery** 929

CHAPTER 27 **Nerve Injury** 946

CHAPTER 28 **Surgery of Hand** 954

CHAPTER 29 **Neck Swelling** 962

CHAPTER 30 **Cleft Lip and Palate** 976

CHAPTER 31 **Anesthesia** 981

CHAPTER 32 **Instrument** 994

CHAPTER 33 **Do's and Dont's in Surgery** 1018

CHAPTER 34 **Miscellaneous (Trials, Terminologies, Classification, Criteria, Scoring, Important Facts, Most Appropriate Investigations)** 1043

Index *1091*

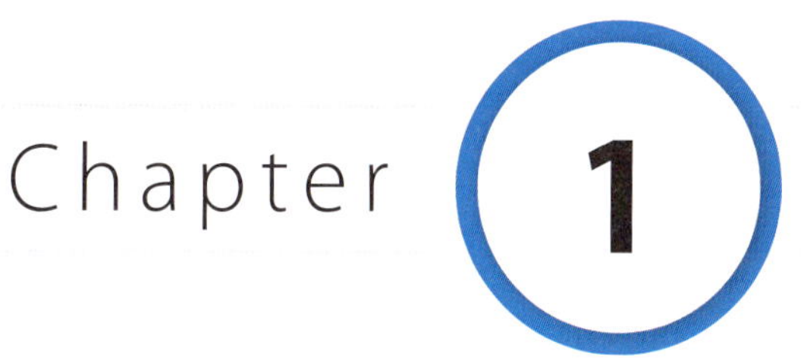

Wound Healing

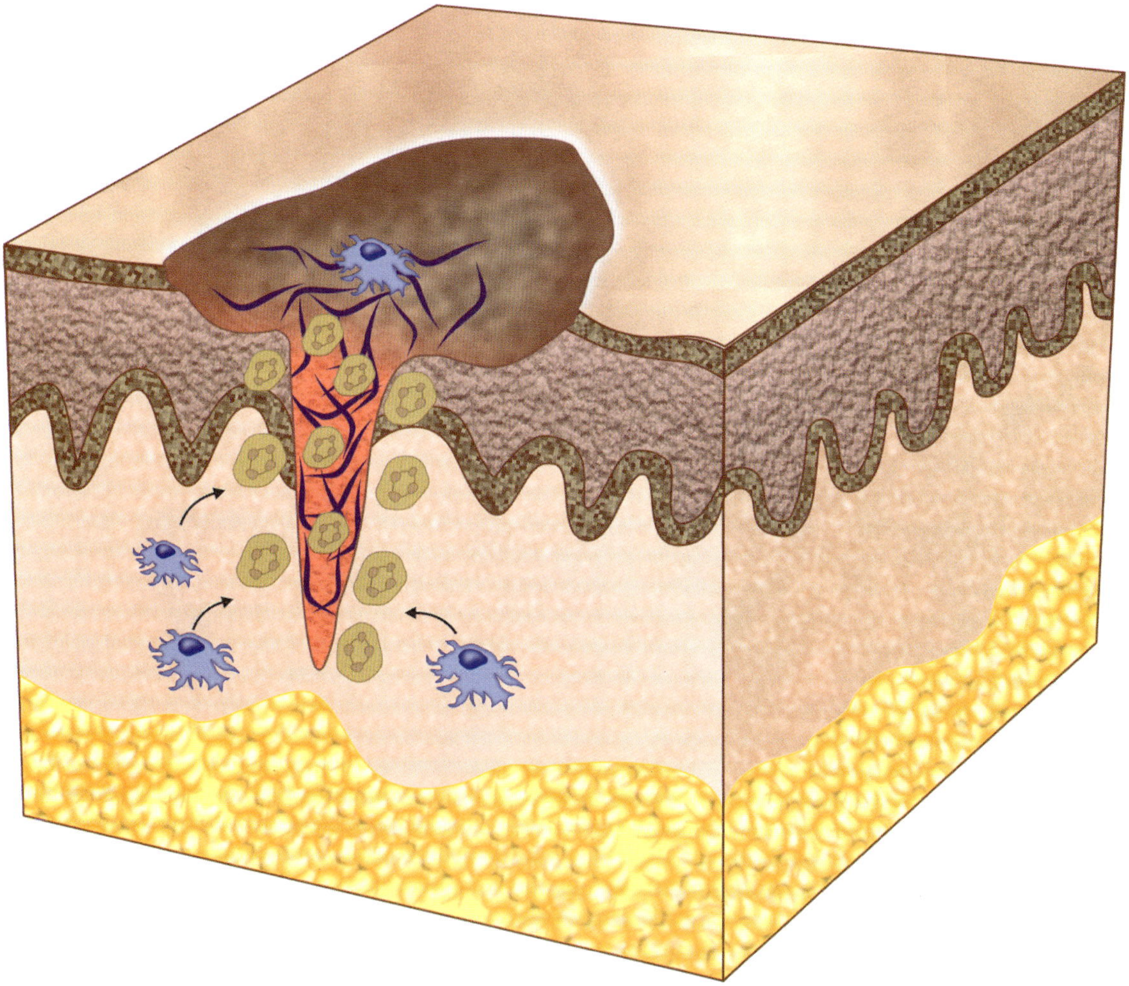

Important Topics

- Classification of Wound
- Phases of Wound Healing
- Factors Affecting Wound Healing
- Complications of Abnormal Wound Healing
- Management of Wound

'It is a most gratifying sign of the rapid progress of our time that our best textbooks become antiquated so quickly.'

Christian Albert Theodor Billroth (1829 –1894)
Austrian Surgeon

Wound Healing

Wound healing is the normal body response to injury (surgical or traumatic) to restore the normal structure and function.

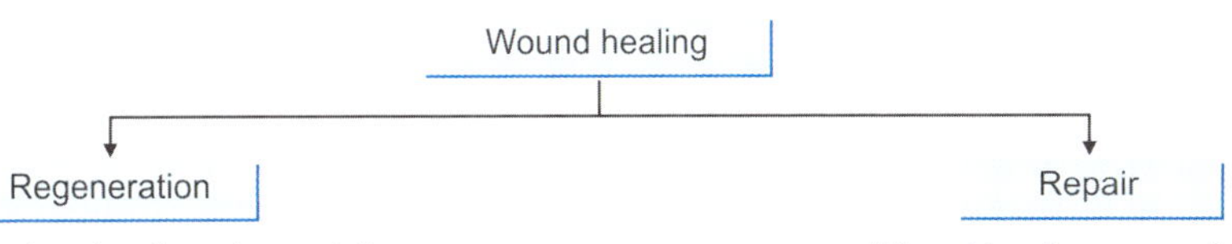

Regeneration

- Perfect restoration of preexisting tissue architecture without scar formation
- In human, regeneration process is limited to epithelium and liver

Repair

- Wound healing occurs by proliferation of connective tissues resulting in fibrosis

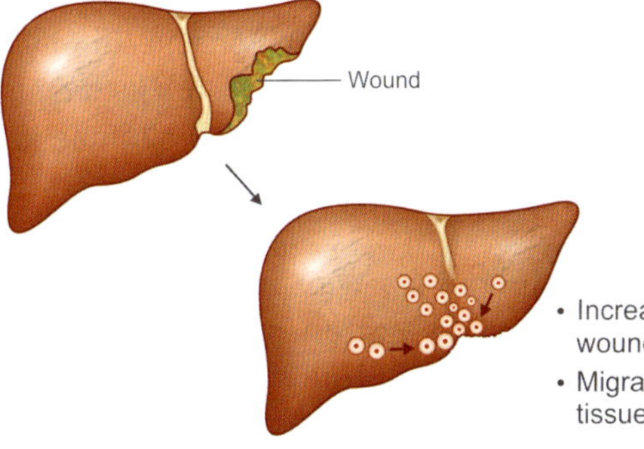

- Increased proliferation of cells in wound site
- Migration of cells into the injured tissue from normal tissue

Characteristics of healing in pediatric wound:

- Increased production of collagen and elastin during healing process.
- Granulation tissue is formed more rapidly than adults.
- Faster healing process.

Characteristics of healing in elderly population:

- Degradation and dysregulation of collagen synthesis impair tissue repair
- Progressive loss of elastic recovery of the skin.
- Slower healing process than adult wound.

Classification of Wound

Rank and Wakefield Classification of Wound

Tidy Wound	Untidy Wound
Incised	Crushed or avulsed
Clean	Contaminated
Healthy tissues	Devitalized tissues
Seldom tissue loss	Often tissue loss
Skin wounds usually single and clean cut	Skin wounds usually multiple and irregular
Fractures are uncommon	Fractures are common and may be multifragmentary
Examples: Surgical incisions, cut injury by glass pieces, knife	*Examples:* Injury from road traffic accident, blast injury, and machinery injury

Classification of Wound According to Wound Healing

Acute wound: Wound that generally proceed through an orderly and timely process of normal healing to produce a healed wound which has anatomic and functional integrity. Example: Surgical incision, incised wound by sharp objects, laceration.

Chronic wound: A wound that fails to progress healing over the normal expected healing over the normal expected healing timeframe (3–4 weeks). The healing process usually delayed in the inflammatory phase. Example: Diabetic ulcer, pressure sore.

Classification According to Integrity of the Skin

Open wound, e.g., Laceration, puncture wound

Closed wound, e.g., Contusion, hematoma

CDC Classification of Surgical Wound

Clean	An uninfected operative wound in which no inflammation is encountered and the respiratory, alimentary, genital, or uninfected urinary tracts are not entered. Operative incisional wounds that follow non-penetrating (blunt) trauma should be included in this category if they meet the criteria.
Clean-contaminated	Operative wounds in which the respiratory, alimentary, genital, or urinary tracts are entered under controlled conditions and without unusual contamination. Specifically, operations involving the biliary tract, appendix, vagina, and oropharynx are included in this category, provided no evidence of infection or major break in technique is encountered.
Contaminated	Open, fresh, accidental wound. In addition, operations with major breaks in sterile technique (for example, open cardiac massage) or gross spillage from the gastrointestinal tract, and incisions in which acute, non-purulent inflammation is encountered including necrotic tissue without evidence of purulent drainage (for example, dry gangrene) are included in this category.
Dirty or infected	Includes old traumatic wounds with retained devitalized tissue and those that involve existing clinical infection or perforated viscera.

Types of Wound Healing

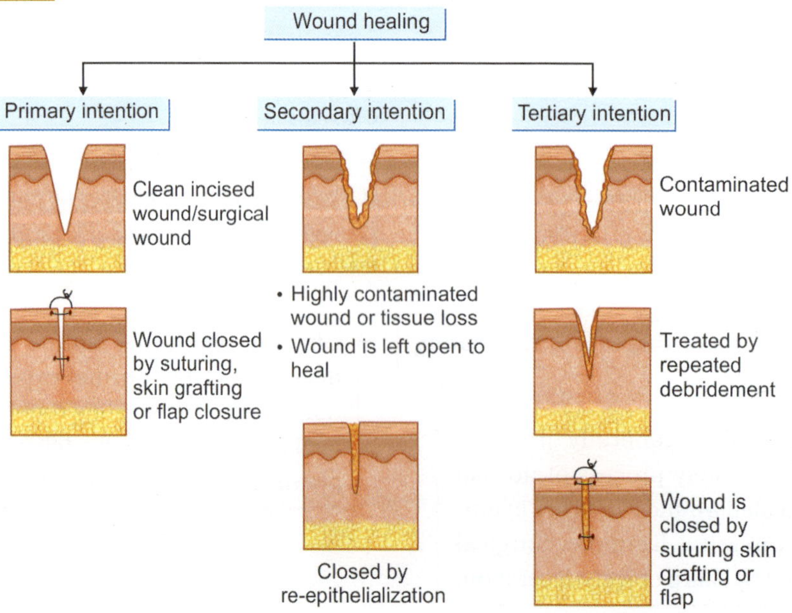

Phases of Wound Healing

Three distinct biological processes: (i) Inflammatory phase; (ii) Proliferative phase; and (iii) Maturational phase. These three phases often overlap.

Inflammatory Phase

Day 1

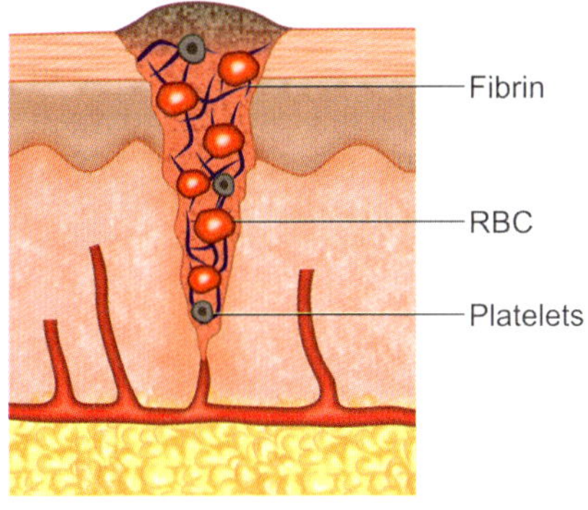

Immediately after injury, blood vessels are disrupted, resulting in exposure of subendothelial collagen to platelets, leads to platelet aggregation and activation of coagulation pathway.

The endproduct of coagulation cascade is fibrin, which plays an important role in clot formation and wound healing. This fibrin acts as scaffold for migration of PMN and monocytes into the wound. It also serves as a reservoir for cytokines.

Platelets and granulocytes release a number of substances, such as platelet derived growth factor (PDGF), transforming growth factor-β (TGF-β), fibronectin, serotonin and histamine.

Day 1–4

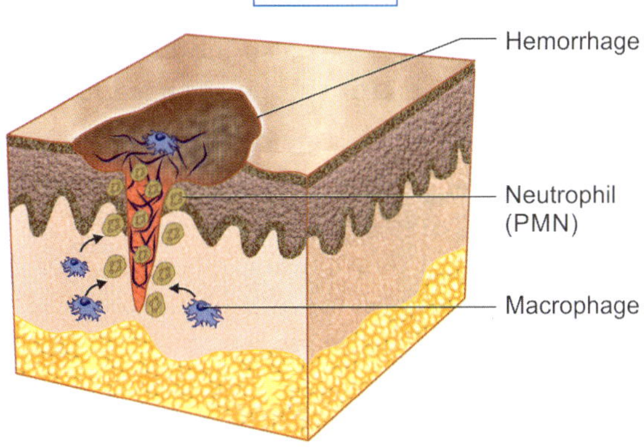

Leukocytes begin to migrate out from the vessels to the wound. The release of histamine and serotonin causes increased vascular permeability and various chemotactic factors facilitate migration.

PMNs are the first inflammatory cells to enter the wound. Increased vascular permeability and presence of chemotactic substances (e.g., IL-1, TNF-α, TGF-β, PDGF) facilitate migration of PMNs. In the first 24–48 hours, neutrophils make about 50% of all cells in the wound.

These PMNs phagocytize bacteria, foreign material and devitalized tissue. They also release TNF-α2 (an important cytokine for angiogenesis and collagen synthesis) and collagenases. Over time, neutrophils are removed by apoptosis or macrophage phagocytosis.

Macrophages start to migrate in the wound after about 48 hours of injury, and present till healing process is completed. Macrophages also participate in phagocytosis. They synthesize oxygen radical and nitric oxide, release cytokines and growth factors such as TGF-β, VEGF, Insulin-like growth factor (IGF), epithelial growth factor (EGF) and thereby regulate cell proliferation, matrix synthesis, remodeling and angiogenesis.

T-lymphocytes also migrate to the wound usually about 5–7 days after injury. They take part in wound healing by producing stimulatory cytokines (e.g., IL-2) and inhibitory cytokines (e.g., TGF-β, TNF-α).

Mast cells are also recruited in this phase. Degranulation of mast cells release histamine, TNF-α, prostaglandins and protease resulting in increased vascular permeability, cellular activation.

Proliferative Phase

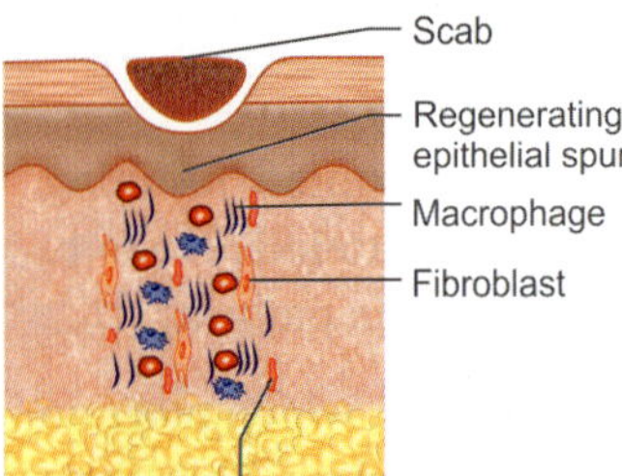

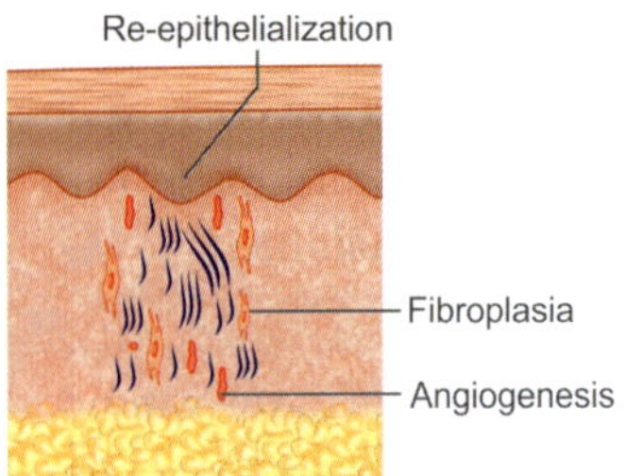

It is the second phase of healing.

This phase involves angiogenesis, fibroplasia and epithelialization, and spans from day 4 to day 12.

Angiogenesis: Endothelial cell migration, its replication and new capillary tube formation result from complex interaction of extracellular matrix material (e.g., fibronectin, hyaluronic acid) and cytokines (e.g., TGF-β, IL-8, VEGF).

The angiogenesis is regulated by TNF-α, TGF-β, VEGF, PDGF those are derived from platelets, macrophages, damaged epithelial cells. Metabolic environment of the wound also influences angiogenesis. Increased lactate, decrease pH and oxygen tension result in reduction of NAD+ inhibitor or angiogenesis.

Fibroplasia: The quiscent fibroblasts are chemoattracted to the injury site, where it replicates and proliferates, being stimulated by macrophage and platelet-derived cytokines (e.g., TGF-β, EGF, IGF-1). *PDGF is the most potent chemotactic and mitogenic factor for fibroblasts.*

The activated fibroblasts now synthesize collagen and other components of extracellular matrix (ECM). ECM consists of fibroblast-derived collagen monomer, proteoglycans and fibronectin. *Two types of collagen are important for wound repair, type I and type III.* Among them, type III collagen plays significant role. *Collagen synthesis significantly begins about 1 week postinjury.* Oxygen, vitamin C, iron are cofactors for cross-linkge of collagen fibers. Fibroblasts also produce matrix metalloproteinases (MMP) which helps to degrade matrix substances resulting in smooth migration of fibroblasts.

Epithelialization: Epithelialization of wound develops due to migration of epithelial cells from the edges of wound, mediated by EGF, TGF-β, PDGF, IGF-1.

Migration of epithelial cells occur at the rate of 1 mm/day and it begins within hours after injury. The attachments between hemidesmosomes of the basal cells and the laminin of the basal lamina are broken down, leading to migration of epithelial cells.

Re-epithelialization is completed within 48 hours in approximated incised wound.

[If epithelium and superficial dermis is only damaged, then the repair process involves re-epithelialization without any fibroplasia (no scar formation at all)]

Maturational Phase

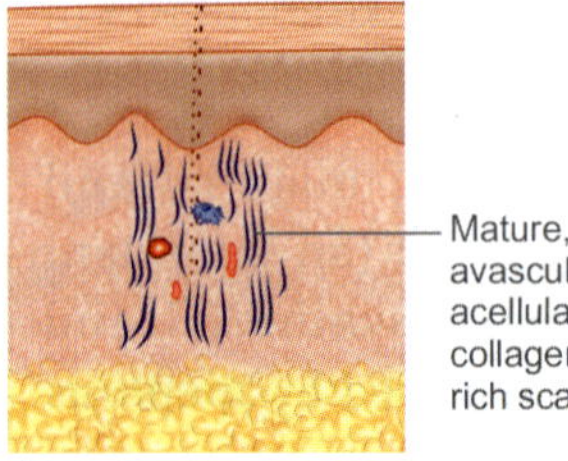

Wound contraction:

This process involves movement of the wound edge toward the center of the wound by the action of myofibroblasts. The process starts 4–5 days after injury and continues for 12–15 days. *Matrix metalloproteinases (MMPs) are important factors for wound contraction.*

Remodeling:

The process begins about 21 days after injury. Collagen synthesis is downregulated, collagen (type III) is broken down by MMPs and replaced by denser collagen (collagen I) that is organized along the lines of stress. An early wound consists of about 30% type III collagen *(uninjured connective tissue composed of 80–90% type I collagen and 10–20% type III collagen). Higher concentration of type III collagen in matrix, more weaker the wound.*

With time, the ratio of type I and III collagen changed to the ratio of intact connective tissue. Cellularity of the wound decreases. As a result, a mature, avascular, acellular collagen rich scar develops. This process reaches a steady state after 12–18 months. *By about 6 months, the wound regains 80% of the strength of an unwounded tissue.*

A well-healed wound never achieves the strength of an unwounded tissue. By 3 weeks, the tissue strength reaches 30% of original strength. After 3 months, the strength reaches the maximum, about 80% of its original strength.

Role of Growth Factors in Healing

Growth Factors	Mechanism of Action
▪ Platelet-derived growth factor (PDGF) ▪ Transforming growth factor α and β (TGF-α, TGF-β) ▪ Fibroblast growth factor (FGF) ▪ Vascular endothelial growth factor (VEGF) ▪ Granulocyte-macrophage colony-stimulating factor (GM-CSF) ▪ Insulin-like growth factor (IGF-1, IGF-2).	▪ Chemotaxis of PMNs, macrophages, fibroblasts ▪ Stimulation of angiogenesis ▪ Stimulation of fibroblasts leads to replication and proliferation ▪ Stimulation of collagen synthesis ▪ Regulation of ECM synthesis

Factors Affecting Wound Healing

Systemic Factors

Malnutrition: Normal healing process is delayed and impaired, leads to weak scar formation.

Hypoxic wound environment: Optimal collagen synthesis for wound healing requires oxygen as a cofactor.

Factors causing hypoxia in wound (e.g., cardiac failure, arterial insufficiency, excessive tension on tissue) affect proper wound healing.

Diabetes mellitus: The lack of insulin (insulin restores collagen synthesis and granulation tissue formation) and hyperglycemia (by affecting the migration and phagocytic function of inflammatory cells and proliferation of fibroblasts and endothelial cells) leads to impaired wound healing.

The micro- and macroangiopathy, associated nephropathy—All adversely affect wound healing.

Diabetic wound also lacks adequate growth factors.

Chronic renal and hepatic disease: Decreased collagen synthesis leads to weak scar formation.

Collagen vascular disease: The disease itself as well as medications are responsible for impaired inflammatory cell migration and collagen deposition.

Smoking: Impairs wound healing by causing cutaneous vasoconstriction, nicotine impairs collagen synthesis.

Steroids and antineoplastic drugs: Steroids inhibit the inflammatory phase of wound healing. It impairs collagen synthesis, inhibit epithelialization and wound contraction. Antineoplastic drugs impair proliferation of fibroblasts as well as inhibit the inflammatory phase of wound healing.

Vitamin and mineral deficiency: Vitamin C deficiency leads to failure in collagen synthesis as well as crosslinking.

Vitamin A increases the inflammatory responses after injury increases the migration of macrophages, helps its activation. It also increases collagen synthesis.

Vitamin A can restore wound healing that are impaired by diabetes, radiation, cyclophosphamide.

Zinc deficiency leads to decreased fibroblast proliferation, delayed epithelialization, decreased collagen synthesis.

Local Factors

Infection: Presence of infection delays wound healing. Infection alters the effects of cytokines, leads to delayed healing.

Wound hypoxia: Local damage to the vessels following trauma, edema around the wound, excessive tension due to suturing lead to wound hypoxia.

Hypoxia leads to impaired fibroblast proliferation and collagen synthesis.

Edema: Leads to increased tendency to skin breach and development of infection.

Ionizing radiation: Leads to abnormal wound healing.

Chemical agents: Chlorhexidine or povidone-iodine *impairs inflammatory cell migration, leads to delayed wound healing.*

Factors Associated with Delayed or Impaired Wound Healing

Local Factors	Systemic Factors
▪ Hypoxia ▪ Infection/contamination ▪ Inflammation ▪ Devitalized or necrotic tissue ▪ Mechanical stress or trauma ▪ Presence of foreign body	▪ Older age ▪ Chronic disease/comorbidity ▪ Immunosuppression ▪ Malnutrition ▪ Connective tissue disorders ▪ Radiation therapy ▪ Medications (e.g., steroids) ▪ Vascular insufficiency

Complications of Abnormal Wound Healing

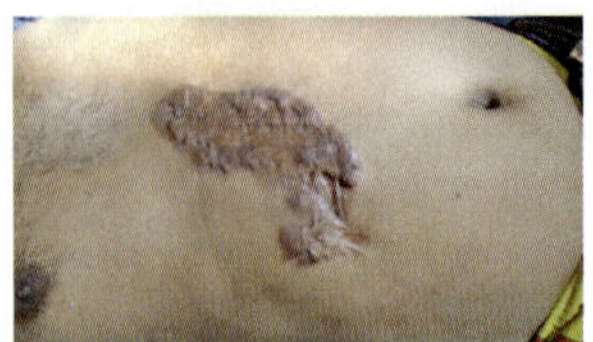
Keloid formation in open cholecystectomy scar.

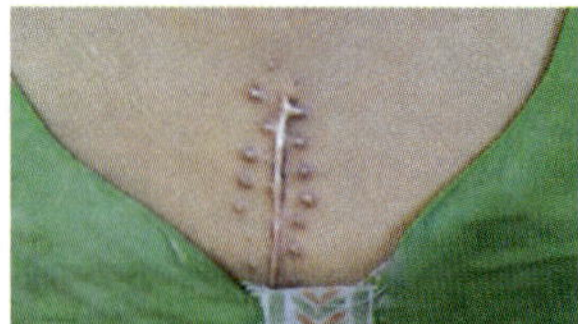
Hypertrophied scar in sternotomy wound.

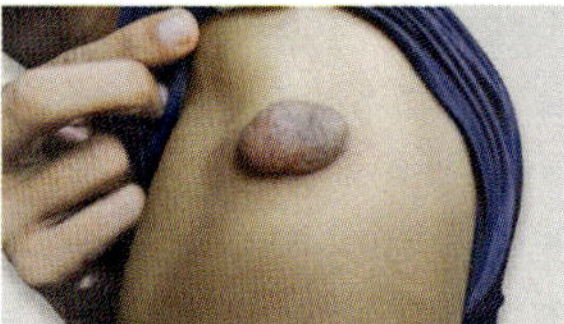
Keloid over the deltoid region.

Poor alignment: When a wound crossed the definite anatomical structure such as vermilion border of lip, without proper alignment during repair, defect in alignment develops.
Contracture: If a linear wound crosses flexor creases vertically, there is development of scar contracture. Deep and extensive burn scar also causes scar contracture.
Altered pigmentation: Most of the scars are hypopigmented. Hyperpigmentation may also occur.
Tattooing: Dirt or soot particles may become implanted in untidy wounds and results in tattooing of scar.
Abnormal skin scar: (i) Hypertrophied scar and (ii) Keloid.
Chronic nonhealing wound, e.g., diabetic ulcer, pressure sore.

Excessive or unaesthetic scar may develop following:
- Surgery
- Burn
- Trauma
- Infection

Different Scar Scale

- Vancouver Scar Scale (VSS)
- Manchester Scar Scale (MSS)
- Patient and Observer Scar Assessment Scale (POSAS)
- Visual Analog Scale (VAS)
- Stony Brook Scar Evaluation Scale (SBSES)

Common Types of Collagen

TYPE I	Skin, bone, scar tissue
TYPE II	Hyaline cartilage
TYPE III	Cardiovascular structures, infant skin, granulation tissue of healing skin wound, scar tissue
TYPE IV	Basement membrane
TYPE V	Basement membrane

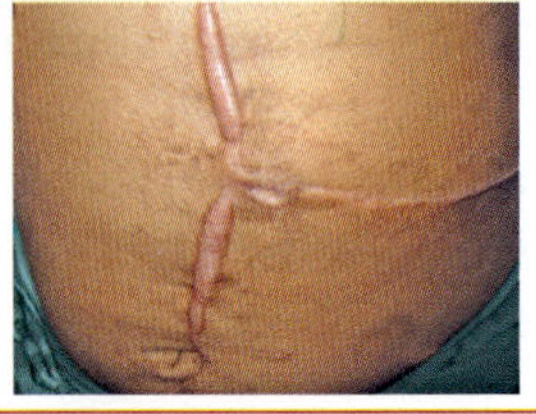

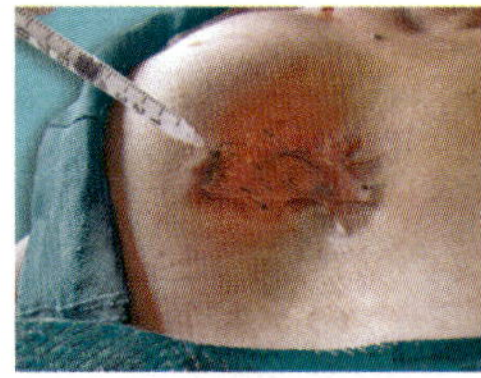

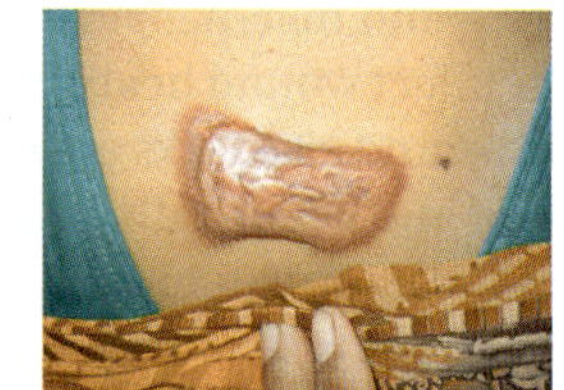

Hypertrophied Scar

- Abnormal skin scar that confines of the original wound.
- Both increased collagen production and collagen breakdown, but the final result is excess collagen in tissue.
- Stretched collagen bundles are aligned in same plane of epidermis, whereas the collagen bundles are randomly arranged and relaxed in normal scar.
- More cellular and vascular than normal scar, also contains aggregates of abundant fibroblasts, vessels, and collagen fibers.
- A hypertrophic scar can develop anywhere in the body and frequently regress spontaneously

Preventive Options for Hypertrophic Scar and Keloids

- Silicone therapy (Silicone sheets and silicone gels)
- Pressure garments
- Avoiding exposure to sunlight
- Continued use of sunscreens with a high to maximum sun protection factor (>50) until scar has matured.

Keloid

- Keloids are proliferative scar that grows beyond the limits of the wound.
- Thicker, more abundant stretched collagen bundles aligned in the same place of the epidermis, as well as acellular.
- Rarely regress spontaneously.
- Genetic predisposition is present.
- More common in darker-pigmented peoples—African and Asian population.
- May develop after surgery, burn, tattoos, ear piercing.
- Certain body parts have increased tendency of keloid formation—presternal, deltoid, earlobe, upper back.

Treatment Options for Abnormal Scars

NONINVASIVE TREATMENT

- Silicone sheets and gels
- Pressure garments
- Massage therapy
- Static and dynamic splints

INVASIVE TREATMENT

- Intralesional corticosteroid injection
- Surgical scar correction and postoperative radiotherapy
- Laser therapy
- Cryosurgery
- Intralesional injection of bleomycin or 5-flurouracil or verapamil

Intralesional Corticosteroid

Most commonly used corticosteroid is triamcinolone acetonide (10–40 mg/mL).

Injected into the papillary dermis every 2–4 weeks until the scar is flattened.

Side effects: (i) Noncompliance (due to pain); (ii) Hypopigmentation; (iii) Atrophy; and (iv) Telangiectasias.

Silicone sheets and gels, pressure garments and Intralesional corticosteroid injection are the evidence-based and recommended treatment for hypertrophic scar and keloids.

Malignant Wound

Mechanisms of wound formation: Tumor cells invade the epithelium, penetrate the epidermis, causing tissue death and necrosis.

Cancers most likely cause malignant wound: (i) Breast cancer; (ii) Head-neck cancer; and (iii) Primary skin malignancies.

Symptoms related to malignant wound: (i) Malodor; (ii) Pain; (iii) Exudate; (iv) Bleeding; and (v) Infection.

Psychological aspects: (i) Body image alteration; (ii) Depression; (iii) Embarassment; (iv) Social isolation; and (v) Problem in sexual relation.

Management of malodor: Bacterial bioburden (mostly anaerobes) is most likely the cause of malodor in malignant fungating wound.

- Topical metronidazole—as gel form
- Crushed metronidazole tablet sprinkled into the wound bed once daily under a nonadherent dressing (e.g. Vaseline gauze) or absorbent foam
- Silver-containing dressings (nanocrystalline silver)
- Honey-based dressing
- Activated charcoal

Management of pain:

- Systemic opiods
- Topical opiods

Management of bleeding:

- Atraumatic dressing change
- Use of nonadherent dressing or nonstick gauze
- Standard hemostatic agent (e.g., Tranexamic acid)
- Thrombin or fibrin spray
- Oxymetazoline nasal spray

Management of Wound

- *Assessment of the patient:* About diabetes mellitus, vascular disorders, drug history, nutritional status
- Assessment of wound
- Wound bed preparation
- Diagnosis of wound infection and management
- Management of biofilm
- Management of wound pain
- Wound cleansing
- Wound dressing
- Adjunctive therapies

Wound Assessment

- Type of wound
- Site and size of the wound
- Etiology
- Condition of the wound bed
- Condition of the wound edge (maceration, dehydration, undermining, rolled) and periwound skin (maceration, excoriation, dry skin, hyperkeratosis, eczema)
- Duration
- Exudate
- Presence of infection

Adjunctive therapies

- Negative pressure wound therapy (NPWT)
- Negative pressure wound therapy with instillation (NPWTi)
- Larval therapy
- Hyperbaric oxygen therapy

Aim of Wound Bed Preparation

- Optimize the wound bed by reducing edema and exudates
- Reducing the bacterial burden
- Correcting the abnormalities contributing to impaired healing

Periwound Skin Protectants

- Petroleum jelly based ointment
- Zinc oxide plus petroleum jelly ointment
- Silicone-based barrier preparations
- Cyanoacrylate formulations
- Alcohol-free barrier film

Wound Exudate

Wound exudate is a normal part of healing.

Exudate helps in the healing process by following mechanisms:

- Provides a moist wound environment.
- Acts as a medium for migration of tissue-repairing cells across wound bed.
- Enables diffusion of immune mediators and growth factors across wound bed.
- Promotes separation of dead or damaged tissue.

Exudate impairs wound healing when it is in wrong amount and of wrong composition.

Types of Wound Exudates

- Serous
- Sanguineous
- Serosanguineous
- Purulent
- Seropurulent
- Hemopurulent
- Hemorrhagic
- Fibrinous

Composition of Exudates

Water	Immune cells	Microorganisms
Fibrin	Protein (albumin, globulin, fibrinogen)	Metabolic waste products
Glucose	Growth factors	Dead cells
Platelets	Proteases	

Wounds with High Level of Exudates	Wounds with Low Level of Exudates
Venous leg ulcer	Ischemic ulcer
Malignant fungating wound	Neuropathic diabetic foot ulcer
Burn	
Dehisced wound	
Rheumatoid ulcer	

Wound infection

Classic Signs of Local Infection	Stages of Wound Infection
▪ Erythema ▪ Increased local temperature ▪ Increasing pain ▪ Increasing malodor ▪ Swelling ▪ Purulent discharge	**Contamination** (presence of non-proliferating organisms within a wound) ↓ **Colonization** (presence of microorganisms within a wound with limited proliferation) ↓ **Local infection** (proliferation of microorganisms causing host reaction) ↓ **Spreading infection** (infection spreads into surrounding tissues) ↓ **Systemic infection** (infection associated with systemic inflammatory response, sepsis, and organ dysfunction)

Factors Associated with Increased Risk of Wound Infection

Patient-related Factors	Wound-related Factors
Uncontrolled or poorly controlled diabetes	Contaminated or dirty wounds
Immunocompromised state (e.g. malignancy, AIDS)	Pre-existing infection
Prior radiation therapy or chemotherapy	Presence of necrotic tissue
Inappropriate antibiotic prophylaxis	Presence of foreign body
Alcohol or drug abuse	Hematoma formation
	Spillage from GI tract
	Anatomically near to a site of potential contamination (e.g., Perineum)

Wound debridement

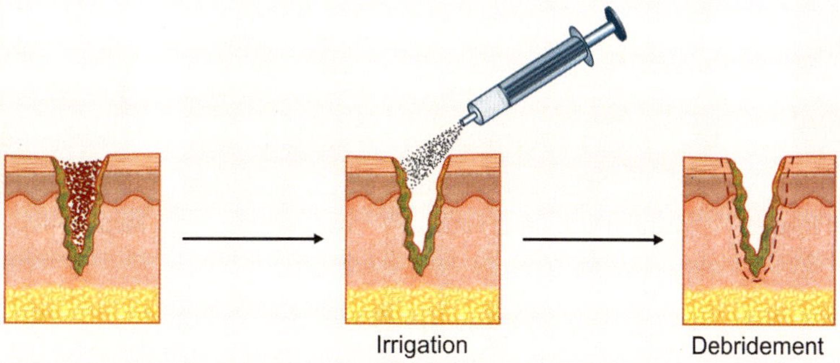

Irrigation

Debridement

Methods of Wound Debridement

SURGICAL	Non-viable tissues are excised by sharp instruments in OT setup to achieve bleeding wound bed.
MECHANICAL	Swab or cotton gauze is used to detach devitalized tissue from wound bed.
ENZYMATIC	Enzymes or chemicals (e.g. Alginogel, enzymatic debriders) are used to soften the devitalized tissues.
LARVAL	Green bottle fly larvae are placed in the wound, larvae ingest devitalized tissues and microorganisms.
ULTRASONIC	Ultrasound energy is used to break-up devitalized tissues.
HYDROSURGICAL	A high-pressure jet of saline is used.
AUTOLYTIC	Slow debridement aided by topical agents (e.g. Cadexomer iodine, honey, etc.)

Wound Dressing

Low-to-moderate exuding wounds	Moderate-to-high exuding wounds	Wounds with eschar, necrotic tissue	Wounds with slough	Dry to low exuding granulating wound	Moderate-to-high exuding granulating wound	Infected or colonized wound
Hydrocolloids	Alginates	Hydrogel, covered by secondary dressing	Alginates	Hydrogel	Alginates	Cadexomer iodine
Hydrogel	Carboxymethyl-cellulose (CMC)	Honey covered by secondary dressing	Hydrocolloids	Low adherent (silicone) dressing	Foam	Silver nanoparticles
Honey	Foams		Hydrogel		CMC	Polyhexamethylene biguanide
Low adherent wound contact layer (silicone)			Honey			
			Polymeric membrane dressings			

Characteristics of Ideal Dressing

- Cost effective
- Permeable to gases and water vapor
- Impermeable to microorganisms
- Comfortable
- Nonirritant
- Minimal pain during change of dressing

Vacuum Assisted Closure (VAC) Therapy

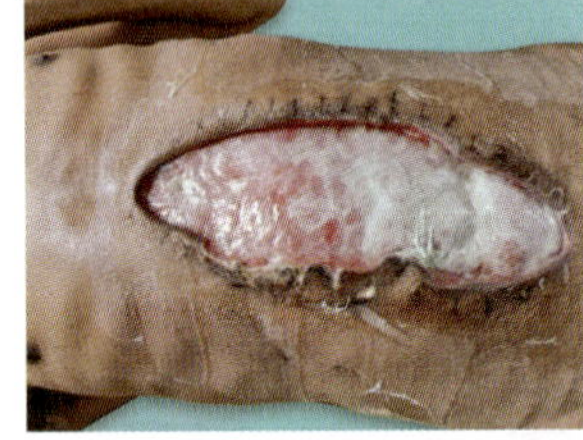

Wound before application of negative pressure wound therapy (NPWT).

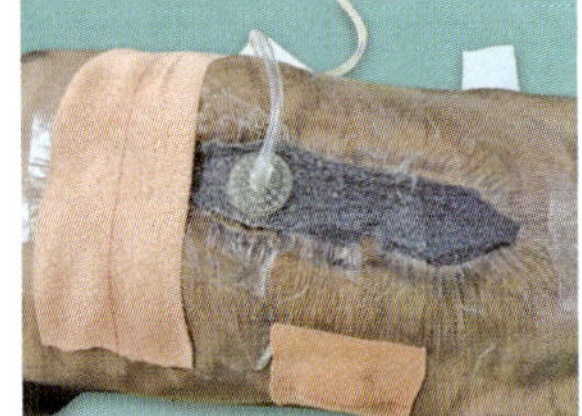

Wound is treating with NPWT.

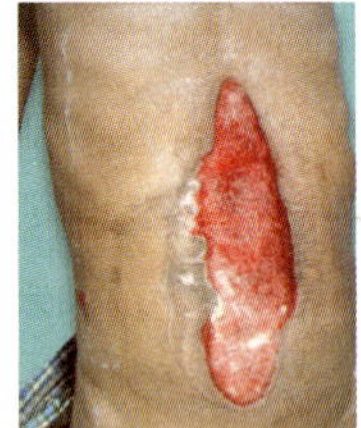

Wound after 5 days of NPWT.

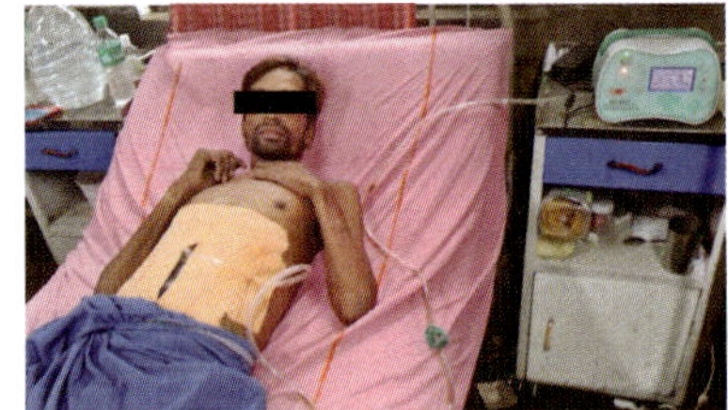

Vacuum-assisted closure (VAC) or negative pressure wound therapy (NPWT)

Mode of Action

- Physical barrier to external contamination
- Remove excess wound exudates
- Facilitate moist wound healing
- Improve tissue perfusion
- Reduce periwound edema
- Formation of granulation tissue
- Wound contraction
- Improves lymphatic drainage

Indications

- Wounds that are failing to heal despite optimal treatment
- Highly exuding wounds
- Non-infected, non-ischemic, deep complex diabetic foot ulcers
- Non-infected inflammatory ulcers (secondary to scleroderma, SLE, rheumatoid arthritis)
- Stage 3 and 4 pressure ulcers
- Dehisced sternal wound following cardiac surgery
- Open abdominal wound
- Complex traumatic wounds

Components of VAC System

(i) Black, hydrophobic polyurethane foam with open pores or white, hydrophilic polyvinyl alcohol foam dressing with denser, smaller pores- introduced into the wound; (ii) Transparent, semi-occlusive adhesive drape-secured over the foam dressing to the healthy skin around the wound margin; (iii) A pad attached to a drainage tube is placed over a small hole cut into the drape. End of the drainage tube is connected to the suction source; (iv) Electrically powered unit- creates negative pressure (- 125 mm Hg); (v) Disposable reservoir- wound fluid is collected under negative pressure; and (vi) A microprocessor- detects any alteration in negative pressure or air leak and triggers an alarm.

Factors Related to Good Response to VAC Therapy

- Healthy, granular wound bed
- Wound size >2 cm wide
- Freshly debrided wound
- Wound with high level of exudates
- Well-perfused wound
- Non-infected wound
- Patient with minimal comorbidities
- Early commencement of VAC therapy

Contraindications to VAC Therapy

- Enteric, non-enteric and unexplored fistula
- Malignant wound
- Wound with eschar and necrotic tissue
- Exposed blood vessels, nerves, bowel
- Untreated osteomyelitis
- Patients with high risk for bleeding

Assessment of Treatment

Within one week of VAC therapy, evidence of granulation tissue arises in a well-perfused wound. Wound area is reduced around 15% after one or two weeks. Also, a beefy, granular appearance of wound bed suggest positive outcome of VAC therapy. If increased inflammation of wound margins after VAC therapy, therapy have to discontinued.

Case 1

History and Physical Examination

A 16-year-old female patient presented in the surgical outpatient department with a swelling in her left ear lobe for last 6 months. Patient had history of ear piercing in her both earlobe 1 year back. Initially, it was small, but now it becomes increasing, and patient was concerned due to cosmesis. She was advised to take opinion from surgeon. Her only significant past history was ear piercing 1 year back.

On clinical examination, the swelling was non-tender, rubbery in consistency, dumb-bell shaped, 2.0 cm in diameter, on the lower part of the helix of left ear. A small swelling was also present on the site of ear piercing on right side.

Diagnosis

Clinical diagnosis was keloid. Keloid is primarily a clinical diagnosis. There is no role of biopsy or imaging for confirmation of diagnosis.

Discussion

In history: Ear piercing of both ear 1 year back and appearance of swelling after 6 months of ear piercing.
On clinical examination: Swelling at the site of ear piercing, rubbery in consistency, growth beyond wound margins.
Both history and clinical findings are in favor of diagnosis of keloid.

Management Algorithm

- Intralesional corticosteroid is one of the recommended treatments. Triamcinolone acetonide injection 2 weeks interval till the swelling decreasing in size or flattened.
- Other treatment options like silicon sheets and gels, surgical scar correction and postoperative radiotherapy, etc. are available, but they are not cost-effective as compared to intralesional corticosteroid.
- Only surgical excision is not preferred as it is associated with high chance of recurrence.

Case 2

History and Clinical Examination

A 55-year-old male patient presented in the surgical outpatient department with a nonhealing ulcer in the right foot for last 4 months. Patient had a history of nail prick following which wound infection developed. No history suggestive of intermittent claudication or rest pain was present. Patient was treated with oral antibiotics, but response was not satisfactory. Patient was taking oral anti-diabetics for last 5 years. He was a chronic smoker for last 20 years.

Physical Examination
Patient is alert, conscious, cooperative
Temperature: 101°F
Pulse: 96/min; BP: 146/90 mm Hg

Examination of the Lower Limb
The left lower limb is normal. On the right foot, a 4 cm × 5 cm ulcer with eschar and necrotic tissues was present on the dorsolateral aspect. Structural deformity of the right foot was evident without any sensory neuropathy. No blackish discoloration or frank gangrenous changes was present. Peripheral pulses are palpable in both lower limbs.

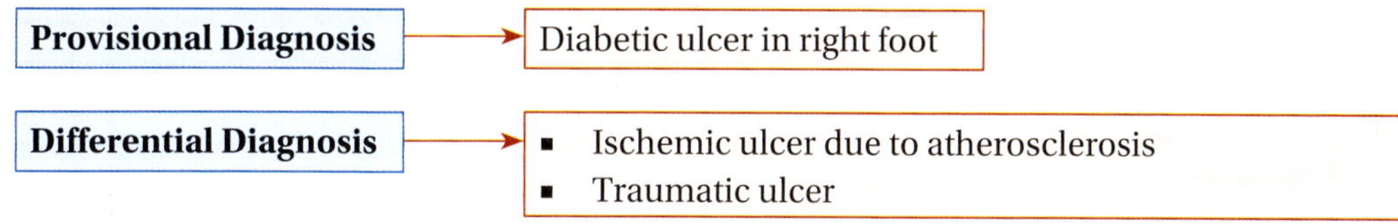

Provisional Diagnosis → Diabetic ulcer in right foot

Differential Diagnosis →
- Ischemic ulcer due to atherosclerosis
- Traumatic ulcer

Investigations

Hb: 10.2 gm%, total leukocyte count: 17,000/cumm, Fasting blood sugar: 224 mg/dL, PPBS: 326 mg/dL, HbA1c: 8.5, Serum creatinine: 1.2 mg/dL, lipid profile—within normal range.
Doppler USG of arterial system of both lower limbs: Mild atherosclerotic changes in both lower limbs with triphasic flow pattern.

Discussion

History of taking oral anti-diabetics for last 5 years and laboratory findings (FBS, PPBS, HbA1c) are suggestive of diabetes, particularly uncontrolled diabetes. History (no history of intermittent claudication or rest pain), physical examination (no gangrenous changes, peripheral pulses are palpable), and Doppler imaging excludes peripheral occlusive arterial disease.

Management Algorithm

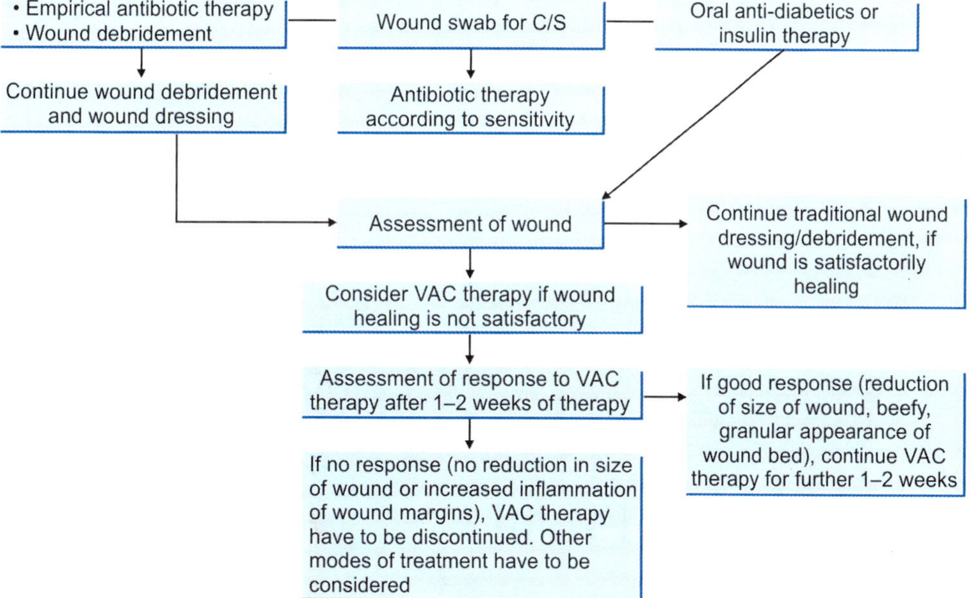

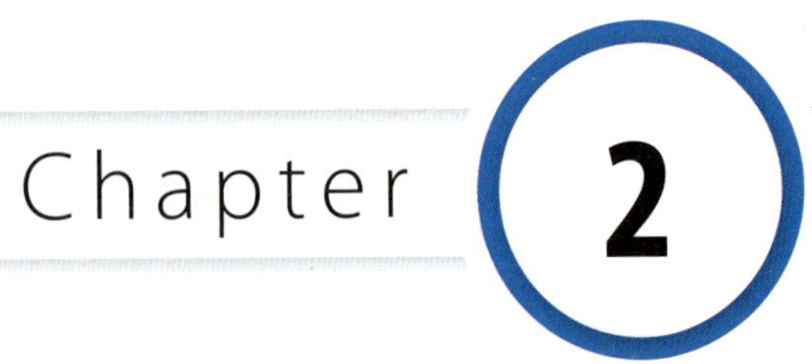

Disorders of Fluid, Electrolyte, and Acid-base Balance

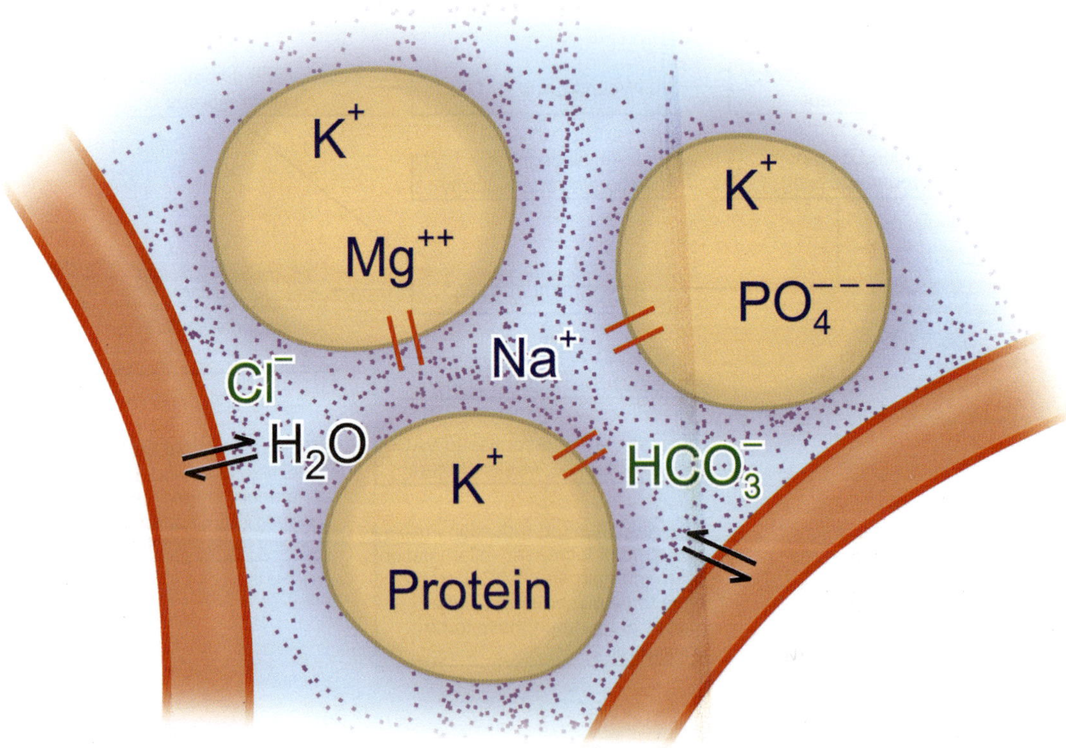

Important Topics

- Composition of Total Body Water
- Disturbances in Fluid Balance and its Management
- Electrolyte Imbalance and its Management
- Acid-base Imbalance and its Management
- Crystalloids and Colloids and their Composition

'There is a strange disparity between the sciences of inert matter and those of life. Astronomy, mechanics, and physics are based on concepts which can be expressed, tersely and elegantly, in mathematical language. ....Those who investigate the phenomena of life are as if lost in an inextricable jungle, in the midst of a magic forest, ... but are incapable of defining in algebraic equations.'

Alexis Carrel (1873 – 1944)
French-born American Surgeon

Total Body Water

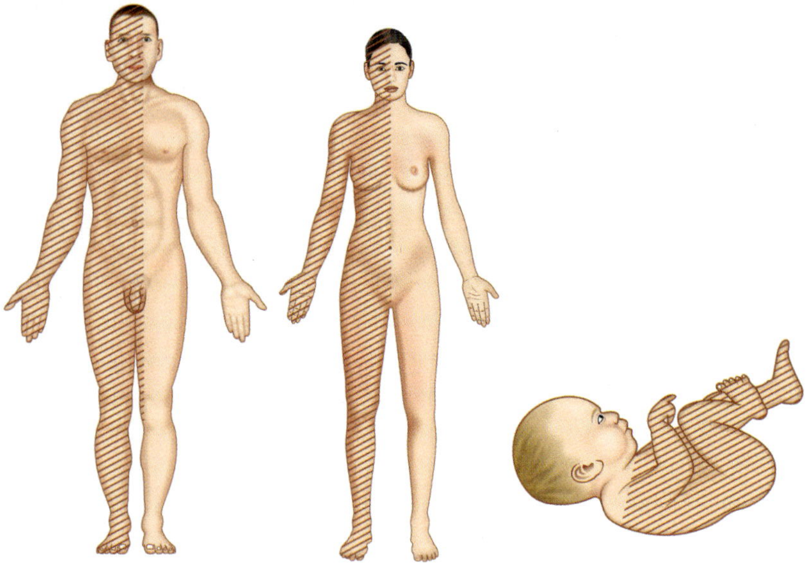

60% 50% 80%

- 50–60% of total body weight.
- Muscles and solid organs have higher water content than fat and bones.
- **In male:** TBW is 60% of total body weight.
- **In female:** TBW is about 50% of total body weight (higher adipose tissue and less muscle mass).
- **In newborn:** TBW is about 80% of total body weight.

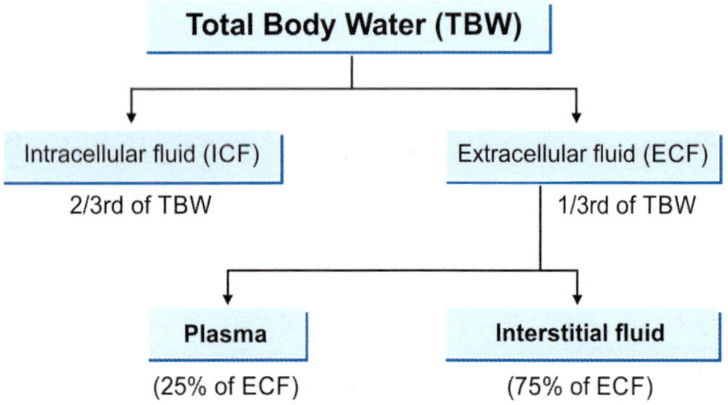

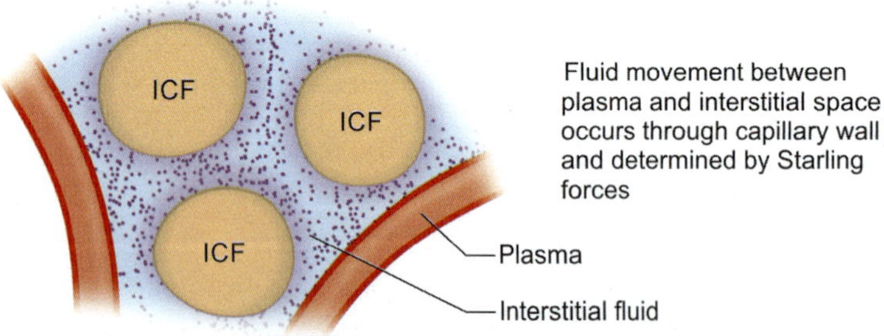

Total Body Water (TBW)
Intracellular fluid (ICF)
2/3rd of TBW
Extracellular fluid (ECF)
1/3rd of TBW
Plasma
(25% of ECF)
Interstitial fluid
(75% of ECF)

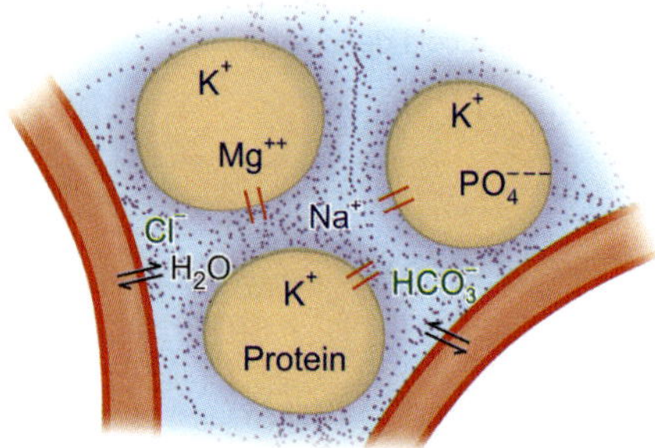

K+
Mg++
Na+
K+
PO4---
Cl-
H2O
K+
Protein
HCO3-

ICF
ICF
ICF
Fluid movement between plasma and interstitial space occurs through capillary wall and determined by Starling forces
Plasma
Interstitial fluid

- Composition of plasma and interstitial fluid are same.
- Major ions in ECF are Na^+, Cl^-, and HCO_3^-.
- Major ion in ICF is K^+.
- More protein in plasma.
- Different transporters, channels, and ATP-driven pumps maintain the specific composition of each compartment.
- Water is freely diffusible, whereas movements of ions and proteins are restricted through the fluid compartments.

Equivalent (Eq) = Atomic weight (g)/Valence

Miligram (mg) = (Miliequivalent (mEq) × Atomic weight)/Valence

Miliequivalent (mEq) = (mg × Valence)/Atomic weight

Milimole (mmol) = mEq × Valence

1 mEq = 1 mmol (for univalent ions)

2 mEq = 1 mmol (for bivalent ions)

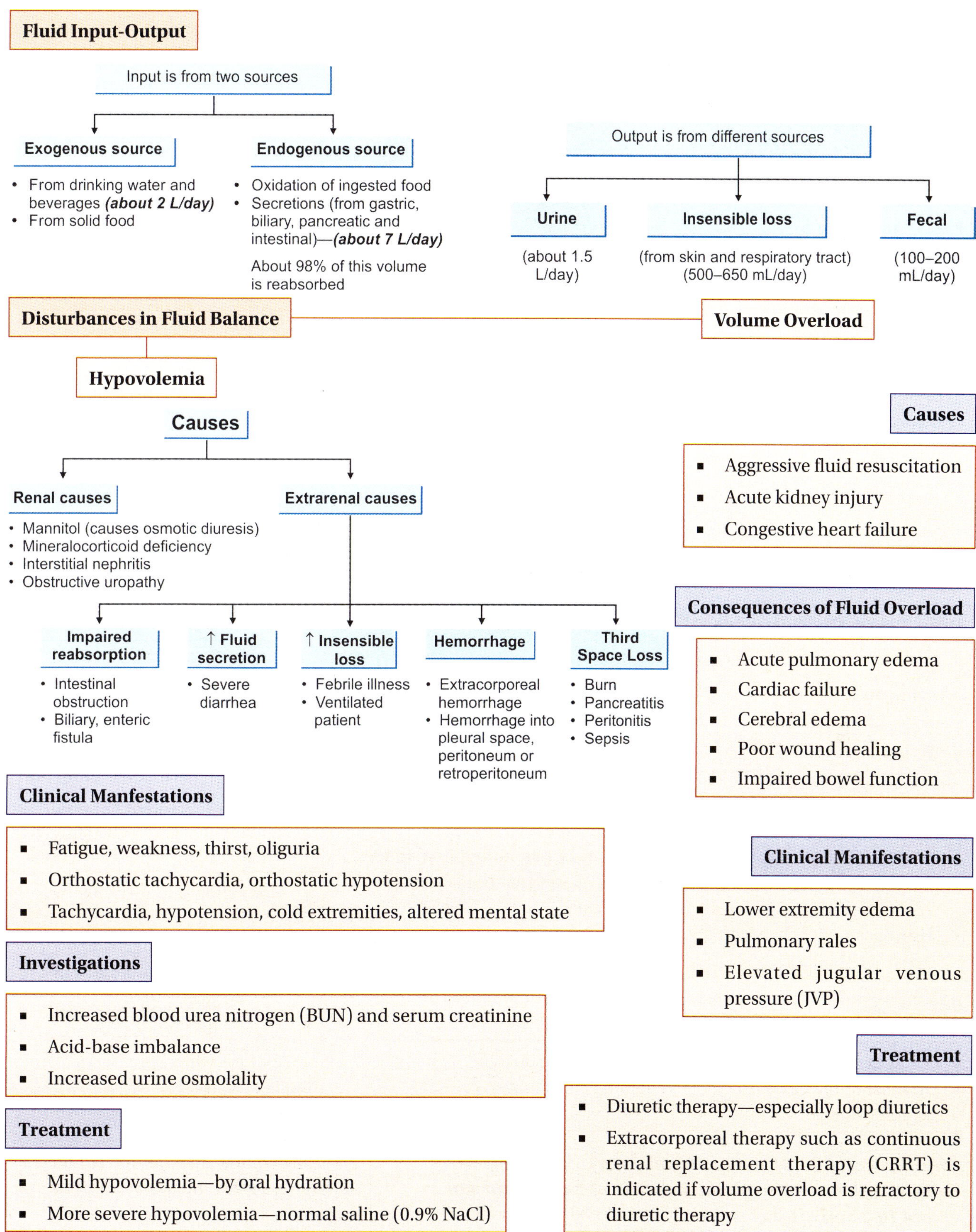

Clinical Manfestations

- Fatigue, weakness, thirst, oliguria
- Orthostatic tachycardia, orthostatic hypotension
- Tachycardia, hypotension, cold extremities, altered mental state

Investigations

- Increased blood urea nitrogen (BUN) and serum creatinine
- Acid-base imbalance
- Increased urine osmolality

Treatment

- Mild hypovolemia—by oral hydration
- More severe hypovolemia—normal saline (0.9% NaCl)

Clinical Manifestations

- Lower extremity edema
- Pulmonary rales
- Elevated jugular venous pressure (JVP)

Treatment

- Diuretic therapy—especially loop diuretics
- Extracorporeal therapy such as continuous renal replacement therapy (CRRT) is indicated if volume overload is refractory to diuretic therapy

Electrolyte Imbalance

Hyponatremia

Hyponatremia is defined as plasma Na^+ concentration <135 mEq/L.

- Sodium is the principal cation in ECF.
- Bone is a major source of sodium.

Causes

Causes

Depletion
- Small intestinal obstruction (loss of gastric, biliary, pancreatic and intestinal secretions)
- Fistula (duodenal, biliary, pancreatic, high intestinal)
- Renal loss (diuretics, renal disease)
- Severe diarrhea

Dilutional
- ↑Oral intake of water
- ↑IV fluid infusion (without Na^+)
- Shifting of water from intracellular space to extracellular space

Drugs Causing Hyponatremia
- Tricyclic antidepressants
- Thiazide diuretics, ACE-inhibitors
- Carbamazepine, SSRIs
- IV immunoglobulin (IVIG)

True hyponatremia: Serum Na^+ <135 mEq/L with low serum osmolality.

Pseudohyponatremia: Serum Na^+ <135 mEq/L with normal serum osmolality.

Clinical Manifestations

- Nausea, headache, vomiting
- Acute cerebral edema, seizures, coma
- Normocapneic or hypocapneic respiratory failure.

Causes of pseudohyponatremia: Marked hyperlipidemia, hyperproteinemia.

Causes of pseudohypernatremia: Severe hypoproteinemia.

Treatment

- Acute symptomatic hyponatremia—hypertonic 3% saline.
- In most of the cases, calculated sodium is administered in isotonic fluid.

Rapid correction of hyponatremia may cause osmotic demyelination syndrome (the increase of Na^+ should not exceed 10–12 mEq/L/hr)

Hypernatremia

Hypernatremia is defined as plasma Na^+ concentration >145 mEq/L

Causes

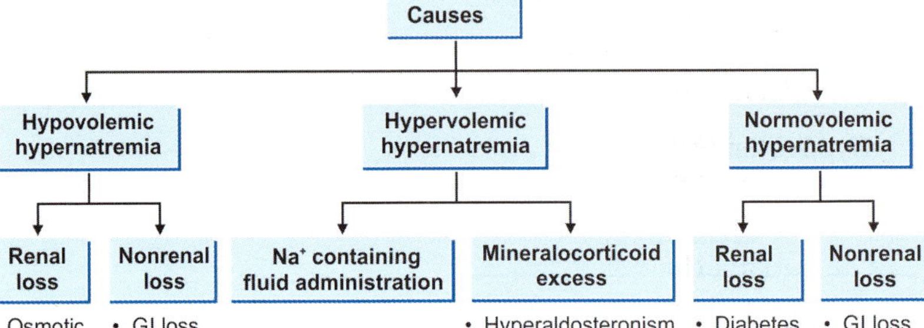

Clinical Manifestations

- Lethargy, mild confusion, coma
- Rhabdomyolysis
- Parenchymal or subarachnoid hemorrhage (in pediatric patients)

Treatment

- Correction of underlying causes (diarrhea, hyperglycemia, hypercalcemia, hypokalemia)
- Oral administration of water or by nasogastric tube
- Hypotonic saline (1/4 or 1/2NS)—depending on patient's clinical condition

Hypernatremia should be corrected slowly (no more than 10 mM/day) to avoid development of cerebral edema.

Hypokalemia

Hypokalemia is defined as plasma K^+ <3.5 mEq/L.

- Kidney plays a major role in potassium homeostasis.
- More than 98% of total-body potassium is intracellular.
- Skeletal muscle is the chief source of potassium in the body.

Causes

Decreased intake: Inadequate dietary intake, potassium-free IV fluid infusion

Increased gastrointestinal loss: Diarrhea, high volume nasogastric suction, high-output biliary and intestinal fistula, chronic laxative use.

Increased renal loss: Diuretics (thiazides), aminoglycosides, amphotericin, primary hyperaldosteronism.

Increased intracellular shift: Metabolic alkalosis, insulin therapy, hyperthyroidism, alcohol withdrawal, severe head injury.

Drugs Causing Hypokalemia

- Bronchodilators, tocolytics—by increasing cellular uptake
- Thiazide diuretics, loop diuretics—by increasing renal potassium excretion.
- Aminoglycosides, amphotericin, cisplatin, ifosfamide (associated with hypomagnesemia)- increased renal potassium and magnesium wasting.

Clinical Manifestations

- Muscle weakness, paralysis, skeletal myopathy
- Intestinal ileus
- Ventricular and atrial arrhythmias
- Acute kidney injury

Characteristic ECG changes

- Broad, flat T-waves
- ST depression
- QT prolongation

Causes of pseudohypokalemia: In vitro uptake of potassium (due to delayed transport of venous blood specimen), acute leukemia (due to profound leukocytosis).

Treatment

Correction of the Cause of Hypokalemia

Potassium supplementation:

Oral supplementation: With food rich in potassium (coconut water, fruit juice, milk, meat extracts, honey) and potassium syrup or effervescent tablet.

Intravenous supplementation: (i) IV potassium should be administered in saline solution, not in dextrose solution; (ii) Potassium concentration in IV solution in peripheral route must be 20–40 mEq/L.

Severe hypokalemia should be managed in intensive care set-up.

Serum magnesium should be measured in all hypokalemic patients as coexistent hypomagnesemia may present.

- Rapid IV supplementation of potassium may cause dysrhythmia and cardiac arrest.
- Serum potassium should be checked daily during IV supplementation.

Hyperkalemia

Hyperkalemia is defined as plasma K^+ >5.5 mEq/L.

Foods rich in potassium
Banana, tomato, citrus fruits

Causes

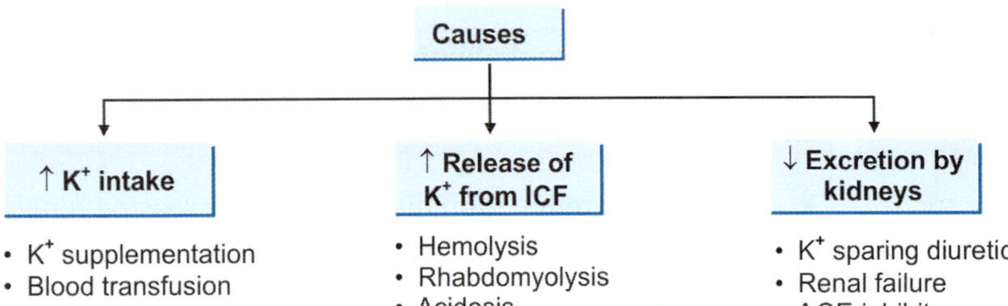

Drugs Causing Hyperkalemia

- ACE inhibitors
- Angiotensin receptor blockers
- Beta-blockers
- NSAIDs
- Spironolactone
- Amiloride, triamterene, trimethoprim

Clinical Manifestations

- Weakness, ascending paralysis
- Cardiac arrhythmias (sinus bradycardia, ventricular tachycardia, ventricular fibrillation, asystole).

Characteristic ECG Changes

- Tall-peaked T-waves
- Loss of P-waves
- Prolongation of PR and QRS intervals
- Sine wave pattern

Treatment

Hyperkalemia is a medical emergency and should be treated urgently if evidenced by ECG findings.

Insulin in dextrose solution— Insulin shifts the K^+ into intracellular compartment. Recommended dose is 10 units of IV regular insulin followed by 50 mL of 50% dextrose followed by 10% dextrose infusion at a rate of 50-75 mL/hr with close monitoring of plasma glucose.

IV calcium gluconate—Calcium raises the action potential threshold and reduces the excitability. Dose is 10 mL of 10% calcium gluconate IV infusion over 2–3 minutes with cardiac monitoring.

IV calcium should be used very cautiously in patients taking digoxin.

Cation exchange resin: Sodium polystyrene sulfonate. Recommended dose is 15–30 gm powder in 33% sorbitol suspension.

Inhaled albuterol: 10–20 mg of nebulized albuterol in 4 mL of normal saline for 10 minutes. This therapy should be used with extreme caution in patients with known cardiac disease.

Hemodialysis (if hyperkalemia is a manifestation of renal failure).

Hypocalcemia

Hypocalcemia is defined as total serum calcium concentration <8.8 mg/dL in the presence of normal plasma protein concentration.

Calcium is an extracellular cation.

Most of the body calcium present within the bone matrix (>90%)

Serum calcium is present in 3 forms:

1. Protein-bound form—about 40% (albumin)
2. Complexed to phosphate or other anions (10%)
3. Ionized form (50%)

The ionized form is responsible for blood coagulation and neuromuscular stability.

The normal serum calcium level is monitored by:

- Vitamin D
- Parathyroid hormone
- Calcitonin.

Normal serum calcium level is 8–10 mg/dL.

Causes

Hypoparathyroidism

- Inadvertent damage to all parathyroid glands during thyroid or parathyroid surgery
- Autoimmune endocrinopathies
- Hypomagnesemia (causes impaired PTH secretion)
- *Parathyroid agenesis:* DiGeorge's syndrome

Secondary hyperparathyroidism

- Nutritional vitamin D deficiency
- Impaired 1,25 $(OH)_2D$ production (secondary to renal insufficiency)
- Acute pancreatitis
- Osteoblastic metastases (prostate cancer)
- Acute rhabdomyolysis

Drugs Causing Hypocalcemia

- Bisphosphonates
- Phenytoin, ketoconazole
- Calcium chelators (Edetic acid, Edetate disodium anhydrous).

Clinical Manifestations

Paresthesias of fingers, toes, perioral region

Chvostek's sign: Twitching of the circumoral muscles in response to tapping over the area of facial nerve anterior to the ear.

Trousseau's sign: Carpal spasm is initiated by inflating blood pressure cuff 20 mm Hg above the patient's systolic blood pressure for 3 min.

Seizure, carpopedal spasm, bronchospasm in severe hypocalcemia

Characteristic ECG Changes

- Prolongation of QT interval
- Terminal T-wave inversion, T-wave flattening (rarely)

Treatment

Acute hypocalcemia: IV Calcium gluconate (10 mL of 10% in 50 mL of 5% dextrose or 0.9% Normal saline over 5 min). Associated hypomagnesemia, if present, should be treated with magnesium supplementation.

Chronic hypocalcemia: Calcium supplements with vitamin D_3 or calcitriol.

Hypercalcemia

Mild hypercalcemia is defined as total serum calcium level is up to 11–11.5 mg/dL.

Moderate hypercalcemia is defined as total serum calcium level is 11.5–14 mg/dL.

Drugs Causing Hypercalcemia

- Thiazides
- Lithium
- Vitamin A and its analogs
- Calcium-containing antacids

Causes

Primary hyperparathyroidism: Adenoma or hyperplasia of parathyroid glands

Tertiary hyperparathyroidism: Secondary to chronic renal failure or vitamin D deficiency

Hypercalcemia of malignancy:

Humoral hypercalcemia of malignancy (due to overproduction of PTHrP)—in many solid tumors (e.g., lung, head and neck, renal carcinoma)

Lytic skeletal metastases—breast carcinoma, multiple myeloma

Excess 1,25 $(OH)_2D$ production:

Vitamin D intoxication, granulomatous disease (tuberculosis, sarcoidosis), Hodgkin lymphoma

Hyperthyroidism, immobilization—due to increased bone resorption

Endocrine disorders: Pheochromocytoma, adrenal insufficiency

Familial hypocalciuric hypercalcemia

Clinical Manifestations

Mild hypercalcemia—usually asymptomatic

More severe hypercalcemia (>12–13 mg/dL)—presents with multisystem manifestations:

Renal: Polyuria, polydipsia, nephrolithiasis, nephrocalcinosis

Skeletal: Bone pain, osteoporosis, pathologic fractures, osteitis fibrosa cystica (in hyperparathyroidism)

Gastrointestinal: Nausea, constipation, anorexia, abdominal pain, peptic ulcer disease, pancreatitis.

Neuropsychiatric: Lethargy and fatigue, personality change, depression, impaired concentration.

Characteristic ECG Changes

- Bradycardia, AV block
- Shortened QT interval

Treatment

- **Mild, asymptomatic hypercalcemia**—immediate treatment is not indicated. Treatment will be dictated by the underlying disease.

Significant, symptomatic hypercalcemia—immediate and aggressive treatment is indicated.

- **Hydration and diuresis**—IV 4–6 L of saline over first 24 hours. Loop diuretics (e.g., frusemide) should be initiated once the intravascular volume is restored to normal.
- **Bisphosphonates** (Zoledronic acid, pamidronate, ibandronate)—indicated for treatment of malignancy-associated hypercalcemia
- **Glucocorticoids** (IV hydrocortisone or oral prednisone)—indicated in hypercalcemia related to excess 1,25$(OH)_2D$
- **Hemodialysis**—indicated in resistant, life-threatening hypercalcemia

Hypomagnesemia

Hypomagnesemia is defined as serum magnesium level below 1.46 mg/dL.

Causes

- **Decreased intake:** Decreased dietary consumption, starvation, TPN without magnesium supplementation, alcohol dependence
- **Increased gastrointestinal loss:** Diarrhea, nasogastric suction, intestinal fistula, malabsorption, small bowel bypass surgery
- **Increased renal loss:** Alcohol dependence, medications (thiazides, aminoglycosides), inherited tubular disorders (Bartter syndrome, Gitelman syndrome), Familial hypomagnesemia with hypercalciuria and nephrocalcinosis.
- **Increased intracellular shift:** Refeeding syndrome, hungry bone syndrome, acute pancreatitis.

Clinical Manifestations

- **Neuromuscular:** Tremor, tetany, positive Chvostek's and Trousseau's sign, fasciculation, seizures, delirium
- **Cardiovascular:** Hypertension, congestive heart failure, atrial and ventricular premature systoles, atrial fibrillation
- **Other electrolyte abnormalities:** Hypokalemia, hypocalcemia

Treatment

- **Mild or asymptomatic hypomagnesemia:** Oral magnesium (magnesium gluconate, magnesium lactate, magnesium chloride, magnesium citrate).
- **Severe and symptomatic hypomagnesemia:** IV magnesium sulfate 1–2 gm given over 1 hour.
- **In non-emergent scenario:** IV magnesium sulfate 4–8 gm over 12–24 hour.
- Any associated electrolyte abnormalities, e.g., hypokalemia or hypocalcemia should be corrected.

Renal function should be considered during in any form of magnesium replacement. In patients with chronic renal disease (creatinine clearance <30 mL/min/1.73 m^2), renal dosing should be done to avoid hypermagnesemia.

- Magnesium is an abundant intracellular cation.
- Normal serum magnesium ranges between 1.46 and 2.48 mg/dL.
- Most of the body magnesium is in storage form (about 99%).
- Bone is the largest store of magnesium in the body.

Drugs Causing Hypomagnesemia

- Thiazide diuretics
- Aminoglycosides
- Amphotericin B
- Cisplatin
- Cyclosporine
- Prolonged PPI use

Characteristic ECG Changes

- Widening of QRS complex
- Peaked T-waves
- PR prolongation
- Torsades de pointes

Foods Rich in Magnesium

- Green leafy vegetables
- Whole grains
- Legumes, nuts, seeds.

- In older adults, serum magnesium should be checked prior to initiation of PPI therapy.
- Periodic checkup of serum magnesium should be done during long-term PPI therapy.

Hypermagnesemia

Hypermagnesemia is defined as serum magnesium level above 2.6 mg/dL.

Causes

- **Increased intake:** Intake of antacids and laxatives containing magnesium (e.g., magnesium oxide) in elderly patients with impaired renal function, administration of bowel preparation agents (e.g., sodium picosulfate magnesium citrate), milk-alkali syndrome, mothers treated with magnesium infusion for eclampsia.
- **Decreased renal excretion:** Acute and chronic kidney disease, lithium-based psychotropic drugs.
- **Increased extracellular shift:** Tumor lysis syndrome, rhabdomyolysis, diabetic ketoacidosis.

Clinical Manifestations

Serum magnesium <7 mg/dL—weakness, nausea, vomiting, dizziness, confusion

Serum magnesium 7–12 mg/dL—decreased deep tendon reflexes, depressed level of consciousness, hypotension

Serum magnesium >12 mg/dL—flaccid paralysis, decreased respiratory rate, arrhythmia, heart block, coma

Characteristic ECG Changes

- Increased P-R interval
- Increased QRS interval
- Atrioventricular block

Treatment

Mild asymptomatic hypermagnesemia—no active management except removal of sources of exogenous magnesium.

Symptomatic hypermagnesemia needs early treatment.

Intravenous normal saline—promotes dilution of extracellular magnesium. Normal saline is better avoided in patients with poor renal function or in presence of pulmonary edema.

Intravenous loop diuretics (e.g., frusemide)—act by promoting increased renal excretion of magnesium.

Intravenous calcium gluconate—antagonizes the neuromuscular and cardiac effects of magnesium.

Metabolic Acidosis

Metabolic acidosis is defined as acid-base imbalance associated with plasma bicarbonate concentration below 20 mmol/L.

Anion gap (AG) = [Na]- ([Cl]+[HCO_3])

Types of Metabolic Acidosis

High-anion Gap Metabolic Acidosis

- Lactic acidosis
- Diabetic ketoacidosis
- Salicylate or methanol-induced acidosis
- Acute and chronic renal failure

Non-anion Gap Metabolic Acidosis

- Diarrhea
- Renal tubular acidosis
- Pancreatic fistula, high-intestinal fistula
- Ureterosigmoidostomy
- Mineralocorticoid deficiency
- *Medications:* Acetazolamide, amphotericin B, spironolactone

Pathophysiology

Increased endogenous acid production: Lactic acidosis, diabetic ketoacidosis

Accumulation of endogenous acids: Renal failure

Loss of bicarbonate: Diarrhea, high-intestinal fistula, pancreatic fistula, acetazolamide use, ureterosigmoidostomy

Clinical Manifestations

- Nausea, vomiting, headache, lethargy, stupor
- Kussmaul respiration

Treatment

- Treatment of the cause of acidosis
- *Sodium bicarbonate:* Intravenous $NaHCO_3$ is indicated for severe acidemia in normal anion gap acidosis.
- Use of IV sodium bicarbonate is controversial in treatment of high anion gap acidosis.

Metabolic Alkalosis

Metabolic alkalosis is defined as arterial blood pH >7.45 due to metabolic causes.

Biological Effects of Metabolic Alkalosis

- Elevated arterial pH
- Increased serum HCO_3^-
- Increased $PaCO_2$

Clinical Manifestations

- Mental obtundation, confusion
- Muscular cramping, tetany
- Seizures

Pathophysiology

GI loss of hydrogen ion: Vomiting, nasogastric aspiration

Increased alkali administration: Parenteral hyperalimentation (acetate load), blood transfusion (citrate load), antacids (aluminium hydroxide)

Renal loss of hydrogen ion: Conn syndrome, loop and thiazide diuretics, Gitelman's syndrome, Barrter's syndrome

Increased bicarbonate synthesis: Primary aldosteronism, Cushing's syndrome

Treatment

- Treatment of the underlying cause
- Infusion of isotonic saline
- Administration of acetazolamide—accelerates the renal bicarbonate excretion

Respiratory Acidosis

Respiratory acidosis is defined as acid-base imbalance characterized by low pH primarily due to rise in $PaCO_2$.

Causes

Acute respiratory acidosis:

- Acute airway obstruction or bronchospasm due to inhalation injury, anaphylaxis, severe asthma
- Depression of the respiratory center due to head injury, sedatives, general anesthetics

Chronic respiratory acidosis:

- Obesity—hypoventilation syndromes
- End-stage obstructive and restrictive lung disease
- Neuromuscular disorders, e.g., poliomyelitis, muscular dystrophies, myasthenia gravis

Clinical Manifestations

Acute hypercapnia: Anxiety, confusion, psychosis, hallucination, lastly progress to coma

Chronic hypercapnia: Loss of memory, personality change, impairment of coordination

Treatment

Acute respiratory acidosis:

- Management of underlying cause, e.g., tracheal intubation and mechanical ventilation
- Properly titrated oxygen administration
- Rapid correction of hypercapnia should be avoided.

Chronic respiratory acidosis:

- Management of underlying cause
- Measures to improve lung function

Respiratory Alkalosis

Respiratory alkalosis is defined as arterial blood pH >7.45 secondary to respiratory causes.

Causes

Acute respiratory alkalosis:

- Mechanical hyperventilation
- Septicemia
- Anxiety—hyperventilation
- Cerebrovascular accident
- Drugs—salicylates, theophylline, aminophylline

Chronic respiratory alkalosis:

- Pregnancy
- Liver failure

Clinical Manifestations

- Dizziness, mental confusion, seizure
- Hypotension and decreased cardiac output (in anesthesized and ventilated patients)

Treatment

- Management of underlying cause
- Reassurance, management of psychological stress in patients with hyperventilation syndrome

Commonly Used Crystalloids for Parenteral Administration

Crystalloid	Composition
Ringer's lactate (Hartmann's solution)	Sodium 130 mEq/L; Potassium 4 mEq/L; Calcium 3 mEq/L; Chloride 109 mEq/L; Lactate 28 mEq/L
0.9% Sodium chloride solution	Sodium 154 mEq/L; Chloride 154 mEq/L
5% Dextrose solution	50g of Dextrose per liter
5% Dextrose and 0.45% Sodium chloride solution	Sodium 77 mEq/L; Chloride 77 mEq/L; 50 gm of dextrose per liter
Plasma-lyte solution	Sodium 140 mEq/L; Potassium 5 mEq/L; Magnesium 3 mEq/L; Chloride 98 mEq/L; Bicarbonate 27 mEq/L
Isolyte P in dextrose solution	Sodium 23 mEq/L; Potassium 20 mEq/L; Magnesium 3 mEq/L; Chloride 29 mEq/L; Acetate 23 mEq/L; Phosphate 3 mEq/L; Dextrose 50 gm/L
Ringer's injection	Sodium 147.5 mEq/L; Potassium 4 mEq/L; Calcium 4.5 mEq/L; Chloride 156 mEq/L
Hypertonic saline 3%	Sodium 513 mEq/L; Chloride 513 mEq/L
Hypertonic saline 5%	Sodium 856 mEq/L; Chloride 856 mEq/L

Alternative Volume Expanders (Colloids)

Colloid	Composition
Gelofusine (MW–30,000)	Succinylated gelatin (modified gelatin)—40 gm/L; Sodium 154 mEq/L; Chloride 120 mEq/L
Dextran 40 (MW–40,000) Dextran 70 (MW–70,000)	10% Dextran (MW 40,000) solution in 0.9% NaCl or 5% glucose 6% Dextran (MW 70,000)
Hydroxyethyl starch (Voluven) MW- 450,000	6% hydroxyethyl starch 130/0.4 in 0.9% sodium chloride injection; hydrochloric acid and water for injection; Sodium 154 mEq/L; Chloride 154 mEq/L
Hextend 6% (MW–670,000)	Hetastarch 60 g/L; Sodium 143 mEq/L; Chloride 124 mEq/L; Lactate 28 mEq/L; Calcium 5 mEq/L; Potassium 3 mEq/L; Magnesium 0.9 mEq/L
Haemaccel (MW–30,000)	Polygeline 35g/L; Sodium 145 mEq/L; Potassium 5.1 mEq/L; Calcium 6.25 mEq/L; Chloride 145 mEq/L

Chapter 3

Hemostasis–Coagulation–Hemorrhage

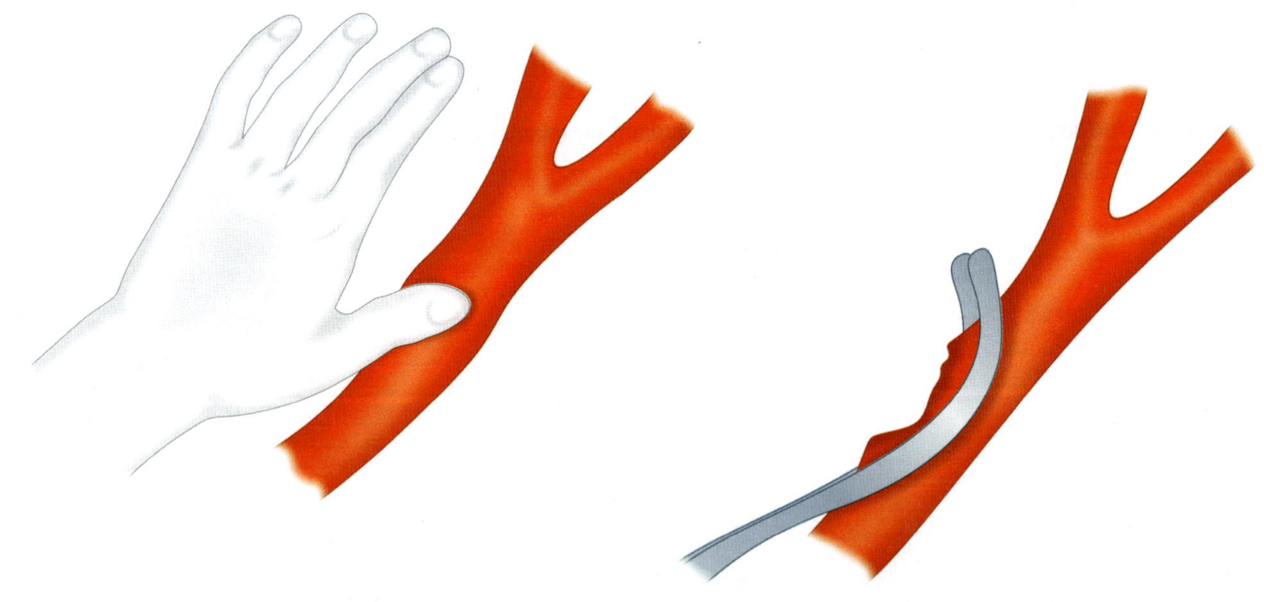

Important Topics

- Physiology of Hemostasis
- Evaluation to Assess Risk of Bleeding
- Hemorrhagic Disorders
- Types of Hemorrhage
- Methods of Hemostasis
- Blood and its Components
- Massive Transfusion

'The best physician is also a philosopher.'

Galen (129 – C. 216)
Greco-Roman Physician

Hemostasis is a complex process that involves four events:

1. Vasoconstriction
2. Platelet plug formation
3. Fibrin formation
4. Fibrinolysis

Endothelial cells, platelets, coagulation factors and anticoagulants are involved in this process.

Chemicals Causing Vasoconstriction

- Thromboxane A2
- Endothelin
- Serotonin
- Bradykinin

Evaluation to Assess Risk of Bleeding During Surgery

History includes:

- Easy bruising
- Spontaneous mucosal bleeding, epistaxis
- Menorrhagia
- Past history of significant bleeding during invasive procedures
- History of liver dysfunction
- Hematologic malignancies, multiple myeloma
- Aspirin, anticoagulant or NSAID intake

Physical examination includes:

- Petechiae
- Ecchymosis
- Lymphadenopathy
- Hepatosplenomegaly

Screening tests:

- For minor operation, operations not requiring extensive dissection, no history suggestive of coagulation difficulties or no family history—Preoperative screening tests are not indicated.
- For major procedures, operations requiring extensive dissections, history, or physical findings suggestive of coagulopathy or positive family history—need preoperative screening tests.

Commonly used screening tests:

- Platelet count
- Activated partial thromboplastin time (aPTT)
- Bleeding time
- Platelet count
- Prothrombin time (PT)

Chemicals Promoting Platelet Aggregation

- Serotonin
- Adenosine diphosphate
- Thromboxane A2

Drugs Causing Platelet Dysfunction

- Aspirin
- Adenosine diphosphate receptor antagonists (e.g., clopidegrel, prasugrel)
- GP IIb/IIIA receptor blockers (e.g., abciximab, eptifibatide, tirofiban)
- NSAIDs
- Volume expanders

- **Warfarin therapy and vitamin K deficiency** prolong the PT.
- **Heparin therapy** causes prolongation of aPTT without alteration of PT.
- **A prolonged PT with normal aPTT** suggests deficiency of vitamin K-dependent factors (factor II, VII, IX, X). *An abnormal aPTT with normal PT* suggests deficiency of proximal intrinsic pathway factors.

Bleeding time—for measurement of primary phase of hemostasis (platelet activation and platelet aggregation)

Clotting time (CT)—measures the time required for formation of first traces of thrombin sufficient to produce a visible clot

Prothrombin time (PT)—measures the activity of both intrinsic and extrinsic pathways

Activated partial thromboplastin time (aPTT)—measures the activity of intrinsic pathway only

INR (International normalized ratio)—The INR is the ratio of measured PT to a mean laboratory control PT

Viscoelastic Assays

- Viscoelastic assays (TEG, ROTEM) measures all dynamic steps of clot formation.
- The devices for all these methods use the same principle based on a cup and pin method. As the blood clots, a graphical representation is made.

Standard TEG (Thromboelastogram)/ROTEM (Rotational thromboelastometry) traces is divided into four main section:

1. **Clot initiation** [R(reaction) time—TEG; CT (clotting time)—ROTEM]
2. **Fibrin polymerization** [K (kinetics) time, α angle—TEG; CFT (clot formation time), α angle—ROTEM]
3. **Clot strength** [MA (maximum amplitude)—TEG; A (amplitude) and MCF (maximal clot firmness)—ROTEM]
4. **Lysis of the clot** [LY30 (lysis at 30 min)—TEG; ML (maximal lysis)—ROTEM]

TEG is a useful assay to identify patients likely to develop thromboembolic complications after injury, predicting early transfusion of RBCs, plasma, platelets and cryoprecipitate.

Hemorrhagic Disorders

Congenital Hemorrhagic Disorders

Hemophilia A: Congenital coagulation disorder (X-linked recessive) characterized by deficiency of factor VIII.

- If affects exclusively in males.
- Laboratory investigation reveals prolonged aPTT with decreased factor VIII: C, normal PT, bleeding time.
- Desmopressin temporarily raise factor VIII level.

Hemophilia B (Christmas disease): Congenital X-linked disorder characterized by deficiency in factor IX.

- Laboratory investigation reveals prolonged aPTT with decreased factor IX, normal PT, platelet count and bleeding time.
- Prothrombin complex concentrate of high-purity factor IX concentrate is the replacement therapy.

von Willebrand's disease:

Most common congenital bleeding disorder characterized by deficiency of von Willebrand factor.

Three types: I, II and III. Inheritance pattern of Type I and II are autosomal dominant and type III is autosomal recessive.

Desmopressin increases plasma levels of vWF.

Acquired Hemorrhagic Disorders

Vitamin K Deficiency

Causes:

- Obstructive jaundice
- Biliary fistula
- Antibiotics (e.g. cephalosporin, quinolones, doxycycline) Vitamin K deficiency is treated by parenteral vitamin K 10 mg once daily for 3–5 days.

Anticoagulant Drugs

Warfarin—acts by inhibiting the synthesis of vitamin K-dependant clotting factors

- Prolongs the PT, slightly prolong aPTT
- Warfarin-induced bleeding is treated by vitamin K, plasma infusion and administration of rF VIIa.

Unfractionated heparin:

- Blocks the activation of factor X
- All coagulation profiles are affected by UFH. aPTT is the most sensitive test to detect it.

Low molecular weight heparin (LMWH): Less bleeding complications than UFH.

- PT is not altered by LMWH therapy.
- If heparin-induced thrombocytopenia develops, fondaparinux is the treatment of choice.

Liver Diseases

- Liver synthesizes all coagulation factors except factor VIII
- Laboratory investigation reveals prolonged PT, slightly increased aPTT.

Thrombocytopenia

- Due to infection (many of the viral and bacterial infections), drugs (e.g., linezolid, piperacillin, vancomycin, etc.) or heparin induced.

Hemorrhage

Types of Hemorrhage

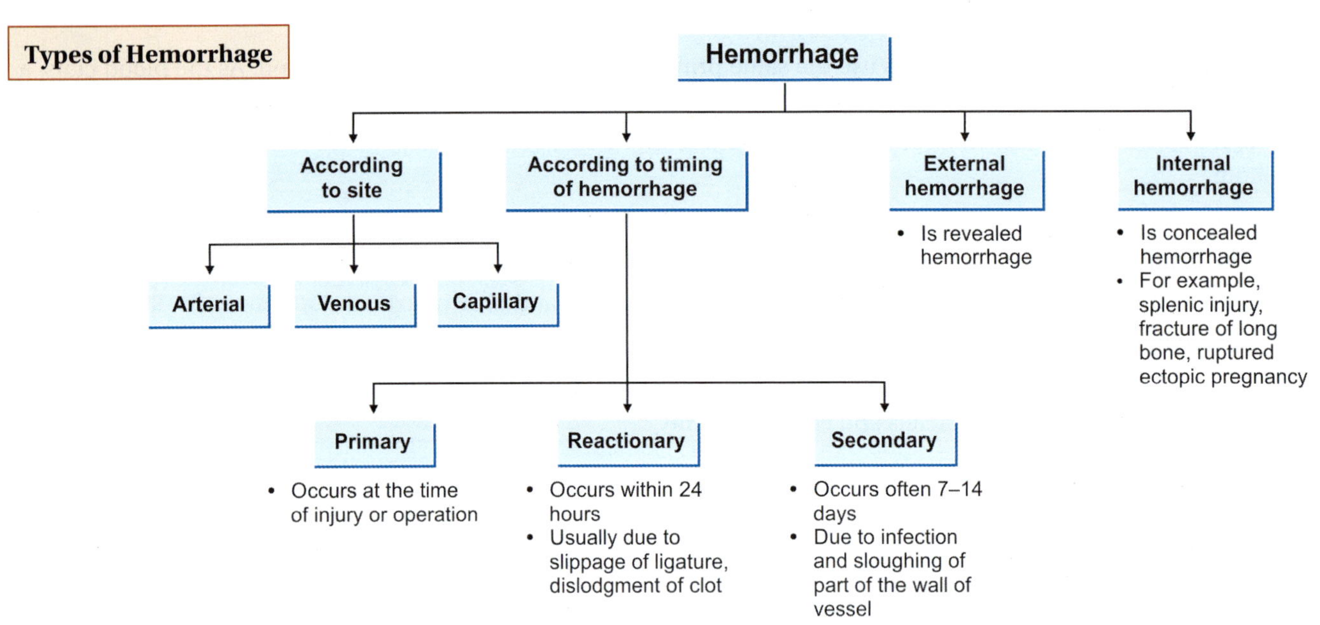

Methods of hemostasis

Mechanical Method

- Direct digital pressure
- Direct pressure by gauze or laparotomy pads
- Application of vascular clamp
- Extremity tourniquet
- Application of suture or clips
- Bone wax (for bleeding from raw surface of bone)

Energy Devices

- *Electrosurgery:* (a) monopolar; (b) bipolar; (c) bipolar vessel sealing device (Ligasure); and (d) Argon beam coagulation.
- Ultrasonic shears (Harmonic shears)

Pharmacological Agents

- Epinephrine
- Tranexamic acid—a synthetic derivative of amino acid lysine that inhibits plasminogen activation, thus preventing impairment of fibrinolysis.

Topical Hemostatic Agents

Passive Agents

- **Gelatin foam (Gelfoam)**—Porcine-derived collagen agents supplied as dry, pliable foam material. They are moistened with saline before use. They provide matrix for clotting initiation. These agents dissolve in 4 to 6 weeks.
- **Oxidized regenerated cellulose (Surgicel)**—Plant-derived agents supplied as mesh sheet. They provide matrix for clotting initiation. These agents dissolve in 1–2 weeks.
- **Microfibrillar collagen (Avitene)**—Bovine-derived collagen agent supplied as sheet or dense powdered form. It helps in platelet adherence and activation. It completely dissolves within 12 weeks.
- **Microporous polysaccharide spheres (Arista)**—Plant-derived starch material supplied as fine powder. It concentrates platelets and proteins of coagulation cascade. It dissolves in 1–2 days.

Active Agents

- **Topical thrombin agents (Evithrom):** Human or bovine-derived agents supplied as liquid form. They may be combined with gelatin matrix (Floseal, Surgiflo) to promote hemostasis.
- **Fibrin sealants (Evicel):** Human-derived liquid preparations of fibrinogen, factor XII, thrombin and calcium. A fibrin-based clot is formed at the site of bleeding after application of this preparation.
- **Tissue adhesives (Bioglue):** Bovine albumin-derived agents supplied as liquid agent. It forms an adhesive matrix and is effective to control bleeding from moderate-sized vessels.

Blood and its Components

Whole blood

- Stored in blood bank in special refrigerators (4°C ± 2°C).
- The shelf life of CPD blood is 3 weeks. During storage, intracellular ADP and 2, 3-DPG is reduced, resulting in shifting of oxygen-Hb dissociation curve, thus decreasing oxygen transport.
- Stored blood is a poor source of platelets, clotting factors (factor V and VIII).
- Recommended rate of transfusion is 150–200 mL/hour.

Packed RBC

- Packed RBC are prepared by certifugation. The supernatant plasma is removed.
- PRBC should be transfused over 90-120 minutes. The transfusion must be completed within four hours of removal from a controlled temperature environment.
- Indicated in pediatric patients, in elderly, patient with chronic anemia.
- Most of the packed RBCs are now leukocyte-reduced to avoid post-transfusion fever, CMV infection, alloimmunization.

Platelet concentrates

- Indicated in both qualitative and quantitative platelet disorders.
- Should be transfused within 120 hours of collection.
- Is prepared either as random donor (RD) platelets or single donor apheresis platelets (SDAP).
- Transfusion time for adult is 30–60 minutes. Platelets should not be transfused through sets that have been used for other blood components.
- Chance of allergic reaction and transmission of infectious diseases are same as whole blood transfusion.

Fresh-frozen plasma

- Is the source of vitamin K-dependent factors and the only source of factor V.
- FFP should be the same group as the patient.
- A unit of FFP is usually administered over 30 minutes.
- FFP once thawed, must not be re-frozen and should be transfused as soon as possible.
- Indicated in congenital hemorrhagic disorders, thrombotic thrombocytopenic purpura, during surgery in patient with liver failure.

Cryoprecipitate

- a leukodepleted plasma product containing concentrated factor VIII, von Willebrand factor and fibronectin.
- Cryoprecipitate is stored at (–25°C). Once thawed, it must not be re-frozen and used within 4 hours.
- Indicated in—bleeding associated with thrombolytic therapy, bleeding patients with both hepatic and renal failure, hypofibrinogenemia due to major hemorrhage and massive transfusion.

Special Blood Components

Prothrombin complex concentrate:

- This concentrate contains either three (II, IX, X) or four (II, VII, IX, X) clotting factors.
- Indicated in acquired factor deficiency and for urgent reversal of warfarin.

Fibrinogen concentrate:

Indicated in bleeding following surgery or trauma and in congenital hypofibrinogenemia.

- Dextrose solution (5%) should not be mixed with any blood components (hemolysis may develop).
- Leukocytes are removed from all blood components to minimize the potential risk of transmission of variant Creutzfeldt-Jakob disease.
- Blood components should be transfused through blood transfusion set with an integral mesh filter (170–200 micron pore size).
- Drugs should not be added to any blood component bag.
- Transfusion set should be changed every 12 hours for a continuing transfusion and on completion of the transfusion.

Complications of Blood Transfusion

Acute Adverse Transfusion Reaction

Reactions occurring within 24 hrs after transfusion

- **Acute immune-mediated reactions**
- **Acute nonimmune-mediated reactions**

Delayed Transfusion Reaction

Reactions occurring after 24 hour or upto months/years after transfusion

- **Delayed immune-mediated reactions**
- **Delayed nonimmune-mediated reactions**

Acute Immune-mediated Reactions

Allergic reaction:

One of the common types of transfusion reactions

Patient develops urticarial rash, itching. Rarely, bronchospasm develops

Treatment involves temporary stopping of the transfusion and administration of antihistaminics and steroids.

Acute immune hemolytic reaction:

- It is due to ABO or Rh-incompatibility.
- Always due to human error (mislabeling the sample or transfusion in a wrong patient).
- Patient presents with fever, chill, discomfort at the infusion site, chest or flank pain, tachypnea, hypotension, hemoglobinuria.
- In anesthetized patient, excessive bleeding from incision or mucus membrane is alarming sign.
- Immediately, the details of the patient and the documents relating to donor blood should be checked.

- Transfusion should be stopped immediately.
- The transfused blood sample and unused blood unit should be sent for analysis and blood bank should be
- informed about the reaction.
- Diuresis should be induced with IV fluids, frusemide, or mannitol.

Febrile nonhemolytic transfusion reaction

- Most common type of reaction associated with transfusion of cellular blood components
- Patient develops chills, rigor and rise of temperature.
- Due to antibodies against donor leukocyte and HLA antigens
- Leukoreduction before storage can prevent this type of reaction.

Anaphylactic reaction

- Patient presents with nausea, vomiting, hypotension, bronchospasm and even shock.
- Transfusion should be stopped immediately. Epinephrine is given subcutaneously. In severe cases, steroid is indicated.

Transfusion-related acute lung injury (TRALI)

- TRALI is defined as new acute lung injury (ALI) that develops during or within six hours of transfusion and no other ALI risk factor is present.
- Patient presents with acute respiratory distress and signs of noncardiogenic pulmonary edema.
- Treatment is supportive and usually patient recovers without any sequelae. Measures for decreasing the incidence of TRALI are use of predominantly male plasma and apheresis platelets.

Acute Nonimmune-mediated Reactions

Transfusion related sepsis

Risk is more in platelet transfusion than PRBC transfusion. Treatment is broad-spectrum antibiotics along with other measures for management of sepsis.

Non-immune hemolytic reactions

RBC hemolysis due to transfusion may develop due to improper storage temperature, improper use of blood warmer, inappropriately small-bore needle, infusion of PRBC through same tubing with hypotonic solution. Management is same as acute immune hemolytic reactions.

Transfusion-associated circulatory overload (TACO)

- TACO is pulmonary edema primarily related to circulatory overload with 3 or more of the following criteria within 12 hours of transfusion: acute respiratory distress, radiographic pulmonary edema, elevated central venous pressure, evidence of left heart failure, elevated B-type natriuretic peptide, and a positive fluid balance.
- Risk factors are patients with extreme age, renal failure or congestive cardiac failure, anemia.
- Clinical presentations include dyspnea, orthopnea, pedal edema, tachycardia.
- Management includes optimization of primary cause, restriction of fluid, and use of diuretics.

Electrolyte imbalance

- Hyperkalemia—Neonates and patient with renal failure are at risk. Fresh or washed RBC are the solution to avoid this complications.
- Hypocalcemia—Citrate (used as anticoagulant in stored blood) chelates calcium and thereby hypocalcemia develops. No definite treatment is required.

Delayed Immune-mediated Reactions

Delayed hemolytic transfusion reactions

- This reaction is due to reactivation of pre-existing antibodies against antigens of transfused RBCs.
- Patient may present with unexplained anemia or no increase in hemoglobin after transfusion.

Alloimmunization

Acute life-threatening anemia may develop in some patients with sickle cell anemia and thalassemia due to presence of alloantibodies.

Transfusion-associated immunomodulation (TRIM)

This immune-mediated reaction is related to transfused leukocytes. Clinical consequences may be increased risk of postoperative infection and transfusion-related multiple organ dysfunction syndrome.

Transfusion-associated graft versus host disease

- Usually develops 8–10 days after transfusion.
- This immune mediated reaction is characterized by fever, maculopapular rash, enterocolitis, elevated liver function test, pancytopenia.
- This reaction is due to engraftment of donor lymphocytes into immunocompromised recipient's bone marrow.

Post-transfusion purpura

- This uncommon reaction predominantly develops in female patients between 1 and 24 days after transfusion.
- Patients present with bleeding from mucous membranes, GI and urinary tract, intracranial hemorrhage.
- Treatment is high-dose IV immunoglobulin.

Delayed Nonimmune-mediated Reaction

Transmission of disease

Viral infections

- Hepatitis C
- Hepatitis B (risk of transmission is more than hepatitis C)
- HIV 1
- Cytomegalovirus (CMV)—Leukocyte-reduced cellular component transfusion can decrease the risk of CMV transmission.

Bacterial infections

- As PRBCs and FFPs are stored at cold temperature, they are not common sources of bacterial contamination (except *Yersinia*, *Acinetobacter*, *Pseudomonas*, *Escherichia* species).
- As platelet concentrates are stored at room temperature, it is a common source of bacterial contamination.

Other infectious diseases

- Malaria
- Babesiosis
- Chagas disease
- Dengue

Iron overload

- Patients with thalassemia, sickle cell anemia and other chronic anemia are at increased risk.
- Can affect hepatic, cardiac, and endocrine system.
- Using alternative therapies (e.g., erythropoietin) and chelating agents (e.g., desferoxamine) are the solution.

Massive Blood Transfusion

Definition: Replacement of one blood volume equivalent (10 units of blood) within 24 hrs or 50% of blood volume equivalent (5 units of blood) in any four hour period in an adult.

Indications: (i) Severe traumatic bleeding; (ii) Ruptured aortic aneurysm; and (iii) Vascular surgical bleeding.

American College of Surgeons (ACS) TQIP (Trauma Quality Improvement Program) Massive Transfusion Protocol (MTP)

Triggers for Initiating Massive Transfusion

- Assessment of Blood Consumption (ABC) score two or more
- Persistent hemodynamic instability
- Active bleeding requiring operation or angioembolization
- Blood transfusion in the trauma bay

→

Blood Product Resuscitation

- Universal blood product (O Rh-negative and O Rh-positive) infusion rather than crystalloids or colloids
- Transfusion of plasma and universal RBC in a ratio of 1:1 or 1:2
- Transfusion of one single donor apheresis or random donor platelet pool for each six units of RBC

Monitoring of Parameters

- INR
- aPTT
- Fibrinogen level
- Hemoglobin or hematocrit
- Platelet count
- Point-of-care testing/thromboelastometry or rotational elastography (if available)
- Ionized calcium
- Blood gas analysis, including base deficit

Resuscitation should be goal directed based on laboratory parameters and clinical evidence of ongoing bleeding.

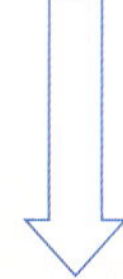

Bleeding is controlled in OR or radiographic and physiologic evidences of bleeding control after angioembolization.

Therapeutic Adjuncts in Massive Transfusion

Tranexemic acid (TXA): 1 gm IV over 10 minutes followed by infusion of 1 gm over 8 hours in injured patients who are actively bleeding and presented within three hours of injury.

Prothrombin complex concentrate (PCC): Only indicated for correction of warfarin-induced coagulopathy in bleeding patients.

Endpoints of Transfusion

- RBC transfusion for hemoglobin ≥10 gm/dL
- Plasma transfusion for prothrombin time <18 seconds
- Plasma transfusion for activated partial thromboplastin time (aPTT) <35 seconds
- Platelet transfusion for platelet count >150 × 10^9
- Cryoprecipitate or fibrinogen concentrate for fibrinogen level >180 g/L

Complications of Massive Transfusion

- Coagulopathy
- Thrombotic complications
- ARDS
- Transfusion-associated circulatory overload (TACO)
- Transfusion-related acute lung injury (TRALI)
- Hemolytic transfusion reaction
- Over-transfusion of RBC

Chapter 4

Gallbladder and Extrahepatic Biliary System

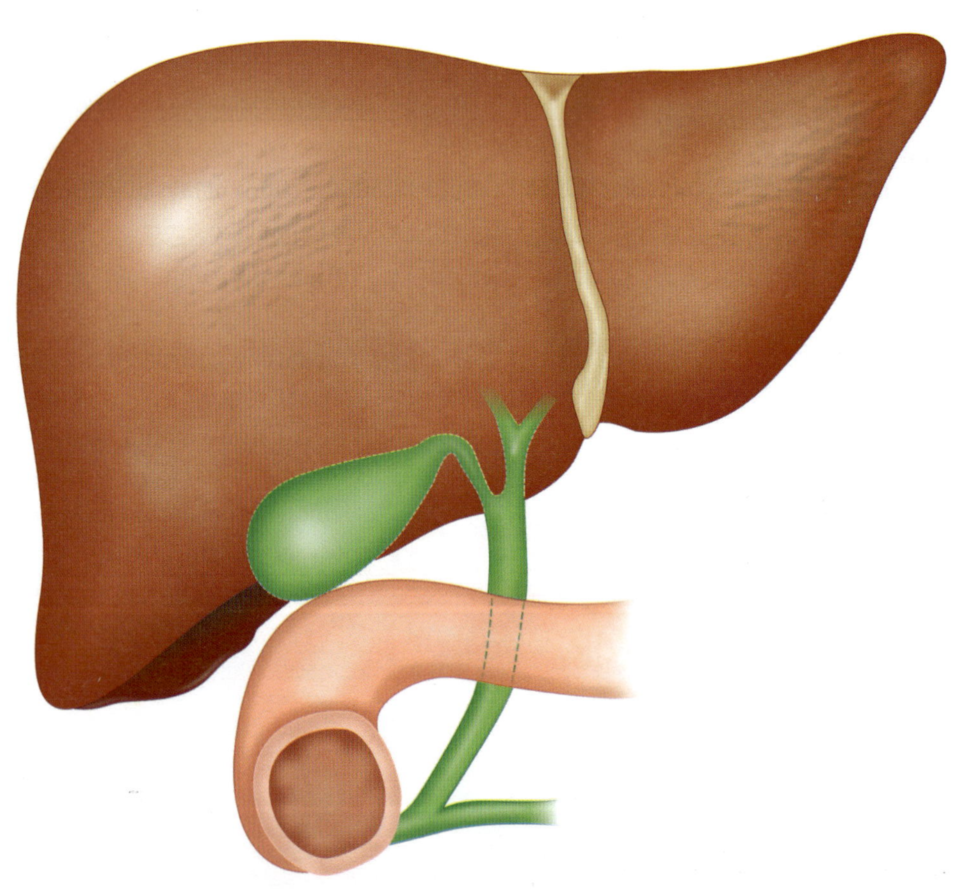

Important Topics

- Surgical Anatomy
- Gallstone and Symptomatic Gallstone Diseases
- Acute Acalculous Cholecystitis
- Biliary Dyskinesia
- Cholecystectomy
- Bile Duct Injury and its Management
- Choledocholithiasis
- Hepatolithiasis
- Biliary Stricture
- Choledochal Cyst
- Recurrent Pyogenic Cholangitis
- Primary Sclerosing Cholangitis
- Gallbladder Polyp
- Gallbladder Carcinoma
- Cholangiocarcinoma
- Biliary Stenting
- Endoscopic Approaches of Biliary System

'Science is not, as so many seem to think, something apart, which has to do with telescopes, retorts, and test tube and especially with nasty smells, but it is a way of searching out by observation, trial and classification, ... its keynote is accuracy and its goal is truth.'

Archibald Garrod (1857– 1936)
British Physician and Biochemist

Anatomy

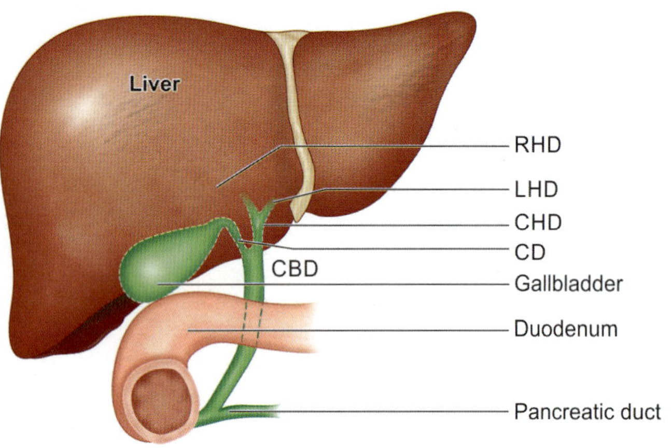

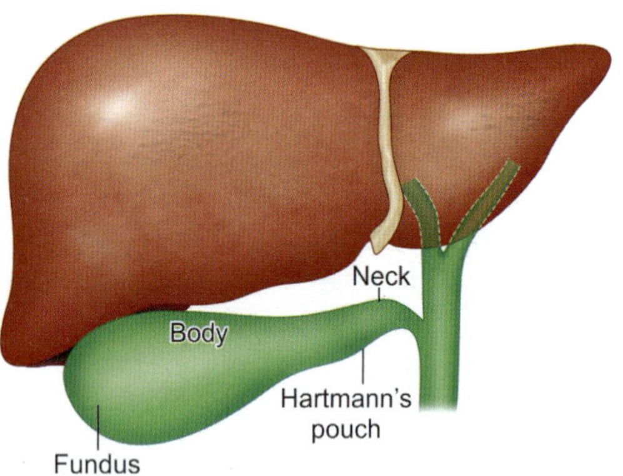

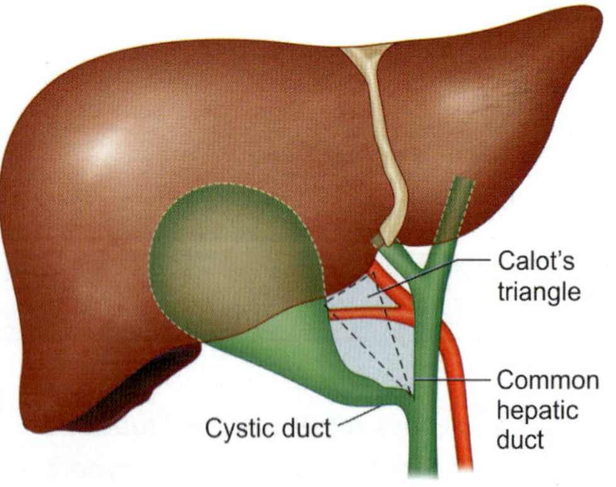

- Gallbladder, **average capacity 30–50 mL,** can distend upto 300 mL.
- Gallbladder is divided into **four anatomic areas:** the fundus, the body, the infundibulum, and the neck.
- The **left hepatic duct is longer** than the right and has a greater propensity for dilatation.
- Gallbladder differs histologically from the rest of the gastrointestinal tract in that **it lacks muscularis mucosa and submucosa.**
- The gallbladder mucosa has the **greatest absorptive power per unit area** than any other structures in the body.
- **About 250–1000 mL of bile** are secreted by hepatocytes everyday.
- Gallbladder is supplied by **cystic artery,** a branch of the right hepatic artery (>90%).
- Course of the cystic artery may vary, but **it nearly always found within the hepatocystic triangle,** the area bound by cystic duct, common hepatic duct and liver margin.
- Gallbladder lymphatics drain into nodes at the neck of the gallbladder. Frequently, a visible lymph node overlies the insertion of cystic artery into gallbladder wall **(Lund's node or Mascagni's lymph node).**
- Common bile duct is about 7–11 cm in length:

Upper third **(supraduodenal part)**

Middle third **(retroduodenal part)**

Lower third **(pancreatic part)**

Contracted sphincter of Oddi

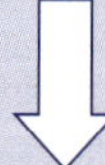

Increased pressure in CBD

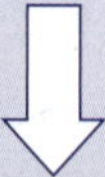

Retrograde flow of bile through cystic duct into the gallbladder

Pathologies of Gallbladder and Biliary System

Gallstone

Risk Factors

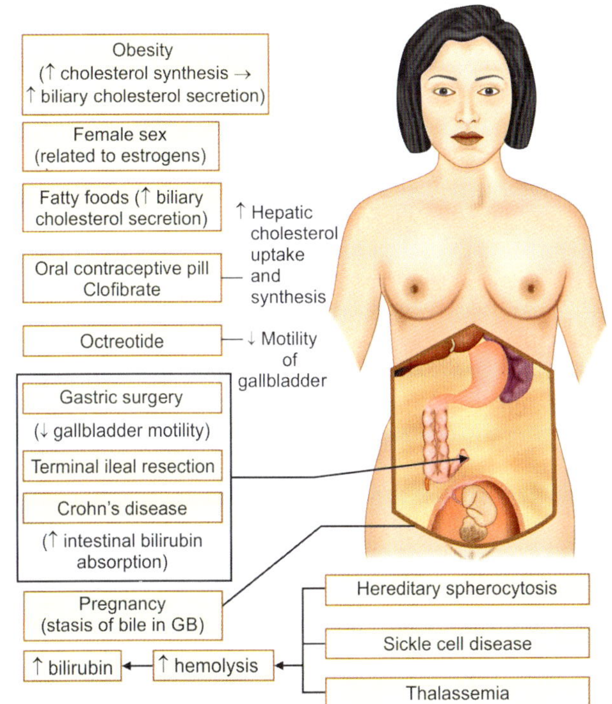

Types of Stone

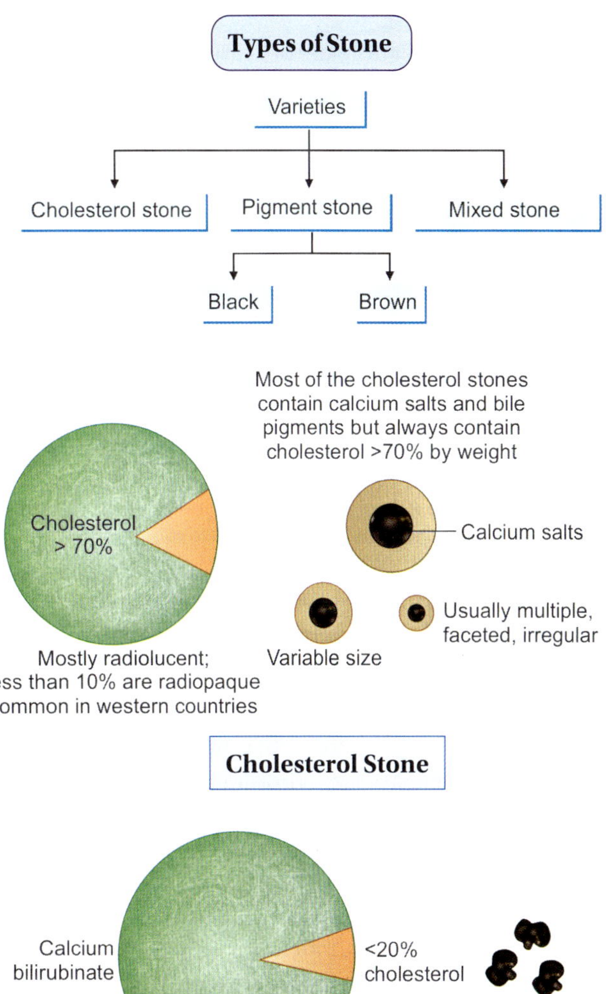

Biliary pseudolithiasis: A rare complication of ceftriaxone therapy, where ceftriaxone-calcium precipitate form sludge. It commonly disappears after discontinuation of therapy.

	Cholesterol stone	Black pigment stone	Brown pigment stone
Composition	≥70% cholesterol with bile pigments and calcium	Calcium bilirubinate, calcium phosphate and calcium bicarbonate	Calcium bilirubinate, calcium palmitate, calcium stearate and cholesterol
Primary event in formation	Supersaturation of bile with cholesterol	Supersaturation of unconjugated bilirubin within the bile	Conjugated bilirubin is degraded by β-glucuronidase (produced by *E. coli*) to unconjugated bilirubin. This bilirubin precipitates with calcium and dead bacteria.
Stone characteristics	Multiple, hard, and faceted	Small, brittle, dark	Small, soft, brownish-yellow, earthy texture
Associated with	Obesity, OCP use	Hemolytic anemia (e.g., hereditary spherocytosis, sickle cell anemia), cirrhosis	Parasitic infection (Ascaris lumbricoides, Clonorchis sinensis), biliary stents, biliary strictures, choledochal cyst.
Found in	Gallbladder	Gallbladder	Mostly in bile duct

Pathogenesis of Cholesterol Stones

Pathogenesis of cholesterol stones involves 3 stages: (i) Cholesterol supersaturation in bile; (ii) Crystal nucleation; and (iii) Stone growth.

↑↑ cholesterol
Bile salt
↓
Precipitation of cholesterol
↓
Nucleation
↓
Cholesterol stone formation

Pathogenesis of Black Pigment Stones

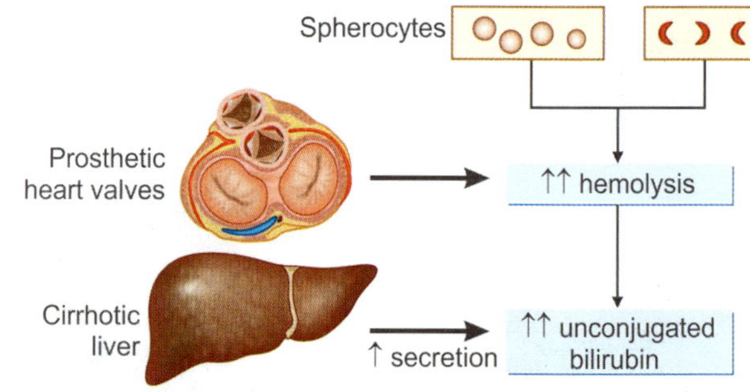

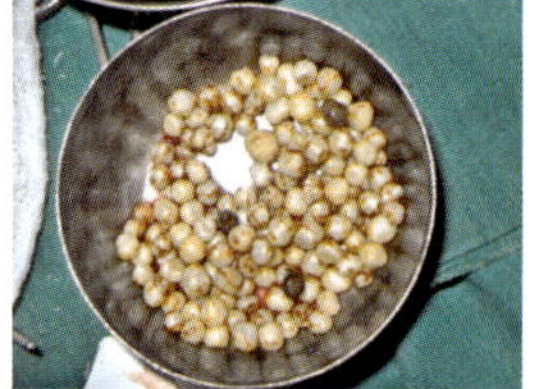

Multiple gallstones removed after cholecystectomy.

Black pigment stones most often secondary to hemolytic disorders such as hereditary spherocytosis, sickle cell disease.

Pathogenesis of Brown Pigment Stones

Brown pigment stones usually occur as primary duct stones, associated with bacterial infection and stasis, parasite infestations (*Clonorchis sinensis, Ascaris lumbricoides*).

E.coli secretes β-glucuronidase that causes hydrolysis of soluble conjugated glucuronide to produce insoluble free bilirubin, which then precipitates with calcium.

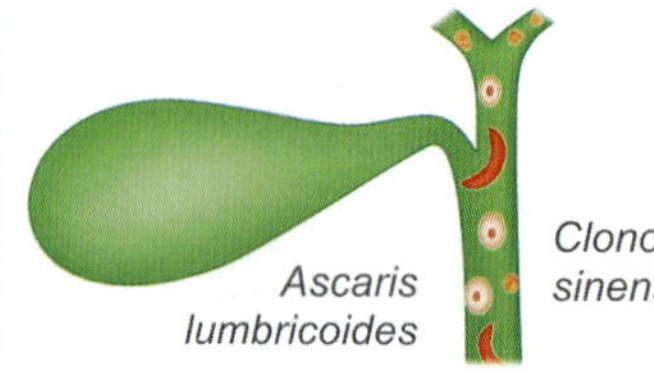

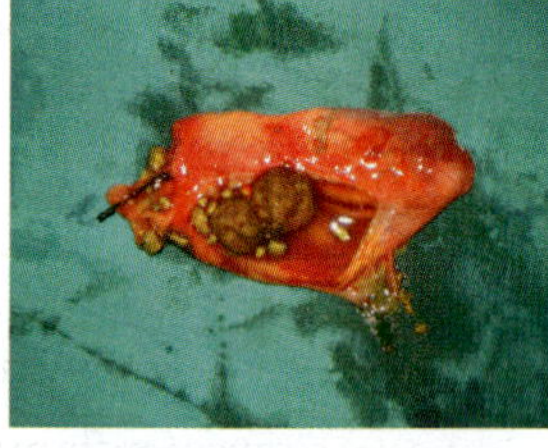

Gallbladder with multiple stones

Biliary Sludge

- Biliary sludge composed of cholesterol monohydrate crystals, calcium bilirubinate and other calcium salts, mucin.
- Clinical conditions associated with biliary sludge formation are pregnancy, rapid weight loss, total parenteral therapy, bone marrow or solid organ transplantation, ceftriaxone therapy.
- Biliary sludge may cause complications—acute pancreatitis, acute cholecystitis, biliary colic.
- On USG, biliary sludge appears as low-amplitude echoes in the dependant part of gallbladder without posterior acoustic shadowing and shift slowly with positioning.
- In asymptomatic patients, expectant treatment may be considered with ursodeoxycholic acid. In patients who develop biliary colic, pancreatitis, cholecystitis, cholecystectomy is the treatment of choice. In patients not fit for surgery, endoscopic sphincterotomy may prevent further episodes of cholangitis, pancreatitis.

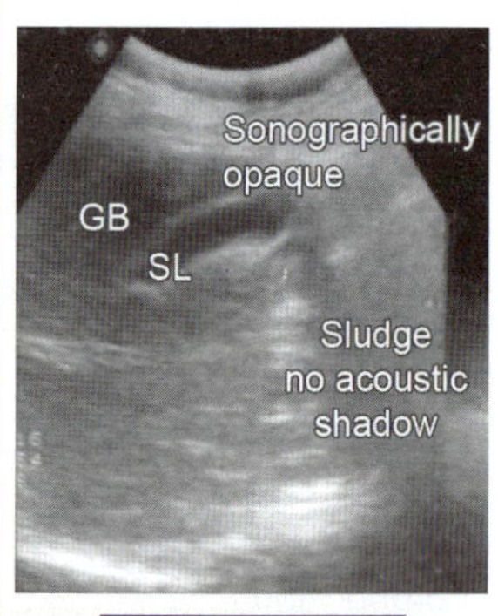

Sludge in gallbladder

Spectrum of Gallstone Disease

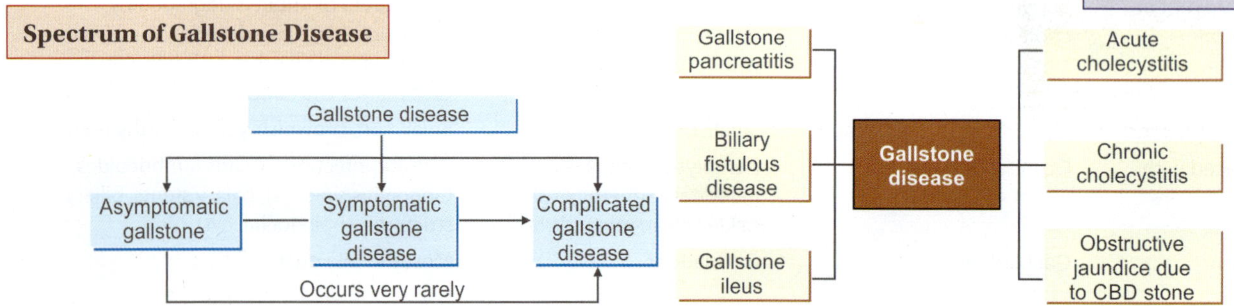

Acute Cholecystitis

Pathophysiology

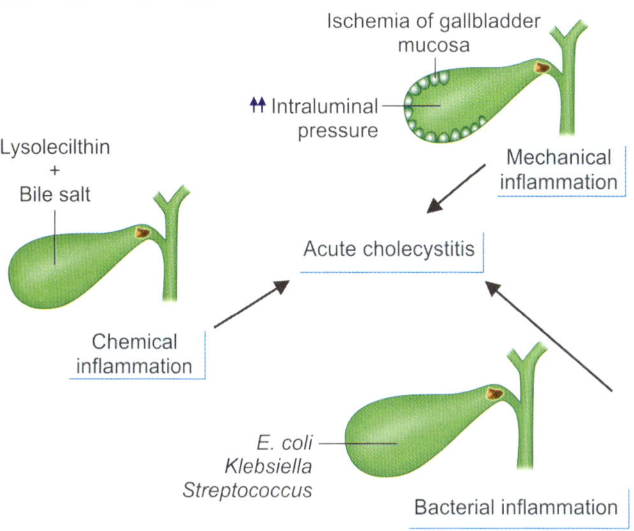

Clinical Manifestations

- Pain in right hypochondrium/epigastrium:
  - May radiate to right upper part of back/interscapular area.
  - Much longer in duration in comparison to previous episodes of biliary colic.
- Nausea and vomiting
- Fever
- Tenderness in right hypochondrium, sometimes associated with guarding
- **Murphy's sign:** In sitting position of the patient, surgeon's fingers are hooked up from behind under the right costal arch and at the height of inspiration, inspiration suddenly ceases.

Diagnosis

Diagnostic Criteria for Acute Cholecystitis (As per Tokyo Guideline 2018)

A. Local signs of inflammation, etc.

(1) Murphy's sign and (2) RUQ mass/pain/tenderness

B. Systemic signs of inflammation, etc.

(1) Fever; (2) Elevated CRP; and (3) Elevated WBC count

C. Imaging findings

Imaging findings characteristics of acute cholecystitis

- *Suspected diagnosis:* One item in A+one item in B
- *Definitive diagnosis:* One item in A+ one item in B+C

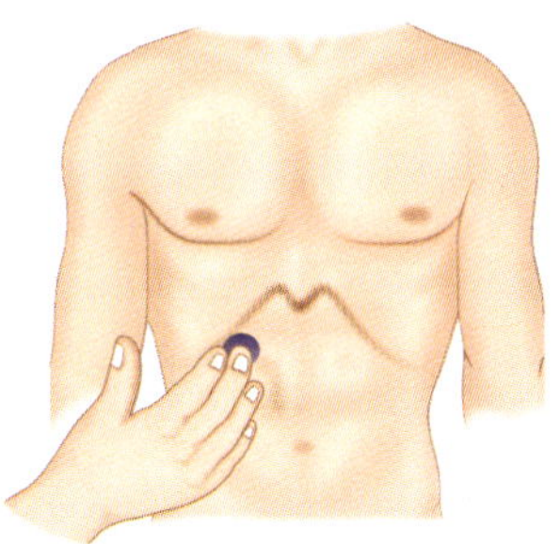

Elicitation of Murphy's Sign

Murphy's sign is highly sensitive and has high predictive value.

Murphy's percussion test: A perpendicular percussion technique for clinical evaluation of acute cholecystitis.

Moynihan's modification of Murphy's sign: Patient is in supine position and surgeon sitting on the edge of the couch, places the left hand over the lower part of the chest so that the thumb lies along the right rib margin. As deep breath is taken, thumb is pressed upwards towards the under surface of the liver.

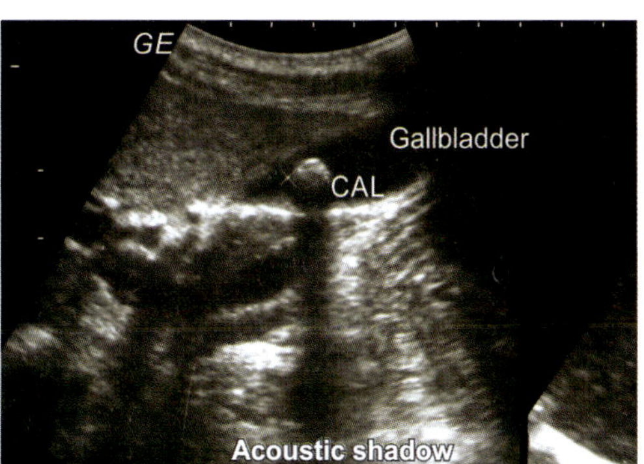

Imaging Findings (USG) Characteristic of Acute Cholecystitis

- Thickened gallbladder wall (>3 mm) and pericholecystic fluid.
- Calculus with acoustic shadow.
- Sonographic Murphy's sign (more sensitive than clinical Murphy's sign because probe is accurately placed over the gallbladder site).

Sonographic Murphy's sign:

Maximal abdominal tenderness from pressure of the USG probe over the visualized gallbladder.

If significant elevation of serum bilirubin, then possibilities are:

- Associated choledochlithiasis
- Mirizzi syndrome

If WBC count is significantly elevated, then possibilities are:

- Gangrenous cholecystitis
- Empyema gallbladder
- Gallbladder perforation

Differential diagnosis:

- Acute gastritis
- Acute pancreatitis
- Subhepatic acute appendicitis
- Pleuritis
- Pneumonia

Severity Grading for Acute Cholecystitis (as per Tokyo Guideline 2018)

Grade III (Severe) Acute Cholecystitis

"Grade III" acute cholecystitis is associated with dysfunction of any of the following organs/systems:

1. *Cardiovascular dysfunction:* Hypotension requiring treatment with dopamine ≥5 μg/kg per min, or any dose of norepinephrine
2. *Neurological dysfunction:* Decreased level of consciousness
3. *Respiratory dysfunction:* PaO_2/FiO_2 ratio <300
4. *Renal dysfunction:* Oliguria, creatinine >2.0 mg/dL
5. *Hepatic dysfunction:* PT-INR >1.5
6. *Hematological dysfunction:* Platelet count <100,000/mm^3

Grade II (Moderate) Acute Cholecystitis

"Grade II" acute cholecystitis is associated with any one of the following conditions:

1. Elevated WBC count (>18,000/mm^3)
2. Palpable tender mass in the right upper abdominal quadrant
3. Duration of complaints >72 hours
4. Marked local inflammation (gangrenous cholecystitis, pericholecystic abscess, hepatic abscess, biliary peritonitis, emphysematous cholecystitis)

Grade I (Mild) Acute Cholecystitis

"Grade I" acute cholecystitis does not meet the criteria of "Grade III" or "Grade II" acute cholecystitis. It can also be defined as acute cholecystitis in a healthy patient with no organ dysfunction and mild inflammatory changes in the gallbladder, making cholecystectomy a safe and low-risk operative procedure.

Treatment

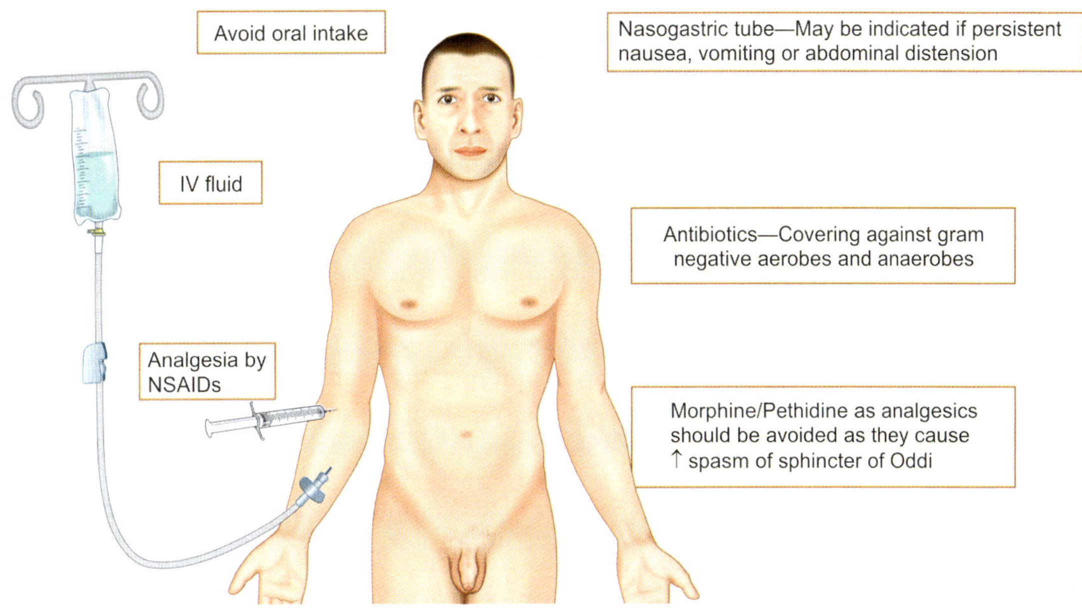

Management of Acute Cholecystitis According to Severity (As per Tokyo Guideline 2018)

1. *In Grade I acute cholecystitis,* laparoscopic cholecystectomy within 7 days (preferably within 72 hours) of onset of symptoms is recommended.
2. *In Grade II acute cholecystitis,* urgent or early laparoscopic cholecystectomy is considered if patient performance status is good and the advanced laparoscopic cholecystectomy technique is available. If the patient's condition is poor, urgent/early biliary drainage, or delayed/elective laparoscopic cholecystectomy can be considered.
3. *In Grade III patients with high surgical risk,* urgent or early biliary drainage should be considered. If any negative predictive factors or favorable organ system failure are not present and patient has good performance status, early laparoscopic cholecystectomy can be considered in advanced centre.

Percutaneous transhepatic gallbladder drainage (PTGBD) is the most preferred method of gallbladder drainage in acute cholecystitis in surgically high-risk patients.

Complications of Acute Cholecystitis

Acute Emphysematous Cholecystitis

- A variant of acute cholecystitis, develops due to secondary infection of the gallbladder wall by gas-forming organisms, e.g., *Clostridium perfringens, E.coli, Bacilis fragilis.*
- It is more common in men, diabetic patients and in patients taking sunitinib (a tyrosine kinase inhibitor).
- CT is the most useful imaging modality for diagnosis (identification of gas in gallbladder wall or lumen).
- Treatment is urgent cholecystectomy. In high-risk patients, percutaneous cholecystostomy is an option.

Gangrenous Cholecystitis

- A life-threatening complication of acute cholecystitis, may develop in elderly and diabetic patients.
- CT is highly specific for diagnosis of acute gangrenous cholecystitis. CT findings suggestive of gangrenous cholecystitis are intramural or intraluminal gas, intraluminal membranes, lack of gallbladder enhancement, and pericholecystic abscess.
- Most common site for necrosis is fundus of the gallbladder.
- Treatment is urgent cholecystectomy.

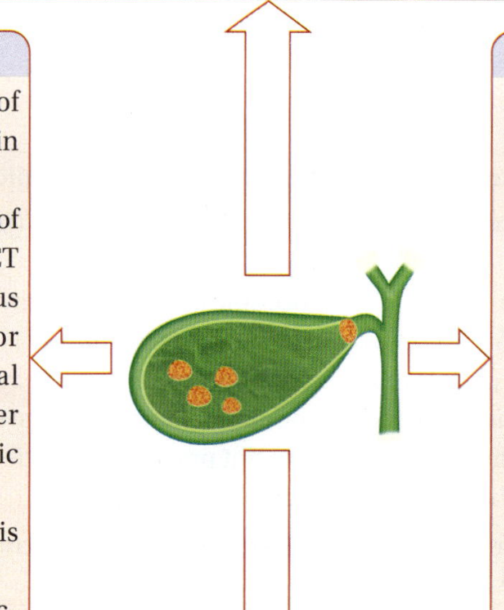

Cholecystoenteric Fistula

- Duodenum is the most common (75–80%) and hepatic flexure of colon (15–20%) is the second most common site of cholecystoenteric fistula.
- Most of the patients are asymptomatic, some of the patients may present with cholangitis or pneumobilia.
- Contrast study of stomach and duodenum shows fistulous connection.
- Often associated with Mirizzi syndrome.

Gallbladder Perforation

- It is one of the severe complications of acute cholecystitis, commonly associated as a sequelae of emphysematous or gangrenous cholecystitis.
- Three types of perforation are described in Niemeier classification.
- Clinical diagnosis is often difficult.
- "Hole sign" (a focal gallbladder defect) in USG or CT is helpful in diagnosis.
- Complications include bile leakage, abscess formation in liver and gallbladder fossa.
- Treatment is drainage of abscess along with cholecystectomy. In type III perforation, besides cholecystectomy, cholecystoenteric fistula have to be managed.

Mucocele of the Gallbladder

- Develops when stone is impacted in the neck of gallbladder, leads to absorption of bile, and replaced by mucus.
- Patient presents with chronic upper abdominal pain and soft, non-tender palpable gallbladder.
- Treatment is cholecystectomy.

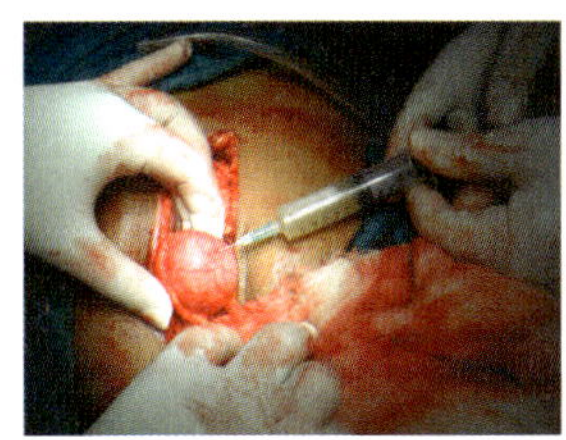

Mucocele of gallbladder

Empyema Gallbladder

- Develops when stone is impacted in neck of gallbladder with superadded infection of the stagnant bile, leads to gallbladder filled with purulent fluid, sometimes frank pus.
- More common in diabetic male patients.
- Patient presents with severe pain in upper abdomen, tender palpable gallbladder, sometimes features of sepsis.
- Treatment is urgent cholecystectomy or urgent decompression under radiological guidance.

Chronic Cholecystitis

Pathophysiology

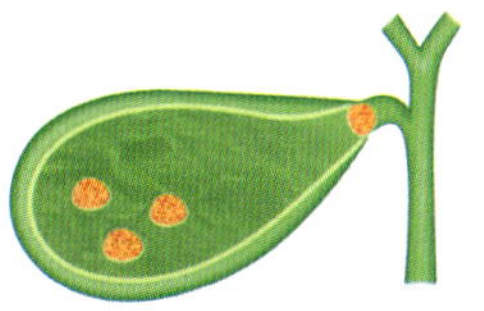

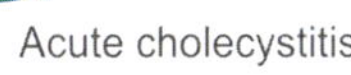

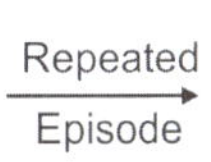

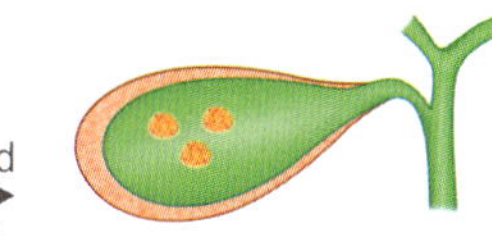

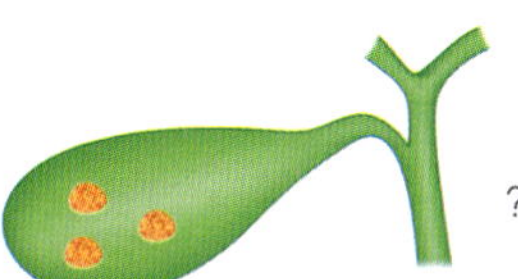

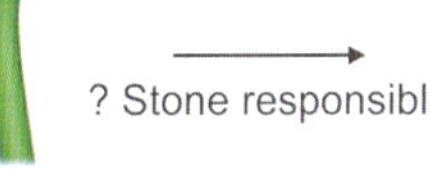

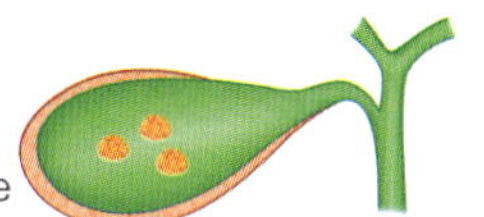

Clinical Manifestations

- Women are more commonly affected.
- One or more episodes of pain in the right hypochondrium or epigastrium.
- Constant, less severe pain for few hours, often self-limiting. Pain usually initiates after taking fatty meal and often self-limited. Radiation of the pain to the right upper back or in between scapula.
- Intolerance to fatty foods
- Nausea, vomiting
- Mild tenderness may be elicited during the pain attack, otherwise no obvious clinical finding.

- Chronic cholecystitis is almost always associated with gallstones.
- Chronic cholecystitis develops either due to recurrent episodes of acute cholecystitis or due to chronic irritation from gallstones.

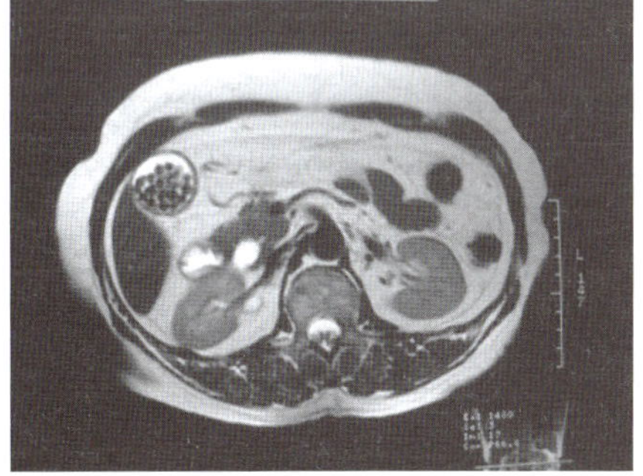

MRI abdomen showing multiple gallstones (MRI is not a routine imaging modality for suspected gallstone disease).

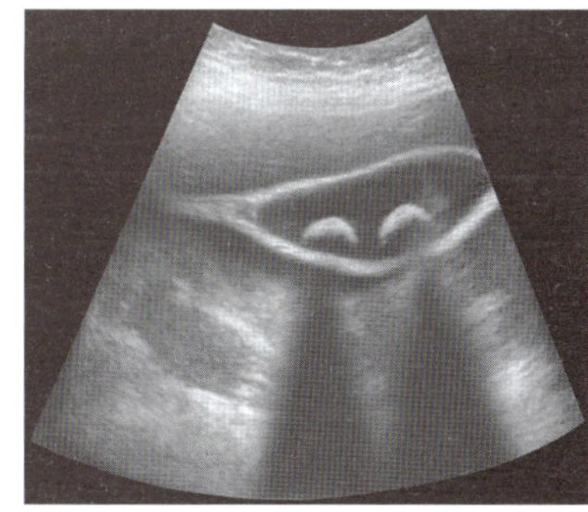

Multiple stones in gallbladder.

Diagnosis

- Ultrasonography of abdomen is the investigation of choice.
- USG findings include contracted or normal appearing gallbladder with calculi, thickened gallbladder wall. Sometimes, only sludge is found.

Treatment

The gold standard treatment of chronic calculus cholecystitis is laparoscopic cholecystectomy.

Laparoscopic cholecystectomy may be performed in any trimester of pregnancy without an increased risk to the mother or fetus.

Preoperative Workup

- Hb%, TC, DC, ESR
- Blood sugar (fasting and postprandial), serum urea, creatinine
- Liver function test
- Serology—HbsAg, HCV-antibody, HIV I&II
- Chest X-ray
- ECG
- Echocardiography (in selected patients)

Principles of Laparoscopic Cholecystectomy in Pregnancy (Adapted from SAGES Guideline)

- Laparoscopic cholecystectomy is the treatment of choice in the pregnant patient with symptomatic gallbladder disease, regardless of trimester.
- Initial abdominal access via subcostal approach using either open (Hassan technique) or closed (Veress needle or optical entry) technique is recommended to avoid the gravid uterus.
- CO_2 insufflation of 10–15 mm Hg can be safely used without increasing adverse outcomes to the patient or fetus.
- Intraoperative CO_2 monitoring by capnography should be used during laparoscopy.
- Venous thromboembolic (VTE) prophylaxis with pneumatic compression devices both intraoperatively and postoperatively and early postoperative ambulation are recommended.

Principles of Laparoscopic Cholecystectomy in Presence of Cirrhosis

- Laparoscopic cholecystectomy is a safe procedure in Child-Pugh class A and B cirrhosis.
- Coagulopathy to be corrected before surgery.
- Preoperative imaging should be considered to detect abdominal wall varices, recanalized umbilical vein.
- Open Hassan approach via infra-umbilical incision is preferred for access to avoid injury of periumbilical varices.
- Subxiphoid port placement to the right of midline to avoid injury of potential collaterals in falciform ligament.
- Excessive cephalad traction of the gallbladder should be avoided during dissection of Calot's triangle.
- Liberal use of energy sources and hemostatic agents.
- If bleeding cannot be controlled, decision for conversion should be taken promptly.
- All port sites should be closed watertight to prevent leakage of ascitic fluid.

Acute Biliary Pancreatitis

Acute pancreatitis caused by gallstone or sludge.

Pathophysiology

Opie's 'common channel' hypothesis: An impacted gallstone at the ampulla of Vater creates a communication between the main pancreatic duct and bile duct, resulting in reflux of bile into the pancreatic duct and initiates pancreatitis.

Duodenal reflux: Passage of gallstone may damage of duodenal sphincter, resulting in reflux of duodenal contents including bile and activated pancreatic juice into the pancreatic duct.

Ductal hypertension: Obstruction of the pancreatic duct at the level of ampulla causes ductal hypertension, resulting in intracellular protease activation that leads to damage of the pancreatic parenchyma.

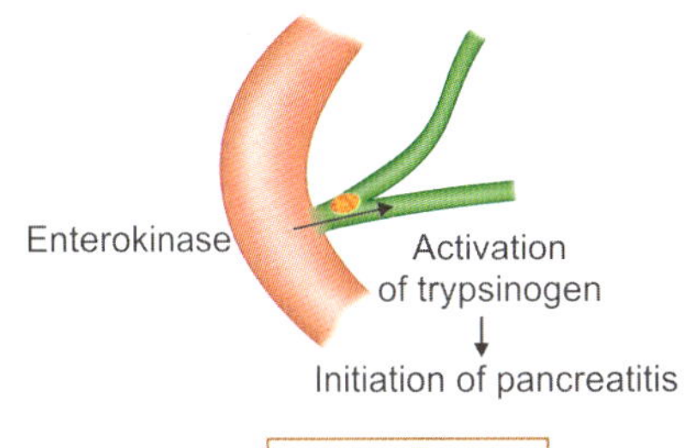

Duodenal reflux

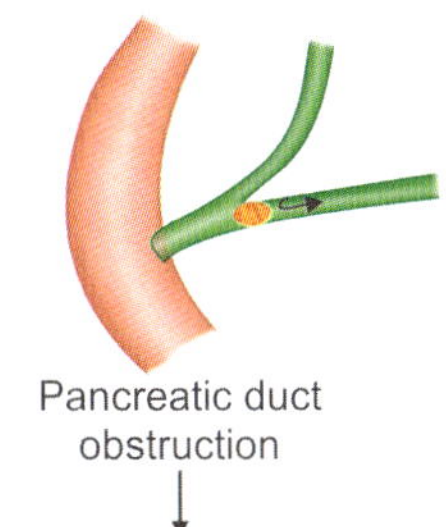

Clinical Presentation

Symptoms

- Pain in epigastrium or right hypochondrium
- Pain radiating to back
- Vomiting

Signs

- Epigastric tenderness
- Guarding in the upper abdomen
- Absent or sluggish IPS
- Diminished breath sound
- Hypotension, tachycardia

Patient previously suffered from biliary colic, previous USG showed multiple stones in gallbladder, now complaining of more severe pain with some systemic manifestations (tachycardia, hypotension, diminished breath sound), **suspect biliary pancreatitis**.

Diagnosis

- Serum lipase and amylase levels above three times the upper level of normal.
- Characteristic findings of acute pancreatitis on abdominal imaging
- Gallstones and/or sludge on imaging (USG/CT scan)

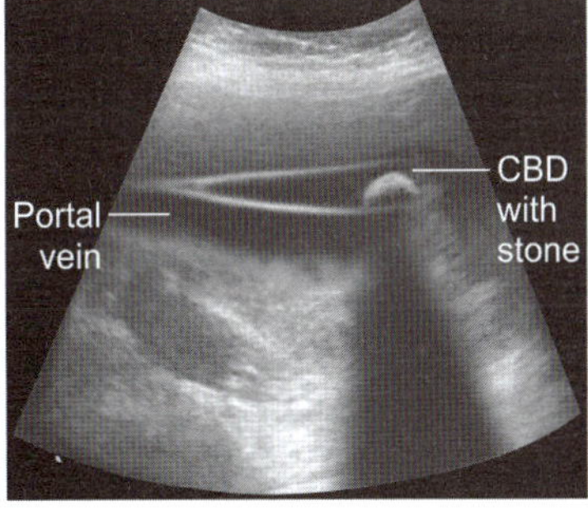

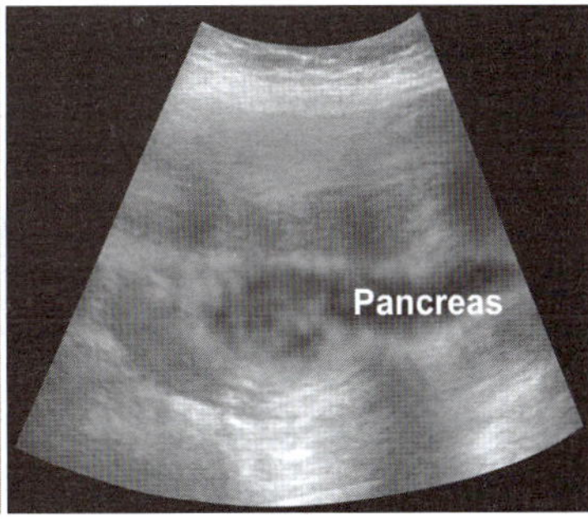

Treatment

In mild biliary pancreatitis, cholecystectomy should be performed during index admission to avoid risk of biliary event recurrence (early cholecystectomy is not associated with increased risk of complications). Biliary tract exploration is performed as required.

In severe biliary pancreatitis (in presence of complications from cholangitis or bile duct obstruction is suspected), emergency endoscopic approach for CBD clearance by (endoscopic sphincterotomy/endoscopic papillary balloon dilation/endoscopic nasobiliary drainage/stenting) followed by cholecystectomy after 4–6 weeks.

Different option of biliary tract exploration

- ERCP prior to laparoscopic cholecystectomy.
- Intraoperative cholangiography during LC and if CBD stone is detected, then either laparoscopic/open CBD exploration.
- ERCP after cholecystectomy.

Gallstone Ileus

A rare type of mechanical intestinal obstruction due to gallstone impaction within the GI tract.

Pathophysiology

- The inflammation of gallbladder causes adhesion with the adjacent gastrointestinal tract.
- The inflammation and the pressure effect of stone causes fistula formation between the gallbladder and the adjacent GI tract.
- The gallstone migrates through the fistula tract and finally impacts anywhere in the GI tract, but commonly in the terminal ileum and causes intestinal obstruction.

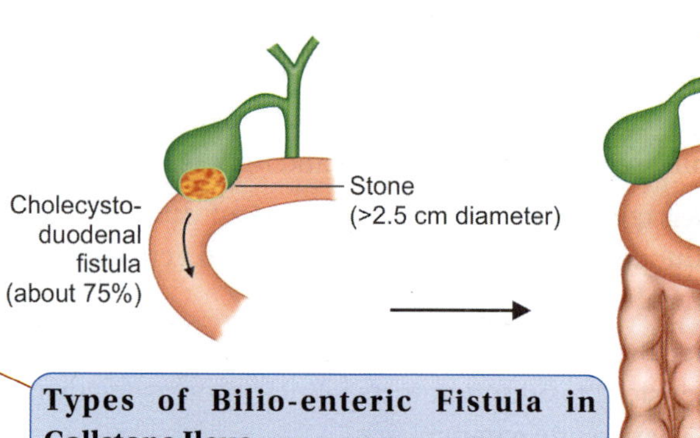

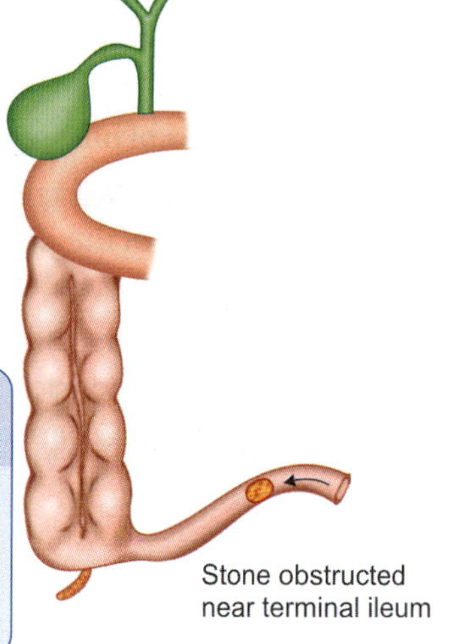

Types of Bilio-enteric Fistula in Gallstone Ileus

- Cholecystoduodenal (most common)
- Cholecystogastric
- Cholecystojejunal
- Cholecystoileal

Clinical Presentation

- History of biliary symptoms
- Chronic episodes (due to passage of gallstone through the GI tract) of intestinal obstruction
- Acute, complete intestinal obstruction (when gallstone definitively becomes impacted)
- Features of acute intestinal obstruction—vomiting, absolute constipation, abdominal distension, high-pitched bowel sound or absent IPS.

Sites of Gallstone Impaction

- Terminal ileum and the ileocecal valve (most common)
- Proximal ileum
- Jejunum
- Duodenum
- Colon

Clinical Presentation

Straight X-ray of abdomen—important role in diagnosis

USG of abdomen—can detect impacted gallstone, pneumobilia, biliary-enteric fistula.

CT abdomen—better imaging modality than straight X-ray or USG for diagnosis of gallstone ileus. Rigler's triad is better observed in CT.

Four Radiographic Signs in Gallstone Ileus (described by Rigler et al.)

1. Partial or complete intestinal obstruction
2. Pneumobilia
3. A gallstone in the bowel
4. Change of position of such gallstone on serial films

Treatment

Surgical Treatment Options

Enterolithotomy: Enterotomy is done proximal to the site of impaction followed by gentle milking of the stone to the enterotomy site is the better option for stone removal. If gallstone is severely impacted and milking of the stone is not possible, enterotomy is done over the stone. Enterotomy is primarily repaired. Resection of intestine is indicated when gut viability is questionable or perforation develops.

Enterolithotomy, cholecystectomy and fistula closure (One-stage procedure) is indicated only in selected patients with good general condition and can tolerate a prolonged operative procedure.

Enterolithotomy followed by cholecystectomy and fistula repair later (Two-stage procedure)—better surgical option for most of the patients.

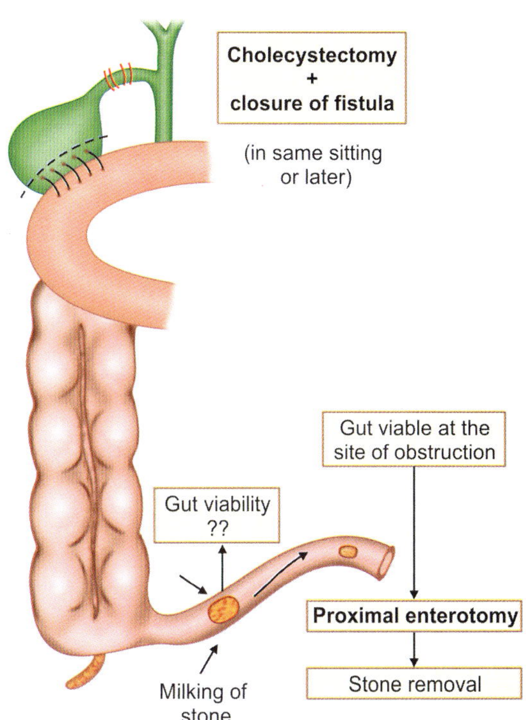

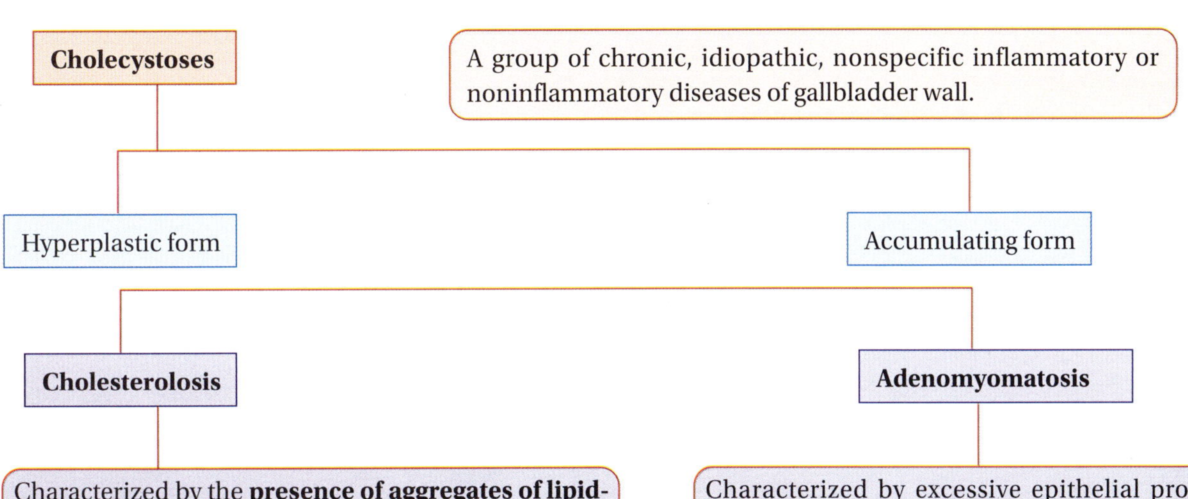

Cholesterolosis

Characterized by the **presence of aggregates of lipid-containing (cholesterol precursors and cholesterol esters)** macrophages in the lamina propria of the gallbladder.

Pathogenesis is unknown. No malignant potential.

Commonly diagnosed after macroscopic examination of the interior of the gallbladder—yellow flecks against a dark-green background **(Strawberry gallbladder)**.

Sometimes, extensive deposits may appear as polypoid excrescences that project into the lumen **(Cholesterol polyp or Cholesterolosis Polyp)**.

Adenomyomatosis

Characterized by excessive epithelial proliferation that leads to epithelial infolding within the underlying muscular layer-formation of epithelial-lined diverticular pouches **(Rokitansky-Aschoff sinuses)**.

Patterns of gallbladder wall involvement: (i) Localized; (ii) Segmental; (iii) Annular; and (iv) Diffuse.

Identification of Rokitansky-Aschoff sinus on imaging is essential for diagnosis of adenomyomatosis.

No malignant potential.

Cholecystectomy is indicated only in symptomatic patients.

Acute Acalculous Cholecystitis

Acute inflammation of the gallbladder without gallstone. About 10% of acute cholecystitis are of acute acalculous type.

Pathophysiology

- Etiology is multifactorial.
- Most likely mechanism is bile stasis or ischemia or both.
- Risk factors related to this pathology may cause bile stasis or hypoperfusion of the gallbladder, resulting in ischemic changes and growth of microorganisms.

Risk Factors

- Extensive trauma
- Severe burn
- Sepsis
- Prolonged parenteral nutrition
- On mechanical ventilation
- After major surgery (e.g., abdominal aortic aneurysm repair, cardiopulmonary bypass).

Clinical Presentation

- Clinical presentations may similar to acute calculous cholecystitis.
- Symptoms and signs related to sepsis may only present.

Diagnosis

- Acute acalculous cholecystitis should be suspected if a critically-ill patient presenting with features of acute cholecystitis.
- USG findings similar to acute cholecystitis except presence of stones.
- HIDA scan—low sensitivity and specificity.

Complications

- Gangrene
- Perforation

Treatment

Percutaneous cholecystostomy: Better treatment option because most of the patients are critically ill. Most of the patients improve within 24 hours.

Cholecystectomy is only indicated if patient not improving after percutaneous cholecystostomy or in presence of gallbladder perforation or gangrene of the gallbladder.

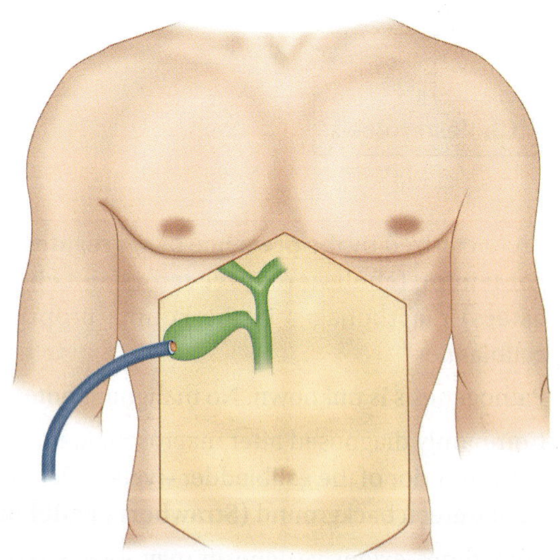

Percutaneous cholecystostomy

Biliary Dyskinesia

Symptomatic functional disorder of the gallbladder of unknown etiology.

Diagnosis

Patient must have **right upper quadrant pain similar to biliary colic** but have normal USG of gallbladder (no stones, sludge, microlithiasis, gallbladder wall thickening, CBD dilation).

Rome III diagnostic criteria for functional gallbladder disorders should be considered.

HIDA (Hepatobiliary iminodiacetic acid) scan: An ejection fraction <35% at 30 minutes is considered abnormal.

Rome III Diagnostic Criteria for Functional Gallbladder Disorder

- Pain episodes that last longer than 30 minutes.
- Recurrent symptoms that occur at variable intervals.
- Pain that is severe enough to interrupt daily activity or lead to ER visits.
- Pain that builds up to a steady level.
- Pain that is not relieved by bowel movements, postural changes, or antacids.
- Exclusion of other structural diseases that could explain the symptoms.
- Other supportive criteria include association of pain with nausea and vomiting, radiation of pain to the infrascapular region, and pain that wakes the patient at the middle of the night.
- Normal liver enzymes, conjugated bilirubin, and amylase/lipase.

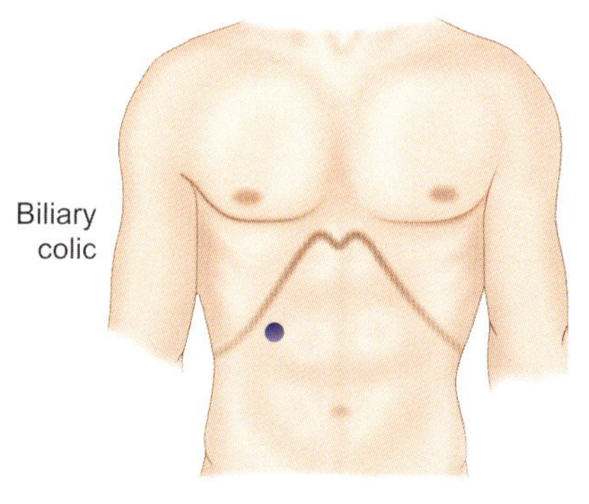

+

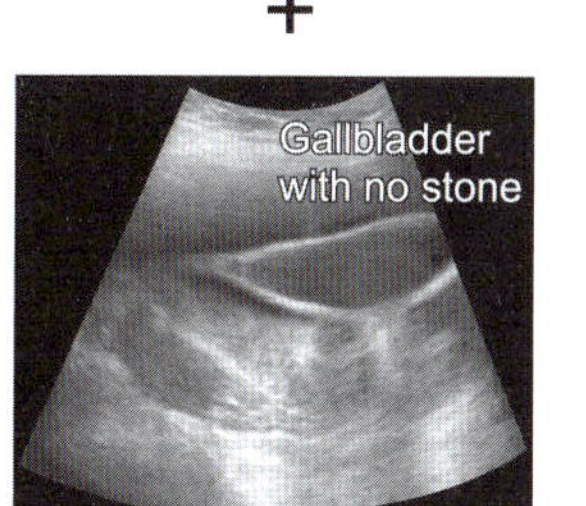

+

Abnormal HIDA scan

1 hour
1.5 hour
2 hour
3 hour
3.5 hours

Treatment

If presence of classic biliary symptoms (Rome III Diagnostic Criteria) with normal USG and abnormal HIDA scan, cholecystectomy should be considered.

Cholecystectomy

Laparoscopic cholecystectomy

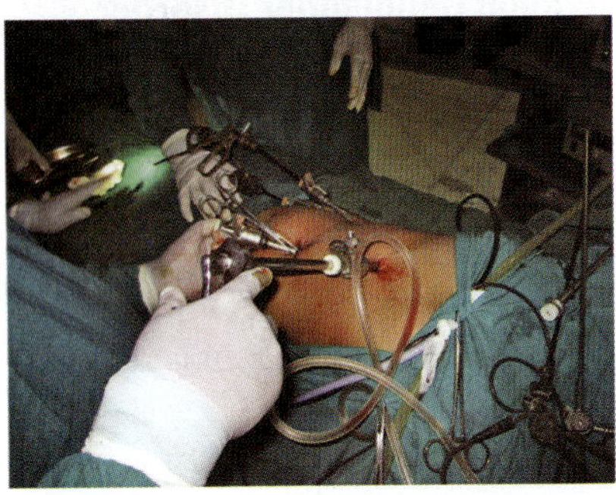

Indications of Laparoscopic Cholecystectomy

- Gallstone with biliary colic
- Chronic calculous cholecystitis
- Acute cholecystitis
- Gallstone pancreatitis
- Asymptomatic cholelithiasis in certain circumstances
- Gallbladder polyp >10 mm

Absolute Contraindications to Laparoscopic Cholecystectomy

- Unable to tolerate GA
- Refractory coagulopathy
- Suspected or confirmed gallbladder carcinoma

Relative Contraindications to Laparoscopic Cholecystectomy

- Frozen upper abdomen due to previous surgery
- Portal hypertension
- Cholecystoenteric fistula
- Chronic obstructive pulmonary disease

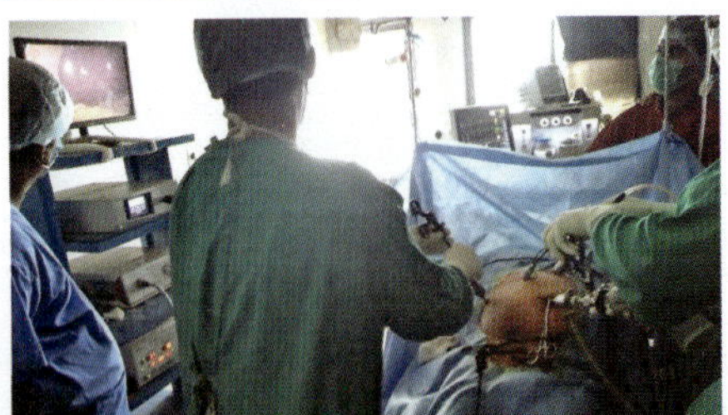

Laparoscopic cholecystectomy (note the position of surgeon, assistants and the monitor)

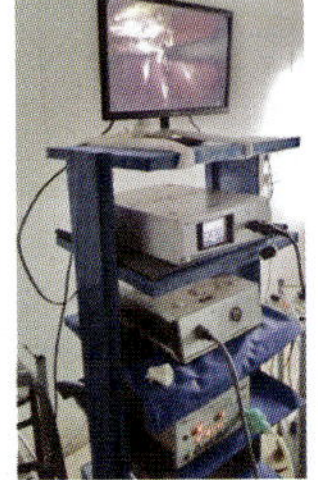
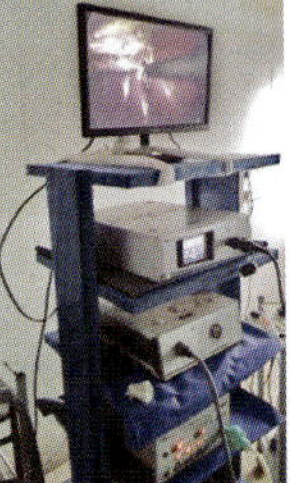

Laparoscopic trolley

Relative Indications of Prophylactic Cholecystectomy

- Patient of sickle cell anemia
- Before or during renal transplantation
- During bariatric surgery

Absolute Contraindications to Cholecystectomy (Laparoscopic or Open)

- Refractory coagulopathy
- Patient not fit for GA
- Severe sepsis causing end organ failure

Open cholecystectomy

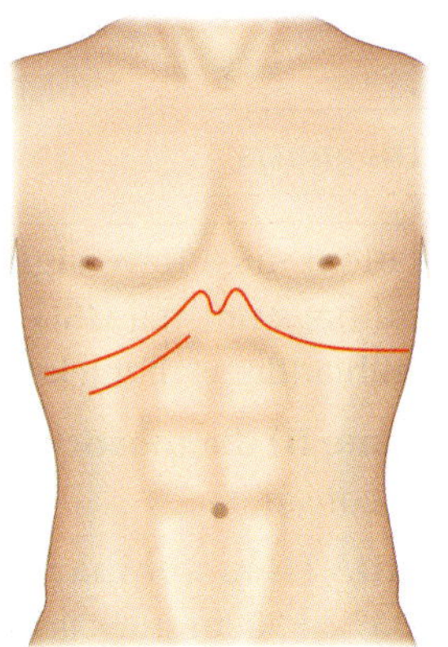

Open cholecystectomy

Indications for Planned Open Cholecystectomy

- Known or suspected gallbladder cancer
- Patient's informed request for open procedure
- Known dense adhesions in upper abdomen
- Planned open CBD exploration.

Operative Room Setup in Laparoscopic Cholecystectomy

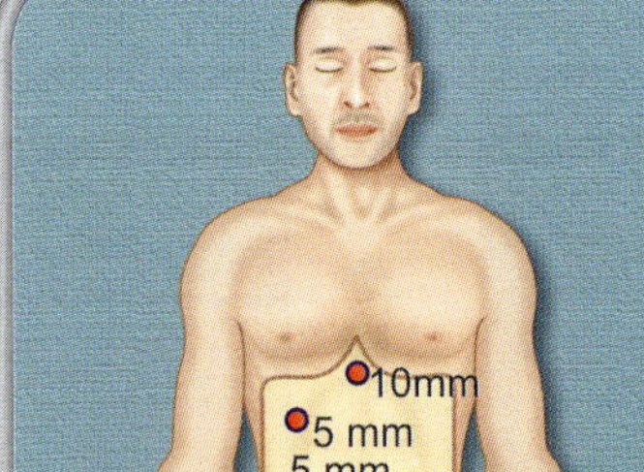

North-American approach

In Europe, Surgeon stands in between legs.

Port Position

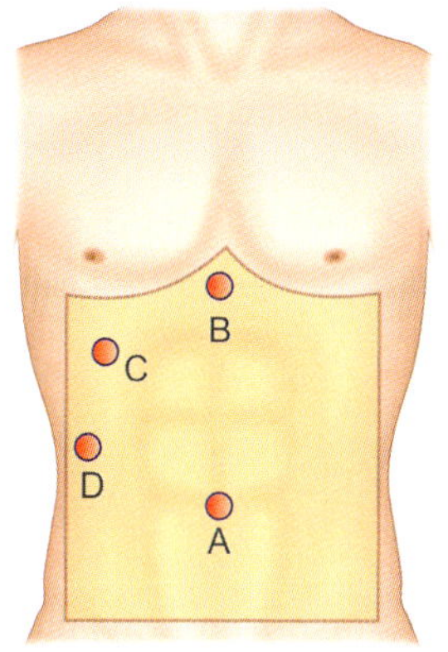

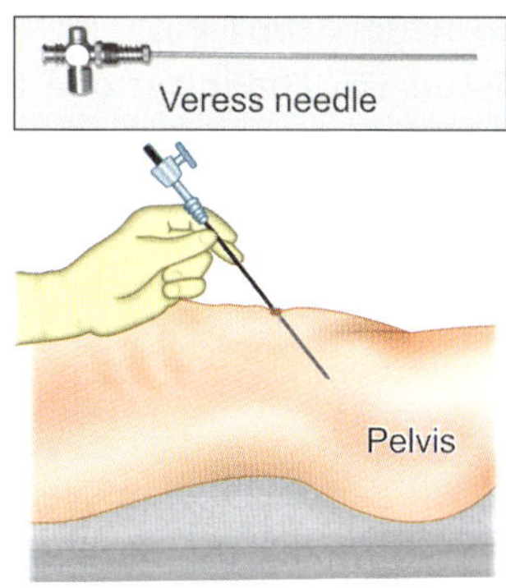

Techniques for Initial Abdominal Access

- Veress needle method
- Open Hasson technique
- Direct trocar placement without prior pneumoperitoneum
- Optical view technique

Hasson's cannula

A: Umbilical port (10 mm): For laparoscope.

B: Epigastric port (10 mm): For surgeon's right hand instrument.

C: Right subcostal port at midclavicular line (5 mm): For surgeon's left hand instrument.

D: Right lateral port at anterior axillary line (5 mm): For gallbladder retraction.

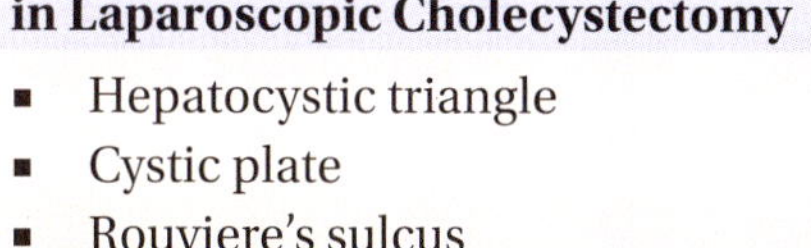

Important Anatomical Landmarks in Laparoscopic Cholecystectomy

- Hepatocystic triangle
- Cystic plate
- Rouviere's sulcus
- Segment 4
- Umbilical fissure

R4U Safety Line

An imaginary line joining the roof of Rouviere's sulcus, base of segment 4 and umbilical fissure. All the dissection during laparoscopic cholecystectomy should be done cephalad to this line.

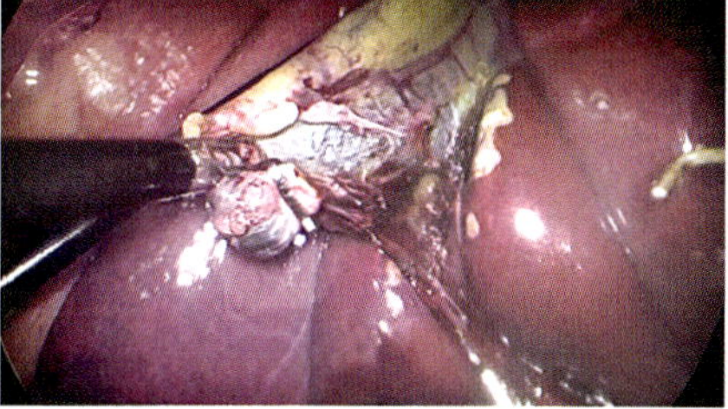

Laparoscopic cholecystectomy in progress (Gallbladder is dissected from the cystic plate).

Cephalad retraction
Instrument through right lateral port
Liver
Instrument through right subcostal port
Instrument through epigastric port
Retraction toward right pelvis

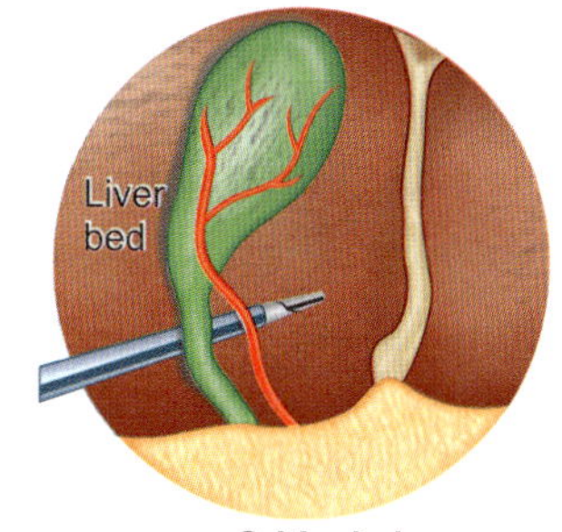

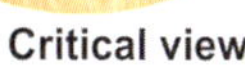

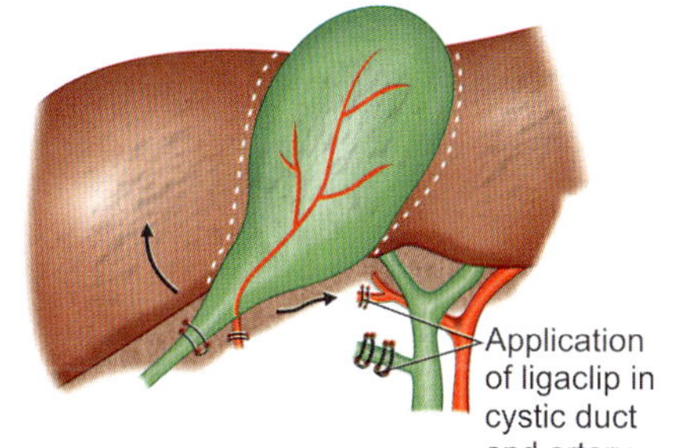

A = **A**nomalous anatomy—Keep in mind the possibility
B = **B**ile duct—Keep away from duct
C = **C**onversion to open—It is not failure, but a wise decision
D = **D**issection—Good dissection to define cystic duct and artery
E = **E**xpect—Expect uneventful postoperative recovery.

SAGES: A Universal Culture of Safety in Cholecystectomy

There are six suggested strategies. Surgeons can employ to adopt a universal culture of safety for cholecystectomy to minimize the risk of bile duct injury.

1. Use the **Critical View of Safety (CVS)** method of identification of the cystic duct and cystic artery during laparoscopic cholecystectomy. **Three criteria are required to achieve the CVS:**
   (i) The hepatocystic triangle is cleared of fat and fibrous tissue; (ii) The lower one-third of the gallbladder is separated from the liver to expose the cystic plate; (iii) Two and only two structures should be seen entering the gallbladder.
2. Understand the potential for aberrant anatomy in all cases.
3. Make liberal use of cholangiography or other methods to image the biliary tree intraoperatively.
4. Consider an intraoperative time-out during laparoscopic cholecystectomy prior to clipping, cutting or transecting any ductal structures.
5. Recognize when the dissection is approaching a zone of significant risk and halt the dissection before entering the zone.
6. Get help from another surgeon when the dissection or conditions are difficult.

Doublet view: CVS should be seen both from the front and back clearly to have complete circumferential visualization of cystic duct and artery.

A bail-out procedure should be chosen if a CVS cannot be achieved to prevent bile duct injury in difficult laparoscopic cholecystectomy for acute cholecystitis.

Bail-out Procedures

(i) Subtotal cholecystectomy

(ii) Fundus first technique

Subtotal cholecystectomy is either fenestrating (Gallbladder is opened and the cystic duct is closed from inside) or reconstituting (closure of the remnant gallbladder wall).

Near-Infrared Fluorescent Cholangiography

This technology involves preoperative intravenous injection of indocyanine green (ICG) and peroperative use of specialized camera system which uses near-infrared light to view the fluorescing ICG. ICG is excreted exclusively in bile, and it emits light when illuminated with near-infrared light. This technology enables real-time identification of cystic duct, common hepatic duct, common bile duct, accessory duct (if any) during cholecystectomy.

Complications of Spilled Gall-stones

- Intra-abdominal abscess
- Abscess in abdominal wall
- Liver abscess
- Fistula

Complications of Cholecystectomy:

- Pneumoperitoneum-related complications
- Perioperative bleeding
- Bile duct injury
- Spilled gallstone and related complications
- Biliary stricture
- Migration of ligaclips

Causes of Perioperative Bleeding in Cholecystectomy

- Bleeding from gallbladder bed
- From cystic artery
- Injury to the right hepatic artery, tributary of middle hepatic vein, portal vein

Complications of Clip Migration

- Choledocholithiasis
- Cholangitis
- Choledochoduodenal fistula

Factors associated with increased conversion rate (from laparoscopic to open):

- Gallbladder wall >4–5 mm on preoperative ultrasound
- Male gender
- Acute cholecystitis (Grade II/III)
- Contracted gallbladder on ultrasound
- Previous abdominal surgery

Reasons for conversion (from laparoscopic to open):

- Inability to correctly identify anatomy of Calot's triangle
- Bile duct injury
- Bleeding or bowel injury that cannot be managed by laparoscopic approach
- Cholecystoduodenal fistula.

Basic Steps in Laparoscopic Cholecystectomy

- The most common site for initial abdominal access is at the midline through the umbilicus or supra- or infraumbilical. The technique of initial abdominal access is either open or closed (by Veress needle) technique.
- After confirming safe peritoneal entry, pneumoperitoneum is created by insufflating CO_2 into the peritoneal cavity through the Veress needle or 1st laparoscopic port (10 mm). In case of closed (Veress needle) technique, Veress needle is replaced by a 10 mm port.
- Through this 10-mm umbilical port, a 10-mm 30° laparoscope is inserted. Patient is placed in reverse Trendelenburg position of 30° and table is rotated to left by 15° (to allow the colon and duodenum to fall away from the liver edge. Another 10-mm port and two 5-mm ports are then placed under direct vision.
- A heavy grasper is introduced through the 5-mm lateral port to grasp the gallbladder fundus and then pushed in a lateral and cephalad direction over the liver edge. The infundibulum is grasped by a grasper (placing lateral traction) through the 5-mm subcostal port by the Surgeon's left hand. Through the 10-mm epigastric port, Surgeon uses the Maryland forceps and diathermy hook for posterior dissection and to dissect the hepatocystic triangle to clear all the fibrofatty tissue for achieving 'Critical View of Safety' (CVS).
- After achieving CVS, cystic duct and artery are clipped with ligaclips (300/400)-one clip on the gallbladder side and two clips on the proximal side of the cystic duct; in cystic artery, two proximally and one on the gallbladder side. Cystic duct and artery are divided by scissors.
- The electrosurgical hook is used to separate the gallbladder from the liver bed. Gallbladder is extracted through umbilical or epigastric port.
- Drain (optional) is placed through the 5-mm lateral port.
- Fascial closure of the umbilical port is done with an absorbable closure. Fascial closure of the epigastric port is optional. Skin closure of all port sites are done by sutures or adhesive strips or skin closure adhesives.

Basic Steps in Open Cholecystectomy

Incision

Right subcostal (Kocher) incision: A finger width below the costal margin. Length of the incision depends on the surgeon.

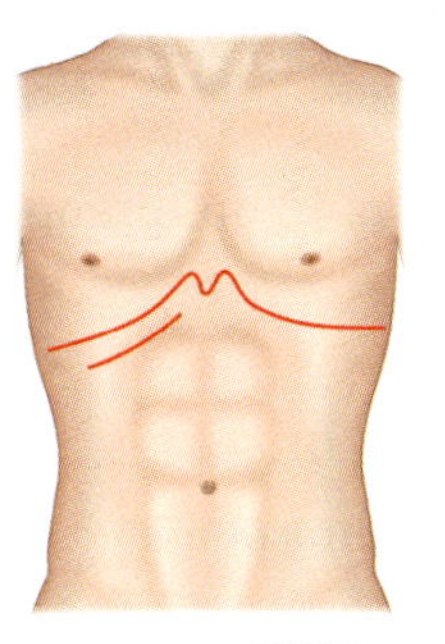

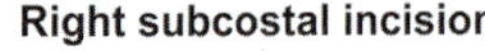

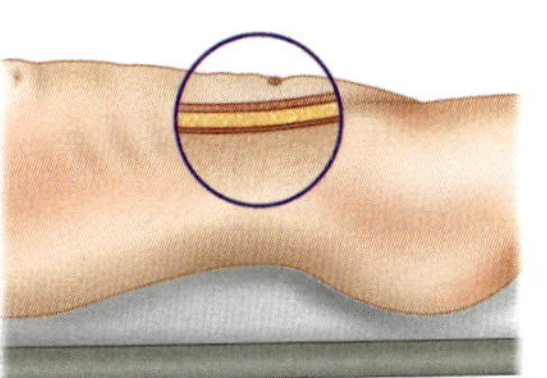

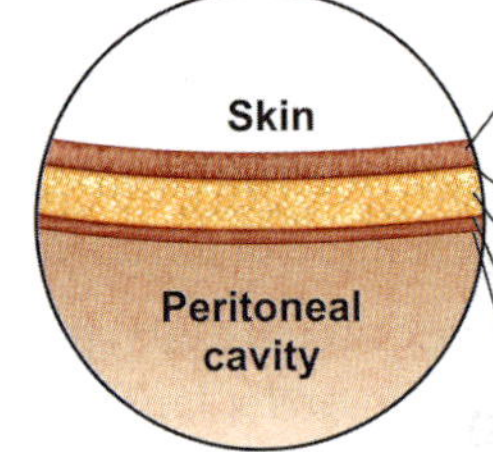

Exposure of the Calot's Traingle

- Retraction of fundus by Moynihan's cholecystectomy forceps—anteriorly and superiorly.
- Retraction of Hartmann's pouch by Moynihan's cholecystectomy forceps—Inferiorly and laterally.
- Laparotomy sponges are placed over the hepatic flexure and over the duodenum. Retraction of duodenum and colon—by Deaver retractor or assistant's left hand over the sponges.

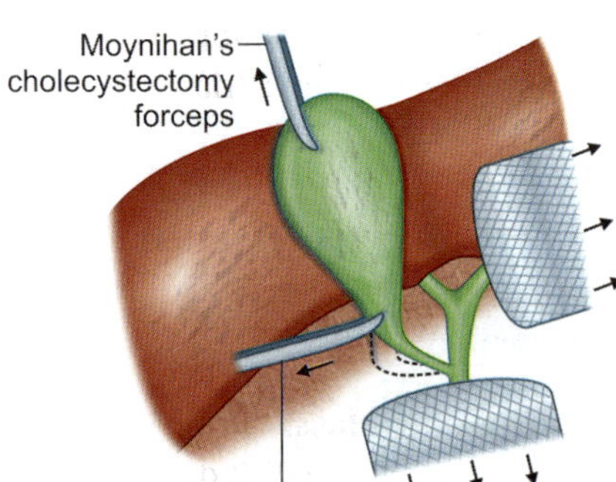

Dissection of Calot's Triangle

- Dissection should be close to gallbladder.
- The junction between gallbladder and cystic duct, not the junction between cystic duct and CBD should be identified.
- Dissection of the cystic artery pathway towards the gallbladder to see its final distribution into gallbladder wall—cystic artery should be ligated close to the gallbladder to avoid unwanted ligature of aberrant right hepatic artery.
- Both duct and artery are ligated with silk sutures. Both duct and artery are divided by scissors.

Dissection of Gallbladder from its Fossa

- Dissection of gallbladder from its fossa by diathermy.
- Dissection should be kept close to gallbladder within the cystic plate.

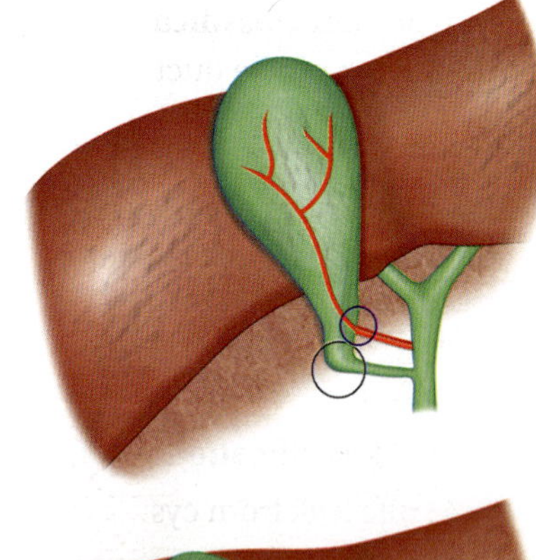

Placement of Drain and Closure

- Evidence-based medicine does not support the use of drain in routine cholecystectomy. Use of drain depends on the surgeon's choice.
- Sheath is closed in one or two layers. Skin is closed with sutures or staples.

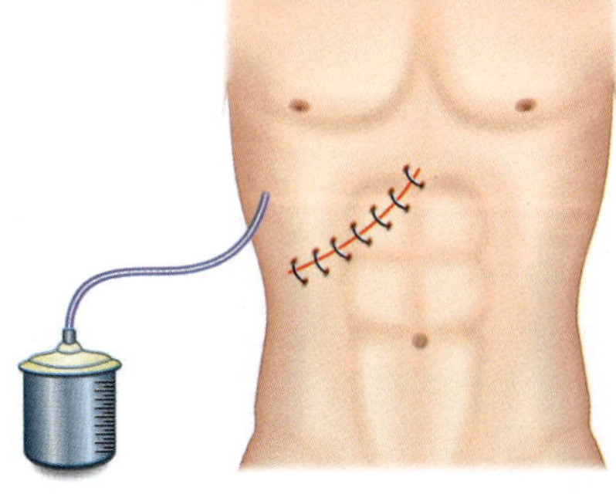

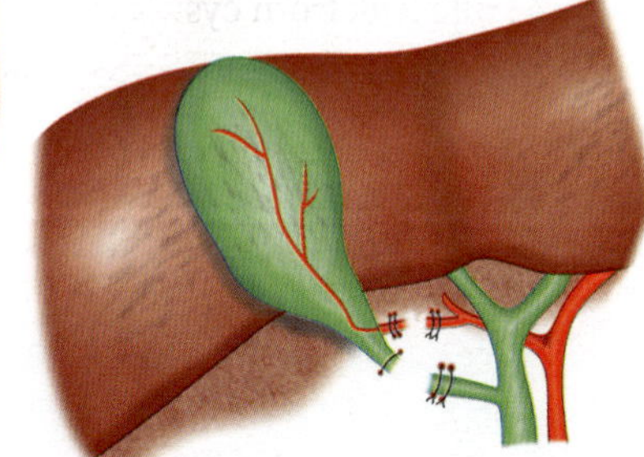

Bile Duct Injury

Factors Responsible

Compromised surgery:

- Insufficient experience
- Inadequate incision and exposure
- Inadequate assistance.

Anomalous anatomy:

- Short cystic duct
- Narrow common bile duct
- Aberrant junction of cystic duct and common hepatic duct.

Inflammatory pathology:

- Chronic inflammation resulting in obscured anatomy of Calot's triangle.

Mistaking the common bile duct for the cystic duct is a frequent visual misperception.

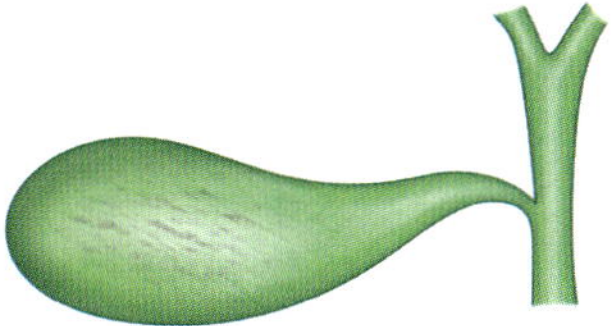

Short cystic duct

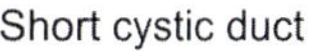

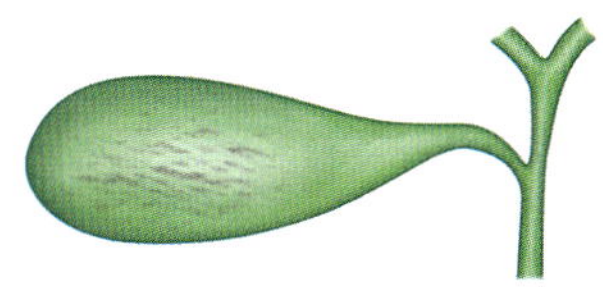

Narrow common bile duct

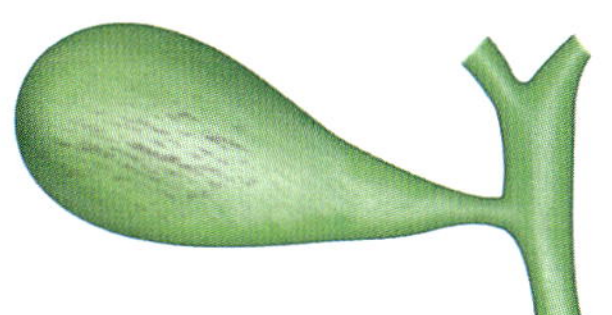

Severe acute cholecystitis resulting in adherence of cystic duct and CBD

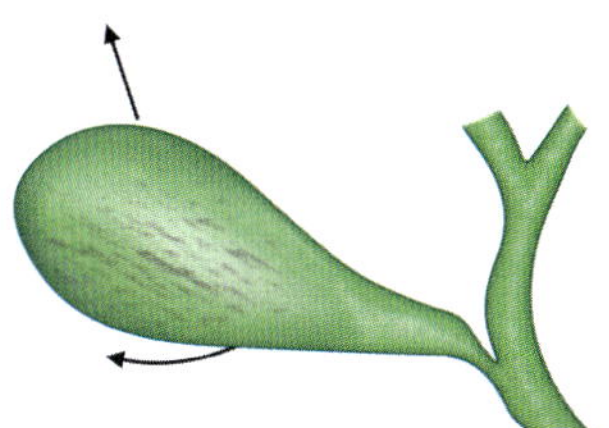

Excessive traction of neck of GB causing tenting of CBD

Classification of Bile Duct Injury

(A) **Bismuth classification (1982):** Based on the location of injury in the biliary tract. This classification includes 5 types, Type I–V. It does not include all spectrum of biliary injuries.

(B) **Strasberg classification (1995):** This classification included Type A to E. Type E is further subclassified into E1-E5, which is analog to Bismuth classification. It does not include any associated vascular injuries.

(C) **McMohan classification (1995):** This classification included two types—minor injury and major injury, based on width of bile duct injury.

(D) **Stewart-Way classification (2003):** This classification included four types, class I to IV. It includes complex bile duct injuries as well as vascular injuries.

(E) **Hannover classification (2007):** This classification included five types—Type A to E with multiple subtypes: [A1,A2]; [B1,B2]; [C1,C2,C3,C4]; [D1,D2,D3,D4}; [E1,E2,E3,E4]. It includes wide variation of bile duct injuries and vascular injuries.

Strasberg Classification

Type A: Bile leak from cystic duct or liver bed without further injury

Type B: Partial occlusion of the biliary tree, most frequently of an aberrant right hepatic duct

Type C: Bile leak from duct (aberrant RHD) that is not communicating with the common bile duct.

Type D: Lateral injury of biliary system, without loss of continuity

Type E: (E1-E5) Circumferential injury of biliary tree with loss of continuity.

Bismuth Classification

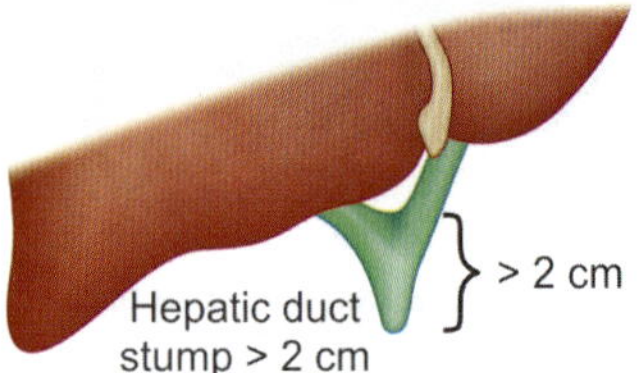

Bismuth type 1

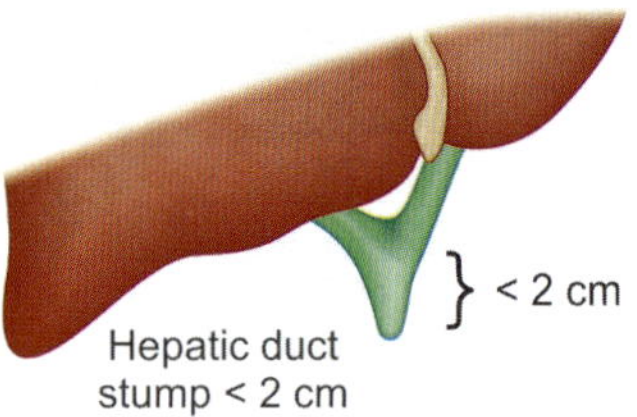

Bismuth type 2

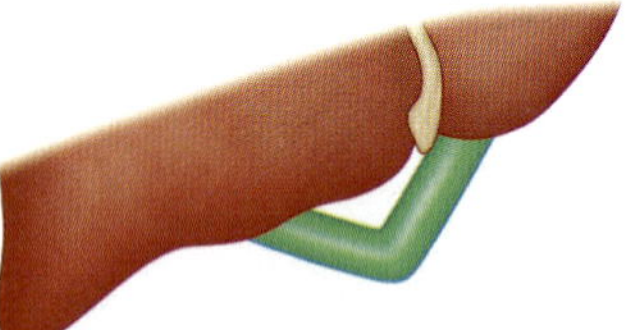

Bismuth type 3

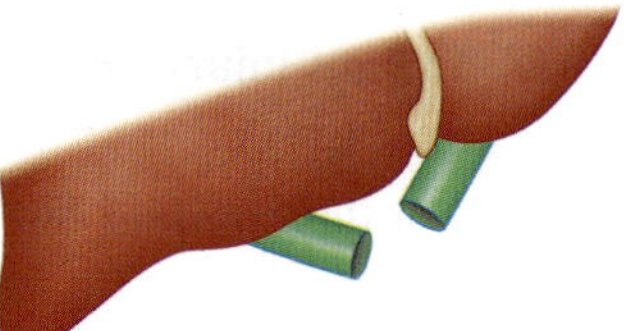

Bismuth type 4

What is bismuth type 5?

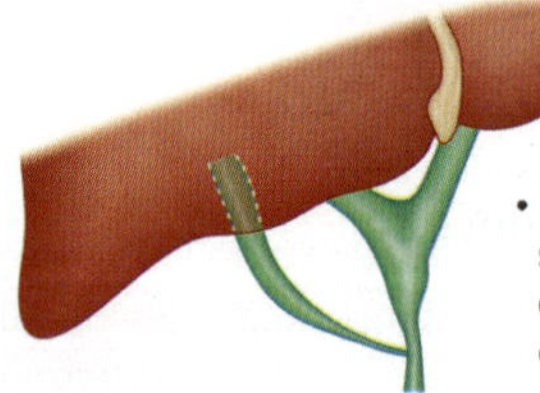

McMahon Classification

Minor Injury: Lacerations under 25% of the common bile duct diameter or cystic-CBD junction

Major Injury: Transection or laceration over 25% of CBD diameter and postoperative bile duct stricture

Hannover Classification

Type A: *Peripheral bile leak (with reconnection to the main bile duct system):*

- A1 Cystic duct leak
- A2 Leak in the region of the gallbladder bed

Type B: *Stenosis of the main bile duct without injury (i.e., caused by a clip):*

- B1 Incomplete
- B2 Complete

Type C: *Tangential injury of the common bile duct:*

- C1 Small punctiform lesion (<5 mm)
- C2 Extensive lesion (>5 mm) below the hepatic bifurcation
- C3 Extensive lesion at the level of the hepatic bifurcation
- C4 Extensive lesion above the hepatic bifurcation

With vascular lesion (i.e., C1d C2, etc.)

- d. right hepatic artery
- s. left hepatic artery
- p. proper hepatic artery
- com. common hepatic artery
- c. cystic artery
- pv. portal vein

Type D: *Completely transected bile duct:*

- D1 Without defect below the hepatic bifurcation
- D2 With defect below the hepatic bifurcation
- D3 At hepatic bifurcation level (with or without defect)
- D4 Above the hepatic bifurcation (with or without defect)

With vascular lesions (i.e. D1d, D2pv, etc.)—d. right hepatic artery; s. left hepatic artery; p. proper hepatic artery; com. common hepatic artery; c. cystic artery; pv. portal vein.

Type E *Strictures of the main bile duct:*

- E1 Main bile duct short circular (<5 mm)
- E2 Main bile duct longitudinal (>5 mm)
- E3 Hepatic bifurcation
- E4 Right main bile duct/segmental bile duct

Stewart-Way Classification	
Class I	CBD mistaken for cystic duct, but recognized. Cholangiogram incision in cystic duct extended into CBD
Class II	Lateral damage to the CHD from cautery or clips placed on duct Associated bleeding, poor visibility
Class III	CBD mistaken for cystic duct, not recognized CBD, CHD, R, L hepatic ducts transected and/or resected
Class IV	RHD mistaken for cystic duct, RHA mistaken for cystic artery, RHD and RHA transected Lateral damage to the RHD from cautery or clips placed on duct.

Management

Injury Recognized at Operation

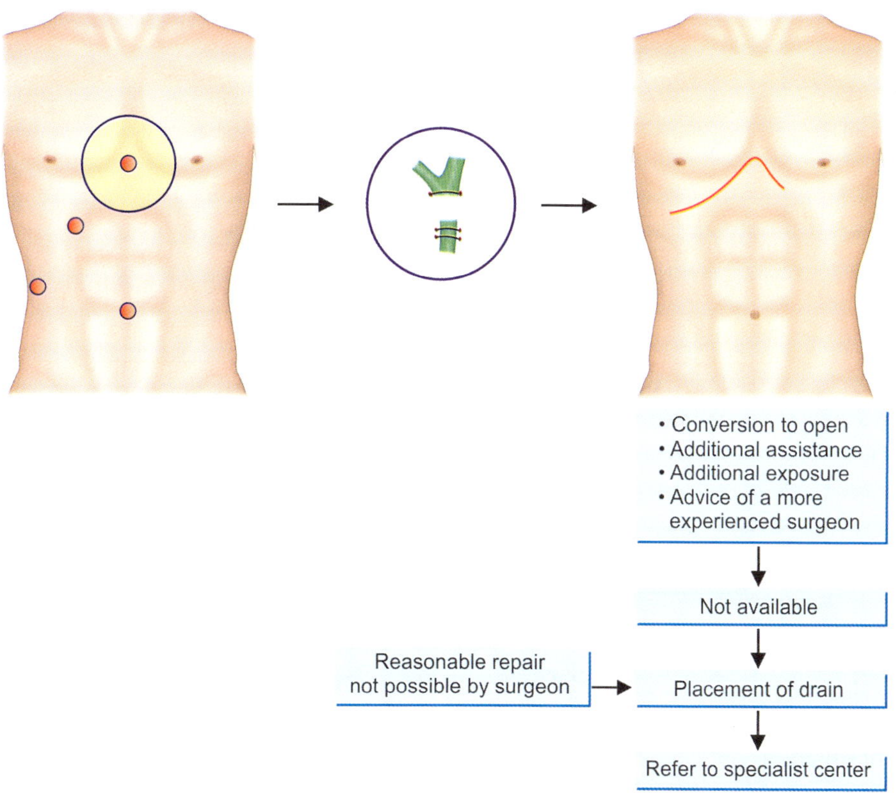

Each failed repair is associated with some loss of bile duct length.

Each failed repair makes further repair more difficult.

Definitive reconstruction should not be attempted if expertise is not available.

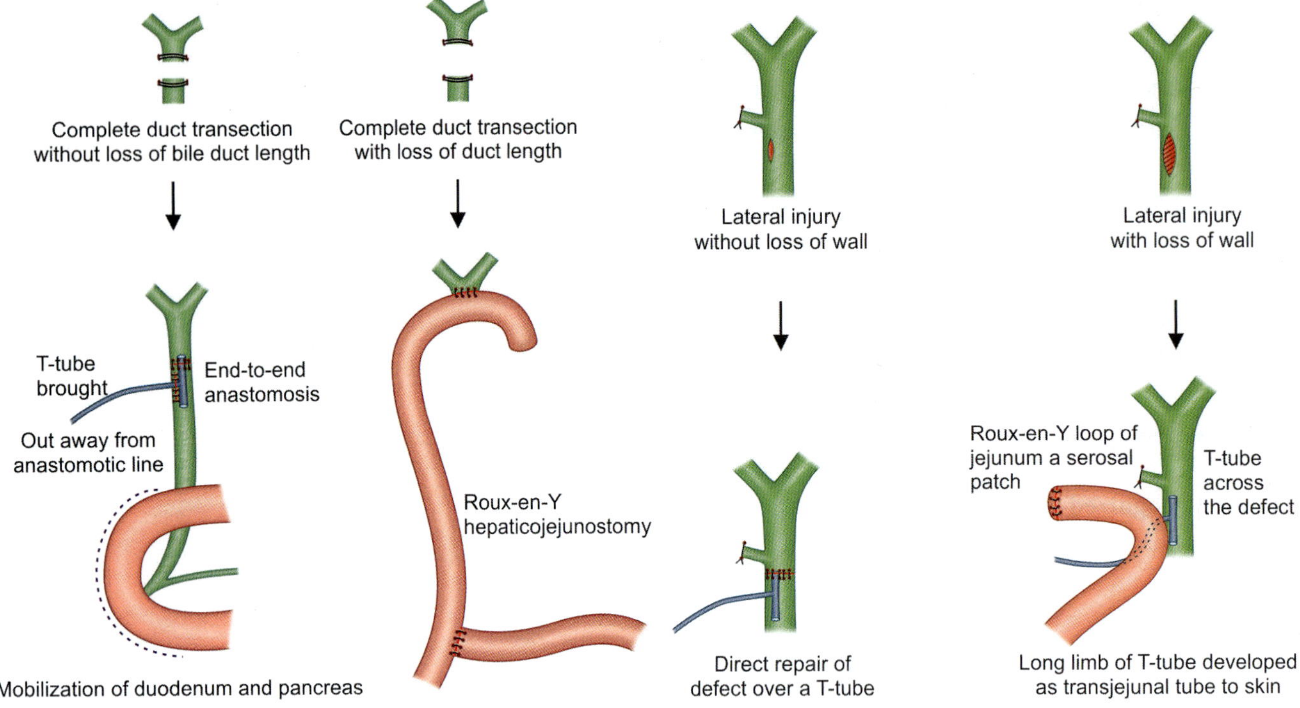

Chance of stricture is more in end-to-end anastomosis.

Long-term outcome is satisfactory in Roux-en-Y hepaticojejunostomy.

Injury Recognized in Immediate Postoperative Period

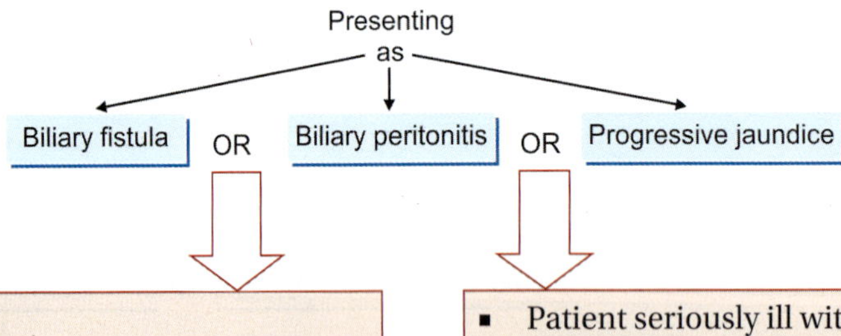

- Avoid early reoperation
- Take control of situation
- Maintain fluid and electrolyte balance
- Maintain nutrition
- Treat infection
- Fistulography
- Wait for at least 2–3 weeks
- Most of the fistulas resolve or output decrease after this period.

- Patient seriously ill with signs of sepsis.
- May present with biloma without sepsis.
- Needs drainage of bile and control of bile leak.
- Delayed definite repair is the best option.

Injuries Presenting at an Interval as Biliary Stricture

Assessment of Stricture → **Surgical Reconstruction**

Cholangiographic evaluation is indicated for defining the Bismuth type of the stricture and extent of ductal dilatation.

MRCP is the gold standard method of cholangiographic evaluation of the biliary system. This imaging modality is also useful for assessment of vascular tree along with atrophy/hypertrophy complex.

PTC is particularly indicated for Bismuth 4 or 5 stricture with undilated ducts.

Technique of repair and outcome after reconstruction depends on the type of injury and stricture location.

A minimum time interval of 4–6 weeks between time of injury and reconstruction is essential for resolution of tissue edema and adequate dilatation of the proximal biliary system.

Roux-en-Y hepaticojejunostomy is the most common method of reconstruction. Principles of hepaticojejunostomy are exposure of a healthy, well-vascularized proximal bile duct followed by mucosa-to-mucosa, tension-free anastomosis between the duct and Roux-en-Y limb of jejunum.

Rarely, in complex strictures, intrahepatic hepaticojejunostomy (Longmire procedure) is indicated.

Partial hepatic resection is indicated in complex biliary injuries associated with vascular injuries or in case where multiple failed repair attempts.

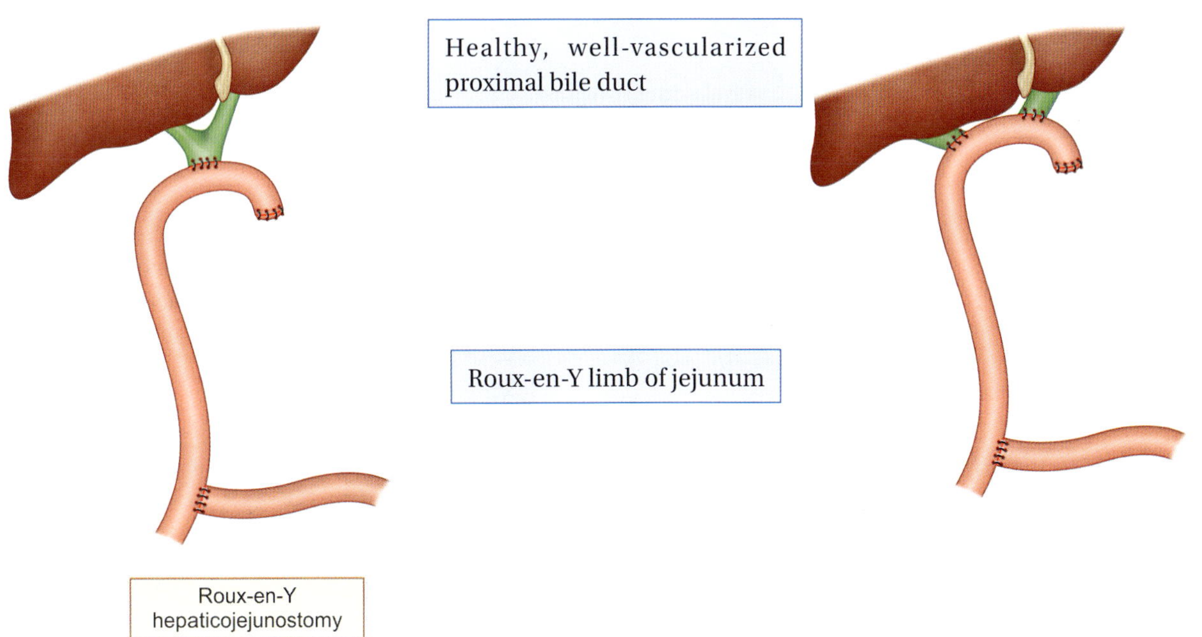

Choledocholithiasis

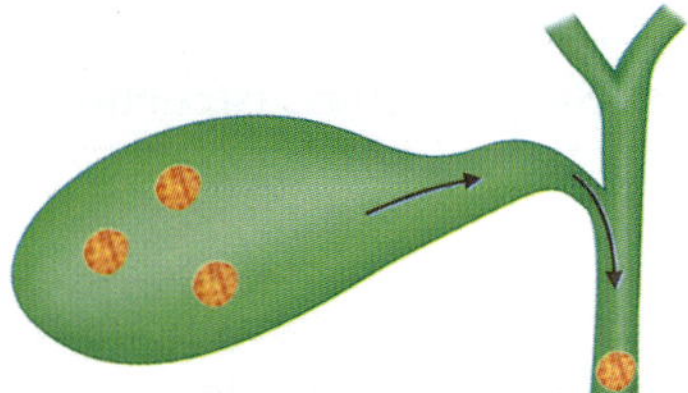

Secondary Bile Duct Stone

- Originates in the gallbladder and migrates into the common bile duct via the cystic duct.
- Cholesterol, mixed or black pigment stones.

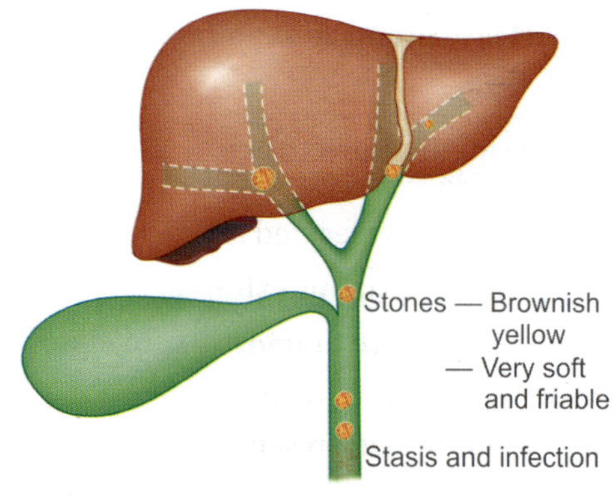

Primary Bile Duct Stone

- Originates de novo within intrahepatic and extrahepatic ducts.
- Associated with benign biliary stricture, sclerosing cholangitis, choledochal cyst.
- Stasis and infection are the main causative factors.
- Usually brown pigment stones.
- Increased chance of stone recurrence.

Clinical Presentation

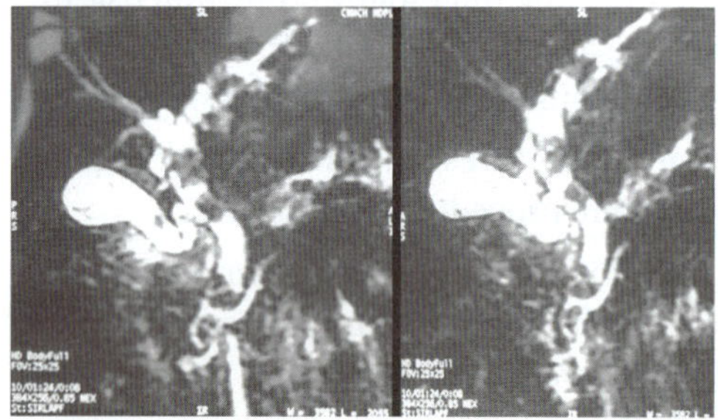

MRCP showing stone in gallbladder, common hepatic duct (CHD) and common bile duct (CBD).

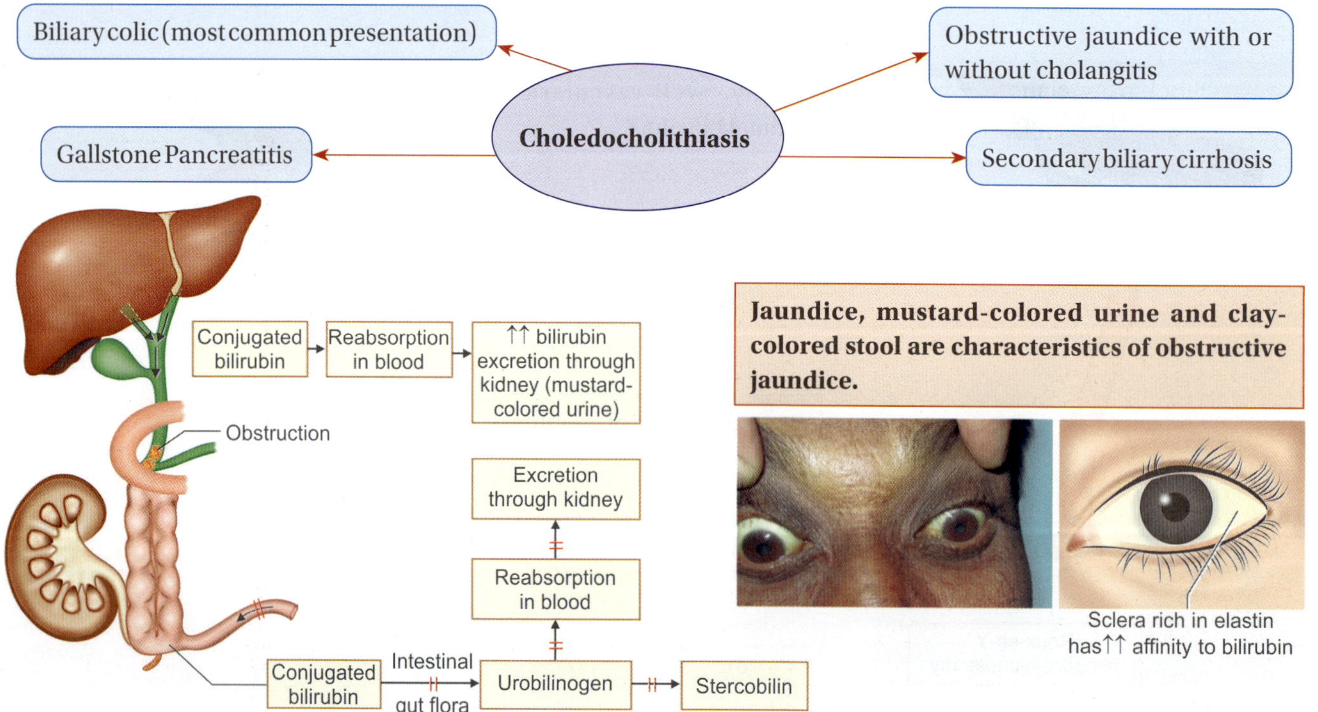

Investigations

Liver function test:

- Conjugated hyperbilirubinemia
- Significantly elevated alkaline phosphatase (atleast three times)

Total leukocyte count: Usually normal, increased when cholangitis develops.

USG is the initial imaging modality of choice.

MRCP or ERCP depending on the possibility of choledocholithiasis based on liver function test, presence of cholangitis, and USG findings.

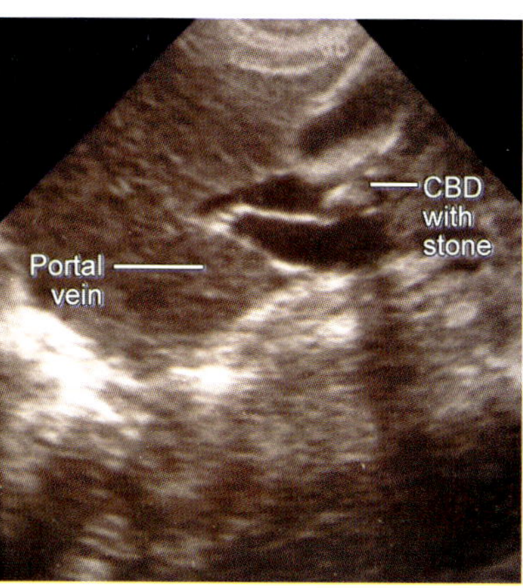

- Stone in CBD is not always visible due to bowel gas.
- Sensitivity of USG for detection of CBD stone is low (about 30–50%).

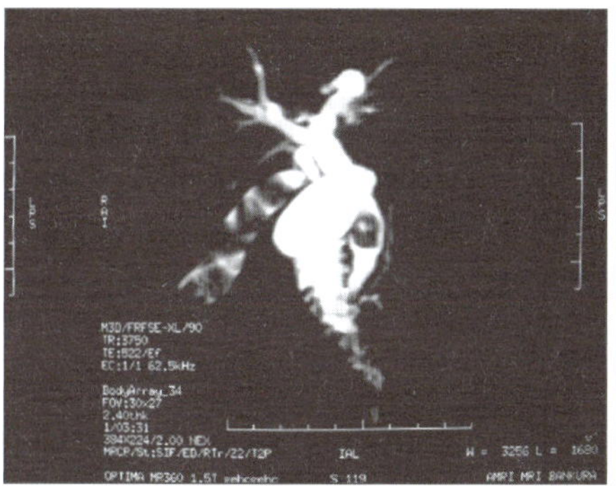

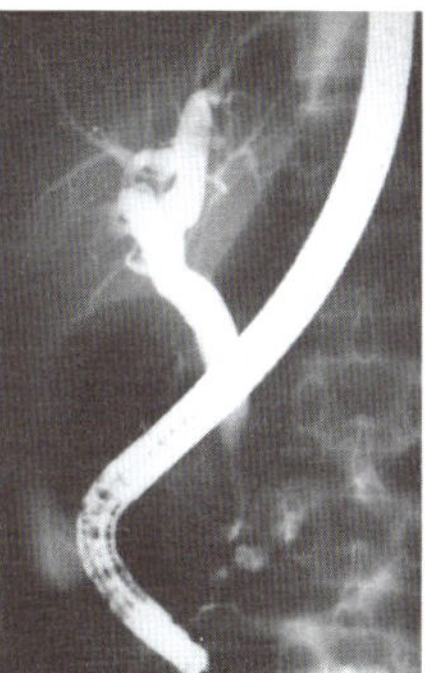

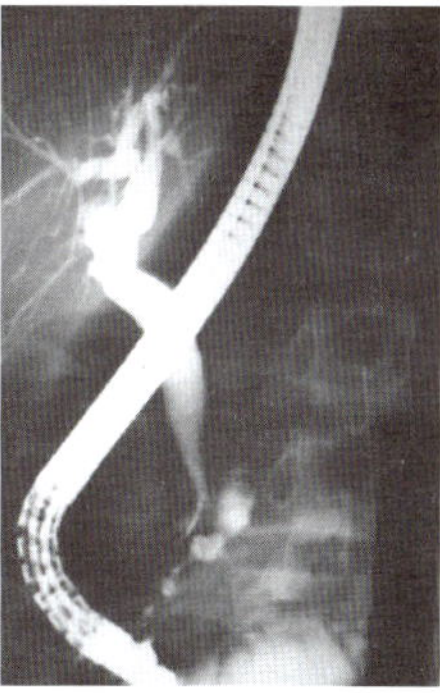

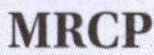

MRCP

- Clear delineation of anatomy of biliary tree.
- High specificity for diagnosis of bile duct stones.
- MRCP is contraindicated in patients having claustrophobia, with cardiac pacemakers, metallic implants, cochlear implants, aneurysm clips.

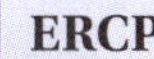

ERCP

- Both diagnostic and therapeutic options.
- Chance of complications, e.g., pancreatitis, cholangitis.

Predictors for Choledocholithiasis and Recommended Strategy [Adapted from ASGE Guideline 2019]

(A) High-risk criteria:

Common bile duct stone on US/cross-sectional imaging Or Clinical ascending cholangitis Or Total bilirubin >4 mg/dL and dilated common bile duct on US/cross-sectional imaging

Recommended strategy: Proceed to ERCP

(B) Intermediate-risk criteria:

Abnormal liver biochemical tests Or Age >55 years Or Dilated common bile duct on US/cross-sectional imaging

Recommended strategy: MRCP, EUS, Laparoscopic IOC or Intraoperative ultrasound

(C) Low-risk criteria:

No predictors present

Recommended strategy: Cholecystectomy with/without IOC or intraoperative ultrasound

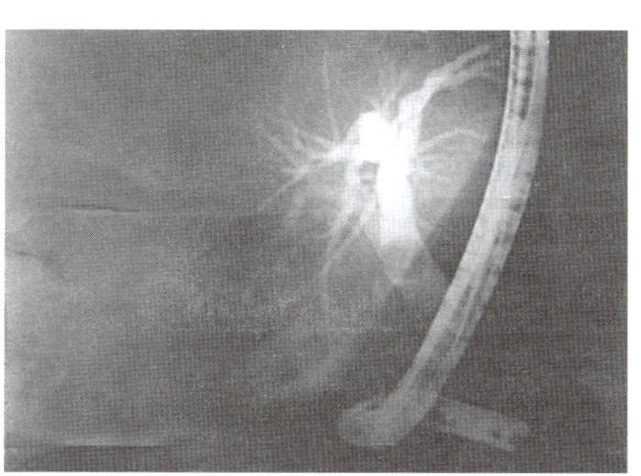

ERCP showing stone in CBD.

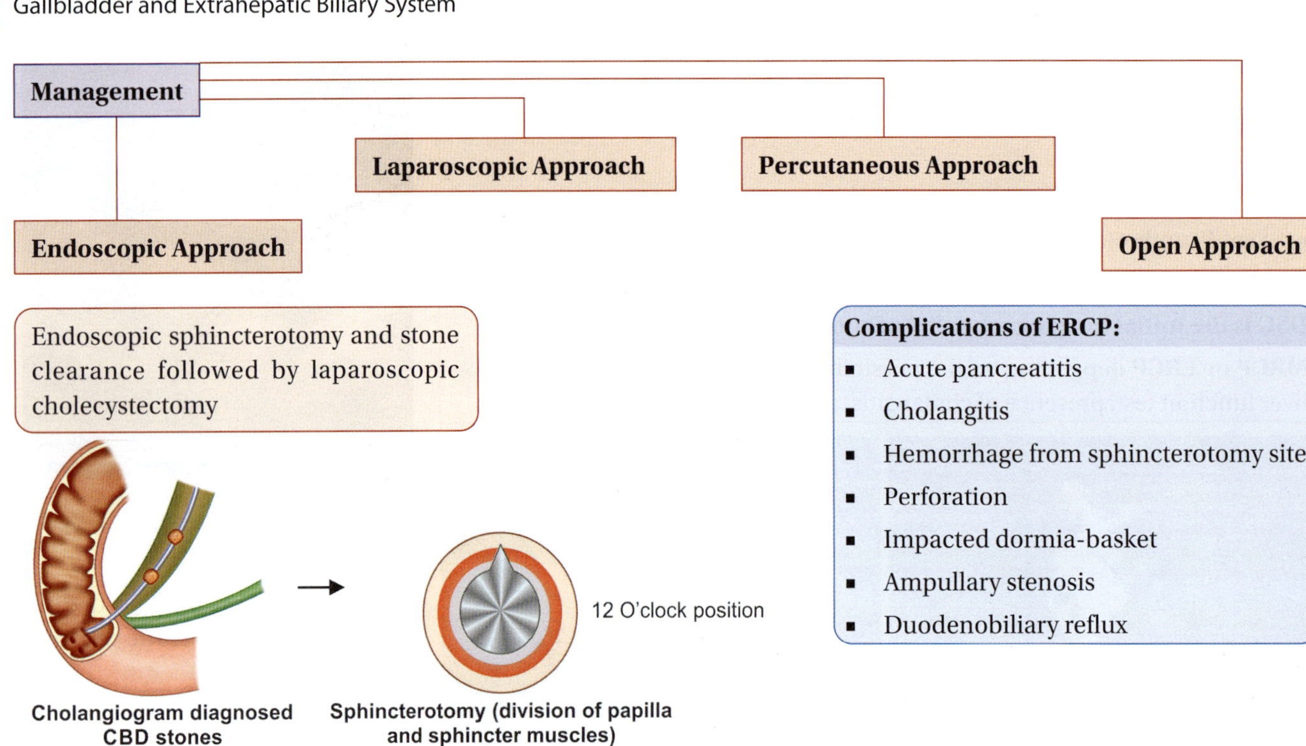

Endoscopic sphincterotomy and stone clearance followed by laparoscopic cholecystectomy

Complications of ERCP:

- Acute pancreatitis
- Cholangitis
- Hemorrhage from sphincterotomy site
- Perforation
- Impacted dormia-basket
- Ampullary stenosis
- Duodenobiliary reflux

Cholangiogram diagnosed CBD stones

Sphincterotomy (division of papilla and sphincter muscles)

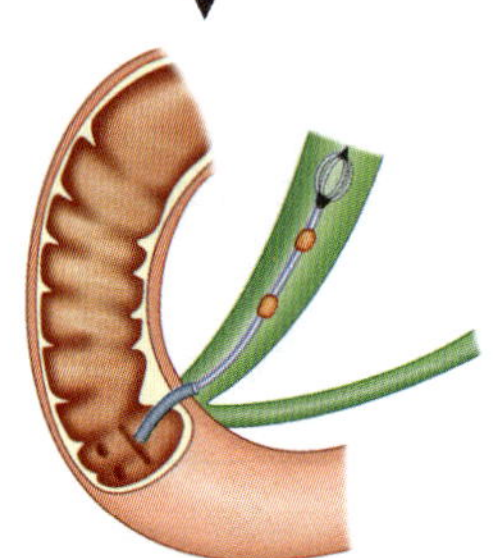

Dormia basket is introduced

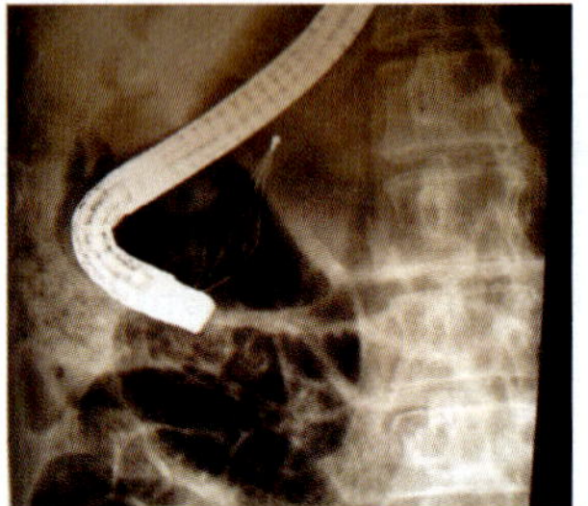

Dormia basket is introduced into in CBD

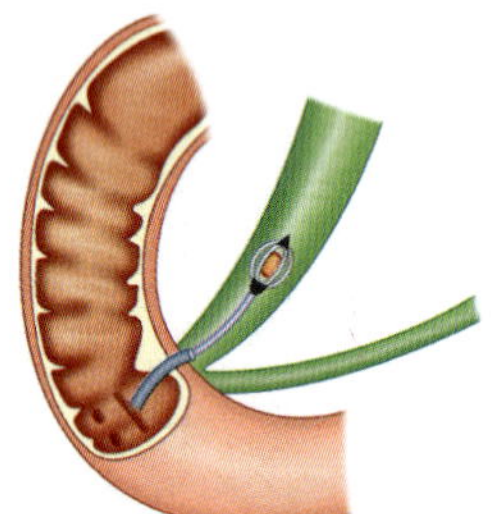

Stone is ensnared in basket

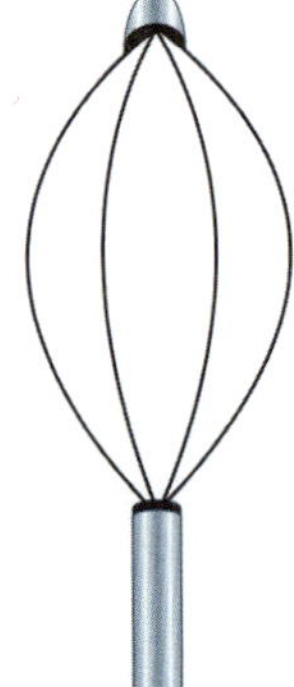

Standard 4 wire Dormia basket

Instruments used for stone extraction after endoscopic sphincterotomy:

- Dormia-type basket
- Fogarty-type balloon catheter (4Fr)
- Duodenobiliary reflux

Various lithotripsy options for biliary stones:

- Mechanical lithotripsy
- Electrohydraulic lithotripsy
- Laser lithotripsy (holmium:YAG laser)
- Extracorporeal shock-wave lithotripsy

"Difficult Stones"- Factors those are responsible for difficulty in cannulation, sphincterotomy and stone extraction:

- Periampullary diverticulum
- Prior surgery such as Roux-en-Y reconstruction or Billroth II partial gastrectomy
- Stone size >1.5 cm
- Numerous, hard stones
- Square, piston-shaped stones tightly fitted within the duct
- Intrahepatic stones
- Stones located proximal to a stricture

If difficulty in stone removal, other options are:

- Lithotripsy
- Stenting (plastic stent)

Laparoscopic Approach

Laparoscopic cholecystectomy with CBD exploration

- Transcystic CBD exploration
- Transcholedochal CBD exploration
- Laparoscopic biliary-enteric bypass

Transcystic CBD Exploration (without choledochoscope)

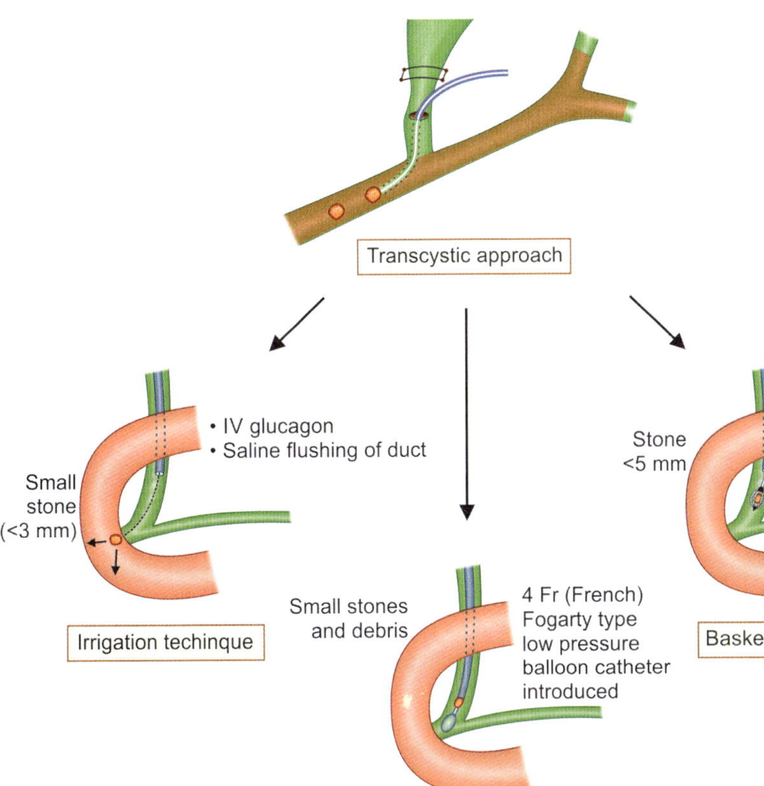

- The cystic duct is exposed for 2–3 cm and incision is made by scissors.
- Cholangiogram catheter is introduced.
- Contrast is injected under fluoroscopy to confirm position and anatomy.

Transcystic approach is not appropriate in:

- Stones >6 mm, intrahepatic stones
- Diameter of cystic duct <4 mm
- Cystic duct entrance to CBD-posterior
- Cystic duct entrance to CBD-distal

Transcystic CBD Exploration (with choledochoscope)

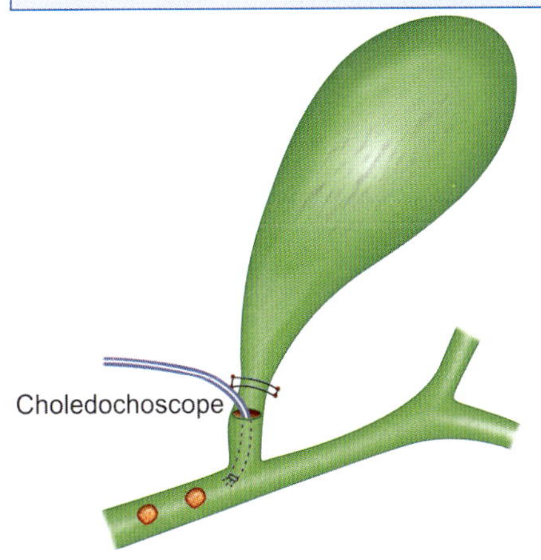

- A guidewire is passed into the CBD through the cystic duct orifice.
- 8-Fr angioplasty balloon is used to dilate the orifice.
- A 12-Fr introducer catheter is placed for repeated passage of choledochoscope.
- Through the choledochoscope, a retrieval basket is introduced under direct vision.

Transcystic CBD Exploration

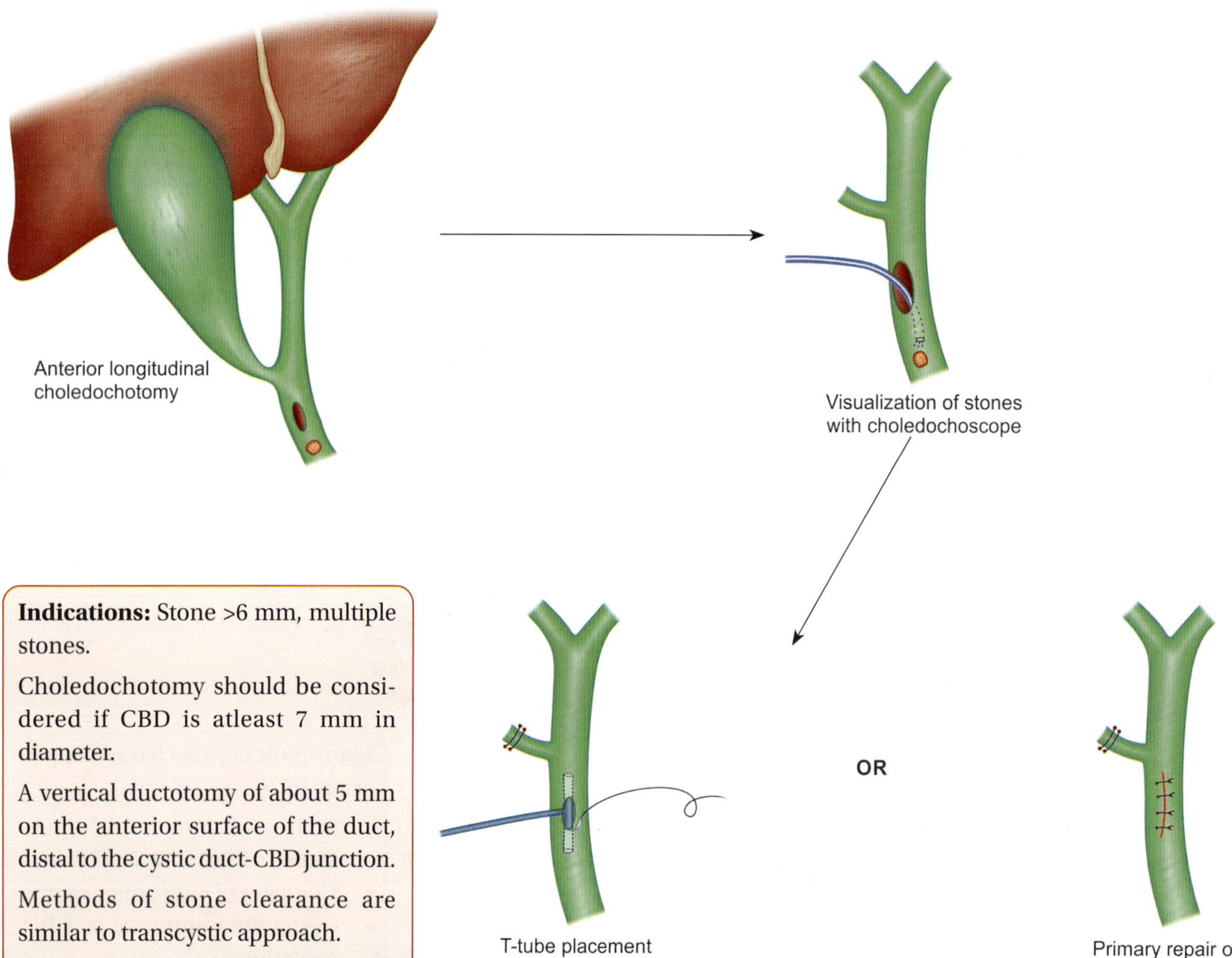

Indications: Stone >6 mm, multiple stones.

Choledochotomy should be considered if CBD is atleast 7 mm in diameter.

A vertical ductotomy of about 5 mm on the anterior surface of the duct, distal to the cystic duct-CBD junction.

Methods of stone clearance are similar to transcystic approach.

Choledochotomy is managed with T-tube placement or primary closure over a stent or only primary closure.

Open Approach

- Open CBD exploration with stone clearance and T-tube placement
- Biliary-enteric bypass
- Transduodenal sphincteroplasty

Indications of Open CBD Exploration

- Large or impacted CBD stone
- Failed endoscopic approach
- Anatomical factors (e.g. duodenal diverticula, post-gastrectomy) preclude endoscopic approach
- Conditions where open cholecystectomy is the preferred approach,eg. Mirizzi syndrome, biliary-enteric fistula, suspected GB carcinoma
- In whom biliary-enteric anastomosis is indicated.
- Other open abdominal procedures in a patient with choledocholithiasis.

Indications of Biliary-enteric Anastomosis for CBD Stone

- Primary CBD stones
- Recurrent CBD stones following ERCP
- Impacted stones at Ampulla of Vater
- Intrahepatic duct stone
- Distal benign biliary stricture
- Associated ampullary stenosis

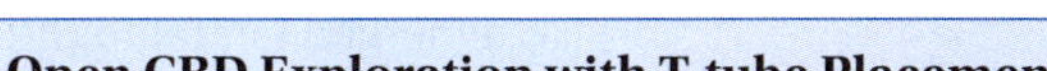

Open CBD Exploration with T-tube Placement

1

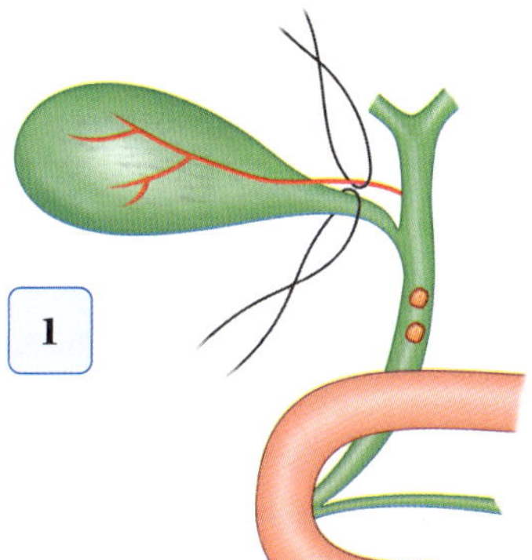

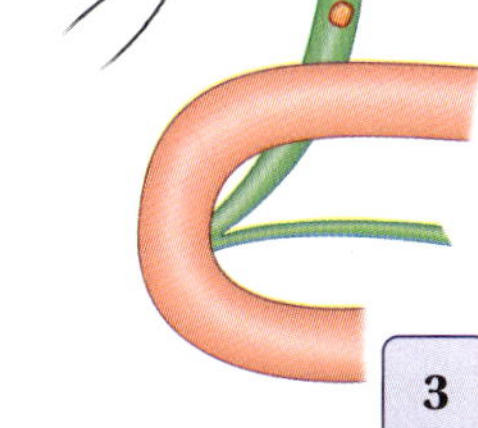

- Calot's triangle is dissected.
- Gallbladder is not removed. Gallbladder can be used as useful aid of retraction.

2

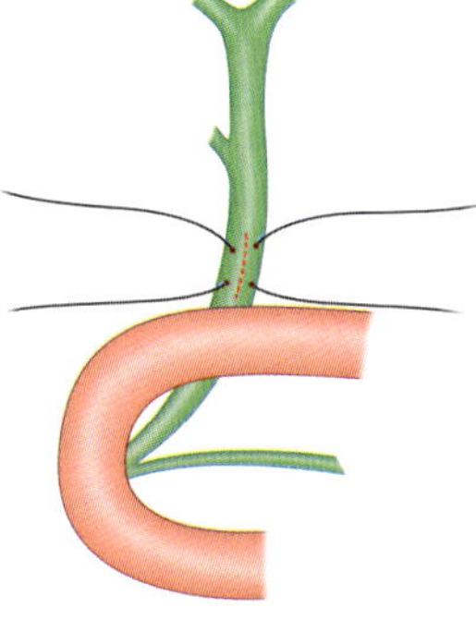

- Site of choledochotomy should be in the lowest part of supraduodenal CBD.
- Needle aspiration to confirm the anatomical structure as bile duct.
- Two stay sutures (3-0 Vicryl) are applied on two sides of the proposed choledochotomy.
- Lifting of the anterior wall minimizes the chance of injury to the posterior wall as well as making the choledochotomy technically more easier.

3

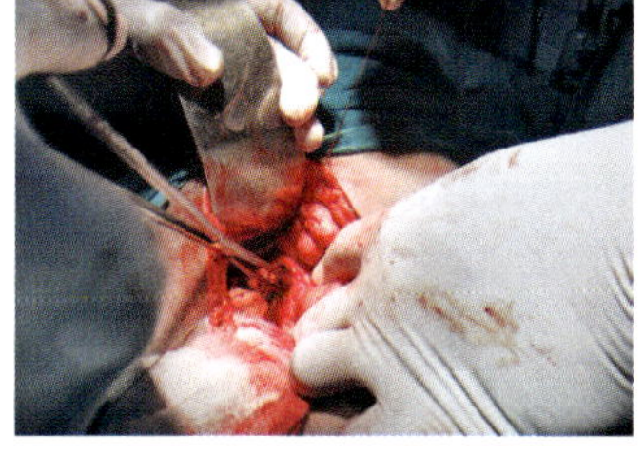

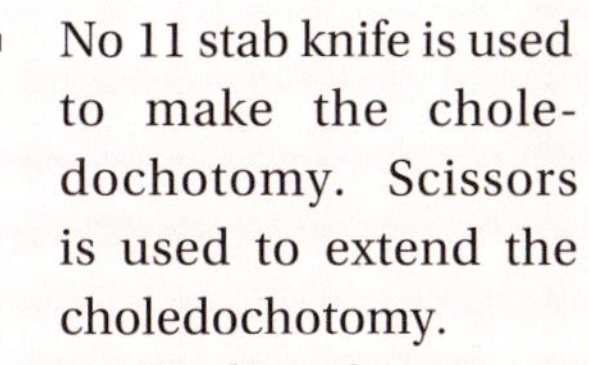

- No 11 stab knife is used to make the choledochotomy. Scissors is used to extend the choledochotomy.
- Desjardins forceps is introduced through the choledochotomy.
- Formed stones are grasped and cleared by Desjardins forceps.

4

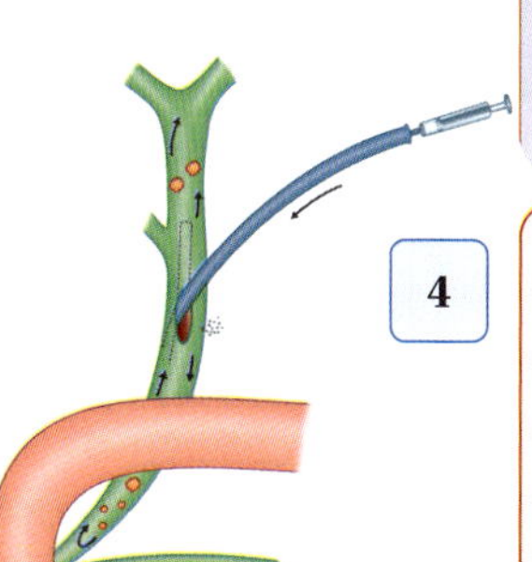

- Rubber catheter is introduced into the duct proximally and distally for flushing with normal saline.
- Flushing with NS clears the duct from smaller stones, sludge.
- Free passage of saline into the duodenum without reflux indicates adequate distal clearance.

5

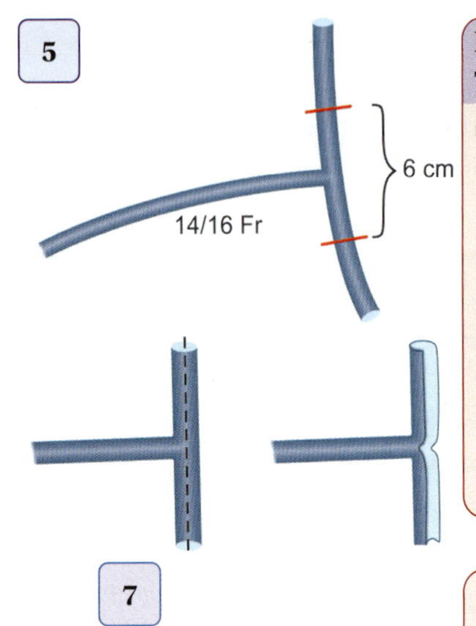

Refashioning of T-tube:

- Vertical limb is refashioned to a total length of 6 cm and a strip of wall (half the diameter) is removed.
- This refashioning prevents blockage of tube and helps easy removal.

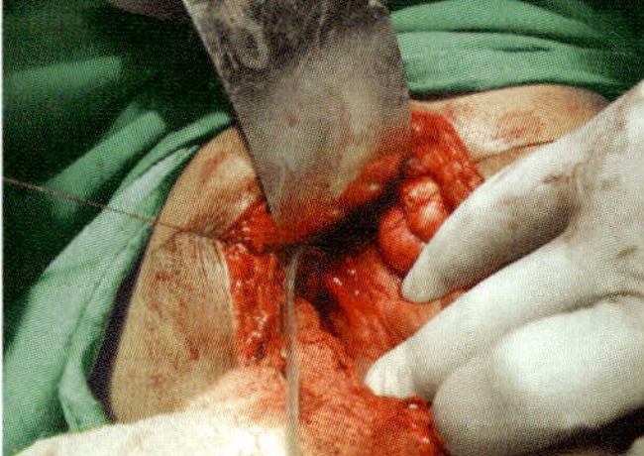

6

Placement of T-tube:

T-tube should be placed in such a manner that upper part should not be beyond the confluence and lower part should not be in the duodenum.

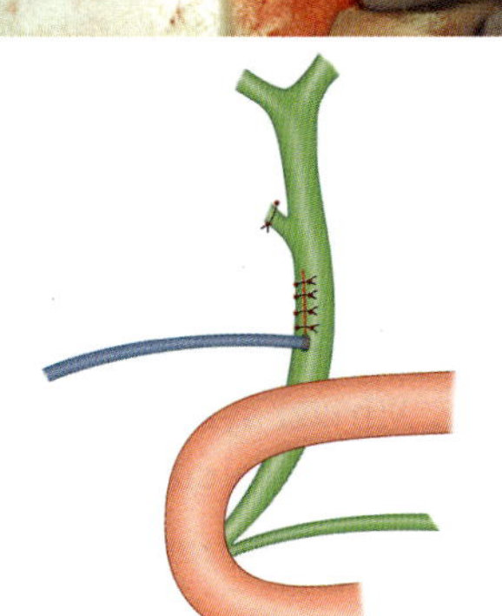

7

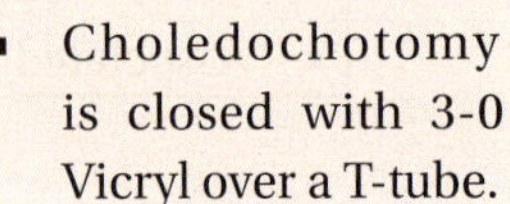

- Choledochotomy is closed with 3-0 Vicryl over a T-tube.
- Care should be taken so that no wall of T-tube is caught in one of the sutures.
- T-tube emerges at the lower end of repair.

8

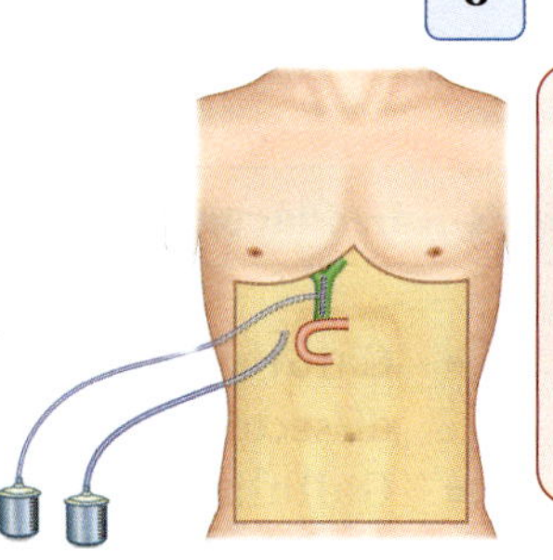

- The T-tube should be emerged lateral to the operative wound.
- This position facilitates radiologic intervention, if necessary.

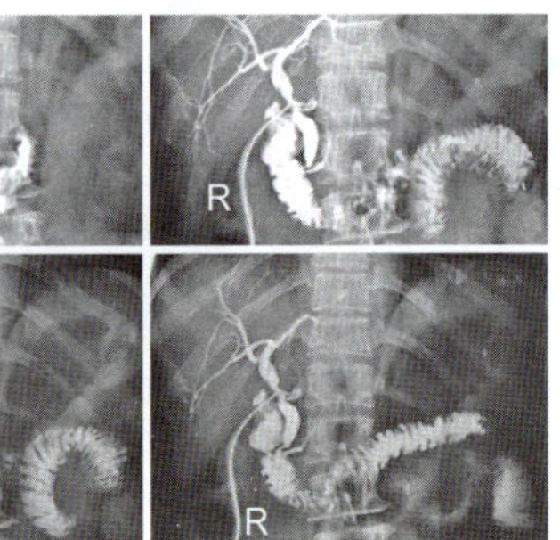

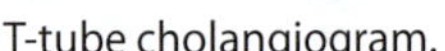

T-tube cholangiogram.

9

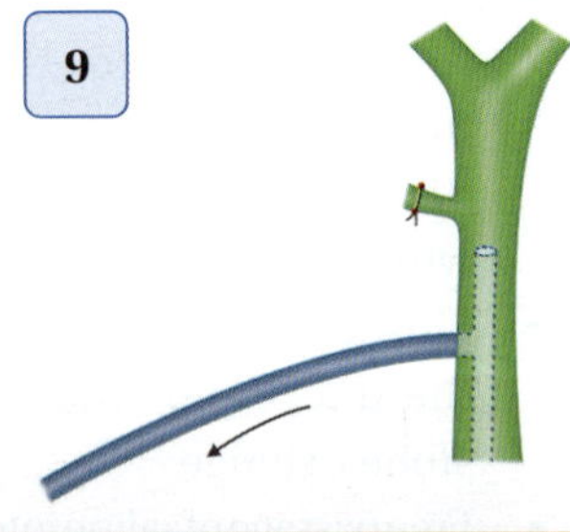

- T-tube cholangiography is done 5–7 days postoperatively.
- If T-tube cholangiogram normal, removal of the tube by smart pull.

Complications of T-tube placement in Choledocholithotomy:

- Premature dislodgement of T-tube
- T-tube obstruction
- Bile leak
- Prolonged fistula
- Delayed biliary stricture

Management of Retained CBD Stone with T-tube

Observation for 4–6 weeks ⇒ Stone is still present ⇒ **Interventional radiology through T-tube tract or endoscopic papillotomy** ⇒ Radiologic or endoscopic approach fails ⇒ **Open CBD exploration.**

Biliary-enteric Bypass

Choledochoduodenostomy is the most common type of biliary-enteric bypass for common bile duct stones.

Choledochoduodenostomy

CBD diameter should be at least 1.2 cm for a choledochoduodenostomy.

1

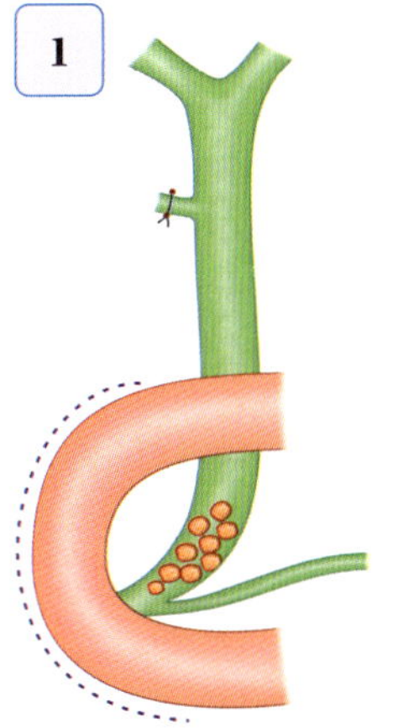

Kocherization of duodenum—for a tension-free anastomosis.

2

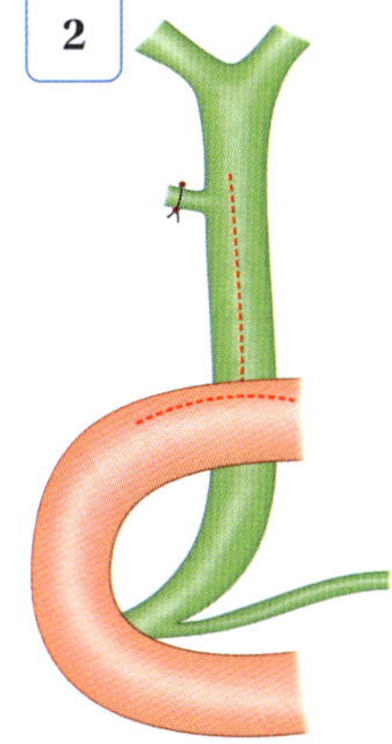

- Incision in CBD about 2.5 cm and extended upto common hepatic duct.
- Incision in postbulbar duodenum is slightly smaller.

3

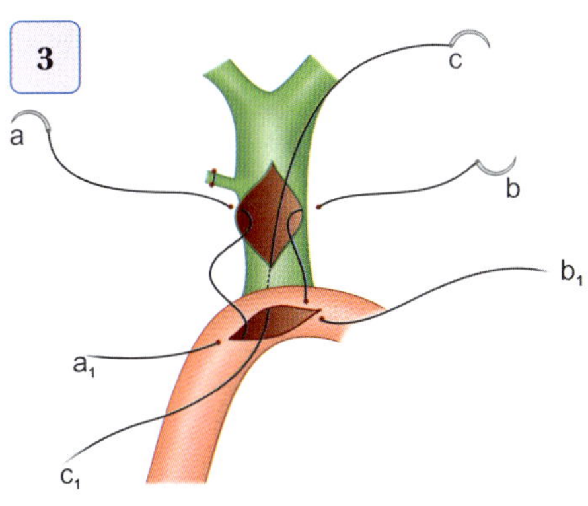

a–a_1 = Midpoint of choledochal incision—Distal corner of duodenal incision.

b–b_1 = Midpoint of choledochal incision—Proximal corner of duodenal incision.

c–c_1 = Lower corner of choledochal incision—Midpoint of duodenal incision.

4

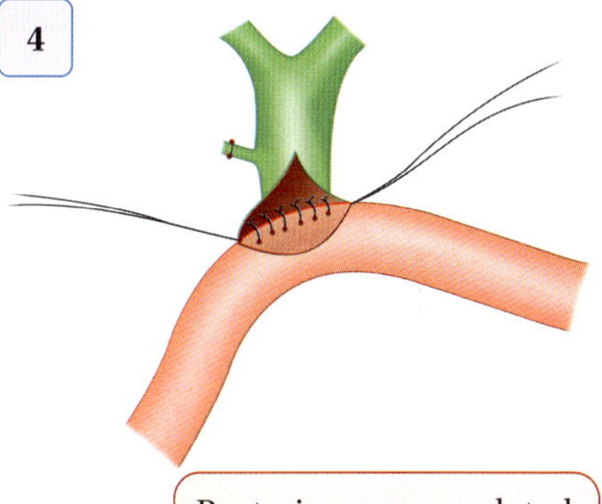

Posterior row completed

5

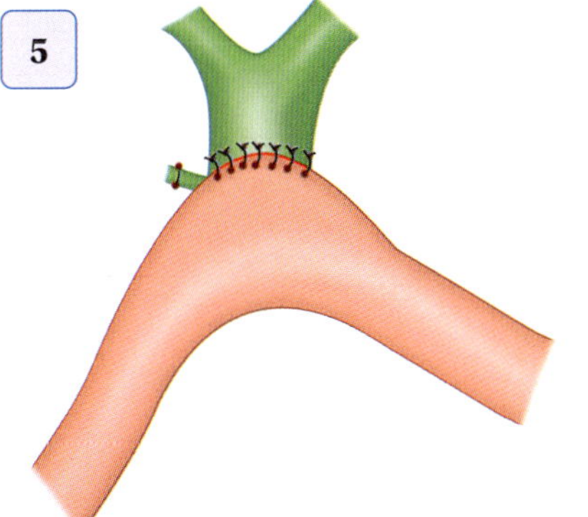

- Stoma size at least 2.5 cm.
- Sutures should be placed close enough so that no evidence of bile leakage.

Complications of Choledochoduodenostomy

- Cholangitis
- Anastomotic leak
- Sump syndrome

Sump Syndrome

A rare complication of side-to-side choledochoduodenostomy. After this anastomosis, the CBD between the anastomosis and the ampulla of Vater acts as a potential sump. Accumulation of food debris, stones, static bile in this reservoir act as a nidus for bacterial proliferation resulting in recurrent cholangitis, pancreatitis, biliary obstruction. Treatment is endoscopic sphincterotomy. If symptoms not improved after endoscopic method, choledochoduodenostomy can be converted to Roux-en-Y choledochojejunostomy.

Transduodenal Sphincteroplasty

Indications:

- Impacted stone at ampulla
- Multiple and recurrent CBD stones
- CBD stones with cholangitis

Contraindications:

- Dilated CBD >2 cm
- Presence of long suprasphincteric stricture
- Presence of duodenal diverticulum.

Management of Retained CBD Stone without T-tube and Recurrent Stone

- Endoscopic sphincterotomy is the first choice.
- If endoscopic therapy fails or not feasible due to altered anatomy, surgical intervention is the alternative. Choledocholithotomy with stone clearance and T-tube placement and completion cholangiography is the optimal management.
- Biliary-enteric drainage (choledochoduodenostomy, transduodenal sphincteroplasty, choledocho-jejunostomy) is only indicated in some specific circumstances.

Management of Primary Duct Stones

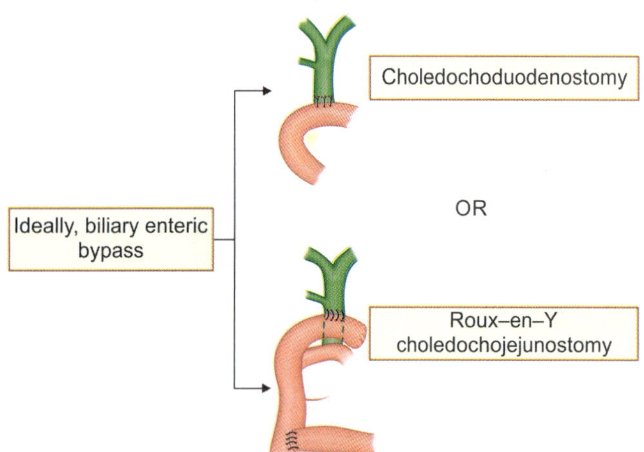

Incomplete Stone Clearance after ERCP

- A **temporary plastic biliary stent** is placed to relieve the obstruction if complete stone clearance is not possible.
- The stent should be changed or removed within 3–6 months to decrease the risk of cholangitis.

Acute Cholangitis

Pathophysiology

Two factors are responsible for development of acute cholangitis: (i) Biliary obstruction resulting in increased intrabiliary pressure; (ii) Bacterial growth in bile.

Elevated intrabiliary pressure allows translocation of bacteria or endotoxin into the vascular system (cholangio-venous reflux).

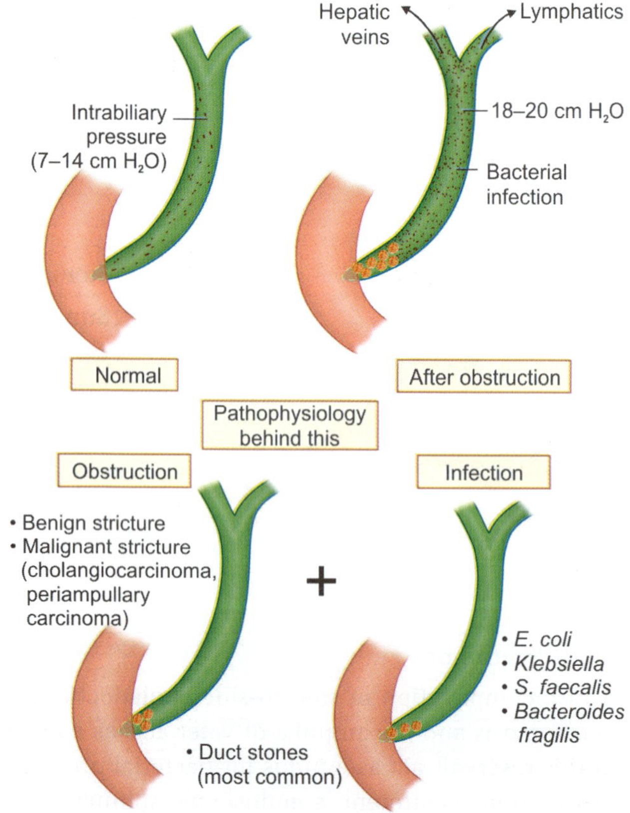

Etiology

- Choledocholithiasis
- Benign biliary stricture
- Stricture of biliary-enteric anastomosis
- Instrumentation of biliary tract
- Sclerosing cholangitis
- Malignant biliary stricture

Clinical Presentation

Charcot's triad

Right upper quadrant pain, intermittent fever accompanied by chills and jaundice. **OR**

Reynold's pentad

Pain abdomen, fever, jaundice, shock and mental obtundation.

Management

Management of Acute Cholangitis According to Severity (as per Tokyo Guideline 2018)

(1) **In Grade I cholangitis**, biliary tract drainage should be considered if no response to the initial treatment (fluid resuscitation, parenteral antibiotics, management of dyselectrolytemia) within 24 hours.

(2) **In Grade II cholangitis**, immediate biliary tract drainage should be considered along with initial treatment. If facility or expertise are not available, patient should be transferred to the institution where biliary tract drainage facility is available.

(3) **In Grade III cholangitis**, urgent biliary tract drainage should be considered along with initial treatment and support of vasopressors, ventilation, etc. If urgent drainage is not feasible, patient should be referred to institution with such facility.

Endoscopic transpapillary biliary drainage is the most preferred drainage method for acute cholangitis (other procedures are surgical, EUS guided or percutaneous transhepatic biliary drainage).

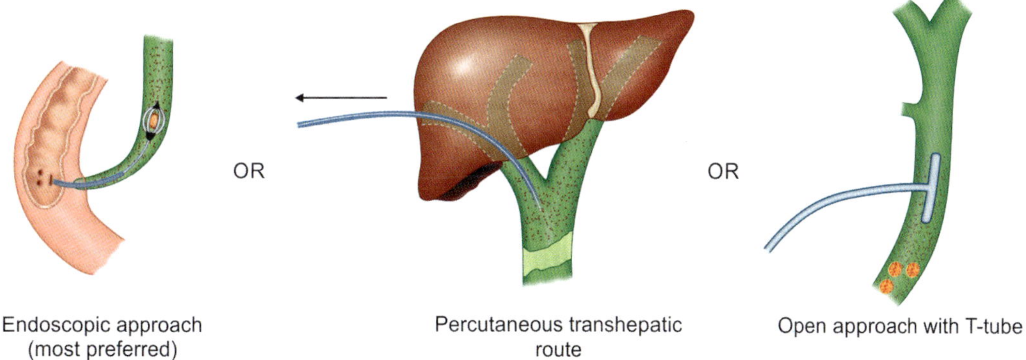

Mirizzi Syndrome

An uncommon complication of symptomatic gallstone disease due to impacted stone at the gallbladder infundibulum, resulting in external compression of bile duct and subsequently different types of fistulous communication between gallbladder and bile duct or GI tract.

Types of Mirizzi Syndrome:

Type I: Impacted gallstone compressing the hepatic duct

Type II: Cholecystocholedochal fistula involving less than one-third of circumference of the bile duct.

Type III: Fistula involving two-thirds of circumference of the bile duct

Type IV: Fistula with complete bile duct destruction

Type V: Cholecystoenteric fistula, with or without gallstone ileus, coexisting with any of the other types of Mirizzi syndrome

Va: Cholecystoenteric fistula without gallstone ileus; **Vb:** Cholecystoenteric fistula complicated by gallstone ileus.

Clinical presentation:

Patients may present with acute cholecystitis or acute cholangitis or obstructive jaundice. Rarely, patient may present with features of gallstone ileus.

Diagnosis:

USG abdomen: Thick-walled contracted gallbladder with a large impacted stone in the infundibulum, dilatation of the hepatic duct above the level of impaction and normal sized CBD—likely findings in Mirizzi syndrome.

MRCP: A useful imaging modality for diagnosis but diagnostic accuracy is low (about 50%).

Most of the Mirizzi syndrome are diagnosed during intraoperative period. Characteristic operative findings are contracted, thick-walled gallbladder or dilated gallbladder with a large stone impacted at neck, distorted and almost obliterated Calot's triangle.

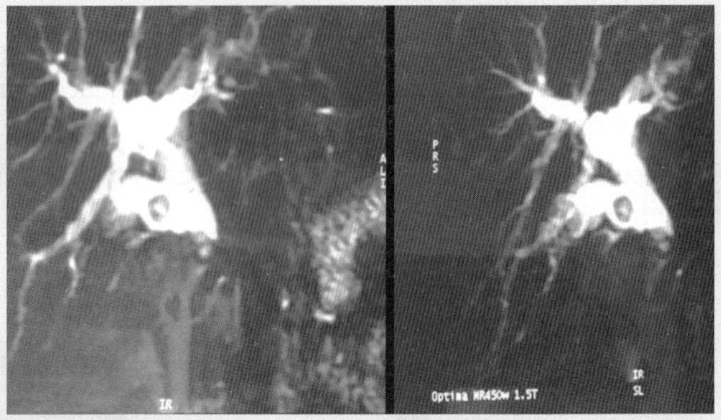

MRCP showing large stone in gallbladder and CBD junction suggestive of Mirizzi syndrome.

Management of Mirizzi syndrome:

Type I: Classic cholecystectomy/Subtotal cholecystectomy.

Type II: Subtotal cholecystectomy with leaving a remnant of gallbladder wall of atleast 5 mm for closure of the bile duct. Bile duct is explored via separate incision to exclude presence of any CBD stone. That choledochotomy incision is closed over a T-tube.

Type III: Subtotal cholecystectomy with leaving a gallbladder wall of atleast 1 cm to repair the duct or bilio-enteric anastomosis.

Type IV: Subtotal cholecystectomy followed by bilio-enteric anastomosis (preferably hepaticojejunostomy).

Type Va: Cholecystectomy along with repair of the fistula.

Type Vb: Treatment of gallstone ileus as initial approach followed by management of gallbladder pathology about 3 months back.

Hepatolithiasis

Presence of stones peripheral to the confluence of right and left hepatic ducts. Intrahepatic stones are of two types: (i) Calcium bilirubinate stones (most common) and (ii) Cholesterol stones.

Etiologies of secondary hepatolithiasis:

(i) Choledochal cyst, particularly type IVA and Caroli's disease; (ii) Biliary stricture; (iii) Anastomotic stricture; and (iv) Roux-en-Y hepaticojejunostomy.

As per Japan Research Group for the study of Hepatolithiasis, intrahepatic stones are classified into:

Type I: Stones only in the intrahepatic bile duct; **Type IE:** Stones in both intrahepatic and extrahepatic bile duct.
Type R: Stones in right side; **Type L:** Stones in left side; **Type LR:** Stones in both right and left side; **Type C**—in caudate lobe.
Calcium bilirubinate stones are characterized by: (i) Present near porta hepatis; (ii) Associated strictures and dilation are common; and (iii) Visualised by CT.
Cholesterol stones are characterized by: (i) Commonly present in segmental and peripheral biliary branches; (ii) Not associated with stricture and dilation; and (iii) Not visualized by CT.

Treatment:

(i) Peroral cholangioscopic lithotripsy; (ii) Percutaneous transhepatic cholangioscopic lithotomy; (iii) CBD exploration followed by T-tube drainage and postoperative cholangioscopy; (iv) Hepatectomy; and (v) Intracorporeal electrohydraulic shock-wave lithotripsy and YAG laser lithotripsy via transhepatic percutaneous approach.

Pneumobilia

Presence of air in the biliary tree.
Causes of pneumobilia:

(i) *Recent instrumentation in the biliary tree:*
- ERCP
- Intraoperative cholangiography

(ii) *Biliary-enteric anastomosis:*
- Choledochoduodenostomy
- Roux-en-Y hepaticojejunostomy

(iii) *Biliary-enteric fistula:*
- Gallstone ileus

(iv) *Incompetent sphincter of Oddi:*
- Patent biliary stent
- Sphincterotomy

Hemobilia

Presence of blood into the biliary tract. Causes of hemobilia:

Trauma: (A) Iatrogenic:
(i) Percutaneous transhepatic biliary drainage;
(ii) Percutaneous transhepatic cholangiography;
(iii) Percutaneous liver biopsy;
(iv) Surgery of the biliary tract; (B) Blunt trauma of liver.

Vascular cause: Hepatic artery aneurysm

Neoplastic lesion: Malignant neoplasms of liver, bile duct, gallbladder when invades the biliary tract.

Parasitic infection: Biliary ascariasis

Bilhemia

Flow of bile into the bloodstream through a communication between biliary tract and hepatic vein or branches of portal vein.

Causes of bilhemia:

- Liver biopsy
- Trauma (accidental or iatrogenic)
- Gallstone erode into the portal vein

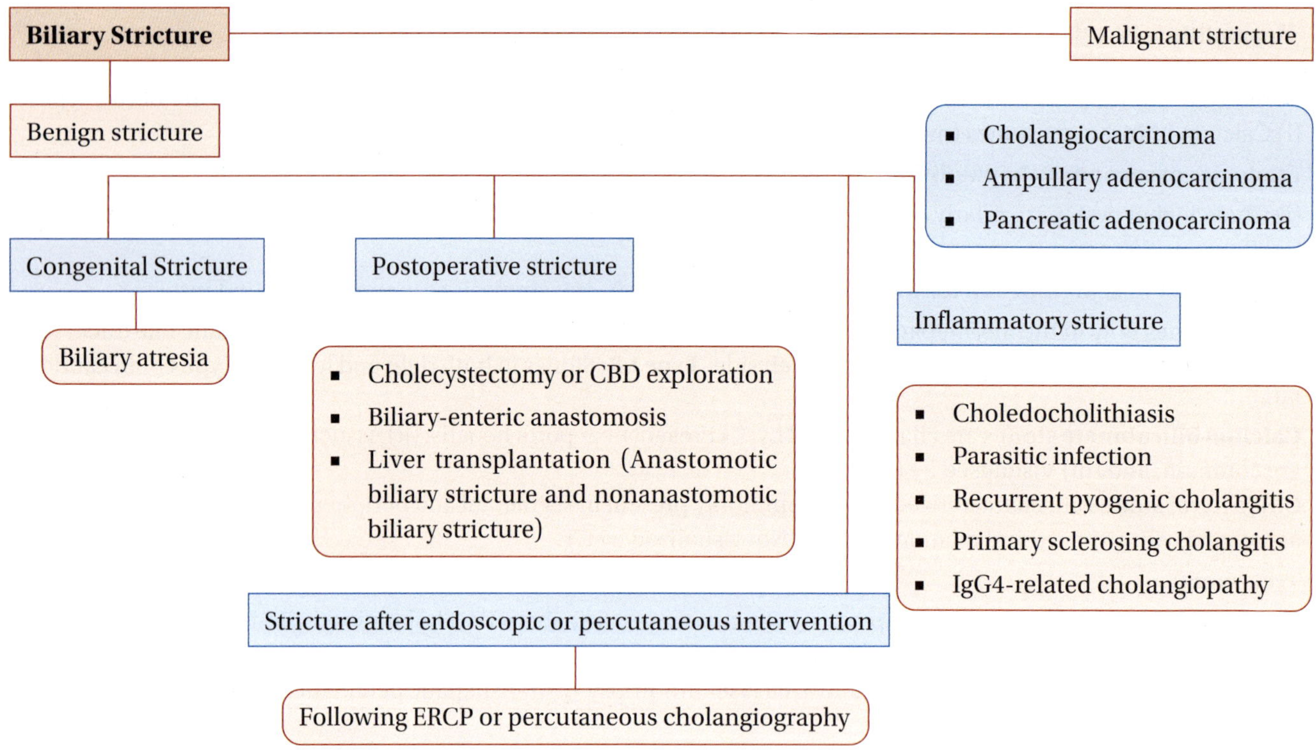

Diagnosis of Biliary Stricture

- **Diagnostic workup** includes history review, cross-sectional imaging (MRCP and multidetector CT) and EUS.
- On MRCP, **benign biliary strictures present as regular,** symmetric, short segment narrowing whereas *malignant strictures* present as irregular, asymmetric, long segment narrowing.
- **For cytohistologic diagnosis,** EUS-FNA or ERCP-guided brush cytology or transpapillary forceps biopsy (TPFB) is indicated.
- If brush cytology or TPFB is inconclusive, intraductal US, per-oral cholangioscopy, confocal laser endomicroscopy may be helpful.

Management of Biliary Stricture

The aim of treatment for benign biliary stricture is to obtain long-term bile duct patency.

Endoscopic approach is the first-line therapeutic approach. Percutaneous approach is indicated if endoscopic approach is not technically feasible. Surgical intervention is indicated when endoscopic and percutaneous approach fail or in postoperative bile duct stricture.

In postoperative bile duct stricture, surgery is the intervention of choice. Alternative option is endoscopic dilation of stricture followed by placement of multiple large-bore plastic stents. In bilioenteric anastomotic stricture, ERCP-guided balloon dilation by balloon-assisted enteroscopy is the preferred approach. In chronic pancreatitis associated biliary stricture, placement of fully covered self-expanding metal stents (FCSEMS) is the ideal treatment option. In postliver transplantation anastomotic biliary stricture, endoscopic approach is the first-line treatment, either endoscopic stricture dilation followed by multiple stent placement or placement of covered SEMSs. In primary sclerosing cholangitis with symptomatic dominant stricture, treatment is balloon or Bougie catheter dilation with or without stent placement.

Choledochal Cyst

Congenital cystic dilatation of the biliary tree.

Pathophysiology

Presence of anomalous biliopancreatic duct junction (APBDJ) resulting in reflux of pancreatic juice into the biliary tree **(Babbitt's theory)** is the most accepted theory.

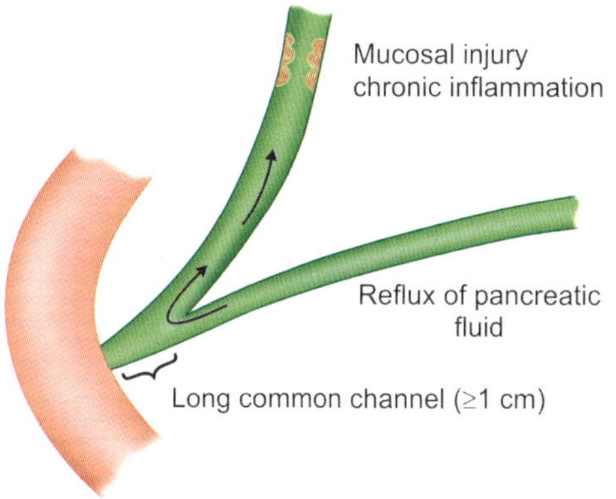

Anomalous pancreatic duct junction (APBDJ) **[most accepted theory]**

Classification of Choledochal Cyst

IA	Cystic dilatation of the common bile duct
IB	Segmental dilatation of the common bile duct
IC	Fusiform dilatation extending to the common hepatic duct
II	True diverticulum in the extrahepatic duct
III	Choledochocele
IVa	Multiple intra- and extrahepatic bile duct cysts
IVb	Multiple extrahepatic bile duct cysts
V	Single or multiple intrahepatic bile duct cysts (Caroli disease)

Todani Modification of Alonso-Lej clasification

Type I — **Most Common**

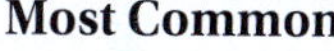

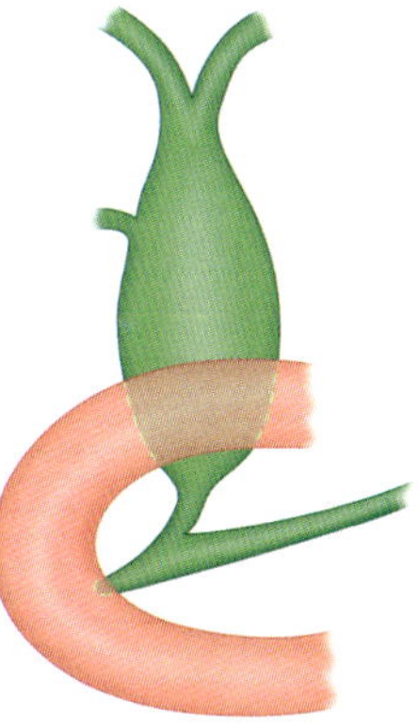

Type II

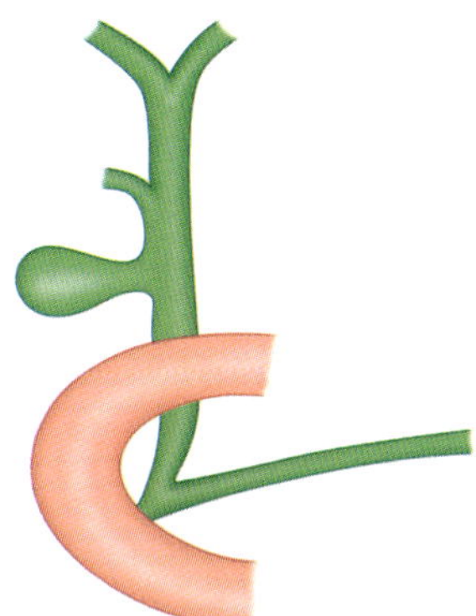

Type III

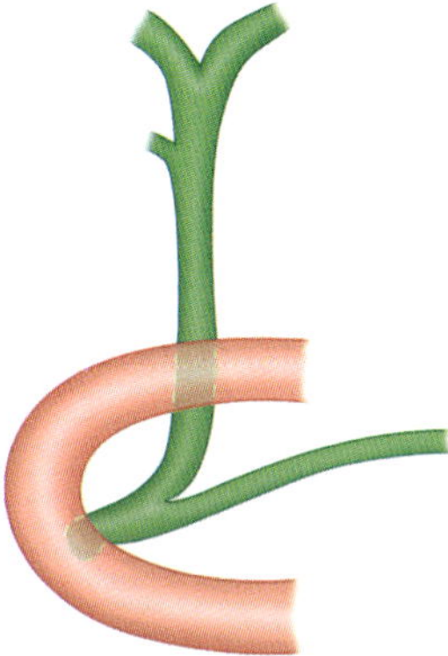

Type IVa

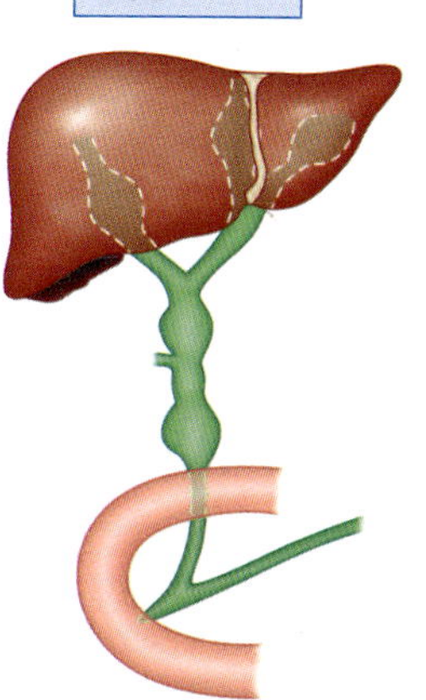

Type IVb

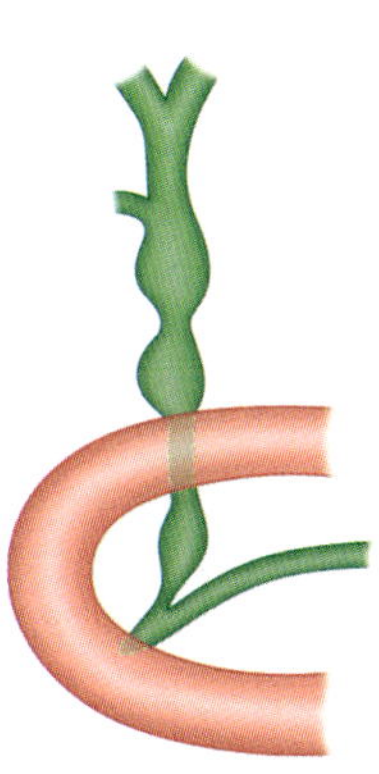

Type V

Caroli Disease

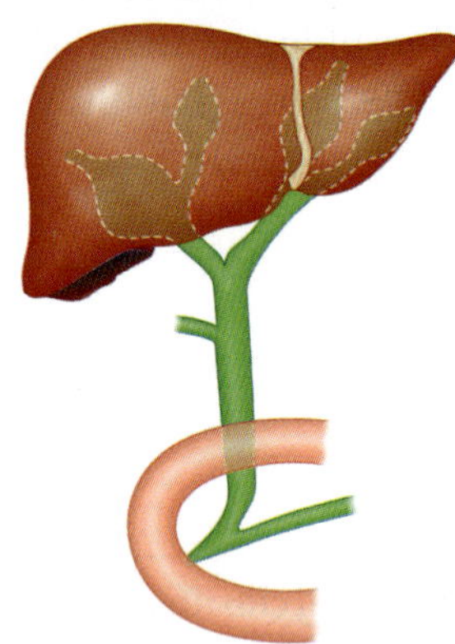

Caroli Syndrome

- Caroli disease when associated with congenital hepatic fibrosis.
- This syndrome is inherited as an autosomal recessive trait and closely related to autosomal recessive polycystic kidney disease.

Clinical Presentation

In pediatric patients, Classic triad (10%)

- Right upper quadrant pain, jaundice, and abdominal mass.

In adult patients

- Abdominal pain, jaundice
- Acute cholangitis, acute pancreatitis

Unusual presentation

- Secondary biliary cirrhosis, carcinoma of bile duct or gallbladder, spontaneous rupture of cyst (in pregnancy)

Diagnosis

USG abdomen—initial imaging modality of choice. This imaging can detect the abnormal cystic dilatation of the extrahepatic and intrahepatic biliary tract. Associated pathologies like cholelithiasis, malignancy can also be detected.

MRCP—the imaging modality of choice for diagnosis of choledochal cyst. This imaging modality can detect the site, size, shape of cystic dilatation and can detect APBDJ. MRCP has limited role in diagnosis of small choledochocele.

ERCP is only indicated if MRCP facility is unavailable or MRCP is contraindicated.

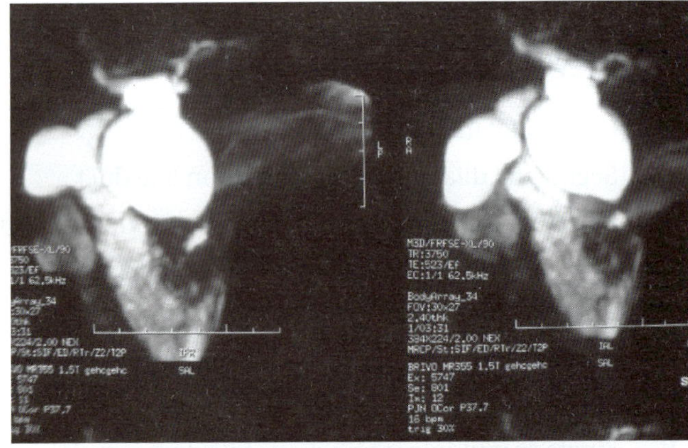

MRCP showing type I choledochal cyst

Treatment

- Surgical treatment of choledochal cyst is aimed to avoid complications or risks associated with the cyst.
- The principle of surgical intervention is complete excision of the cyst followed by reconstruction. Cholecystectomy is also carried out due to increased risk of gallbladder carcinoma.

Lilly's procedure: Due to recurrent cholangitis, sometimes posterior wall of the choledochal cyst is densely adhered to the underlying portal vein and hepatic artery. In this situation, the cyst epithelium is dissected from the posterior fibrotic wall, leaving behind only the posterior fibrotic wall.

Risks associated with choledochal cyst:

- Stone formation (hepatolithiasis, cholelithiasis)
- Recurrent cholangitis
- Pancreatitis
- Malignant transformation (gallbladder, bile duct)
- Spontaneous rupture (in pregnancy)

Type I cyst

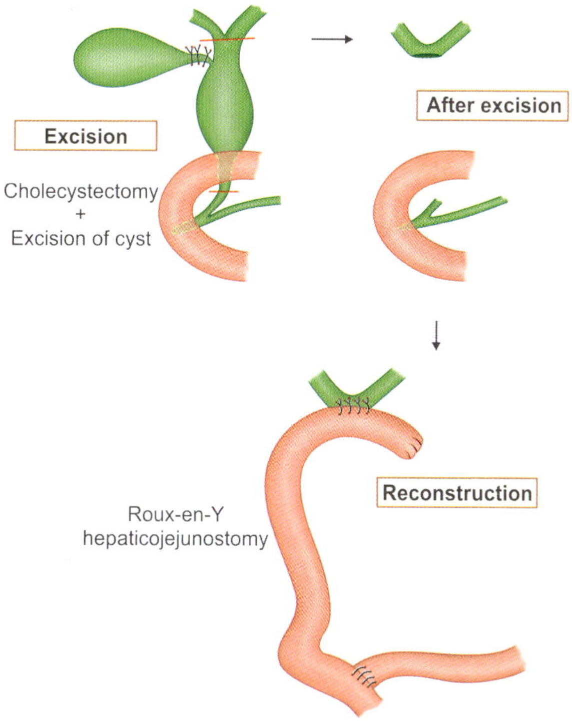

Excision

Cholecystectomy
+
Excision of cyst

After excision

Reconstruction

Roux-en-Y
hepaticojejunostomy

Type II cyst

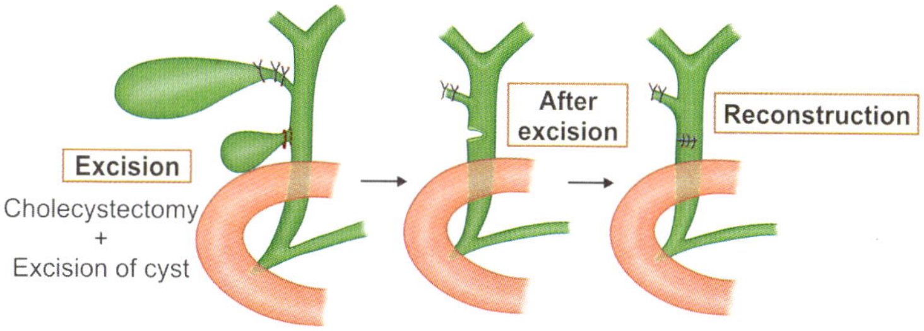

Excision

Cholecystectomy
+
Excision of cyst

After excision

Reconstruction

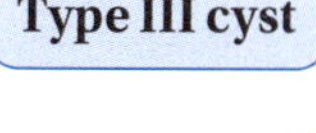

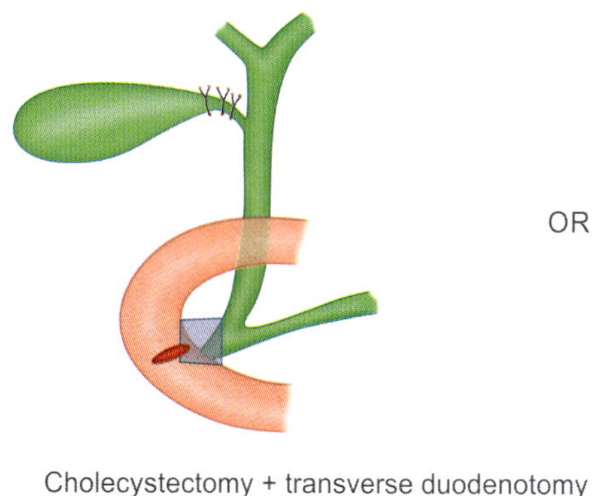

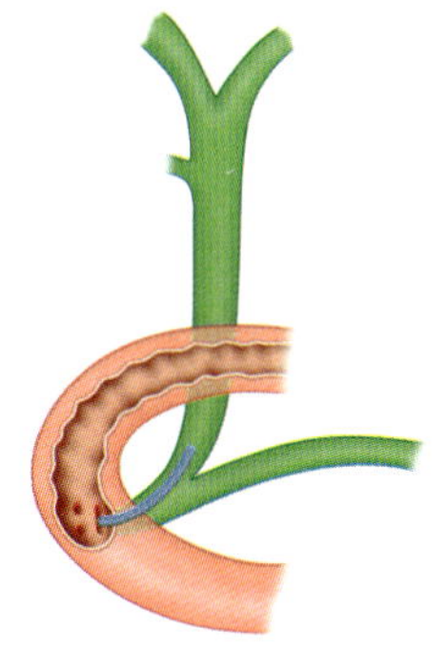

Cholecystectomy + transverse duodenotomy
↓
Excision of cyst

OR

Endoscopic sphincterotomy
and cyst unroofing

Type IV cyst

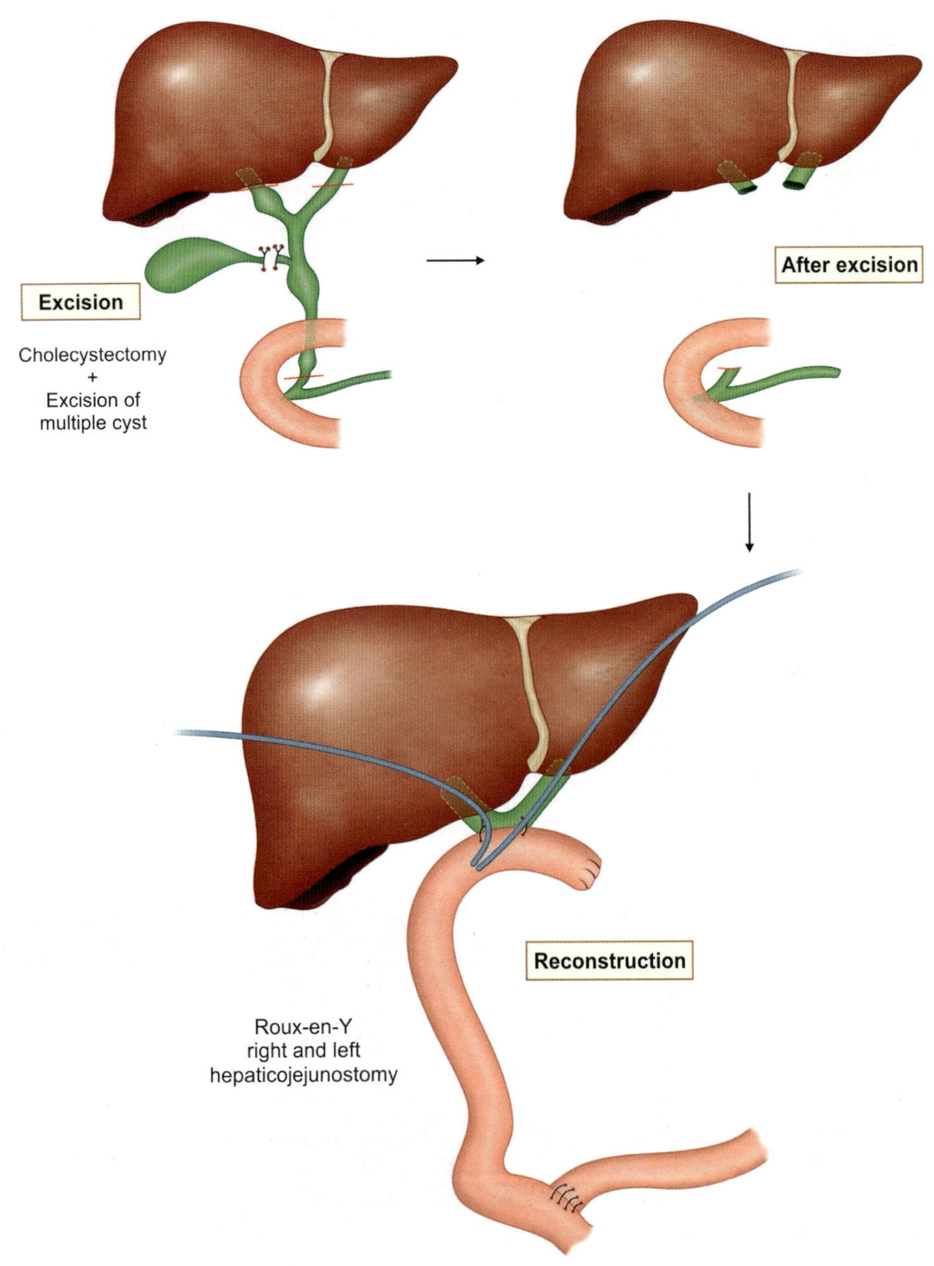
Excision
Cholecystectomy
+
Excision of
multiple cyst
After excision
Reconstruction
Roux-en-Y
right and left
hepaticojejunostomy

Type V cyst

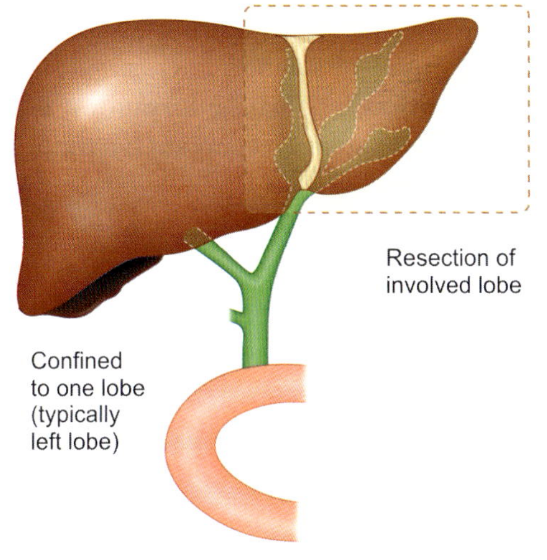

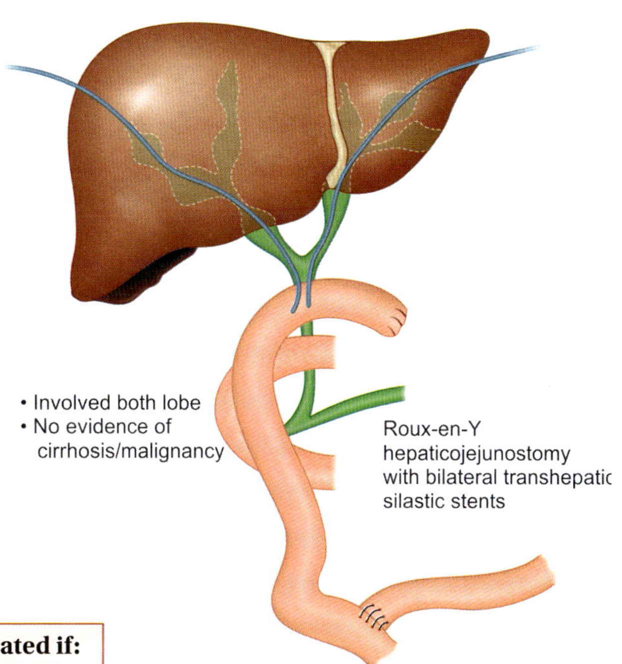

In Caroli's disease, orthotopic liver transplantation is indicated if:
(i) Bilateral Caroli's disease with cholangitis and (ii) Malignant transformation

Follow-up

- Risk of malignancy exists even after complete cyst excision.
- Lifelong follow-up is recommended because of increased risk of cholangiocarcinoma.

Recurrent Pyogenic Cholangitis (Oriental Cholangiohepatitis)

A clinical syndrome characterized **by recurrent bacterial cholangitis, intrahepatic pigment stone** and **biliary strictures** and prevalent in Asian population.

Pathophysiology

- Exact pathophysiology is not known.
- Chronic infestation of the biliary tract by **parasites** (*Clonorchis sinensis, Ascaris lumbricoides*) lead to inflammatory changes of the bile duct, resulting in **stricture formation,** bile stasis, **formation of stone (brown pigment stone), recurrent bacterial cholangitis.**

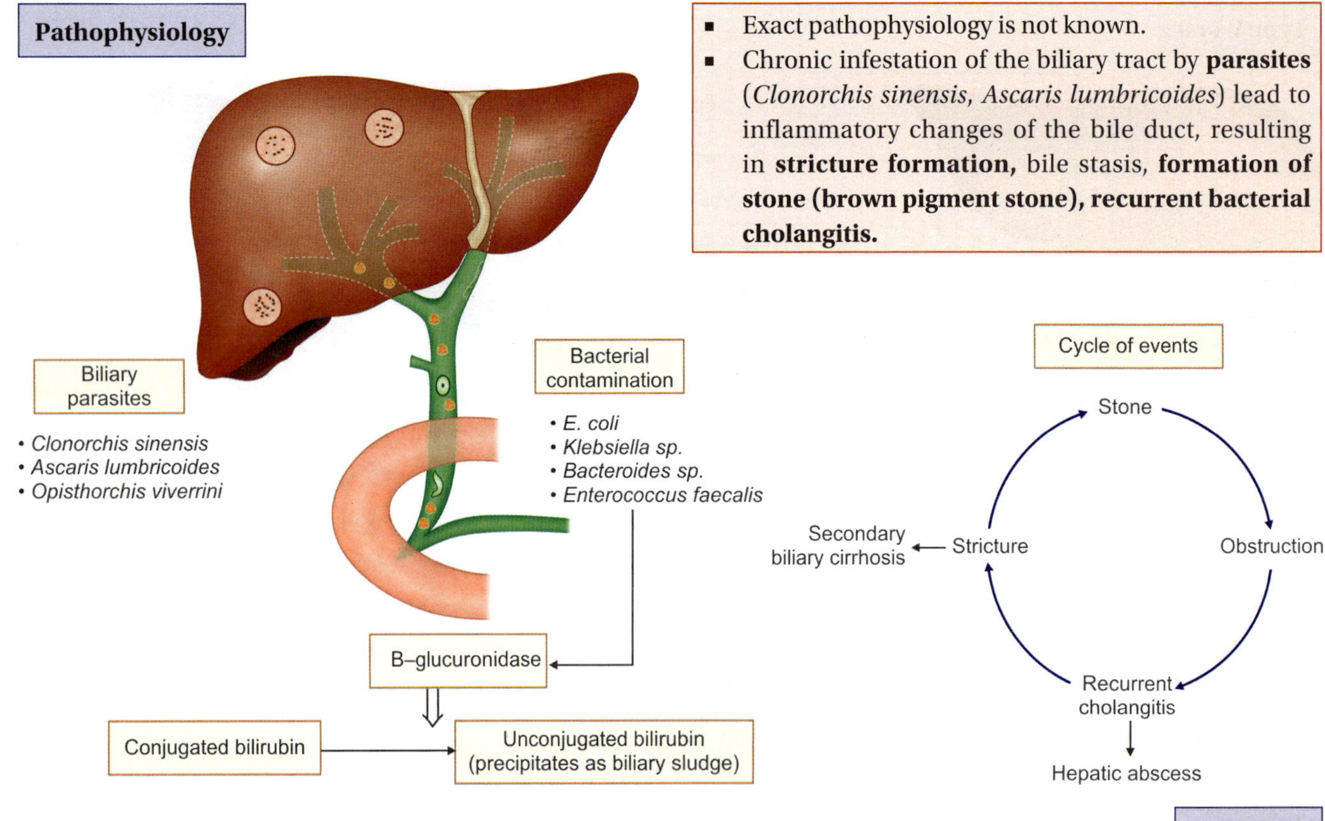

Clinical Presentation

Recurrent upper abdominal pain with fever and jaundice.

Clinical presentation of hepatic abscess may be present.

In long standing disease process, patient may present with clinical features of secondary biliary cirrhosis, portal hypertension.

Complications

- Hepatic abscess—commonly multiple, multiseptate and present in right lobe of liver.
- Segmental liver atrophy
- Secondary biliary cirrhosis
- Portal vein thrombosis
- Cholangiocarcinoma

Diagnosis

Diagnosis is made by characteristic imaging findings.

USG—dilatation of the both intrahepatic and extrahepatic ducts with mural irregularity. Intrahepatic stones and pneumobilia are also the common findings in recurrent pyogenic cholangitis.

CT abdomen—dilated biliary ducts, intrahepatic stones and pneumobilia are common findings. Complications like segmental liver atrophy can be detected by CT scan.

MRCP—highly specific imaging modality for detection of focal biliary strictures, dilated ducts and intrahepatic stones.

ERCP—indicated only when associated therapeutic procedure (biliary decompression) is planned.

Management

The goal of management is to complete clearance of stones from both intrahepatic and extrahepatic bile ducts, to prevent recurrent attacks of cholangitis.

Initial management—management of cholangitis with antibiotics and biliary drainage.

Definitive management includes endoscopic approach, drainage through percutaneous transhepatic approach, biliary-enteric bypass, segmental liver resection, orthotopic liver transplantation.

Endoscopic approach: ERCP is the preferred approach for clearance of stones in extrahepatic bile ducts and intrahepatic ducts but technically difficult for stones in left lateral segment of liver.

Biliary-enteric bypass: This treatment option reduces the risk of recurrent stone formation. Different options include choledochoduodenostomy, Roux-en-Y choledocho-jejunostomy, Roux-en-Y choledochojejunostomy with Hutson loop.

Segmental liver resection is indicated when stones in segmental ducts is associated with segmental liver atrophy.

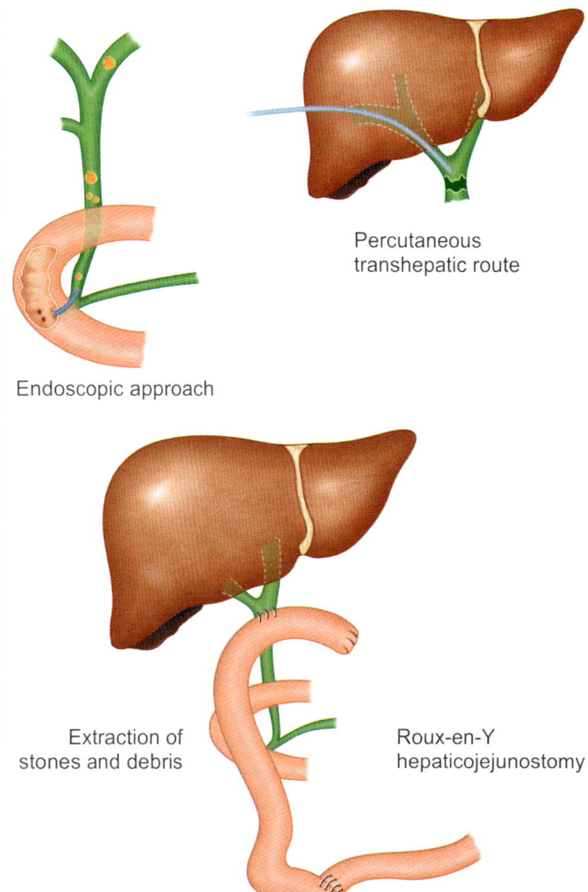

Primary Sclerosing Cholangitis

Primary sclerosing cholangitis is an **immune-mediated chronic cholestatic disease** of liver and biliary tract characterized by inflammation, fibrosis of the intra- and extrahepatic bile ducts resulting in stricture formation that cannot be ascribed to another cause.

Pathophysiology

Exact pathophysiology is not known. The strong association between primary sclerosing cholangitis and inflammatory bowel disease indicates a possible role of **autoimmunity**.

Characteristic association between **human leukocyte antigen haplotype** and the disease have been recognized.

Clinical Presentation

Persistently abnormal liver function test without any specific symptoms.

Cyclic remissions and exacerbations of abdominal pain, jaundice, pruritus and fatigue are typical presentations.

Jaundice with fever associated with chill, suggestive of cholangitis.

Symptoms of associated inflammatory bowel disease.

Advanced disease may present with variceal bleeding or ascites due to portal hypertension.

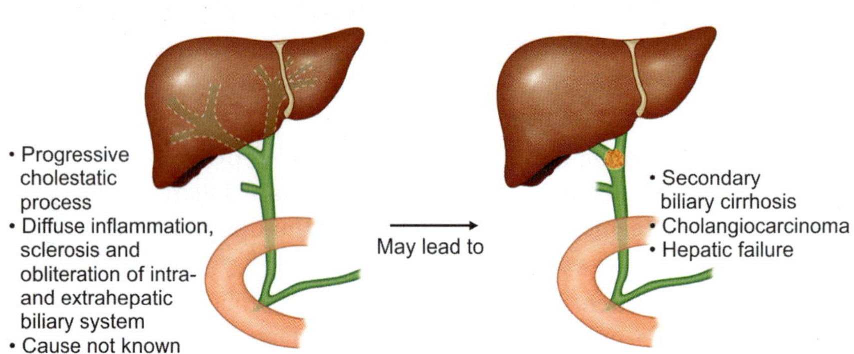

Diagnosis

Diagnosis of PSC is based on: (i) Cholestatic liver biochemistry; (ii) Typical cholangiographic features; and (iii) Absence of other causes of secondary sclerosing cholangitis.

MRCP—the preferred imaging modality for diagnosis of suspected PSC.

ERCP is indicated if any therapeutic intervention is indicated or tissue acquisition is required (dominant stricture seen on imaging) to exclude cholangiocarcinoma.

USG—transabdominal USG is not helpful for diagnosis of PSC but can detect associated choledocholithiasis, GB polyp or portal hypertension.

CT abdomen—CECT is particularly used for diagnosis and staging of suspected cholangiocarcinoma.

Liver biopsy is indicated if diagnosis is uncertain or suspected possible small duct PSC or any overlap variants.

Colonoscopy Full colonscopy with biopsy is recommended regardless of the presence of symptoms.

Investigations to exclude secondary causes of sclerosing cholangitis IgG4, antinuclear antibodies (ANA), antimitochondrial antibodies (AMA), smooth muscle antibodies (SMA), HIV antibodies.

Causes of Secondary Sclerosing Cholangitis

- IgG4-associated cholangitis
- Recurrent pyogenic cholangitis
- Cholangiocarcinoma
- Choledocholithiasis
- HIV cholangiopathy
- Chronic biliary infestation (ascaris, liver flukes)

Characteristic Cholangiographic Findings in PSC:

- Focal stricturing and secular dilatation of bile ducts
- Beading
- Peripheral duct pruning
- Pseudodiverticula

Characteristic Findings in Liver Biopsy

- 'Onion skin' periductal fibrosis
- Periportal inflammation
- Periportal fibrosis
- Ductopenia and bridging fibrosis

Other Immune-mediated Diseases associated with PSC

- Inflammatory bowel disease
- Celiac disease
- Riedel's thyroiditis
- Type 1 diabetes mellitus
- Systemic sclerosis
- Retroperitoneal fibrosis
- Rheumatoid arthritis
- Sarcoidosis

Dominant Stricture

At cholangiography, stenoses measuring <1.5 mm in the common bile duct or <1.0 mm in the hepatic ducts.

Treatment

Medical treatment: Treatment with ursodeoxycholic acid is not recommended for treatment of PSC.

Endoscopic approach: ERCP with balloon dilatation is recommended for PSC with dominant stricture with pruritus and/or cholangitis. Stent insertion (single or multiple plastic stents) is recommended when balloon dilatation is unsuccessful.

Percutaneous transhepatic approach is indicated if endoscopic therapy fails or ERCP is technically not feasible due to altered anatomy (e.g., Roux-en-Y choledochojejunostomy, Roux-en-Y gastric bypass).

Surgical management: Surgical management includes biliary-enteric drainage and liver transplantation. Liver transplantation is favored over surgical drainage due to favorable outcome of transplantation and associated significant risk of complications of surgical drainage (cholangitis, postoperative scarring).

Liver transplantation is the definitive treatment in PSC with decompensated cirrhosis.

In gallbladder polyp associated with PSC

Cholecystectomy is suggested for polyps >8 mm, to prevent the risk of development of gallbladder adenocarcinoma.

Complications of Primary Sclerosing Cholangitis

- Cholangitis
- Cirrhosis, portal hypertension
- Cholangiocarcinoma
- Osteopenia, osteoporosis
- Dediciency of fat-soluble vitamins

Inflammatory Bowel Disease (IBD) Associated with Primary Sclerosing Cholangitis (PSC)

- IBD presents earlier in life than in patients without PSC.
- IBD is often asymptomatic and have a quiescent course.
- Involvement of right-sided colon is common with relative sparing of rectum.
- 'Backwash ileitis' is more common.

Gallbladder Polyp

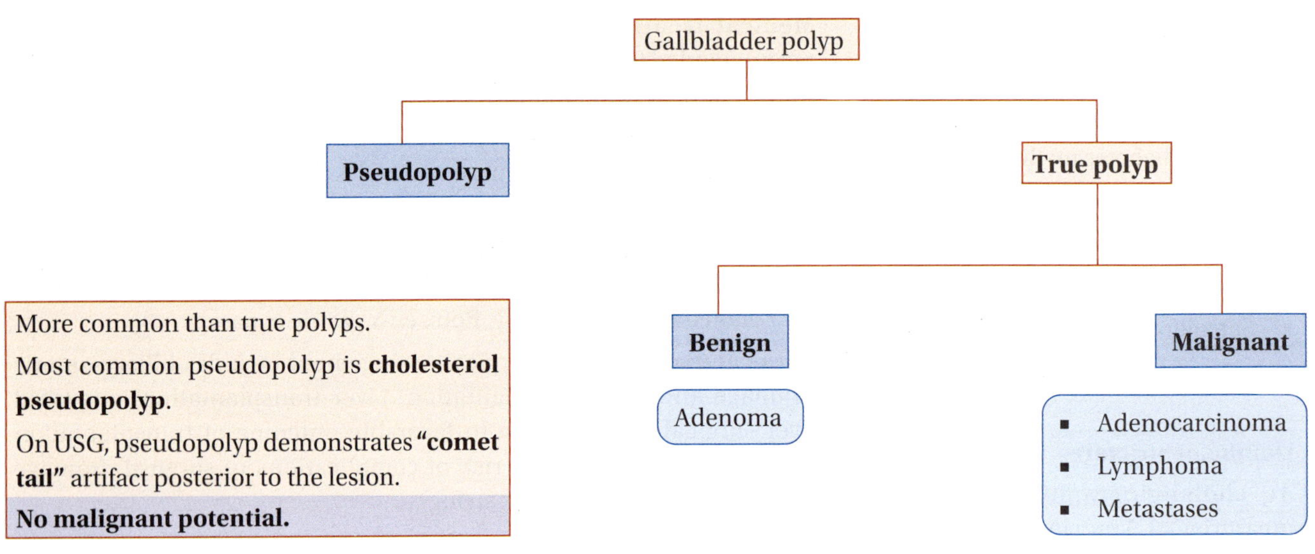

More common than true polyps.

Most common pseudopolyp is **cholesterol pseudopolyp**.

On USG, pseudopolyp demonstrates **"comet tail"** artifact posterior to the lesion.

No malignant potential.

Diagnosis

USG abdomen is the investigation of choice. Routine use of other imaging modalities are not recommended.

In difficult cases, **EUS** may be helpful in decision making.

Treatment (as per ESGAR Guideline)

If polypoidal lesion of the gallbladder is **10 mm or more**, then cholecystectomy is recommended if the patient is fit for and accepts surgery.

Polypoidal lesion of the gallbladder with patient's **symptoms attributable to the gallbladder:** Cholecystectomy is suggested if the patient is fit for and accepts surgery.

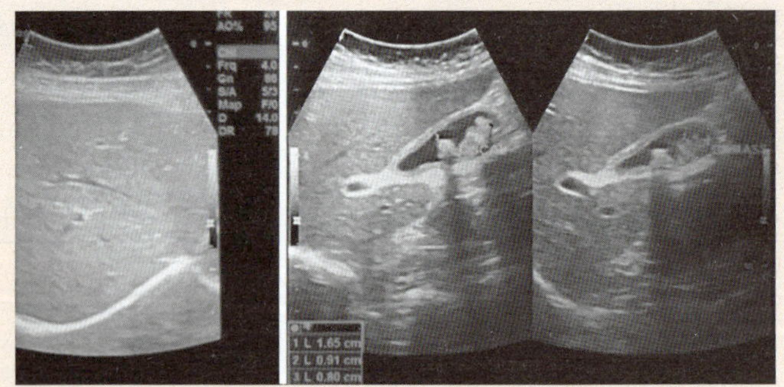

USG showing stone and polypoidal lesion in gallbladder.

If patient has risk factors for gallbladder malignancy (e.g., age >50, history of primary sclerosing cholangitis, Indian ethnicity, sessile polyp including focal gallbladder wall thickening >4 mm) and a polyp 6–9 mm, cholecystectomy is recommended.

If the patient has **no risk factors for gallbladder malignancy** and a gallbladder **polyp of 6–9 mm**, follow-up USG of the gallbladder is recommended at 6 months, 1 year and then yearly upto 5 years.

If the patient has **no risk factors for malignancy** and a gallbladder **polyp of 5 mm or less**, followup is advised at 1 year, 3 years, and 5 years.

During follow-up: (i) Gallbladder polyp reaches 10 mm, cholecystectomy is advised; (ii) Polyp increases by 2 mm or more, cholecystectomy is advised; and (iii) If polyp disappears, discontinue follow-up.

Gallbladder cancer

Most common biliary tract cancer

Women are 2–6 times more likely to develop this cancer.

Risk factor

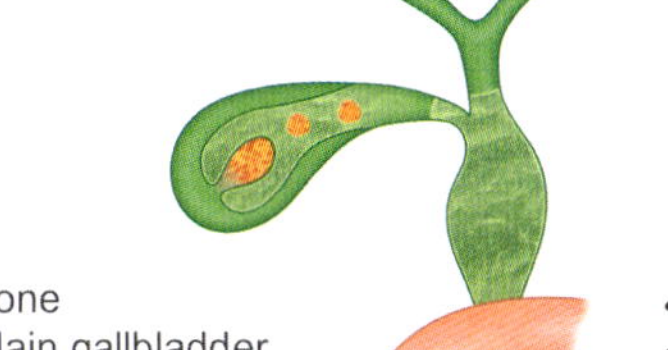

- **Gallstones are the strongest risk factor.** The risk increases with stone size.
- Adenomyomatosis of the gallbladder as risk factor is controversial.

Pathology

Histology

- **Adenocarcinoma (most common):** (i) Papillary adenocarcinoma; (ii) Nonpapillary adenocarcinoma; and (iii) Mucinous adenocarcinoma.
- Squamous cell carcinoma
- Adenosquamous carcinoma
- Oat cell carcinoma

Papillary adenocarcinoma is prognostically better than other histologic types.

Spread of tumor

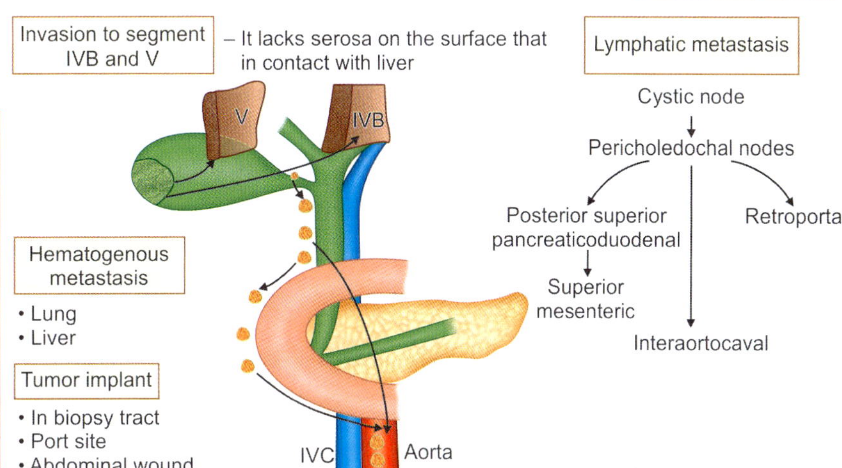

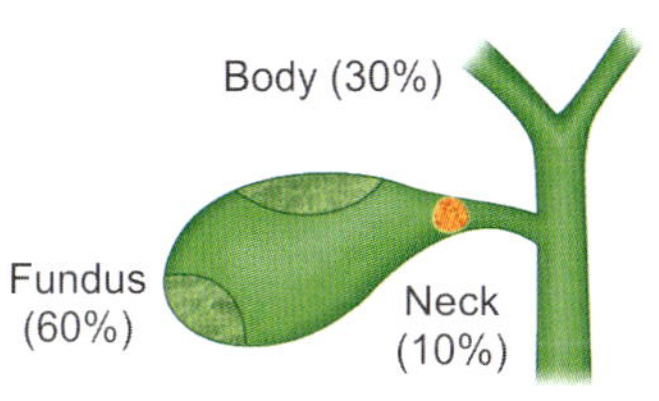

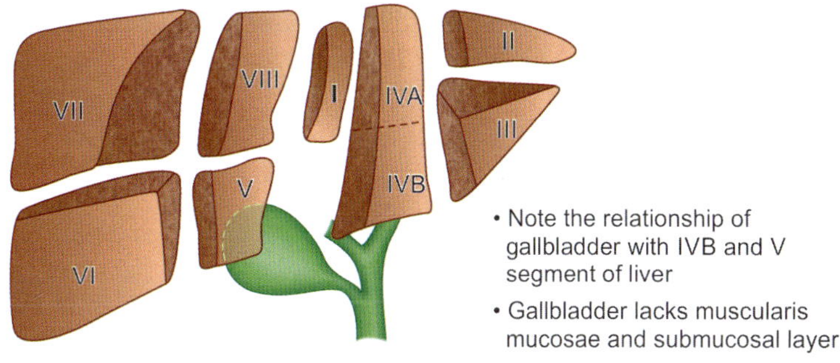

Tumors in fundus and body involve the segment IVB and V early whereas tumors in infundibulum early involve the cystic duct and CBD.

Gallbladder has single muscle layer, so tumor spreads early to major lymphatic and vascular channels. Therefore, gallbladder cancer is associated with early lymphatic spread and hematogenous metastases.

Clinical presentation

- Pain in upper abdomen—similar to chronic cholecystitis or biliary colic.
- In advanced disease, jaundice and palpable mass in right hypochondrium.

Genetics associated with Gallbladder Cancer

- K-ras and p53 mutation
- Microsatellite instability-high (MSI-H)
- HER2/neu overexpression

Diagnosis

Factors responsible for diagnosis of gallbladder cancer at an advanced stage commonly: (i) Clinical presentation is almost similar to chronic cholecystitis; (ii) Often asymptomatic in early stage; and (iii) aggressive biologic behavior.

Initial work-up: Liver function test, estimation of CEA and CA 19-9. These serum markers are not specific for gallbladder cancer.

USG can detect gallstone and gallbladder wall thickening, polypoid mass (nonspecific findings for gallbladder cancer). Discontinuous gallbladder mucosa, echogenic mucosa are USG findings suggestive of gallbladder cancer.

Contrast-enhanced CT abdomen and pelvis—to evaluate tumor penetration through the gallbladder wall, assessment of tumor invasion into adjacent organs/major vessels, evaluation of lymphatic spread and distant metastases.

MRCP is indicated in patients presenting with jaundice to evaluate the biliary invasion of tumor.

ERCP or PTC is indicated only if any therapeutic intervention is planned. In that cases, bile should be collected for cytology.

Biopsy: In imaging, if mass is suspicious for gallbladder cancer and definite resection is planned, biopsy is not indicated. Biopsy should be considered if the tumor is not considered for definite resection. Different options for obtaining tissues are percutaneous fine-needle aspiration, core needle biopsy and EUS-directed fine needle aspiration. **The EUS-directed fine needle aspiration is the best option for tissue retrieval**.

Treatment

Carcinoma incidentally detected after routine cholecystectomy

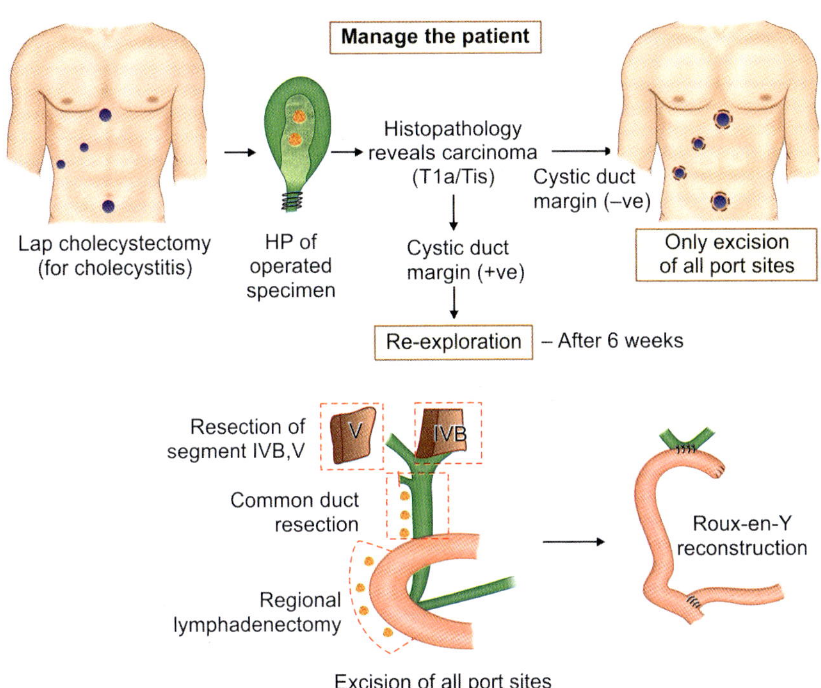

Prophylactic port excision is not associated with improved survival or disease recurrence.

Gallbladder carcinoma suspected peroperatively

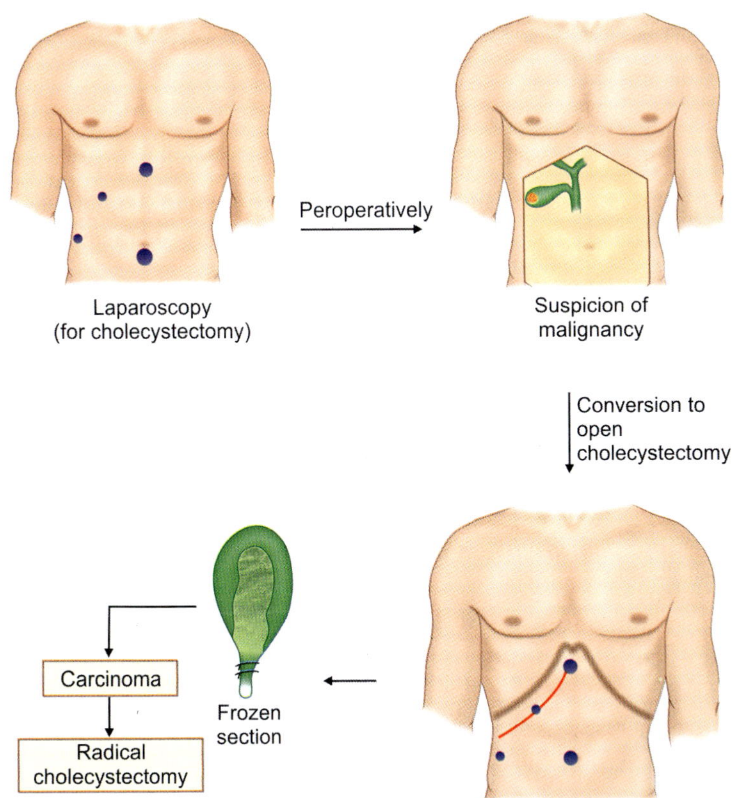

If gallbladder carcinoma is detected by frozen section peroperatively, curative resection (cholecystectomy, en bloc hepatic resection, lymphadenectomy) should be planned.

If expertise is not available, patient should be transferred to a facility where hepatobiliary surgeon is available.

Suspicious Mass Detected on Imaging

After staging work-up, if tumor seems to be resectable, no need of preoperative image-guided biopsy for tissue diagnosis. Diagnostic laparoscopy before definitive resection should be considered to detect radiologically occult disseminated disease, thereby unnecessary laparotomy can be avoided.

T1b or greater lesions—**Cholecystectomy** with **en bloc hepatic resection (segment IVB and V)** and **lymphadenectomy** (lymph nodes in the porta hepatis, gastrohepatic ligament and retroduodenal regions) with or without bile duct excision.

Extended hepatic resection and **common duct resection** may be considered depending on the stage and location of the tumor.

Absolute Contraindications for Resection

- Lymph node metastases beyond the porta hepatis (nodes along celiac axis, aortocaval groove)
- Local invasion of porta hepatis
- Presence of distant metastases

Relative Contraindication for Resection

- Jaundice

Locally Advanced, Node-positive Disease

- Neoadjuvant chemotherapy (gemcitabine/cisplatin, gemcitabine/oxaliplatin, gemcitabine/capecitabine)
- *Palliation of jaundice in unresectable disease:* ERCP stenting or percutaneous approach. Surgical approaches (e.g., Segment III bypass, Longmire operation) are less preferred approach nowadays.

Cholangiocarcinoma

Tumors arising from epithelium of the bile duct

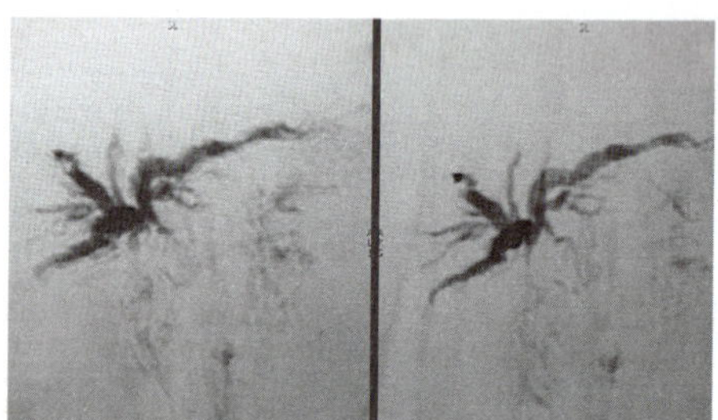

MRCP showing hilar cholangiocarcinoma.

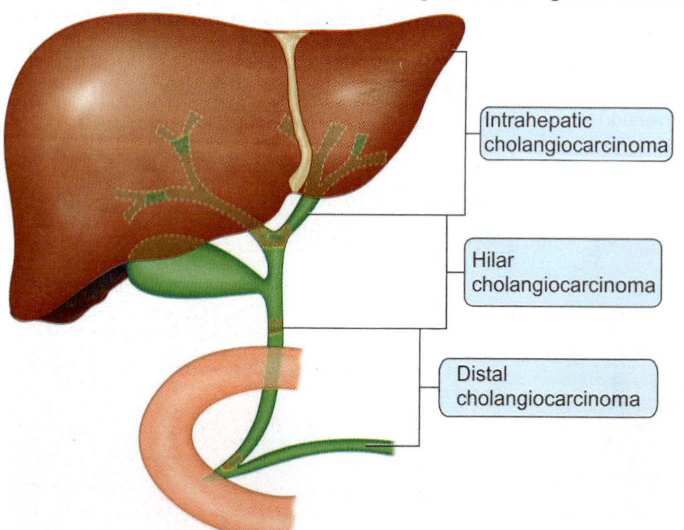

- Also called 'peripheral cholangiocarcinoma'
- Present as liver mass

- Also called **Klatskin tumor**.
- At or near the junction of right and left hepatic duct
- Most common type

- Distal to the junction of right and left hepatic duct and above the ampulla of Vater.

Classification of Hilar Cholangiocarcinoma

Modified Bismuth-Corlette staging system
- Classifies hilar cholangiocarcinoma into four types based on extent of biliary involvement.
- *Limitations of this staging system:* (i) Does not include parameters like vascular involvement, lymph node involvement; and (ii) Cannot predict resectibility or survival.

The Blumgart staging system
- Classifies hilar cholangiocarcinoma into three stages based on the location and extent of bile duct involvement, portal venous invasion and hepatic lobar atrophy.
- *Advantages of this staging system:* Can predict resectability, likelihood of metastases and survival.

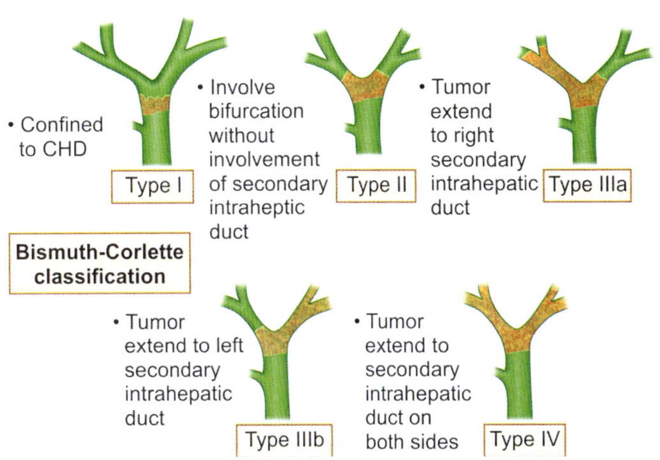

Pathology

Histological Types
- Adenocarcinoma (>90%)
- Squamous cell carcinoma
- Small cell cancer
- Sarcoma
- Lymphoma

Risk Factors

Well established risk factors
- Primary sclerosing cholangitis
- Hepatolithiasis
- Choledochal cyst
- Liver fluke infections (*Opisthorchis viverrini, Clonorchis sinensis*)

Other risk factors

HBV infection, hepatitis C infection, HIV infection, cirrhosis, diabetes, obesity, anomalous pancreatic-biliary junction. alcohol, tobacco.

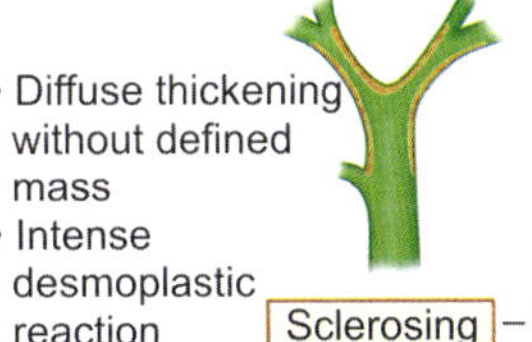

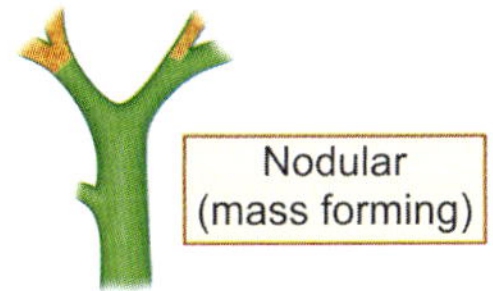

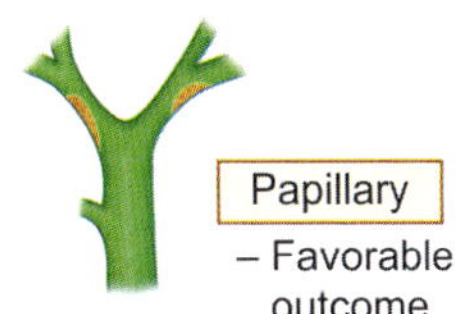

Molecular Profiling of Cholangiocarcinoma

Intrahepatic cholangiocarcinoma: Mutations in IDH 1/2, FGFR, NRAS, BAP1, TGFBR2, TP53
Extrahepatic cholangiocarcinoma: Mutations in KRAS, TP53, ARID1A, HER2

Clinical Presentation

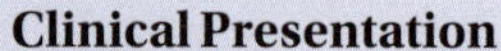

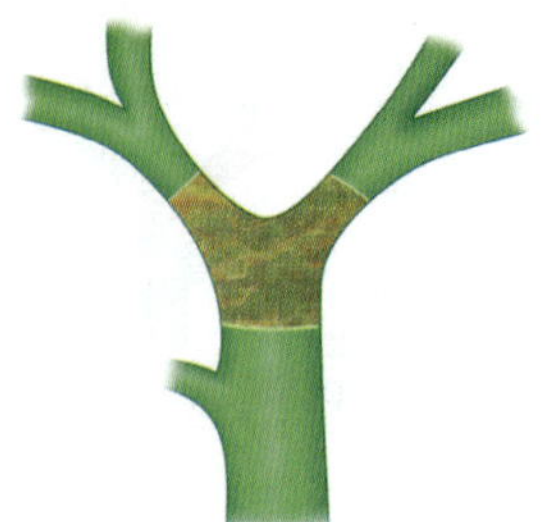

Hilar Cholangiocarcinoma and **Distal cholanagiocarcinoma**

- **Painless progressive jaundice** (most common presentation)
- Pruritus
- Abdominal pain
- Weight loss
- Cholangitis
- Palpable gallbladder (in distal cholangiocarcinoma)

Patient with cholangiocarcinoma causing obstruction of right or left hepatic duct usually not presenting with jaundice.

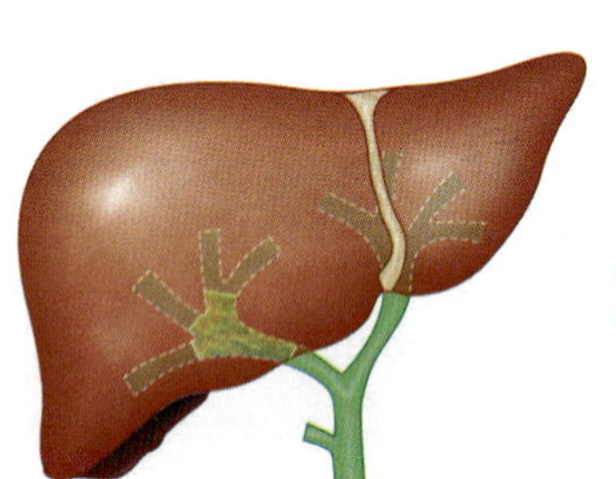

Intrahepatic Cholangiocarcinoma

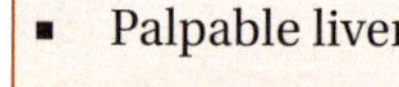

- Palpable liver
- Abdominal pain
- Weight loss

Common Causes of Painless Jaundice

- Carcinoma of head of pancreas
- Hilar or distal cholangiocarcinoma
- Parenchymal liver tumors

Diagnosis

Initial workup includes liver function tests, CEA, CA 19-9.

USG—initial imaging modality. USG findings include dilated intrahepatic biliary radicles, dilatation of the biliary tree proximal to the obstruction, no stone in CBD.

Multiphasic CT/MRI with IV contrast is the investigation of choice to determine tumor resectability, its relationship to adjacent major vessels and biliary tree, presence of satellite lesions, lymph node involvement, and liver metastases. LI-RADS is also helpful to differentiate between HCC and intrahepatic cholangiocarcinoma.

Upper GI endoscopy and colonoscopy should be included as initial workup of suspected intrahepatic cholangiocarcinoma (this intrahepatic lesion may be metastatic).

EUS—an useful imaging modality for distal cholangiocarcinoma and for directed biopsies (if indicated).

ERCP is indicated in distal cholangiocarcinoma which is irresectable or stenting is required.

Serum IgG4 estimation should be considered if diagnosis of extrahepatic cholangiocarcinoma is not certain (IgG4-associated cholangiopathy may mimic extrahepatic cholangiocarcinoma).

Transperitoneal biopsy is contraindicated in patients with hilar cholangiocarcinoma if resection is planned or patient is a potential transplant candidate. In irresectable cholangiocarcinoma, direct cholangiography with directed biopsies is the ideal modality for workup.

Treatment

In resectable hilar cholangiocarcinoma, resection of the involved biliary tract and en bloc liver resection (major hepatectomy involving the right or left liver with caudate lobe) along with regional lymphadenectomy of the porta hepatis is the treatment of choice.

In resectable mid bile duct tumors not involving the liver or pancreas, bile duct excision with frozen section assessment of proximal and distal bile duct margins and pancreaticoduodenectomy with regional lymphadenectomy is the treatment of choice.

Intrahepatic cholangiocarcinoma—hepatic resection with negative margin.

For unresectable or metastatic extrahepatic cholangiocarcinoma, biliary stenting (silastic stent or metallic stent) is the preferred approach for biliary drainage. Surgical bypass is rarely used. Photodynamic therapy with biliary stenting is a new treatment approach for unresectable cholangiocarcinoma.

Curative resection is contraindicated in:

(i) Presence of liver or peritoneal metastases

(ii) Lymph nodes beyond the porta hepatis (for proximal tumors) or head of the pancreas (for distal tumors).

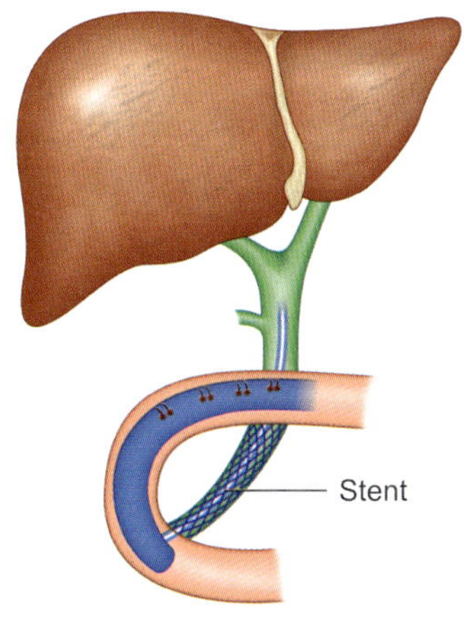

Biliary stenting for unresectable distal cholangiocarcinoma.

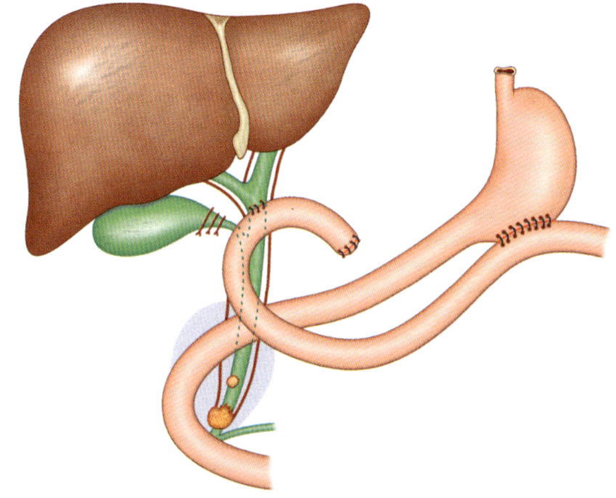

Surgical bypass (hepaticojejunostomy) for unresectable distal cholangiocarcinoma.

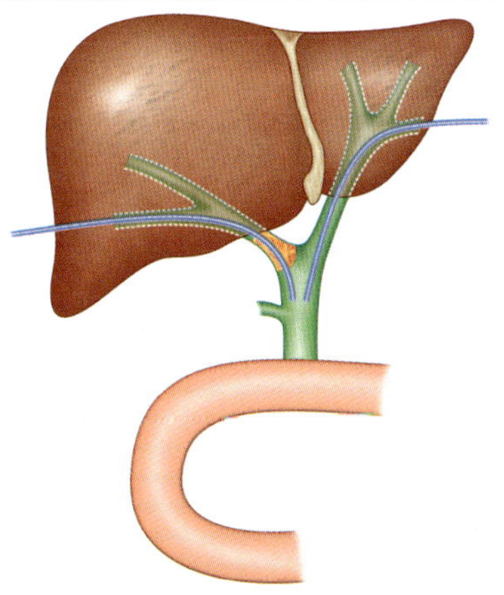

PTC-placed stent for unresectable hilar cholangiocarcinoma.

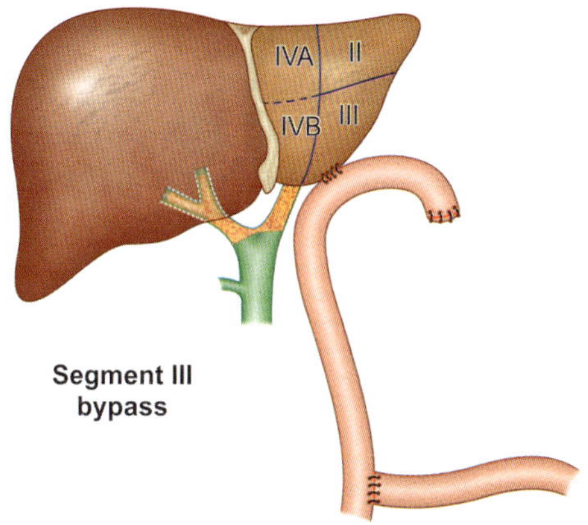

Segment III bypass for unresectable hilar cholangiocarcinoma.

Biliary Stenting

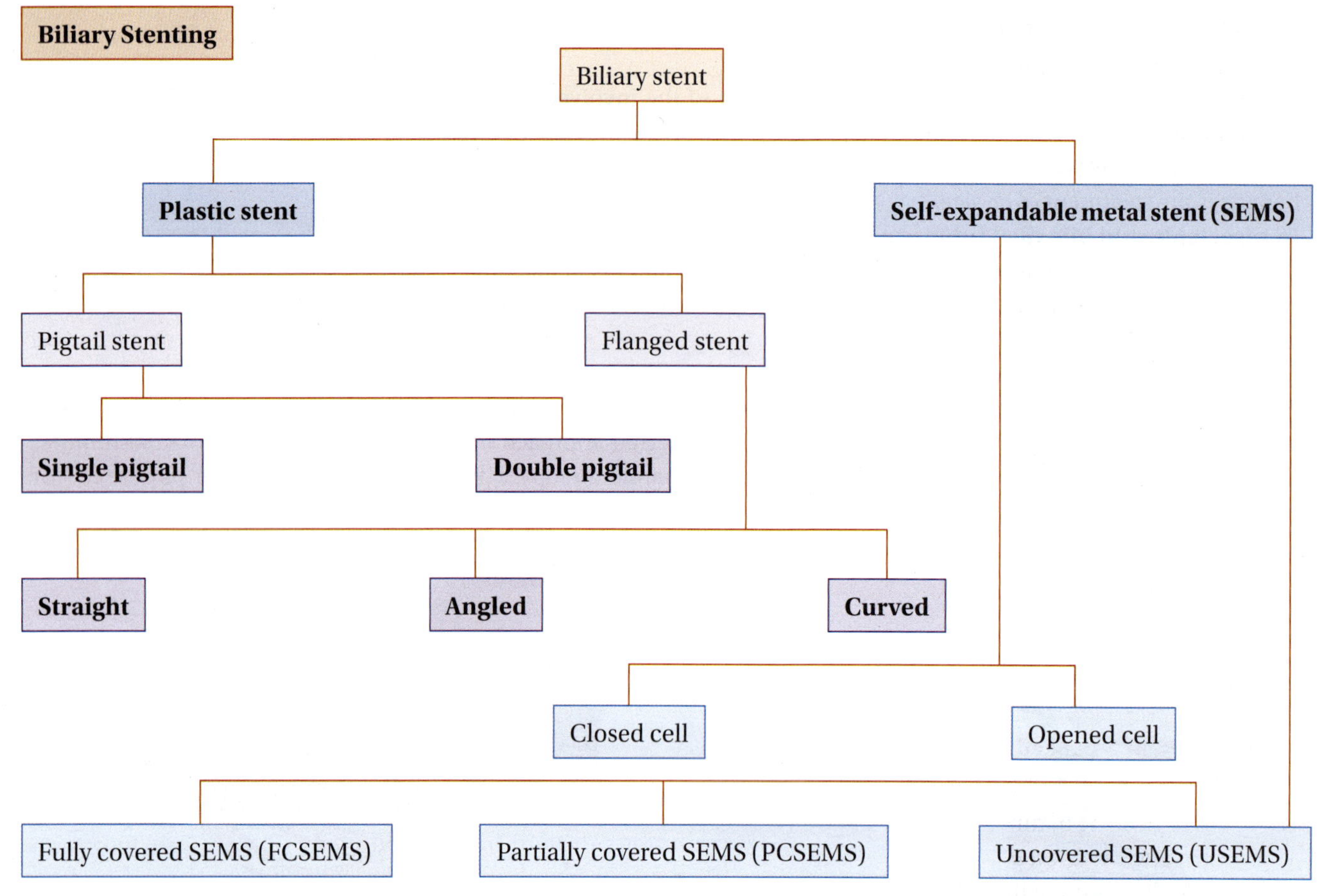

Composition of plastic stent: Polyethylene/ Polyurethane/Teflon

Diameter of plastic stent: 5-Fr to 12-Fr

Length: 1–18 cm

Plastic biliary stents are radiopaque.

Approaches of Biliary Stenting

(i) Stenting via ERCP; (ii) EUS-guided biliary drainage; and (iii) Percutaneous transhepatic biliary drainage (PTBD).

Composition of SEMS: Nitinol (Nickel-titanium)/Stainless steel (Cobalt-chromium)

Composition of coverings in covered SEMS: Silicon/ Polytetrafluoroethylene

Diameter of SEMS: 6–10 mm (when expanded)

Length: 4–12 cm

SEMS are radiopaque.

SEMS with specific designs: (i) SEMSs with antireflux valve; (ii) SEMS with antimigration system; (iii) Radioactive stent; and (iv) Paclitaxel-eluting stent.

Indications of Biliary Stenting

1. **Palliation of malignant obstruction of CBD** by plastic stent (if life expectancy <4 months) or by SEMS (if life expectancy >4 months)
2. **Preoperative stenting in potentially resectable malignant CBD obstruction:** Plastic stent/short intrapancreatic stent/covered SEMS
3. **Malignant hilar stricture:** Plastic stent/uncovered SEMS
4. **Benign CBD stricture:** Multiple plastic stents/fully covered SEMS
5. **Bile leak:** Plastic biliary stent
6. **Irretrievable biliary stones:** Plastic stent

Complications of Biliary Stenting

(1) **Early:** Cholangitis, pancreatitis, bleeding, perforation, early stent migration
(2) **Late:** Stent dysfunction (stent migration and stent occlusion), cholecystitis, duodenal perforation

Among different biliary stents, fully covered SEMS most commonly migrate, least is uncovered SEMS. After distal migration, most of the plastic stents are spontaneously eliminated.

Stent occlusion is caused by sludge (in plastic stents) and by tissue ingrowth or overgrowth (in SEMS)

Ingrowth is growing of tumor between the mesh lines of the stent and *overgrowth* when tumor blocks either proximal or distal end of the stent.

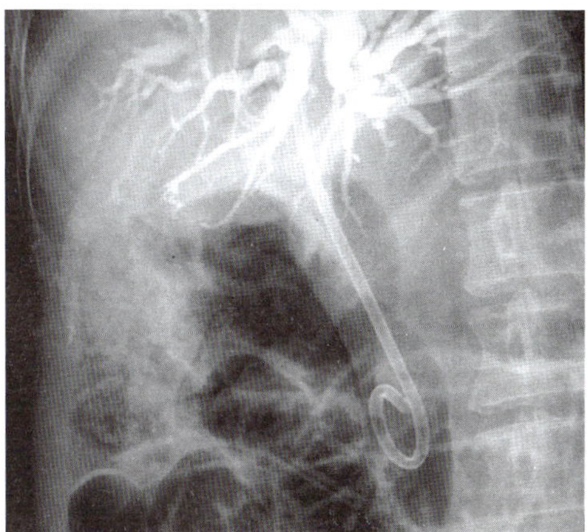

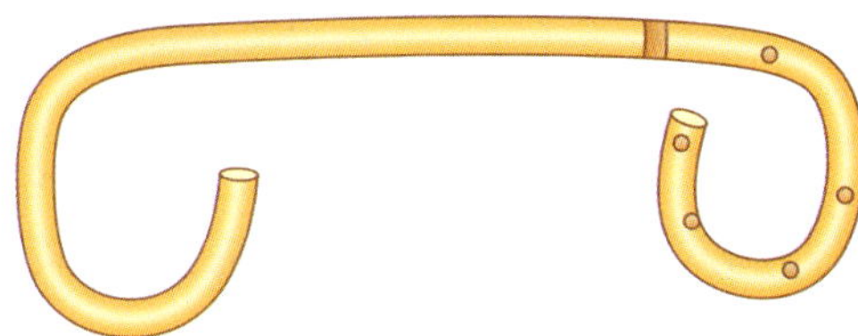

Plastic (polyethylene) stent

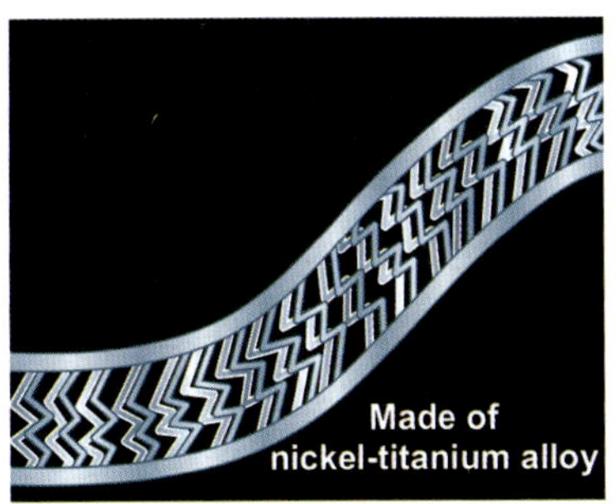

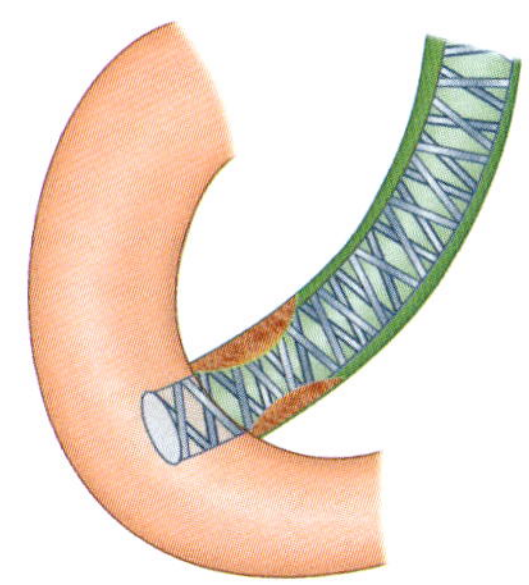

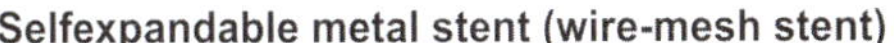

Selfexpandable metal stent (wire-mesh stent)

Endoscopic Therapeutic Approaches of Biliary System

Percutaneous Transhepatic Approach

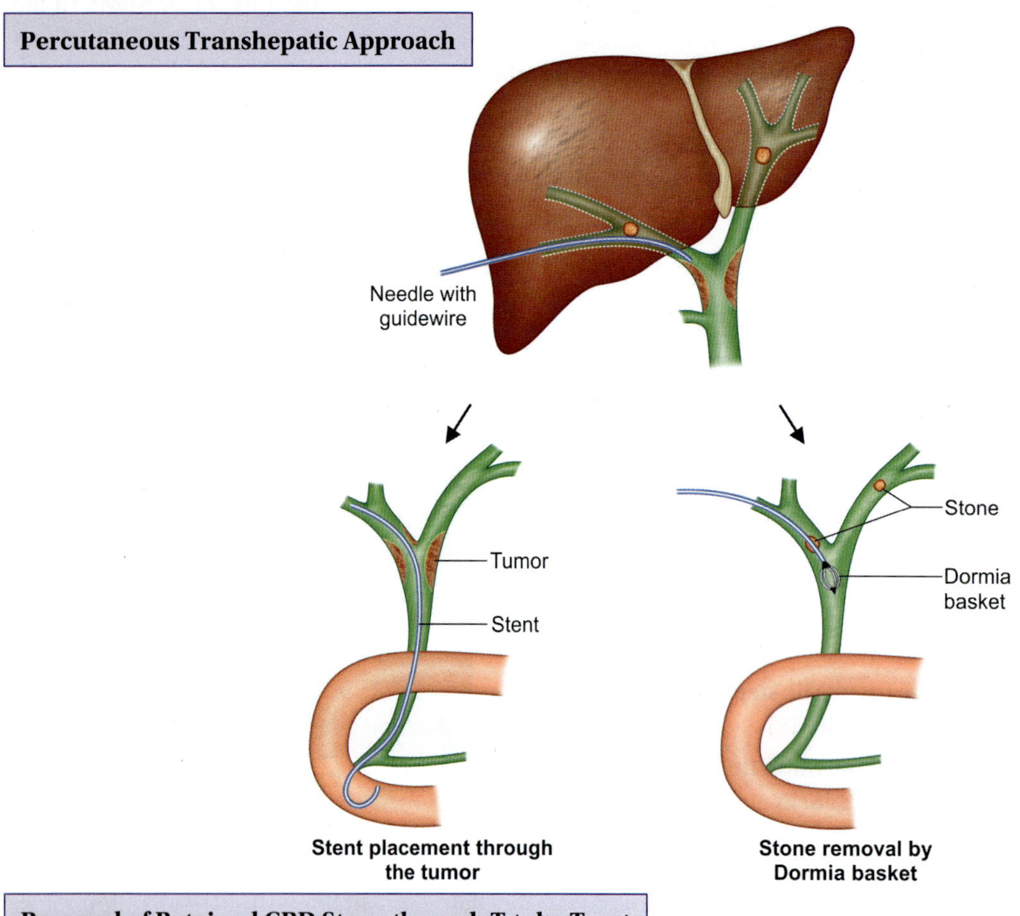

Stent placement through the tumor

Stone removal by Dormia basket

Removal of Retained CBD Stone through T-tube Tract

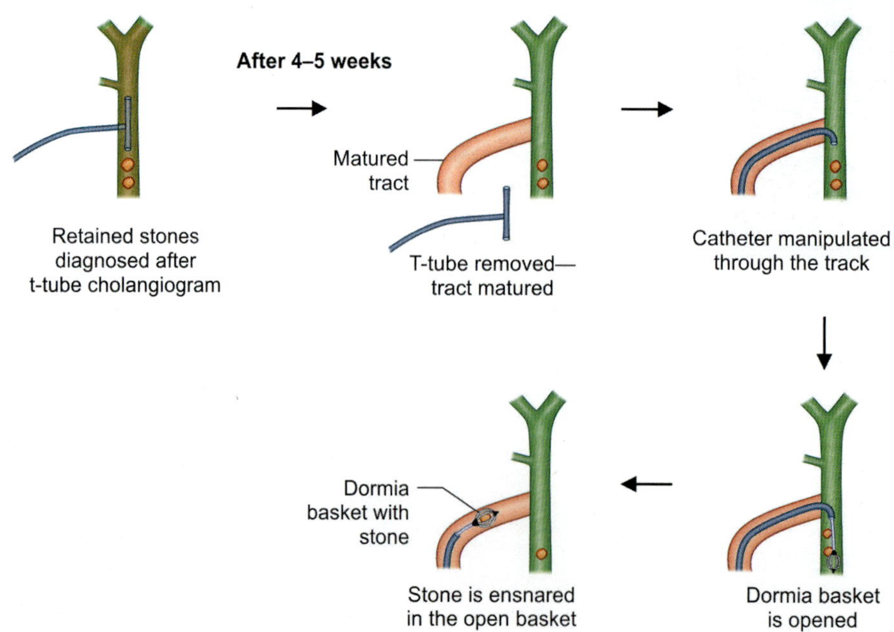

Removal of CBD Stones by Endoscopic Sphincterotomy

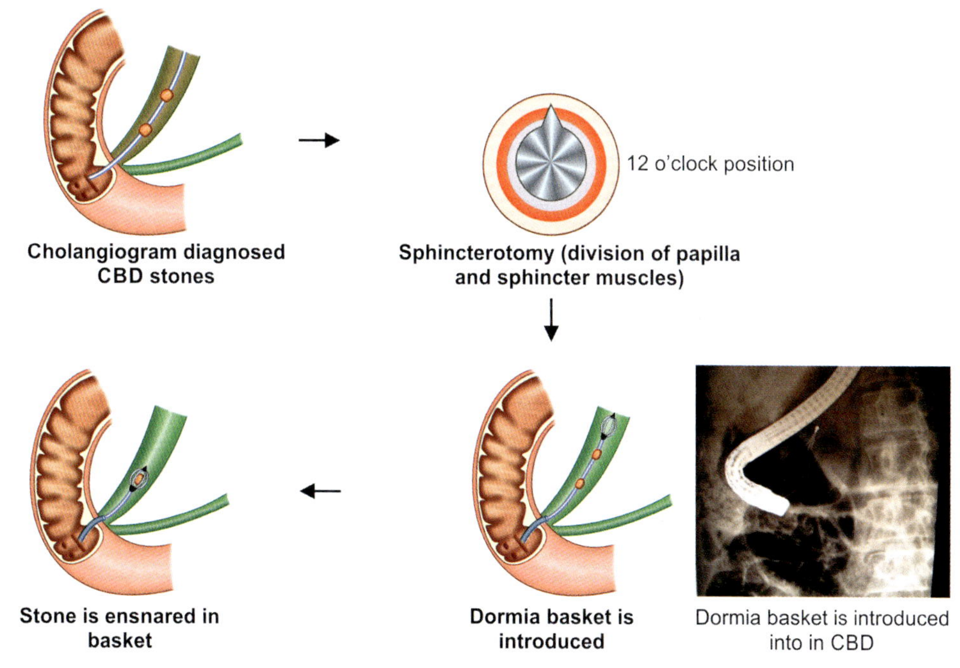

Anomalous Anatomy of Gallbladder and Biliary System

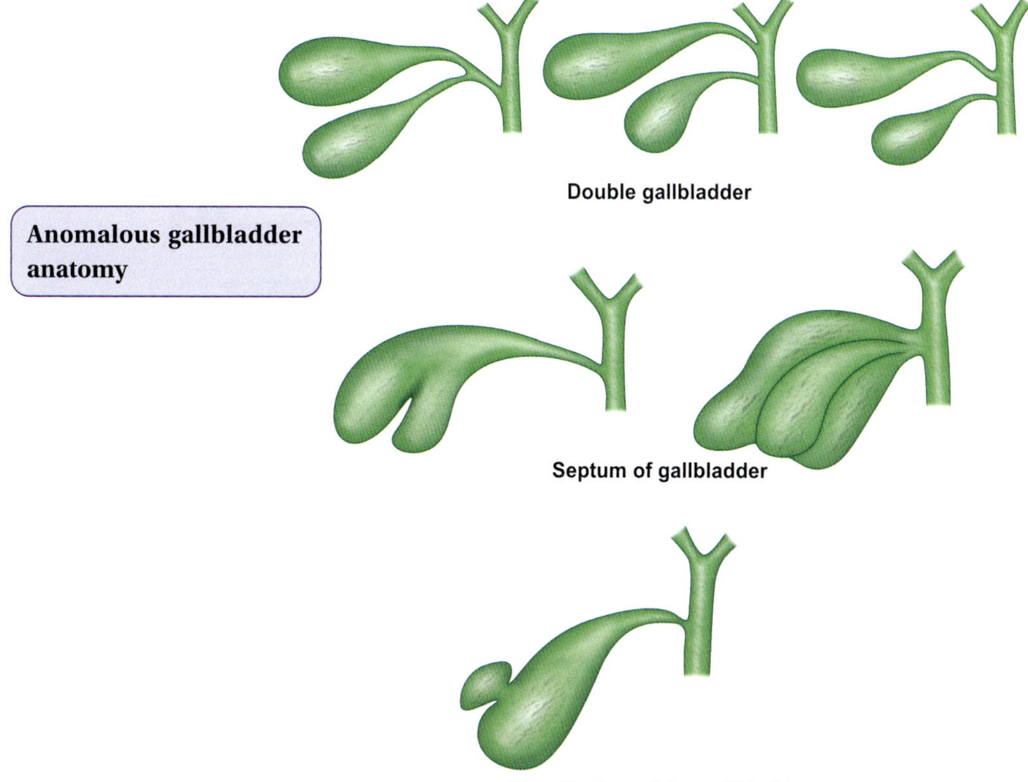

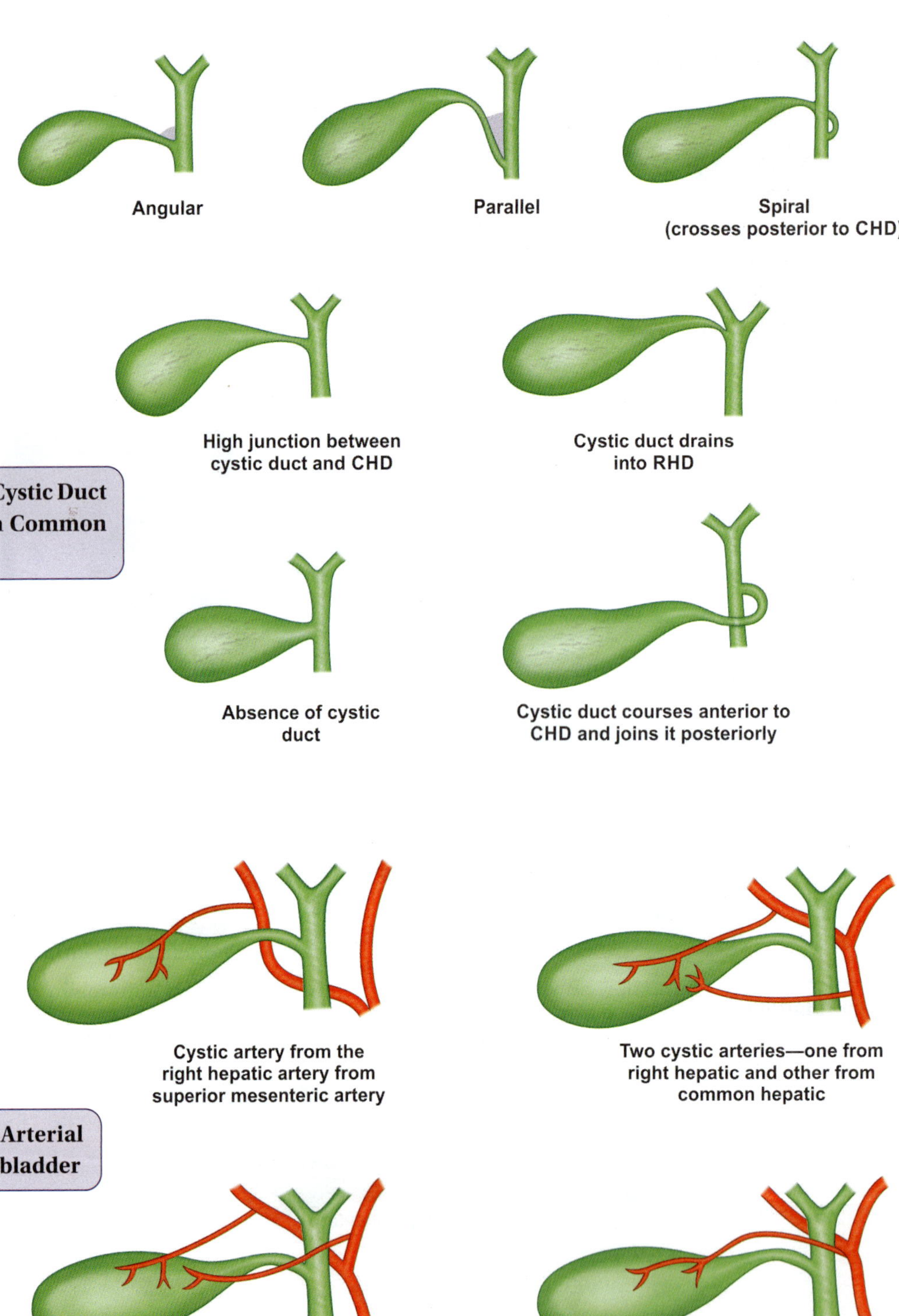
Angular
Parallel
Spiral
(crosses posterior to CHD)
High junction between
cystic duct and CHD
Cystic duct drains
into RHD
Variations of Cystic Duct
Insertion with Common
Hepatic Duct
Absence of cystic
duct
Cystic duct courses anterior to
CHD and joins it posteriorly
Cystic artery from the
right hepatic artery from
superior mesenteric artery
Two cystic arteries—one from
right hepatic and other from
common hepatic
Variations in Arterial
Supply of Gallbladder
Two cystic arteries,
One from right hepatic other
from left hepatic
Cystic artery arising
from right hepatic, running
anterior to CHD

Case 1

History and Physical Examination

A 45-year-old female patient presented with acute onset pain in the right upper abdomen for last 2 days along with repeated episodes of vomiting. Patient was treated with oral antibiotics and antispasmodics by local physician, but pain was not relieved.

No history of similar type of pain or jaundice in the recent past. No history of hematemesis or melena. Patient is hypertensive but non-diabetic. History of taking OCP for last 20 years.

Physical examination

Patient alert, conscious, cooperative

Temperature 101°F, Pulse 110/min, BP 142/90 mm Hg

Examination of abdomen:

Tenderness and guarding in the right hypochondrium, Murphy's sign positive

IPS: sluggish

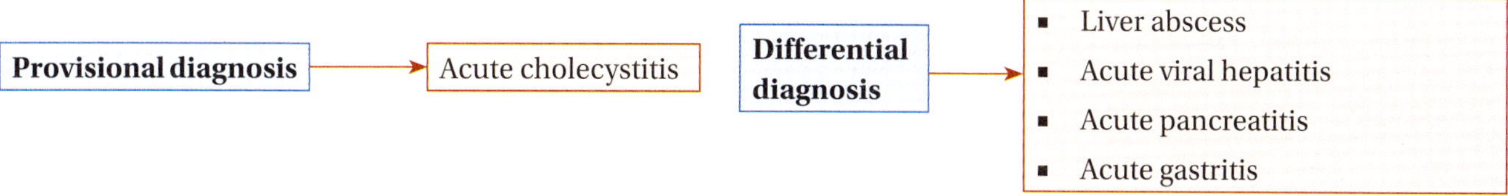

Investigations

Hb: 11.2 gm%; Total leukocyte count 17,000/cumm; Fasting sugar 82 mg/dL; Serum creatinine 0.9 mg/dL; Liver function test (LFT)—within normal limit.

USG abdomen: Multiple stones in gallbladder, thickened gallbladder wall, pericholecystic fluid present, sonographic Murphy's sign also presents, CBD not dilated, no intraluminal pathology.

Diagnosis

In history, middle-aged female patient suffering from acute onset right upper abdominal pain for last 2 days not responding to oral antibiotics and antispasmodics.

Physical examination: (i) Tenderness and guarding in the right hypochondrium; and (ii) Murphy's sign positive.

Both history and clinical findings were suggestive of acute cholecystitis. USG findings confirmed the provisional diagnosis. No need of other investigations for confirmation.

Management Algorithm

IV fluid, IV antibiotics (coverage against gram-negative aerobes and anaerobes), analgesics

Assessment of severity of acute cholecystitis (Grade I/II/III)

↓

Decision of early/delayed laparoscopic cholecystectomy or urgent biliary drainage depends on time interval between onset of symptoms and admission and severity of cholecystitis

↓

Early cholecystectomy

- Grade I (mild) cholecystitis and patient presents within 72–96 hours of the onset of symptoms.
- Grade II (moderate) cholecystitis, patient presents within 72–96 hours, patient's performance status is good, advanced technique and proper expertise is available.

Delayed cholecystectomy

- Grade I or II cholecystitis and patients present after 72–96 hours
- Grade II cholecystitis, patient presents within 72–96 hours but proper expertise and advanced technique are not available.

Urgent biliary drainage (Cholecystostomy or percutaneous transhepatic gallbladder drainage)

- Grade III cholecystitis in surgically high-risk patients
- Grade II cholecystitis with poor performance status

↓

Delayed cholecystectomy (after 6–10 weeks)

As this is a patient of grade I (mild) acute cholecystitis (as per Tokyo Guideline 2018), early laparoscopic cholecystectomy is the recommended treatment.

Case 2

History and Physical Examination

A 40-year-old female patient presented in the surgical outpatient department with history of recurrent attacks of pain in the right upper abdomen for last 6 months. The pain persisted for few hours, often associated with nausea. The pain often radiated to the right upper back. She also recalled that most of the times the pain was initiated after intake of fatty meals. No history of jaundice, hematemesis or melaena. Patient is normotensive and non-diabetic.

Physical examination

Patient alert, conscious, cooperative

Temperature 98.4°F, Pulse 82/min, BP 140/82 mm Hg

Examination of abdomen

No tenderness in right hypochondrium or epigastrium

No lump palpable in the right upper abdomen

Provisional diagnosis → Chronic calculous cholecystitis

Differential diagnosis →

- Peptic ulcer disease
- Amebic liver abscess
- Chronic hepatitis
- Gallbladder carcinoma

Investigations

Hb 13.0 gm%; Total leucocyte count 7,000/cumm; Fasting sugar 82 mg/dL; Serum creatinine 0.9 mg/dL; Liver function test (LFT)—within normal limit.

USG of upper abdomen: Multiple stones in gallbladder, contracted gallbladder, CBD not dilated, no intraluminal pathology.

Discussion

A middle-aged female patient suffering from recurrent attacks of right upper abdominal pain that was often initiated after taking fatty meals and radiation to the right upper back—suggestive of chronic calculous cystitis. Unremarkable clinical examination and normal laboratory values are also in favor of the diagnosis.

USG abdomen confirmed the diagnosis by revealing stones in contracted gallbladder. No need of other imaging.

Management Algorithm

- Preoperative work-up
- Hb%, TC, DC, ESR
- Blood sugar (Fasting and Postprandial)
- Serum urea, creatinine
- Liver function test
- Viral markers (HbsAg, HCV antibody, HIV I & II)
- Chest X-ray, ECG

→ Laparoscopic cholecystectomy

Case 3

History and Physical Examination

A 43-year-old female patient presented with yellowish discoloration of eyes and urine for last 1 month. Patient experienced recurrent attacks of right upper abdominal pain along with nausea and vomiting for last 3 months. She also complained of clay-colored stool and itching all over the body. No history of fever with chill and rigor. No history of hematemesis or melena. No history of blood transfusion. Patient is diabetic but normotensive.

Physical examination

Patient alert, conscious, cooperative

Jaundice—present

Temperature: 99°F, Pulse 68/min, BP: 130/80 mm Hg

Examination of abdomen—Mild tenderness in the right hypochondrium, no lump palpable.

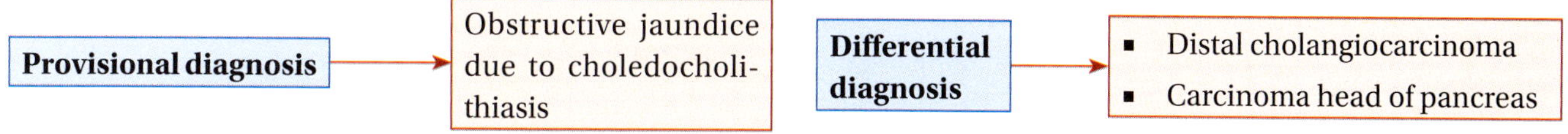

Provisional diagnosis → Obstructive jaundice due to choledocholithiasis

Differential diagnosis →
- Distal cholangiocarcinoma
- Carcinoma head of pancreas

Investigations

Hb: 11.5 gm%; Total leucocyte count: 7,000/cumm; Fasting sugar: 114 mg/dL; Serum creatinine: 0.9 mg/dL; Liver function test (LFT)—Total bilirubin 7.5 mg/dL (conjugated: 5.2 mg/dL; unconjugated: 2.3 mg/dL); alkaline phosphatase: 625 IU/L; INR: 1.5

USG abdomen: Multiple stones in gallbladder, contracted gallbladder, CBD: 8.5 mm, multiple stones in CBD.

Discussion

Patient presented with jaundice, clay-colored stool and itching, all suggestive of obstructive jaundice. As patient's recurrent right upper abdominal pain suggestive of biliary colic and no lump was not palpable in the right hypochondrium, the provisional diagnosis was in favor of obstructive jaundice due to common bile duct stone.

Laboratory investigations also confirmed the diagnosis of obstructive jaundice (conjugated hyperbilirubinemia and more than three times elevated level of alkaline phosphatase).

USG abdomen revealed the dilated CBD as well as etiology of biliary obstruction. No need of further investigations for treatment.

Management Algorithm

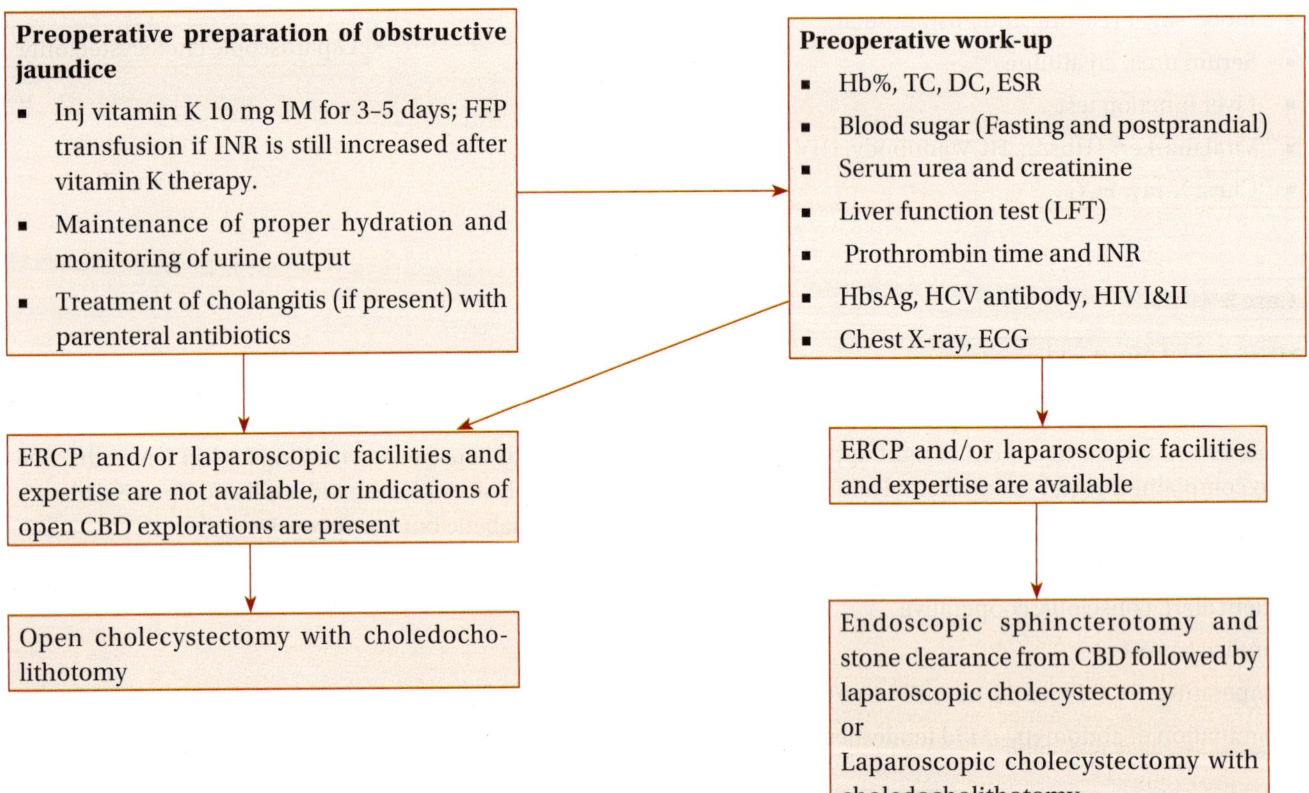

Case 4

History and Physical Examination

A 56-year-old female patient presented with vague right upper abdominal pain along with nausea and occasional vomiting for last 3 months. Patient was treated conservatively with oral medications by the local physician. For last 1 month, patient also complained of decreased appetite. No history of jaundice, hematemesis, melena. No history of blood transfusion. Patient is diabetic and hypertensive.

Physical Examination

Patient alert, conscious, cooperative

Pallor—present; Jaundice—not present

Temperature 99°F, Pulse 78/min, BP 130/80 mm Hg

Examination of abdomen—Mild tenderness in the right hypochondrium, no lump palpable

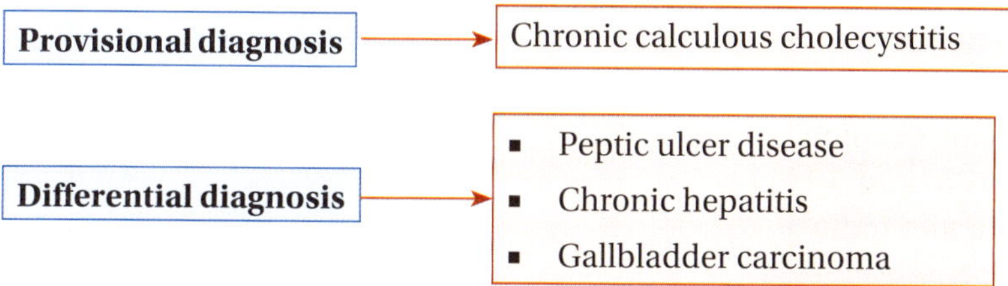

Investigations

Hb 11.5 gm%; Total leukocyte count 7,000/cumm; Fasting sugar 114 mg/dL; Serum creatinine 0.9 mg/dL; Liver function test (LFT): Total bilirubin 1.2 mg/dL; alkaline phosphatase 207 IU/L, AST and ALT—within normal limit

USG of abdomen: Irregular wall thickening of gallbladder with multiple stones, a polypoidal mass lesion in the fundus region, CBD 4.3 mm, no intraluminal pathology.

Contrast-enhanced CT abdomen: Focal mass within the gallbladder; No local infiltration into adjacent liver parenchyma (T2), multiple pericholedochal lymph nodes

CEA: 10 ng/mL; CA19-9: 55 units/mL.

Discussion

History and clinical findings in favor of chronic calculous cholecystitis, but USG findings suspicious of gallbladder carcinoma. CT abdomen findings are also suggestive of gallbladder carcinoma. Elevated CEA and CA19-9 level also suggestive of gallbladder cancer. MRCP was not required as jaundice was not present. As the staging, work-up suggests it as a potentially resectable tumor, CT-guided biopsy from the suspicious gallbladder lesion was not planned. Extended cholecystectomy was planned by open approach.

Management Algorithm

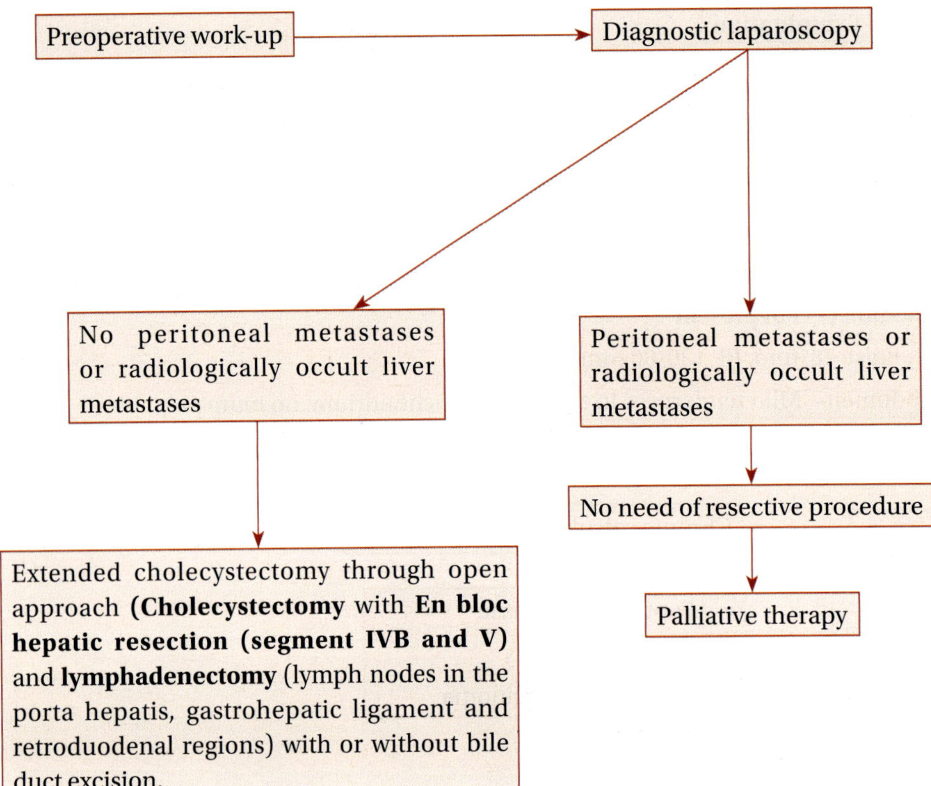

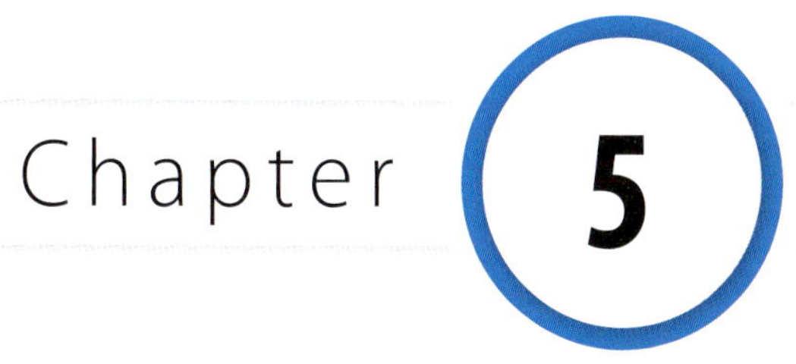

Diseases of the Liver

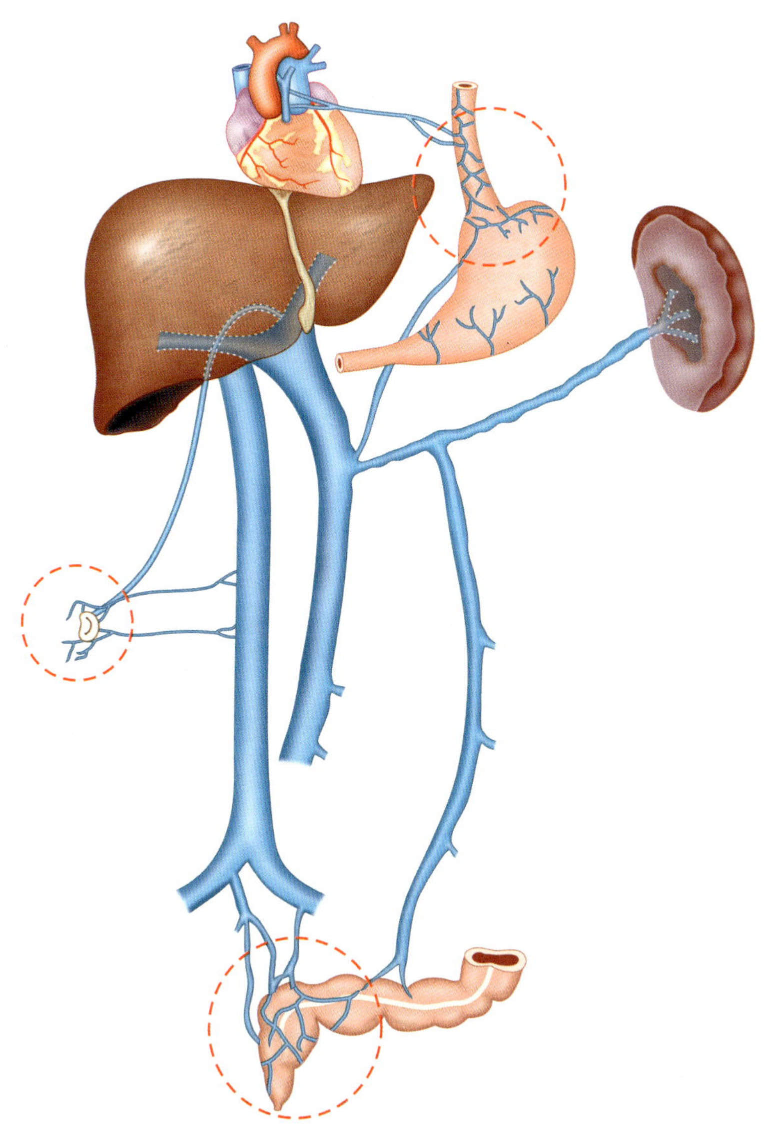

Important Topics

- Surgical Anatomy
- Pyogenic Liver Abscess
- Amebic Liver Abscess
- Hydatid Cyst
- Cystic Lesions of Liver
- Neoplasms of Liver
- Liver Transplantation
- Portal Hypertension
- Cirrhosis of Liver

'Medicine is a science of uncertainty and an art of probability.'

William Osler (1849 –1919)
Canadian Physician

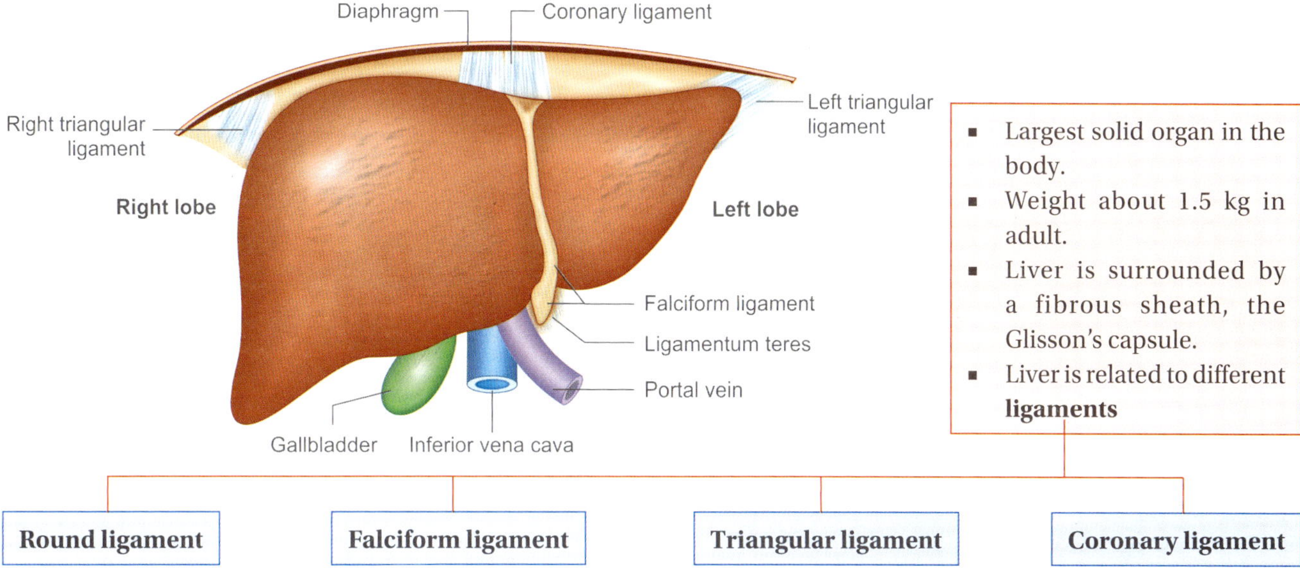

- Largest solid organ in the body.
- Weight about 1.5 kg in adult.
- Liver is surrounded by a fibrous sheath, the Glisson's capsule.
- Liver is related to different **ligaments**

Round ligament | **Falciform ligament** | **Triangular ligament** | **Coronary ligament**

Round ligament (ligamentum teres): A remnant of obliterated left umbilical vein. In portal hypertension, this vascular channel may open up to form collateral channel. This ligament is a guide to identify the segment III hepatic duct during hepaticojejunostomy.

Falciform ligament: Liver is attached in front with the anterior abdominal wall by falciform ligament. The ligamentum teres runs in the lower free border of the falciform ligament.

Triangular ligament: Right and left triangular ligaments anchor the two sides of the liver to the diaphragm.

Coronary ligament: Coronary ligament is formed by reflection of the peritoneum from the diaphragm to the posterior surfaces of the right lobe of liver. Right coronary ligament anchors the liver to the right retroperitoneum.

Couinaud System of Segmental Nomenclature

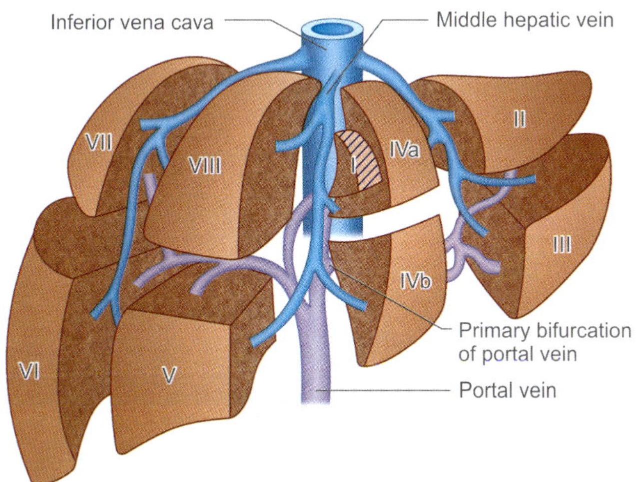

- The plane of the middle hepatic vein and the primary bifurcation of the portal vein divide the liver into right and left lobe.
- Right lobe (V, VI, VII, VIII)
- Left lobe (II, III, IV)
- Caudate lobe

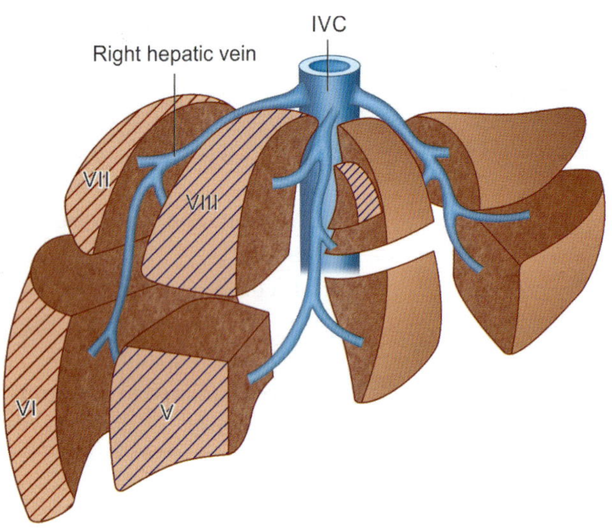

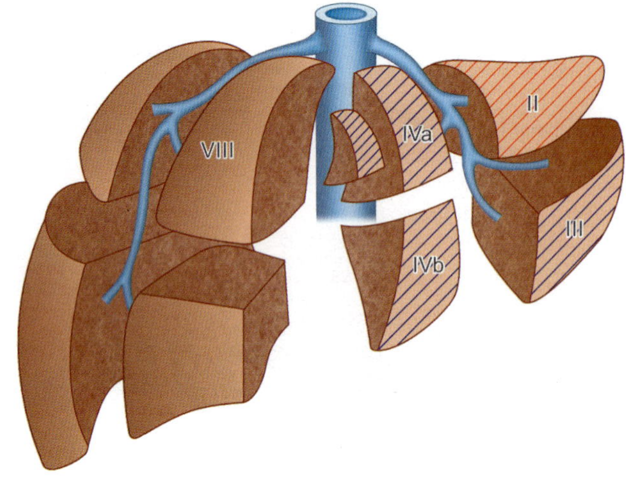

- Right lobe is divided into anterior and posterior sectors by the plane of right hepatic vein.
- Right anterior sector (V, VIII)
- Right posterior sector (VI, VII)

- Left lobe is divided into medial and lateral sectors by the plane of left hepatic vein.
- Left medial sector (IV)
- Left lateral sector (II, III)

Couinaud's 'sectors' are now termed as 'sections' in Brisbane Terminology of Liver Anatomy and Resections.

Segmental Anatomy of the Liver by CT Scan

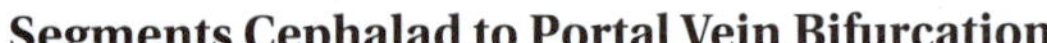

Segments Cephalad to Portal Vein Bifurcation

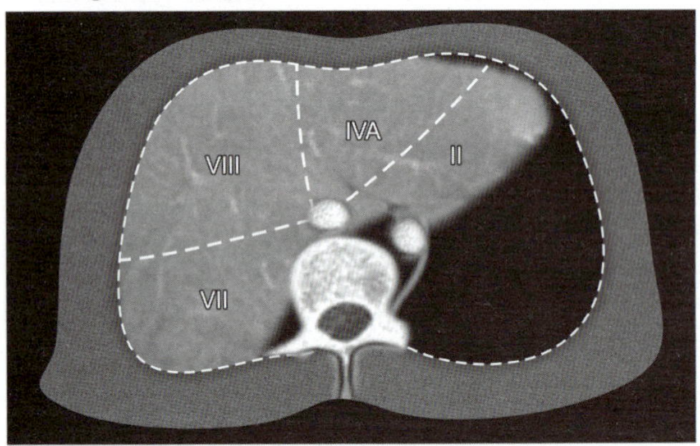

Segments Caudal to Portal Vein Bifurcation

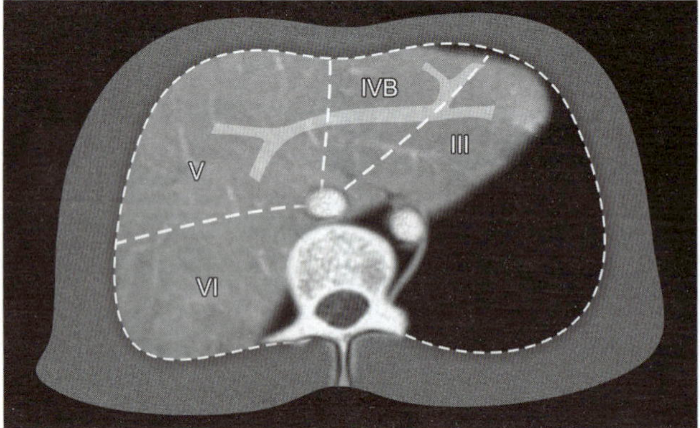

Cysts
- Congenital cyst
- Polycystic liver disease
- Bile duct cyst
- Hydatid cyst

Infective
- Pyogenic liver abscess
- Amebic liver abscess

Benign tumor
- Adenoma
- Focal nodular hyperplasia
- Hemangioma

Benign Pathology

Primary
- Hepatocellular carcinoma
- Hepatoblastoma
- Angiosarcoma

Secondary
- Metastases from colorectal cancers, neuroendocrine tumors, etc.

Malignant Pathology

Pyogenic Liver Abscess

Etiology and Pathophysiology

Biliary Route *Biliary etiologies:* (i) Malignant biliary obstruction; (ii) Intrahepatic stones; and (iii) Intervention in the biliary tract

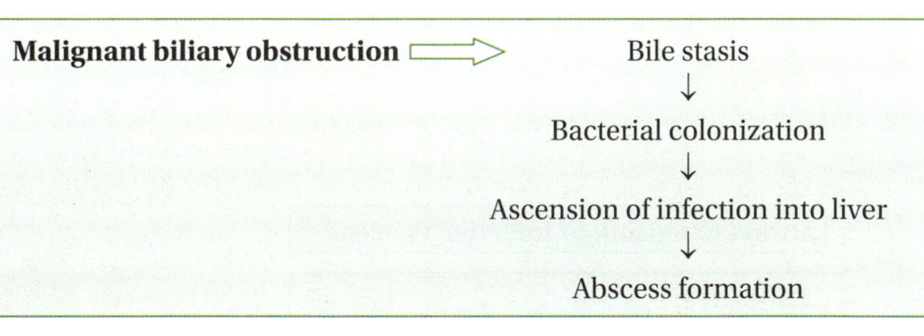

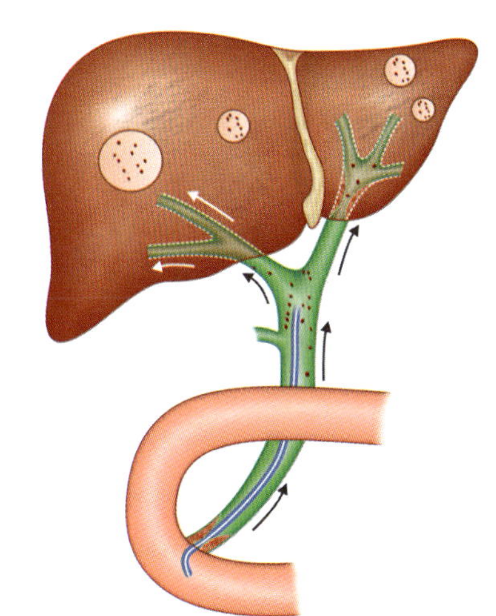

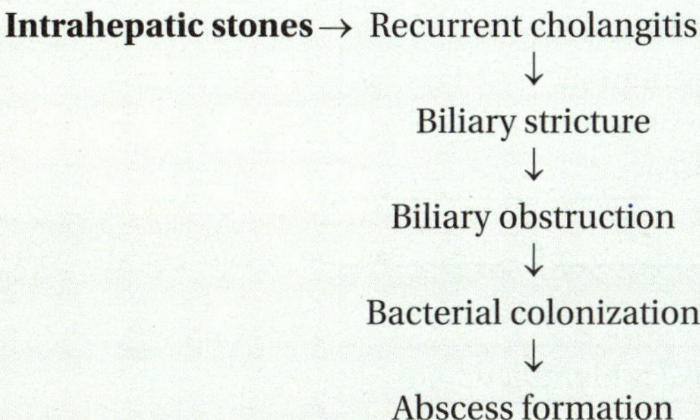

Intervention in the Biliary Tract
- Percutaneous transhepatic cholangiography
- Stenting
- Biliary-enteric anastomosis

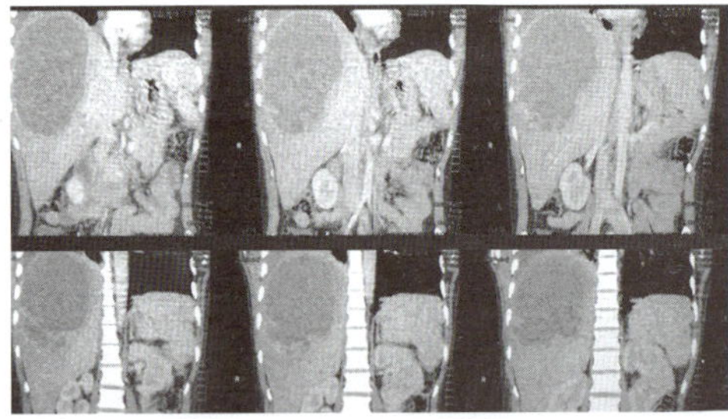

CECT abdomen showing large liver abscess in right lobe of liver with elevated right hemidiaphragm.

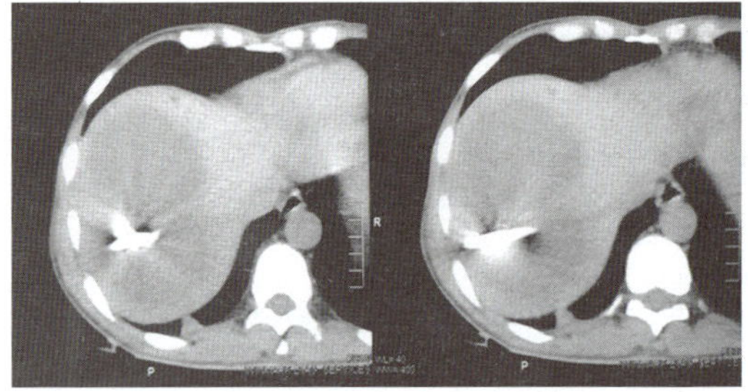

Pigtail catheter drainage of liver abscess.

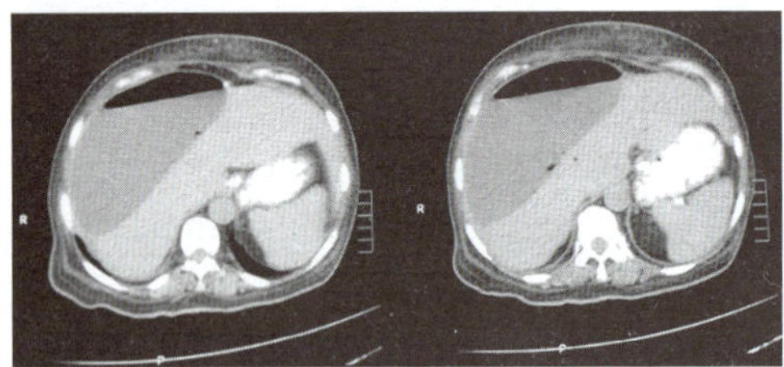

CT abdomen showing liver abscess.

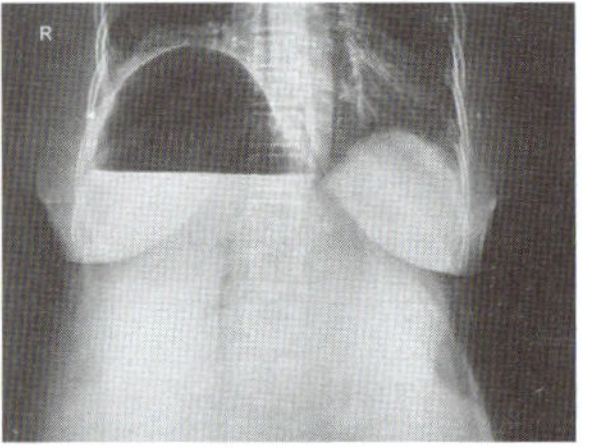

X-ray abdomen findings suggestive of liver abscess.

Portal Venous Route

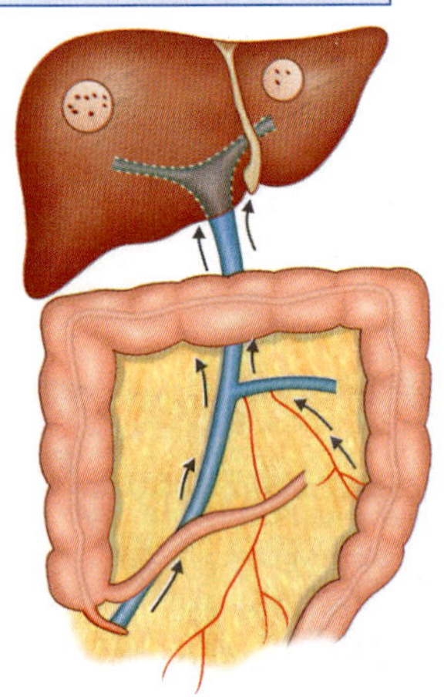

Etiologies

- Acute appendicitis
- Diverticulitis
- Perforated viscus
- Pelvic inflammatory disease
- Anorectal suppuration
- Colonic cancer
- Gastric cancer

Hepatic Artery Route

Etiologies:

- Osteomyelitis
- Endocarditis
- Pneumonia
- IV drug abuse

Traumatic

Etiologies:

- Blunt or penetrating liver trauma
- Following liver resection
- Percutaneous ethanol injection
- Radiofrequency ablation
- Transarterial chemoembolization

Direct Extension of Infective Process

Etiologies:

- Subphrenic abscess
- Empyema of gallbladder
- Gallbladder perforation
- Intestinal perforation
- Perinephric abscess

Cryptogenic

No underlying cause is identified.

Characteristic Features

- Mostly right lobe is involved **(due to preferential mesenteric and portal venous flow)**.
- Left lobe is next common **(associated mostly with intrahepatic stones)**.
- Multiple abscesses and bilateral lobe involvement are also common **(usually associated with biliary or hepatic arterial route).**
- Large, solitary abscess may present **(abscess formation via portal venous route or traumatic).**

Miliary type: Mostly associated with fungal infection and immunosuppressive state

↑

MICROABSCESS (abscess less than 2 cm in diameter)

↓

Cluster pattern: Commonly associated with coliform and enteric organisms

Clinical Features

Symptoms

- Fever with chill and rigor
- Pain abdomen
- Cough
- Respiratory distress

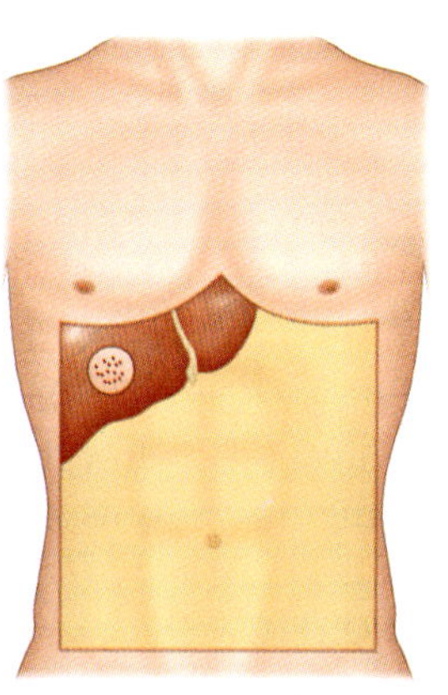

Signs

- Rise of temperature
- Intercostal tenderness
- Tenderness in right hypochondrium
- Hepatomegaly
- Jaundice
- Diminished breath sound on right side

***Klebsiella pneumoniae*-associated liver abscess** (distinct clinical presentation)

- **Polymicrobial** liver abscess
- **Monomicrobial** cryptogenic **noninvasive** liver abscess
- **Monomicrobial** cryptogenic **invasive** liver abscess

Monomicrobial cryptogenic invasive liver abscess

- Also called monomicrobial cryptogenic invasive *K.pneumoniae*-associated liver abscess (CIKPLA) syndrome.
- Diabetic patients are typically affected.
- Predominantly found in South-east Asia region.
- Characterized by distant septic seeding →
  - Endophthalmitis (most common septic lesion)
  - Lung abscess
  - Meningitis
  - Osteomyelitis
  - Septic arthritis
  - Septic epidural abscesses

Investigation

Laboratory Test

- Leukocytosis
- Increased level of alanine transferase
- Increased level of alkaline phosphatase, gamma-glutamyl transferase.

NOT DIAGNOSTIC

X-ray of Chest and Abdomen

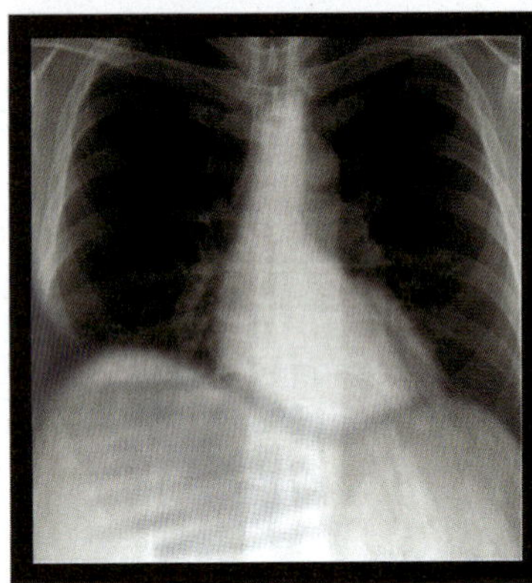

- Elevated right hemidiaphragm
- Atelectasis
- Right-sided pleural effusion
- Enlargement of liver shadow
- Air-fluid level just below the right hemidiaphragm (if gas-forming organisms are present)

NOT DIAGNOSTIC

USG of Abdomen

- Round or oval areas of hypoechoic lesion
- Smooth wall

DIAGNOSTIC IMAGING MODALITY

Most common predisposing conditions for PLA

- Can detect **pathology of biliary tract and gallbladder**
- Can guide for aspiration of pus from abscess.

Contrast-enhanced CT Abdomen

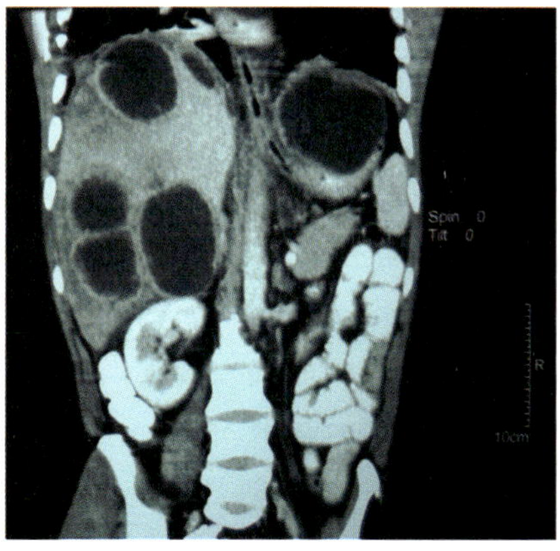

DIAGNOSTIC IMAGING MODALITY

- Target-like sign is characteristic in CT abdomen → Central hypodense region and peripheral contrast enhancement
- CT can detect other intra-abdominal pathologies (e.g., acute appendicitis, acute diverticulitis) → May be the predisposing conditions for PLA
- Can detect complications of pyogenic liver abscess →
  - Rupture of abscess into peritoneal cavity
  - Pleural effusion
  - Vascular complications
- Useful to guide percutaneous aspiration and drainage of abscess.

MR Cholangiopancreatography — Indicated if biliary origin is suspected after CT evaluation.

Treatment — **Initial management**

Broad-spectrum Parenteral Antibiotics **AND** **USG or CT-guided Aspiration of Pus**

Coverage against:

- Gram-negative bacilli
- Anaerobes
- Microaerophilic streptococci

Pus is to send for aerobic and anaerobic culture

Possible Isolated Microorganisms

Gram-negative aerobes:

- *Escherichia coli*
- *Klebsiella pneumoniae*
- *Pseudomonas aeruginosa*
- *Proteus* spp.

Gram-positive aerobes:

- *Streptococcus milleri*
- *Staphylococcus aureus*
- *Enterococcus* spp.

Gram-negative anaerobes:

- *Bacteroides* spp.
- *Fusobacterium* spp.

Selection of antibiotics according to sensitivity

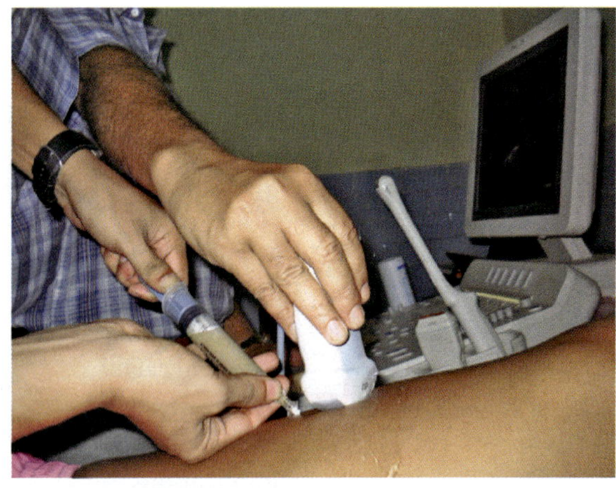

If patient is immunosuppressive, then culture for mycobacteria and fungus should be considered.

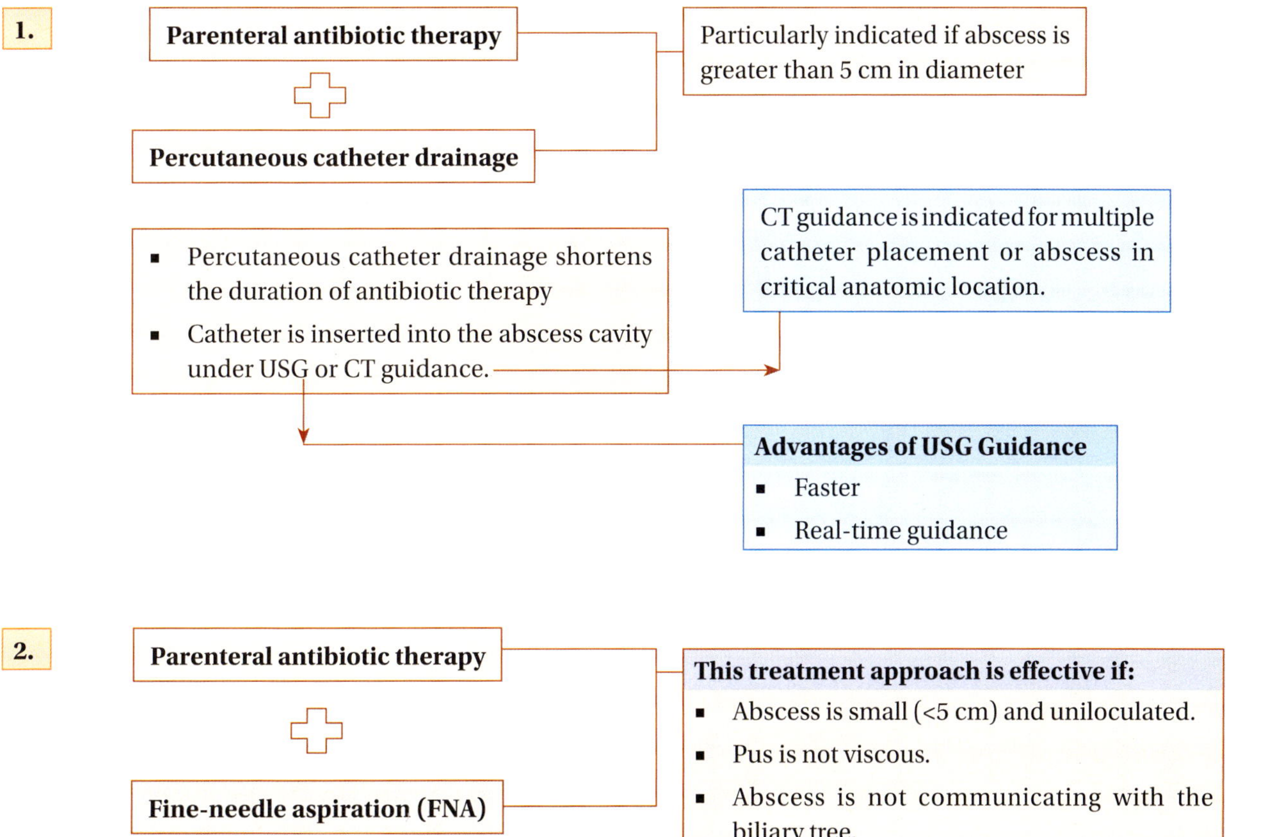

Antibiotic Therapy in Pyogenic Liver Abscess

- Initially, broad-spectrum parenteral antibiotic therapy should be initiated.
- Choice of antibiotics based on coverage against gram-negative bacilli, anaerobes.
- Changing of antibiotics according to culture-sensitivity report of aspirated pus.
- Oral antibiotic therapy can be started when patient becomes afebrile and WBC count become normal.
- Antibiotic therapy should be prolonged in pyogenic liver abscess.

3. Surgical Management

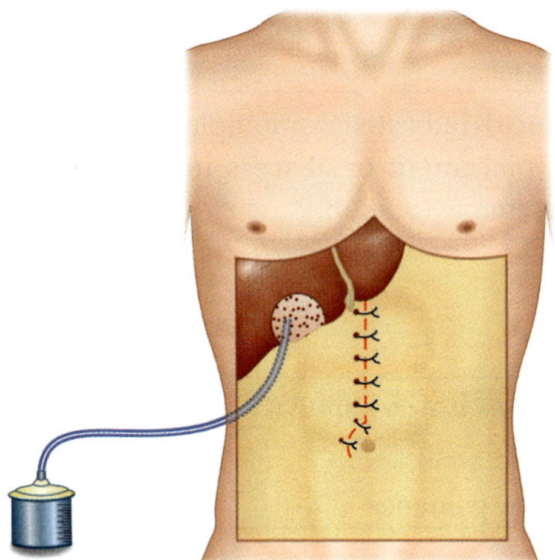

Indications of Surgical Drainage

- Not responding to percutaneous catheter drainage
- Intraperitoneal rupture of abscess
- Complications (e.g., bleeding) develop following catheter drainage.

If abscess is multiloculated with thick pus

Approaches for Surgical Drainage

- Open approach
- Laparoscopic approach

Indications of Liver Resection in Pyogenic Liver Abscess

- Rarely indicated
- Multiple abscesses resulting in destruction of surrounding liver parenchyma
- Abscesses associated with intrahepatic strictures or intrahepatic stones.

Amebic Liver Abscess

Pathophysiology

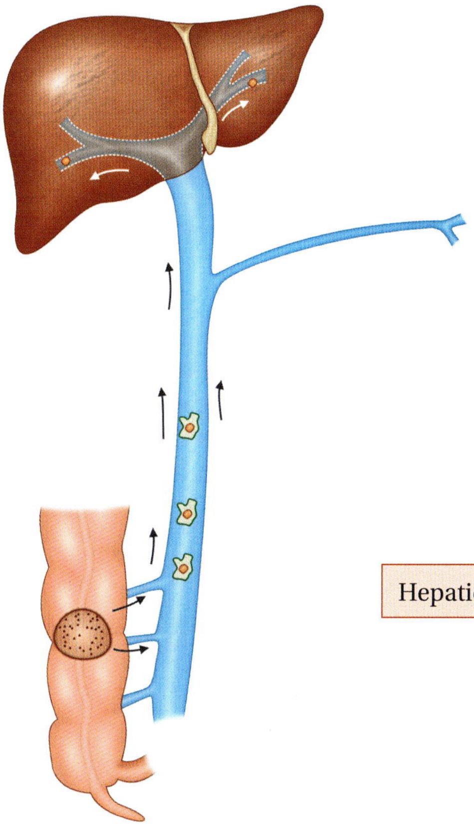

Most common extraintestinal form of invasive amebiasis

From the base of amebic ulcer in large intestine (mostly cecum and ascending colon)

- Cecum is the most common site of amebic colitis
- Right colon is drained by right portal branch
- Right lobe of liver is most commonly affected by amebic liver abscess

↓

Trophozoites of *E. histolytica* enter as emboli in the radicles of portal vein

↓

Trophozoites enter periportal sinusoids and lobules

↓

Multiplication in liver cells

↓ (two branches)

- Hepatic cytolysis
- Thrombosis of portal venules by ameba

↓

Focal necrosis of liver cells (Liquefaction necrosis)

About the Abscess

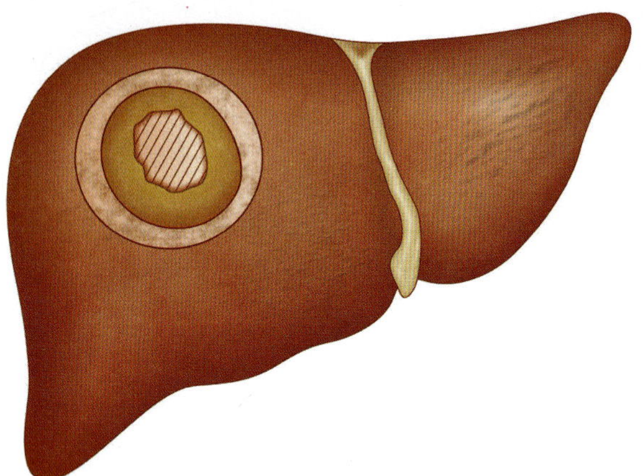

- Mostly solitary abscess.
- Commonly in the right lobe of liver.
- Left lobe abscesses are less common but more prone to rupture.
- Abscess cavity may be traversed by **vascular and biliary structures.**
- Abscess wall is ill-defined with minimal fibrosis.

These structures are covered by Glisson's capsule. This capsule is resistant of liquefaction necrosis.

About the Pus of Amebic Liver Abscess

- Contains liquefied liver tissue and blood
- Color varies from grayish yellow to chocolate-resembles anchovy sauce
- Sterile
- Free of amebae
- No odor

Clinical Features

More common in adult males

Rarely affected group but also increased risk group:

- Neonates
- Pregnant women
- Women in postpartum period

Symptoms

- Pain abdomen (dull, constant, localized in right upper quadrant)
- Anorexia
- Nausea and vomiting
- Fever with rigor
- Weight loss

Signs

- Tender, soft hepatomegaly
- Intercostal tenderness
- Jaundice
- Basal lung signs (in right side)

Differential Diagnosis

- Acute cholecystitis
- Acute viral hepatitis
- Pyogenic liver abscess

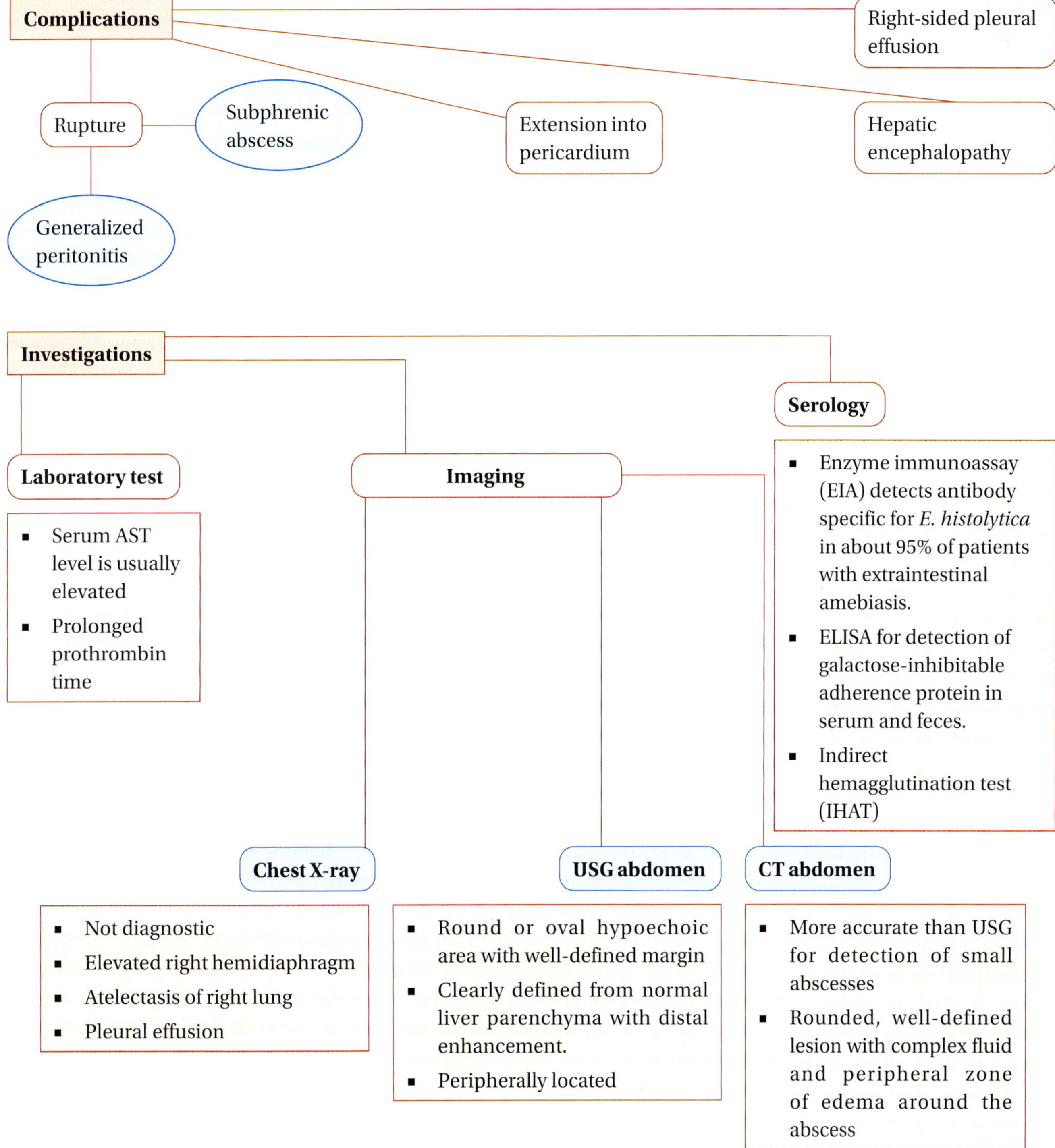
Complications
Right-sided pleural effusion
Rupture
Subphrenic abscess
Extension into pericardium
Hepatic encephalopathy
Generalized peritonitis
Investigations
Serology
Enzyme immunoassay (EIA) detects antibody specific for E. histolytica in about 95% of patients with extraintestinal amebiasis.
ELISA for detection of galactose-inhibitable adherence protein in serum and feces.
Indirect hemagglutination test (IHAT)
Laboratory test
Serum AST level is usually elevated
Prolonged prothrombin time
Imaging
Chest X-ray
Not diagnostic
Elevated right hemidiaphragm
Atelectasis of right lung
Pleural effusion
USG abdomen
Round or oval hypoechoic area with well-defined margin
Clearly defined from normal liver parenchyma with distal enhancement.
Peripherally located
CT abdomen
More accurate than USG for detection of small abscesses
Rounded, well-defined lesion with complex fluid and peripheral zone of edema around the abscess

Management

Chemotherapy

- Metronidazole is the drug of choice.
- Metronidazole achieves high concentration in the intestine and liver.
- Can cross placenta and blood-brain barrier.
- Contraindicated during first trimester of pregnancy and during breastfeeding.
- Oral dose—*in adults:* 500–750 mg three times daily for 7–10 days; *in children:* 35–50 mg/kg in three divided doses for 10 days.
- IV dose is 500 mg every 6 hours.
- Improvement in symptoms within 72–96 hours of administration
- Tinidazole, ornidazole, secnidazole are also effective

Not responding in 48–72 hours

Metronidazole + Emetine or dehydroemetine

- Intramuscular or deep subcutaneous injection
- *Dose:* 1 mg/kg/day for 10 days
- *Side effects:* Myositis, hypotension, tachycardia, T-wave inversion, prolonged Q-T interval
- Contraindicated in renal, cardiac and muscular diseases.

Percutaneous Aspiration and Catheter Drainage

- Indicated if no improvement of symptoms after 7 days of chemotherapy.
- Abscess is more than 10 cm in diameter.
- Left lobe abscess
- Impending rupture of a large abscess
- If differential diagnosis is pyogenic liver abscess and investigations are not in favor of amebic liver abscess.

Surgical Intervention

- Rupture of abscess into the peritoneal cavity
- Suspected fistulization (hepatogastric, hepatoduodenal, hepatocolonic fistula)

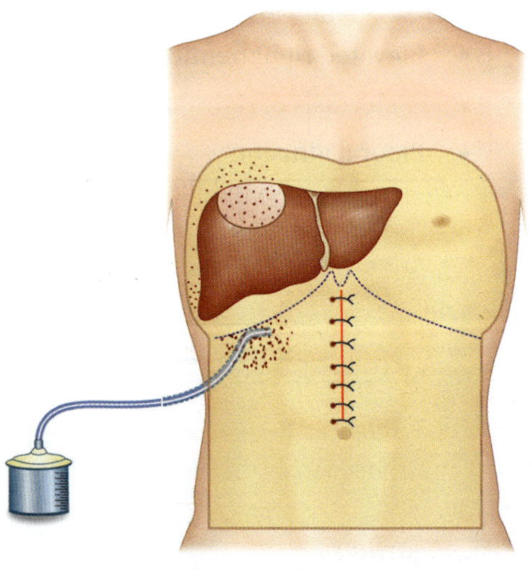

Hydatid Cyst

Ingestion of embryonated egg (contact with dog/ingestion of contaminated water or vegetable)

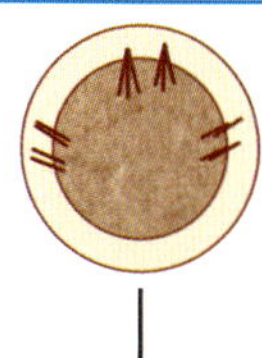

The protective chitinous layer is lost in duodenum

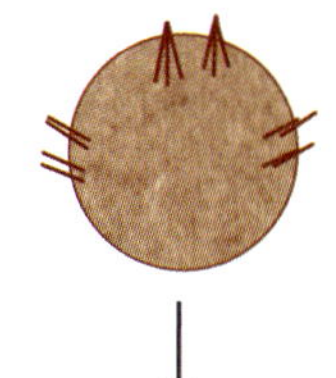

Hexacanth embryo (oncosphere) passes through the intestinal wall

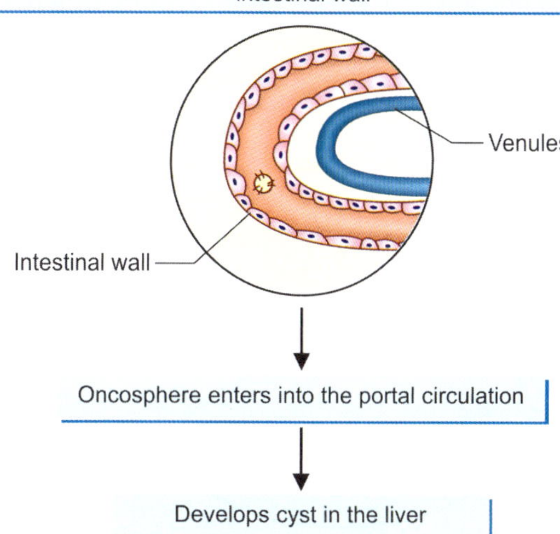

Oncosphere enters into the portal circulation

Develops cyst in the liver

Human echinococcosis or hydatid disease is a zoonosis caused by **larval forms (metacestodes)** of *Echinococcus tapeworms* found in small intestine of carnivores. Among different species of *Echinococcus*, two are of clinical importance—***E. granulosus*** and ***E. multilocularis***.

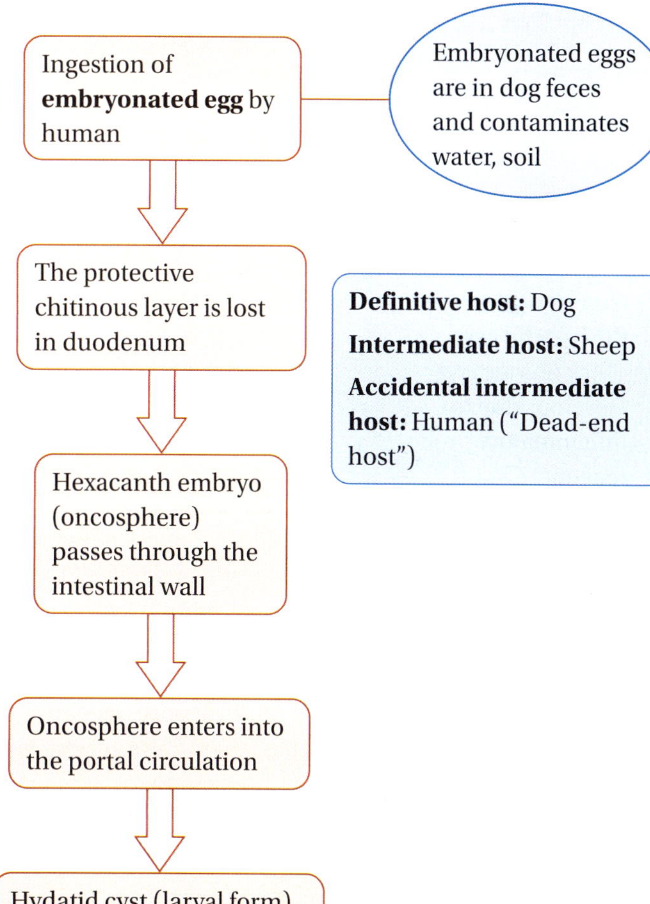

Definitive host: Dog

Intermediate host: Sheep

Accidental intermediate host: Human ("Dead-end host")

Persons at increased risk of hydatid cyst:

- Close contact with pet dog
- Veterinary workers
- Shepards
- Butchers

Species of *Echinococcus*

- *E. granulosus* → **Cystic echinococcosis**
- *E. multilocularis* → Alveolar echinococcosis
- *E. vogeli* → Polycystic hydatid disease (rare)
- *E. oligarthus* → Polycystic hydatid disease (rare)

- Hydatid cyst can develop in almost any organ—liver, lung, brain, bone, spleen, kidney, skeletal muscle.
- **Liver is the most commonly involved organ.**
- Up to 80% patients have single organ involvement.

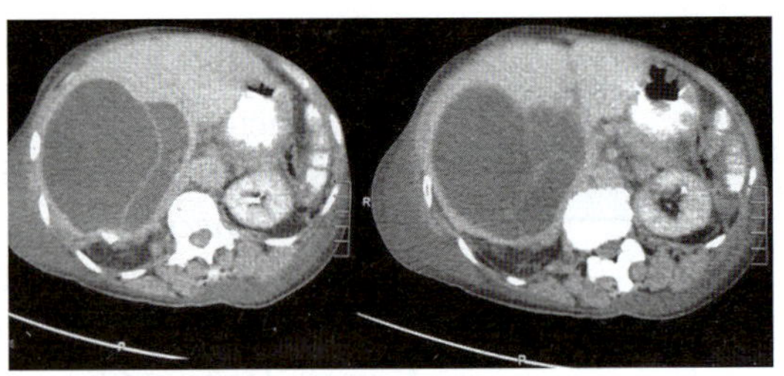

CT abdomen showing hydatid cyst of liver.

About the Cyst

Pericyst

Ectocyst (laminated membrane)

Endocyst (germinal membrane)

Daughter cyst

Brood capsule

Scolex

Hydatid sand

Ectocyst (Pericyst)

- Outermost layer of the hydatid cyst
- Thick fibrous layer
- Develops due to inflammatory reaction
- Develops from host tissue
- Acts as a mechanical support of the cyst
- No anatomical plane exists between the ectocyst and host parenchyma

- Ectocyst is present in hydatid cyst of liver and spleen.
- Ectocyst is absent in hydatid cyst of lungs and brain.

Laminated Membrane

- The layer between the pericyst and germinal layer.
- Acellular layer of the cyst.
- Protects the cyst from host enzymes, bacteria.

Germinative Membrane (Germinal Layer)

- Germinative membrane is the living component of the parasite.
- Responsible for formation of protoscolices, brood capsules, cyst fluid, **daughter cysts**.

Endogenous daughter cyst

Develops by endogenic vesiculation

Exogenous daughter cyst ("Satellite hydatid cyst")

Develops when ectogenic vesiculation develops through a defect in the laminated membrane.

About the Cyst Fluid

- Clear, colorless, odorless, sterile fluid
- Secreted by the germinal membrane
- Fluid is antigenic.
- Bile-stained cyst fluid indicates cystobiliary communication.

Both mother and daughter cysts have similar structure (laminated membrane, germinative membrane, cyst fluid, brood capsules, protoscolices) except adventitial layer (ectocyst), which is absent in daughter cyst.

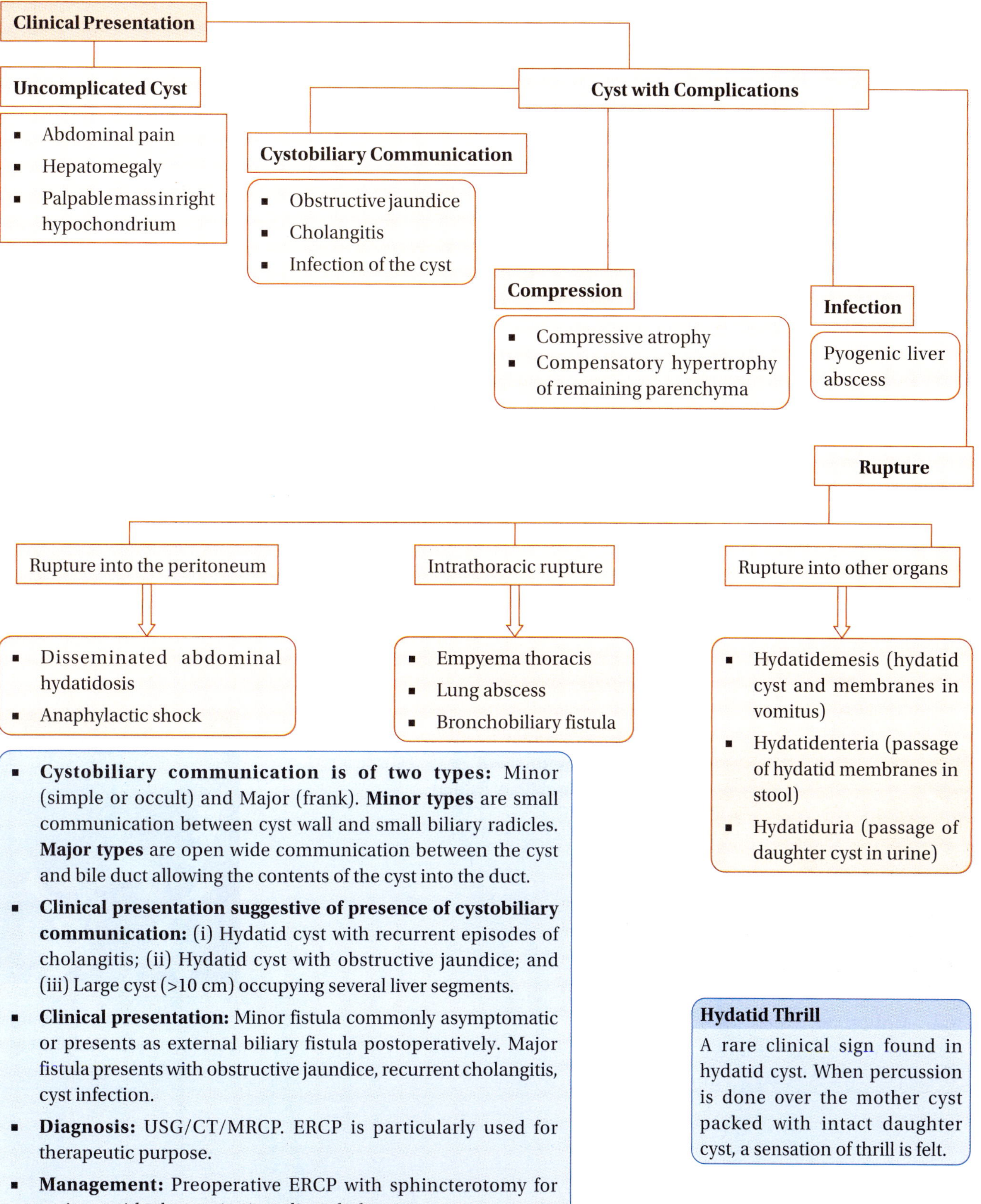

- **Cystobiliary communication is of two types:** Minor (simple or occult) and Major (frank). **Minor types** are small communication between cyst wall and small biliary radicles. **Major types** are open wide communication between the cyst and bile duct allowing the contents of the cyst into the duct.
- **Clinical presentation suggestive of presence of cystobiliary communication:** (i) Hydatid cyst with recurrent episodes of cholangitis; (ii) Hydatid cyst with obstructive jaundice; and (iii) Large cyst (>10 cm) occupying several liver segments.
- **Clinical presentation:** Minor fistula commonly asymptomatic or presents as external biliary fistula postoperatively. Major fistula presents with obstructive jaundice, recurrent cholangitis, cyst infection.
- **Diagnosis:** USG/CT/MRCP. ERCP is particularly used for therapeutic purpose.
- **Management:** Preoperative ERCP with sphincterotomy for patients with obstructive jaundice, cholangitis.

Hydatid Thrill

A rare clinical sign found in hydatid cyst. When percussion is done over the mother cyst packed with intact daughter cyst, a sensation of thrill is felt.

Investigation

Serology

- **IgG-ELISA** — **Most useful immunodiagnostic test for human cystic echinococcosis**
- Indirect hemagglutination antibody test (IHAT)
- Latex agglutination test (LAT)

- False-negative result in cysts of brain, eye, calcified cyst, in young children.
- False-positive result in patients with other helminthic diseases.

Imaging

USG

- Basis of cystic echinococcosis diagnosis in abdominal organs.
- Can evaluate number of cysts, its stage (active, degenerating, inactive).
- Can detect cyst-related complications.

CT scan

- CT scan accurately reveals information about location of cyst(s) in relation to liver segments.
- CT scan can detect exogenous daughter cysts.
- Also indicated when suspicion of disseminated disease, abscess, cystobiliary fistula.

MR and MRCP

Indicated in:

- Subdiaphragmatic location
- Disseminated disease
- Complicated cysts (abscess, cystobiliary fistula)

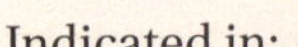

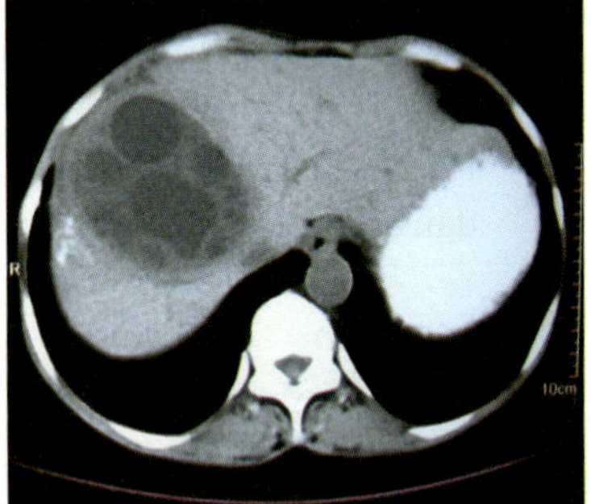

CT abdomen showing hydatid cyst with multiple daughter cysts in liver.

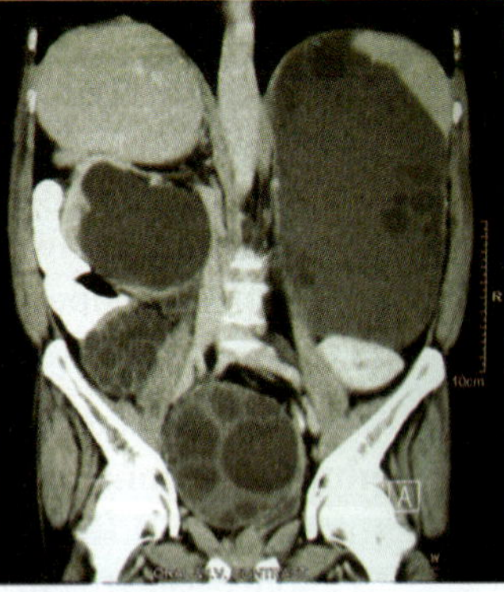

CT abdomen showing hydatid cysts in different abdominal organs.

WHO-IWGE Classification (Ultrasound Classification)

Type CL

- Unilocular, simple cyst with uniform anechoic content.
- Cyst may show fine echoes due to shifting of brood capsules which is often called hydatid sand (**'snowflake sign'**)
- Cyst wall is visible

Status—Active

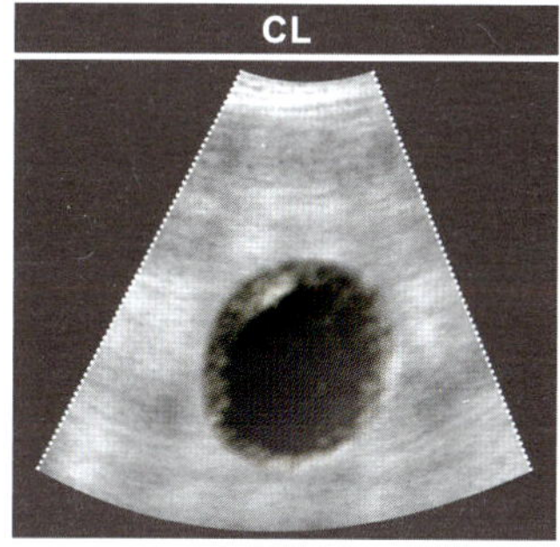

Type CE4

- Heterogeneous hypoechoic or hyperechoic degenerative contents.
- No daughter cysts.
- **'ball of wool' sign**—indicative of degenerating membranes.
- **Status—Inactive**

Type CE1

- Uniform anechoic content in unilocular cystic lesion(s)
- Normally round, may be oval
- No cyst wall
- **Status—Active**

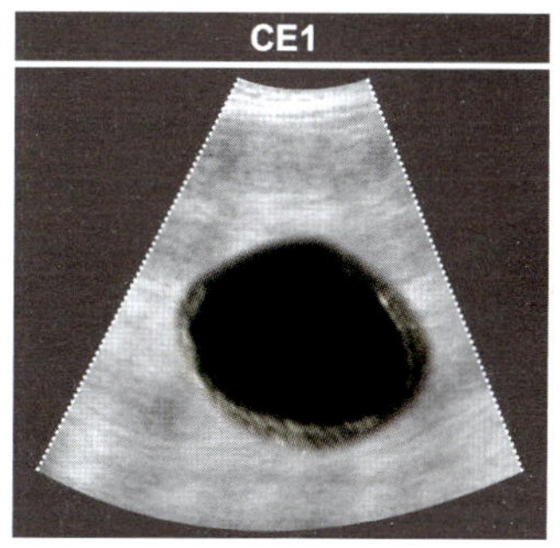

Type CE5

- Cysts characterized by thick calcified wall
- Degree of calcification varies from partial to complete.
- **Status—Inactive**

Type CE2

- Mulivesicular, multiseptated cysts, cyst septations produce 'wheel-like' structures, daughter cysts is indicated by 'honey-comb' like structures.
- Cyst wall visible.
- **Status—Active**

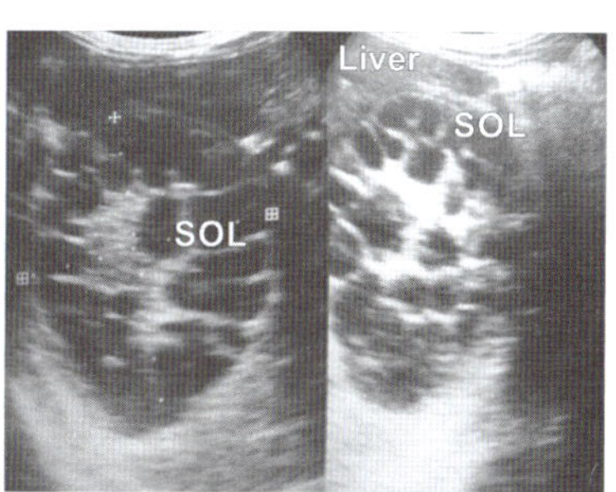

Active cyst—CL, CE1, CE2

Transitional—CE3a and CE3b

Inactive cyst—CE4 (Degenerative cyst) and CE5 (Partial or totally calcified cyst).

Type CE3

- Unilocular cyst, may contain daughter cysts.
- Anechoic content with detachment of laminated membrane from the cyst wall visible as floating membrane—**'water-lily sign'**.
- **Status—Transitional**

CE3 can be differentiated into CE3a (with detached endocyst) and CE3b (predominantly solid with daughter vesicles).

Gharbi Classification (1981)

Type I—Pure fluid collection

Type II—Fluid collection with a split wall

Type III—Fluid collection with septa

Type IV—Heterogeneous appearance

Type V—Reflecting thick walls

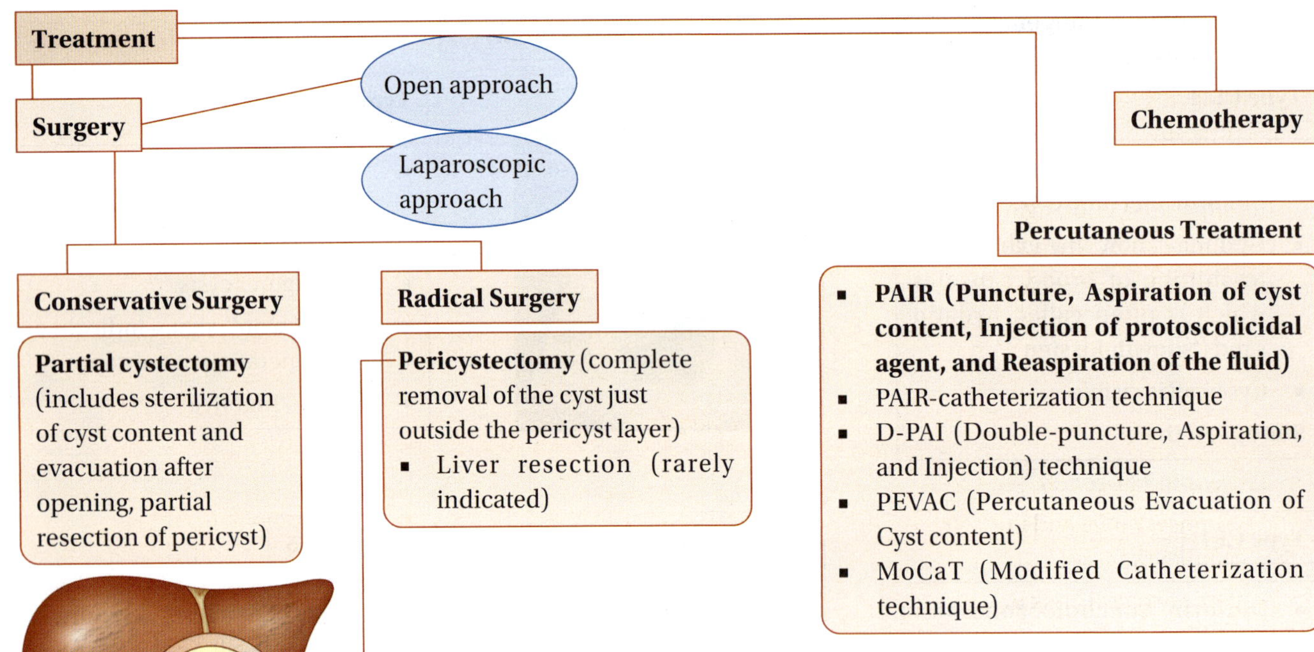

Closed Total Pericystectomy

Complete removal of the cyst without opening it

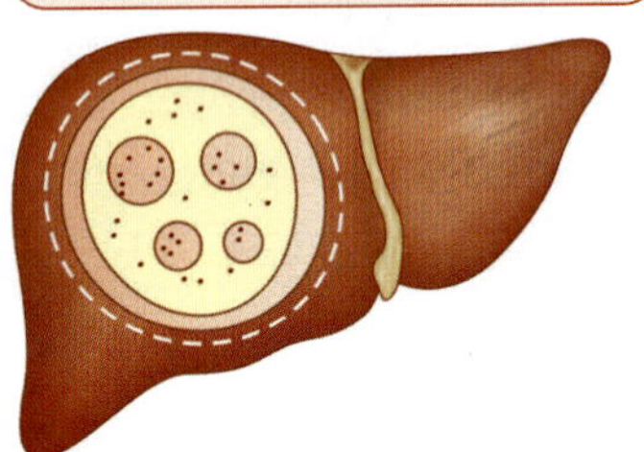

Open Total Pericystectomy

Includes sterilization of metacestode with protoscolicidal agents, evacuation of cyst content and then removal of pericystic tissue

Protoscolicidal agents	Minimum contact time
20% hypertonic saline	15 minutes
10% povidone-iodine solute	10 minutes
0.5% cetrimide solution	05 minutes
3% hydrogen peroxide	15 minutes

Indications of Surgery

- Complicated hydatid cyst (infection, cystobiliary communication)
- Large CE2, CE3b cysts with multiple daughter vesicles
- Single cyst, situated superficially, with increased chance of rupture.
- Cysts exerting pressure on adjacent vital organs.

Contraindications of Surgery

- Inactive, asymptomatic cyst
- Cyst difficult to access
- Very small cysts or multiple cysts
- Patient not fit for surgery.

Basic Operative Principles of Partial Cystectomy

- Generous incision (either right subcostal with proximal midline extension or bilateral subcostal incision)[Midline incision—for cyst in left lobe or abdominal hydatidosis].
- **Prevention of intraoperative spillage** of cyst content.
- **Protection of peritoneal tissues and organs** with protoscolicide-soaked surgical drapes.
- **Injection of protoscolicide into the cyst** before opening it (if aspirated cyst fluid is not bile-stained).
- Removal of laminated membrane and daughter cysts after opening the cyst.
- Detection of any **cystobiliary communication** and its management, if present.
- Management of **residual cavity**.

Intraoperative Management of Cystobiliary Communication

- Leaving a white gauze on the inner surface of the cyst for few minutes, with gentle pressure on the gallbladder.
- Intraoperative cholangiography—in suspected cystobiliary communication.
- In small fistula—simple suturing is effective.
- For larger one- Roux-en-Y hepaticojejunostomy is better option.

Management of Residual Cavity

- **Omentoplasty (best option)—**mobilization of the greater omentum to pack the cyst cavity.
- Capitonnage (no longer used)—infolding the redundant cyst wall into the depth of the cyst with successive layers of sutures.

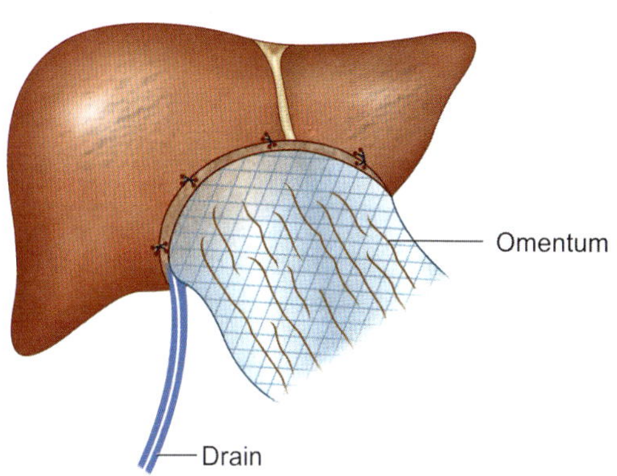

Laparoscopic Approach

- Both conservative and radical surgery is safe in selected patients.
- Major drawback is risk of spillage.
- Specialized devices have been used for safe insertion of cyst, effective evacuation of cyst contents.

Complications of Conservative Surgery

- Liver abscess
- Biliary fistula
- Biliary stricture
- Recurrence

Causes of Recurrence Following Conservative Surgery

- Local recurrence
- Secondary hydatidosis due to intraoperative rupture
- Cysts in other organs not detected during imaging or peroperative period
- Reinfestation

Surgical Options for Cystic Echinococcosis of Lung

- Lobectomy
- Pericystectomy
- Extrusion of cyst (Barrett's technique)

PAIR (Puncture, Aspiration, Injection, Re-aspiration)

Indications
- Inoperable patients
- Patient refuses surgery
- Relapse after surgery
- CE1> 5 cm, CE3a >5 cm

Contraindications
- CE2, CE3b, CE4, CE5
- Presence of cystobiliary communication
- Inaccessible location
- Superficial location.

Techniques of PAIR
- Albendazole (15 mg/kg daily in two divided doses) atleast 4 days before and 4 weeks after PAIR.
- Percutaneous transhepatic cyst puncture (transhepatic cyst puncture prevents peritoneal spillage) under USG/CT guidance.

↓

- 30–50% of the cyst volume is aspirated

↓

- To detect cystobiliary communication, either aspirated fluid is sent for analyzing presence of bilirubin or injection of contrast medium into cyst cavity

↓

- If no cystobiliary communication

↓

- Injection of protoscolicidal agent (20% NaCl or 95% Ethanol)

↓

- Reaspiration after 15–20 minutes (as much fluid as possible)

Risks
- Anaphylactic shock or other hypersensitivity reactions
- Secondary hydatidosis (due to spillage)
- Sclerosing cholangitis (if presence of cystobiliary communication)
- Biliary fistula may develop (due to sudden intracystic decompression)
- Persistence of satellite daughter cyst.

Benefits
- Cost-effective in comparison to surgery or chemotherapy alone
- Minimally invasive procedure
- Removal of large number of protoscolices with the aspirated fluid.

Modified PAIR techniques are indicated for large volume cysts, cyst with multiple daughter cysts

PAIR Catheterization

A catheter is placed in the cyst cavity

↓

Aspiration of cyst content

↓

Injection of protoscolicidal agent

↓

Reaspiration

↓

Catheter is left for 24 hours

↓

95% alcohol is injected (if drain amount is less than 10 mL and no bile)

↓

Fluid reaspirated

↓

Catheter is withdrawn

If drain amount is more than 10 mL or presence of bile, catheter is placed until drain amount is less than 10 mL.

PEVAC (Percutaneous Evacuation of Cyst Content)

Catheter is placed in the cyst cavity

↓

Aspiration of cyst content

↓

Catheter is replaced by 14–18 Fr sheath

↓

Suction catheter and special cutting instrument are introduced through the sheath for evacuation and fragmentation of contents of cyst along with irrigation of protoscolicidal agent

↓

Sheath is removed and catheter is placed (if no bile or minimal drain)

↓

Catheter is removed

Chemotherapy — Mebendazole or Albendazole — **Albendazole is the drug of choice**

Indications

- Inoperable patients with liver or lung CE
- Multiple cysts in two or more organs
- CE1 and CE3a cysts in liver and lung
- Prevention and management of secondary hydatidosis
- Prevention of recurrence following surgery or PAIR.

Contraindications

- Cysts at risk of rupture
- In early pregnancy
- Severe chronic liver disease
- Bone marrow depression.

Principles of Chemotherapy

- Albendazole 10–15 mg/kg/day, in two divided doses, with fat-rich meal, for 3–6 months continuous treatment.
- No need of monthly treatment interruption.
- Leukocyte count should be measured at 2-week intervals during the first 3 months (leukopenia may develop in early phases of chemotherapy).
- Peri-interventional prophylaxis (PAIR procedure) with albendazole 4 days before the procedure and atleast 4 weeks thereafter.
- Perioperative prophylaxis with albendazole 1 week before the procedure and post-treatment prophylaxis for 3–8 weeks.

Watch and Wait Approach — In uncomplicated CE4 and C5 cyst

CL cyst should not be treated, until its parasitic status is not confirmed.

Simple Cyst of the Liver

Aberrant bile duct lost communication with biliary tree

Formation of simple cyst

Progressive dilation

Pathophysiology

Aberrant bile duct lost communication with the biliary tree
↓
Progressive dilation
↓
Formation of simple cyst

Features of a Simple Cyst

- Unilocular cyst
- Contains serous fluid
- No communication with the intrahepatic biliary tree
- Size ranges from few mm to more than 20 cm
- In about 50% cases, solitary cyst
- Female to male ratio is 9:1 in symptomatic or complicated cysts

Clinical Features

- Most of the patients are asymptomatic.
- Abdominal pain
- Early satiety
- Palpable abdominal mass

Complications

- Rapid growth
- Intracystic hemorrhage
- Spontaneous rupture into the peritoneal cavity

Large cyst in female patient of 50 years or more—think of simple cyst of liver.

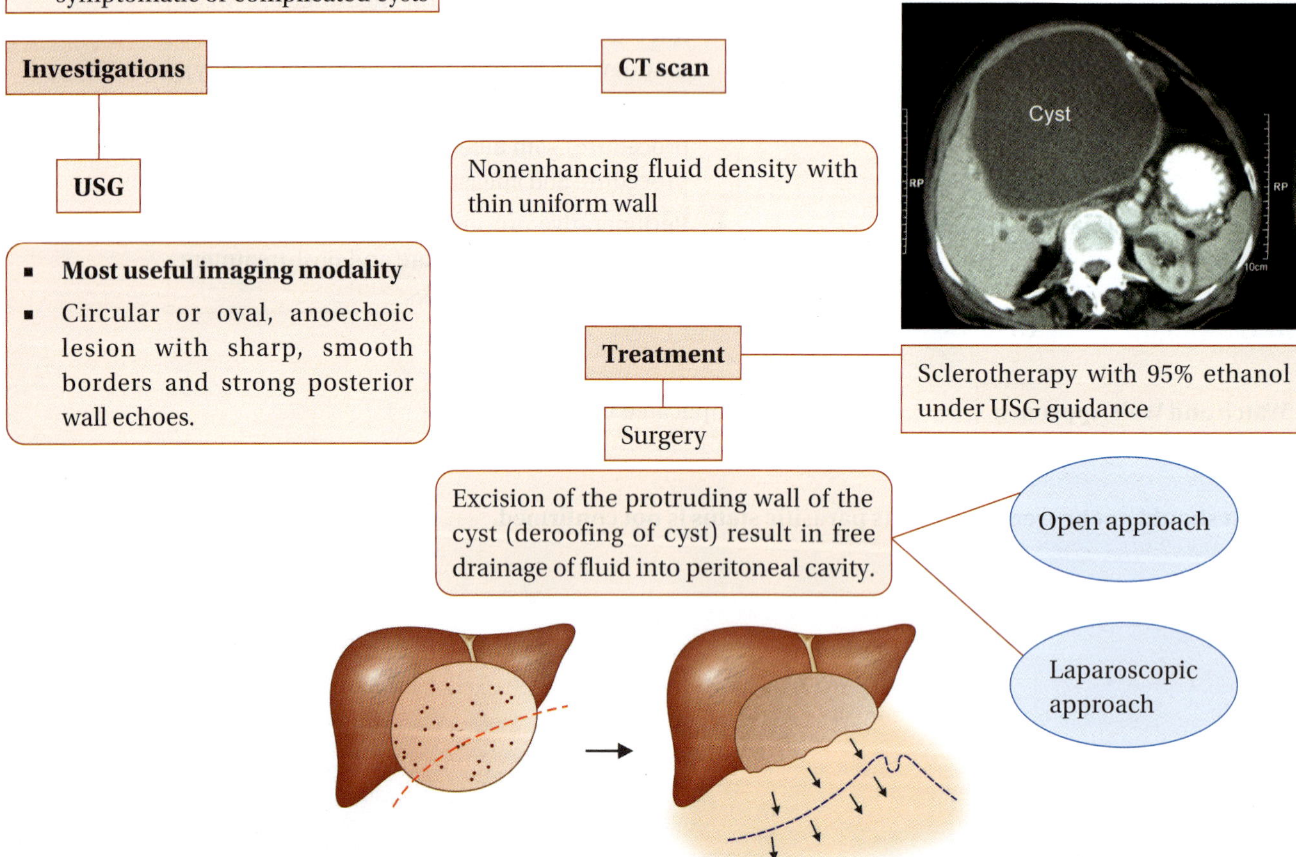

Polycystic Liver Disease

Polycystic liver disease (PCLD) associated with autosomal dominant polycystic kidney disease (ADPKD)

- Autosomal dominant transmission
- Mutations in either *PKD1* or *PKD2* gene

Isolated PCLD (without ADPKD)

- Autosomal dominant transmission
- Mutations in *PRKCSH* or *SEC63* or *LRP5* genes.

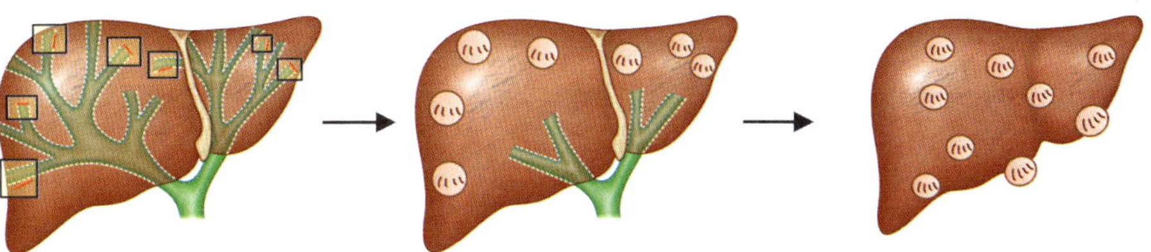

Pathophysiology

Von Meyenburg complexes (biliary microhamartoma)
⇩
Lost communication with biliary tree
⇩
Cystic dilation of hamartoma
⇩
Cyst formation

Features of Liver Cysts

- Cysts are unilocular
- Contain serous fluid
- Lined by single-layered epithelium
- Not communicate with intrahepatic biliary tree
- Hepatic parenchymal volume is preserved.

Clinical Features

- Most of the patients are asymptomatic
- Abdominal pain or discomfort
- Early satiety
- Palpable liver

Complications

- Intracystic hemorrhage
- Cholestasis due to compression
- Infection.

Investigation

- **CT scan**
- **USG**: Multiple round or oval hypoechoic lesion with sharp margin

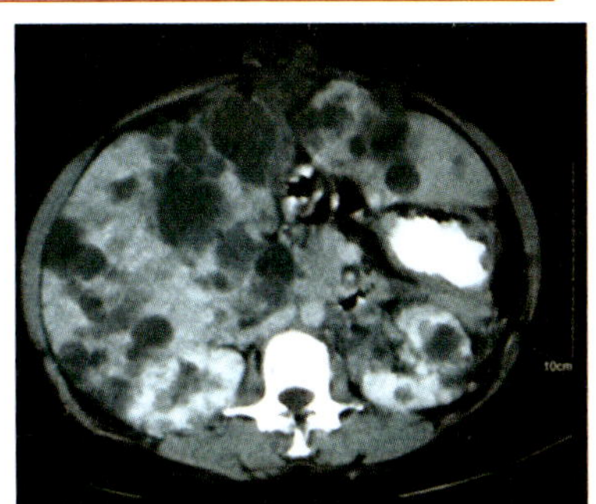

CECT abdomen showing multiple cyst in liver and kidneys.

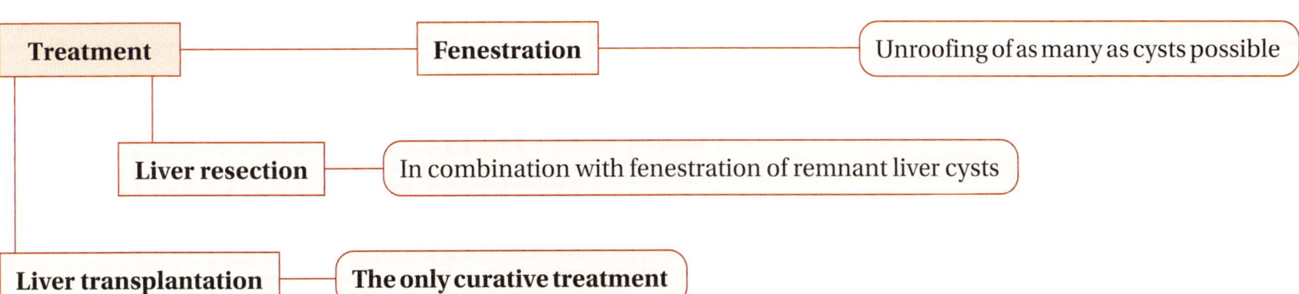

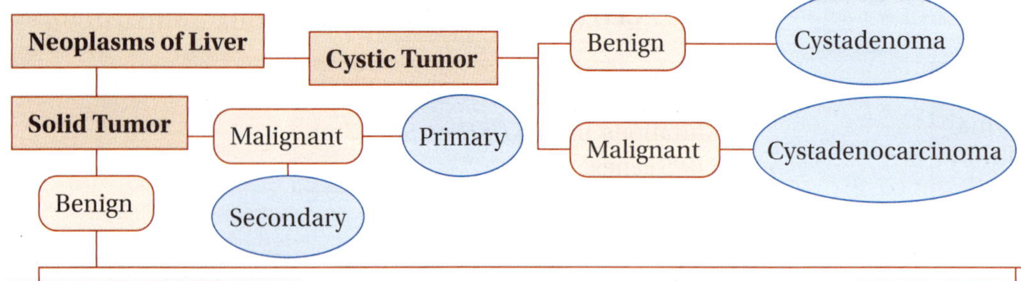

Hepatic Hemangioma

- Most common benign liver tumor of unknown etiology.
- Predominantly found in women (5:1 ratio)
- Sizes ranges from <3 cm ("capillary hemangioma") to up to 10 cm ("cavernous or giant hemangiomas").
- Mean age is 50 years, equal distribution in the right and left lobe of liver.
- Giant hemangiomas are commonly associated with fibrosis, thrombosis, and calcifications. Small hemangiomas may become entirely fibrous, appears as solitary fibrous nodule, and occasionally misdiagnosed as a malignant fibrous tumor.
- **Syndromes associated with this tumor:** (i) Kasabach-Merritt syndrome; (ii) Klippel-Trenaunay-Weber syndrome; (iii) Osler-Weber-Rendu syndrome; and (iv) von Hippel-Lindau syndrome.
- Most of the hemangiomas are asymptomatic, typically detected during imaging. Larger lesions may present with right upper quadrant pain or epigastric mass. Rarely, giant hemangiomas may present with consumptive coagulopathy (known as **Kasabach-Merritt syndrome**) that manifests as thrombocytopenia, disseminated intravascular coagulation, and systemic bleeding.
- USG, CT and MRI are useful imaging modality for diagnosis of hepatic hemangioma. **MRI is the preferred modality** and contrast-enhanced US, if available, can increase both the sensitivity and specificity of US.
- **Two common imaging atypias are:** (i) Rapidly filling hemangioma and (ii) Giant hemangioma.
- Pregnancy, use of OCP or anabolic steroids are not contraindicated in patients with hemangioma.
- Biopsy should be avoided due to risk of bleeding.
- Regardless of the size, no intervention is required for asymptomatic hemangiomas. Indications for treatment are severe symptoms or development of complications. Treatment is surgery (enucleation or anatomic liver resection).

Focal Nodular Hyperplasia

- Second most common benign tumor of the liver.
- Predominantly found in women (9:1 ratio).
- Most FNH and their surrounding liver parenchyma express estrogen receptors. FNH is considered a hyperplastic reaction to an aberrant dystrophic artery.
- Pregnancy and OCP are not associated with development or progression of FNH.
- **Molecular profiles are:** (i) Upregulation of extracellular matrix genes associated with activation of the transforming growth factor-β signaling pathway and (ii) Overexpression of Wnt/β-catenin target gene, including GLUL, coding for glutamine synthase. A typical map-like pattern of glutamine synthase expression on immunohistochemistry is specific for FNH.
- Typically, FNH is a solitary lesion. Multiple FNH may be associated with Budd-Chiari syndrome, hereditary hemorrhagic telangiectasia, obliterative portal venopathy.
- FNH is typically a solitary, well-circumscribed, unencapsulated mass, showing a central fibrous scar, which contains dystrophic arterial vessels. **Atypical forms of FNH are:** (i) FNH without a central scar and (ii) FNH with significant steatosis.
- On cross-sectional imaging, "spoke wheel pattern" is characteristic of FNH. With use of hepatobiliary MR contrast agents (e.g., Gadoxetic acid, GD-BOPTA), the sensitivity and diagnostic accuracy is highly increased.
- Liver biopsy is not routinely indicated to confirm the diagnosis.
- Asymptomatic FNH does not require intervention. Intervention is indicated if the lesion is pedunculated or exophytic or having symptoms. Surgery (partial hepatic resection) is the treatment of choice. Embolization or radiofrequency ablation are other treatment options.

Hepatocellular Adenoma

- A rare, benign liver neoplasm with strong female predominance (9:1 ratio).
- **Risk factors:** (i) Use of OCP; (ii) Anabolic androgenic steroid therapy; (iii) Glycogen storage disease Ia and III; (iv) Obesity; (v) Metabolic syndrome (Diabetes mellitus, insulin resistance, dyslipidemia); and (vi) McCune-Albright syndrome. The risk of transformation to HCC is more in male patients and patients with metabolic syndrome.
- **Clinical variants:** (i) Liver adenomatosis (multiple adenomas, >3 and ≥10 lesions, same clinical, histological and radiological features) and (ii) Telangiectatic hepatocellular adenoma (commonly associated with OCP use, androgenic steroid therapy, obesity).
- **Molecular classification (based on mutations in oncogenes and tumor suppressor genes):** (i) HNF1α-mutated HCAs (H-HCA)- inactivation of HNF-1α; (ii) Inflammatory adenomas (I-HCA)- mutations of gp130, FRK, STAT3, GNAS and JAK1; (iii) β-catenin activated HCA (β-HCA); and (iv) Unclassified. B-HCA exhibit the highest risk of transformation into HCC.
- **Risk factors associated with malignant transformation:** (i) Male patient; (ii) HCA patients with metabolic syndrome; (iii) HCA >5 cm; and (iv) β-HCA molecular subtype.
- **Risk factors associated with hemorrhage:** (i) Size >5 cm; (ii) IHCA subtype; (iii) Exophytic growth; and (iv) Tumor in left lateral liver.
- **Complications of HCA:** (i) Hemorrhage and (ii) Malignant transformation.
- Among CEUS, CT or MRI, MRI enhanced with gadoxetate disodium or gadobenate dimeglumine is highly useful imaging modality to differentiate HCA from FNH and other focal lesions of liver, also useful for identify the subtypes of HCA based on imaging patterns.
- Liver biopsy is not routinely indicated.
- In women with HCA, pregnancy is not discouraged if tumor size <5 cm in diameter with no intratumoral bleeding and frequent US surveillance is feasible.
- In male patients, resection should be considered regardless of size (due to high risk of malignancy). In female patients, initial management of HCAs <5 cm includes discontinuation of OCPs and control of body weight. Reassessment after 1 year and then annual screening.
- Resection is the first-line of curative treatment. Embolization or ablation (RFA) may be considered in poor surgical candidates.
- Liver transplantation is rarely indicated in following situations: (i) Multiple unresectable lesions in men; (ii) Patient with glycogen storage disorders unresponsive to medical treatment; and (iii) Large HCA associated with intrahepatic venous shunt.

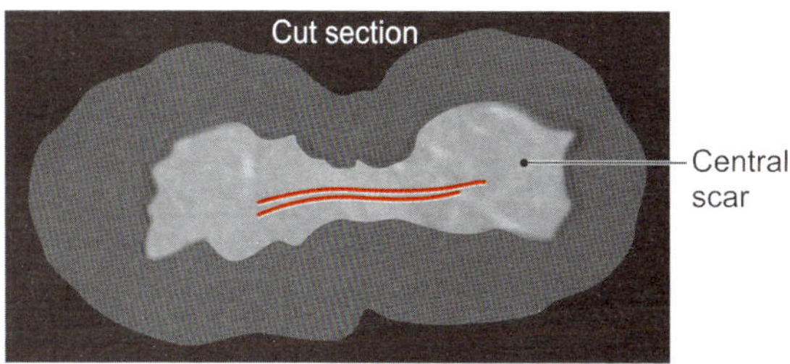

Cut section of focal nodular hyperplasia showing central scar with dystrophic arterial vessels.

Hepatocellular Carcinoma

Risk Factors

Viral Infections

- Hepatitis B infection
- Hepatitis C infection

High HBV DNA and HCV RNA load in blood are independent risk factors

Cirrhosis

- Alcoholic cirrhosis
- Cirrhosis secondary to HbsAg carrier state

Environmental Exposure to Aflatoxin

- Aflatoxin is produced by *Aspergillus flavus, Aspergillus parasiticus.*
- Aflatoxin B1 is most hepatotoxic.
- Others are B2, G1, G2

Inherited Errors of Metabolism

- Hereditary hemochromatosis
- Wilson's disease
- Porphyria cutanea tarda
- α 1-antitrypsin deficiency
- Stage IV primary biliary cirrhosis.

Metabolic Disorders

- Obesity
- Diabetes
- Nonalcoholic fatty liver disease

Pathophysiology

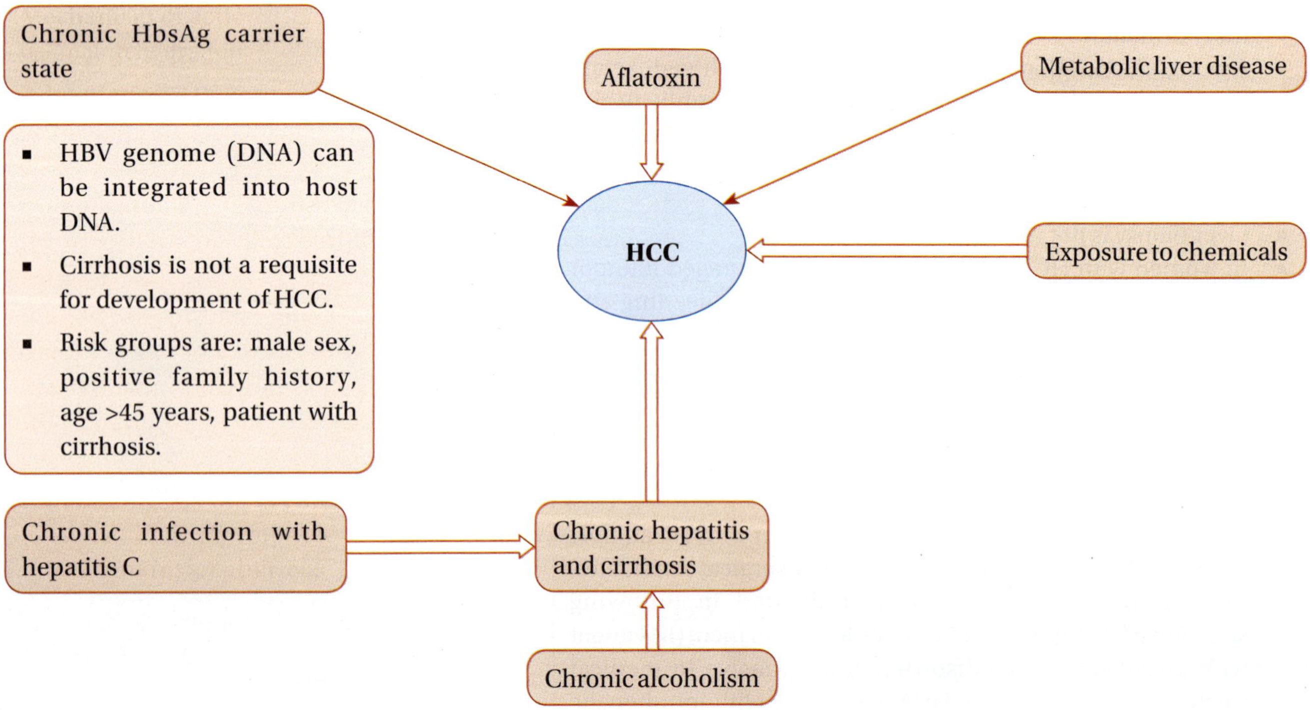

Chronic HbsAg carrier state → HCC

- HBV genome (DNA) can be integrated into host DNA.
- Cirrhosis is not a requisite for development of HCC.
- Risk groups are: male sex, positive family history, age >45 years, patient with cirrhosis.

Aflatoxin → HCC

Metabolic liver disease → HCC

Exposure to chemicals → HCC

Chronic infection with hepatitis C → Chronic hepatitis and cirrhosis → HCC

Chronic alcoholism → Chronic hepatitis and cirrhosis

Fibrolamellar Hepatocellular Carcinoma

- A variant of hepatocellular carcinoma.
- Patients are younger.
- Rarely associated with hepatitis, cirrhosis.
- Alpha fetoprotein level is not elevated.
- Better prognosis than HCC.
- A molecular target, DNAJB1-PRKACA chimera, is identified in 79–100% cases.
- Complete resection is the only curative option.

Combined Hepatocellular Cholangiocarcinoma

- Rare type of hepatobiliary tumor.
- AFP or CA19-9 level may be elevated.
- Imaging findings consisting of features of both HCC and cholangiocarcinoma.
- Resection is the only curative treatment option.

HCC Screening—"at risk" Population

- Liver cirrhosis induced by hepatitis B and C
- Alcoholic cirrhosis
- Cirrhosis due to genetic hemochromatosis, NAFLD or NASH, stage IV primary biliary cirrhosis
- Cirrhosis due to α 1-antitrypsin deficiency
- Hepatitis B carriers.

- Screening USG every 6 months with or without AFP estimation
- If AFP is elevated or liver mass nodule more than 10 mm on USG, then multiphasic CT or MRI.

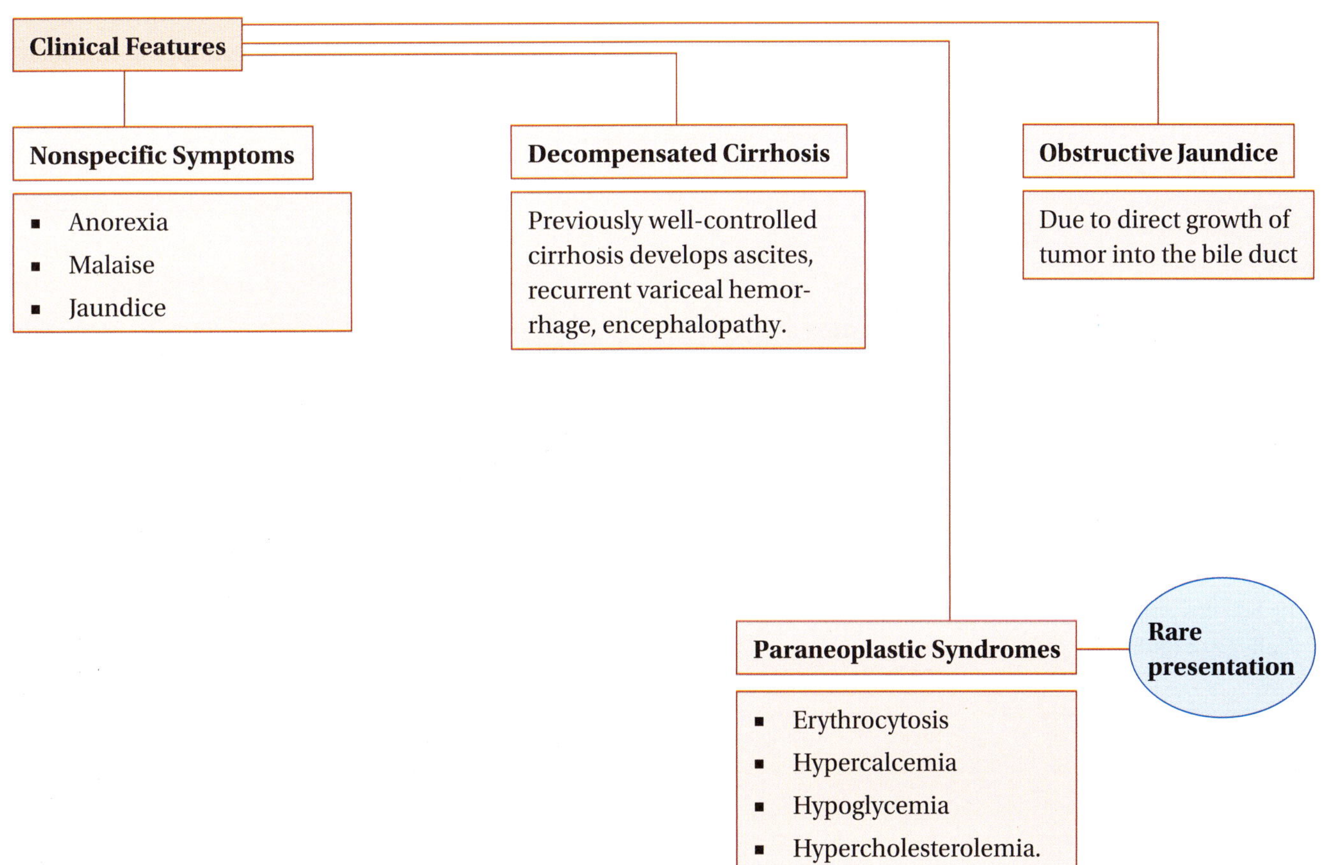

Investigations

Imaging

Muliphasic liver protocol CT with IV contrast

- Contrast enhancement in arterial phase followed by contrast washout in the delayed nonperipheral venous phase—**typical pattern of HCC**.
- Can detect size and site of lesion.
- Can evaluate the relationship of tumor with portal and hepatic vein.
- Can assess biliary involvement and nodal metastases.

Sites of Metastases from HCC

- Lungs
- Bones
- Lymph nodes
- Adrenals, peritoneum

Multiphasic contrast-enhanced MRI

Serum biomarkers

- AFP is the most commonly used serum biomarker for HCC.
- AFP level is not a sensitive or specific diagnostic test for HCC.
- **AFP level may be elevated in**—(i) Chronic hepatitis; (ii) Intrahepatic cholangiocarcinoma; and (iii) Germ cell tumors.
- **Other serum biomarkers are**—(i) Protein induced by vitamin K absence or antagonist II (PIVKA II) and (ii) Lens culinaris agglutinin-reactive AFP (AFP-L3)-an isoform of AFP.

Biopsy

- Biopsy is not indicated if imaging features are suggestive of HCC.

Biopsy is indicated:

- Lesion is suspicious for malignancy but multiphasic CT or MRI findings not indicative of HCC.
- In patients who are not considered high risk for developing HCC (patients not having cirrhosis, previous history of HCC or chronic HCV).
- In conditions where nonmalignant liver nodules may develop and may be confused with HCC in imaging (i.e., cardiac cirrhosis, congenital hepatic fibrosis, Budd-Chiari syndrome, hereditary hemorrhagic telengiectasia).

LI-RADS (Liver Imaging Reporting And Data System)—a comprehensive system for standardizing the terminology, interpretation, reporting and data collection of liver observations of CT, MRI and CEUS in individuals at high risk for hepatocellular carcinoma.

LI-RADS system is supported and endorsed by American College of Radiology (ACR).

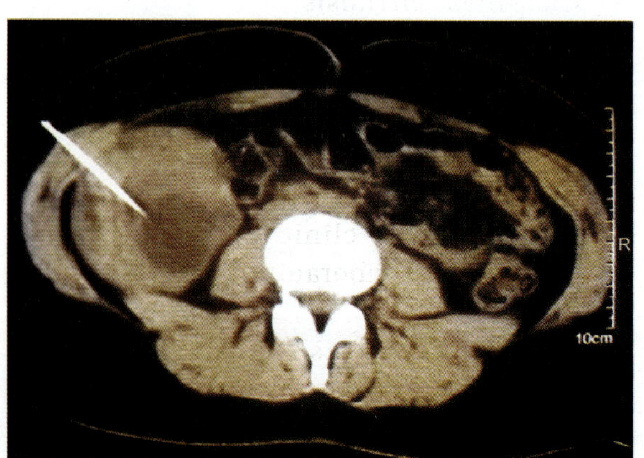

CT-guided FNAC from liver SOL.

Workup (After Diagnosis)

Detection of Hepatitis B and C Infection

- HbsAg
- Hepatitis B surface antibody
- Hepatitis B core antibody
- HCV antibody
- Assessment of viral load if positive for HbsAg, HbcAb-IgG

Assessment of Hepatic Function

- Serum bilirubin, AST, ALT, ALP
- Prothrombin time
- Serum albumin
- Platelet count

Assessment of Hepatic Functional Reserve

- The Child-Pugh scoring
- Model for End-stage Liver Disease (MELD)
- Albumin-Bilirubin (ALBI) grade
- Indocyanine green (ICG) clearance test

Imaging

- Multiphasic contrast-enhanced CT or MRI (if not already done)—to assess metastatic disease and nodal involvement.
- Chest CT (lung is common site of metastasis in HCC)
- Bone scan (if bone metastases is suspected).

The Child-Pugh Scoring

- This scoring system is used for assessment of hepatic functional reserve in cirrhotic patients.
- Score includes: (i) Albumin (g/dL); (ii) Bilirubin (mg/dL); (iii) Prothrombin time; (iv) Ascites; and (v) Encephalopathy.
- Classifies cirrhosis as compensated (Class A) and decompensated (Class B and C).
- *Advantages:* (i) Bedside tool and (ii) Parameters include both clinical findings and laboratory investigations.
- *Drawback:* Signs of clinically significant portal hypertension (varices, splenomegaly, etc.) are not included.

Model for End-stage Liver Disease (MELD)

- MELD is a system for evaluation of hepatic reserve in patients of 12 years or older.
- It is derived using three parameters: (i) Serum bilirubin; (ii) Serum creatinine; and (iii) INR.
- MELD is a numerical scale ranging from 6 (less ill) to 40 (gravely ill).
- This scoring system is used to stratify patients on the liver transplantation waiting list according to their risk of death within 3 months.

ICG Clearance Test

- This test is used for assessment of liver function prior to hepatic resection in patients associated with cirrhosis.
- ICG retention rate of 14% at 15 minutes after IV injection of the dye is the cut-off value.

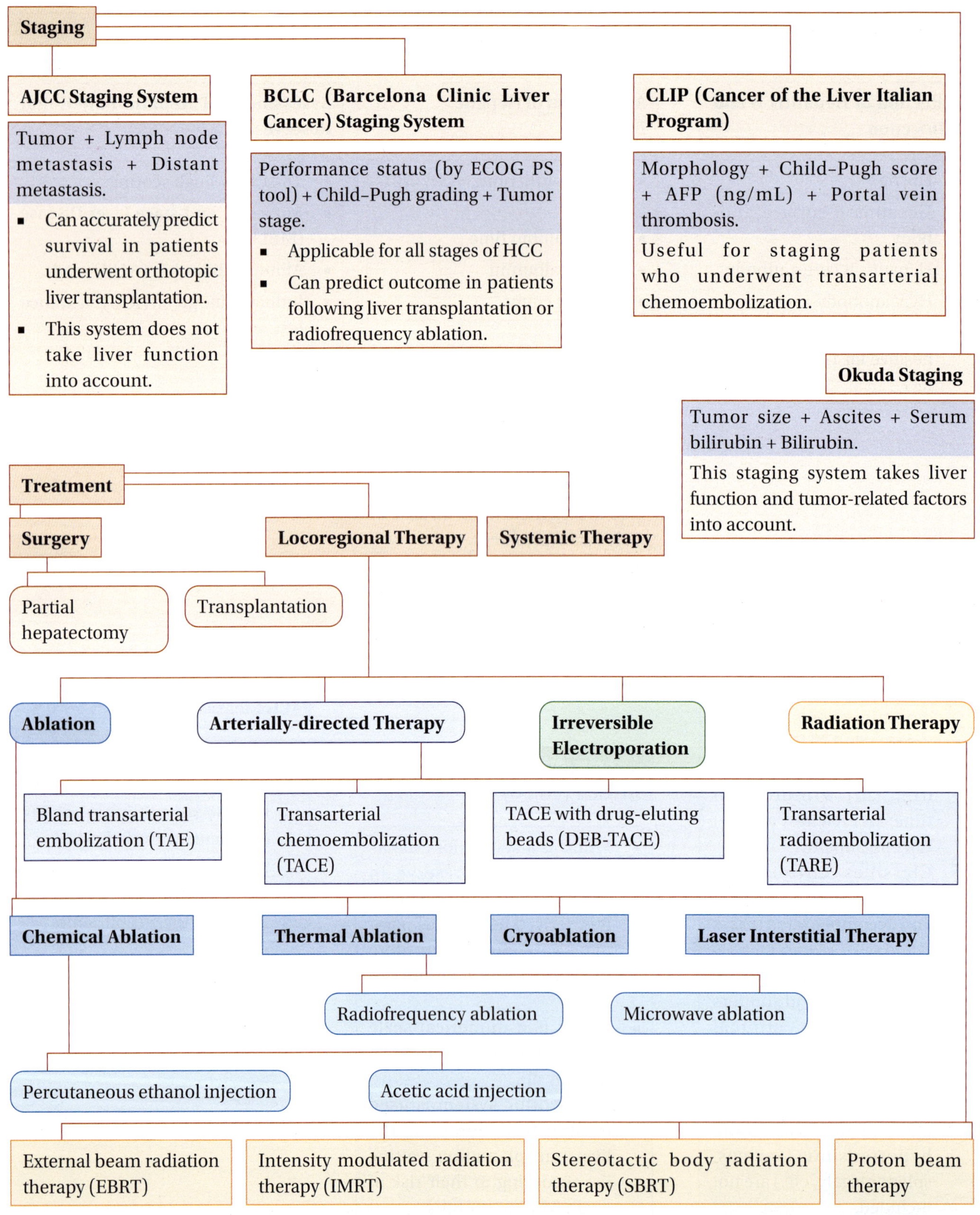
Staging
AJCC Staging System
Tumor + Lymph node metastasis + Distant metastasis.
Can accurately predict survival in patients underwent orthotopic liver transplantation.
This system does not take liver function into account.
BCLC (Barcelona Clinic Liver Cancer) Staging System
Performance status (by ECOG PS tool) + Child-Pugh grading + Tumor stage.
Applicable for all stages of HCC
Can predict outcome in patients following liver transplantation or radiofrequency ablation.
CLIP (Cancer of the Liver Italian Program)
Morphology + Child-Pugh score + AFP (ng/mL) + Portal vein thrombosis.
Useful for staging patients who underwent transarterial chemoembolization.
Okuda Staging
Tumor size + Ascites + Serum bilirubin + Bilirubin.
This staging system takes liver function and tumor-related factors into account.
Treatment
Surgery
Locoregional Therapy
Systemic Therapy
Partial hepatectomy
Transplantation
Ablation
Arterially-directed Therapy
Irreversible Electroporation
Radiation Therapy
Bland transarterial embolization (TAE)
Transarterial chemoembolization (TACE)
TACE with drug-eluting beads (DEB-TACE)
Transarterial radioembolization (TARE)
Chemical Ablation
Thermal Ablation
Cryoablation
Laser Interstitial Therapy
Radiofrequency ablation
Microwave ablation
Percutaneous ethanol injection
Acetic acid injection
External beam radiation therapy (EBRT)
Intensity modulated radiation therapy (IMRT)
Stereotactic body radiation therapy (SBRT)
Proton beam therapy

Partial Hepatectomy

Indications

- Solitary tumor of any size with no evidence of gross vascular invasion
- Early stage HCC with Child-Pugh Class A

Principles of Resection

- Resection of tumor with free margin of atleast 5 mm
- Minimal blood transfusion
- Maximal preservation of nontumorous liver

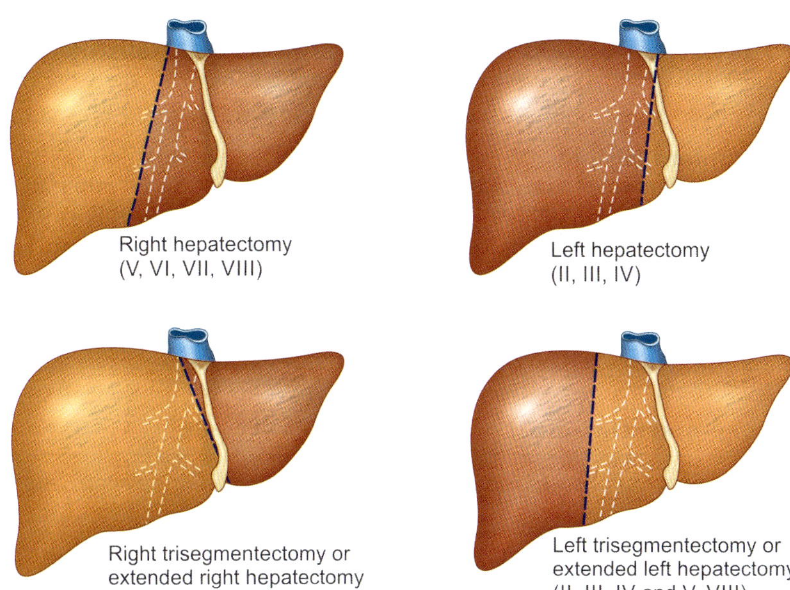

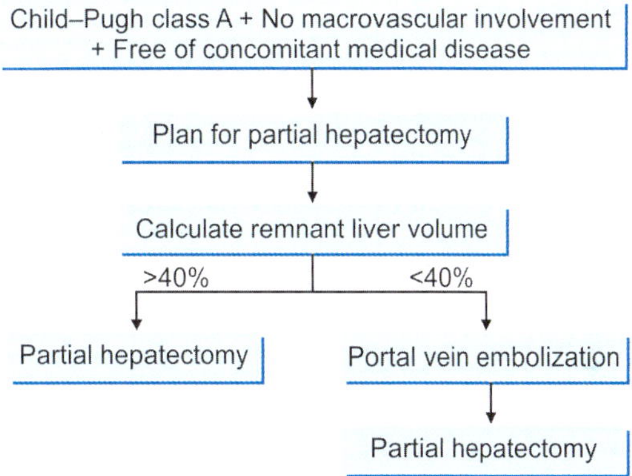

Indications of Liver Resection in Malignant Conditions

- Hepatocellular carcinoma
- Hilar cholangiocarcinoma
- Gallbladder carcinoma
- Metastatic tumors in liver (arising from colorectal cancers, neuroendocrine tumors)

Complications of Liver Resection

- Hemorrhage
- Bile leakage
- Posthepatectomy liver failure
- Hepatorenal syndrome.

Indications of Liver Resection in Benign Conditions

- Caroli disease
- Intrahepatic stones associated with pyogenic cholangitis
- Intrahepatic biliary strictures
- Recurrent pyogenic cholangitis
- Hemangioma
- Cystadenoma
- Focal nodular hyperplasia
- Hydatid cyst of liver
- Polycystic liver disease
- Liver trauma

The Brisbane 2000 Terminology of Hepatic Anatomy and Liver Resections

First-order Division

- *Right hemiliver or right liver:* Segments 5-8 (+/- segment 1), resection of these segments is termed as Right hepatectomy or Right hemihepatectomy (stipulate +/-segment 1)
- *Left hemiliver or left liver:* Segments 2-4 (+/-segment 1), resection of these segments is termed as Left hepatectomy or Left hemihepatectomy (stipulate+/-segment 1)

Second-order Division

- *Right anterior section:* Segments 5, 8, Resection of these segments is termed as Right anterior sectionectomy.
- *Right posterior section:* Segments 6, 7, Resection of these segments is termed as Right posterior sectionectomy.
- *Left medial section:* Segment 4, Resection of this segment is termed as Segmentectomy 4 or Left medial sectionectomy.
- *Left lateral section:* Segment 2, 3, Resection of these segments is termed as Bisegmentectomy 2, 3 or Left lateral sectionectomy.
- *Right hemiliver plus left medial section:* Segment 4-8, Resection of these segments is termed as Right trisectionectomy or Extended right hepatectomy or Extended right hemihepatectomy.
- *Left hemiliver plus right anterior section:* Segment 2-4, 5, 8, Resection of these segments is termed as Left trisectionectomy or Extended left hepatectomy or Extended left hemihepatectomy.

Third-order Division

- *Segments 1-9:* Any one of segment 1 to 9, Segmentectomy (e.g., Segmentectomy 6)
- *Two contiguous segments:* Any two of segment 1 to 9 in continuity, Bisegmentectomy

Addendum Alternative Second-order Division (Second-order Division based on Portal Vein)

- *Right anterior sector or right paramedian sector:* Segment 5, 8, Resection of these segments is termed as Right anterior sectorectomy or right paramedian sectorectomy.
- *Right posterior sector or right lateral sector:* Segment 6, 7, Resection of these segments is termed as Right posterior sectorectomy or Right lateral sectorectomy.
- *Left medial sector or left paramedian sector:* Segment 3, 4, Resection of these segments is termed as Left medial sectorectomy or Left paramedian sectorectomy.
- *Left lateral sector or left posterior sector:* Segment 2, Resection of this segment is termed as Left lateral sectorectomy or Left posterior sectorectomy or Segmentectomy 2.

Liver Transplantation

- Living donor liver transplantation
- Cadaveric liver transplantation

Ideal Candidate

Patient meeting UNOS (United Network for Organ Sharing) criteria:

(i) Radiologic evidence of a single lesion ≥2 cm and ≤5 cm in diameter, or 2–3 lesions ≥1 cm and ≤3 cm in diameter.

(ii) No evidence of macrovascular involvement or extrahepatic disease.

Early-stage HCC with Child-Pugh Class B and C.

MELD Score and Liver Transplantation

MELD score was adopted by UNOS:

(i) To estimate of risk of death within 3 months for patients in the waiting list for cadaveric liver transplant.

(ii) To prioritize the allocation of the liver transplants.

MELD score 17 or more are considered for candidates for liver transplantation.

Methods to calculate liver volume for living donor transplantation

- CT volumetry
- Urata formula

Absolute Contraindications to Liver Transplantation

- Severe cardiopulmonary disease
- Active alcohol and substance abuse
- Active extrahepatic malignancy
- AIDS
- Active infection outside of the hepatobiliary system
- Lack of adequate psychosocial support.

Locoregional Therapies

Percutaneous Ethanol Injection

Mechanism of action: Injection of 95% ethanol causes coagulative necrosis and fibrous reaction in tumor tissue.

Indications: Unresectable HCC and metastatic liver tumors close to liver hilum and major vessels.

Advantages: (i) Cost-effective than RFA and (ii) Safer ablation technique.

Contraindications: (i) Low platelet count (<40,000); (ii) Patient with coagulation disorders; and (iii) Obstructive jaundice.

Disadvantages: (i) Needs multiple session therapy

Complications: (i) Liver abscess; (ii) Subcapsular hematoma; and (iii) Hemobilia.

Radiofrequency Ablation (RFA)

Mechanism of action: The alternating radiofrequency current (300–500 KHz) around the ablation electrode produces heat to denature cell protein, causing cell death.

Indications: (i) Unresectable HCC; (ii) Unresectable colorectal liver metastases; (iii) Recurrent HCC; (iv) As a bridge therapy to transplantation; and (v) Intrahepatic cholangiocarcinoma.

Advantages: (i) Adequate local control of tumors ≤3 cm; (ii) widely available; and (iii) safe procedure.

Disadvantages: (i) "Heat-sink effect" in perivascular tumors and (ii) Risk of thermal injury to important structures.["heat sink effect"—during ablation therapy, major vessels close to the tumor can absorb most of the heat generated. This effect may decrease the effectiveness of therapy].

Complications: (i) Postablation syndrome (e.g., low-grade fever, fatigue); (ii) Biloma; (iii) Biliary fistula; (iv) Ascites; (v) Liver abscess; and (vi) Pleural effusion.

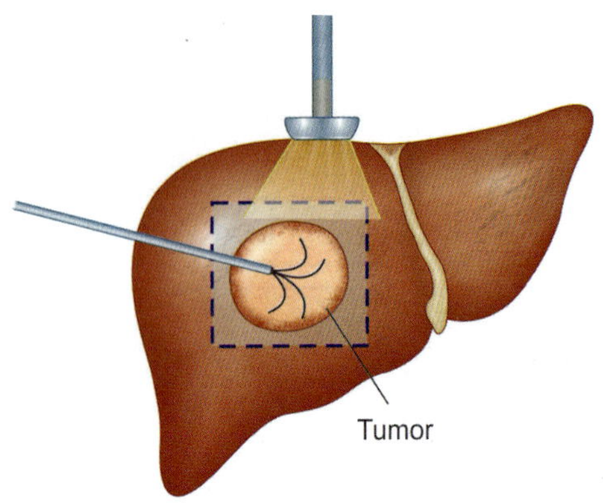

Radiofrequency Ablation

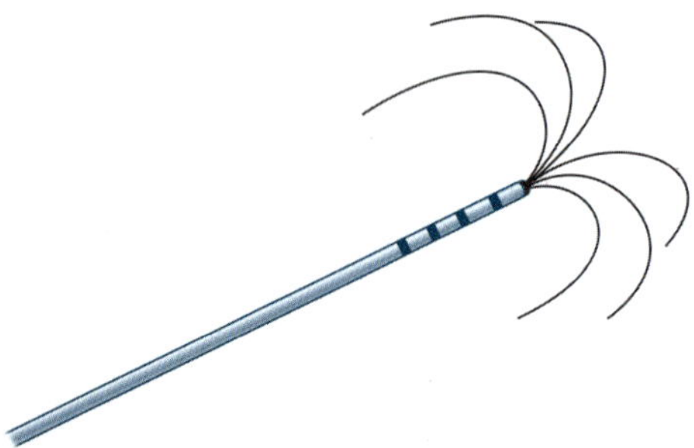

Multiple Array Needle Electrode

Cryoablation

Mechanism of action: Cryoablation causes cell death by cellular dehydration.

Advantages: (i) Periprocedural imaging of ice-ball formation can be done and (ii) Multiple probes can be activated at a same time.

Complications: (i) Hemorrhage; (ii) Cracking of iceball; (iii) Cryoshock; (iv) Biliary fistula; and (v) Myoglobinuria.

Bland Transarterial Embolization (TAE)

Mechanism of action: Tumor ischemia by embolization of feeding artery and more distal small vessels via hepatic artery catheterization.

Embolizing agents are: (i) Nonspherical polyvinyl alcohol (PVA) and (ii) Hydrophilic microspheres (Tris-acyl gelatin microspheres, Spherical PVA, Polyphosphazene-coated polymethylmethacrylate microspheres.

Complications: (i) Postembolization syndrome; (ii) Nontargeted embolization; (iii) Liver failure; and (iv) Liver abscess.

Microwave Ablation

Mechanism of action: The point application of electromagnetic microwave radiation causes oscillation of water molecules of tissue, causing heat production.

Advantages: (i) Tumors > 3 cm can be treated and (ii) Multiple probes can be activated at same time.

Disadvantages: Risk of thermal injury to critical structures.

Complications: (i) Liver abscess and (ii) Skin burn at needle track.

Laser Interstitial Thermal Therapy (LITT)

Mechanism of action: Nd:YAG laser (wavelength 1064 nm) is delivered by flexible quartz fibers and heat is produced by conversion of absorbed light. Laser is delivered under real-time MR imaging guidance.

Complications: (i) Severe pain; (ii) Post-procedural fever; and (iii) Asymptomatic pleural effusion.

Transarterial Radioembolization (TARE)

^{90}Y, a pure β-emitter is the most commonly used radioactive element for radioembolization. ^{131}I (a β and γ-emitter) labeled Iodized oil is also used. TARE technique is based on catheter-based administration of glass or resin microspheres embedded with yttrium-90.

Indications: (i) As a bridge therapy in patients with HCC waiting for orthotopic liver transplantation; (ii) for downstaging HCC; (iii) Unresectable metastatic colorectal carcinoma; and (iv) Unresectable metastatic neuroendocrine tumors.

Complications: (i) Radiation-induced liver disease; (ii) Portal hypertension; and (iii) Radiation pneumonitis.

Transarterial Chemoembolization (TACE)

Mechanism of action: Tumor ischemia by embolization along with intra-arterial chemotherapy.

Principles of TACE: (i) delivers a highly concentrated dose of chemotherapeutic agent to tumor cells; (ii) prolongation of contact time between chemotherapeutic agent and tumor; and (iii) minimal systemic toxicity of chemotherapy.

Chemotherapeutic agents used in TACE: (i) Doxorubicin (most commonly used); (ii) Cisplatin; (iii) Epirubicin; (iv) Mitoxantrone; and (v) Mitomycin C. Embolic agents used: (i) Gelatin sponge particles (most commonly used); (ii) Polyvinyl alcohol articles (PVA); (iii) Starch microspheres; and (iv) Absolute ethanol.

Indications: (i) Unresectable HCC; (ii) As a bridge therapy in patients waiting for liver transplantation; (iii) Metastatic NETs and GISTs; and (iv) Spontaneous rupture of HCC (emergency indication).

Contraindication: Child-Pugh Class C

Complications: (i) Postembolization syndrome; (ii) Liver failure; (iii) Nontargeted embolization; and (iv) Liver abscess.

TACE with Drug-eluting Beads (DEB-TACE)

Mechanism of action: Microspheres loaded with chemotherapeutic agent delivers the drug within the target tissue for an extended period of time.

Drug-eluting beads are: (i) PVA-based microspheres and (ii) Superabsorbent polymer microspheres. Chemotherapeutic agents are: (i) Doxorubicin and (ii) Irinotecan.

Advantages: Toxicity of chemotherapeutic agents lower in comparison to conventional TACE.

Irreversible Electroporation

Mechanism of action: Pulses of direct current can perforate the cell by disrupting electrical potential across the cell membranes.

Advantages: (i) No risk of thermal injury; (ii) Safe approach for tumors close to major biliary vascular structures; and (iii) No heat-sink effect.

Disadvantages: Needs general anesthesia.

Complications: (i) Hemorrhage and (ii) Biliary fistula.

Liver Metastases

Liver Metastases

- **Colorectal Liver Metastases**
  - Colorectal Cancer
- **Neuroendocrine Metastases**
  - Carcinoid tumors
  - Pancreatic endocrine tumors
  - Other NETs (pheochromocytoma, neuroblastoma, medullary thyroid carcinoma)
- **Noncolorectal, Non-neuroendocrine Metastases**
  - Breast cancer
  - Renal cell carcinoma
  - Melanoma
  - Nonsmall cell lung carcinoma
  - Gastrointestinal stromal tumor

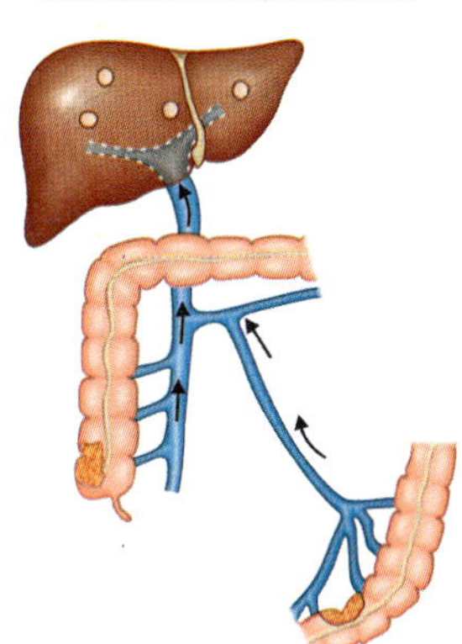

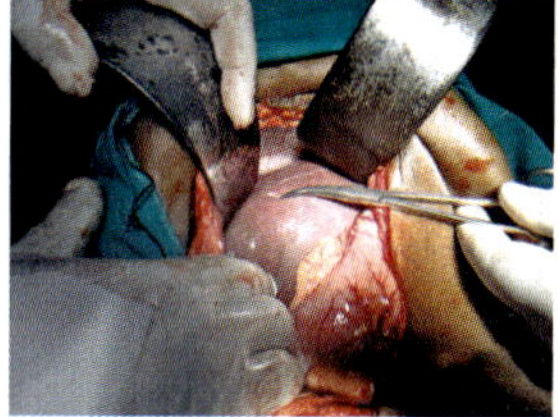

Peroperative picture of liver metastases.

Diagnosis

- Triphasic MDCT is a useful imaging modality.
- Hypodense lesion in portal venous phase is suggestive of metastases from colorectal cancers.
- Homogeneous enhancement in early arterial phase with isoattenuation in portal venous phase is suggestive of neuroendocrine metastases or noncolorectal, non-neuroendocrine metastases.

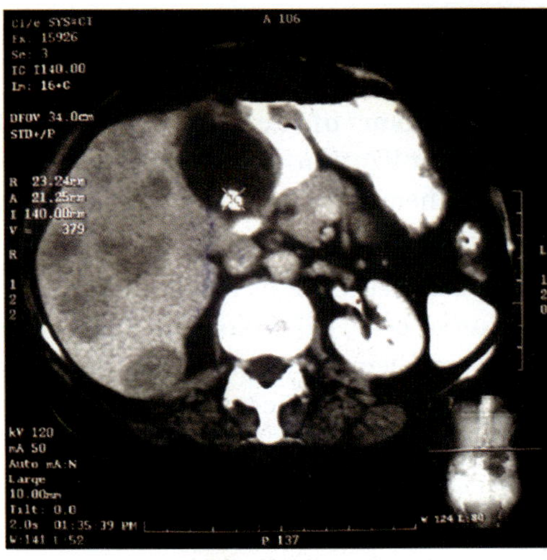

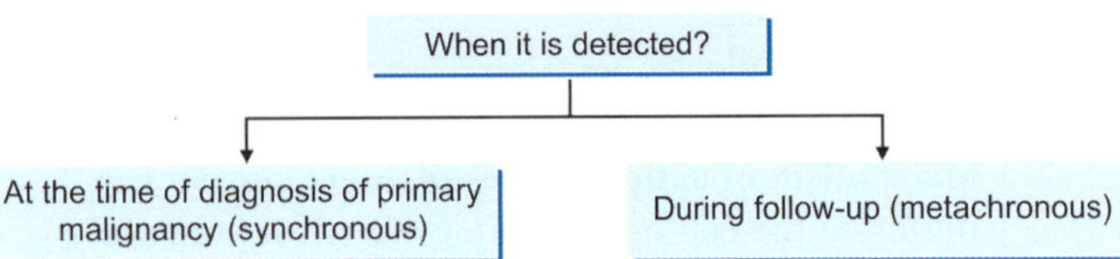

Treatment

Treatment approaches of synchronous resectable colorectal metastases

Classic Approach

- A staged approach where colorectal cancer is treated before the metastases.
- Not practiced nowadays.

Combined or Synchronous Approach

- Most common approach for resectable, synchronous colorectal metastases.
- Indicated in symptomatic colorectal cancer with low-volume metastases (four or fewer, less than three segments involved, or all in the same lobe) in a low-risk surgical patient.

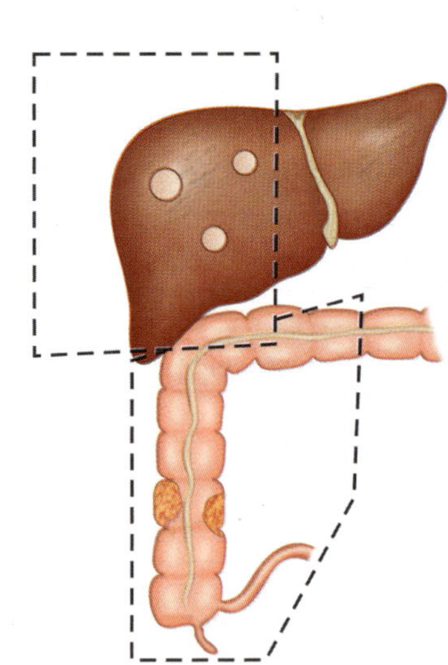

Combined or synchronous approach.

Ablation therapies (e.g., radiofrequency ablation, ethanol injection are other alternative approaches.

Reversed Approach

- A staged approach where metastatic disease is treated before the primary tumor.
- Indicated in patients with asymptomatic rectal cancer with high-volume metastatic disease.

Portal Hypertension — Elevated pressure (more than 10 mm Hg) in portal venous system due to resistance to portal blood flow.

Normal portal pressure is 5–10 mm Hg.

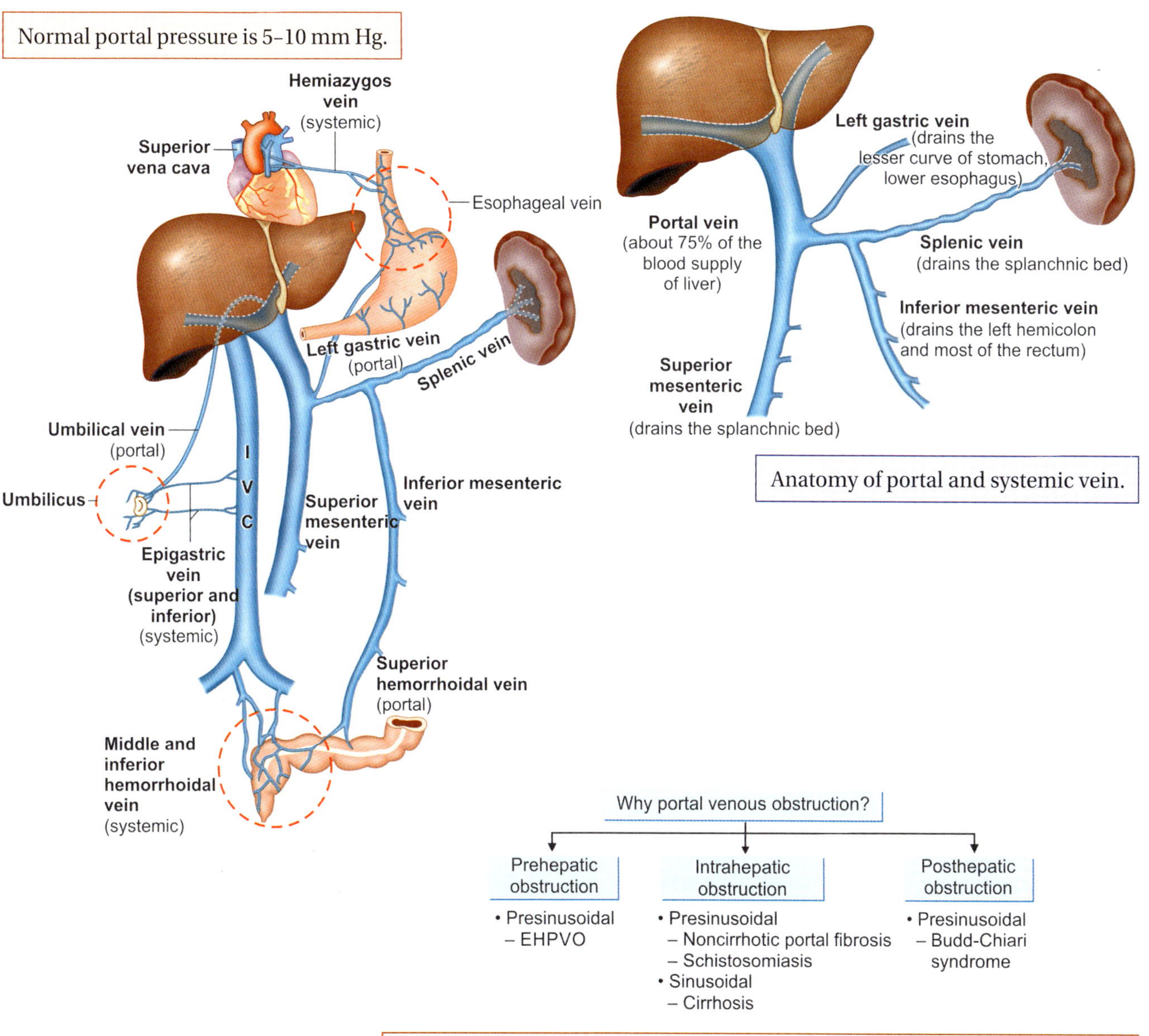

Anatomy of portal and systemic vein.

Why portal venous obstruction?

- Prehepatic obstruction
  - Presinusoidal
    - EHPVO
- Intrahepatic obstruction
  - Presinusoidal
    - Noncirrhotic portal fibrosis
    - Schistosomiasis
  - Sinusoidal
    - Cirrhosis
- Posthepatic obstruction
  - Presinusoidal
    - Budd-Chiari syndrome

- **In western countries**, the most common cause of portal hypertension is cirrhosis.
- **In India**, noncirrhotic portal fibrosis and extrahepatic portal venous obstruction account for about 50% of cause of portal hypertension.

Extrahepatic Portal Vein Obstruction (EHPVO)

- Portal vein replaced by multiple branches — Portal cavernoma.

About 75% of children with portal hypertension having EHPVO.

Common causes:

- Neonatal peritonitis
- Umbilical vein catheterization
- *Hypercoagulable states:*
  - P. rubra vera
  - Myelofibrosis
  - Protein C deficiency
  - Protein S deficiency

Noncirrhotic Portal Fibrosis

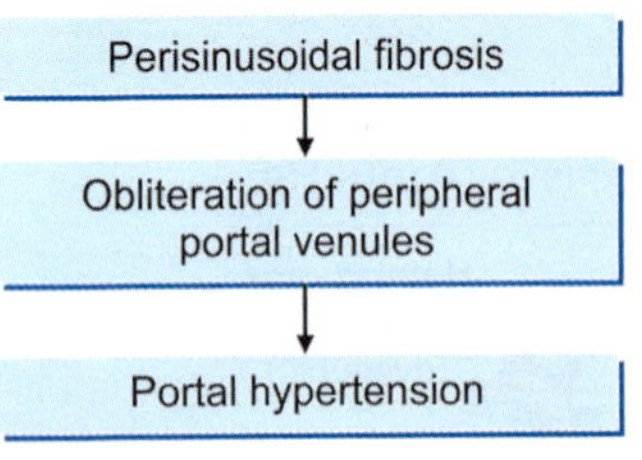

Etiology—Not known

Budd-Chiari Syndrome

Causes of Budd-Chiari syndrome:

In western countries

- Primary myeloproliferative disorders
- Paroxysmal nocturnal hemoglobinuria
- Protein C, protein S, antithrombin III deficiency

In India

- Pregnancy related hypercoagulability
- Infections
- IVC web or membrane

Type I: Major hepatic vein obstruction, Patent IVC

Type II: IVC obstruction above the level of hepatic venous opening

Type III: IVC obstruction, hepatic vein obstruction

Cirrhosis

Cirrhosis is classified into two prognostic stages depending on presence or absence of clinically evident decompensating events: Compensated and Decompensated.

Etiology

- Chronic alcoholism
- Posthepatitis B and C
- Primary biliary cirrhosis

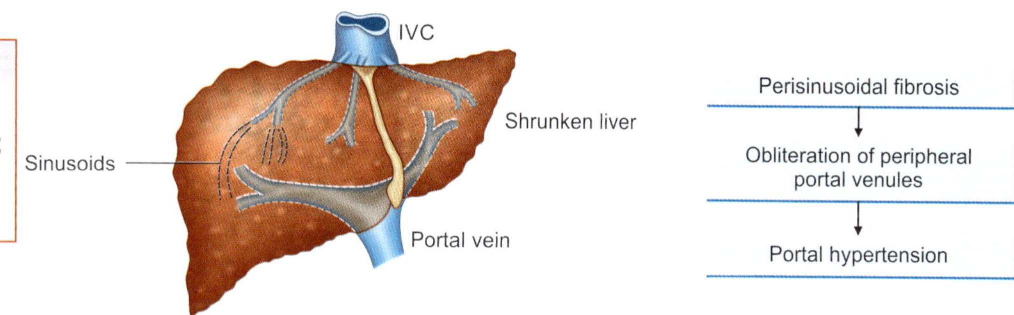

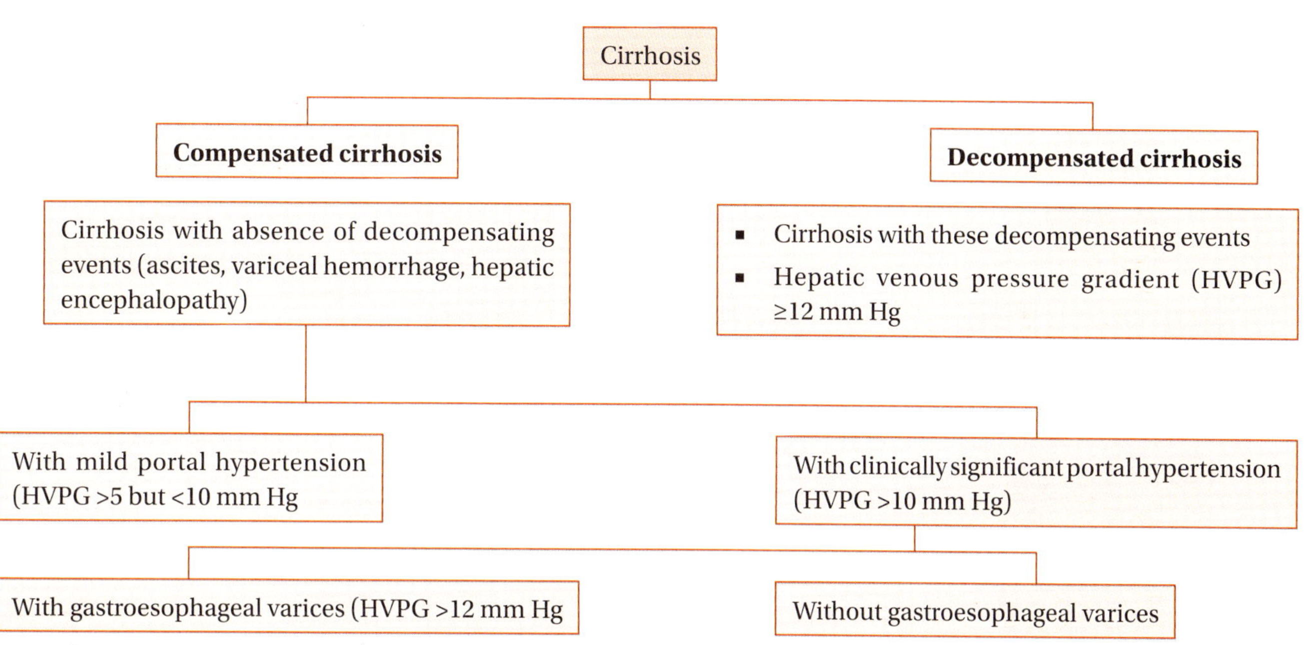

Left-sided Portal Hypertension (Sinistral Hypertension)

- Rare, but life-threatening cause of upper gastrointestinal bleeding.
- It usually develops as a result of isolated obstruction of the splenic vein.
- Pathologies commonly responsible for splenic vein thrombosis or obstruction are—chronic pancreatitis, pancreatic pseudocysts, pancreatic neoplasm.
- Commonly gastric varices develop in this type of portal hypertension.

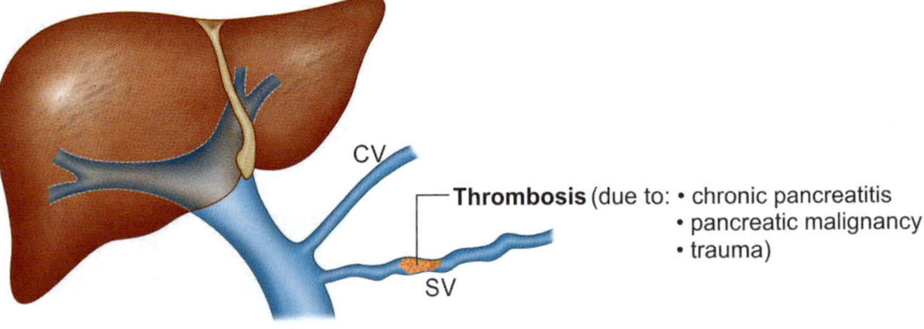

Clinical Presentation

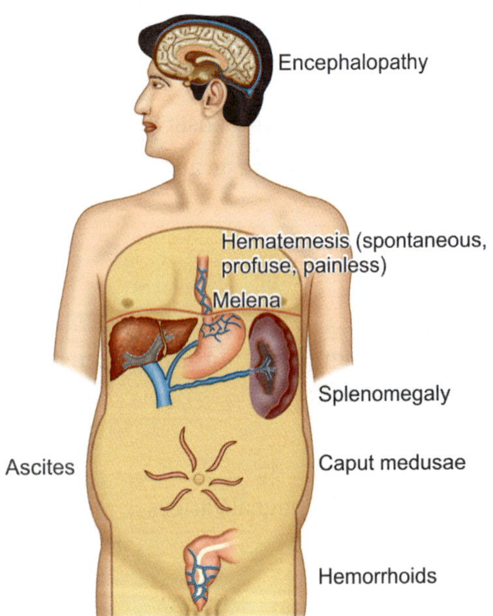

Investigations

Investigations

Laboratory evaluation
- Hematological (to rule out hypersplenism)
- Liver function test
- Coagulation profile
- Viral markers

Imaging
- **Ultrasonography:**
  - To demonstrate presence of ascites, splenomegaly
  - Differentiates EHPVO from intrahepatic PHT
  - In EHPVO, it shows the extent of thrombosis in PV, SV, SMV
- **Doppler USG:**
  - To detect the direction of blood flow
  - Helps in establishing diagnosis of Budd-Chiari syndrome by showing obstruction in hepatic veins and or IVC
- **Spiral CT angiography:**
  - Gives excellent information before planning shunt surgery

Endoscopy
- **Upper GI endoscopy:**
  - To visualize the presence of varices
  - To grade the varices
  - To detect nonvariceal causes of PHT
  - To detect other causes of hematemesis

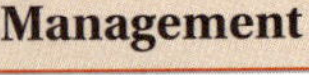

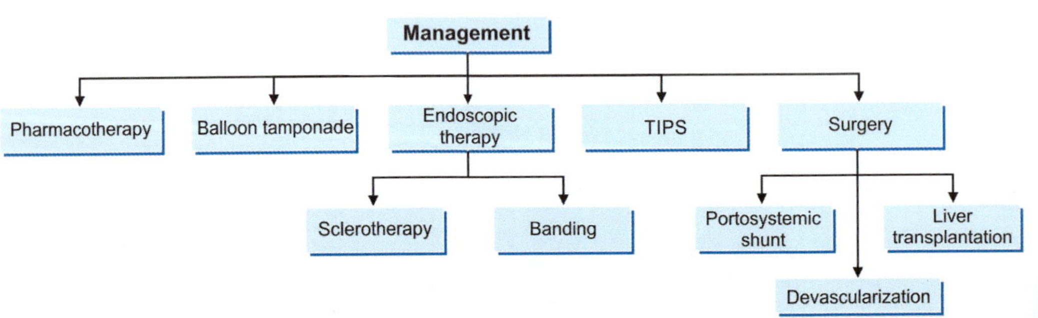

Pharmacotherapy

Splanchnic Vasoconstrictors (↓ Portal Blood Flow)

- **β-blockers**
  - Propranolol causes
  - Splanchnic arteriolar vasoconstriction
    - ↓ portal venous inflow → Venous
    - ↓ heart rate, ↓ cardiac output → ↓ portal venous inflow
- **Vasopressin and its Analog**
  - Terlipressin
  - Glypressin
  - Splanchnic arteriolar vasoconstriction → ↓ portal inflow
- **Hormones**
  - Somatostatin and its analog (e.g., octreotide) → ↓ azygos blood flow

Balloon Tamponade

Indications

- Used in acute life-threatening bleeding from esophageal or gastric varices that not responding to medical therapy, endoscopic hemostasis.
- Immediate endoscopic sclerotherapy not possible due to excessive bleeding obscuring the view.

By Balloon Tamponade System

- Sengstaken-Blakemore tube
- Minnesota tube
- Linton-Nachlas tube

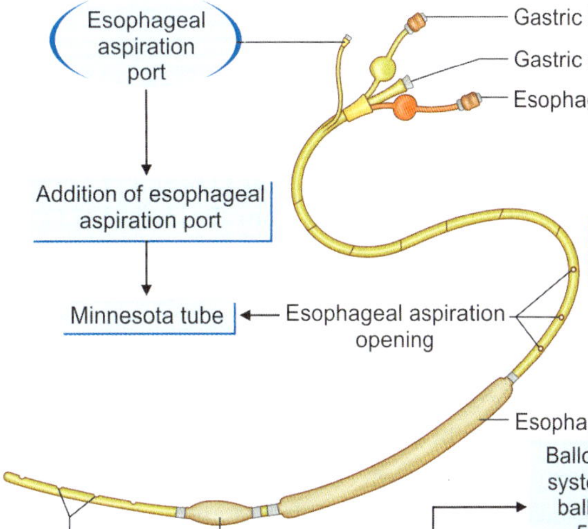

Esophageal aspiration port → Addition of esophageal aspiration port → Minnesota tube ← Esophageal aspiration opening

Gastric balloon → Balloon tamponade system with gastric balloon (capacity 500 mL) only → Linton-Nachlas tube

How balloon tamponade system works?

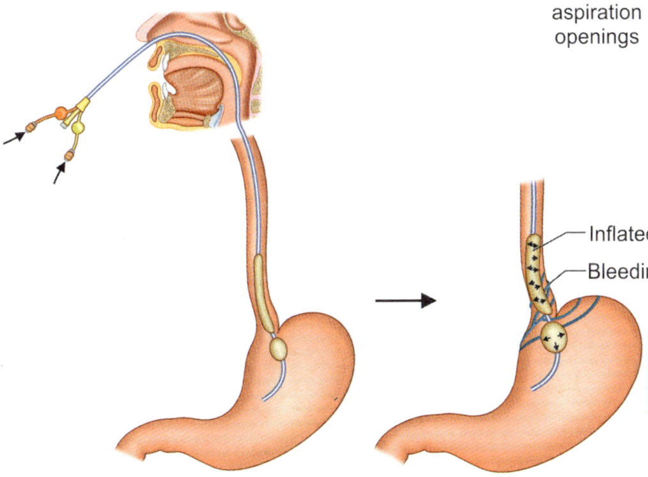

Inflated balloon exerts direct pressure on the varices → Controls bleeding

Endoscopic Treatment

Endoscopic treatment

- Variceal sclerosis
- Variceal ligation

① ②

1. Intravariceal injection
2. Paravariceal (submucosal) injection
3. Intravariceal + paravariceal injection

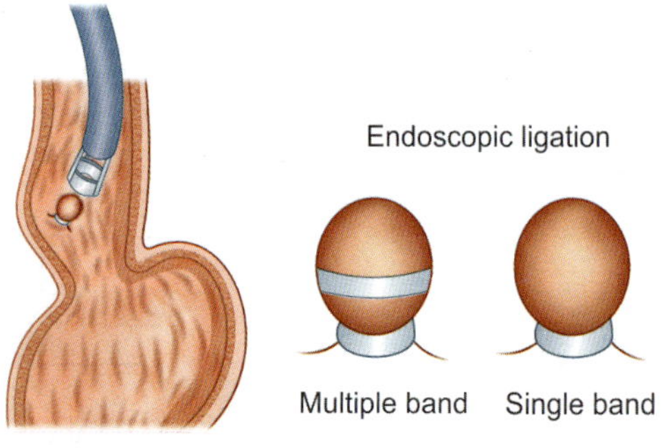

Sclerosants for Variceal Sclerosis

- 1.5% sodium tetradecyl sulfate
- 0.5–1.0% polidocanol
- 5% sodium morrhuate

Transjugular Intrahepatic Portosystemic Shunt (TIPS)

Transjugular intrahepatic portosystemic shunt (TIPS) is a percutaneous method of shunting blood from the portal vein to hepatic vein by placing self-expanding stent graft within the portosystemic tract, thereby reducing the portosystemic pressure gradient. It is an effective method to treat the complications of portal hypertension (e.g., uncontrolled variceal hemorrhage, refractory ascites, hepatic hydrothorax) and as a bridge to liver transplant.

Indications: (i) Uncontrollable variceal hemorrhage; (ii) Current or prior variceal hemorrhage that is not amenable to initial or continued endoscopic therapy; (iii) Prophylaxis against recurrent variceal bleed in high-risk patients; (iv) Portal hypertensive gastropathy or intestinopathy; (v) Refractory ascites; (vi) Hepatic hydrothorax; (vii) Hepatopulmonary syndrome; and (viii) Decompression of portosystemic collaterals prior to abdominal surgical procedures.

Contraindications: *Absolute contraindications*—(i) Congestive cardiac failure; (ii) Multiple hepatic cysts; (iii) Uncontrolled sepsis; and (iv) Severe pulmonary hypertension. *Relative contraindications*—(i) Hepatoma, especially if central; (ii) Obstruction of all hepatic veins; (iii) Portal vein thrombosis; (iv) Severe coagulopathy (INR >5); and (v) Thrombocytopenia (<20,000/cm^3).

Complications: (i) TIPS dysfunction (due to occlusion/ stenosis); (ii) Transcapsular puncture; (iii) Encephalopathy; (iv) Stent migration; (v) Hemolysis; and (vi) Sepsis.

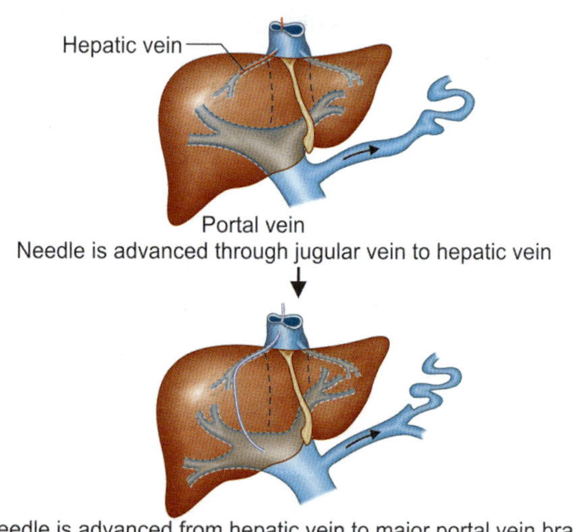

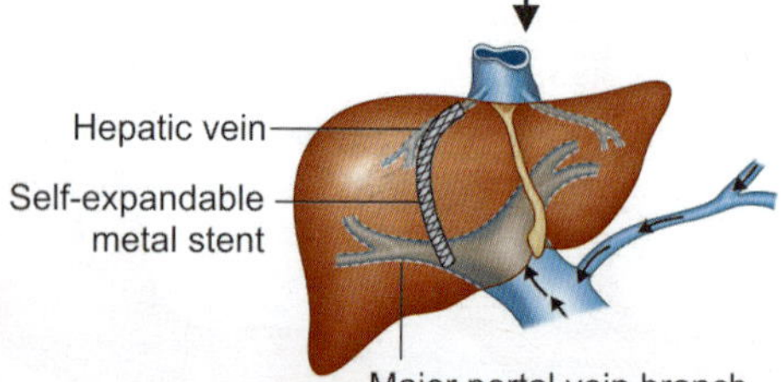

Metal stent is placed between middle hepatic vein and major portal vein branch

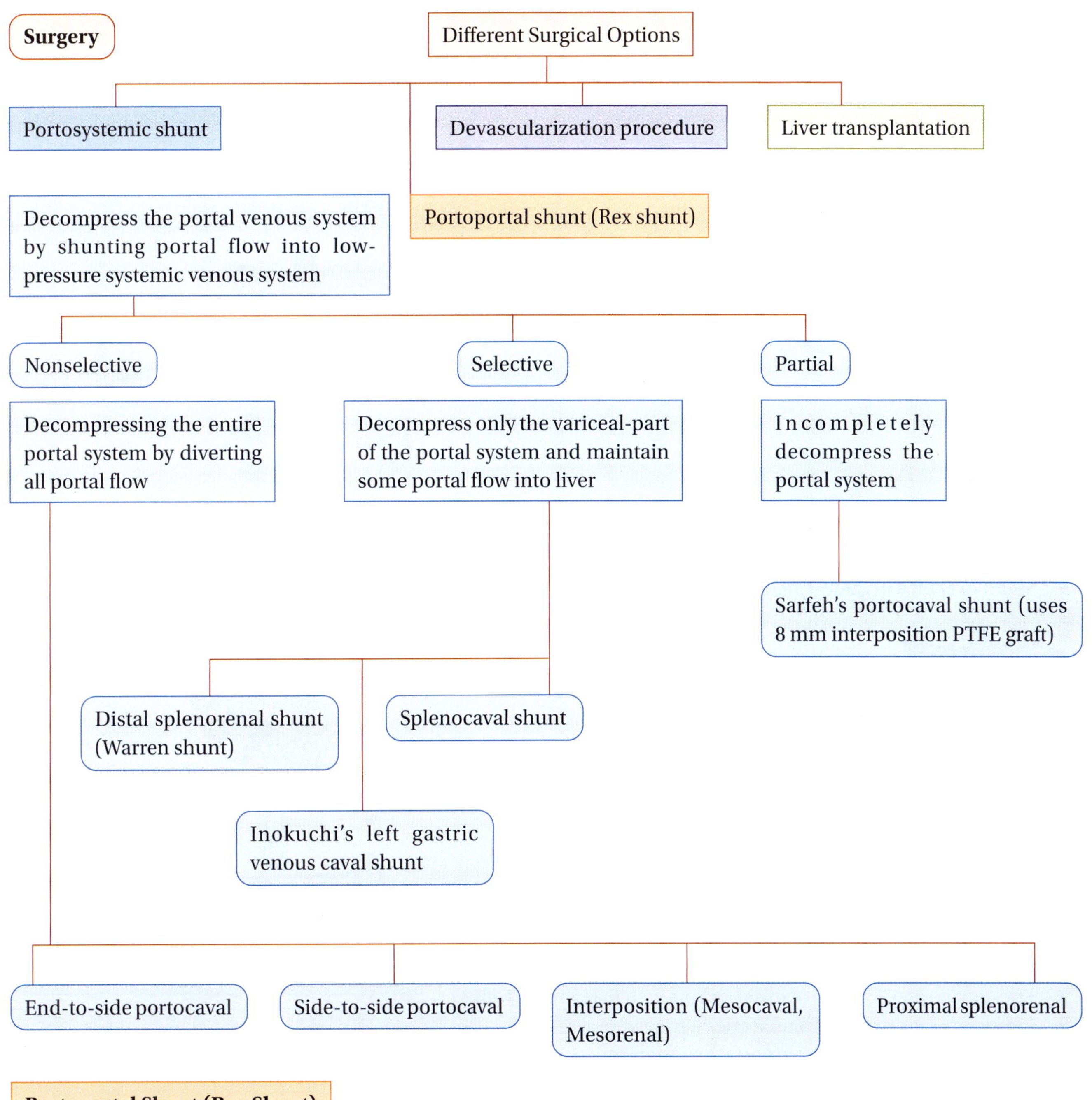

Portoportal Shunt (Rex Shunt)

- Connection between superior mesenteric vein and left portal system at the recessus of Rex
- Indicated in extrahepatic portal vein obstruction

End-to-side Portocaval Shunt

- Portal vein is divided
- End of portal vein is anastomosed to side of IVC

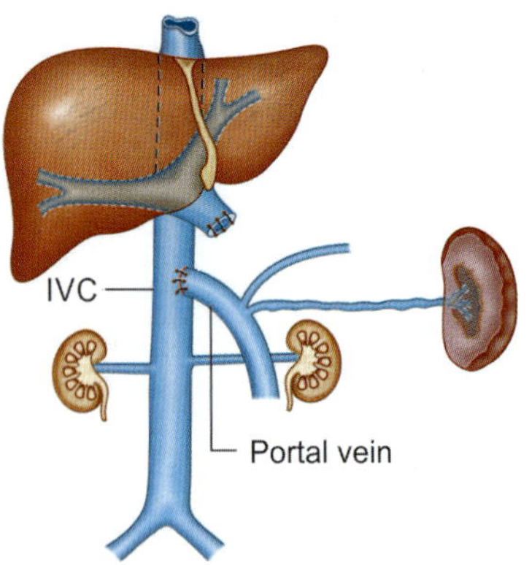

Side-to-side Portocaval Shunt

- Maintain the continuity of portal vein
- Shunt of choice in Budd-Chiari syndrome

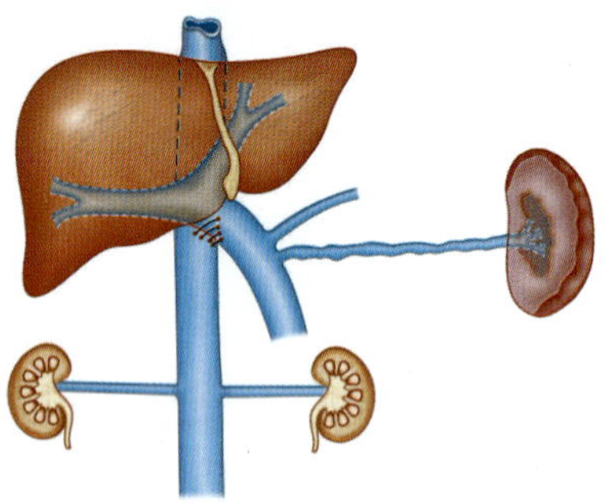

Distal Splenorenal Shunt (Warren Shunt)

- Most common type of selective shunt
- End-to-side anastomosis of distal splenic vein to left renal vein
- Ligation of coronary and pancreatic vein
- Shunt of choice in idiopathic portal hypertension

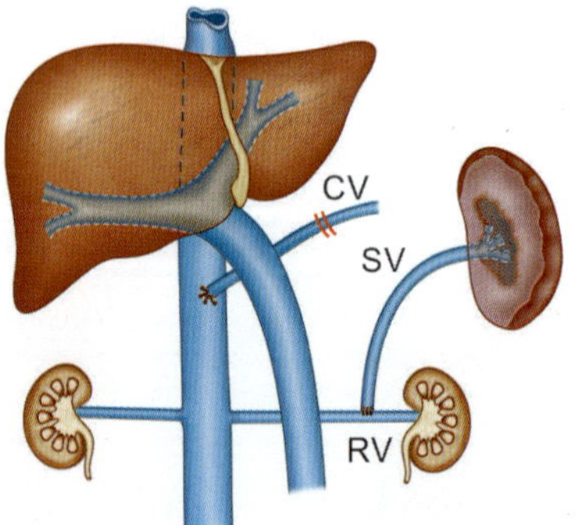

Interposition (Mesocaval, Mesorenal) Shunt

- Interposing a conduit of autologous vein graft or synthetic graft between superior mesenteric vein and IVC (mesocaval) or renal vein (mesorenal)
- Internal jugular vein as autologous vein graft
- Dacron or PTFE as synthetic graft

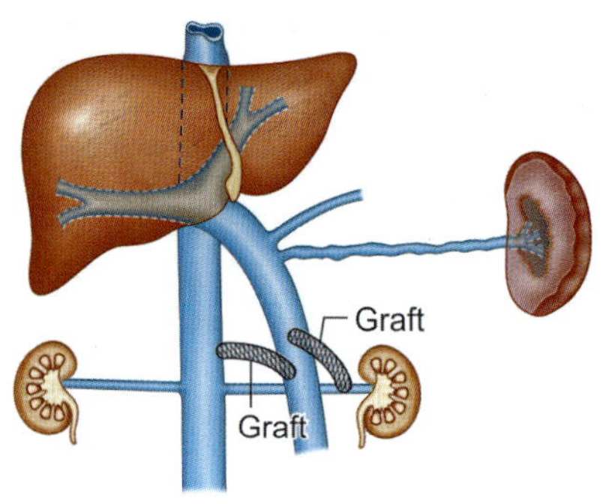

Proximal Splenorenal Shunt

- Splenectomy is done
- Hilar end of splenic vein is anastomosed to renal vein

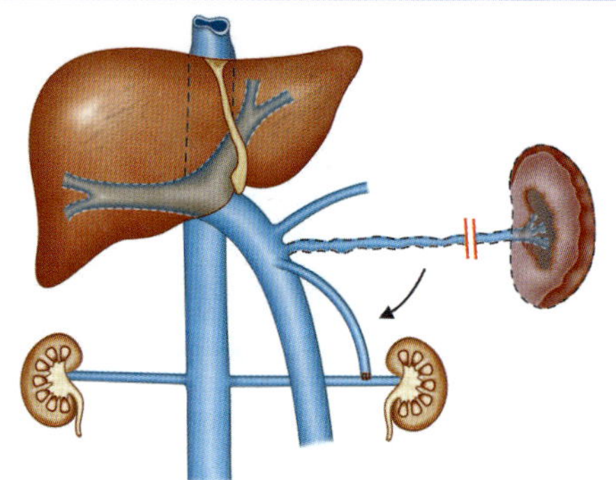

Sarfeh's Portocaval Shunt

Shunt between portal vein and IVC using 8 mm interposition PTFE graft

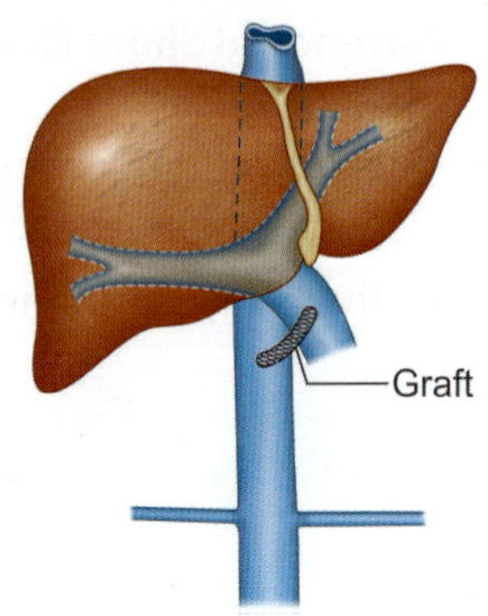

Esophagogastric Devascularization Procedures

Indications:
In patients with esophageal varices but with an unsuitable anatomy for portosystemic shunt.

Sugiura procedure

Most commonly practiced devascularization procedure.
Comprises distal esophagus and proximal gastric devascularization, esophageal transection followed by end-to-end anastomosis, splenectomy

Modified Hassab procedure

Comprises devascularization of distal esophagus and proximal esophagus, vagotomy with pyloroplasty, splenectomy.

Johnston procedure

Esophageal transection and reanastomosis

Mathur procedure

Devascularization of distal esophagus and proximal stomach, esophageal transection and reanastomosis, Nissen fundoplication with or without splenectomy.

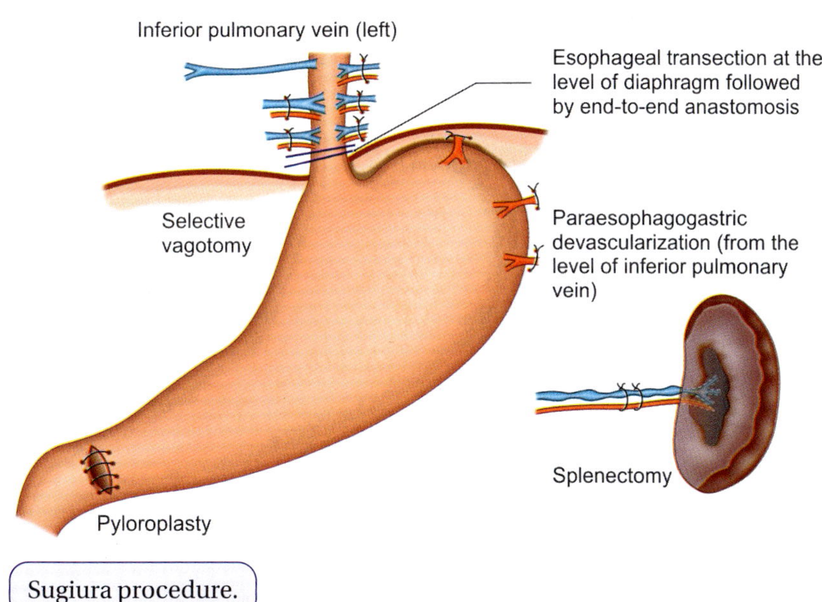

Sugiura procedure.

Management of Variceal Hemorrhage (based on AASLD Guideline)

Prevention of first variceal hemorrhage

High-risk small esophageal varices

By nonselective beta-blockers (propanolol, nadolol)

Medium or large varices

Nonselective beta-blockers, Carvedilol or endoscopic variceal ligation

Management of Acute Variceal Hemorrhage

- "Restrictive" PRBC transfusion (hemoglobin threshold of 9 g/dL and maintaining it at 9–11 g/dL)
- Antibiotic prophylaxis with ceftriaxone (1 g/day) for maximum 7 days
- Vasoactive drugs as IV infusion (somatostatin, octreotide, terlipressin, vasopressin)

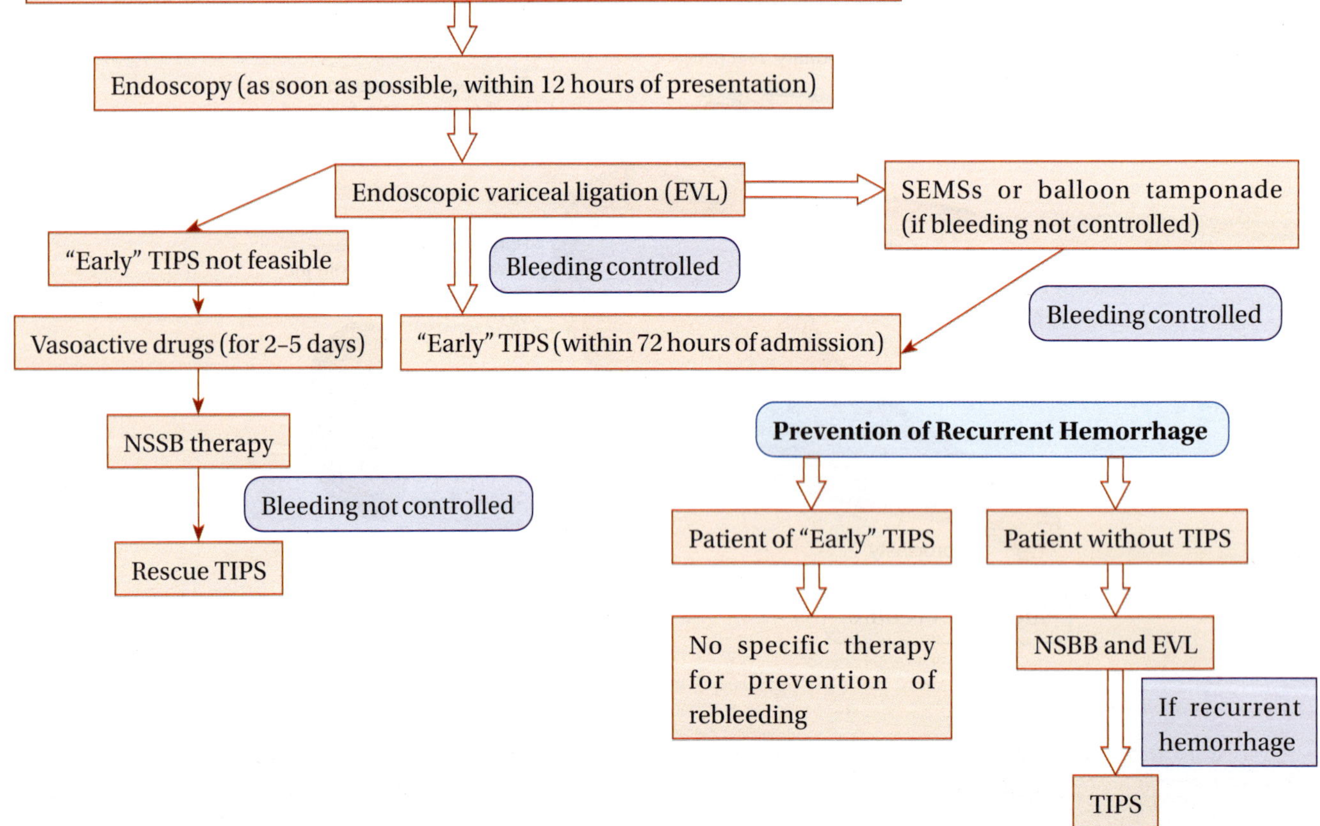

Case 1

History and Physical Examination

A 40-year-old male patient presented in the emergency department with complain of pain in right upper abdomen with fever with chill and rigor. The pain and fever started 4 days back. He consulted with local physician and started oral antibiotics, but no such improvement.

No history of similar abdominal pain. No history of any surgical intervention or blood transfusion.

Patient was a chronic smoker (20 biris/day), occasional drinker, but no history of drug abuse.

Physical examination

Patient alert, conscious

Temperature—102°F

Pulse—110/min, BP—116/84 mm Hg, Respiratory rate—22/min

Examination of abdomen:

- Tenderness in right hypochondrium, local guarding
- Intercostal tenderness—present
- On auscultation, diminished breath sound on right side, IPS—normal

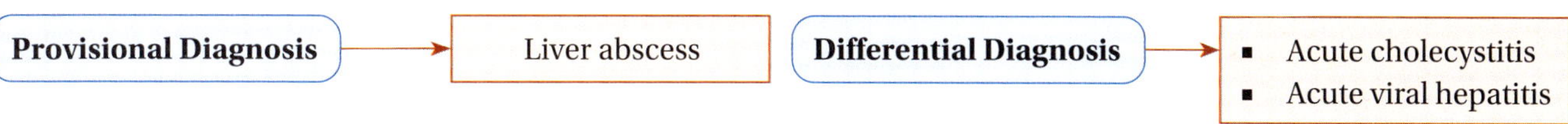

Investigations

Hb—10.2 gm%, Total leukocyte count—18,000/cumm, Fasting sugar—88 mg/dL, Serum creatinine—0.9 mg/dL, AST and ALT—within normal limit, INR—1.2

USG abdomen—a 6.0 × 5.4 × 5.0 cm abscess in right lobe of liver.

CT abdomen—a 6.5 × 5.2 × 5.4 cm abscess involving segment VII and VIII. Another 2.0 × 2.0 × 3.5 cm abscess in segment V.

Discussion

In history—Pain in right upper abdomen with fever with chill and rigor.

Physical examination—(i) Tenderness in right hypochondrium; (ii) Presence of intercostal tenderness; and (iii) Diminished breath sound on right side.

Both history and clinical findings in favor of liver abscess (pyogenic/amebic). Laboratory findings—Leukocytosis (18,000/cumm)—in favor of pyogenic abscess.

USG and CT findings—suggestive of abscess in liver.

Management Algorithm

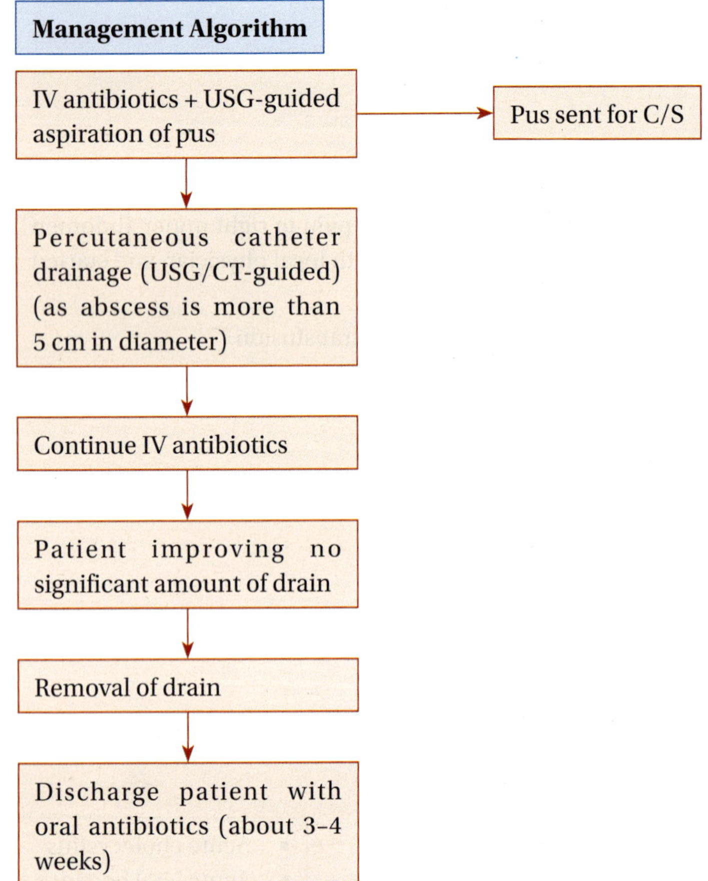

Case 2

History and Physical Examination

A 37-year-old female patient presented with intermittent pain in the right upper abdomen with occasional fever. The pain was dull aching in nature, not associated with any type of food intake. No history of vomiting. No history of jaundice.

No history of hospital admission, hypertension, diabetes.

No history of addiction. History of OCP use for last 10 years.

Physical examination

Temperature—98.4°F

Pulse—86/min, BP—110/82 mm Hg, Respiratory rate—16/min

Examination of abdomen:

- Mild tenderness in right hypochondrium
- A 3 × 3 cm firm lump palpable in right hypochondrium that moves with respiration.

Investigations

Laboratory findings: Hb—11.3 gm%, Total leukocyte count—7,000/cumm, Fasting sugar—72 mg/dL, Serum creatinine—0.8 mg/dL, AST and ALT—within normal limit.

Imaging

USG abdomen: Multivesicular cyst with 'honeycomb appearance' in right lobe of liver 4.0 × 3.2 × 4.2 cm (WHO CE2 type)

CT abdomen: Cyst in right lobe of liver with multiple daughter cysts.

Serological test: IgG—ELISA—Positive.

Discussion

- In history—suggestive of pathology related to liver or gallbladder.
- Physical examination—Firm lump in right hypochondrium—most likely related to liver or gallbladder
- Laboratory findings—not suggestive.
- USG and CT abdomen—both imagings suggestive of hydatid cyst of liver.
- Serological test—also confirmatory

Management Algorithm

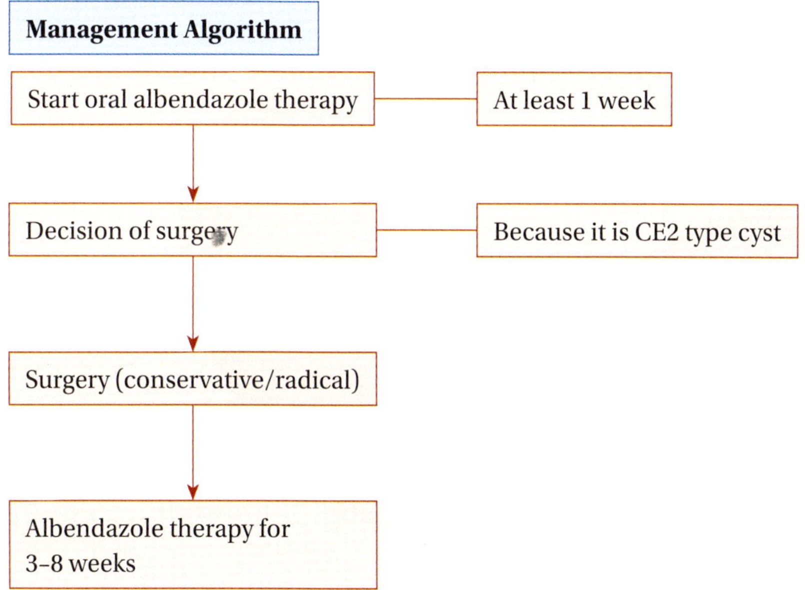

Chapter 6

Diseases of Pancreas

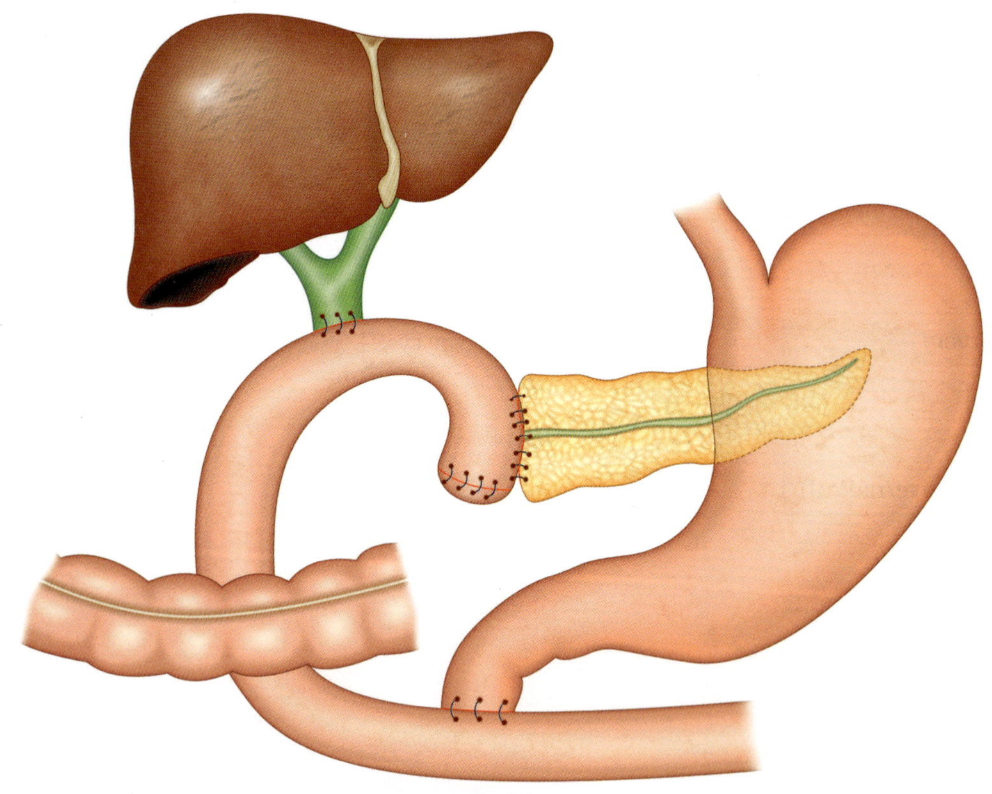

Important Topics

- Acute Pancreatitis
- Chronic Pancreatitis
- Cystic Neoplasms of the Pancreas
- Pancreatic Carcinoma
- Pancreatic Stent
- Endoscopic Ultrasound

'Seeing is an experience. A retinal reaction is only a physical state .... People, not their eyes, see. Cameras and eye-balls, are blind .... there is more to seeing than meets the eyeball.'

Norwood Russell Hanson (1924–1967)
American Philosopher of Science

Acute Pancreatitis

Etiology

- **Gallstone (most common cause)**
- Alcohol abuse
- Idiopathic **(often due to occult microlithiasis)**
- Hypertriglyceridemia
- Drugs
- Trauma
- Anatomical abnormalities of pancreas **(Annular pancreas)**
- Post-ERCP
- Infectious
- Hypercalcemia
- Genetic **(cystic fibrosis gene—*CFTR* gene)**
- Malignancy **(particularly IPMN)**

Drugs Causing Acute Pancreatitis

- Azathioprine
- 6-mercaptopurine
- Tetracycline
- Didanosine
- Valproic acid
- Pentamidine

Infections Causing Acute Pancreatitis

Viral infection (mumps, coxsackie, hepatitis B, cytomegalovirus, herpes simplex, varicella- zoster)

Bacterial infection (*Legionella, Mycoplasma, Salmonella, Leptospira*)

Fungal infection (Aspergillus)

Parasitic infection (*Toxoplasma, Cryptosporidium*)

Post-ERCP Pancreatitis

"New or worsened abdominal pain with lipase at least three times the upper limit of normal at more than 24 hours after the ERCP, requiring hospital admission or prolongation of planned admission".

Risk Factors: (1) *Patient related:* (i) Female patient; (ii) Previous episode of pancreatitis; and (iii) Suspected sphincter of Oddi dysfunction; (2) *Procedure related:* (i) Cannulation attempts duration >10 min; (ii) Pancreatic guidewire passages >1; and (iii) Injection of contrast medium into pancreatic duct.

Prophylaxis: (i) Diclofenac or indomethacin 100 mg rectally immediately before or after ERCP; and (ii) Prophylactic stent placement (for high-risk ERCPs).

Pathophysiology

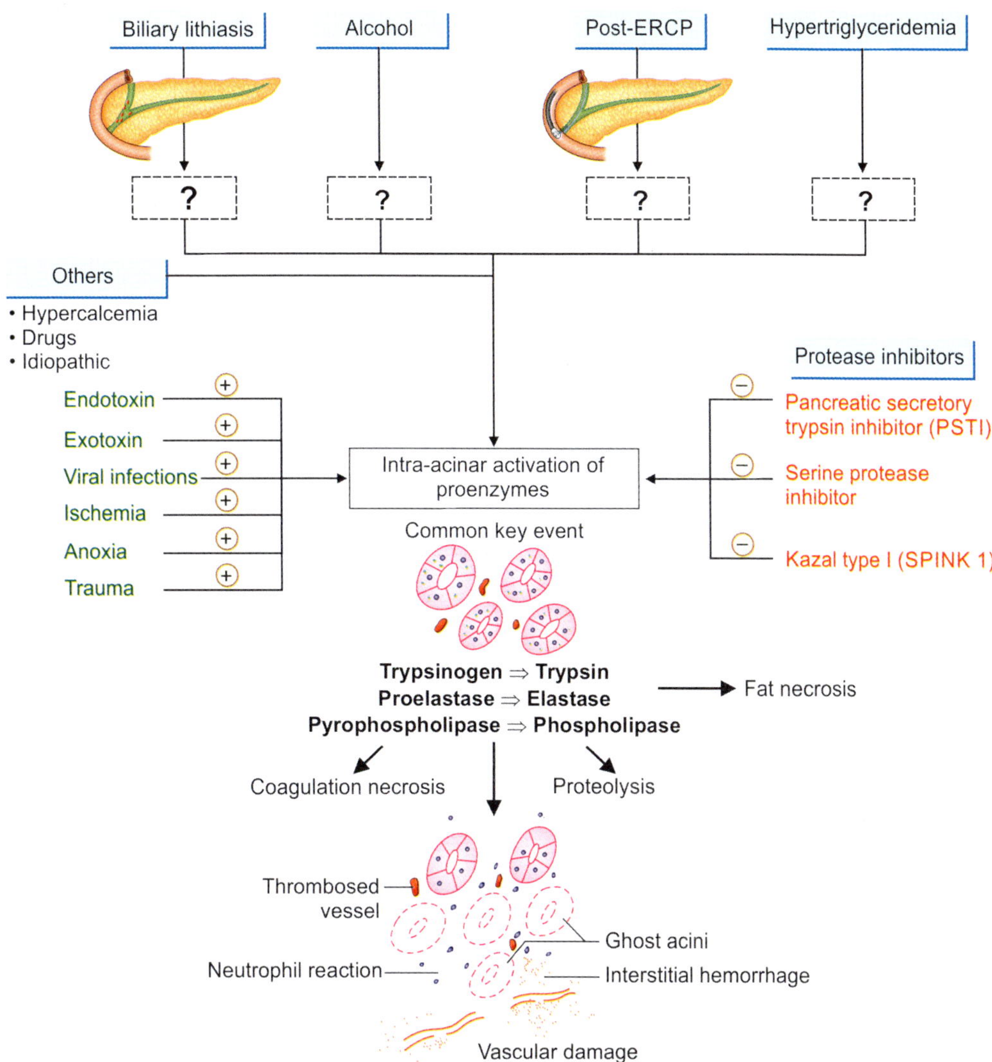

Definition of Acute Pancreatitis

The definition of acute pancreatitis is based on fulfillment of two out of three criteria:

1. Abdominal pain consistent with acute pancreatitis (acute onset, severe epigastric pain often radiating to the back)
2. Serum lipase or amylase at least three times greater than the upper limit of normal.
3. Characteristic findings of acute pancreatitis on contrast-enhanced CT and less commonly MRI or transabdominal ultrasonography.

Classification of Acute Pancreatitis and their Complications

Based on Revised Atlanta Consensus Classification, 2012

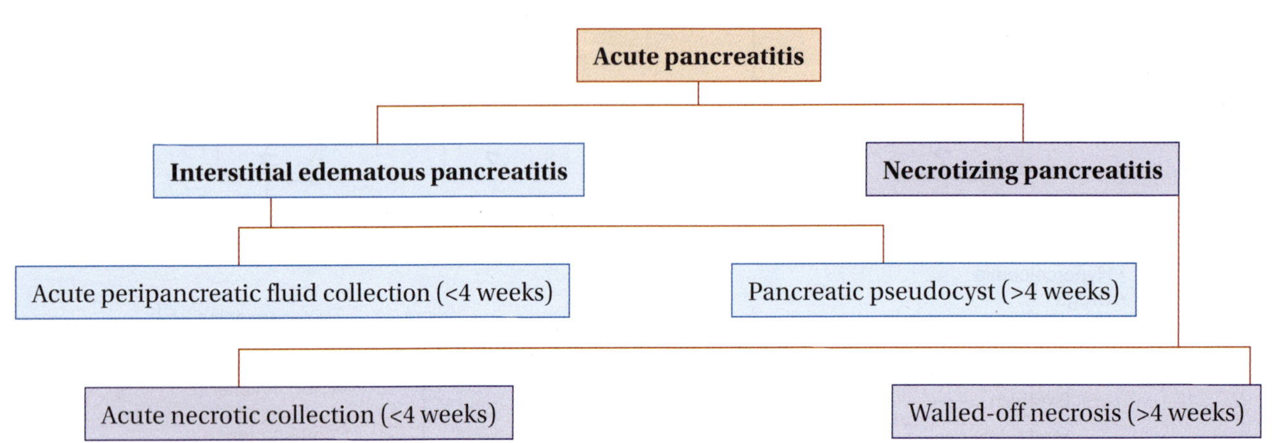

Interstitial edematous pancreatitis: Acute inflammation of the pancreatic parenchyma and peripancreatic tissues, but without recognizable tissue necrosis.

Necrotizing pancreatitis: Inflammation associated with pancreatic parenchymal necrosis and/or peripancreatic necrosis.

Acute peripancreatic fluid collection (APFC): Peripancreatic fluid associated with interstitial edematous pancreatitis with no associated peripancreatic necrosis, seen within the first 4 weeks after onset of pancreatitis and without the features of a pseudocyst.

Pancreatic pseudocyst: An encapsulated collection of fluid with a well-defined inflammatory wall usually outside the pancreas with minimal or no necrosis, occurs more than 4 weeks after onset of interstitial edematous pancreatitis to mature.

Acute necrotic collection (ANC): A collection containing variable amounts of both fluid and necrosis associated with necrotizing pancreatitis; the necrosis can involve the pancreatic parenchyma and/or the peripancreatic tissues.

Walled-off necrosis (WON): A mature, encapsulated collection of pancreatic and/or peripancreatic necrosis that has developed a well-defined inflammatory wall, usually occurs >4 weeks after onset of necrotizing pancreatitis.

Phases of Acute Pancreatitis

Early phase: Usually lasts for the first week, may extend into the second week.

Late phase: Persists for weeks to months

Clinical Presentation

- Acute onset, severe epigastric pain, often radiating to the back, aggravated by movement, coughing and relieved by leaning forward position.
- Anorexia, nausea, vomiting
- Localized epigastric tenderness of variable intensity
- Tender, distended abdomen
- Reduced bowel sound (if associated paralytic ileus)
- Tachycardia, hypotension
- Reduced breath sound (due to pleural effusion)
- Hemorrhagic pancreatitis (rare) may present with ecchymoses of the periumbilical skin (Cullen sign), in flanks (Grey-Turner's sign) or over the inguinal ligament (Fox's sign).

In acute pancreatitis, pleural effusion commonly present on left side.

Signs in Acute Pancreatitis

- **Cullen sign**
- **Grey Turner's sign**
- **Fox's sign**
- **Colon cut-off sign** in straight X-ray of abdomen, abrupt cut-off of colonic gas shadow beyond the splenic flexure.
- **"Sentinel loop" sign** in straight X-ray of abdomen, isolated distended loop of bowel due to underlying inflamed organ.

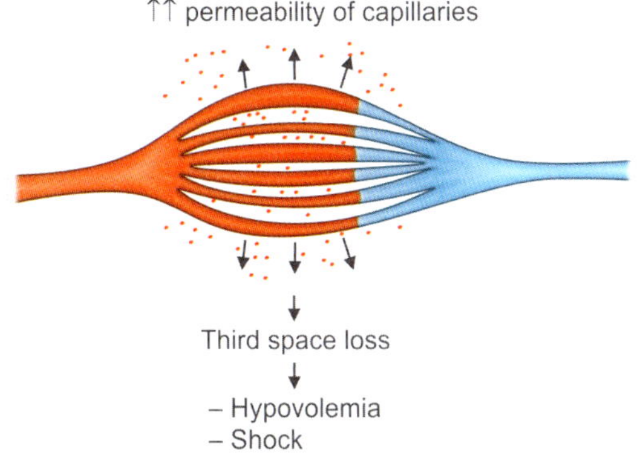

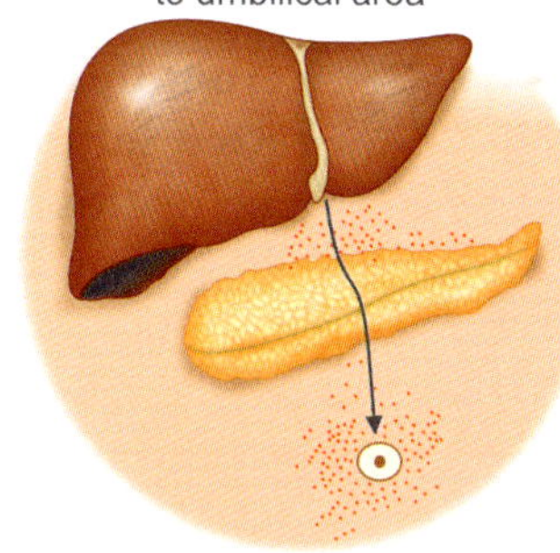

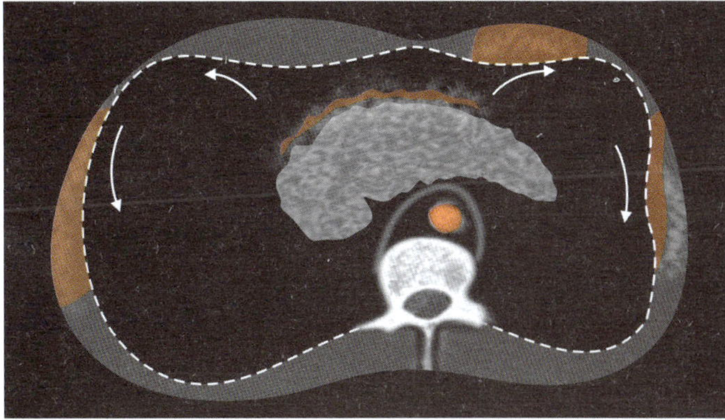

Diagnosis

Any two of the three

Classic clinical presentation

Acute onset, severe epigastric pain often radiating to the back

Serum lipase (or amylase) activity

At least three times greater than the upper limit of normal

Imaging

- Contrast-enhanced CT abdomen
- Magnetic resonance imaging
- Transabdominal USG

Elevated lipase or amylase level do not predict prognosis or severity of pancreatitis.

Serum amylase is elevated in other acute abdominal (e.g., peptic perforation) and extra-abdominal pathologies (e.g., sialadenitis).

Serum lipase is elevated within 4–8 hour, peaks at 24 hour and return to normal level over the next 8–14 days.

Serum amylase commonly elevated within 6–24 hours, reaches peak at 48 hours and return to normal level within 3–7 days.

Serum lipase level may not be raised in: (i) Severe necrotizing pancreatitis; and (ii) Acute on chronic pancreatitis

Imaging study is usually not required for diagnosis.

CT is indicated for diagnostic purposes if: (i) prolonged period between onset of symptoms and presentation; and (ii) suspicion of duodenal perforation.

Initial Investigations to Determine the Etiology

- Serum triglycerides
- Serum calcium
- Transabdominal USG of upper abdomen

Serum lipase is more reliable and specific diagnostic marker of acute pancreatitis than serum amylase.

Indications and Timing of Initial CT in Acute Pancreatitis

- Diagnosis is uncertain
- Patient not responding to conservative management
- Patient clinically deteriorating
- Confirmation of severity assessed by clinical predictors
- Optimal timing is at least 72–96 hours after onset of symptoms

Why early CT is not recommended in acute pancreatitis?

Pancreatic and peripancreatic necrosis become obvious in CT after 72 hours of onset of acute pancreatitis.

CT scoring system is not superior to clinical staging system in predicting prognosis and severity of disease.

For discriminating between viable and nonviable pancreatic tissue, pancreatic and portal venous phase in CT are sufficient.

To distinguish between pseudocyst and walled-off necrosis, MR is the preferred imaging modality.

Endoscopic ultrasonography (EUS) is indicated for occult microlithiasis, neoplasms and chronic pancreatitis in idiopathic acute pancreatitis. Secretin-stimulated MRCP and CT are indicated if EUS is negative.

Assessment of Severity

Predictive scoring systems: (i) APACHE II (1989); (ii) Ranson (1974); (iii) Modified Glasgow Score (2003); and (iv) BISAP (2008).

SIRS at admission and **Persistent SIRS at 48 hours** [As per IAP/APA guideline]

Persistent (>48 hours) organ failure [As per Revised Atlanta Classification]

Single serum markers: (i) C-reactive protein; (ii) Procalcitonin; (iii) Hematocrit; and (iv) Blood urea nitrogen

CT scoring system (Mortele modified CT severity index, Balthazar CT severity index)

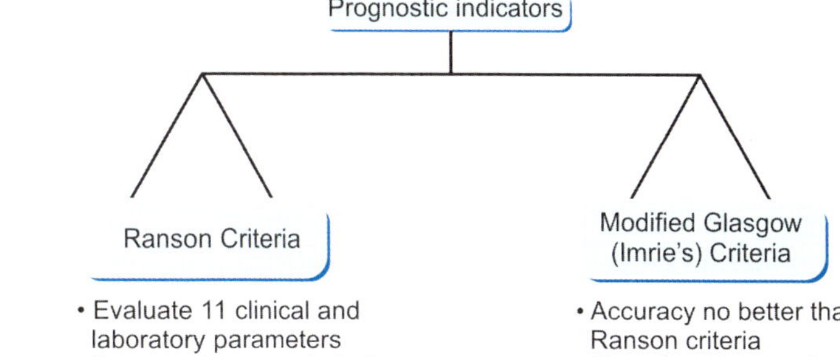

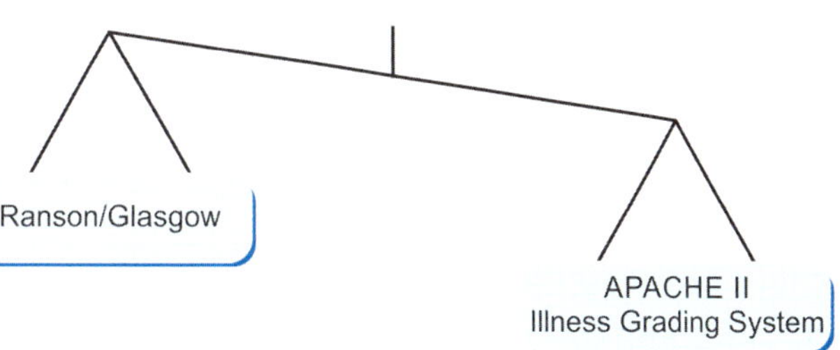

- Allocates three sets of points: A, B, C
  - **A** – Assessment of clinical parameters, e.g., vital signs, electrolytes, arterial blood gas
  - **B** – Points allocated in accordance with age
  - **C** – Points allocated for comorbid disease or chronic health of patient
- Can be employed throughout the courses of the disease to follow progression and response to therapy

SIRS (Systemic inflammatory response syndrome) is defined by two or more of the following four criterias

(i) Temperature <36°C (96.8°F) or >38°C (100.4°F)

(ii) Heart rate >90/min

(iii) Respiratory rate >20/min

(iv) White blood cells (<4 × 10^9/L, >12 × 10^9/L) or 10% bands

Modified Glasgow (Imrie's) criteria

At 48 hours after admission

- PaO_2 <59.3 mm Hg
- Age >55 years
- WBC >15 × 10^9/L
- Calcium <8 mg/dL
- BUN >44.4 mg/dL
- LDH >600 IU/L
- Albumin <3.2 g/dL
- Glucose >180 mg/dL

Modified Ranson criteria (for gallstone pancreatitis)

On admission

- Age >70 years
- WBC >18,000/cumm
- Blood glucose >220 mg/dL
- Serum AST >250 IU/L
- Serum LDH >400 IU/L

At 48 hours

- Serum calcium <8 mg/dL
- Hematocrit fall greater than 10% from admission
- BUN increase >2 mg/dL
- Base deficit >5 mg/dL
- Fluid needs >4 L

Total 10 parameters, maximum score 10.

Ranson criteria (for non-gallstone pancreatitis)

On admission

- Age >55 years
- WBC >16,000/cumm
- Blood glucose >200 mg/dL
- Serum AST >250 IU/L
- Serum LDH >350 IU/L

At 48 hours

- Serum calcium <8 mg/dL
- Hematocrit fall greater than 10% from admission
- BUN increase >5 mg/dL
- Arterial PaO_2 <60 mm Hg
- Base deficit >4 mg/dL
- Fluid needs >6 L

Total 11 parameters, each positive parameter is assigned with 1 point. Maximum score is 11.

Grading of Severity of Acute Pancreatitis (as per revised Atlanta classification)

Mild acute pancreatitis: (i) No organ failure; and (ii) No local or systemic complications

Moderately severe acute pancreatitis: Organ failure that resolves within 48 hours (transient organ failure) and/or local or systemic complications without persistent organ failure.

Severe acute pancreatitis: Persistent organ failure (>48 hours), either single organ failure or multiple organ failure.

Organ failure is defined as a score of 2 or more for one of these organ systems (respiratory, cardiovascular, and renal) using the modified Marshall scoring system

Grading of Severity of Acute Pancreatitis (Determinant-based classification)

Mild acute pancreatitis: No organ failure AND No (peri) pancreatic necrosis

Moderate acute pancreatitis: Transient organ failure AND/OR Sterile (peri) pancreatic necrosis

Severe acute pancreatitis: Persistent organ failure OR Infected (peri) pancreatic necrosis

Critical acute pancreatitis: Persistent organ failure AND Infected (peri) pancreatic necrosis

Mortele Modified CTSI Scoring (2004)

Normal pancreas	0 point
Intrinsic pancreatic abnormalities with or without inflammatory changes in peripancreatic fat	2 points
Pancreatic or peripancreatic fluid collection or peripancreatic fat necrosis	4 points

Necrosis absent	0 point
<30% necrosis	2 points
>30% necrosis	4 points

To the above score, 2 points are added for the presence of extrapancreatic finding (pleural effusion, ascites, vascular complications, parenchymal complications or gastrointestinal tract involvement).

Total score is then categorized as:

Mild pancreatitis	Score 0–2
Moderate pancreatitis	Score 4–6
Severe pancreatitis	Score 8–10

Balthazar CT Severity Index (1990)

Balthazar original grading system + Presence and extent of pancreatic necrosis

Necrosis absent	0 point
<30% necrosis	2 points
30–50% necrosis	4 points
>50% necrosis	6 points

Balthazar CTSI is calculated by adding the score of Grade A–E and score of necrosis. Total score is then categorized as:

Mild pancreatitis	CTSI score 0–3
Moderate pancreatitis	CTSI score 4–6
Severe pancreatitis	CTSI score 7–10

Balthazar Original Grading System (1985)

Grade A	Normal pancreas	0 point
Grade B	Focal or diffuse enlargement of pancreas	1 point
Grade C	Intrinsic pancreatic abnormalities with inflammatory changes in peripancreatic fat	2 points
Grade D	Single ill-defined fluid collection (phlegmon)	3 points
Grade E	Two or multiple, poorly defined fluid collections or presence of gas in or adjacent to the pancreas	4 points

Management

Fluid Resuscitation

Recommended fluid: Ringer's lactate. **Optimal infusion rate** for initial fluid resuscitation 5–10 mL/kg/h

Resuscitation goals: Heart rate <120/min; Mean arterial pressure 65–85 mm Hg; Urinary output >0.5–1 mL/kg/h; hematocrit 35–44%. Measuring stroke volume variation, intrathoracic blood volume determination are newly emerging invasive approach to monitor response to fluid resuscitation in critical care settings.

Early fluid resuscitation can reduce the risk of SIRS, organ failure, in-hospital mortality but cannot prevent development of necrosis.

Antibiotic Prophylaxis

Routine antibiotic prophylaxis is not recommended. Prophylactic antibiotics in acute pancreatitis are not associated with significant mortality or morbidity.

Systemic antibiotic (coverage against both aerobic and anaerobic gram-negative and gram-positive organisms) should be given if strong clinical suspicion of infection of necrotizing pancreatitis.

Nutritional Support

Enteral nutrition or parenteral nutrition: Enteral nutrition is associated with decreased systemic complications, multiorgan failure, need for surgical intervention and mortality.

Oral feeding or enteral tube feeding: Enteral tube feeding is indicated in patients with predicted severe acute pancreatitis requiring nutritional support.

Timing of restarting oral feeding: Once abdominal pain is decreasing and inflammatory markers are improving.

Enteral tube feeding (Nasogastric or Nasojejunal): Nasojejunal feeding is indicated when patient cannot tolerate nasogastric feeding.

Indications of parenteral nutrition: (i) Patient cannot tolerate enteral tube feeding; (ii) Nutritional goals cannot achieved with enteral feeding; and (iii) Enteral nutrition is contraindicated.

Management of Abdominal Compartment Syndrome

(1) Medical management:

- Nasogastric drainage
- Prokinetics
- Rectal tube placement
- Adequate analgesia and sedation
- Fluid resuscitation on demand

(2) Invasive decompression:

- Percutaneous catheter drainage of ascites
- Midline laparostomy
- Bilateral subcostal laparostomy
- Subcutaneous linea alba fasciotomy

Management of Biliary Pancreatitis

Mild Biliary Pancreatitis

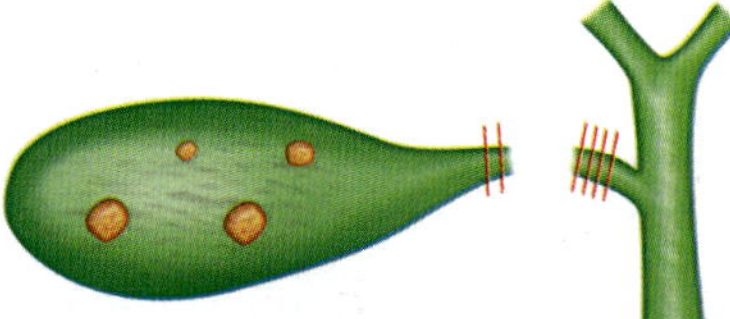

Biliary Pancreatitis with Cholangitis

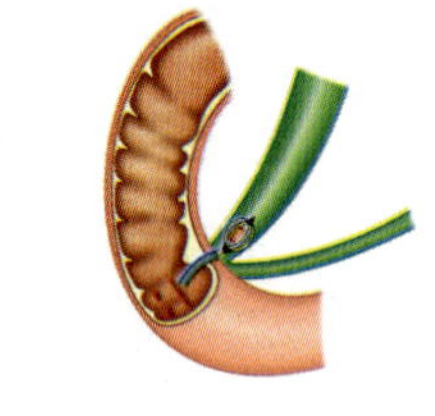

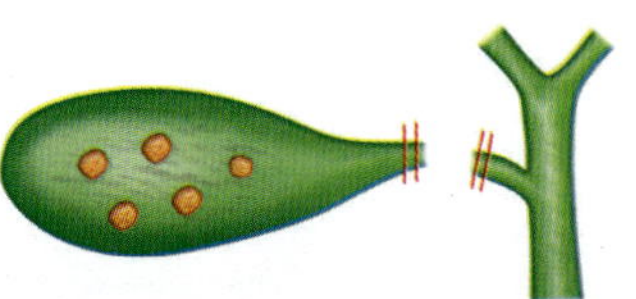

Urgent ERCP (<24 hours) is indicated in acute cholangitis.

Management of Necrotizing Pancreatitis

Indications for Intervention in Necrotizing Pancreatitis

- Clinically suspected (i.e., persistent fever, elevated inflammatory markers, gas in peripancreatic collections on CT) or documented (by FNA) infected necrotizing pancreatitis with clinical deterioration
- Ongoing organ failure for several weeks with associated walled-off necrosis (WON)
- Gastric outlet obstruction or biliary obstruction due to mass effect of large WON

Management of Infected Pancreatic Necrosis or Walled-off Necrosis (WON)

Principles of management: Early organ support and nutritional optimization followed by delayed intervention (>4 weeks) by minimally invasive intervention with a step-up approach.

Different methods of intervention:

- Percutaneous catheter drainage
- Video-assisted retroperitoneal debridement (VARD)
- Minimally invasive retroperitoneal (MIRP) necrosectomy
- Endoscopic transluminal necrosectomy
- Open surgical necrosectomy with open packing/with closed packing/with continuous closed postoperative lavage/programmed open necrosectomy

Timing of intervention: About 4 weeks after onset of symptoms, when walled-off necrosis (with full encapsulation) is documented on CECT [Early intervention in first 2 weeks increases the risk of mortality and morbidity (e.g., bleeding, perforation)].

Percutaneous Catheter Drainage (PCD)

The least invasive technique for management of infected pancreatic necrosis.

Under CT or USG guidance, a pigtail catheter is placed (by Seldinger or Trocar technique) in the most dependent part of the collection.

Advantages: (i) Technically not demanding; and (ii) Facility widely available

Complications: (i) Dislodging or clogging of catheter; (ii) Intestinal perforation; and (iii) External pancreatic fistula.

Video-assisted Retroperitoneal Debridement (VARD)

VARD is always a part of "Step-up approach".

A left subcostal incision (4–5 cm) is given one or two fingers below the left costal margin over the midaxillary line, near the percutaneous drain.

A zero-degree laparoscope is introduced through the incision and necrosis is removed by the ring forceps (introduced parallel to the videoscope) under full videoscopic vision. Only loose necrotic part is removed to avoid complication of bleeding. Two large bore surgical drains are placed into the collection.

Complications: (i) Bleeding; (ii) Pancreatic fistula; (iii) Perforation of intestine; and (iv) Incisional hernia.

Minimally Invasive Retroperitoneal Necrosectomy (MIRP)

- Modification of open lateral approach.
- Access is achieved by placing ports at the site of percutaneous catheter. Debridement is performed using instruments through the working port. A pigtail catheter is introduced into the acute necrotic collection after debridement of pancreatic and peripancreatic necrosis.

Endoscopic Transluminal Necrosectomy

Under EUS guidance, through the stomach wall, the necrotic collection is punctured. Two pigtail drains and one nasocystic catheter are placed in the collection.

If no clinical improvement within 72 hours, endoscopic necrosectomy is performed through this tract.

Open Necrosectomy

Indications: (i) Lack of expertise and instrumentation related to minimally invasive or endoscopic approach; and (ii) Presence of complications like perforation or necrosis.

- In open necrosectomy with **open packing approach**, abdomen is left open after debridement and packing the cavity.
- In open necrosectomy with **closed packing approach**, abdomen is closed after thorough debridement and packing.
- In open necrosectomy with **continuous closed postoperative lavage approach**, large-bore drains are placed in a closed peripancreatic compartment for postoperative continuous lavage.
- In **programmed open necrosectomy approach**, limited debridement every 48 hours through the abdomen (closed by zipper or mesh to the fascial edges of the wound).

Management of Pseudocyst

Indications for treatment of pseudocyst:

Symptomatic (e.g., abdominal pain, gastric outlet obstruction, early satiety, jaundice): Presence of complications (infection, bleeding, rupture, fistulization to adjacent hollow organs)

Treatment options for pseudocyst: (i) Percutaneous drainage; (ii) Endoscopic transpapillary drainage; (iii) Endoscopic transmural drainage; (iv) Open cyst-gastrostomy; (v) Open cyst-duodenostomy; (vi) Open cyst-jejunostomy; and (vii) Laparoscopic pancreatic pseudocyst drainage.

Causes of Pseudocyst

- Acute pancreatitis
- Chronic pancreatitis
- Pancreatic trauma

Factors associated with less likelihood of spontaneous resolution:

- Cyst presenting for more than 6 weeks
- Cyst greater than 6 cm in diameter
- Cyst associated with chronic pancreatitis

Complications of Pseudocyst

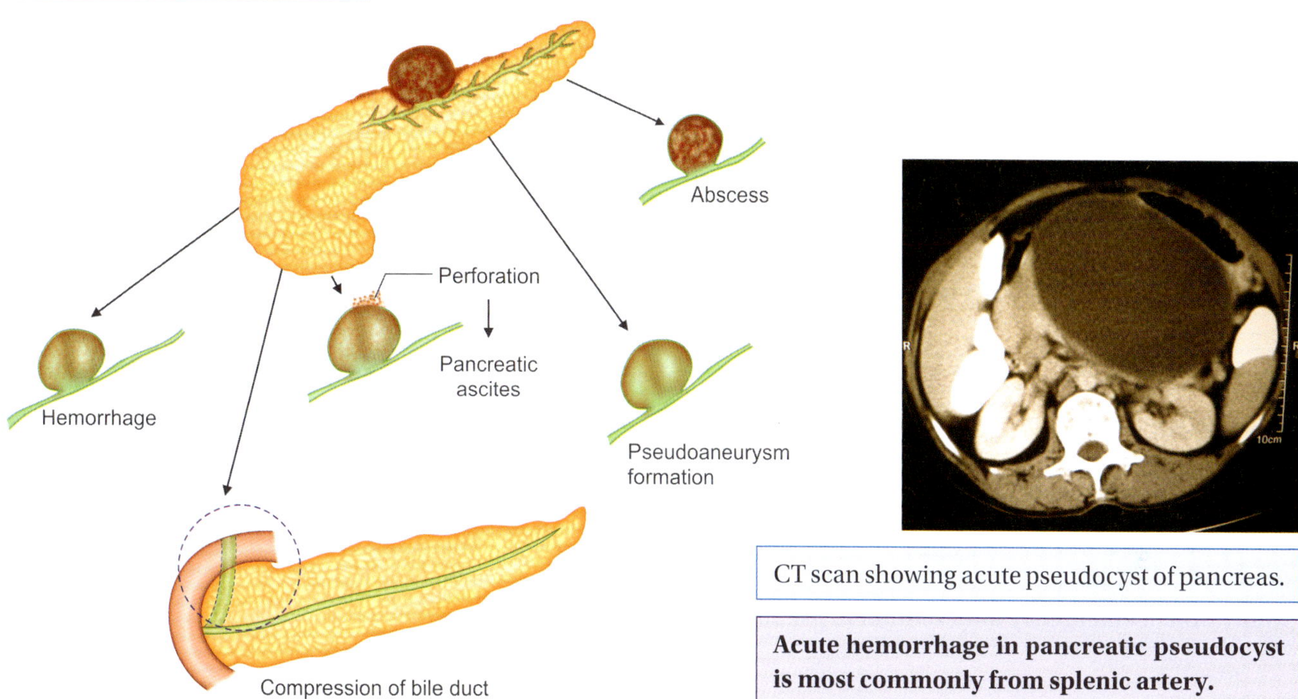

CT scan showing acute pseudocyst of pancreas.

Acute hemorrhage in pancreatic pseudocyst is most commonly from splenic artery.

Percutaneous Drainage

Not a preferred method for treatment of pseudocyst.

Indications: (i) Endoscopic or surgical drainage is not feasible due to co-morbidities; and (ii) Infected pseudocyst.

Complications of percutaneous drainage: (i) External pancreatic fistula; (ii) Secondary infection of the cyst; and (iii) Drain infection.

Endoscopic Transpapillary Drainage

- Preferred endoscopic treatment option when pseudocyst communicating with the main pancreatic duct.
- Opacification of both biliary and pancreatic ductal system by ERCP.
- Sphincterotomy of bile duct and pancreatic duct.
- A 7-Fr stent is introduced into the pseudocyst through pancreatic duct.

Endoscopic Transmural Drainage

- Preferred endoscopic treatment option in pseudocysts with visible indentation of the enteric lumen.
- Drainage is done under either esophagogastroduodenoscopy-directed or EUS-guided using multiple plastic stents or single fully covered self-expanding metal stent or *lumen apposing metal stent (LAMS).*
- EUS-guided drainage is safer and better technical success rate than EGD-directed drainage.

Complications of Endoscopic Drainage

(i) Pseudocyst wall perforation; (ii) Pseudocyst infection; (iii) Stent blockage; (iv) Bleeding; and (v) Recurrence

Other Uses of Lumen Apposing Metal Stent (LAMS)

(i) Endoscopic transmural drainage of WON (Walled-off necrosis); (ii) EUS-guided choledochoduodenostomy and gallbladder drainage; and (iii) EUS-guided gastroenterostomy

Indications of open surgery for pseudocyst: (i) Refractory to endoscopic or laparoscopic drainage; (ii) Recurrent pseudocysts; and (iii) Pseudocyst with associated biliary and/or duodenal stenosis.

Cystogastrostomy

Indicated for pseudocysts in the body and/or tail of the pancreas and bulges into the posterior wall of the stomach.

Cystoduodenostomy

Indicated for pseudocysts in the head of pancreas.

Cystojejunostomy

Indicated in: (i) Pseudocysts extend well into the transverse mesocolon; and (ii) Large pseudocysts (>10 cm). Most dependent surgical drainage procedure.

Laparoscopic drainage

Indicated: (i) Pseudocyst with solid component; and (ii) Pseudocyst with portal hypertension.

Different laparoscopic approaches are: Intragastric cyst-gastrostomy approach, anterior transgastric cyst-gastrostomy approach, cyst-gastrostomy through lesser sac approach, cyst-jejunostomy approach.

Pancreatic resection

Indicated in: (i) Diagnosis of cystic neoplasm cannot be ruled out; (ii) Pseudocyst in the tail of pancreas with a pancreatic duct cut-off; and (iii) Pseudocyst with inflammatory mass in the head of pancreas.

Indication of emergency intervention in pseudocyst: Massive bleeding from pseudoaneurysm.

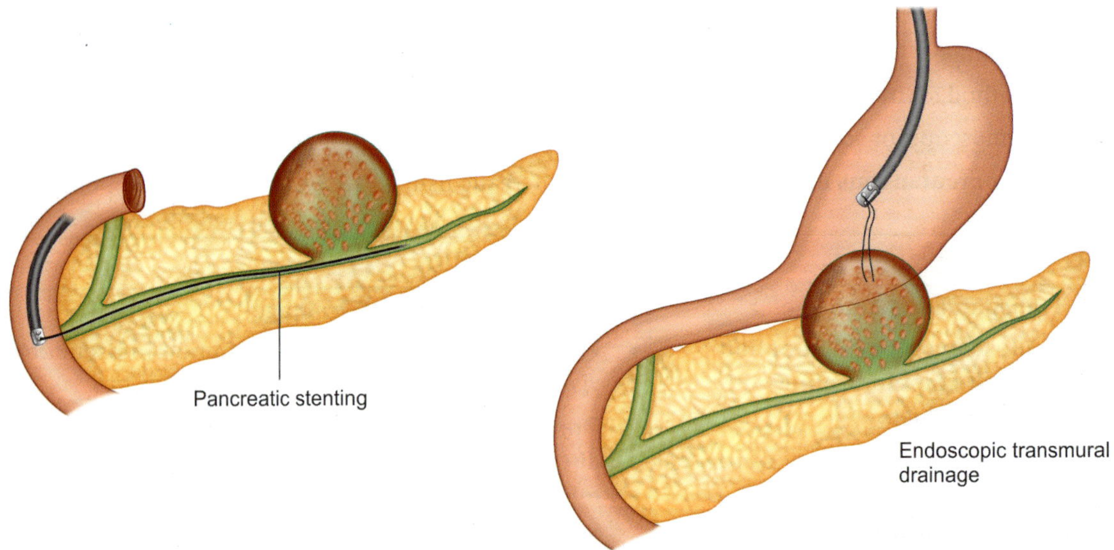

Cystogastrostomy

Pseudocyst adheres to the stomach and indenting it.

Cystoduodenostomy

Pseudocyst adherent to duodenum and indenting it.

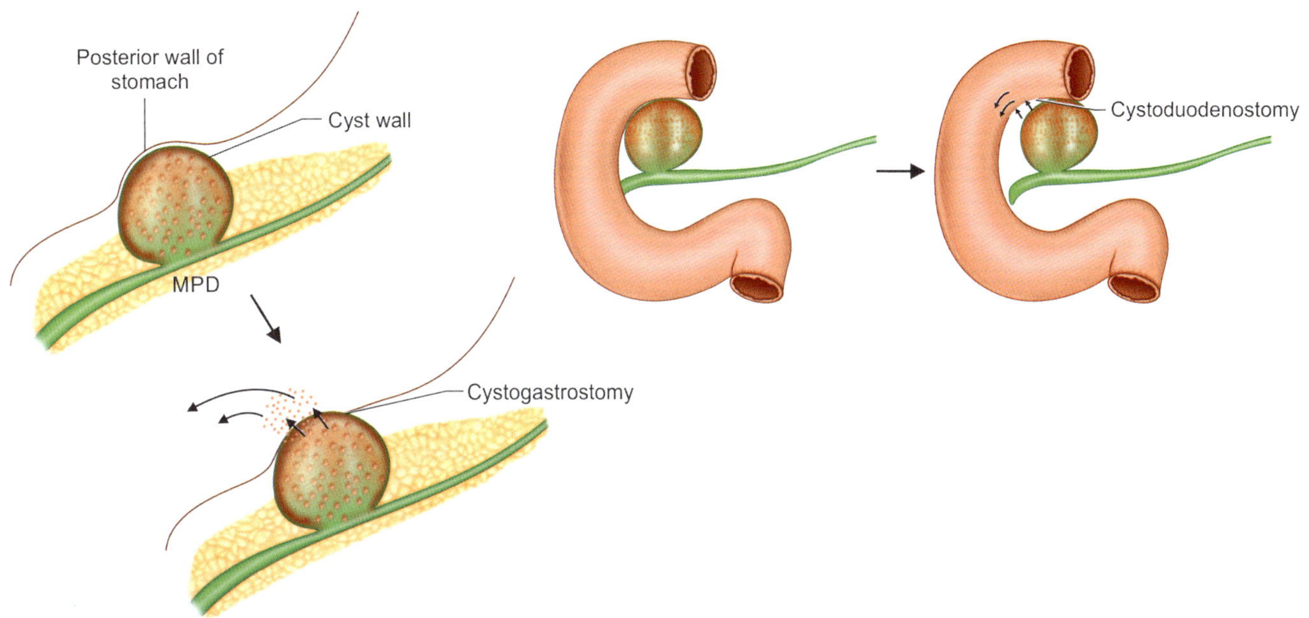

Operative Pictures of Cystogastrostomy

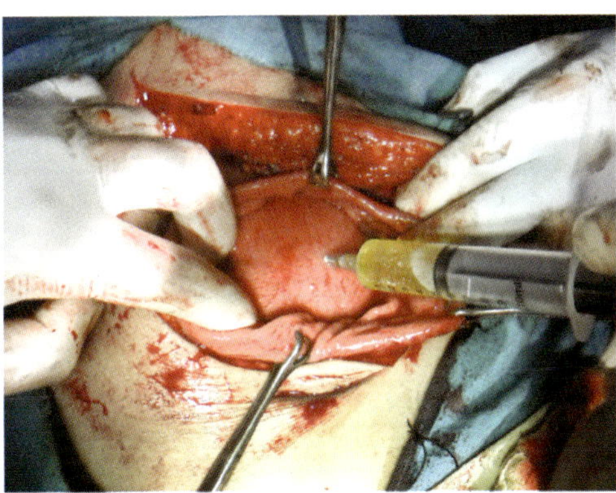

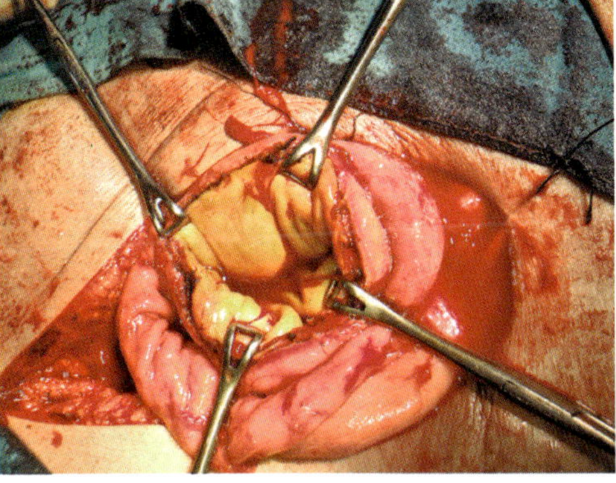

Cystojejunostomy

Pseudocyst arising from body and tail of pancreas and bulging through left transverse mesocolon.

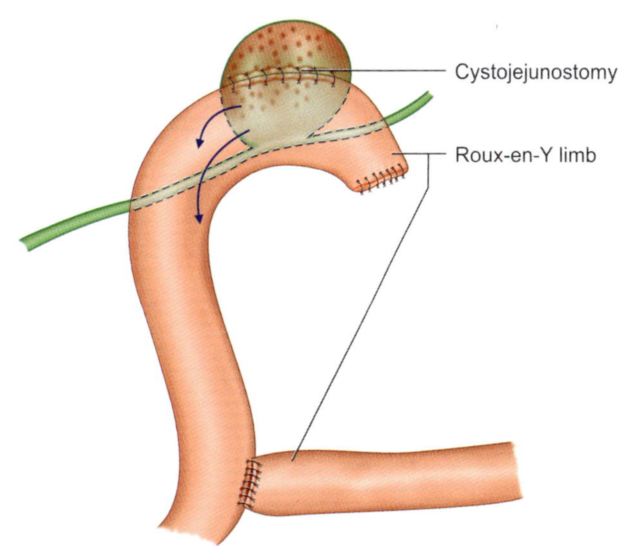

Pseudocyst of pancreas	Walled-off necrosis
Complication of acute interstitial edematous pancreatitis	Complication of acute necrotizing pancreatitis
Homogeneous fluid density	Heterogeneous fluid density
Absence of solid components	Presence of solid components
Treatment is drainage of cyst	Treatment is debridement of necrosis

Pseudocyst of pancreas	Cystic neoplasm of pancreas
Epithelial lining is absent	Epithelial lining is present
No malignant potential	Some of the lesions have malignant potential or malignant
Secondary to acute pancreatitis, chronic pancreatitis, pancreatic trauma	Pathophysiology unknown
On imaging, usually unilocular cyst with no solid component	On imaging, thick wall, lobulated margins, internal septa, solid component, mural nodules may be demonstrated
Cyst fluid analysis usually shows high amylase content	Cyst fluid analysis usually show high CEA or CA19-9 but low amylase
Most of the patients develop spontaneous resolution of cyst	No chance of spontaneous resolution
Treatment is drainage of cyst either by endoscopic or laparoscopic or open approach.	Treatment is resection.

Nealon Classification: Categories of Ductal Abnormalities in Patients with Pseudocyst (ERCP)

Type I: Normal duct/no communication with cyst

Type II: Normal duct with communication

Type III: Otherwise normal duct with stricture and no duct-cyst communication

Type IV: Otherwise normal duct with stricture and duct-cyst communication

Type V: Otherwise normal duct with complete cut-off

Type VI: Chronic pancreatitis, no duct-cyst communication

Type VII: Chronic pancreatitis with duct-cyst communication.

Chronic Pancreatitis

Definition

Cambridge definition: "A continuing inflammatory disease of the pancreas, characterized by irreversible morphologic change, and typically causing pain and/or permanent loss of function".

APA definition: "Chronic, progressive pancreatic inflammation and scarring, irreversibly damaging the pancreas, and resulting in loss of exocrine and endocrine function".

Mechanistic definition (2016): "Chronic pancreatitis is a pathologic fibro-inflammatory syndrome of the pancreas in individuals with genetic, environmental and/or other risk factors who develop persistent pathologic responses to parenchymal injury or stress". In addition,' Common features of established and advanced CP include pancreatic atrophy, fibrosis, pain syndromes, duct distortion and strictures, calcifications, pancreatic exocrine dysfunction, pancreatic endocrine dysfunction and dysplasia".

Classification of Chronic Pancreatitis (Based on Etiology and Risk Factors)

Traditional Classification

- Alcohol
- Idiopathic
- Hereditary
- Obstructive
- Hyperlipidemia

TIGAR-O Classification

- **Toxic-metabolic:** Alcohol, tobacco smoking, hypercalcemia, hyperlipidemia, chronic renal failure, medications, toxins.
- **Idiopathic:** Early onset, late onset, Tropical
- **Genetic mutations:** *PRSS1, CFTR, SPINK1*, other.
- **Autoimmune:** Isolated, syndromic
- **Recurrent and Severe Acute Pancreatitis Associated Chronic Pancreatitis:** Post-necrotic (severe acute pancreatitis), vascular disease/ischemic, post-irradiation
- **Obstructive:** Pancreas divisum, Sphincter of Oddi disorders, duct obstruction (e.g., Tumor), Post-traumatic pancreatic duct scars.

M-ANHEIM

M-multiple risk factors including:

- *Alcohol consumption:* Excessive (>80 g/day), increased (20–80 g/day), moderate (20 g/day)
- Nicotine consumption
- *Nutritional factors:* High calorie proportion of fat and protein, hyperlipidemia
- *Hereditary factors:* Hereditary, familial, idiopathic (early-onset, late-onset, tropical)
- *Efferent duct factors:* Pancreas divisum, annular pancreas, and other congenital abnormalities of the pancreas, pancreatic duct obstruction (e.g., tumors), post-traumatic pancreatic duct scars, sphincter of Oddi dysfunction
- *Immunological factors:* Autoimmune pancreatitis
- *Miscellaneous and rare metabolic disorders:* Hypercalcemia, hyperparathyroidism, chronic renal failure, drugs, toxins.

Pathophysiology

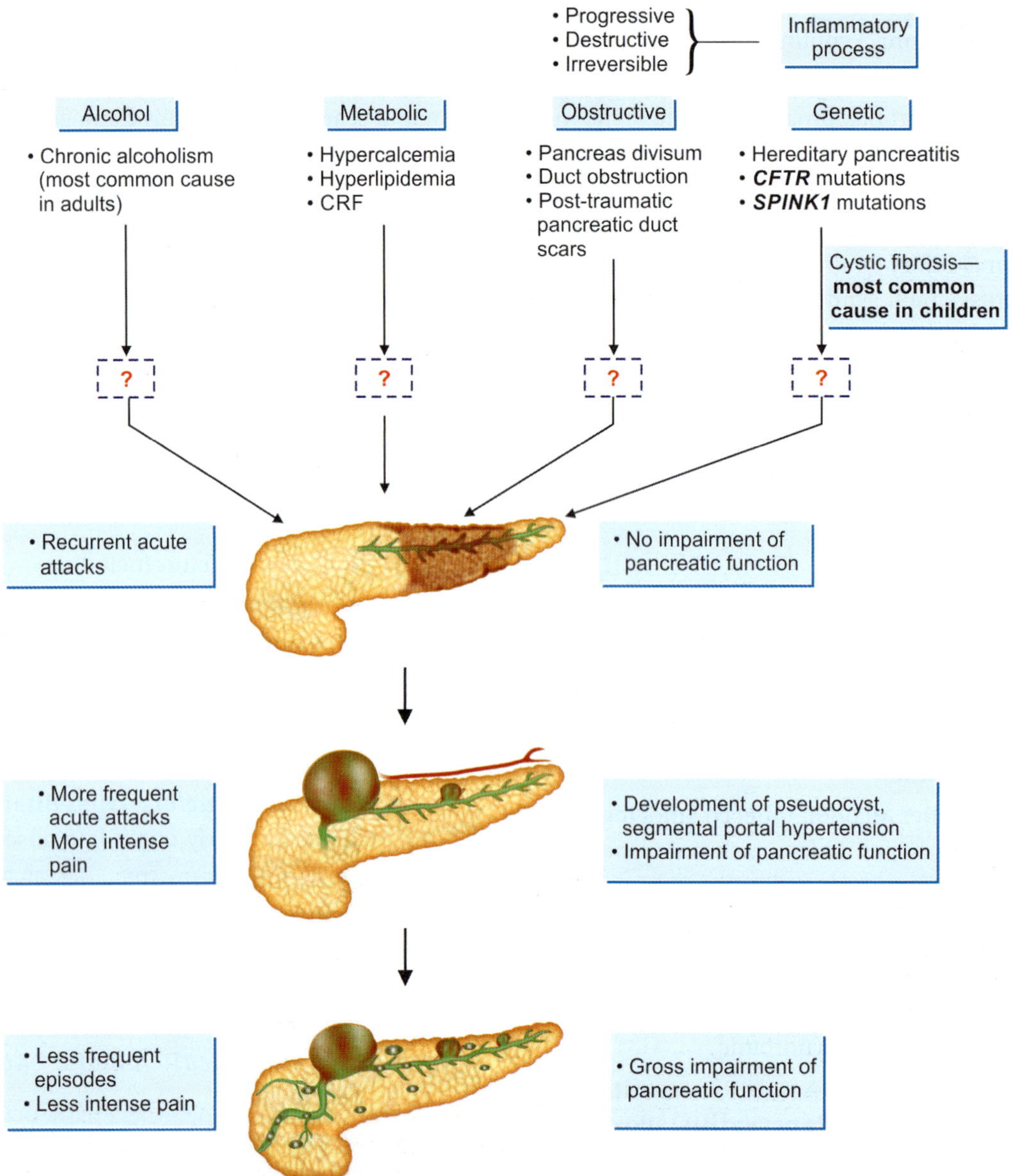

Theories of Chronic Pancreatitis Pathogenesis

- Toxic-metabolic theory
- The oxidative-stress hypothesis
- The stone and duct obstruction theory
- Primary duct hypothesis
- The necrosis-fibrosis hypothesis
- Sentinel acute pancreatitis event hypothesis

Genetic variations associated with chronic pancreatitis:

(i) PRSS1; (ii) CFTR; (iii) CTRC; (iv) PRSS2; (v) SPINK1; and (vi) CASR

Typical Gross Changes in Chronic Pancreatitis

- Decrease in size of the pancreas
- Loss of lobular pattern (in areas of scarring)
- Presence of stones in main pancreatic duct

Typical Ductal Findings in Chronic Pancreatitis

- Enlargement of main pancreatic duct
- Intraductal calcifications
- Dilated side branch radicals
- Beaded and irregular main pancreatic duct

Typical Histologic Changes in Chronic Pancreatitis

- Atrophy of acinar tissue
- Fibrosis (perilobular/interlobular/intralobular)

Typical Changes at Cellular Level

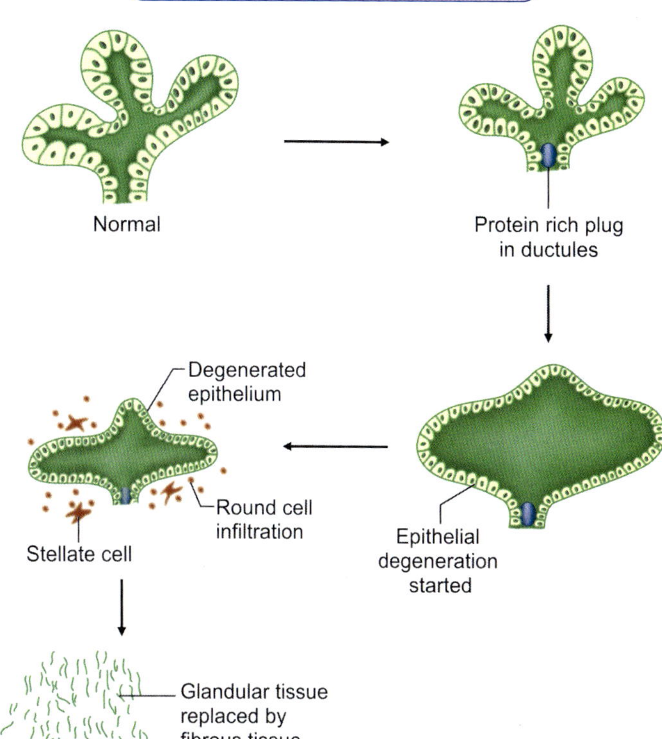

Stages of Chronic Pancreatitis

Early Stage

- Recurrent acute attack of pain
- Normal pancreatic endocrine and exocrine function
- No development of complications

Moderate Stage

- Frequency of attack of pain increases with increased intensity
- Impairment of pancreatic function, steatorrhea rarely develops
- *Complications:* Pseudocyst, cholestasis.

Advanced Stage

- Pain decreases (due to "burnout' of the pancreas)
- Severe impairment of pancreatic function, steatorrhea, diabetes mellitus
- *Complications:* Pseudocyst, cholestasis, segmental portal hypertension

Clinical Presentation

Patient presents with
- Abdominal pain
- Malabsorption and steatorrhea
- Pancreatogenic diabetes

- **Abdominal pain is the most common symptom**
- Usually epigastric in location with radiation to back
- Pain typically steady and boring
- Persists for hours or days, taking food or alcohol usually exacerbate pain
- Patient with pain typically sit in a bending forward position or lie on their side in a fetal position

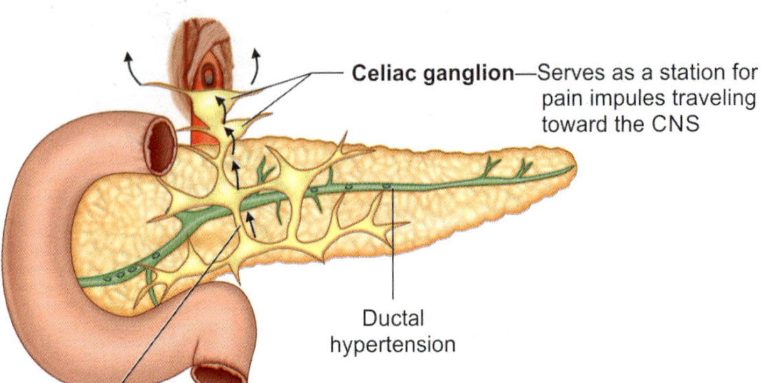

Mechanism of Pain in Chronic Pancreatitis

- Ductal hypertension
- Altered nociception
- Local inflammation
- Pancreatic nerve hypertrophy and intra-/perineural inflammation

Types of Pain in Chronic Pancreatitis

- **A-type pain:** One or more discrete episodes of pain interspersed with pain-free intervals
- **B-type-pain:** Persistent (i.e., daily) pain over prolonged period of time and/or closely clustered exacerbations of severe pain

Assessment of Pain in Chronic Pancreatitis

- **One-dimensional scale** (e.g., Visual analog scale)
- **Multidimensional scale** (e.g., The Brief Pain Inventory, The McGill Pain Questionnaire, The Izbicki pain score)

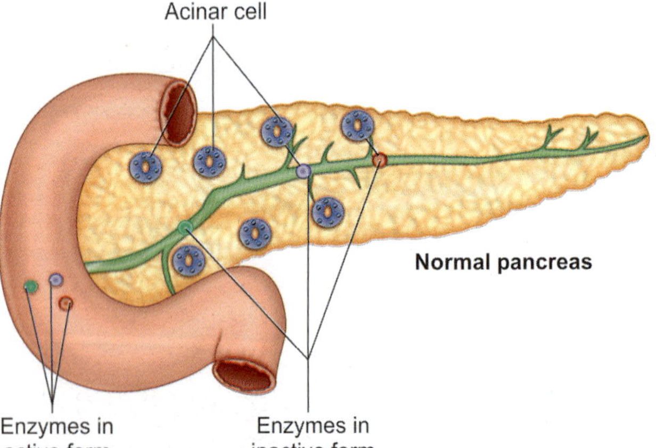

Chronic pancreatitis

Acinar cells replaced by fibrous tissue

↓↓ secretion of pancreatic enzymes → Malabsorption of protein and lipid

Pancreatic enzymes:

- Pancreatic amylase
- Pancreatic lipase
- Phospholipase A2
- Trypsin
- Chymotrypsin
- Elastase

Malabsorption and steatorrhea are due to pancreatic exocrine insufficiency.

Steatorrhea

Bulky, foul smelling, loose stool, pale in color and float on the surface of water.

Causes of pancreatic exocrine insufficiency

- Chronic pancreatitis
- Cystic fibrosis
- Hereditary hemochromatosis
- Zollinger-Ellison syndrome
- Pancreatic resection

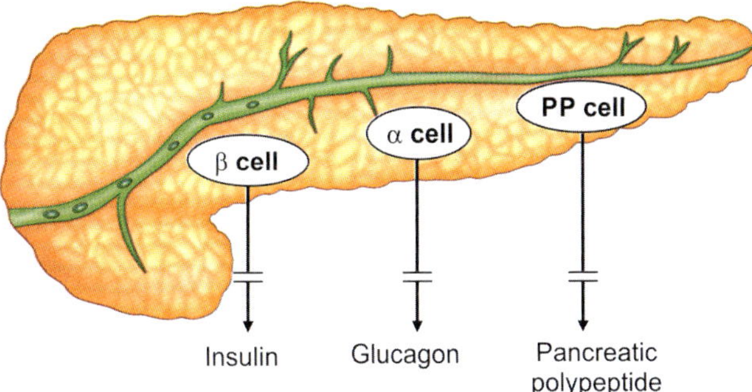

Pancreatogenic diabetes mellitus is classified as **Type3c** diabetes mellitus (by ADA and WHO).

It refers to diabetes due to diseases of the exocrine pancreas: Pancreatitis (acute, relapsing, or chronic pancreatitis of any etiology), pancreatectomy/trauma, neoplasia, cystic fibrosis, hemochromatosis, and fibrocalculous pancreatopathy. **Most common underlying disease is chronic pancreatitis.**

Enhanced peripheral sensitivity to insulin and decreased hepatic sensitivity to insulin.

Patients become hyperglycemic when insulin replacement is insufficient (due to unsuppressed hepatic glucose production).

Patients become hypoglycemic when insulin replacement is barely excessive (due to enhanced peripheral insulin sensitivity and a deficiency of pancreatic glucagon secretion to counteract the hypoglycemia).

Diagnostic Criteria of T3cDM (proposed by Ewald and Bretzel)

Major Criteria (all must be fulfilled)

- Presence of exocrine pancreatic insufficiency (according to the monoclonal fecal elastase-1 test or direct function tests)
- Pathological pancreatic imaging (endoscopic ultrasound, MRI, CT)
- Absent of type 1 diabetes mellitus associated autoimmune markers.

Minor Criteria

- Impaired beta-cell function (e.g., HOMA-B, C-peptide/glucose ratio)
- No excessive insulin resistance (e.g., HOMA-IR)
- Impaired incretin secretion (e.g., GLP-1, pancreatic polypeptide)
- Low serum level of lipid soluble vitamins (A, D, E, and K)

Complications

- **Duodenal obstruction**
- **Bile duct obstruction**
- **Pseudocyst**
- Splenic vein thrombosis
- Arterial pseudoaneurysms
- Pancreatic carcinoma
- Pancreatico-pleural fistula
- Osteoporosis

Characteristic Features of Pseudocyst Associated with Chronic Pancreatitis

- Multiple, small cysts
- Communication with the ductal system is usually present.
- Less chance of spontaneous resolution

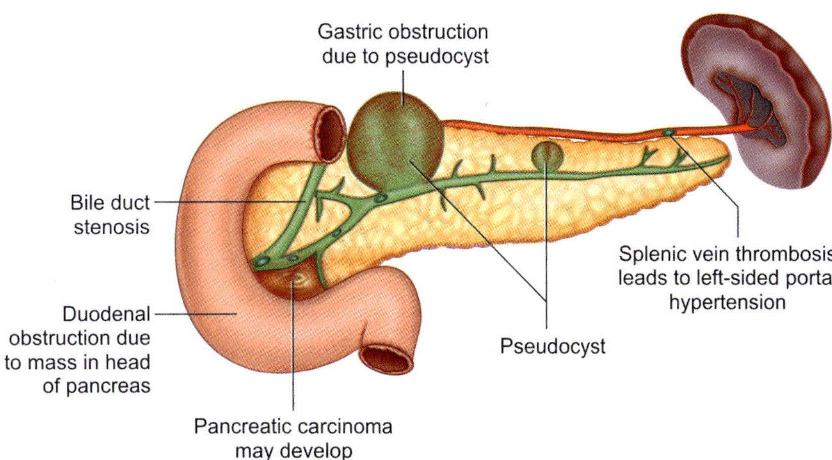

Investigations

Pancreatic Function Test

Indirect pancreatic function test is used to quantify the degree of insufficiency.

- Serum trypsinogen
- Fecal elastase
- Fecal fat measurement
- 13C-mixed triglyceride test

Direct pancreatic function test: High sensitivity for late chronic pancreatitis

- CCK stimulation test (acinar cell stimulation measuring trypsin and/or lipase)
- Secretin stimulation test (ductal cell stimulation measuring bicarbonate)
- Endoscopic pancreatic function test (ePFT)

Endoscopic US

- Can detect small neoplasm in the setting of chronic inflammation.
- Small intraductal lesion, intraductal mucus, cystic lesions, subtle ductular abnormalities are detected.
- Tissue samples can be obtained under image guidance.

Imaging

Transabdominal USG—not sensitive or specific in the diagnosis of CP.

CT scan—best initial imaging modality.

MRI—more sensitive than USG and CT. Also help in diagnosis of early CP by secretin-enhanced MRCP.

EUS—if diagnosis is in question after cross-sectional imaging.

Secretin-enhanced MRCP is indicated if cross-sectional imaging and EUS are not diagnostic.

Endoscopic retrograde pancreatography provides useful information, but rarely used as diagnostic modality.

Typical CT findings in Chronic Pancreatitis

- Dilatation of main pancreatic duct and secondary radicals
- Pancreatic calcification (intraductal or parenchymal or both)
- Pancreatic parenchymal atrophy
- Beaded and irregular MPD
- Presence of "duct-penetrating"sign (dilated duct or branches which penetrate an apparent mass)

ERCP

- Is indicated only if diagnosis is uncertain despite use of other imaging modalities.
- Placement of pancreatic duct stent to relieve obstruction
- For draining pseudocyst
- For taking biopsy or brushing for cytology

Cambridge Classification (Based on Ductal Changes in Pancreatogram)

Grade	Main pancreatic duct	Branch ducts
Normal	Normal	Normal
Equivocal (Cambridge 1)	Normal	<3 Abnormal
Mild (Cambridge 2)	Normal	≥3 Abnormal
Moderate (Cambridge 3)	Abnormal	>3 Abnormal
Severe (Cambridge 4)	Abnormal*	>3 Abnormal

*including large cavity >10 mm, intraductal filling defects, duct obstruction (stricture), duct dilation or irregularity, calculi/pancreatic calcification, or contiguous organ invasion.

Rosemont Classification (based on EUS Findings)

Major Criteria (A and B)	Minor Criteria
Parenchymal Major A Criteria • Hyperechoic foci with shadowing • Well-circumscribed lobularity	*Parenchymal Minor Criteria* • Cysts • Stranding • Non-shadowing hyperechoic foci • Lobularity with noncontiguous lobules
Ductal Major A Criteria MPD calculi	*Minor Ductal Criteria* • Dilated ducts (body ≥3.5 mm and tail ≥1.5 mm) • Irregular MPD contour • Dilated side branches ≥1 mm • Hyperechoic duct margin
Parenchymal Major B Criteria Lobularity with honey-combing	

- The diagnosis of CP is **consistent**, if: 1 Major A criteria + ≥3 minor criteria or 1 Major criteria + Major B criteria or 2 Major A criteria
- The diagnosis of CP is **suggestive** if: 1 Major A criteria + <3 minor criteria or 1 Major B criteria + ≥3 minor criteria or ≥5 minor criteria
- The diagnosis of CP is **indeterminate** if: 3 or 4 minor criteria with no major criteria or Major B criteria alone or with <3 minor criteria.

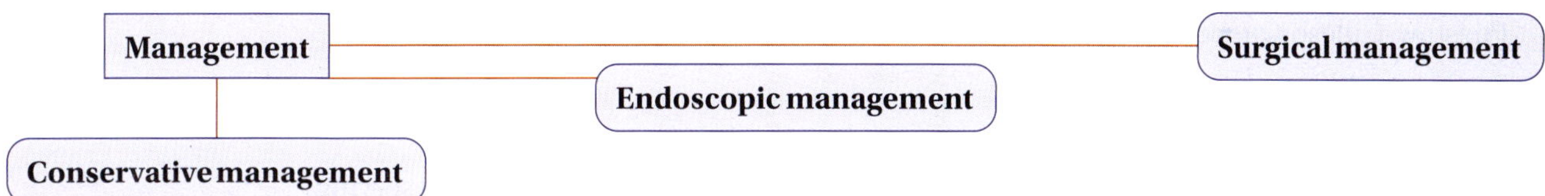

- Abstinence from smoking and alcohol
- Six small low-fat meals during the day
- Increase intake of fluid
- Diet should be rich in carbohydrates, 30–40% of calories must be come from fat
- Medium-chain triglycerides are preferred.
- *Oral pancreatic enzyme supplementation (with meals):* Preparations are: (i) Uncoated preparation; (ii) Coated preparation; and (iii) Enteric-coated microsphere preparation

Management of pain: NSAIDs → Weaker narcotics (e.g., tramadol) → Stronger narcotics (e.g., morphine) → Neuromodulating agents (e.g., pregabalin). Neurolytic therapy includes: (i) Celiac plexus nerve block (USG/CT/EUS guided); and (ii) Thoracoscopic denervation of splanchnic nerves.

Endoscopic Management

Indications: (i) Pancreatic ductal obstruction by calculi or stricture; (ii) Bile duct stenosis; and (iii) Symptomatic pseudocysts with no ductal obstruction.

Management of pancreatic stone: (i) ESWL for radiopaque, obstructive MPD stones >5 mm located in head/body of pancreas; and (ii) ERCP for radiolucent MPD stones ≤5 mm.

Management of pancreatic stricture: (i) Single 10-Fr plastic stent for painful dominant MPD stricture and (ii) For refractory stricture, multiple side-by-side plastic stents or SEMS or surgery.

Management of biliary stricture: Temporary insertion of multiple side-by-side plastic stents or FCSEMS.

Management of pseudocysts: (i) Transpapillary drainage for small (<5 cm) pseudocysts communicating with the MPD in the head and body of pancreas and (ii) Transmural drainage for other CP-related pseudocysts (EUS-guided/conventional access)

Surgical Management

Indications

(i) Intractable abdominal pain; (ii) Presence of secondary complications (e.g., pseudocyst, biliary stricture, internal pancreatic fistula, suspected pancreatic neoplasm); and (iii) Unsuccessful endoscopic therapy

Types of Surgery

Drainage procedure:

- Partington and Rochelle modification of Puestow procedure
- Puestow-Gillesby procedure
- Duval procedure

Resection:

- *Partial pancreatoduodenectomy:* Kausch-Whipple procedure (Classic/Pylorus-preserving)

Duodenum-preserving Pancreatic Head Resection (DPPHR):

- Beger procedure
- Frey procedure
- Berne modification of Beger procedure
- Hamburg modification of Frey procedure (Izbicki procedure)

Pancreatic left resection

Total pancreatectomy with islet autotransplantation (TPIAT)

Duval's Procedure (1954)

- It is a drainage procedure for chronic pancreatitis.
- It involves: (i) Drainage of duct of pancreatic tail by Roux-en-Y pancreaticojejunostomy; and (ii) Distal pancreatectomy and splenectomy
- Not practiced nowadays

Puestow-Gillesby Procedure (1958)

- It is a drainage procedure.
- It involves: (i) Drainage of the entire pancreatic duct by Roux-en-Y pancreaticojejunostomy; and (ii) Distal pancreatectomy and splenectomy
- Not practiced nowadays

Partington and Rochelle Modification of Puestow Procedure (1960)

- It involves: Drainage of the entire pancreatic duct by retrocolic side-to-side pancreaticojejunostomy (Lateral pancreaticojejunostomy)
- Most commonly performed drainage procedure.
- About 80% patients with dilated MPD experience relief of pain but long-term outcome is poor.
- This procedure is justified if: (i) MPD dilated (>7 mm); (ii) Absent of any dominant mass in head of pancreas; and (iii) Absence of obstructive symptoms (e.g., CBD or duodenal obstruction)
- *Advantages:* (i) All ductal stones can be removed and (ii) No loss of pancreatic tissues.

Partington and Rochelle Modification of Puestow Procedure

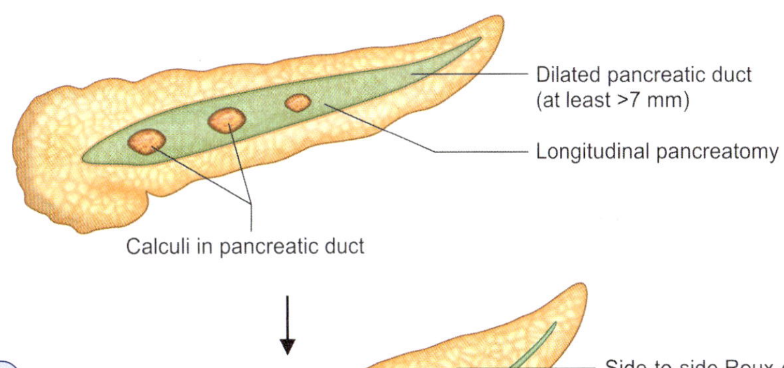

Puestow-Gillesby Procedure

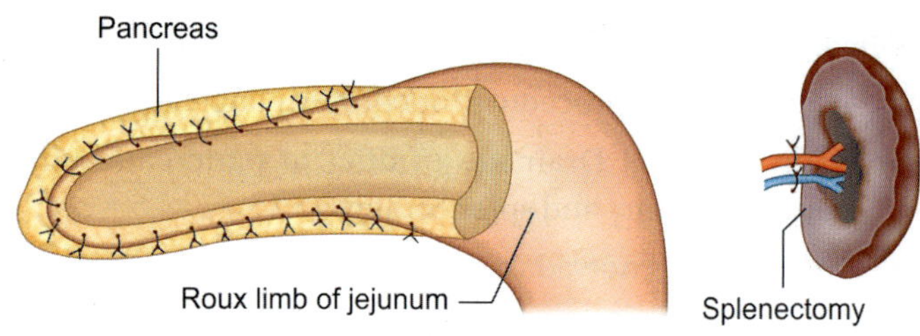

Partial Pancreatoduodenectomy

- Kausch-Whipple procedure (PD) and Pylorus-preserving PD (ppPD) described by Traverso and Longmire (1978)
- *Indications:* (i) Enlarged head of the pancreas with cysts and calcifications and (ii) Suspicion of malignancy in pancreatic head
- *Advantages:* (i) Reasonable short-term pain relief and (ii) Complications related to pancreatic head can be managed.
- *Disadvantages:* (i) Postoperative morbidity and mortality is higher in comparison to other surgical procedures for CP and (ii) Long-term occurrence of exocrine and endocrine insufficiency.
- Not a preferred surgical option for chronic pancreatitis.

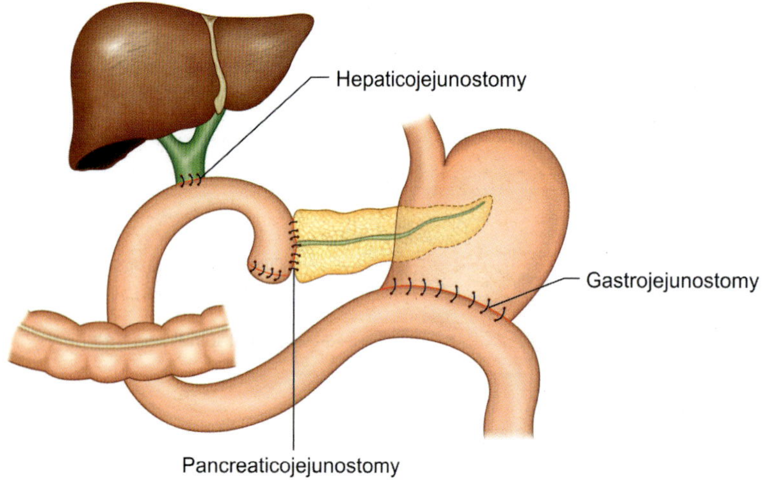

Pylorus Preserving Pancreaticoduodenectomy

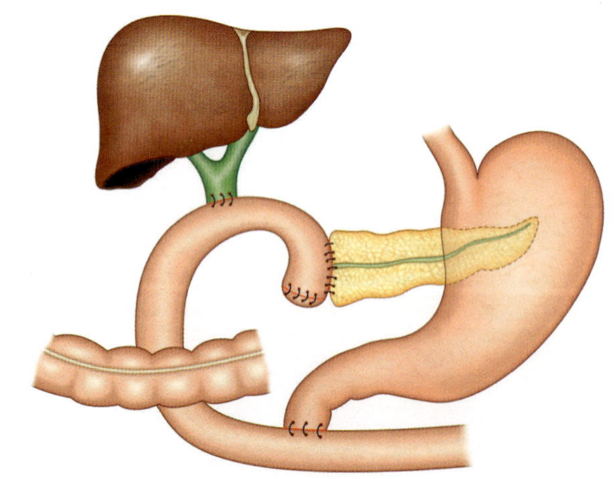

Beger Procedure (1972)

- *It involves-* (i) Division of the neck of pancreas on the level of portal vein; (ii) Pancreatic head is excavated and the duodenum is preserved with a thin layer of pancreatic tissue; and (iii) Reconstruction is done by means of a Roux-en-Y jejunal loop with an end-to-side anastomosis to the distal pancreas and a side-to-side anastomosis to the excavated pancreatic head.
- *Advantages:* (i) Significant relief of pain; (ii) Decompression of the duodenum and neighboring vessels; (iii) Preservation of the duodenum; (iv) Decompression of bile duct; and (v) Presence of any malignancy can be ruled out.
- *Disadvantages:* (i) Distal ductal stones, if present, cannot be managed and (ii) Loss of pancreatic tissue
- Beger's DPPHR is superior to PD and ppPD in terms of significant weight gain, pain relief and endocrine function.

Berne DPPR (2001)

- In this technique, advantages of Beger's and Frey's operations are combined.
- The pancreatic head is not transected, rather, the anterior capsule of the pancreatic head is incised, and inflammatory mass is almost removed, leaving only a thin rim of pancreatic tissue. Reconstruction is done by a single side-to-side anastomosis between excavated pancreatic head and Roux-en-Y jejunal loop.

Frey Procedure (1985)

- This technique includes: (i) Duodenum-sparing resection of the pancreatic head, without division of the neck and (ii) Lateral pancreaticojejunostomy (as described by Partington and Rochelle).
- This procedure is particularly indicated if an obstruction is present in the left-sided pancreatic duct along with less severe inflammation in head of the pancreas.
- Advantages: (i) Stones anywhere from the duct can be managed; (ii) Duodenum is preserved; and (iii) Malignancy can be ruled out.

Hamburg Modification of Frey Procedure (Izbicki Procedure)

- This procedure is particularly effective in small duct disease (Wirsungian ductal diameter <3 mm)
- This procedure includes: (i) Longitudinal V-shaped excision of the ventral aspect of the pancreas (allows sufficient drainage of secondary and tertiary pancreatic ducts) and (ii) Reconstruction by Roux-en-Y pancreaticojejunostomy sewn to the capsule of pancreas

Pancreatic Left Resection

- *Indications:* (i) Pseudocyst and fistula in the tail and (ii) MPD stenosis at the tail of pancreas.
- Pancreatic left resection can be done with or without splenectomy.
- Pancreatic left resection with splenectomy is indicated for perisplenic pseudocyst or fibrotic encasement of splenic vessels.

Frey Procedure

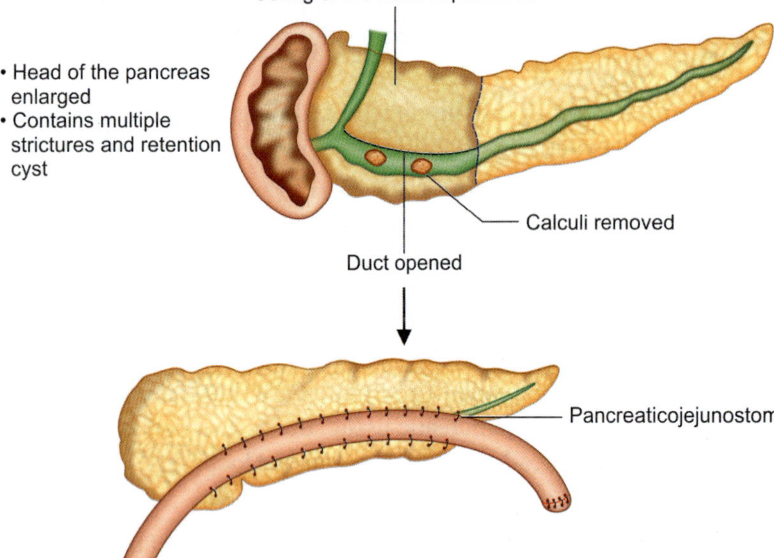

Pancreatic Left Resection

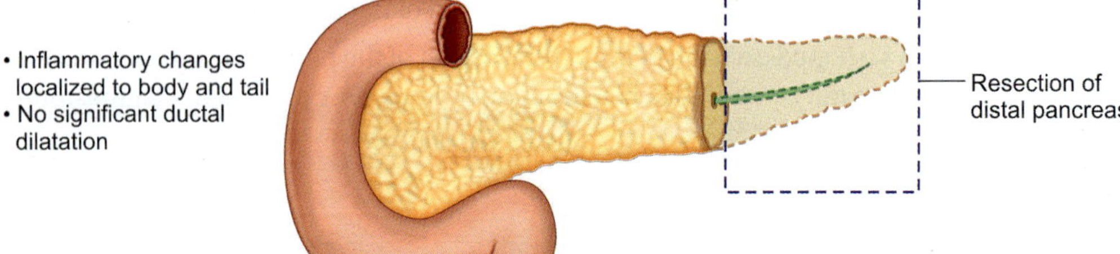

Total Pancreatectomy with Islet Autotransplantation

- This technique includes: (i) Pancreatectomy; (ii) Isolation of islets by digestion of pancreas; and (iii) Islet infusion (via portal vein or umbilical vein)
- *Indications:* (i) Hereditary chronic pancreatitis; (ii) Small duct chronic pancreatitis; and (iii) Failure of conventional surgical procedures
- *Contraindications:* (i) Patient with type 1 or 3 diabetes; (ii) Portal hypertension; and (iii) Portal vein thrombosis

Cystic Neoplasms of the Pancreas

Serous Cystadenoma

- Benign cystic neoplasm of pancreas
- Classified as: (i) Microcystic; (ii) Macrocystic (oligocystic); and (iii) Mixed
- Predominant in women
- These cystic lesions present as a pancreatic mass with numerous, small fluid-filled or solid appearing grape-like cysts. Rarely in communication with pancreatic duct.
- Characteristic imaging features are: (i) Microcystic or honeycomb appearance and (ii) Central scar
- Cyst fluid analysis reveals: (i) Low viscosity; (ii) Low CEA; and (iii) Low amylase
- For asymptomatic patients: Observation. Resection is indicated for larger lesions (≥4 cm) or symptomatic patients.

Mucinous Cystic Neoplasm

- These cystic neoplasms are mucin-producing tumors with malignant potential.
- Develop almost exclusively in women.
- Most common location is body or tail of the pancreas, no communication with the pancreatic duct.
- An ovarian-like stroma surrounding the columnar epithelium is diagnostic.
- Lesions are unilocular or multilocular, macrocystic; not communicating with pancreatic duct.
- Cyst fluid analysis reveals: (i) High viscosity; (ii) Elevated CEA; and (iii) Low amylase
- Imaging findings suggestive of malignancy: (i) Presence of septations; (ii) Larger size (>6 cm); (iii) Irregularity or thickening of cyst wall; and (iv) Mural nodularity.
- Due to its malignant potential, all MCNs must be resected.

Intraductal Papillary Mucinous Neoplasm (IPMN)

- IPMN can be classified into three types: (i) Main duct—IPMN (MD-IPMN); (ii) Branch duct—IPMN (BD-IPMN); and (iii) Mixed type, based on imaging and/or histology.
- *MD-IPMN* is characterized by segmental or diffuse dilation of the main pancreatic duct of >5 mm without other causes of obstruction.
- *BD-IPMN* is characterized by pancreatic cysts >5 mm in diameter that communicate with the MPD.
- *Mixed type* has both the criteria of MD-IPMN and BD-IPMN.
- Dedicated MRCP is the imaging of choice for evaluating a pancreatic cyst.
- "Worrisome features" on imaging: (i) Cyst ≥3 cm; (ii) Enhancing mural nodule <5 mm; (iii) Thickened-enhanced cyst walls; (iv) MPD size 5–9 mm; (v) Abrupt change in the caliber with distal pancreatic atrophy; (vi) Lymphadenopathy; (vii) Elevated serum level of CA 19-9; and (viii) Rapid rate of cyst growth >5 mm/2 years. Patients with "worrisome features" should be evaluated by EUS (Doppler EUS/Contrast-enhanced harmonic EUS) to further stratify the lesion.
- "High-risk stigmata" on imaging(CT/MRI or EUS): (i) Obstructive jaundice in a patient with a cystic lesion of the pancreatic head; (ii) Enhanced mural nodule ≥5 mm; and (iii) MPD ≥10 mm. Cysts with "high-risk stigmata" should undergo resection without further work-up.
- Patients with cysts ≤3 cm without "worrisome features" should undergo surveillance according to size.
- In MD-IPMN, resection is recommended for all surgically fit patients with "high-risk stigmata" on imaging. In BD-IPMN, absolute indications for resection are: (i) Cytology positive for high-grade dysplasia and (ii) Presence of mural nodules.
- Types of resection (e.g., pancreatoduodenectomy, left pancreatectomy, total pancreatectomy along with lymph node dissection) depends on the site and extent of the lesion.

Solid Pseudopapillary Neoplasm (Frantz Tumor or Hamoudi Tumor)

- Solid pseudopapillary neoplasm is rare tumor of pancreas with low-grade metastatic potential.
- It is more common in females in their second or third decade of life.
- These tumors have both cystic and solid components with areas of hemorrhage and calcification.
- Tumors less likely to invade other adjacent organs.
- *Clinical presentation:* Palpable abdominal mass, abdominal discomfort, weight loss are common presentations.
- *Diagnosis:* Contrast-enhanced ultrasound (CEUS), contrast CT and MRI are useful imaging modalities for diagnosis. EUS-FNA with immunohistochemistry is helpful for more definitive diagnosis of SPN (SPN is positive for beta-catenin, vimentin, CD10)
- *Management:* Surgical resection is the treatment of choice. Based on the location of the tumor, pylorus preserving pancreaticoduodenectomy or central pancreatectomy or distal pancreatectomy have to considered.

Mucin-producing Cystic Lesions

- Intraductal papillary mucinous neoplasms (IPMNs)
- Mucinous cystic neoplasms

Elevated CEA is a marker that distinguishes mucinous from nonmucinous cyst. KRAS and GNAS mutations are commonly associated with significant mucinous cysts.

Cysts with no Communication with Pancreatic Duct

- Serous cystadenoma
- Mucinous cystic neoplasms

Facts must be keep in mind

- Solid component in a cystic lesion, septations in a cyst—think of cystic neoplasm.
- Pseudocysts should be biopsied at the time of internal drainage—to rule out benign or malignant neoplastic lesion.
- Dilated pancreatic duct should be biopsied at the time of decompression procedure to rule out ductular neoplasm.
- In a patient without history of pancreatitis, cystic lesion in pancreas is a cystic neoplasm until proved otherwise.

Cystic Lesions with Malignant Potential

- Intraductal papillary mucinous neoplasms (IPMNs)
- Mucinous cystic neoplasms (MCNs)
- Solid-pseudopapillary epithelial neoplasm (SPEN)
- Pancreatic neuroendocrine tumors

Pancreatic Carcinoma

Pathophysiology

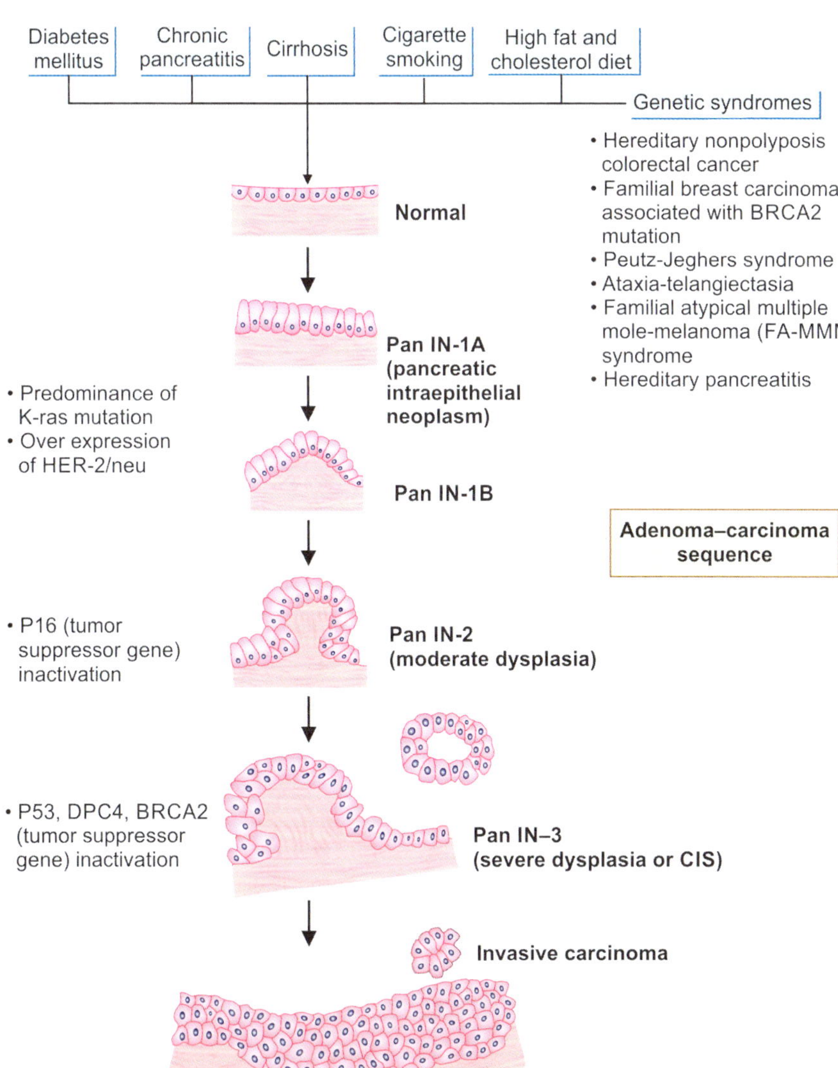

Risk Factors

- Cigarette smoking
- Heavy alcohol consumption
- Exposure to chemicals and heavy metals (e.g., beta-napthylamine, benzidine, benzene, asbestos, pesticides, chlorinated hydrocarbons)
- Increased BMI
- Diabetes mellitus
- Chronic pancreatitis
- Genetic syndromes

Periampullary Cancers

- Cancers arising out of or within 1 cm of the papilla of Vater.
- It includes ampullary, pancreatic, bile duct, and duodenal cancer.

Pancreatic Cancer Screening (as per International CAP Consortium Guidelines) of High-risk Individuals

- First-degree relatives of patients with pancreatic cancer from familial kindreds
- Carriers of P16 or BRCA2 mutations with an affected first-degree relative
- Patients with Peutz-Jeghers syndrome
- Patients with Lynch syndrome
- Affected first-degree relative with pancreatic cancer
- Screening is done with EUS and/or MRI/MRCP

Pathology

Ductal adenocarcinoma is the most common histologic type (about 85%)- arises from ductal epithelial cells.

Other histologic types:

- Acinar cell carcinoma—presents as larger tumor but a better prognosis
- Adenosquamous carcinoma
- Undifferentiated carcinoma with osteoclast-like giant cells
- Colloid carcinoma
- Signet ring cell carcinoma

Premalignant tumors of pancreas

Mucinous cystic neoplasms (MCNs)

Intraductal papillary mucinous neoplasms (IPMNs)

Ductal adenocarcinomas infiltrate along nerve sheath (perineural growth), lymphatics.

Lymph node metastasis and distant metastasis (e.g., liver) are commonly present.

Fibrosis is a characteristic finding in both chronic pancreatitis and ductal adenocarcinoma. Image-guided tissue biopsy is therefore often misleading and inconclusive.

Clinical Presentation

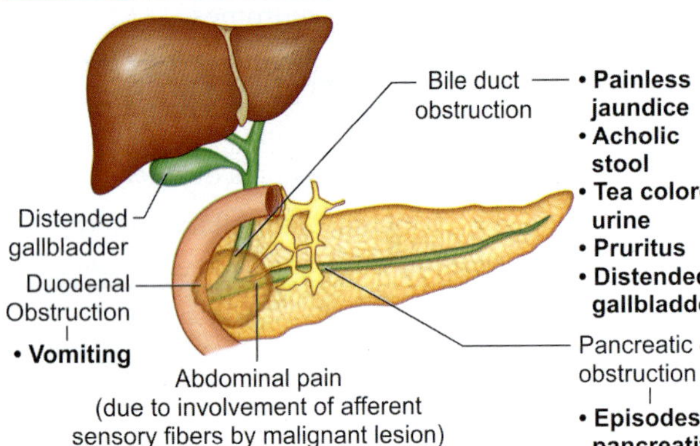

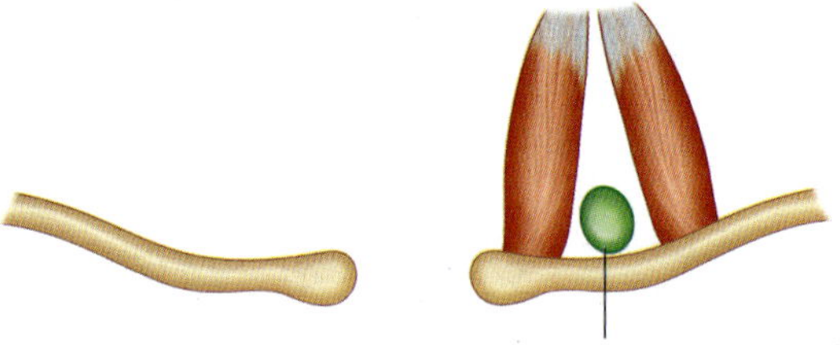

Recent-onset diabetes in elderly patient especially associated with vague abdominal pain and continuous weight loss—suspect pancreatic carcinoma.

Cancer involving body or tail of pancreas presents with only abdominal pain and weight loss.

Thomas sign

Passage of "silver stools" (color of oxidized silver or aluminum paint) is diagnostic of cancer of Ampulla of Vater. This is a combination of clay-colored stool of obstructive jaundice and melena.

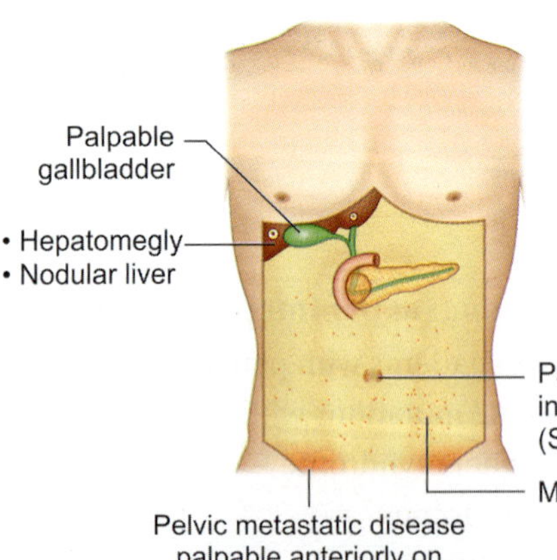

Investigations

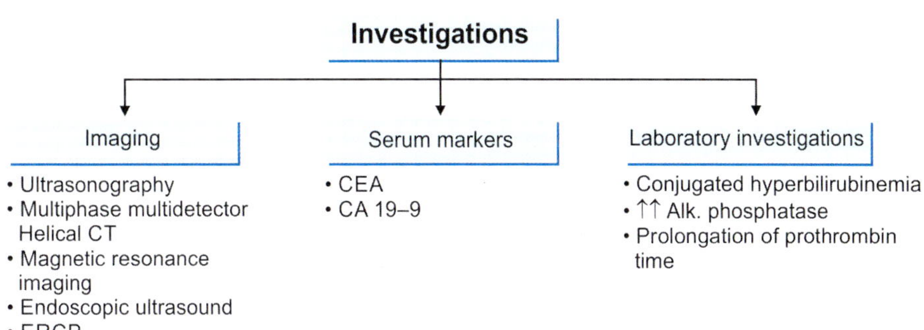

CA 19-9 (a sialylated Lewis A blood group antigen) is the most useful biomarker for early detection, staging, prognostic marker after resection and predictive marker for response to chemotherapy.

CA 19-9 should be measured in:

- Resectable disease prior to surgery.
- Following surgery immediately prior to administration of adjuvant therapy.
- Borderline resectable disease prior to neoadjuvant therapy
- Borderline resectable disease after neoadjuvant therapy

Lewis negative individuals do not express CA 19-9 antigen, so CA 19-9 level may be undetectable in these group of patients.

CA 19-9 is also elevated in:

- Cholangitis
- Biliary obstruction
- Autoimmune pancreatitis
- Cirrhosis
- Cholangiocarcinoma
- Colon cancer

A dedicated pancreatic-protocol CT abdomen is recommended in all patients with clinical suspicion of pancreatic carcinoma.

In pancreatic-protocol CT, neutral oral contrast medium (e.g., water) and intravenous contrast medium are used. This dedicated pancreatic protocol CT includes: (i) Early arterial phase; (ii) Pancreatic phase (late arterial phase); and (iii) Portal venous phase (hepatic phase).

Early arterial phase (17–25 seconds after contrast injection): Images of the aorta and superior mesenteric artery.

The pancreatic phase (35–40 seconds after contrast injection): (i) Differentiates hypoattenuating tumors (e.g., pancreatic adenocarcinoma) or hyperattenuating tumors (e.g., neuroendocrine tumors) against normal pancreatic parenchyma; (ii) Better delineation of pancreatic duct and intrapancreatic CBD; and (iii) Variations of arterial anatomy (e.g., aberrant or replaced right hepatic artery).

The portal venous phase (after 70 seconds of contrast injection): (i) Delineates tumor-venous relationship (e.g., abutment or encasement of portal vein); (ii) Delineation of variations of venous anatomy; and (iii) Detects hepatic metastases.

Endoscopic ultrasonography (EUS) is not recommended for staging evaluation.

EUS is indicated when tissue diagnosis is necessary for neoadjuvant therapy or palliative chemoradiotherapy.

Endoscopic retrograde cholangiopancreatography (ERCP) is indicated for biliary stenting (for preoperative biliary decompression or as a palliative measure) and for tissue diagnosis.

Advantages of EUS-guided FNA

- Better diagnostic yield
- Less risk of peritoneal seeding
- Less risk of bleeding or infection

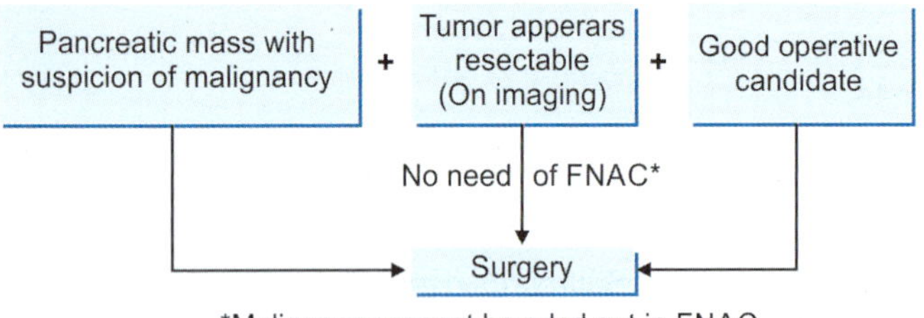

*Malignancy cannot be ruled out in FNAC

Indications of tissue diagnosis:

- Neoadjuvant therapy is planned
- Before starting therapy in metastatic diseases

Different methods of biopsy:

- EUS-guided FNA (preferred option)
- CT-guided FNA
- Endoscopic cholangioscopy
- Pancreatic ductal brushings

Diagnostic staging laparoscopy

- The aim of diagnostic laparoscopy is to avoid unnecessary laparotomy in patients with peritoneal or serosal implants or liver metastasis that may not be detected in cross-sectional imaging.
- This modality may be considered in patients with resectable disease but with increased risk of disseminated disease (markedly elevated CA 19-9, large tumor, large regional lymph nodes) and in patients with borderline resectable disease prior to neoadjuvant therapy.

Treatment

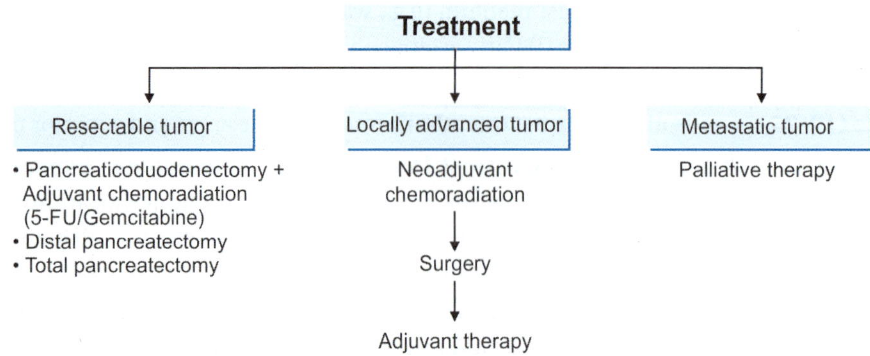

Criteria Defining Resectability Status

Resectable

Arterial: No arterial tumor contact (celiac axis, superior mesenteric artery, common hepatic artery)

Venous: No tumor contact with the superior mesenteric vein or portal vein or ≤180° contact without vein contour irregularity.

Borderline Resectable

Arterial

Pancreatic head/uncinate process:

- Solid tumor contact with CHA without extension to CA or hepatic artery bifurcation
- Solid tumor contact with the SMA of ≤180°
- Solid tumor contact with variant arterial anatomy (e.g., accessory right hepatic artery, replaced right hepatic artery, replaced CHA and the origin of replaced or accessory artery)

Pancreatic body/tail:

- Solid tumor contact with the CA of ≤180°
- Solid tumor contact with the CA of >180° without involvement of the aorta and with intact and uninvolved gastroduodenal artery.

Venous

- Solid tumor contact with the SMV or PV >180°, contact of ≤180° with contour irregularity of the vein or thrombosis of the vein but with suitable vessel proximal and distal to the site of involvement allowing for safe and complete resection and vein reconstruction.
- Solid tumor contact with the inferior vena cava.

Locally Advanced

Arterial

Head/uncinate process:

- Solid tumor contact with SMA >180°
- Solid tumor contact with the CA >180°

Pancreatic body/tail:

- Solid tumor contact of >180° with the SMA or CA
- Solid tumor contact with the CA and aortic involvement

Venous

- Unreconstructable SMV/PV due to tumor involvement or occlusion (can be due to tumor or bland thrombus)

Cancers of head of pancreas and uncinate process: Pancreaticoduodenectomy (Whipple procedure)

Cancers of body of pancreas and tail: Distal pancreatectomy with En bloc splenectomy

Cancers of neck of pancreas: Extended pancreaticoduodenectomy (pancreaticoduodenectomy extending to the left of SMV) or extended distal pancreatectomy (distal pancreatectomy extending to the right of the SMV) or total pancreatectomy depending on the extent of involvement.

Lymphadenectomy

Standard lymphadenectomy must involve the removal of ≥15 lymph nodes for adequate pathologic staging. Extended lymphadenectomy is not recommended.

Standard lymphadenectomy for cancer of head of pancreas:

- Suprapyloric (station 5)
- Infrapyloric (station 6)
- Anterosuperior group along the common hepatic artery (station 8a)
- Along the bile duct (station 12b)
- Around the cystic duct (station 12c)
- On the posterior aspect of superior and inferior portion of the head of pancreas (station 13a)
- On the right lateral side of SMA (station 14a and 14b)
- On the anterior surface of the superior (station 17a) and inferior portion of the head of pancreas (station 17b)

Standard lymphadenectomy for cancer of body and tail of pancreas:

- At the splenic hilum (station 10)
- Along the splenic artery (station 11)
- The inferior margin of pancreas

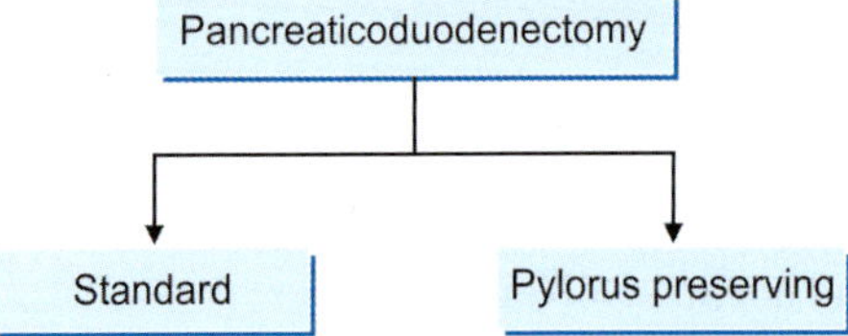

Classic Whipple is developed by **Walther Kausch** and later perfected by **Allen O Whipple**.

Ideal candidates of classic Whipple are periampullary tumors involving the first part of duodenum or distal stomach.

Classic Whipple involves En bloc resection of the pancreatic head, the duodenum, the distal common bile duct, the gallbladder, and the distal stomach.

Pylorus preserving pancreaticoduodenectomy (PPPD) popularized by **Traverso and Longmire**.

Ideal candidates of PPPD are periampullary tumors not involving the proximal duodenum, pylorus, or distal stomach.

PPPD preserves the distal stomach, pylorus and the first part of duodenum.

Advantages: Decreased blood loss, shorter operative time, improved postoperative weight gain, morbidity and mortality are almost similar to classic Whipple.

Disadvantages: Increased incidence of delayed gastric emptying

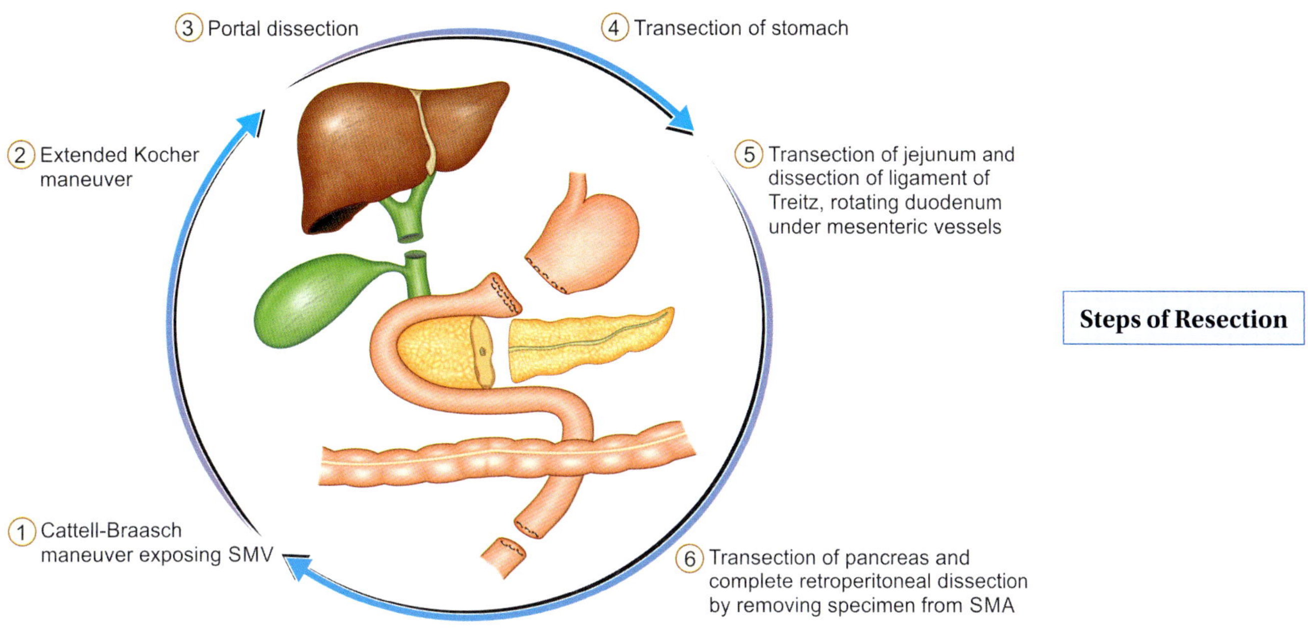

Steps of Resection

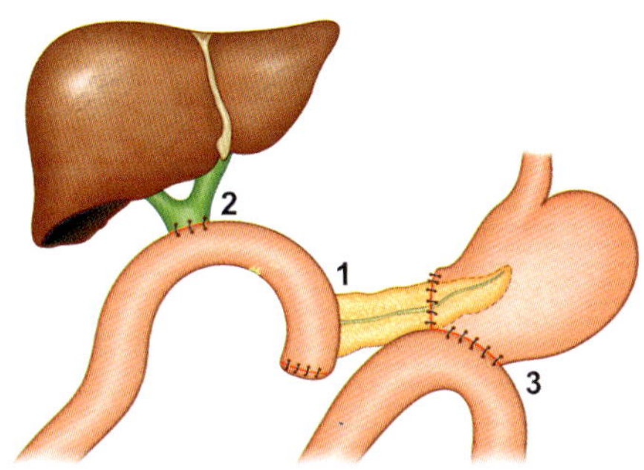

Steps of Reconstruction

Techniques of Pancreaticojejunostomy

- Duct-to-mucosa pancreaticojejunostomy
- Invaginating end-to-side pancreaticojejunostomy
- End-to-end dunking/invaginating pancreaticojejunostomy

Techniques of Pancreaticogastrostomy

- Duct-to-mucosa pancreaticogastrostomy
- Invaginating end-to-side pancreaticogastrostomy
- Binding pancreaticogastrostomy

Margins Analyzed Pathologically in Whipple Specimen

- SMA (retroperitoneal/uncinate) margin
- Posterior margin
- Portal vein groove margin
- Portal vein margins (if partial or complete vein resection is done)
- Pancreatic neck (transection) margin
- Bile duct margin
- Proximal and distal enteric margins
- Anterior surface

Complications of Pancreaticoduodenectomy

- Delayed gastric emptying
- Hemorrhage
- Postoperative pancreatic fistula
- Biliary leak
- Intra-abdominal collection

Postoperative Pancreatic Fistula (POPF)

A POPF is defined as a drain amylase of over three times that of the serum amylase at or beyond postoperative day 3 (proposed by International study group on pancreatic fistula).

Grade A POPF: A short-lived fistula with no clinical symptoms but with higher drain amylase levels with minimal clinical effect that requires no significant alterations in management protocols.

Grade B POPF: Clinical symptoms and radiographic imaging may depict peri-pancreatic fluid collections. The management includes at least one of the following: antibiotic administration, supplemental nutrition, placement of a postoperative percutaneous drain, or readmission to the hospital.

Grade C POPF: The most severe class with patients being clinically unstable. It is associated with sepsis, organ dysfunction, and death; therefore, re-operation and exploration may be required.

Factors that affect rate and grade of POPF: (i) Techniques of reconstruction (Roux-en-Y reconstruction with isolated pancreatic drainage/conventional loop reconstruction; Pancreaticojejunostomy/Pancreaticogastrostomy); (ii) Placement of stent; (iii) Duration of drain; and (iv) Use of somatostatin analogs.

Palliative Management

Palliation of Gastric Outlet Obstruction and Obstructive Jaundice

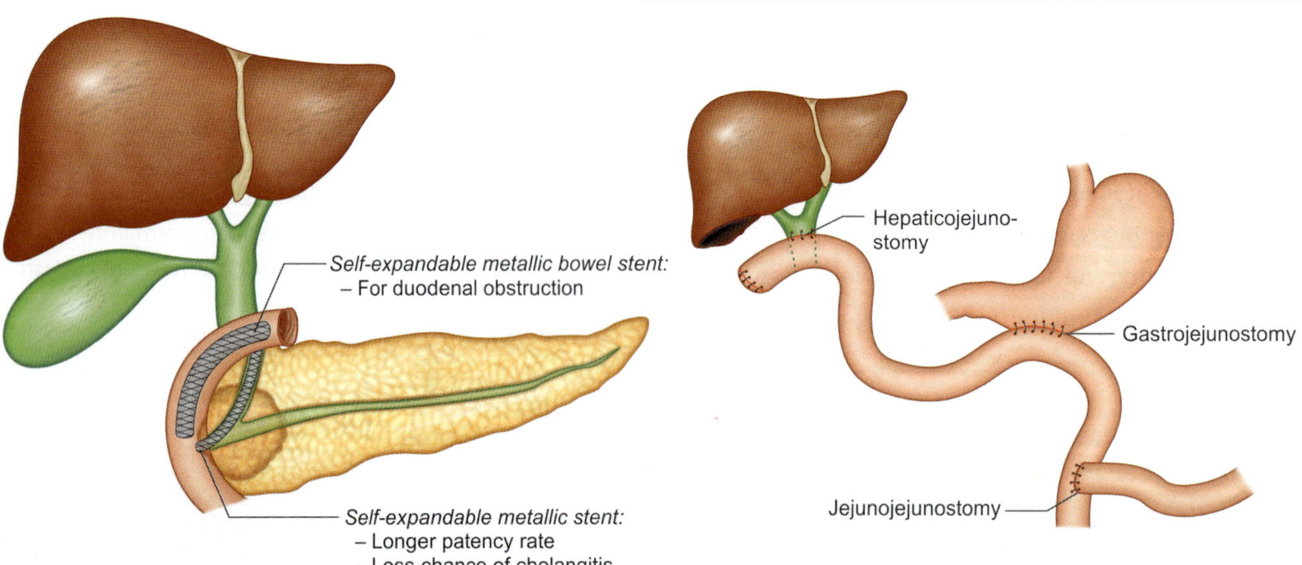

- In endoscopic biliary stenting, *SEMS* are used. Among different methods of biliary-enteric bypass, *choledochojejunostomy or hepaticojejunostomy* is preferable.
- If patient has short life expectancy or poor performance status, *endoscopically placed duodenal stent* is preferred for GOO management. If patient having more than 3–6 months life expectancy and good performance status, *open or laparoscopic gastrojejunostomy* with or without jejunostomy tube placement is the preferred approach.
- Open or laparoscopic gastrojejunostomy provides better and durable palliation than enteral stenting.

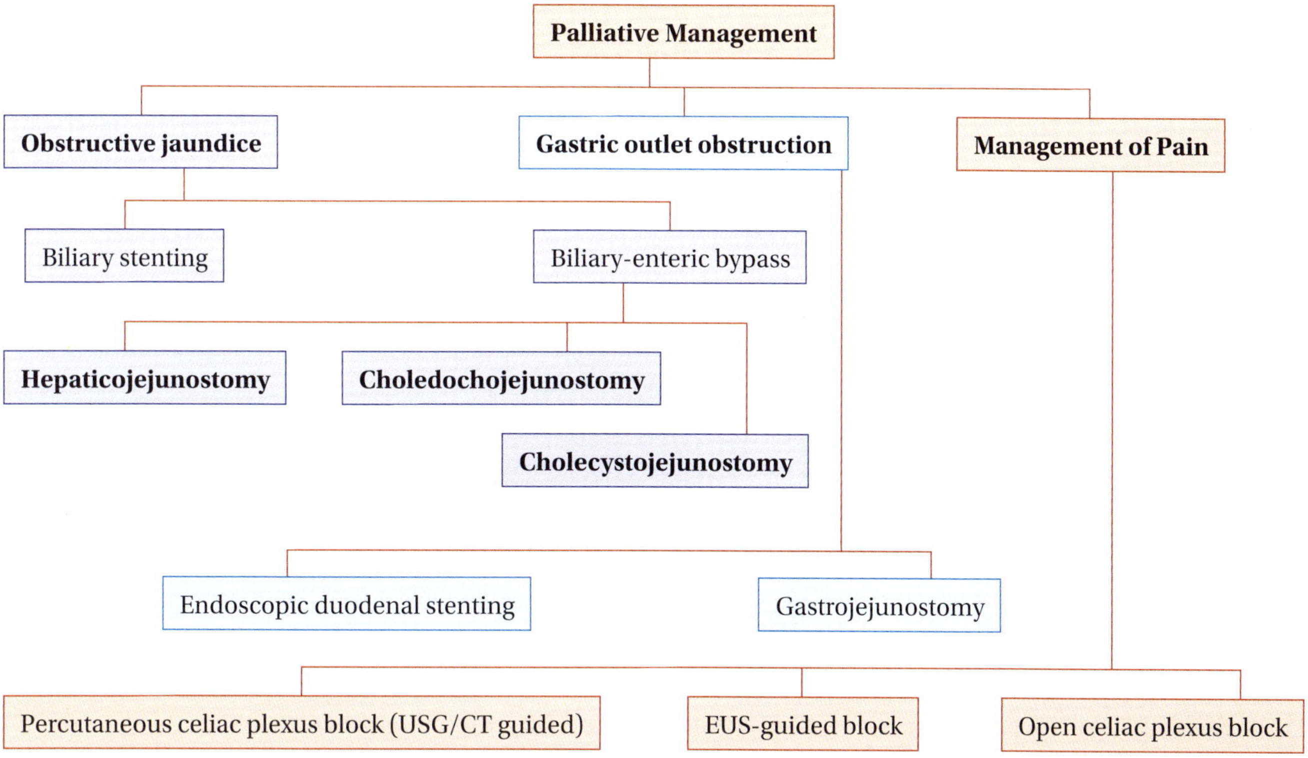

Palliative Management

- **Obstructive jaundice**
  - Biliary stenting
  - Biliary-enteric bypass
    - **Hepaticojejunostomy**
    - **Choledochojejunostomy**
    - **Cholecystojejunostomy**
- **Gastric outlet obstruction**
  - Endoscopic duodenal stenting
  - Gastrojejunostomy
- **Management of Pain**
  - Percutaneous celiac plexus block (USG/CT guided)
  - EUS-guided block
  - Open celiac plexus block

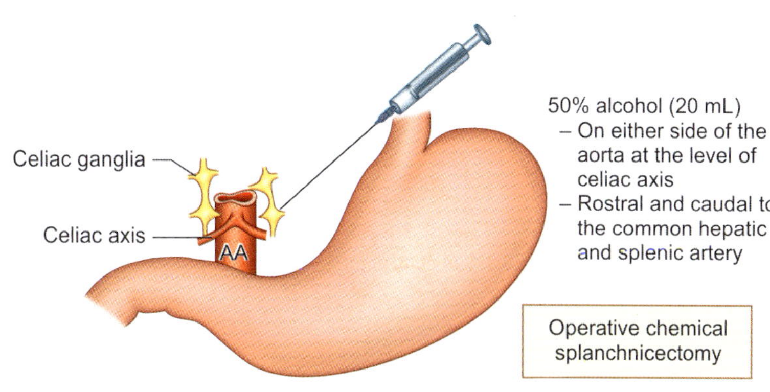

Pancreatic Stents

Types: (i) Plastic stent and (ii) SEMS. Plastic stent is made of polyethylene, length ranges from 2–25 cm, diameter ranges from 3 F to 11.5 F. Different types of plastic stents are straight, curved, wedge, single pigtail, with distal flange, winged. Sideholes are present throughout the length of the stent to facilitate drainage of the pancreatic side ducts.

Indications

- Pancreatic duct strictures (in chronic pancreatitis)
- Pancreatic duct leak (following trauma, pancreatic surgery, as a complication of severe acute pancreatitis)
- Chronic pancreatitis in pancreas divisum
- Prevention of post-ERCP pancreatitis in high-risk patients (e.g., difficult cannulations, pancreatic sphincterotomy, precut sphincterotomy)
- Pancreatic pseudocyst with ductal communication.

Complications: (i) Stent migration; (ii) Stent occlusion; (iii) Stent-induced pancreatic ductal changes; and (iv) Pancreatitis.

Endoscopic Ultrasound (EUS)

Endoscopic ultrasound uses dedicated echoendoscopes. Echoendoscopes are of two types: (i) Radial scanning and (ii) Curvilinear-array (CLA). EUS-FNA is performed by CLA echoendoscopes.

Indications

(i) EUS-guided sampling for biochemical analyses as well as cytopathological examination in pancreatic cystic lesions

(ii) EUS-guided sampling in pancreatic solid lesions and pancreatic mass associated with chronic pancreatitis

(iii) EUS-guided sampling for the diagnosis of indeterminate biliary strictures

(iv) EUS-guided core biopsy for diffuse esophageal or gastric wall thickening after failure of standard biopsy techniques.

EUS-guided sampling for the assessment of regional lymph nodes in T1 adenocarcinoma of esophagus

EUS-guided celiac plexus neurolysis (with absolute alcohol)

EUS-guided biliary and pancreatic access (if conventional ERCP fails to achieve pancreaticobiliary access due to altered anatomy)

Complications

(i) Perforation; (ii) Infection; (iii) Pancreatitis; (iv) Hemorrhage; (v) Tumor seeding; and (vi) Biliary seeding (rare).

Case 1

History and Physical Examination

A 26-year-old male patient presented with acute onset upper abdominal pain along with nausea and vomiting for last 2 days. The pain was severe and often radiating to the back. No history of similar episodes of pain abdomen in the recent past. No history of hematemesis or melena. Patient is a chronic smoker and alcoholic for last 5 years.

Physical Examination

Patient alert, conscious, cooperative

Temperature 100°F; Pulse 116/min; BP 100/60 mm Hg; Respiratory rate 18/min

Examination of abdomen: Tenderness and guarding in the epigastrium; abdomen mildly distended

IPS: Sluggish

Systemic examination: Diminished breath sound on left side.

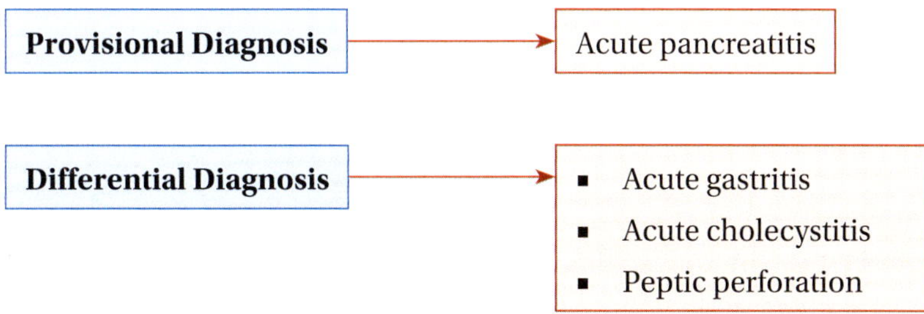

Investigations

Serum amylase 412 U/L; Serum lipase 1024 U/L

Hb 11.2 gm%; Total leukocyte count 17,000/cumm; Fasting sugar 82 mg/dL; Serum creatinine 0.9 mg/dL; Liver function test (LFT)—within normal limit

Discussion

A chronic alcoholic male patient presented with severe acute upper abdominal pain (with radiation to the back) along with tachycardia, hypotension, tenderness and guarding in epigastrium, sluggish IPS and diminished breath sound on left side (acute pancreatitis related pleural effusion is commonly left-sided) are highly suggestive of acute pancreatitis. Significantly elevated serum lipase and amylase level suggestive of acute pancreatitis. As two of the three diagnostic criteria are fulfilled, no need of any imaging for diagnosis.

Management Algorithm

- Fluid resuscitation
- Pain management
- Other supportive measures
- No role of prophylactic antibiotics

→ Assessment of severity as per Revised Atlanta classification (mild, moderate, severe)

↓

Monitoring of clinical and laboratory parameters

← Patient's condition improving → Initiation of oral feeding

↓ Patient's clinical parameters and inflammatory markers are not improving

↓ Contrast-enhanced CT scan (to detect local complications)

Case 2

History and Physical Examination

A 43-year-old male patient presented in the surgical OPD with dull aching upper abdominal pain with early satiety for last 3 weeks. Patient also noticed a swelling in the upper abdomen. About 2 months back, patient was admitted for about 7–8 days with symptoms of acute onset upper abdominal pain along with vomiting. No history of jaundice, hematemesis or melena. Patient is chronic alcoholic for last 15 years.

Physical Examination

Patient alert, conscious, cooperative

Temperature 98.4°F; Pulse 86/min; BP 110/80 mm Hg; Respiratory rate 18/min

Examination of abdomen:

A 4 cm × 4 cm non-tender, cystic, intra-abdominal lump palpable in the epigastrium.

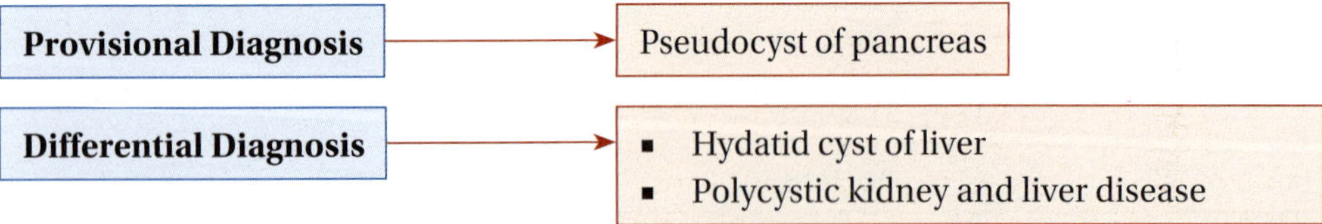

Investigations

Hb 13.2 gm%; Total leukocyte count 7,000/cumm; Fasting sugar 82 mg/dL; Serum creatinine 0.9 mg/dL; Liver function test (LFT)—within normal limit.

USG of abdomen: A cystic lesion with well-demarked margin, no solid component and related to pancreas.

CT scan abdomen: A cystic lesion measuring 7.0 cm × 5.2 cm × 6.4 cm with thickened wall without any solid component, related to body of pancreas.

Discussion

A chronic alcoholic male patient presented with upper abdominal lump and dull aching pain. About 2 months back, the clinical presentations were suggestive of acute pancreatitis. So, the abdominal lump is most likely related to acute pancreatitis. Clinical findings also confirmed a lump in the epigastric region. Both US and CT also confirmed the presence of cystic lesion (without solid component) related to pancreas. Based on history, clinical and imaging findings, the diagnosis was pseudocyst of pancreas. No need of any further imaging for confirmation of diagnosis.

Management Algorithm

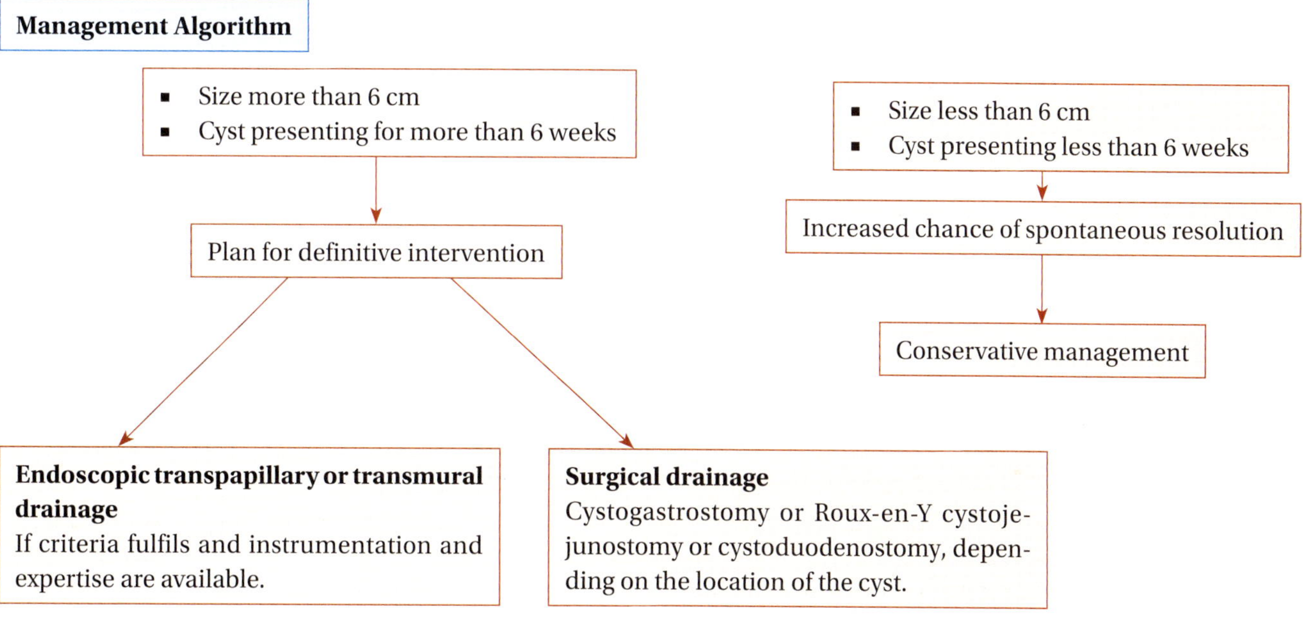

Case 3

History and Physical Examination

A 55-year-old male patient presented with jaundice, clay-colored stool, and pruritus for last 2 months. Patient also complained of repeated episodes of vomiting. History of loss of appetite and significant weight loss also present. Patient had no history of abdominal pain, jaundice in the recent past. No history of melena. No history of blood transfusion.

Physical Examination

Patient alert, conscious, cooperative

Jaundice—present

Temperature 98.4°F; Pulse 66/min; BP 110/80 mm Hg; Respiratory rate 18/min

Examination of abdomen: Non-tender gallbladder lump palpable

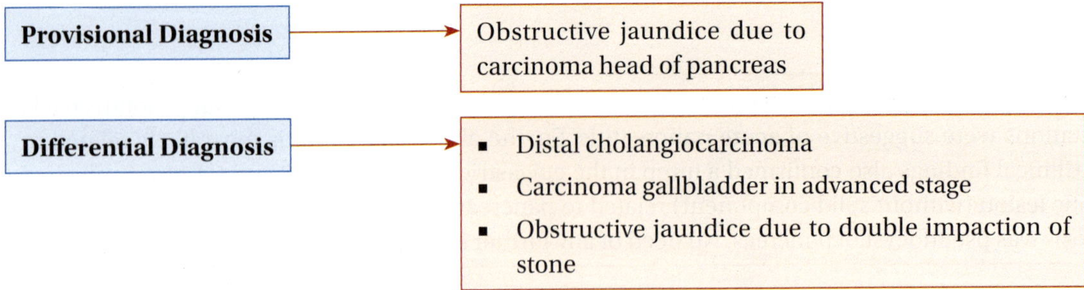

Provisional Diagnosis

Obstructive jaundice due to carcinoma head of pancreas

Differential Diagnosis

- Distal cholangiocarcinoma
- Carcinoma gallbladder in advanced stage
- Obstructive jaundice due to double impaction of stone

Investigations

Hb 10.2 gm%; Total leukocyte count 7,000/cumm; Fasting sugar 82 mg/dL; Serum creatinine 1.2 mg/dL; Liver function test (LFT): Total bilirubin 11.6 mg/dL; Alkaline phosphatase 1102 IU/L

CA 19-9 150 U/mL (normal range 0–37 U/mL)

USG of abdomen: Heterogeneous, hypoechoic mass in pancreatic head region

Pancreatic-protocol CT scan abdomen: Hypoattenuating mass lesion in pancreatic head region with no arterial tumor contact with celiac axis, superior mesenteric artery, common hepatic artery and no tumor contact with superior mesenteric vein or portal vein.

Discussion

A 55-year-old patient presented with clinical features of obstructive jaundice along with loss of appetite and weight loss. History of repeated episodes of vomiting also present. Clinical examination revealed a non-tender gallbladder lump. All these findings are in favor of obstructive jaundice due to periampullary cancer.

Laboratory findings were also in favor of obstructive jaundice, elevated CA 19-9 level was highly suggestive of pancreatic cancer. Imaging findings confirmed the presence of mass lesion in head of pancreas. Pancreatic-protocol CT abdomen also assessed the resectability of the tumor. As the tumor is resectable, preoperative biopsy was not done. Pancreaticoduodenectomy was planned.

Management Algorithm

Preoperative workup

↓

Diagnostic laparoscopy

↙ ↘

No peritoneal metastases or liver metastases (not detected in CT) → Pancreaticoduodenectomy

Peritoneal metastases or liver metastases (not detected in CT) → Palliative therapy

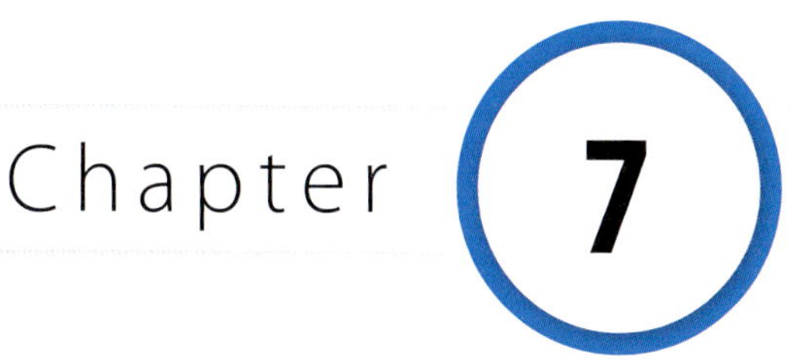

Chapter 7

Spleen

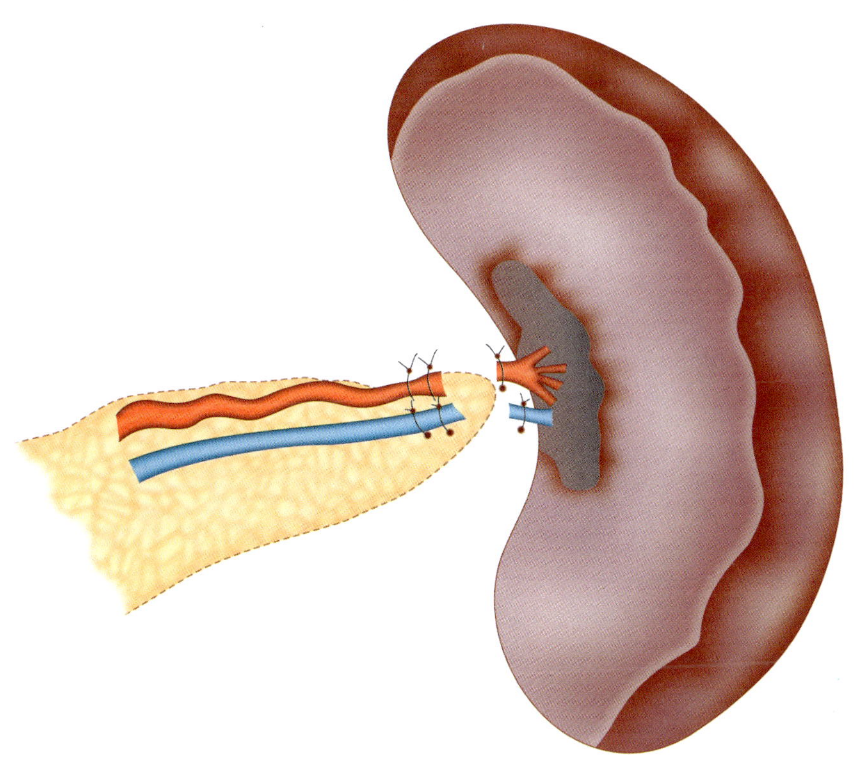

Important Topics

- Surgical Anatomy
- Functions of Spleen
- Accessory Spleen, Splenosis
- Indications of Splenectomy
- Miscellaneous Splenic Pathologies
- Hypersplenism
- Splenectomy

'I would never use a long word, even, where a short one would answer the purpose. I know there are professors in this country who 'ligate' arteries. Other surgeons only tie them and it stops the bleeding just as well.'

Oliver Wendell Holmes (1809–1894)
American Writer, Physician and Physiologist

Anatomy

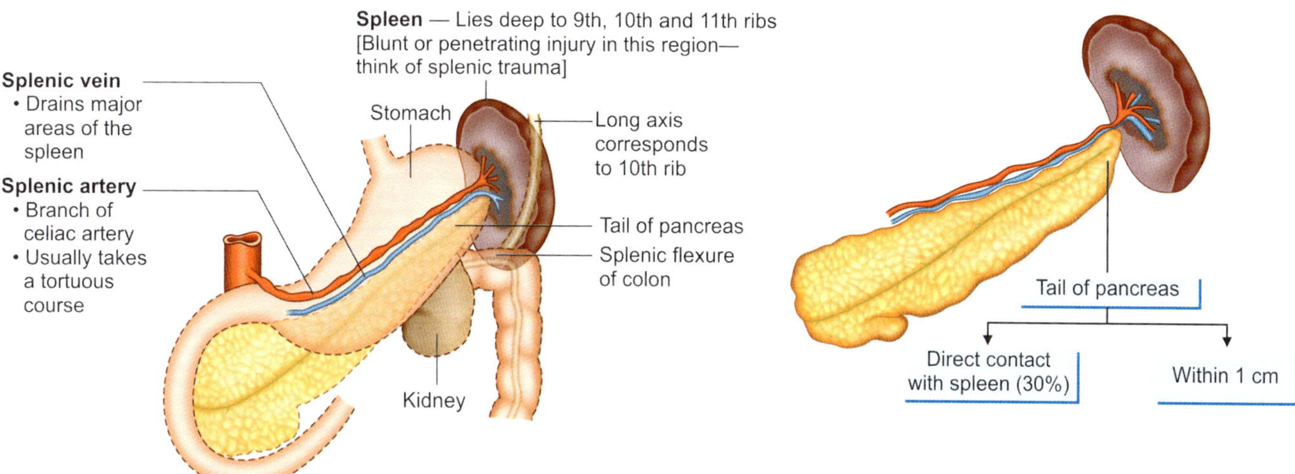

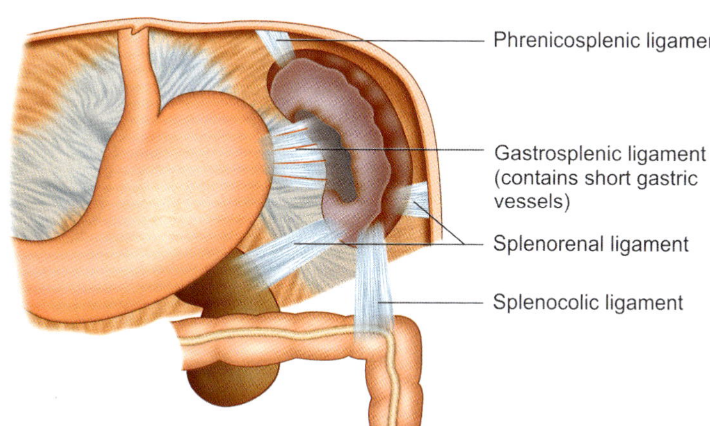

Ligaments with surgical importance:

- Gastrosplenic ligaments (contain short gastric vessels)
- Splenocolic ligaments (contains atleast two small vessels)
- Splenorenal ligament (Avascular)
- Phrenosplenic ligament (Avascular)

In portal hypertension, the avascular ligaments become vascular.

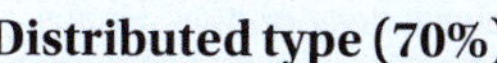

Distribution of splenic artery

Magistral type (30%)

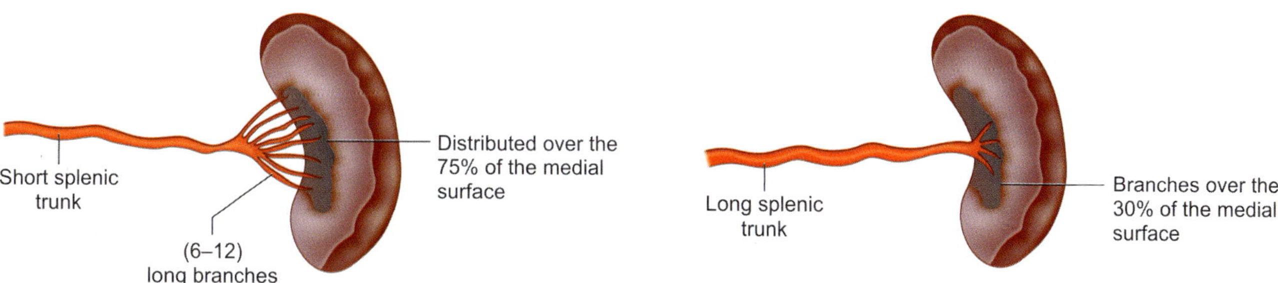

Functions of Spleen

Spleen is the largest secondary immune organ

Spleen is composed of two major units—**Red pulp and white pulp**.

1. **Red pulp** is composed of large number of venous sinuses and splenic cords (Cords of Billroth). Red pulp contains reticular cells, macrophages, monocytes, lymphocytes, plasma cells.
2. **White pulp** is composed of periarteriolar lymphoid sheaths (PALS) and lymphoid nodules. White pulp contains T- and B-lymphocytes.
3. **The marginal zone** lies between red pulp and white pulp. This zone is composed of sinuses and loose lymphoid tissues and contains lymphocytes and macrophages.

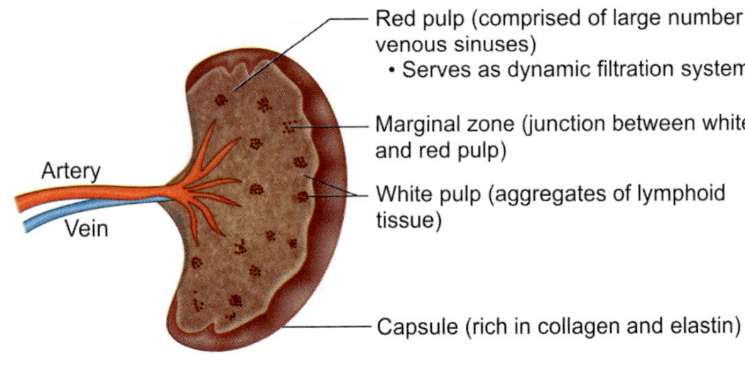

Howell-Jolly bodies are remnants of RBC nuclei.

Heinz bodies are denatured hemoglobin in RBC.

Functions of Spleen

Pitting: RBC inclusion bodies (Parasites, Howell-Jolly bodies, Heinz bodies) are pinched off during passing through slits of splenic cord in red pulp.

Culling: Abnormal, senescent RBCs are phagocytosed by macrophages in sinuses in red pulp.

Synthesis of antibodies: IgM, tuftsin, opsonin, interferon are synthesized in the white pulp.

Opsonization of bacteria: Opsonization of the encapsulated bacteria by the opsonizing antibodies are important for effective removal of bacteria from the circulation.

Extramedullary hematopoiesis

Reservoir of RBC and platelets

Iron metabolism: Macrophages in red pulp are involved in recycling of iron from senescent and damaged red blood cells.

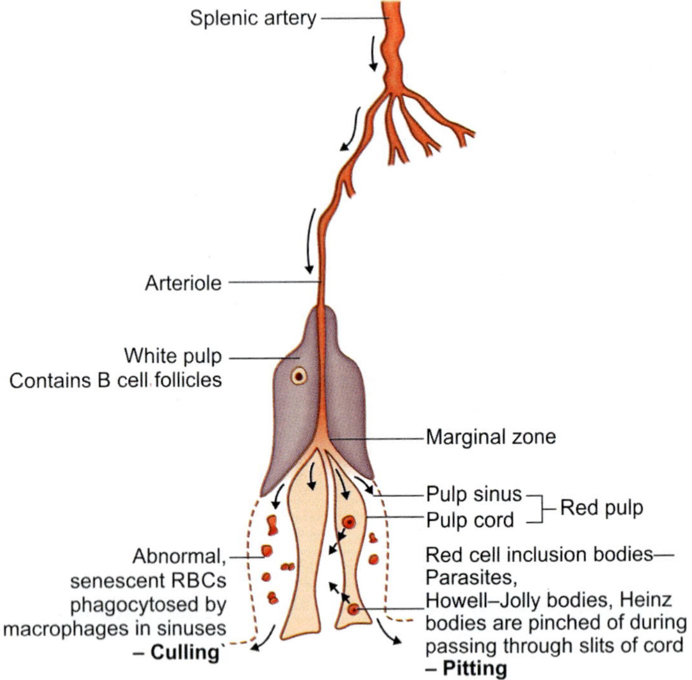

Splenic hematopoiesis in following conditions:

- In fetal life
- Myeloproliferative disorders
- Chronic hemolytic anemia

Accessory Spleen

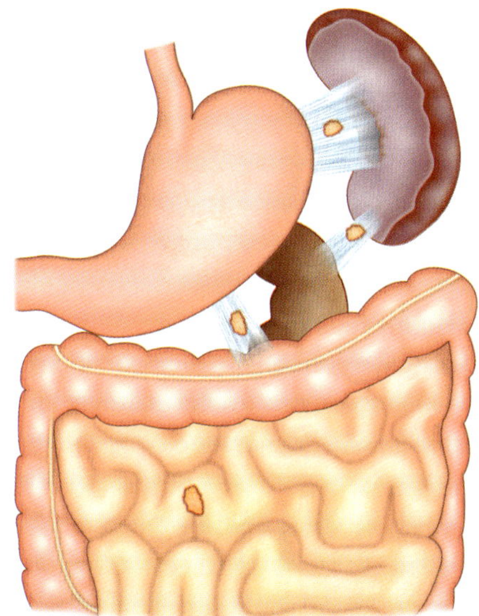

Accessory spleen is a congenital anomaly characterized by ectopic splenic tissue completely separated from original spleen.

Accessory spleen is similar to original spleen in structure and immunological function.

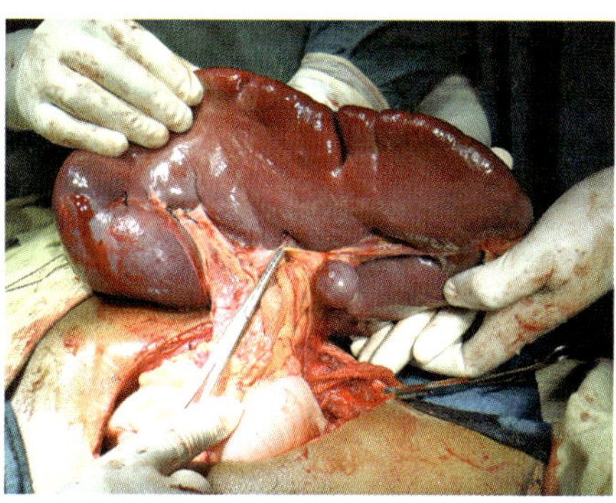

Location of Accessory Spleen

- A region of splenic hilum and vascular pedicle **(most common)**
- Gastrocolic ligament
- Tail of the pancreas
- The greater omentum
- Greater curvature of stomach
- Splenocolic ligament
- Small and large bowel mesentery

Failure to identify accessory spleen may lead to recurrence of some hematological diseases for which splenectomy is performed.

Splenosis

Splenosis is autotransplantation of splenic tissue usually following traumatic rupture.

The splenic implants are numerous and located within the peritoneal cavity.

Derives their blood supply from neighboring tissues.

Differential diagnosis includes accessory spleen, metastatic cancer, hemangioma.

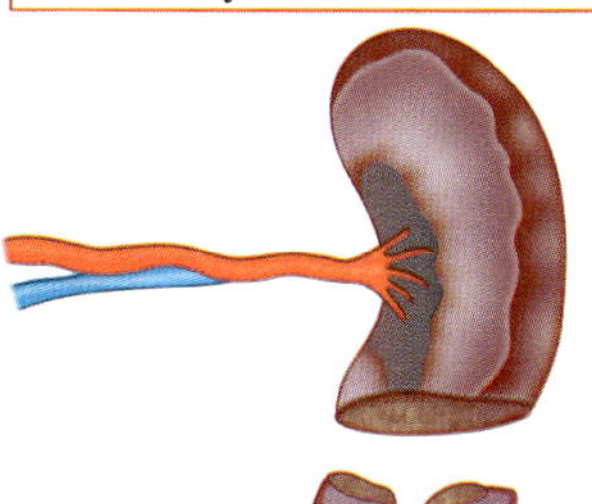

Peritoneal seeding of splenic fragments (not connected to portal circulation)

Differences between Accessory spleen and Splenosis

- Accessory spleen is a congenital condition whereas splenosis is an acquired condition.
- Accessory spleen is more common.
- Accessory spleen is supplied by the splenic artery whereas splenosis is supplied from neighboring tissues.
- Accessory spleen is few in number whereas splenosis are numerous.

Wandering Spleen

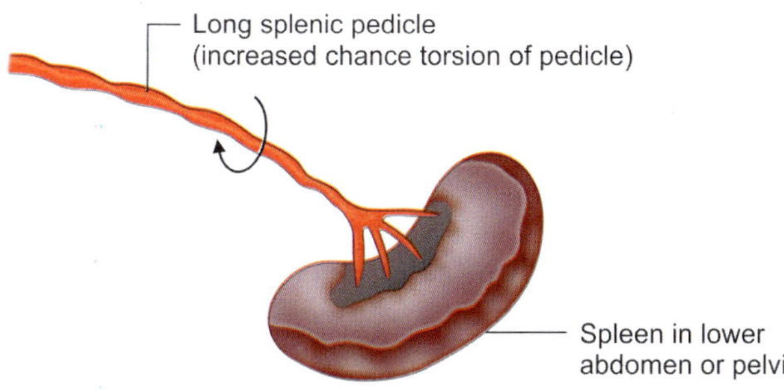

Wandering spleen is due to failure of development of suspensory ligaments of spleen.

- This clinical entity is characterized by migration of spleen from its normal anatomical position to any other abdominal or pelvic position and long splenic pedicle.
- Wandering spleen is at **increased risk of torsion**, resulting in partial or complete infarction.
- **Splenectomy** is indicated for splenic infarction and **Splenoplexy** is indicated in patients without pedicle torsion.

Indications of Splenectomy

- Diffuse enlargement of spleen by neoplastic disorders, hemopoietic disorders, metabolic and storage disorders
- Autoimmune disorders
- Trauma to the spleen
- Splenic vein thrombosis and splenic artery aneurysm
- Cyst, tumor, abscess in spleen
- Iatrogenic splenectomy
- Incidental splenectomy
- Staging splenectomy

Splenectomy as Curative Treatment in:

- Idiopathic thrombocytopenic purpura (ITP)
- Thrombotic thrombocytopenic purpura (TTP)
- Hairy cell leukemia
- G6PD deficiency
- Abscess of the spleen
- Splenic artery aneurysm
- Parasitic and nonparasitic cysts
- Splenic trauma

In Hereditary Spherocytosis:

- Splenectomy is the treatment even the patient is asymptomatic and anemia is compensated.
- If associated cholelithiasis (pigment stone), cholecystectomy should be performed along with splenectomy.
- Unless the clinical manifestations are severe, splenectomy should be delayed until age 6.
- Children under age 5 with high transfusion requirements, partial splenectomy (80%) may correct while maintaining normal immune functions.
- Splenectomy cures the anemia and jaundice in all patients.

In Idiopathic Thrombocytopenic Purpura:

Splenectomy is indicated in:
- Patients who do not respond to steroids
- Relapse after an initial remission on steroids
- Steroid-dependent patients
- Patients develop steroid toxicity

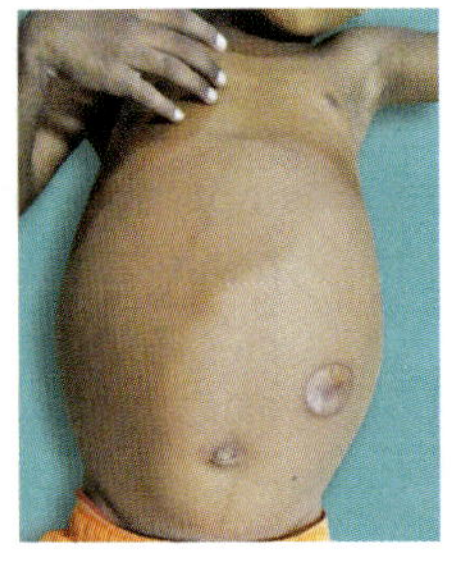

Massive splenomegaly in thalassemia

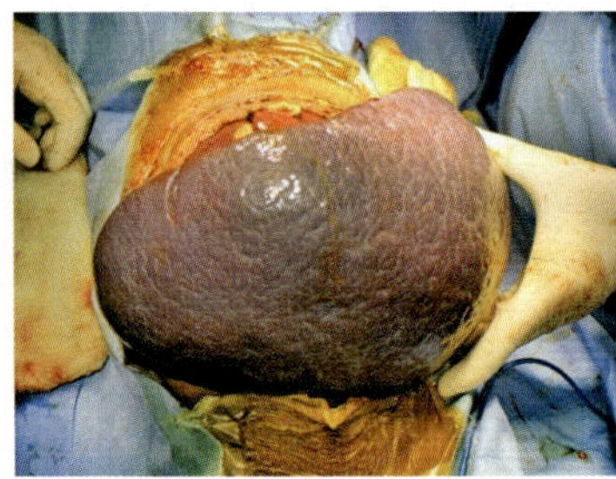

Peroperative picture of thalassemic spleen

Common Indications of Splenectomy

- Trauma
- Hematological disorder (e.g., thalassemia)
- Malignancy
- Iatrogenic injury

Role of Splenectomy in:

Sickle cell disease—for relief of symptoms (e.g., acute sequestration crises, splenic abscess, hypersplenism)

Thalassemia: (i) Decrease the frequency of transfusion; (ii) to relief the discomfort due to splenomegaly; and (iii) to relief painful splenic infarction

Hereditary spherocytosis—improves anemia and other symptoms (e.g., leg ulcers, growth retardation, skeletal changes)

Acute myeloid leukemia—improves symptoms like abdominal pain, early satiety.

Hairy cell leukemia and prolymphocytic leukemia: (i) Significant tumor regression in bone marrow and other sites and (ii) Correction of thrombocytopenia and anemia in most of the patients.

In Thalassemia Major:

Splenectomy is indicated for:
- Transfusion requirements >200 mL/kg/year
- Discomfort
- Painful splenic infarction
- Massive splenomegaly (Spleen is palpable >8 cm below the costal margin and/or weight >1000 g)

In Idiopathic Myelofibrosis:

Splenectomy is indicated in:
- Major hemolysis unresponsive to medical management
- Massive splenomegaly causing symptoms
- Life-threatening thrombocytopenia
- Portal hypertension with variceal hemorrhage

Incidental Splenectomy

Removal of spleen during surgical procedures adjacent to spleen, either to facilitate exposure or due to disease involvement or uncontrolled bleeding from capsular tear.

Chance of injury during left adrenalectomy, left nephrectomy, left colectomy.

Splenectomy is indicated: (i) If cancer of distal pancreas with lymph node involvement of splenic hilum and (ii) Renal cell carcinoma or left adrenal tumor infiltrating spleen.

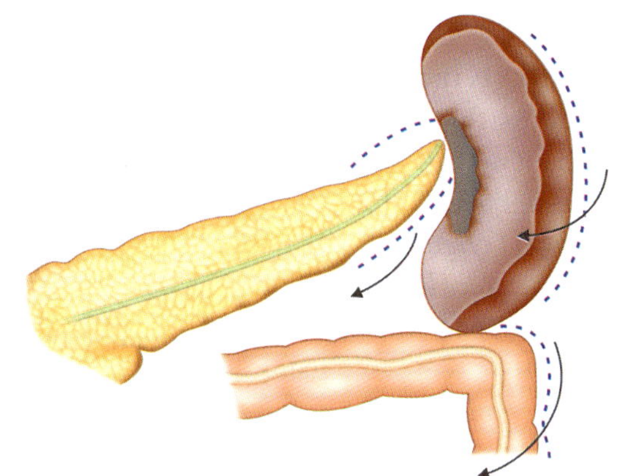

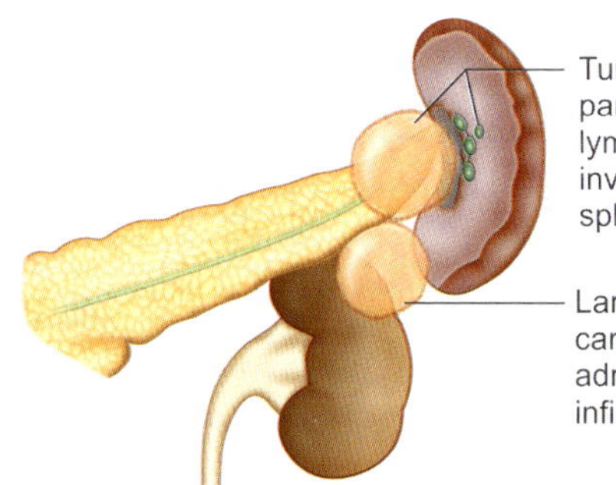

Splenic Artery Aneurysm

This is the *most common visceral artery aneurysm* and the third most common site of intra-abdominal aneurysm (after abdominal aorta and iliac arteries).

Risk factors include: (i) Atherosclerosis; (ii) Hypertension; (iii) Portal hypertension; (iv) Collagen vascular diseases; and (v) Pregnancy. *Risk factors for pseudoaneurysm:* (i) Blunt and penetrating trauma; (ii) Iatrogenic trauma during instrumentation; and (iii) Chronic pancreatitis.

Risk of rupture is increased in: (i) Pregnancy (3rd trimester); (ii) Pseudoaneurysm; (iii) Portal hypertension; (iv) Diameter of aneurysm more than 2 cm; and (v) Liver transplantation.

Most of the splenic artery aneurysms are asymptomatic. Clinical presentation of ruptured aneurysm is sudden onset left upper quadrant pain, hypovolemic shock and gastrointestinal bleeding.

MDCT with IV contrast is the imaging modality of choice. Direct catheter angiography is the most specific imaging modality but associated with more procedural risk.

Surgical intervention is indicated for all symptomatic aneurysms. In asymptomatic and incidental aneurysms, surgical intervention is indicated if diameter of aneurysm is more than 2 cm, patient is pregnant or of child-bearing potential.

Surgical approach depends on location of aneurysm. *Distal aneurysms* are managed by aneurysmectomy and splenectomy. *Proximal aneurysms* are managed by resection of aneurysm with interposition graft. Endovascular and laparoscopic approach may be considered in selected patients.

Splenic Abscess

Splenic abscess is a rare clinical condition.

Risk factors: (i) Immunosuppression (congenital or acquired immunodeficiency states, use of immunosuppressive drugs); (ii) Endocarditis (hematogenous seeding of bacteria); (iii) Trauma (secondarily infected hematoma); (iv) Diabetes; (v) Intravenous drug abuse; and (vi) Embolization for splenic artery pseudoaneurysm.

Clinical presentation includes fever, left upper quadrant tenderness, splenomegaly, leukocytosis.

CT scan is the gold standard imaging modality for diagnosis.

The gold standard treatment is splenectomy. Percutaneous drainage may be considered in unilocular abscess with a complete thick wall and no internal septations.

Splenic Vein Thrombosis

Chronic pancreatitis is the most common cause of splenic vein thrombosis. Other causes are acute pancreatitis, pancreatic pseudocyst, pancreatic carcinoma.

Most of the patients are asymptomatic. SVT may present with gastrointestinal bleeding due to isolated gastric varices or gastroesophageal varices as a result of localized portal hypertension, termed as *sinistral portal hypertension or left-sided portal hypertension*.

The investigation of choice is venous-phase celiac angiography.

Wait and watch policy is followed in asymptomatic patients without gastric varices. In symptomatic patients, *splenectomy* is the treatment of choice.

Cysts and Tumors of Spleen

Cysts of Spleen

- Congenital (epithelial) cyst
- Pseudocyst—secondary to trauma, infection, infarction
- Hydatid cyst

Tumors of Spleen

- Hemangioma (most common benign neoplasm of spleen)
- Lymphangioma
- Littoral cell angioma
- Lymphoma (most common tumor of spleen)
- Angiosarcoma
- Metastases (from carcinoma of breast and lung, melanoma)

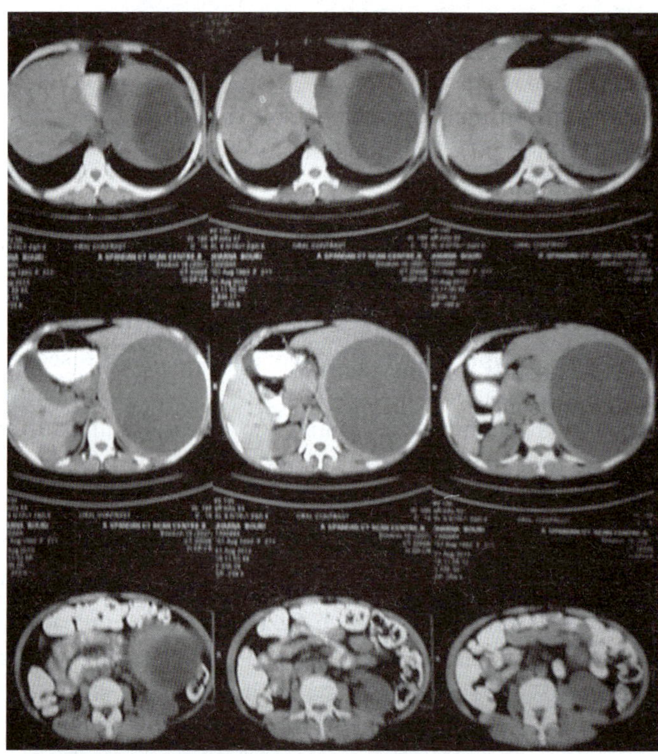

Littoral Cell Angioma

A vascular tumor unique to the spleen, arises from the lining cells (Littoral cell) of the splenic red pulp sinuses.

Hypersplenism is characterized by:

- Splenomegaly
- Cytopenia(s)
- Normal or hyperplastic bone marrow
- Response to splenectomy.

Hypersplenism is classified into three categories based on etiology: (i) Primary hypersplenism; (ii) Secondary hypersplenism; and (iii) Occult hypersplenism.

Causes of Hyposplenism

- Sickle cell anemia
- Celiac disease
- Bone marrow transplantation
- Inflammatory bowel disease
- Alcoholic liver disease

Mild splenomegaly: 300–500 g

Moderate splenomegaly: 500–1000 g

Massive splenomegaly: >1000 g

Peliosis of Spleen

Sinusoidal dilation leading to multiple cyst-like blood-filled cavities within the splenic parenchyma.

Splenectomy

Open Splenectomy

Indications of Open Splenectomy

- Grade IV and V splenic injury
- Massive splenomegaly
- Portal hypertension
- Extensive splenic irradiation
- Splenic abscess

Laparoscopic Splenectomy

Indications of Laparoscopic Splenectomy

- Benign hematologic diseases
- Malignant hematologic diseases
- Splenic cyst

Relative Contraindications

- Splenomegaly (weight >1000 g or maximal diameter >15 cm)
- Traumatic spleen
- Portal hypertension

Minimally Invasive Approaches of Splenectomy

- Laparoscopic splenectomy
- Hand-assisted laparoscopic splenectomy
- Single-port laparoscopic splenectomy
- Robot-assisted laparoscopic splenectomy
- Natural orifice transluminal endoscopic surgery for splenectomy

Partial Splenectomy

Indications of Partial Splenectomy

- Grade II, III splenic injury with hemodynamic stability or absence of other intra-abdominal injury
- Splenomegaly in hereditary spherocytosis and Gaucher's disease
- Non-parasitic cyst in spleen
- Hamartoma and other benign splenic tumors

Contraindications of Partial Splenectomy

- Inability to maintain >25% of splenic mass for adequate splenic function
- Inability to mobilize the spleen and tail of the pancreas to the midline.

Operative Steps in Elective Open Splenectomy

Incision

Left subcostal incision

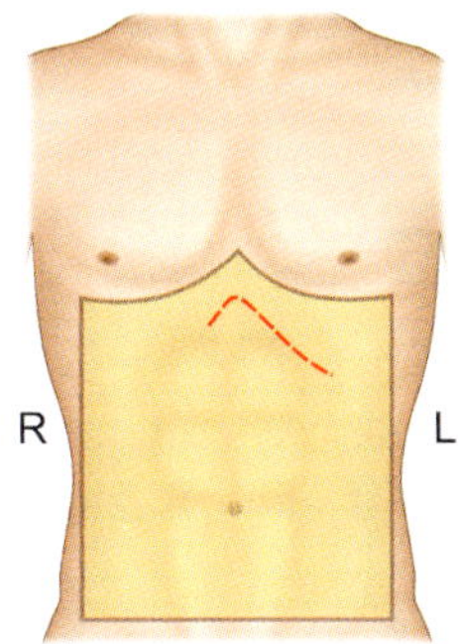

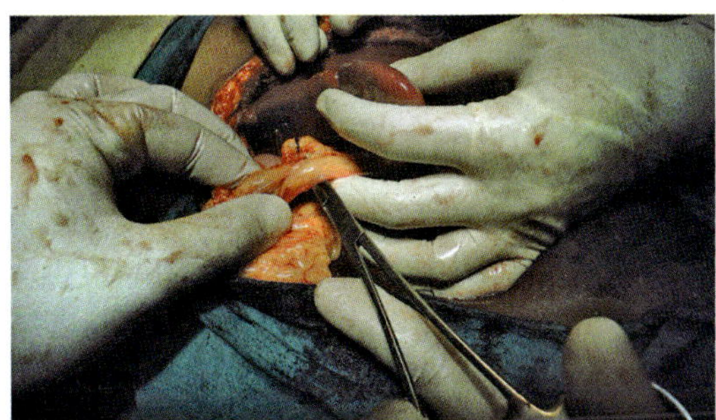

Operative picture showing ligation of short gastric vessels.

Division of Short Gastric Vessels

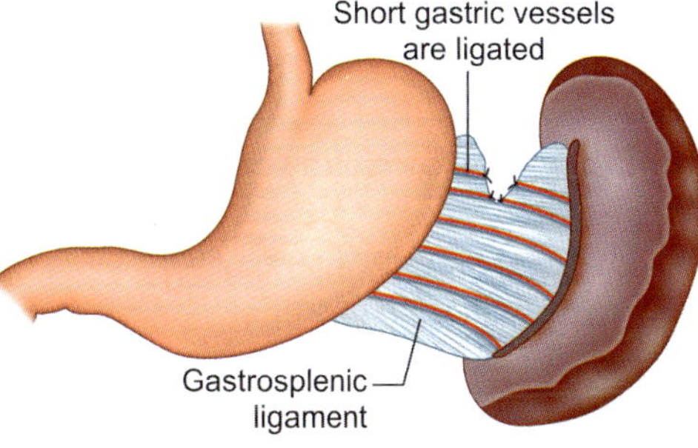

- Short gastric vessels are divided by sutures or energy device.
- The vessels high on the stomach are most difficult to divide and chance of injury to stomach is more.

Ligation of Splenic Artery

In massive splenomegaly, splenic artery is isolated above the pancreas through the lesser sac and then ligated.

Division of Ligamentous Attachments

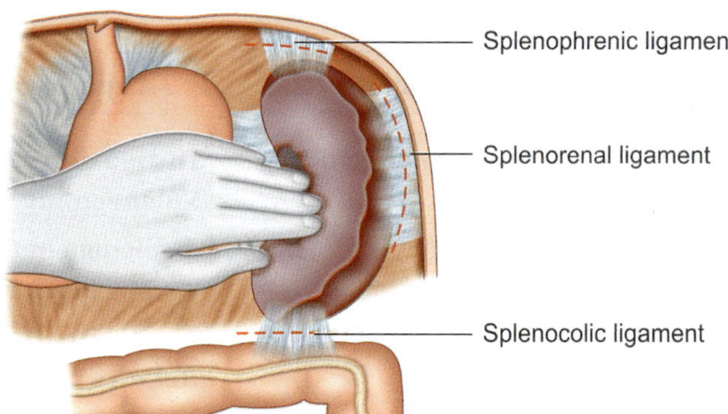

Ligation of Splenic Pedicle

- The splenic artery and vein are individually ligated. The vessels are doubly ligated proximally.
- Care must be taken to avoid injury to the tail of pancreas during ligation of the pedicle.

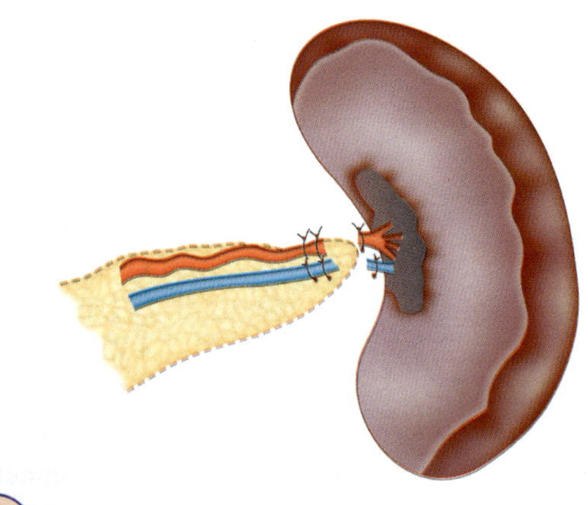

Observation to Check Hemostasis

Three areas to be checked for bleeding: (i) Inferior surface of the diaphragm; (ii) Greater curvature of stomach; and (iii) Hilar region

Thorough exploration for any accessory spleen.

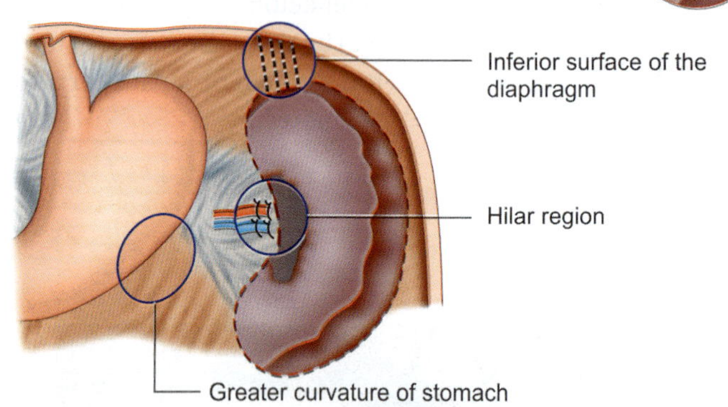

Complications of Splenectomy

- Hemorrhage—primary/reactionary
- Acute dilatation of stomach, necrosis of greater curvature
- Acute pancreatitis, pancreatic fistula
- Atelectasis
- Subphrenic abscess
- Thrombocytosis—may lead to thromboembolic complications
- **Overwhelming post-splenectomy infection (OPSI)**
- Diaphragmatic rupture, abdominal wall hematoma *(unique complications in laparoscopic splenectomy).*

Post-splenectomy Blood Picture

Immediate blood picture:
Leukocytosis, thrombocytosis. Within 2–3 weeks, counts and survival of each lineage become normal

Permanent blood picture:
- Anisocytosis
- Poikilocytosis
- Howell-Jolly bodies (nuclear remnant)
- Heinz bodies (denatured Hb)
- Basophilic stippling

Overwhelming Post-splenectomy Infection (OPSI)

- *OPSI is defined as* 'septicemia and/or meningitis, usually fulminant but not necessarily fatal, occurring at any time after removal of the spleen.'
- *Patients at risk:* (i) Extremes of age; (ii) Immunocompromised patients; and (iii) Splenectomy for hematologic disorders (e.g., hemoglobinopathy, myelodysplasia, malignancy).
- *S. pneumonia is the most common causal organism*, followed by *H. influenza* type B and *N. meningitidis*. Increased susceptibility to parasites (e.g., Babesia microti) and malaria parasites are noted in endemic areas.
- Overall lifetime risk of OPSI is low (<1–5%).
- The risks of OPSI and associated death are highest in the first year after splenectomy.
- OPSI is a life-threatening complication and early diagnosis, and treatment is key to reduce morbidity and mortality.
- Treatment is immediate administration of broad-spectrum intravenous antibiotics.

Prevention of OPSI

Vaccination

Vaccination is indicated to prevent the most extreme infectious complication, OPSI, caused by encapsulated bacteria (e.g., *Streptococcus pneumoniae*, *H. influenzae* type b, *Neisseria meningitidis*, *Capnocytophaga canimorsus*) in asplenic patients.

In elective splenectomy, vaccination should be given 14 days prior to surgery. *In emergency splenectomy*, vaccination should not be less than 14 days after splenectomy (suboptimal immune response if given before that) but if patient is discharged before 14 days, then vaccination just before discharge.

Vaccines: (1) Pneumococcal vaccine—Pneumococcal polysaccharide vaccine (PPV23), Pneumococcal conjugate vaccine (PCV13) in children <2 years [*S. pneumoniae*-total 90 serotypes]; (2) *Haemophilus influenzae* b vaccine (Hib); and (3) Meningococcal C vaccine [coverage against 5 serotypes of *N. meningitidis* among 6 serotypes]

Patient should be informed that vaccination can only reduce the risk of OPSI.

Revaccination of pneumococcal and meningococcal vaccine every 5 years; *H. influenzae* vaccine every 10 years and influenza vaccination yearly.

Antibiotic Prophylaxis

"High-risk patients" should receive lifelong antibiotic prophylaxis. All other patients should receive an emergency supply to be started for sudden acute severe illness prevention [as per British Committee for Standards in Hematology (BCSH) recommendation].

Education of the Patient

- Education of the asplenic patient and their family members about the potential infection risk is important.
- Asplenic patients should always carry a medical alert in the form of a laminated card or bracelet and up-to-date vaccination card.

Case 1

History and Physical Examination

A 5-year-old boy with a diagnosis of thalassemia major referred from medicine department to surgical OPD for consideration of splenectomy. History revealed that the patient requires repeated blood transfusion. Patient also complained of discomfort and early satiety for last 1 year.

Physical Examination

- Pallor—present
- Examination of abdomen—massive splenomegaly

Investigations

Hb: 7.2 gm%; Total WBC count: 5,000/cumm; Platelet count: 70,000/cumm
Total serum bilirubin: 4.6 mg/dL (Unconjugated: 3.4 mg/dL, Conjugated: 1.2 mg/dL)
Viral markers: HbsAg—nonreactive; HCV antibody—reactive; HIV I & II—non-reactive

Discussion

A 5-year-old boy with thalassemia major presented with history of repeated blood transfusion (more than 200 mL/kg/year) and early satiety. On clinical examination, massive splenomegaly was present. On laboratory findings, features of hypersplenism (leukopenia, thrombocytopenia) were also present. These transfusion requirement and massive splenomegaly are the indications of splenectomy in thalassemic patient.

Management Algorithm

Preoperative Work-up
Vaccination against *S. pneumonia*, *H. influenzae* type b, *N. meningitides* 14 days prior to surgery.

→ Elective splenectomy taking universal precautions (patient was HCV positive)

↓

Education of the parents of the patient about the potential risk of infection after splenectomy.

Case 2

History and Physical Examination

A 45-year-old male patient admitted in the surgical emergency ward with a history of blunt trauma abdomen following road traffic accident.

Physical Examination:

Patient—alert, conscious, cooperative; GCS—15/15
Pallor—present; Pulse—110/min, BP—100/70 mm Hg; Respiratory rate—18/min
Examination of abdomen—Bruise marks over the left hypochondrium, abdomen soft, no specific point of tenderness

Provisional Diagnosis → Splenic injury due to blunt trauma

Investigations

FAST revealed moderate amount of free fluid in the peritoneal cavity.

Discussion

A 45-year-old male patient presented with pallor, tachycardia and hypotension along with bruise marks over the left hypochondrium following RTA. FAST also revealed free fluid in the peritoneal cavity. So, the provisional diagnosis was splenic injury.

Management Algorithm

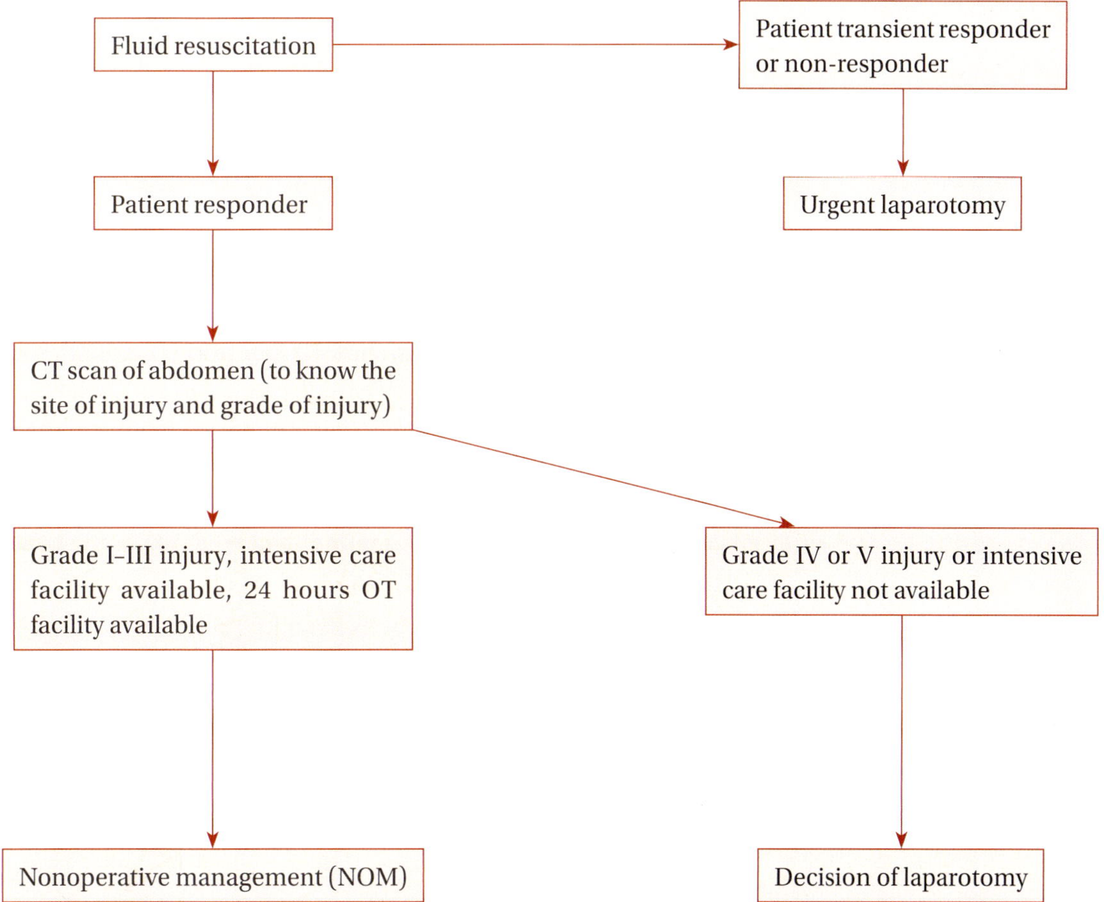

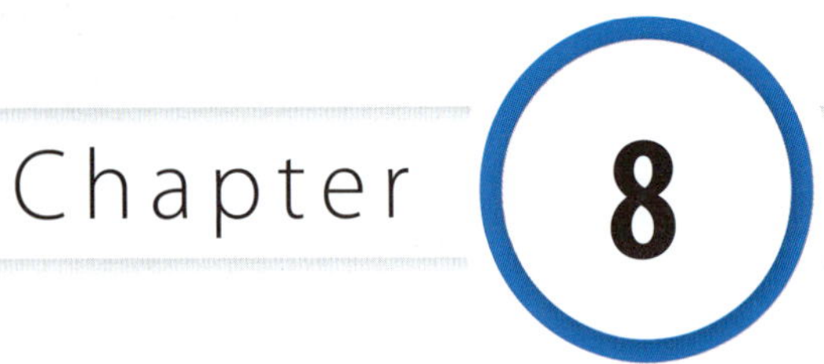

Chapter 8

Abdominal Wall, Peritoneum, Mesentery, and Retroperitoneum

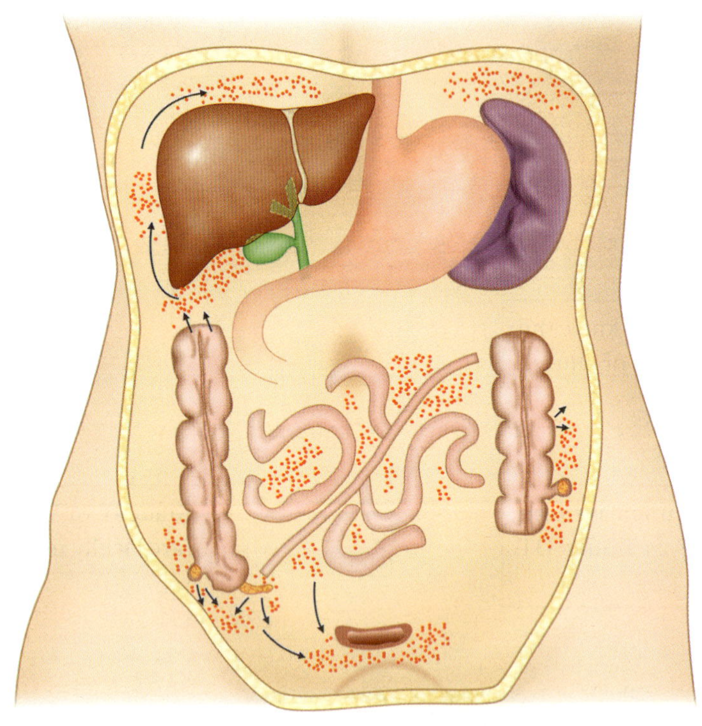

Important Topics

- Congenital Abdominal Wall Defects
- Vitellointestinal Duct Anomalies
- Patent Urachus
- Diastasis of Rectus Abdominis
- Rectus Sheath Hematoma
- Desmoid Tumor
- Surgical Anatomy of Peritoneum
- Intra-abdominal Abscess
- Mesothelioma
- Pseudomyxoma Peritonei
- Mesenteric Cyst
- Nonspecific Mesenteric Lymphadenitis
- Retroperitoneal Pathologies

'Every one is fond of comparing himself to something great and grandiose, ..., I am a mere street scavenger (chiffonier) of science. With my hook in my hand and my basket on my back, I go about the streets of science, collecting what I find.'

Francois Magendie (1783–1855)
French Physician and Physiologist

Abdominal Wall

Congenital Abdominal Wall Defects

Exomphalos (Omphalocele)

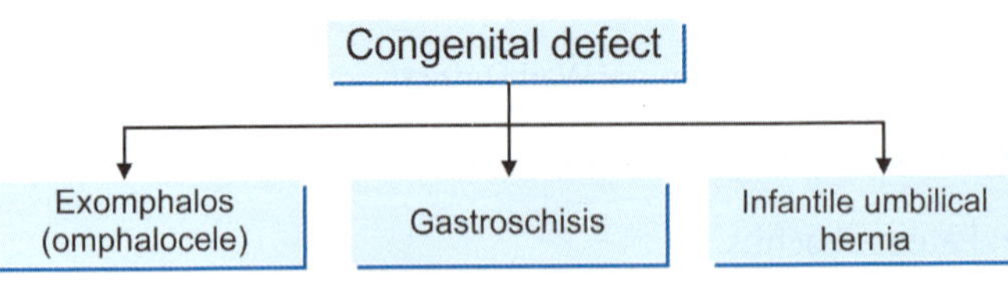

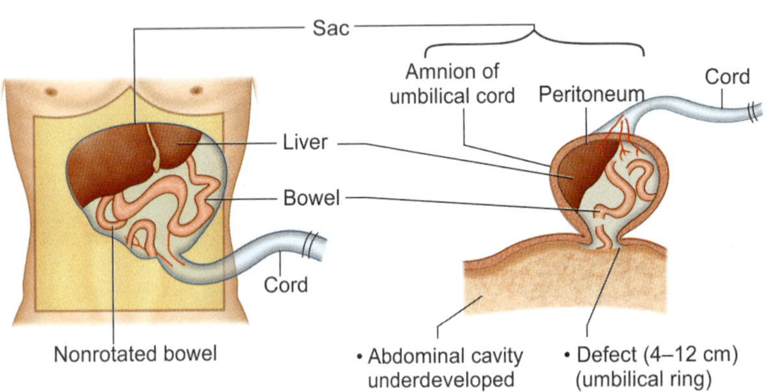

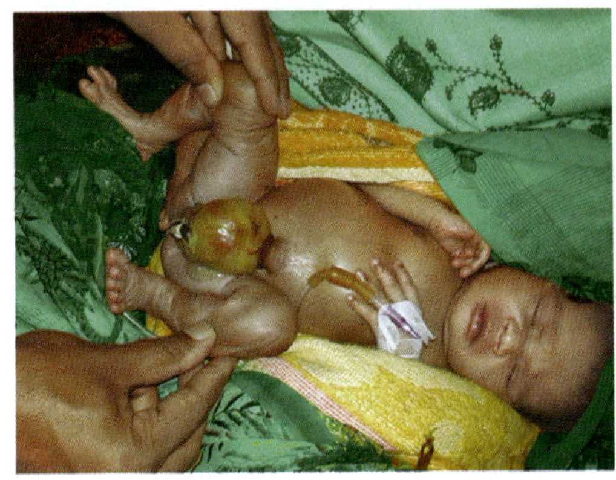

Exomphalos (Omphalocele) is a common congenital abdominal wall defect characterized by herniation of the abdominal visceras into the umbilical cord. The herniated visceras are contained within the omphalocele sac (sac consists of amnion, Wharton's jelly and peritoneum). The umbilical cord is attached to the sac.

Development

Omphalocele develops when the intestine fails to return to the abdominal cavity after normal embryonic herniation into the umbilical cord (during the 6th week of development) due to delayed closure of the lateral folds.

Perinatal Care

Once exomphalos is detected by antenatal USG, further investigations, e.g amniocentesis and fetal echocardiography should be done to exclude other associated congenital anomalies. Elective cesarean section is preferred in large omphaloceles due to increased risk of sac rupture or liver injury during vaginal delivery. All infants with this defect should be delivered in a center where both neonatal and pediatric surgical expertise is available.

Neonatal Resuscitation

Neonates with exomphalos, particularly with ruptured sac, are highly susceptible to significant fluid loss. The intact sac is protected with saline-soaked gauze. In case of ruptured exomphalos, the herniated intestine/viscera is covered with a waterproof cellophane bowel bag and the neonates should be nursed in the right lateral position with the bowel supported.

Herniated Visceras in Omphalocele

- Intestine
- Liver, bladder and stomach
- Ovary, and testis

Associated Congenital Anomalies

- **Cardiac anomalies** (tetralogy of Fallot, atrial septal defect)—most common
- **Chromosomal abnormalities**—trisomies 13, 18, and 21
- **Beckwith-Wiedemann syndrome—**macrosomia, macroglossia, pancreatic islet cell hyperplasia, and omphalocele
- **Pentalogy of Cantrell**
- **Pulmonary hypoplasia**
- **Lower midline syndrome—**cloacal exstrophy, imperforate anus, vertebral anomalies, omphalocele, and meningomyelocele

Evaluation of associated congenital anomalies particularly cardiac defects and pulmonary hypoplasia and if present, management should be considered depending on the associated anomalies.

Nasogastric tube should be inserted for bowel decompression.

Surgical Management

A small defect can be repaired in a single stage. Staged repair (silastic pouch and gradual reduction/sequential ligation of the sac) is indicated for larger defects.

Postoperative Care

Most of the patients with primary repair need mechanical ventilation for a few days during the postoperative period.

Types of omphaloceles (according to the site of the defect):

- Epigastric omphalocele
- Central omphalocele
- Hypogastric omphalocele

Types of omphalocele (according to the size of the sac):

- Minor omphalocele
- Giant omphalocele (>5 cm)

Gastroschisis

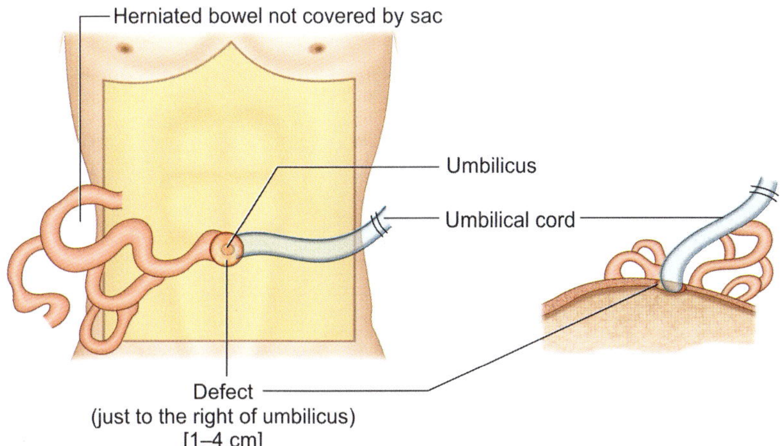

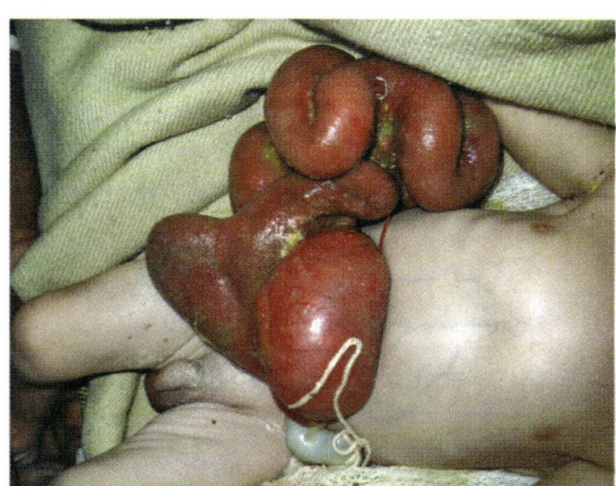

Gastroschisis is a common congenital abdominal wall defect characterized by a defect just to the right of umbilicus and herniated intestine without any sac. This condition is less commonly associated with congenital anomalies than omphalocele. The herniated bowel is usually covered with inflammatory peel and may be associated with foreshortening, necrosis and perforation.

Development

Exact cause is not known. Most common postulated hypothesis is a in-utero vascular event involving the omphalomesenteric artery.

Perinatal Care

Gastroschisis is diagnosed by routine antenatal USG. Early delivery (~37 weeks gestation) is preferred by some obstetricians to minimize the bowel damage from exposure to amniotic fluid. All infants with this defect should be delivered in a center where both neonatal and pediatric surgical expertise is available.

Herniated Visceras in Gastroschisis

- Intestine (most common)
- Liver, testes, and ovary (less commonly involved)

Associated Congenital Anomalies

- Intestinal atresia (most common)
- Intestinal duplication
- Meckel's diverticulum
- Limb-body wall defect syndrome (rare association)

Neonatal Resuscitation

Neonates with gastroschisis are susceptible to significant heat and fluid loss due to exposed bowel. To prevent this fluid loss, the bowel is covered with a waterproof cellophane bowel bag. Fluid resuscitation should be started to maintain the fluid deficit. The neonate should be nursed in the right lateral position to prevent kinking of the mesentery. Nasogastric tube should be inserted for bowel decompression.

Thorough evaluation of the neonate is indicated to exclude any associated congenital anomalies (particularly bowel atresia) and any evidence of malrotation, bowel necrosis or perforation.

Surgical Management

Principles of surgical management are: (i) Returning of the herniated viscera with minimal injury and (ii) Careful inspection of the bowel to search for obstructing bands, atresia or perforation and management of these pathologies before abdominal closure.

Surgical options include: (i) Primary reduction with fascial closure and (ii) Use of silastic pouch (spring-loaded silo/pre-formed silo), serial reduction and then delayed fascial closure.

Postoperative Care

As most of the neonates have associated intestinal hypomotility and defective intestinal absorption, total parenteral nutrition should be continued for a few weeks during the postoperative period.

Long-term Outcome

Most of the neonates achieve normal growth and development.

Infantile Umbilical Hernia

- Umbilical hernia develops as a result of incomplete closure or weakness at the umbilical ring.
- This hernia is more common in **premature and low-birth-weight babies** and more commonly associated with trisomy 18, 21, Marfan syndrome, Beckwith -Wiedemann syndrome, and mucopolysaccharidoses.
- Parents notice a bulging of the umbilicus when the baby cries or strains.

Most of the umbilical hernias spontaneously resolve within 2–3 years

- **Surgery is indicated:** (i) Patient developing complications (incarceration, strangulation) and (ii) Hernia persisting beyond 4–5 years of age.
- **Suture repair with a nonabsorbable suture** under general anesthesia is the primary surgical management.

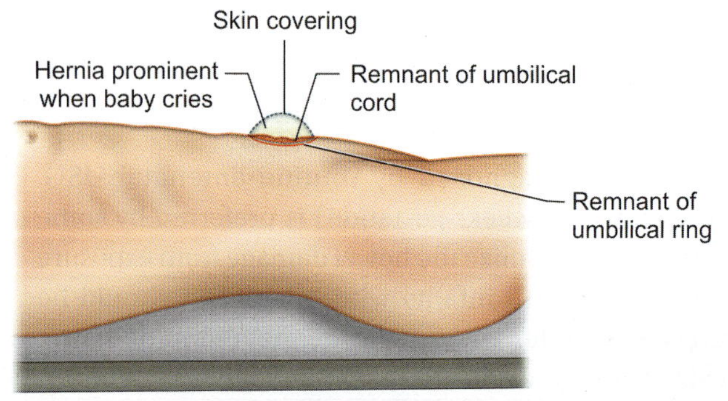

Vitellointestinal Duct (Omphalomesenteric duct) Anomalies

- During fetal development, midgut connects to the yolk sac through the vitellointestinal duct. Normally the duct obliterates.
- Failure of obliteration of this duct result in various anomalies.

If entire duct remains patent:

- Patient presents with feculent umbilical discharge.
- Treatment is early laparotomy followed by excision of the fistulous tract.

Distal part of the duct (near umbilicus) remains unobliterated:

- **Umbilical sinus** is formed from the unobliterated duct, and the epithelial lining of the sinus becomes everted to form adenoma. The obliterated duct is replaced by a fibrous band.
- Treatment is excision of the umbilicus along with the band.

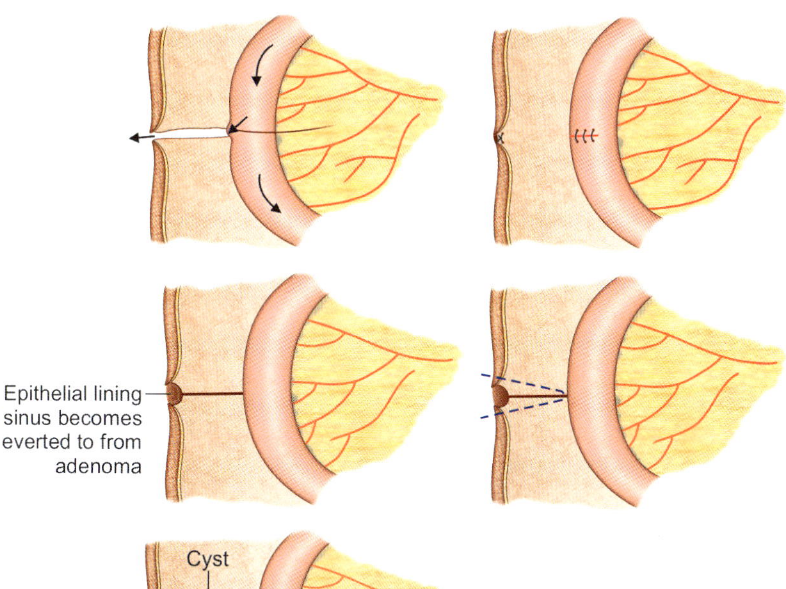

Mid part of the duct remains unobliterated:

- The unobliterated part becomes a cystic swelling *(vitelline cyst)* and the obliterated proximal and distal duct is replaced by fibrous band.
- Treatment is excision of the cyst along with the fibrous band.

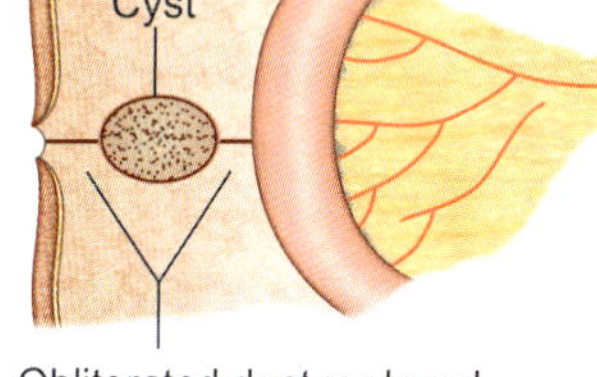

Proximal part of the duct remains unobliterated:

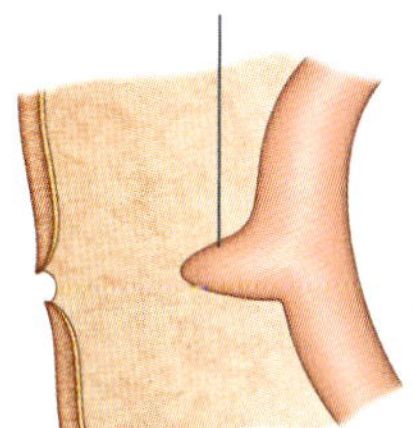

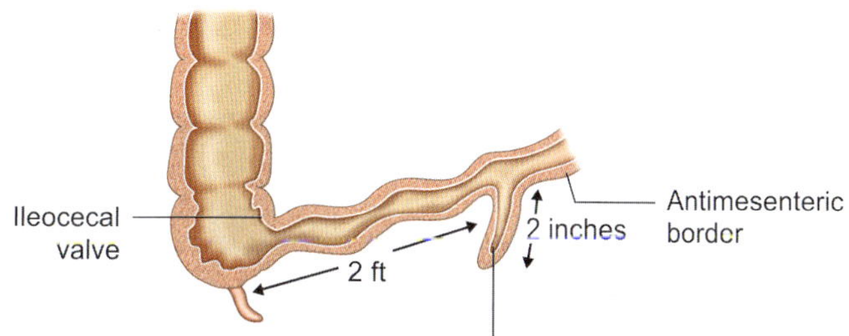

- **Meckel's diverticulum** develops when proximal part of the vitellointestinal duct becomes unobliterated. It is a true diverticulum. It is located in the antimesenteric border of the terminal ileum within 2 ft of the ileocecal valve.
- Patient may present with GI bleeding, and diverticulitis, band obstruction (band presenting from tip of the diverticulum to the umbilicus.
- Treatment is excision of the diverticulum along with fibrous band (if present).

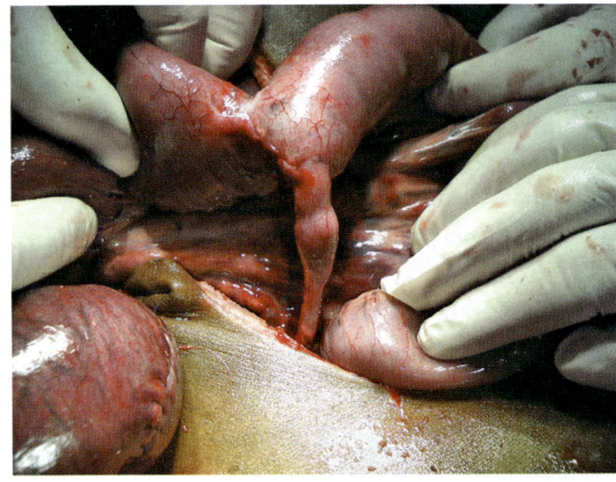

Umbilical Granuloma

- Umbilical granuloma is the commonest umbilical anomaly in neonates and infants.
- It develops due to overgrowth of granulation tissue at the base of the umbilical cord after its separation.
- Neonate presents with discharging moist, erythematous mass in the umbilicus.
- Most commonly used treatment is application of 75% silver nitrate. Other treatment options are double ligature technique, application of salt, steroid.

Patent Urachus

- Patent urachus develops when embryologic tissues connecting the developing urinary bladder and the umbilicus fail to resolve.
- **Total failure of obliteration** leads to a patent, tubular connection between urinary bladder and the umbilicus. Patient presents with discharge of urine from umbilicus, recurrent UTI and dermatitis around umbilicus. These manifestations usually present in presence of associated distal urinary obstruction.
- **Unobliteration of the distal part of urachus** results in persistent umbilical discharge, and recurrent omphalitis.
- **Unobliteration of the proximal part of the urachus** results in bladder diverticulum.
- **Urachal cyst** develops when midpart of the urachus becomes patent and the proximal and distal urachus obliterates.
- **Treatment** is resection of urachus with part of the bladder followed by closure of the bladder in two layers.

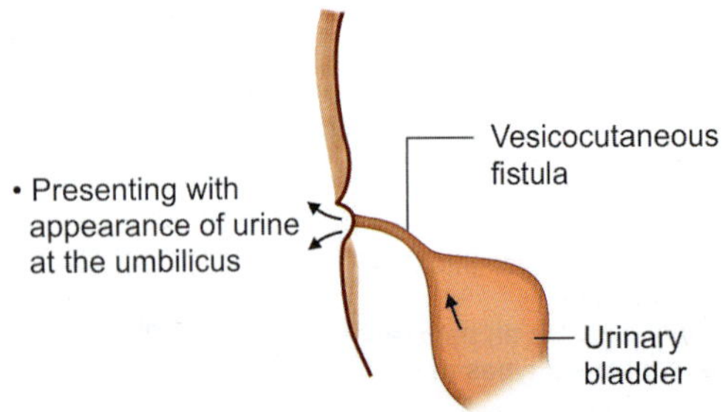

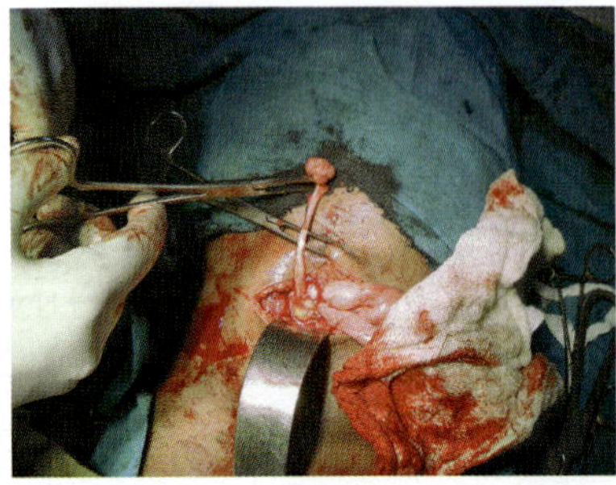

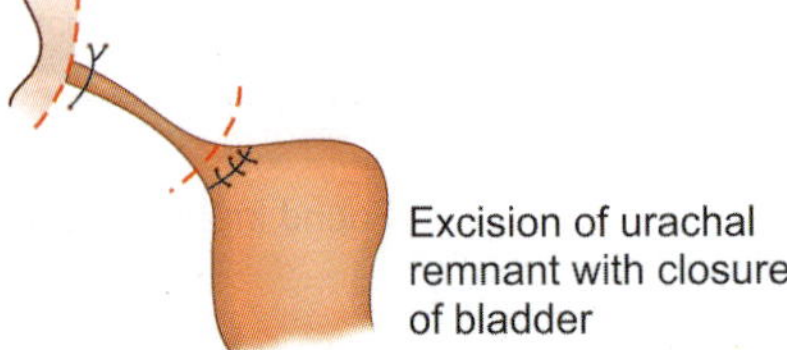

Diastasis of the Rectus Abdominis Muscles (DRAM)

- Diastasis of the rectus abdominis muscles is characterized by separation of the rectus abdominis muscle pillars along with the widening of the linea alba.
- This condition typically presents during the postpartum period, may present in advanced age, obese individuals.

Clinical Presentation

Patients present with characteristic bulging of the abdominal wall (without any fascial defect) in the midline on straining or straight leg raising. Umbilical hernia is often associated with diastasis recti.

Diagnosis

For diagnosis, no imaging is necessary. CT or MRI is indicated to evaluate the inter-rectus distance.

Indications for surgery:

- Cosmesis
- Discomfort with movement
- Associated umbilical hernia.

Different Surgical Options

- Abdominoplasty
- Midline plication of the linea alba
- Midline plication with mesh repair
- Endoscopic/laparoscopic approach.

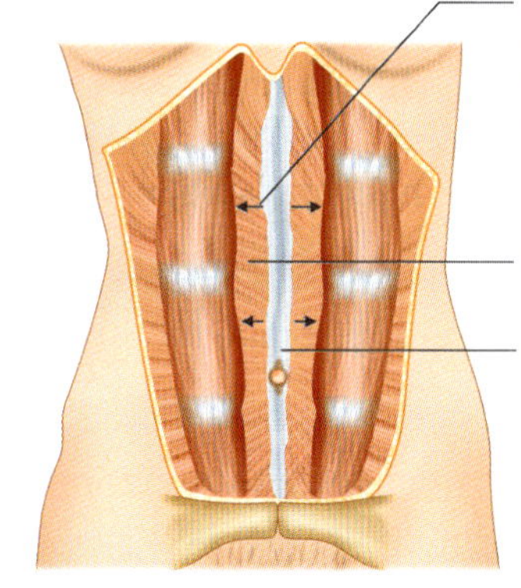

Classification System for Diastasis Recti

- The Nahas classification (based on etiology and myofascial deformity)
- The Rath classification (based on the level of attenuation relative to the umbilicus and the patient age)
- The Beer classification (based on the normal width of the linea alba).

Endoscopic/Laparoscopic Approaches for Diastasis Recti

- **Subcutaneous onlay laparoscopic approach (SCOLA):** An approach for umbilical hernia associated with concomitant diastasis recti.
- **Endoscopic-assisted linea alba reconstruction (ELAR):** A new operative approach for diastasis recti and concomitant umbilical, trocar or epigastric hernia.
- **Endoscopic-assisted linea alba reconstruction plus mesh augmentation (ELAR plus):** For treatment of diastasis recti and concomitant primary ventral hernia.

Rectus Sheath Hematoma

Rectus sheath hematoma develops as result of tearing of the terminal branches of superior or inferior epigastric arteries or its perforating branches within the rectus sheath.

Pathophysiology

Direct abdominal trauma or sudden forceful contraction of the abdominal muscles (following coughing, sneezing, any vigorous physical activity) in at risk individuals (on anticoagulation therapy, thin elderly women) causes tearing of the epigastric vessels.

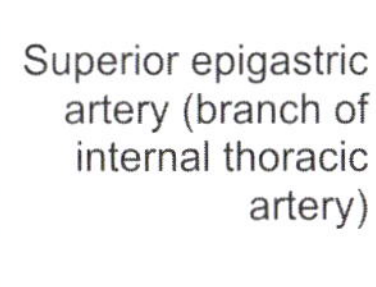

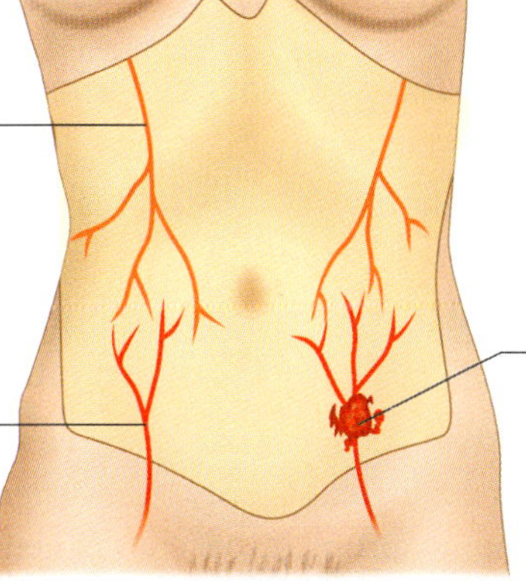

Clinical Presentation

Acute, severe, persistent abdominal pain associated with palpable abdominal mass (usually at the level of arcuate line). The abdominal mass remains palpable when patient contracts the abdominal wall muscles by lifting the head in supine position **(Fothergill's sign)**. Other uncommon findings include abdominal ecchymosis, features of hypotension.

Diagnosis

Both USG and CT are useful imaging modalities. CT is the most definitive investigation for establishing the diagnosis.

Management

Most of the rectus sheath hematomas are self-limiting. Bed rest, analgesics and discontinuation of anticoagulant therapy are effective measures in most patients. If expanding hematoma or clinical deterioration, endovascular embolization or surgical intervention (evacuation of hematoma and ligation of bleeding vessel) must be considered.

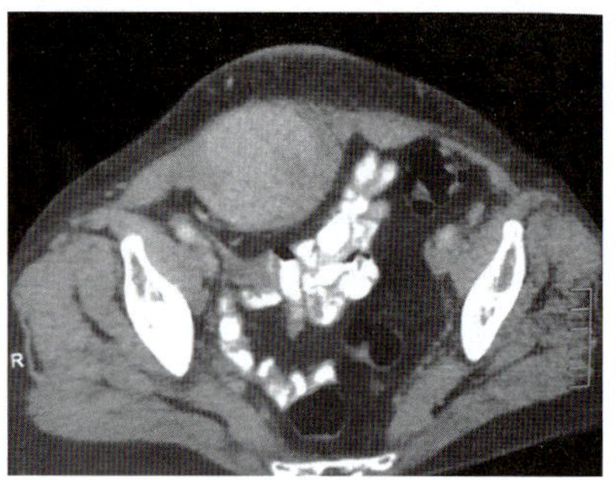

CT abdomen showing desmoid tumor.

Desmoid Tumor (Aggressive Fibromatoses)

Desmoid tumors are defined as "clonal fibroblastic proliferations that arise in the deep soft tissues and are characterized by infiltrative growth and a tendency toward local recurrence but an inability to metastasize"(WHO definition). Desmoid tumors are locally malignant, nonmetastasizing mesenchymal neoplasms. These tumors are characterized by aggressive fibroblastic proliferation and high recurrence rate. Extra-abdominal (e.g., shoulder girdle), abdominal wall and intraabdominal (mesenteric and pelvic) are the different sites of desmoid tumor. Sporadic abdominal wall desmoid tumors occur particularly in young women during gestation or within 1 year of childbirth.

Genetics

Mutation in the *CTNNB1* gene encoding the β-catenin pathway in sporadic desmoid tumors.

Workup:

(i) Imaging of the tumor (CT/MRI); (ii) Biopsy (may not indicated if complete resection is planned); and (iii) Evaluation for Gardner's syndrome/FAP.

Treatment

- **"Wait and see" approach:** If tumors are asymptomatic and not located in an area that may lead to functional limitations if tumor increases in size.
- **Resection:** For resectable tumors, R0 resection is the treatment of choice. If R1 resection, then observation or re-resection may be considered.
- **Radiotherapy:** It is indicated for unresectable tumors in extremity, head-neck or superficial trunk; but not recommended for unresectable retroperitoneal or intraabdominal desmoid tumors.

For unresectable, progressive, recurrent aggressive tumors, treatment options are: (i) NSAIDs (sulindac or celecoxib); (ii) Hormonal or biological agents (tamoxifene, toremifine, low-dose interferon); (iii) Chemotherapy (methotrexate and vinblastine, doxorubicin-based regimens); and (iv) Tyrosine kinase inhibitors (imatinib, sorafenib).

Peritoneum and Peritoneal Cavity

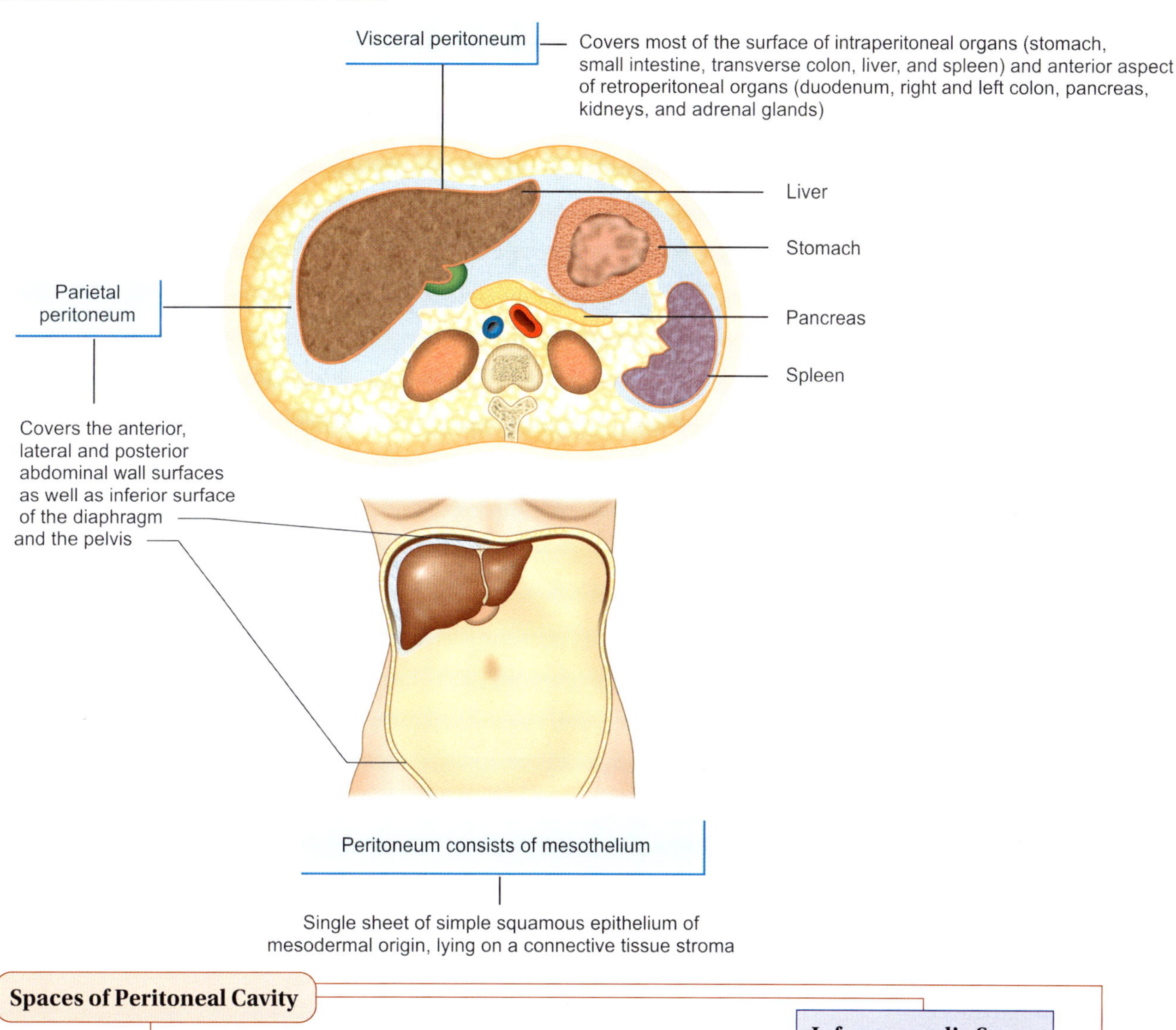

Peritoneum consists of mesothelium

Single sheet of simple squamous epithelium of mesodermal origin, lying on a connective tissue stroma

Spaces of Peritoneal Cavity

Supramesocolic space

Right Supramesocolic Space

- Right subphrenic space
- Anterior right subhepatic space
- Posterior right subhepatic space (Morison pouch)
- Lesser sac

Left Supramesocolic Space

- Anterior left subhepatic space
- Posterior left subhepatic space
- Anterior left subphrenic space
- Posterior left subphrenic space

Inframesocolic Space

- Right inframesocolic space
- Left inframesocolic space
- Right and left paracolic gutters

Pelvic Spaces

- Paravesical spaces
- Rectovesical pouch
- Rectouterine pouch (Pouch of Douglas)

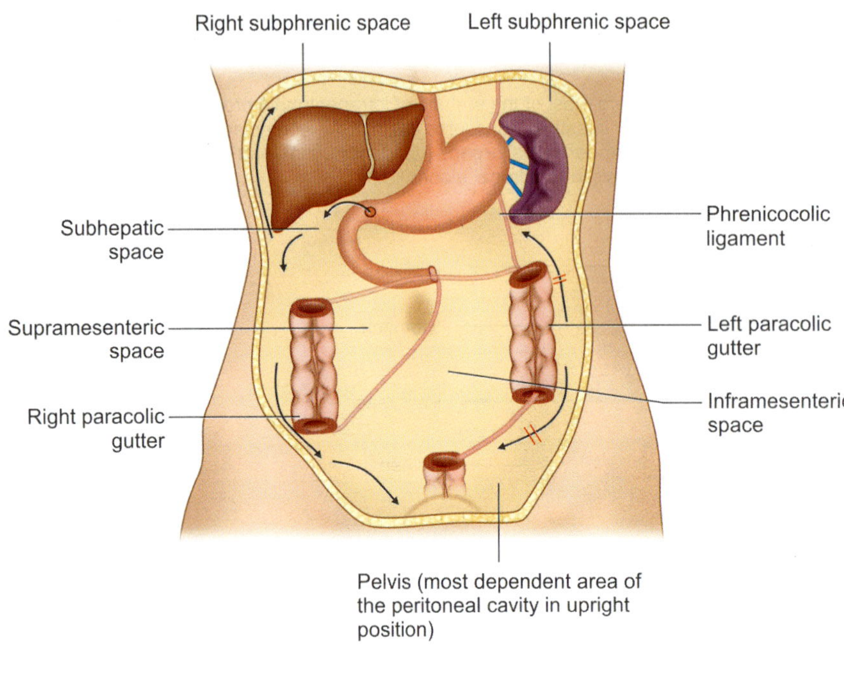

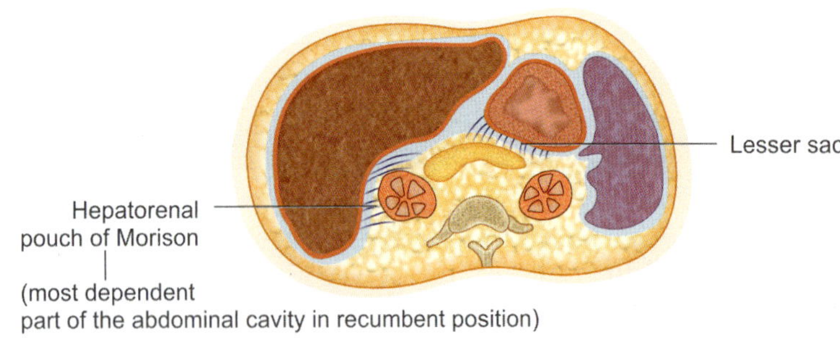

- Knowledge about the peritoneal space helps to predict the route of infection.
- The transverse mesocolon divides the peritoneal cavity into supramesocolic and inframesocolic spaces.
- Communication from the left paracolic gutter with the pelvis is limited due to the sigmoid colon.
- Communication from the left paracolic gutter with the left subphrenic space is limited due to phrenicocolic ligament.
- The right paracolic gutter communicates freely with the right subphrenic space.
- In male, rectovesical space is the most gravity-dependent area for fluid accumulation; in female, it is the rectouterine pouch.

Intra-abdominal Abscess

Types

(i) Intraperitoneal abscess; (ii) Retroperitoneal abscess; and (iii) Visceral abscess.

- **Intraperitoneal abscess:** It develops following resolution of diffuse peritonitis or perforation of hollow viscus or rupture of visceral abscess. For examples, Pelvic abscess and subphrenic abscess.
- **Retroperitoneal abscess:** It develops following hematogenous spread of organisms, from traumatic duodenal injury/perforation or from ruptured renal abscess.
- **Visceral abscess:** It develops following hematogenous or lymphatic spread of microorganisms into visceral parenchyma. For examples, liver abscess and splenic abscess.

Microbiology

The bacteriology of intraperitoneal, retroperitoneal and visceral abscesses are mainly polymicrobial—gram negative and positive, aerobic and anaerobic.

Different Intraperitoneal Abscesses

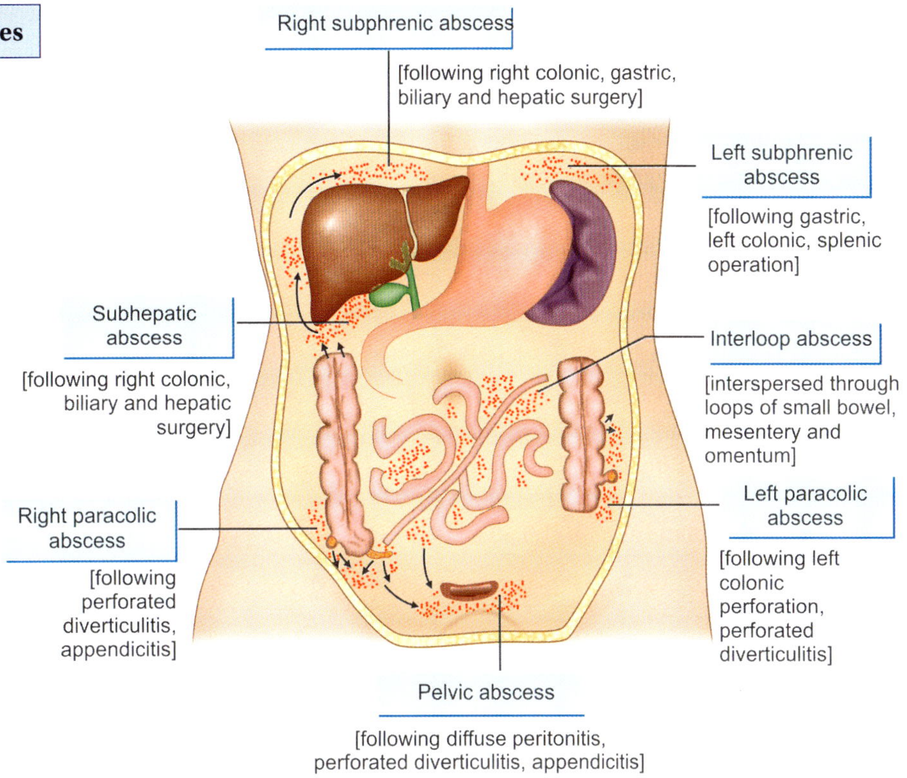

Right subphrenic abscess
[following right colonic, gastric, biliary and hepatic surgery]
Left subphrenic abscess
[following gastric, left colonic, splenic operation]
Subhepatic abscess
[following right colonic, biliary and hepatic surgery]
Interloop abscess
[interspersed through loops of small bowel, mesentery and omentum]
Right paracolic abscess
[following perforated diverticulitis, appendicitis]
Left paracolic abscess
[following left colonic perforation, perforated diverticulitis]
Pelvic abscess
[following diffuse peritonitis, perforated diverticulitis, appendicitis]

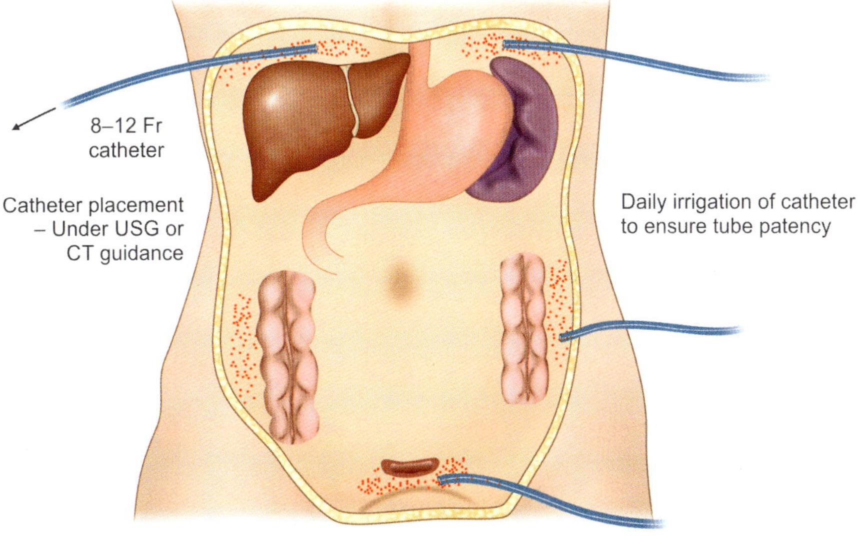

8–12 Fr catheter
Catheter placement – Under USG or CT guidance
Daily irrigation of catheter to ensure tube patency

Diagnosis

- Both USG and CT are useful imaging modality for site and size of the abscess as well as can guide percutaneous drainage.
- USG is more accurate for abscesses in right upper abdomen and pelvis. Staples, dressing and stoma may impede the USG image. USG cannot differentiate abscess from hematoma, seroma, biloma, and lymphocele.
- CT scan can differentiate between simple and complex abscess, more accurate for detection of retroperitoneal abscess.

Management

Percutaneous drainage or open surgical drainage—depends on the nature and site of abscess.

Percutaneous drainage is more effective if:

- Simple and single abscess
- Abscess content is not thick
- No communication with bowel
- No loculations in abscess cavity
- Subphrenic abscess, paracolic abscess, and superficial pelvic abscess

Surgical drainage is first choice in:

- Interloop abscess
- Multiple abscesses
- Abscess cavity communicates with bowel
- Ill-defined abscess

Pelvic Abscess

Pathophysiology

Pelvic abscess develops:

i. As a sequel of any diffuse peritonitis or anastomotic leakage following bowel or rectal surgery
ii. As a complication of pelvic inflammatory disease, inflammatory bowel disease, diverticulitis, and appendicitis.

Clinical Presentation

The patient presents with high-grade fever, lower abdominal pain, passage of mucus in the stool in the postoperative period, palpable pelvic mass. Per rectal examination reveals a bulging of the anterior rectal wall.

Diagnosis

USG (transabdominal/transvaginal) and CT scan are useful imaging modalities for diagnosis.

Management

USG (TRUS or TVS) or CT guided drainage with concomitant antibiotic therapy is the treatment of choice. Open surgical drainage (through rectum or posterior fornix) is another treatment option.

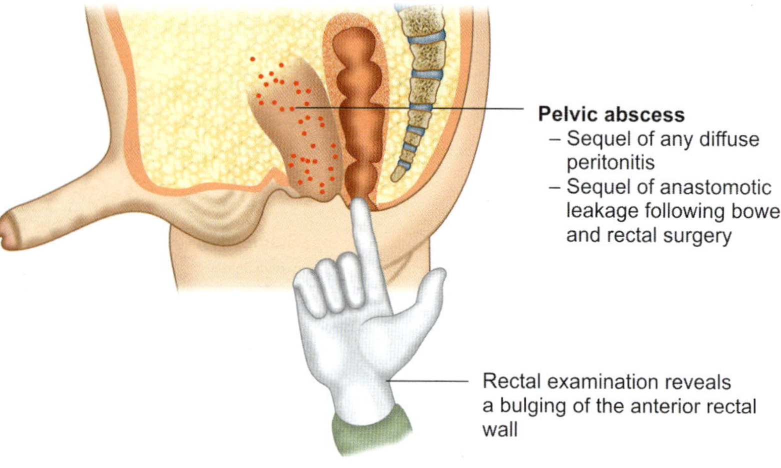

Malignant Peritoneal Mesothelioma

- **Most common primary malignant peritoneal neoplasm**
- Malignant mesothelioma shows male predominance.
- Patient presents with abdominal pain, ascites and weight loss.
- 50–70% of patients have a history of asbestos exposure.
- This tumor presents as hard, whitish nodules scattered over the peritoneal surfaces. Local invasion of liver, intestine and abdominal wall is common.
- Complete surgical resection is technically demanding and requires peritonectomy with resection of involved organs.

Pseudomyxoma Peritonei

- Pseudomyxoma peritonei is characterized by diffuse gelatinous ascites **("jelly belly")** with mucinous implants on peritoneal surfaces and omentum.
- This rare clinical entity develops due to rupture of mucinous neoplasm of appendix. Tumor cells are most commonly implanted in the right hemidiaphragm, greater and lesser omentum (due to 'redistribution phenomenon'), rectovesical pouch, pouch of Douglas.
- **Clinical presentation:** In the initial stage, non-specific symptoms and signs are present. In the advanced stage, patients present with ascites, intestinal obstruction, and pelvic mass.
- **Diagnosis:** Contrast-enhanced CT of abdomen and pelvis is the imaging modality of choice for diagnosis.
- **Treatment:** Cytoreductive surgery (bilateral parietal and diaphragmatic peritonectomies, right hemicolectomy, radical greater omentectomy with splenectomy, cholecystectomy and liver capsulectomy, pelvic peritonectomy, bilateral salpingo-oophorectomy with hysterectomy in females) with hyperthermic Intra-peritoneal chemotherapy (HIPEC).

Mesenteric Cyst

Mesenteric cyst can develop from any part of the mesentery of the bowel from the duodenum to the rectum. Most commonly found in small bowel mesentery (mostly in ileal mesentery) followed by large bowel mesentery.

Types: (i) Chylolymphatic cyst; (ii) Enterogenous cyst; (iii) Urogenital remnant cyst; and (iv) Dermoid cyst.

Chylolymphatic Cyst

- Most common type of mesenteric cyst.
- Benign proliferation of ectopic lymphatics, which lack communication with the main lymphatic system.
- The wall of the cyst is thin, lined by flat endothelium, contains clear lymph or chyle.
- Commonly solitary and unilocular.
- Blood supply of the cyst is independent from that of adjacent bowel.
- Treatment is enucleation of the cyst.

Enterogenous Cyst

- Developed by sequestration from the intestinal canal during development
- The wall of the cyst is thicker, lined by mucous membrane, content is mucinous.
- The cyst and the adjacent bowel have a common blood supply.
- Treatment is resection of cyst along with adjacent segment of intestine.

Urogenital Remnant

- Developed from a remnant of the wolffian duct.
- Clinically present as retroperitoneal mass.
- Cyst may be unilocular or multilocular.
- Treatment is resection.

Tillaux's Triad

(i) A fluctuating swelling near the umbilicus; (ii) A swelling freely mobile in the direction perpendicular to the attachment of mesentery **(Tillaux's sign)**; and (iii) Zone of resonance around the swelling.

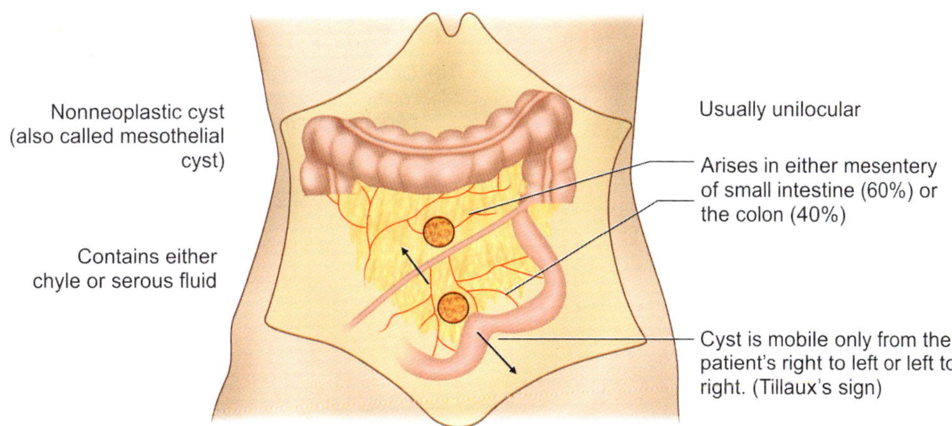

Acute Nonspecific Mesenteric Lymphadenitis

- Acute nonspecific mesenteric lymphadenitis is a **self-limiting inflammation of mesenteric lymph nodes**.
- This clinical condition usually develops in **children and young adults**.
- It usually follows after an upper respiratory tract infection.
- **Patient presents** with fever, pain in right lower abdomen and tenderness in right iliac fossa.
- **USG abdomen** is the imaging modality of choice for diagnosis.
- **Management** includes pain management and reassurance of patient and family.

Acute pain in right lower quadrant

Diagnosis is made after exploration with a clinical diagnosis of acute appendicitis

Most commonly in children and young adults

Yersinia enterocolitica is particularly associated with this syndrome in children

Normal appendix

Mesenteric lymph node enlargement

Differential Diagnosis

- Acute appendicitis
- Meckel's diverticulitis
- Intussusception
- Torsion of the ovarian cyst

Omental Graft and Transpositions

- The omentum is rich with vascular and lymphatic plexuses.
- Uses of omental graft and transpositions:
  - Repair of gastroduodenal perforation
  - Repair of vesicovaginal and vesicocolic fistulas
  - Reconstruction of chest and mediastinal defects following chest wall resection
  - Closure of full thickness defects of esophagus
  - Reconstruction of scalp defects.

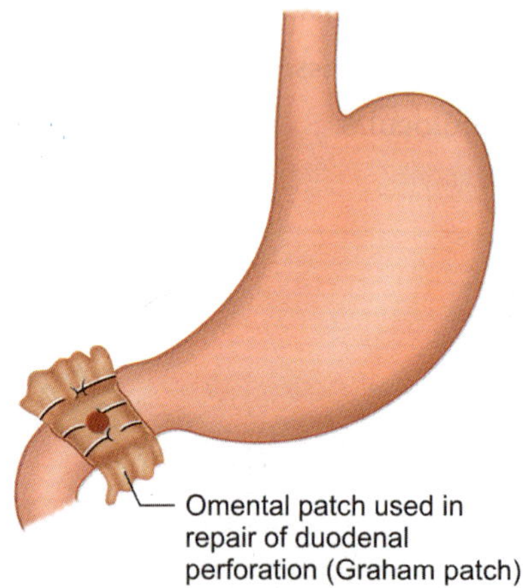

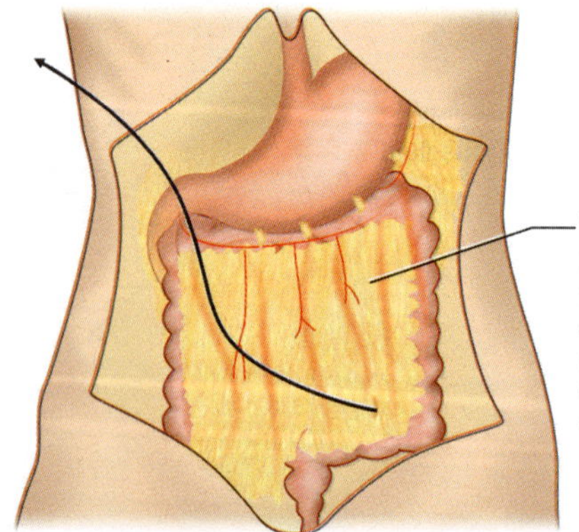

Functions of the Omentum

- Localizes infection in the abdominal cavity
- Helps in neovascularization
- Helps in transport of phagocytes into the peritoneal cavity.

Retroperitoneal Abscess

Retroperitoneal abscess is a rare clinical condition and difficult to diagnose due to insidious onset.

Etiology

- Genitourinary infection (e.g., pyelonephritis)
- Gastrointestinal infection (appendicitis, diverticulitis, pancreatitis)
- Tuberculosis of the spine.

Clinical features

Abdominal or flank pain, fever with chill, malaise and weight loss.

Diagnosis

CT is the investigation of choice.

Treatment

- Antibiotics and CT guided drainage in unilocular abscess.
- Antibiotics and open drainage in multilocular abscess.

GI infections (appendicitis, diverticulitis, and pancreatitis)

Tuberculosis of the spine

Infections originating from kidney

P. mirabilis
E. coli

- *E. coli*
- *Enterobacter*
- *Enterococci*
- *Bacteroides*

Retroperitoneal abscess

Retroperitoneal Hematoma

Etiology

- Blunt and penetrating abdominal trauma
- Percutaneous interventions
- Endovascular procedures

Clinical Presentation

Significant flank, groin or abdominal pain following an interventional procedure, and hemodynamic instability

Diagnosis

Multi-slice CT is the investigation of choice.

Management

- Fluid resuscitation, blood transfusion, correction of coagulopathy.
- Endovascular treatment includes selective intra-arterial embolization or placement of stent-graft over the punctured vessel.
- Open approach is indicated if failure of endovascular procedure or facility is not available or if patient is unstable.

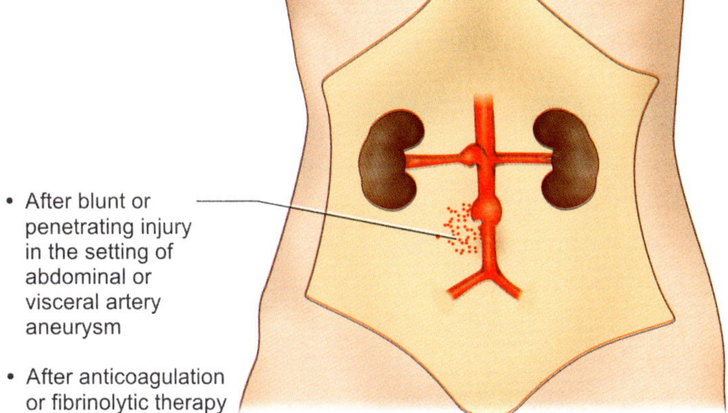

Spontaneous retroperitoneal hematoma is related to:

- Anticoagulation therapy
- Coagulopathy
- Rupture of angiomyolipoma, and renal cell carcinoma.

Retroperitoneal Fibrosis

Retroperitoneal fibrosis is a rare fibro-inflammatory condition characterized by proliferation of fibrous tissue in the retroperitoneum.

Etiology

(i) Idiopathic (70%) and (ii) Secondary to malignancies, autoimmune disorders, infections, drugs and other conditions.

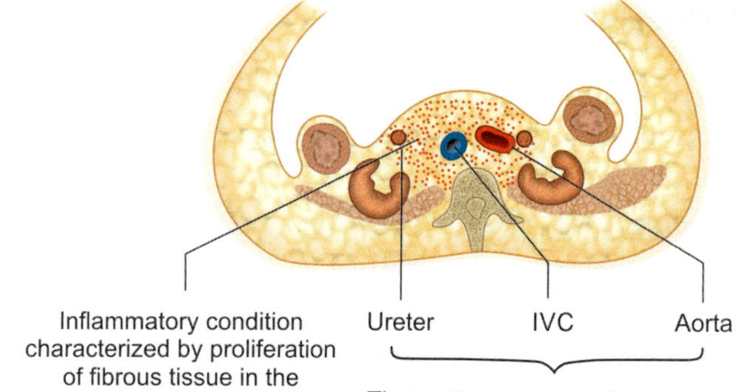

Retroperitoneal fibrosis secondary to:

- **Drugs** (methysergide, β-blockers, hydralazine, α-methydopa, entacapone, anti-TNFα therapy)
- **Infections**
- **Trauma**
- **Retroperitoneal hemorrhage.**
- **Radiation therapy.**
- **Autoimmune disorders** (ankylosing spondylitis, SLE, Wegener's granulomatosis, polyarteritis nodosa).
- **Malignancies** (prostate, NHL, sarcoma, carcinoid tumor, and gastric carcinoma).

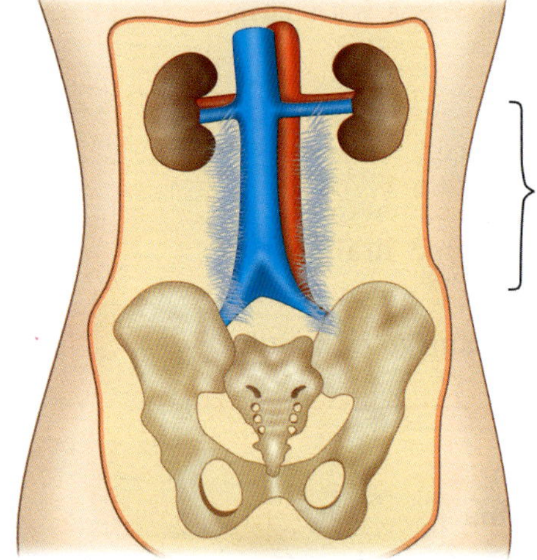

Idiopathic Retroperitoneal Fibrosis (Ormond Disease)

- Idiopathic retroperitoneal fibrosis is a rare disease usually involves the adventitia of abdominal aorta and iliac arteries, surrounding retroperitoneum and ureter.
- This clinical condition mainly affects men in the fifth or sixth decades of life.

Clinical Presentation

- Nonspecific symptoms including abdominal or flank pain, weight loss, loss of appetite, and malaise.
- In advanced stage of the disease, bilateral ureteric obstruction leads to renal failure.
- Hypertension may be present.

Diagnosis

- CT or MRI is the imaging modality of choice for diagnosis. CT shows fibrous plaque (isodense or slightly hyperdense compared with surrounding muscle) surrounding the anterolateral sides of the abdominal aorta, encasement of the IVC, medial ureteral deviation and/or obstruction.
- Retroperitoneal biopsy (CT/laparoscopic or open) is indicated to rule out malignancy.

Associated Autoimmune Disorders

- Autoimmune thyroiditis
- Rheumatoid arthritis
- Ankylosing spondylitis
- Systemic lupus erythematosus

Associated Fibro-inflammatory Conditions

- Riedel's thyroiditis
- Sclerosing cholangitis
- Mediastinal fibrosis
- Peyronie's disease
- Sclerosing sialoadenitis

Management

- **Glucocorticoids** are the first-line therapy. In patients without renal impairment or with mild ureteral obstruction, no ureteral drainage is indicated.
- In patients with moderate or severe hydronephrosis, **ureteral drainage** (by double J-stent or nephrostomy placement) followed by medical therapy is indicated.
- **Methotrexate** is effective as steroid-sparing agent in patients with multiple relapses.
- **Surgical ureterolysis with intraperitonealization and omental wrapping of the ureters** is the last option for chronic residual hydronephrosis.

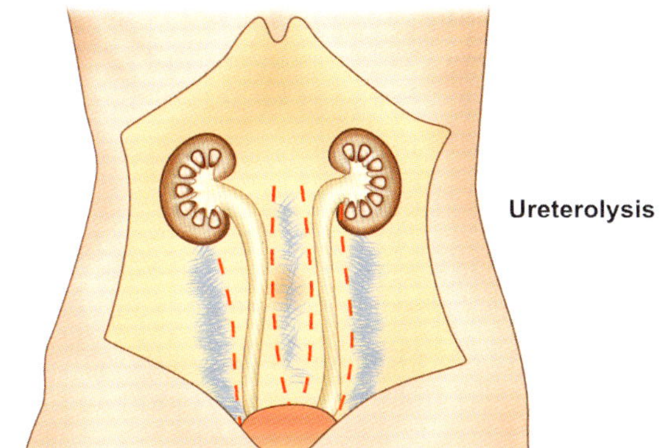

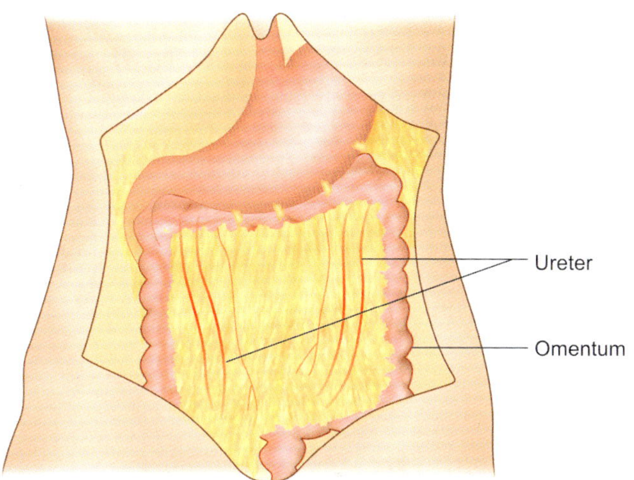

Retroperitoneal Neoplasm

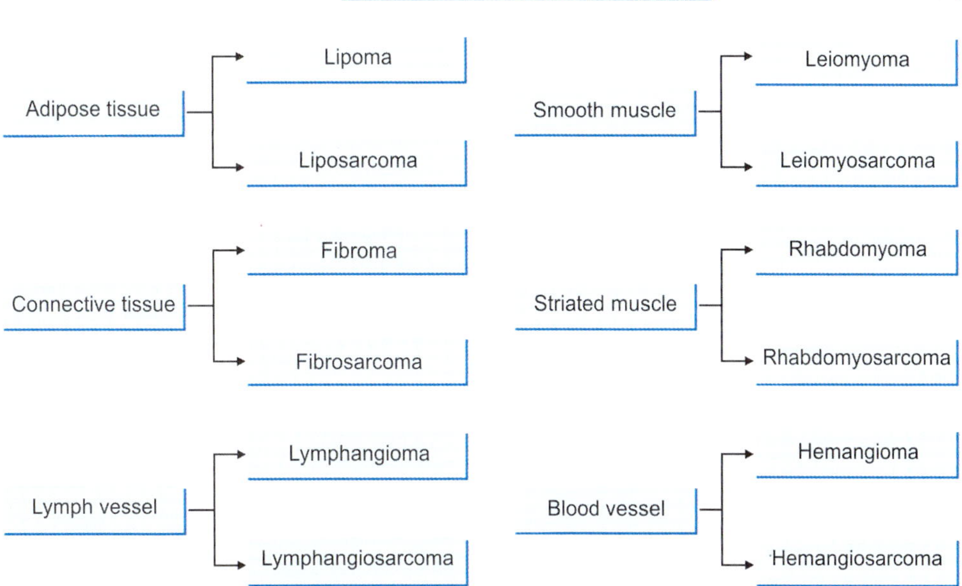

- Most of the retroperitoneal neoplasms are malignant, among them two-third tumors are mesenchymal in origin.
- Sarcomas comprise about one-third of retroperitoneal tumors. Liposarcoma is the most common type of retroperitoneal sarcoma followed by leiomyosarcoma.
- Patients with Von Recklinghausen's disease and Li-Fraumeni syndrome have an increased incidence of sarcoma.
- Mutations of *p53* and *RB-1* genes have a predilection for the development of sarcoma.

Clinical Presentation

- Most patients present with asymptomatic abdominal mass.
- Abdominal pain, GI hemorrhage, early satiety, nausea, vomiting, weight loss, and lower extremity swelling are usual clinical manifestations in symptomatic group of patients.

Diagnosis

- **Contrast-enhanced CT scan of abdomen and pelvis** is the imaging modality of choice. CT scan is helpful to determine the site, size, relationship to adjacent organs and major vessels, presence or absence of metastases.
- **Preoperative biopsy (core needle biopsy)** is indicated if distant metastases is present or tumor seems unresectable or chemo-sensitive tumor (e.g., lymphoma) is suspected.

Management

- Treatment is en bloc resection of the tumor and any involved organs. Radical lymphadenectomy is not indicated.
- Local recurrence even after complete resection is common.

Case 1

History and Physical Examination

A 5-year-old boy presented with a history of appearance of swelling over the umbilicus when crying or straining. As per his mother, the swelling becomes prominent for last 6 months. No history of appearance of swelling in the groin region. From the obstetric history, it was revealed that the baby was born prematurely and also low-birth weight baby.

Physical examination

- Build, and nutrition—average
- Examination of abdomen—A swelling appears on straining over the umbilicus. A fascial defect of 2 cm × 1.5 cm is revealed after reduction of the swelling.

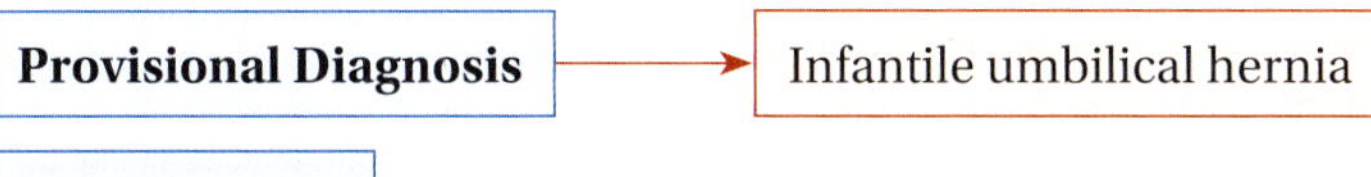

Investigations

Clinical diagnosis is sufficient for taking the decision of proper management. Imaging is indicated not for confirmation of diagnosis, but for accurate delineation of the defect.

Discussion

A 5-year-old boy presented with history and clinical features suggestive of infantile umbilical hernia. As the age of spontaneous resolution (2–3 years) has over, surgery is indicated for this patient.

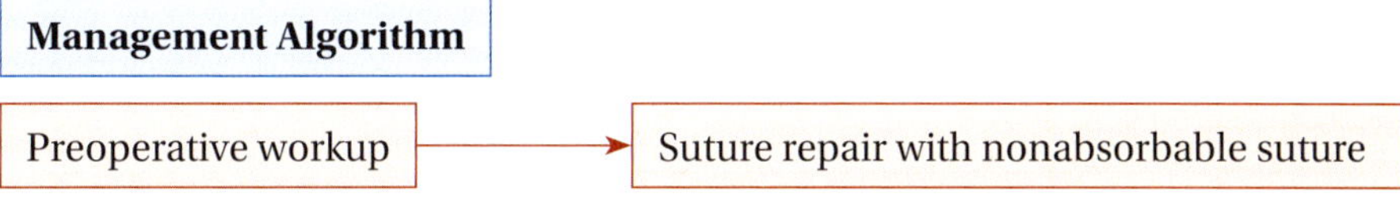

Case 2

History and Physical Examination

A 28-year-old female patient presented with mid-abdominal swelling for last 1 year. The swelling gradually increasing in size and associated with vague abdominal pain. No history of vomiting or bowel irregularities. History of loss of appetite but no history of weight loss. Menstrual and obstetric histories were normal.

Physical examination

Pallor–present

Examination of the abdomen—A nontender, cystic, mobile swelling in the mid-abdomen measuring 6 cm × 5 cm. The swelling is freely mobile perpendicular to the attachment of mesentery. No other significant clinical findings.

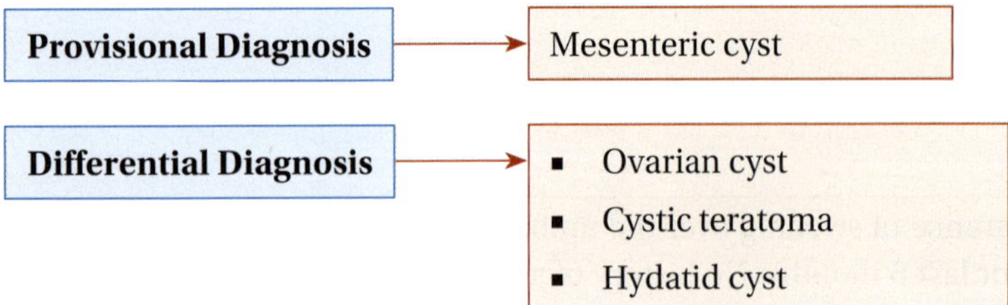

Investigations

- Laboratory reports are within normal limit.
- *USG abdomen:* A cystic lesion measuring 6.8 cm × 5.6 cm in the lower abdomen.
- *CT scan abdomen:* A cystic lesion measuring 7.1 cm × 6.2 cm × 6.0 cm in the right lower abdomen, displacing the small intestine and colon to the left side.

Discussion

History and clinical findings suggestive of an abdominal cystic lesion. Though the provisional diagnosis was mesenteric cyst, imaging findings cannot confirm the diagnosis as well as cannot exclude the differential diagnosis. So, laparotomy was planned.

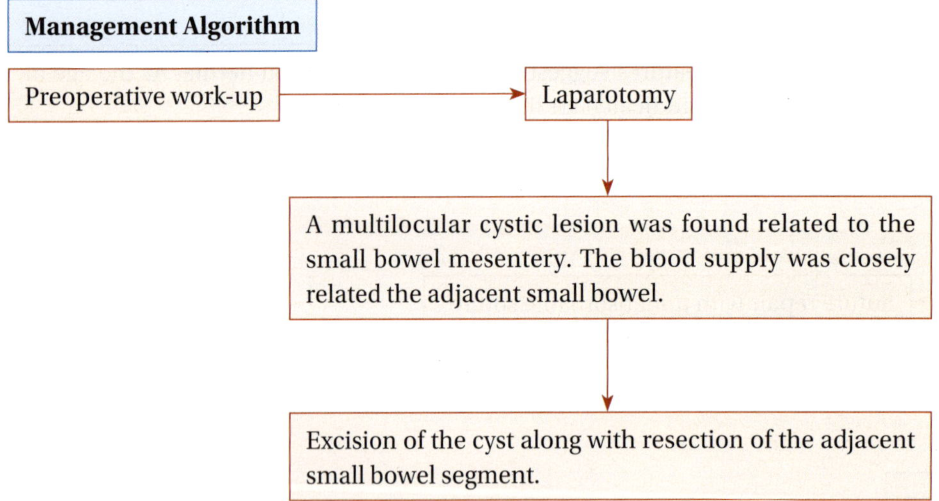

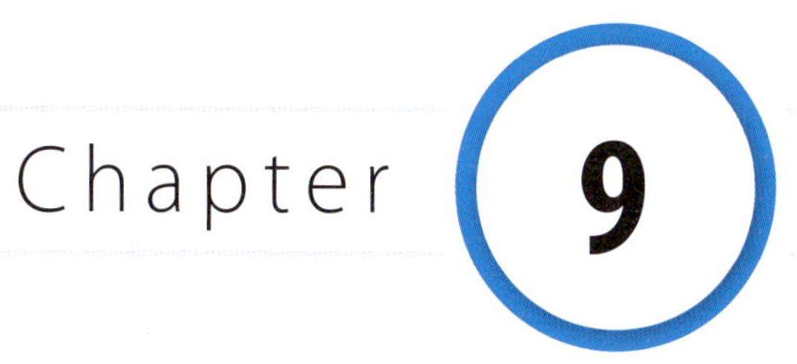

Chapter 9

Diseases of the Stomach

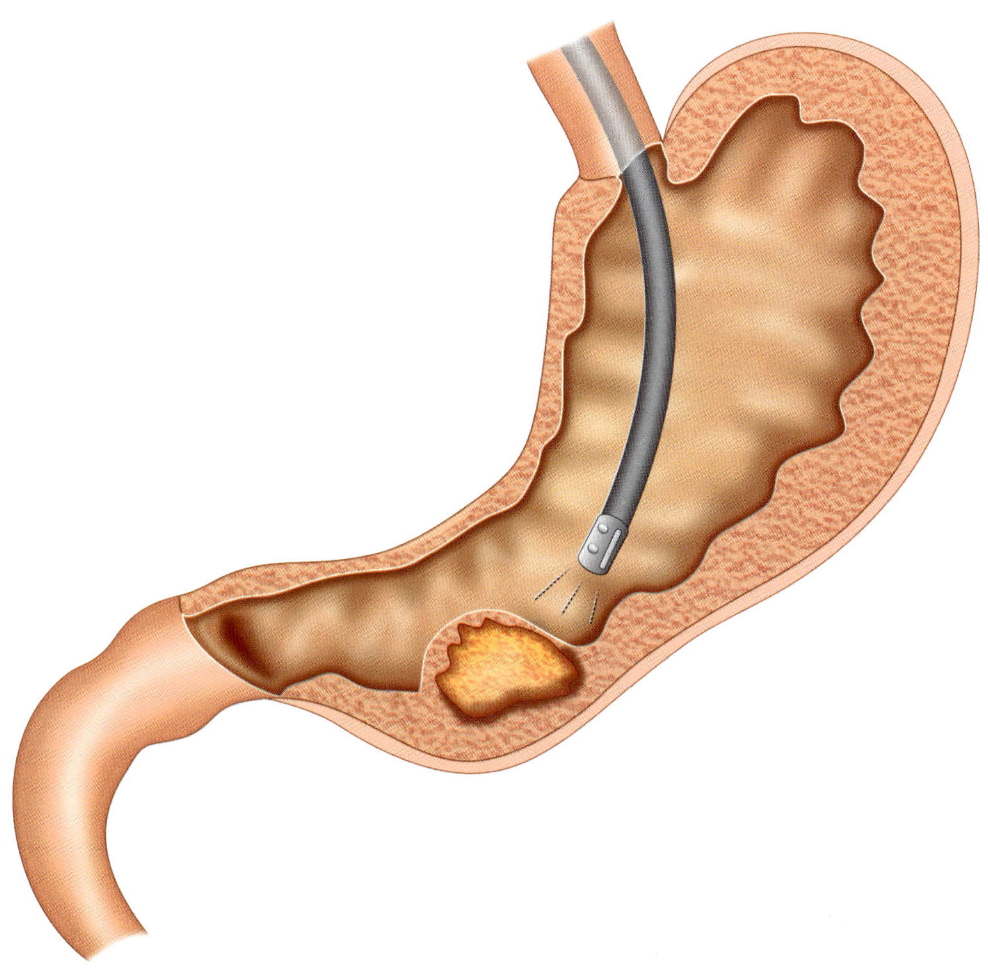

Important Topics

- Peptic Ulcer Disease
- Gastritis
- Adenocarcinoma of Stomach
- Gastrointestinal Stromal Tumor
- Gastric Lymphoma
- Other Lesions of Stomach
- Postvagotomy Syndromes
- Postgastrectomy Syndromes

'The extraordinary development of modern science may be her undoing. Specialism, now a necessity, has fragmented the specialities, themselves in a way that makes the outlook hazardous. The workers lose all sense of proportion in a maze of minutiae.'

William Osler (1849–1919)
Canadian Physician

Peptic Ulcer Disease

Peptic ulcer disease commonly develops in the **stomach** and **proximal duodenum**.

Other Sites of Peptic Ulcer

- Lower end of esophagus
- Meckel's diverticulum
- Gastrojejunostomy stoma (in the jejunal mucosa)

Etiopathogenesis

Common causes

- *Helicobacter pylori* infection
- NSAIDs

Rare causes

- Medications
- Smoking
- Zollinger-Ellison syndrome
- Burn injury (Curling's ulcer)
- Head injury (Cushing ulcer)
- Antral G cell hyperplasia
- Hyperparathyroidism

Medications Causing Peptic Ulcer

- NSAIDs
- Corticosteroids
- Bisphosphonates
- Potassium chloride
- 5-fluorouracil

Chronic Diseases Associated with Increased Risk of Peptic Ulcer Disease

- Crohn's disease
- Cystic fibrosis
- Systemic mastocytosis
- Chronic renal failure
- Polycythemia vera
- Cirrhosis of liver

H. pylori is also found in:

- Heterotopic gastric mucosa in proximal esophagus and Barrett's espophagus
- Gastric metaplasia in duodenum
- Meckel's diverticulum
- Heterotopic gastric mucosa in the rectum

H. pylori infection may also lead to:

- Gastritis
- Gastric MALT lymphoma
- Gastric cancer

Role of *H. pylori*

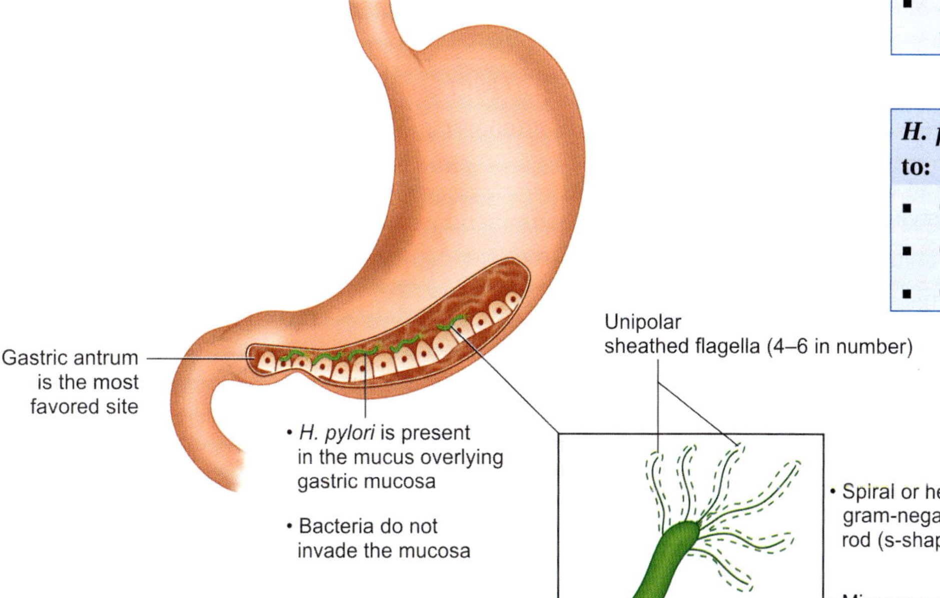

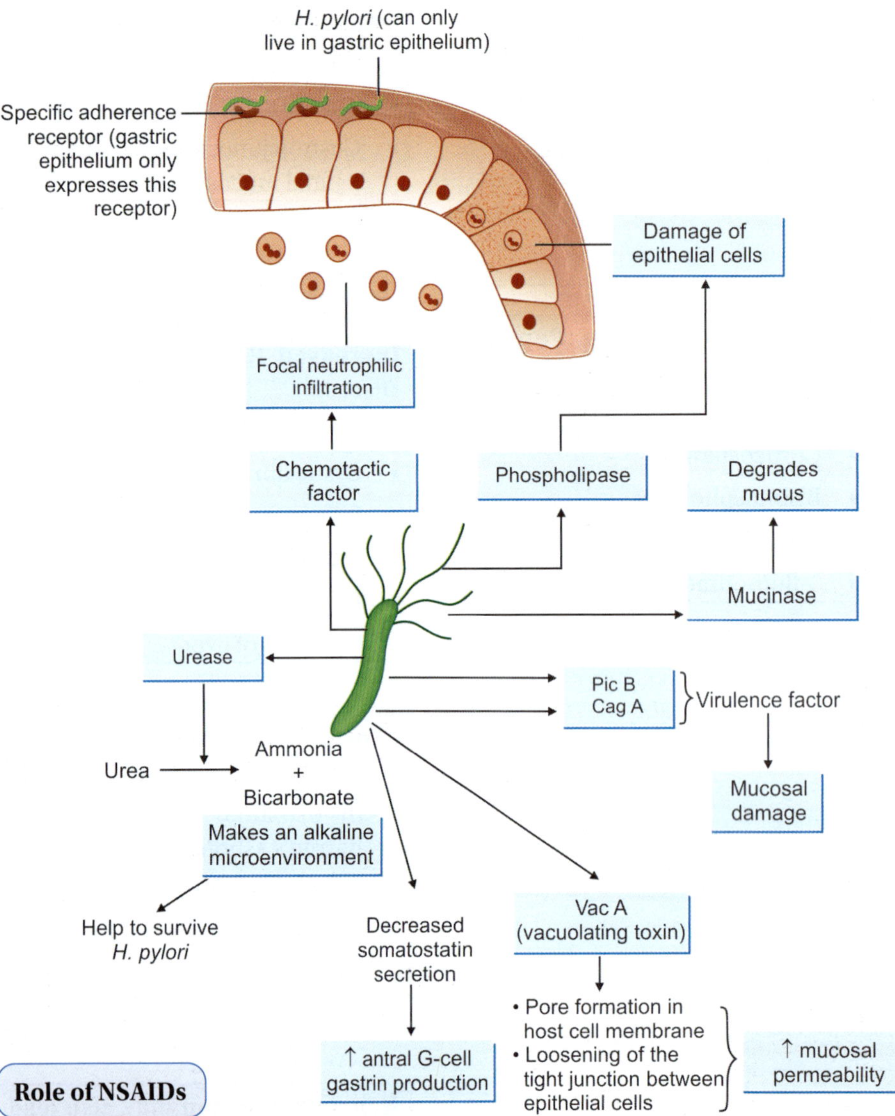

Virulence Factors of *H. pylori*

- Vacuolating toxin (VacA)
- Cytotoxin-associated antigen (CagA)
- Urease
- Blood group antigen-binding adhesin (BabA)

Role of NSAIDs

NSAIDs decrease the prostaglandin synthesis by inhibiting the **COX-1 enzyme.**

Prostaglandins inhibit gastric secretion, stimulate bicarbonate secretion, and increases gastric mucosal blood flow.

Risk factors for NSAIDs-related GI complications:

- Age >65 years
- Concomitant use of anticoagulants, corticosteroids
- Use of low-dose aspirin
- *H. pylori* infection
- History of complicated peptic ulcer

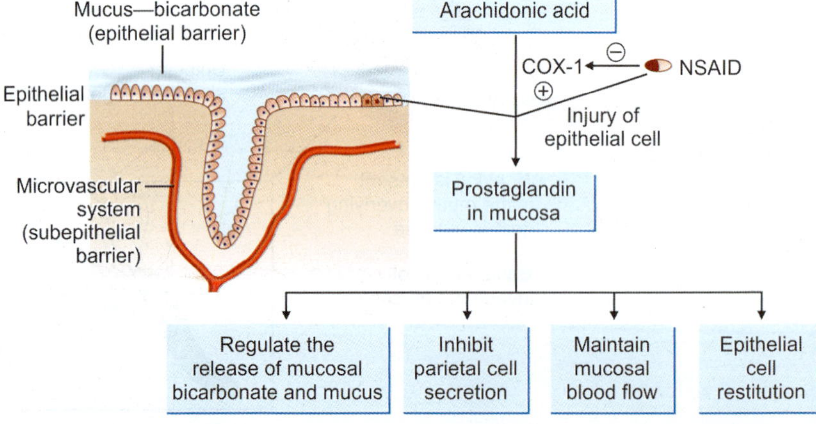

Pathophysiology of Duodenal Ulcer

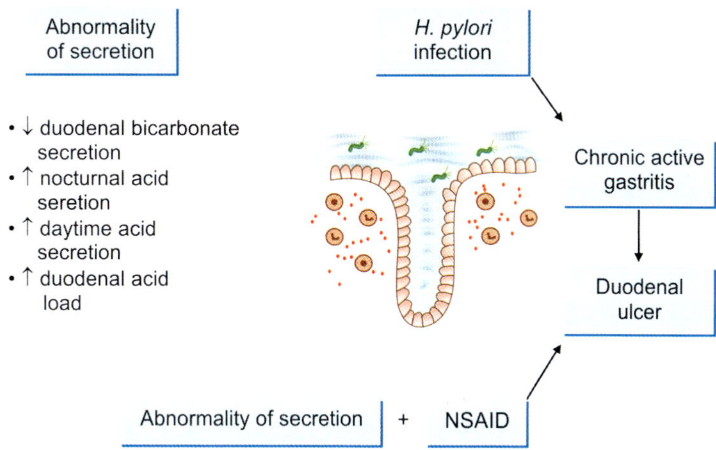

Pathophysiology of Gastric Ulcer

Gastric ulcer is classified into type I to V based on location of ulcer and acid secretion **(Modified Johnson classification)**

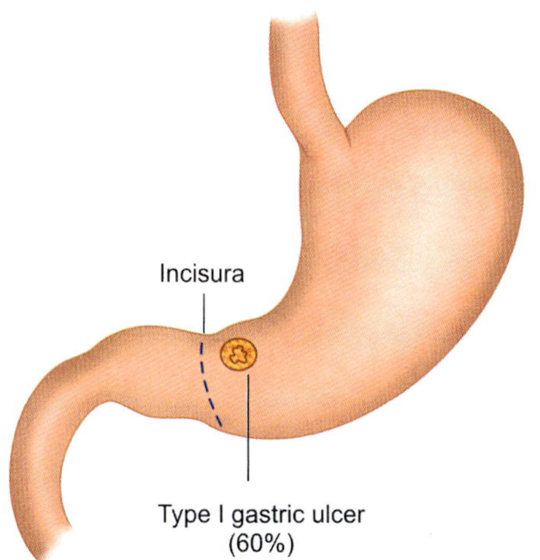

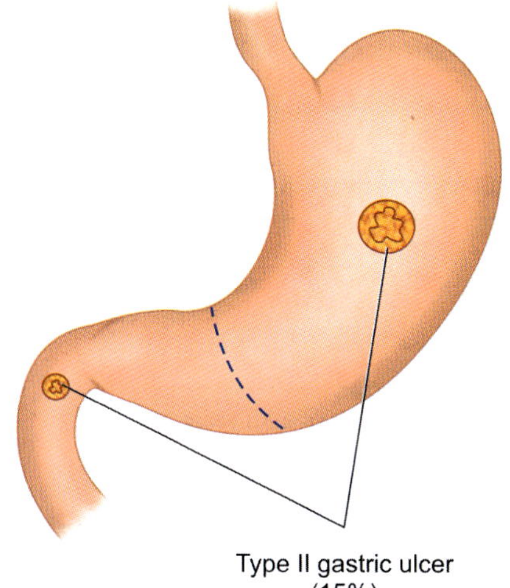

Type I Gastric Ulcer

- Ulcer on the lesser curvature near the incisura
- Low acid output
- Ulcer develops due to impaired mucosal defense

Type II Gastric Ulcer

- Ulcer at the body of the stomach associated with duodenal ulcer
- Increased acid secretion

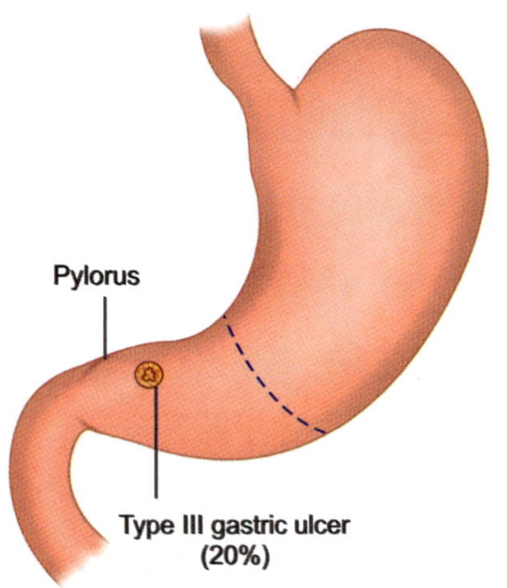

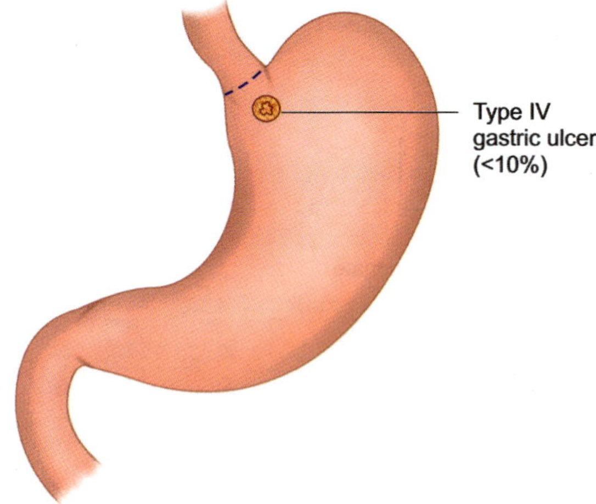

Type III Gastric Ulcer

- Ulcer on the prepyloric region (within 2–3 cm of pylorus)
- This ulcer behaves like duodenal ulcer
- Increased acid secretion

Type IV Gastric Ulcer

- Ulcer on the lesser curvature near the GE junction
- Low acid secretion
- Impaired mucosal defense
- Exact pathogenesis not known

Type V Gastric Ulcer

- Ulcer anywhere in the stomach
- Induced by medication
- Low acid secretion

Clinical Presentation of Peptic Ulcer

Clinical Presentation of Duodenal Ulcer

Epigastric pain

- Occurs 90 minutes to 3 hours after meal
- Pain relieved by antacids or food
- Pain awakens the patient from sleep

Nausea/vomiting

Weight gain

Clinical Presentation of Gastric Ulcer

Epigastric pain

- Precipitated by food

Nausea/vomiting

Weight loss

Other Symptoms and Signs

- Hematemesis
- Melena
- Anemia

Complications of Peptic Ulcer

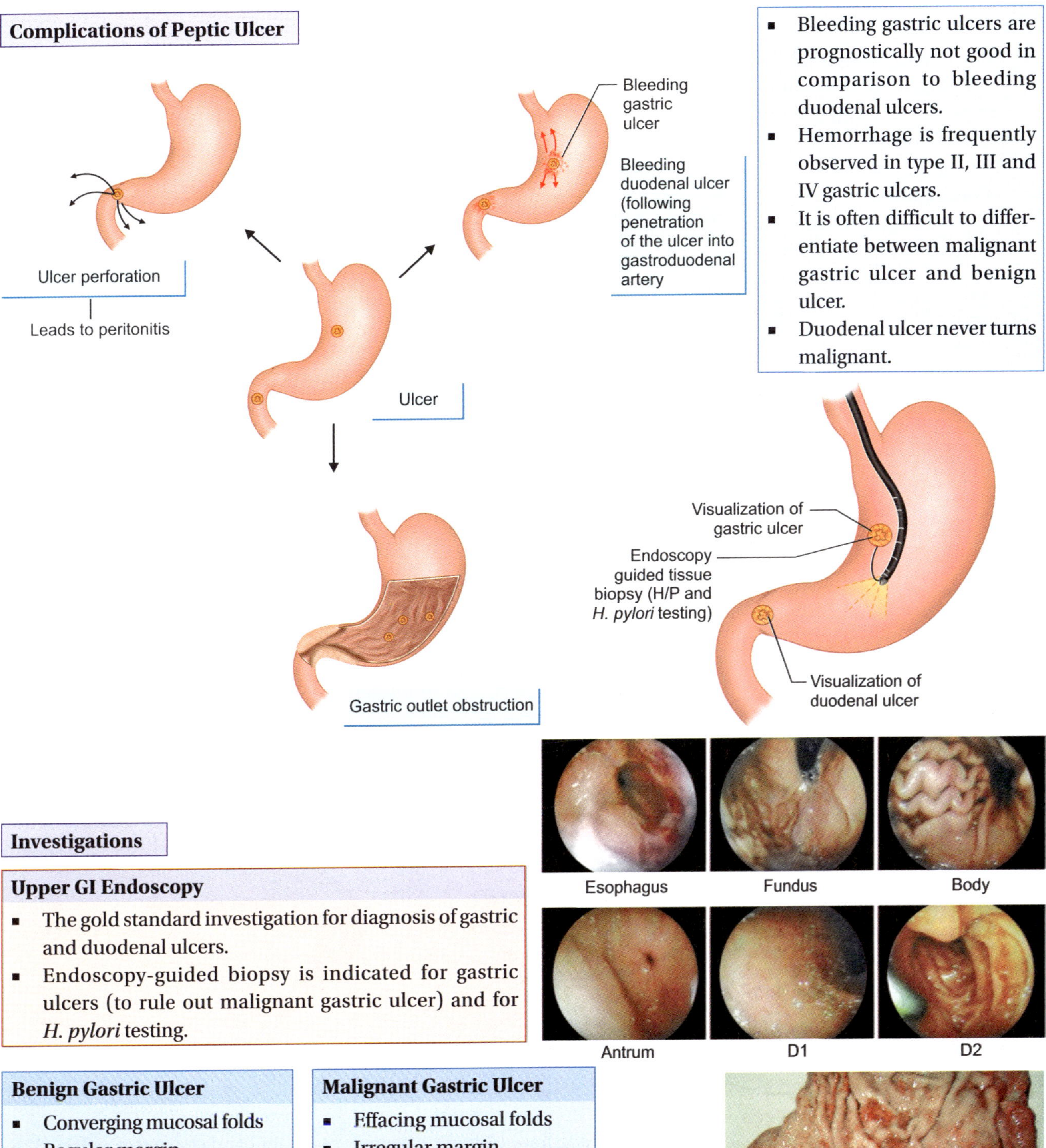

- Bleeding gastric ulcers are prognostically not good in comparison to bleeding duodenal ulcers.
- Hemorrhage is frequently observed in type II, III and IV gastric ulcers.
- It is often difficult to differentiate between malignant gastric ulcer and benign ulcer.
- Duodenal ulcer never turns malignant.

Investigations

Upper GI Endoscopy

- The gold standard investigation for diagnosis of gastric and duodenal ulcers.
- Endoscopy-guided biopsy is indicated for gastric ulcers (to rule out malignant gastric ulcer) and for *H. pylori* testing.

Benign Gastric Ulcer

- Converging mucosal folds
- Regular margin
- Punched out edges
- Surrounding area normal
- Small in size

Malignant Gastric Ulcer

- Effacing mucosal folds
- Irregular margin
- Everted edges
- Surrounding area irregular
- Large in size

Resected specimen of stomach showing malignant gastric ulcer.

H. pylori Testing

- **Noninvasive tests:** (i) Serology (ELISA, Latex agglutination test, Immunochromatographic tests); (ii) Urea breath test (UBT); and (iii) *Helicobacter pylori* Stool antigen test (HpSA).
- **Invasive tests:** Endoscopic tissue biopsy—(i) Histological examination; (ii) Rapid urease test; and (iii) Culture.

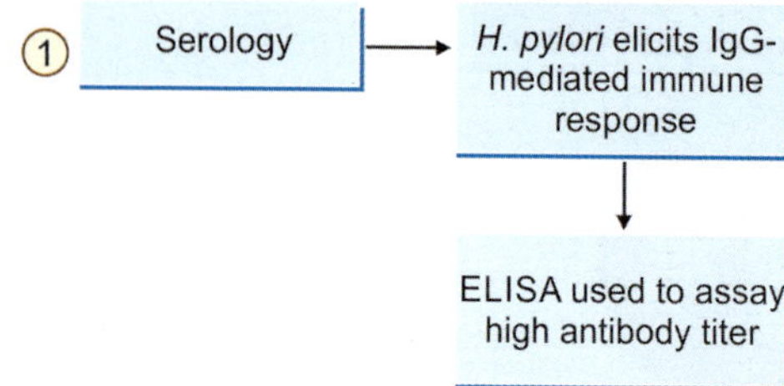

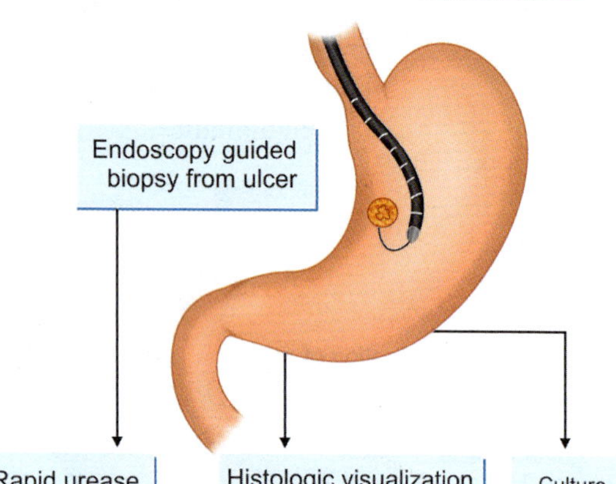

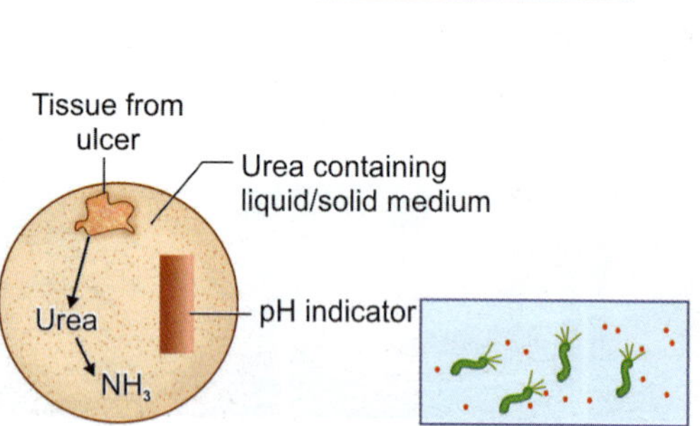

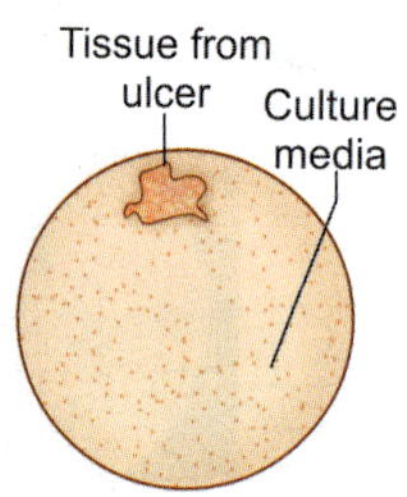

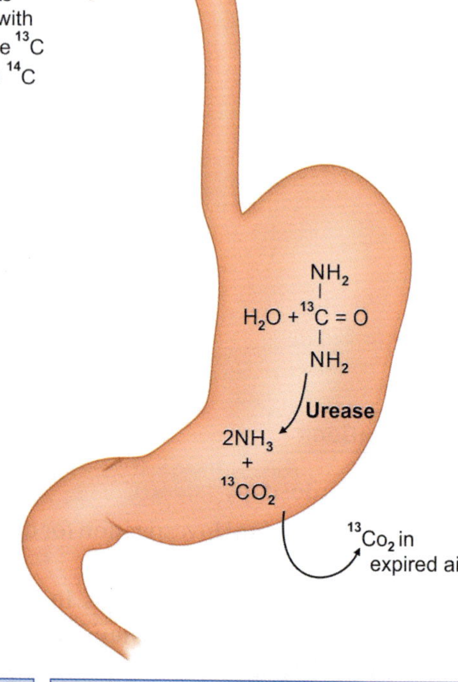

Tissue from ulcer

Culture media

- High sensitivity and specificity
- Results available within hours

- With routine hematoxylin and eosin stain or silver, Giemsa or Genta stain (for improved visibility)
- High sensitivity and specificity

- Culture media not widely available
- Expensive
- For result, 3–5 days is required

Stool Antigen Test

- This test is based on direct identification of bacterial antigen in stool
- The stool antigen test is less costly than urea breath test, easy to perform, good sensitivity and specificity. It is effective for diagnosis and for monitoring effectiveness of therapy

Urea Breath Test (UBT)

- UBT is a highly sensitive and specific non-invasive test
- Highly accurate test and easy to perform.
- The test should be performed atleast 4 weeks after antibiotic therapy and 2 weeks after PPI or H_2-blocker therapy

Serological Testing

- Most widely available non-invasive test
- Rapid and cheap test
- Effective for screening populations and in patients with bleeding ulcer or on antibiotic therapy where other tests may be equivocal

Treatment

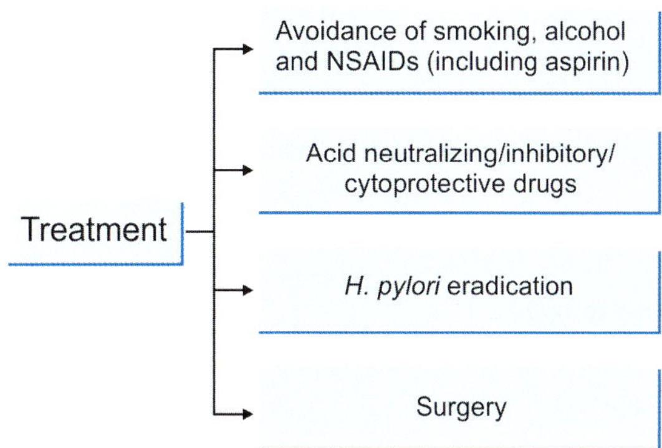

Acid Neutralizing/Inhibitory/Cytoprotective Drugs

H_2 blockers

Proton Pump Inhibitor

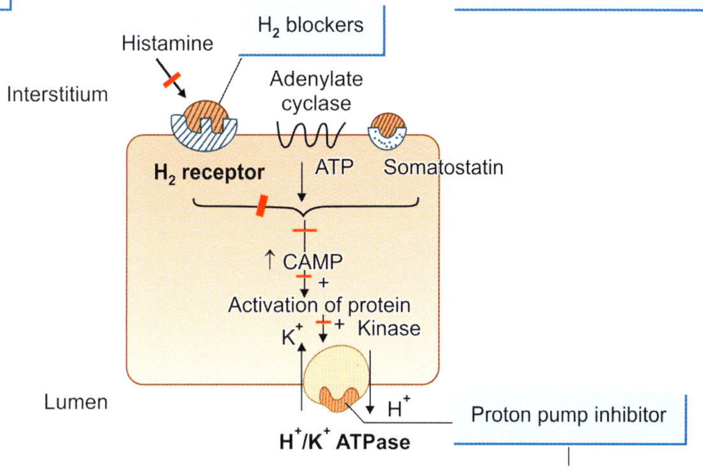

H_2 blockers

Histamine

Interstitium

Adenylate cyclase

Somatostatin

H_2 receptor

ATP

↑ CAMP

Activation of protein Kinase

K^+

H^+

Lumen

H^+/K^+ ATPase

Proton pump inhibitor

Irreversible inhibition of H^+/K^+ ATPase resulting in inhibition of all types of acid secretion from all types of secretogogues

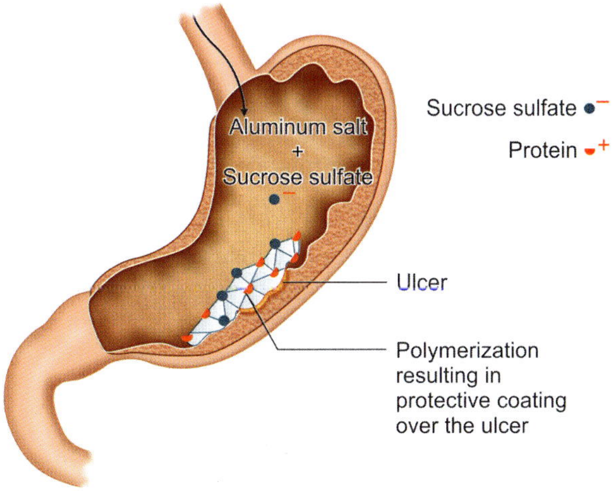

Aluminum salt + Sucrose sulfate

Sucrose sulfate •–

Protein •+

Ulcer

Polymerization resulting in protective coating over the ulcer

Sucralfate → (Salt of sucrose + sulfated aluminium hydroxide)

↓ Acidic environment

Polymerization

Sucrose sulfate (–) + Aluminium salt

\+

Protein (+) in base of ulcer

Other mechanisms by which Sucralfate helps in ulcer healing:

- Stimulates the synthesis and release of gastric mucosal prostaglandins
- Stimulates bicarbonate and mucus secretion
- Concentrate fibroblast growth factor

Other indications for *H. pylori* testing and eradication therapy:

- A past history of peptic ulcer disease (no documented evidence of eradication therapy)
- Low-grade gastric MALT lymphoma
- After endoscopic resection of early gastric cancer
- Patients initiating chronic treatment with NSAIDs

***H. pylori* Eradication Therapy**

Clarithromycin triple therapy: Consisting of amoxicillin, clarithromycin and PPI for 14 days if clarithromycin resistance is less than 15% and no previous history of macrolide exposure.

Bismuth quadruple therapy: Consisting of PPI, bismuth, tetracycline, and a nitroimidazole for 14 days. This therapy is particularly indicated if patient had previous macrolide exposure or allergic to penicillin.

If first-line therapy with Clarithromycin triple therapy fails, Bismuth quadruple therapy or levofloxacin-containing salvage regimens are the preferred options.

If first-line therapy with Bismuth quadruple therapy fails, Clarithromycin triple therapy or levofloxacin-containing salvage regimens are the preferred treatment options.

Tests to prove eradication: Urea breath test or stool antigen test or biopsy-based test at least 4 weeks after antibiotic therapy and after PPI therapy withheld for 1–2 weeks.

Surgery

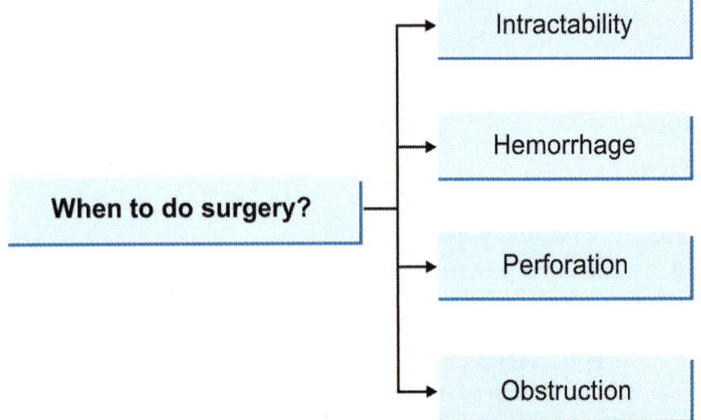

Intractable or Refractory Peptic Ulcer

Endoscopically proven ulcers that fail to heal despite 8–12 weeks of antisecretory therapy.

Recurrent Peptic Ulcer

Endoscopically proven ulcer greater than 5 mm in diameter that develops within 12 months following complete ulcer healing documented by repeat endoscopy.

Surgery for Intractable Duodenal Ulcer

- Proximal gastric vagotomy (Highly selective vagotomy).
- Truncal Vagotomy and drainage procedure.
- Truncal vagotomy and antrectomy followed by reconstruction (Billroth I reconstruction/Billroth II/ Roux-en-Y reconstruction).

Conditions Associated with Intractable or Refractory Ulcer

- Noncompliance
- Persistence of *H. pylori* infection
- Continuous consumption of NSAIDs
- Zollinger-Ellison syndrome

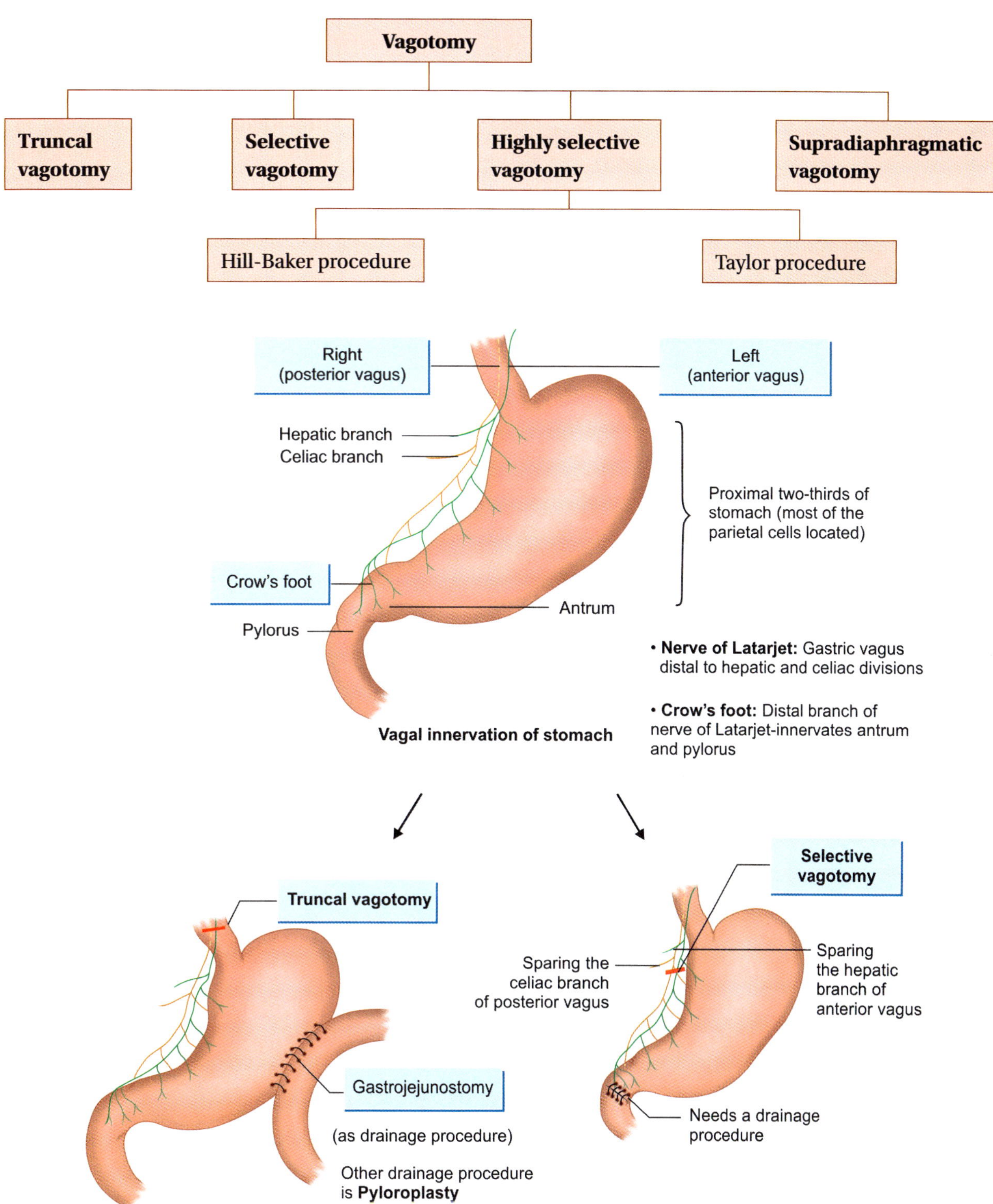

Vagal innervation of stomach

Truncal Vagotomy and Drainage Procedure

Selective Vagotomy and Drainage Procedure

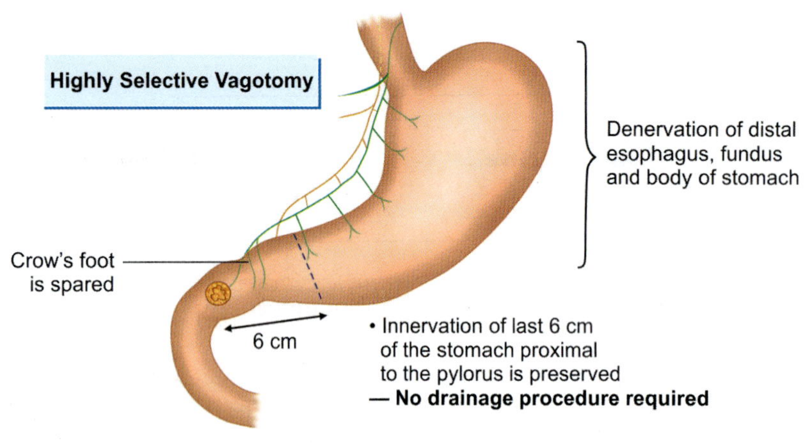

Highly selective vagotomy is also called **proximal gastric vagotomy** or **parietal cell vagotomy**.

Hill-Baker procedure is posterior truncal vagotomy with anterior parietal vagotomy. **Taylor procedure** is posterior truncal vagotomy with Anterior lesser-curve seromyotomy.

Supradiaphragmatic vagotomy (via minimally invasive thoracoscopy) is indicated in recurrent peptic ulcer in whom previously vagotomy was performed.

Drainage procedures for truncal and selective vagotomy

- **Pyloroplasty**
  - **Heineke-Mikulicz pyloroplasty**
  - **Finney pyloroplasty**
- **Jaboulay gastroduodenostomy**
- **Gastrojejunostomy**

Pyloroplasty → Heineke-Mikulicz pyloroplasty

Pyloroplasty → Finney pyloroplasty

Recommended technique of pyloroplasty

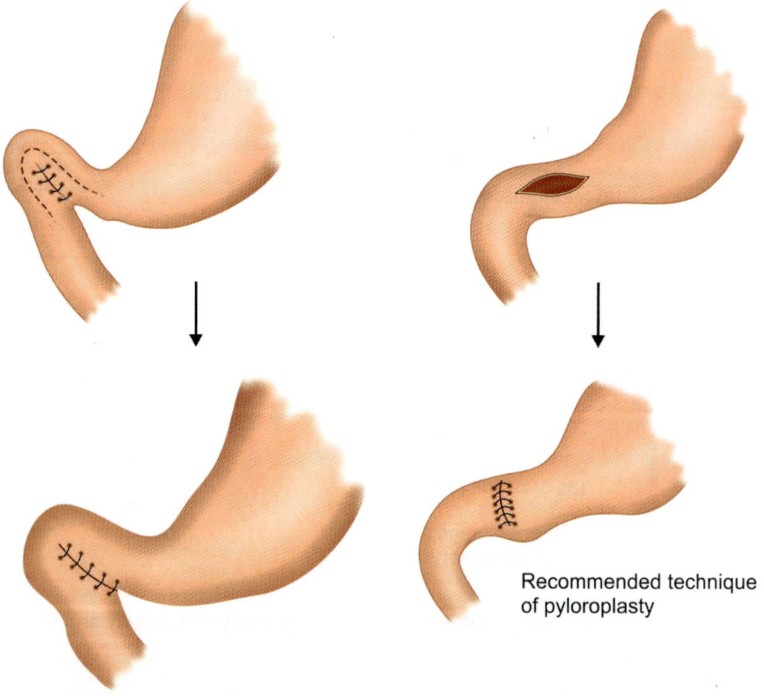

Finney pyloroplasty
(not recommended)

Heineke-Mikulicz pyloroplasty
(commonly performed technique)

Surgery for Intractable Gastric Ulcer

Type I Ulcer

Vagotomy is not recommended because acid output is normal or low.

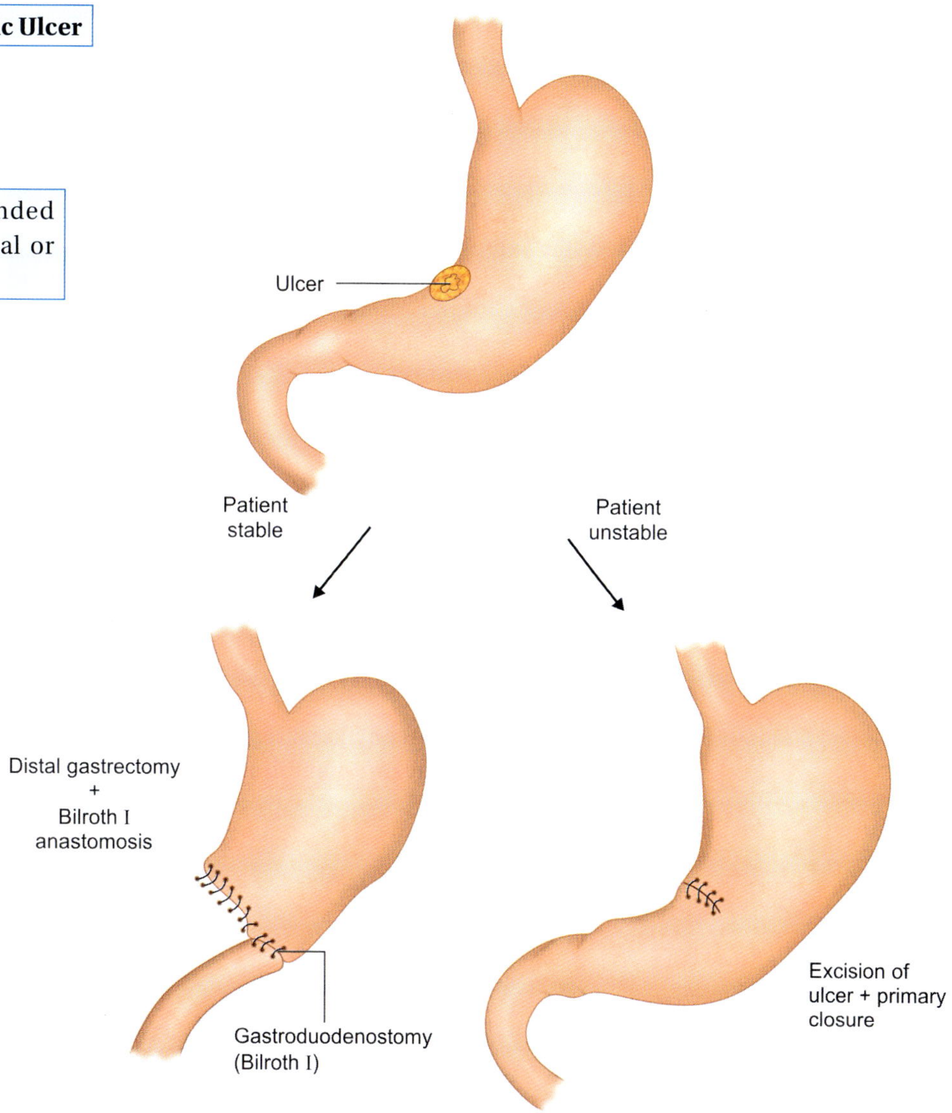

Ulcer
Patient stable
Patient unstable
Distal gastrectomy + Bilroth I anastomosis
Gastroduodenostomy (Bilroth I)
Excision of ulcer + primary closure

Types II and III Ulcer

Highly selective vagotomy is not recommended.

Truncal vagotomy + Excision of ulcer
If patient unstable
Truncal vagotomy + Distal gastrectomy
If patient stable

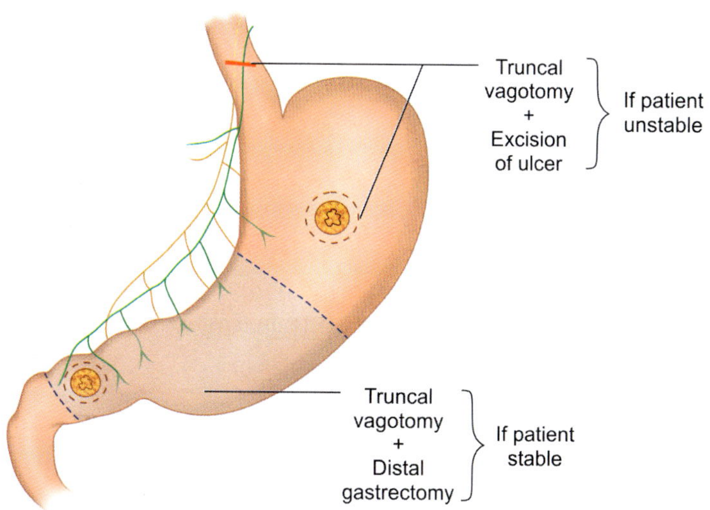

Type IV Ulcer

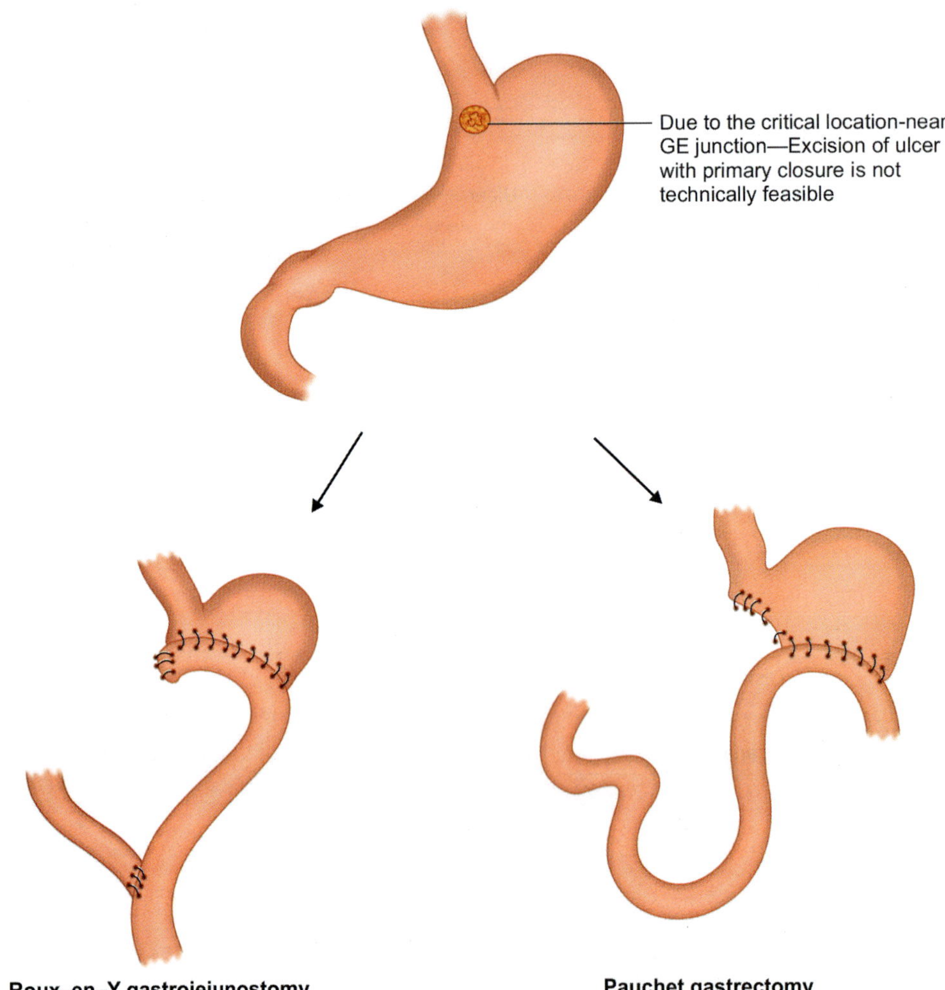

Perforated Peptic Ulcer

Risk factors for perforation

H. pylori infection, use of NSAIDs or steroids, smoking, previous history of peptic ulcer disease, Zollinger- Ellison syndrome.

Clinical presentation

- Sudden onset, severe upper abdominal pain, abdominal distension
- Abdominal tenderness, card-board rigidity, obliterated liver dullness, absent or sluggish peristaltic sound, tachycardia. Features of peritonitis may be minimal or absent in contained and/sealed leak.
- Features of sepsis or septic shock.

Diagnosis

Imaging for diagnosis:

- X-ray of chest and abdomen (Erect/left lateral)
- CT scan of abdomen (greater sensitivity than X-ray)
- Contrast study (by administration of water-soluble contrast via nasogastric tube)—when both CT and X-ray are inconclusive.

CT scan abdomen is now the preferred imaging modality in suspected peptic ulcer perforation due to: (i) Its higher sensitivity in detecting free air; (ii) Ability to characterize the site and size of perforation; and (iii) To exclude other abdominal pathologies.

CXR (upright)/left lateral decubitus view of abdomen

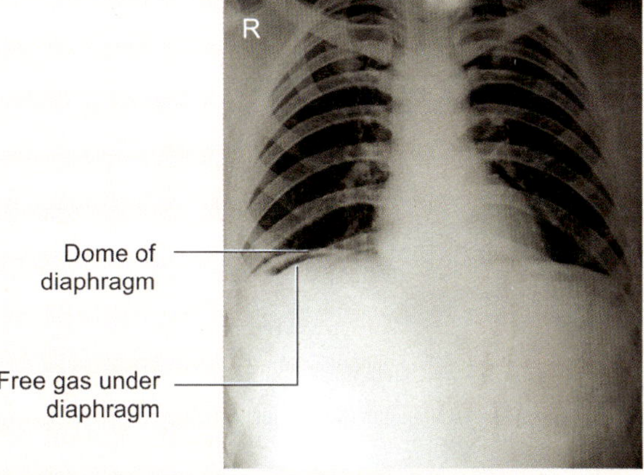

- Diagnostic accuracy of erect and left lateral decubitus views are same.
- Left lateral decubitus is better tolerated by patients presenting with peritonitis.

CT Findings Suggestive of Perforation

- Pneumoperitoneum
- Intraperitoneal fluid
- Extraluminal contrast extravasation
- Bowel wall thickening

- Free air is absent in X-ray in about 30% of patients with peptic perforation. So, absence of free gas cannot exclude the diagnosis of perforation.
- A patient with sudden onset of severe upper abdominal pain associated with pneumoperitoneum in X-ray, the diagnosis is perforated peptic ulcer primarily duodenal, until proved otherwise.

Scoring Systems (Used for Predicting Mortality and Morbidity)

(i) Boey score; (ii) New Pulp score; and (iii) ASA score. The Boey score is most commonly used, followed by ASA score. The predictability of New Pulp score and ASA score are better than Boey score.

Treatment

- Assessment of the patient (stable or unstable, presence of sepsis/septic shock or not)
- Fluid resuscitation with IV crystalloids
- Nasogastric decompression by Ryle's tube
- Urinary catheterization—to monitor urine output, so that fluid resuscitation can be properly monitored. Invasive hemodynamic monitoring, if indicated.

Nonoperative Management

Criteria that have to be fulfilled for trial of nonoperative management (NOM):

- Radiologically undetected leak
- No signs of peritonitis or sepsis
- Adequate monitoring facility available
- Facility of renal and respiratory support
- Round-the-clock OT facility available

Nonoperative management includes:

(i) Nil per mouth; (ii) Fluid resuscitation; (iii) Decompression by nasogastric tube; (iv) IV antibiotics (coverage against gram negative, gram positive and anerobic bacteria); (v) PPI therapy; and (vi) Follow-up endoscopy at 4–6 weeks. If subhepatic or subdiaphragmatic abscess develops following NOM, USG, or CT-guided drainage of abscess is indicated.

Operative Management

Indications for surgery:

- Signs of peritonitis
- Significant pneumoperitoneum
- Significant extraluminal contrast extravasation
- Delayed presentation
- Older age

Surgical interventions for perforated duodenal ulcer:

- Laparoscopic simple repair
- Laparoscopic omental patch technique
- Graham's omentopexy (placing the omentum as a plug over the perforation without any attempt for primary closure of perforation)
- Modified Graham's omentopexy (primary closure with interrupted sutures covered with a pedicled omentum on the top of the repair)

Surgical intervention for perforated gastric ulcer:

Distal gastrectomy with Bilroth I anastomosis if patient is stable. Biopsy of the ulcer followed by omental patch closure if patient is unstable.

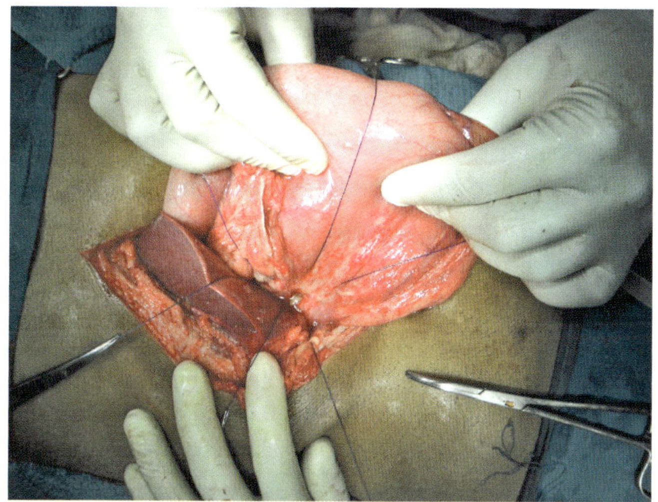

Operative picture showing perforation at D1.

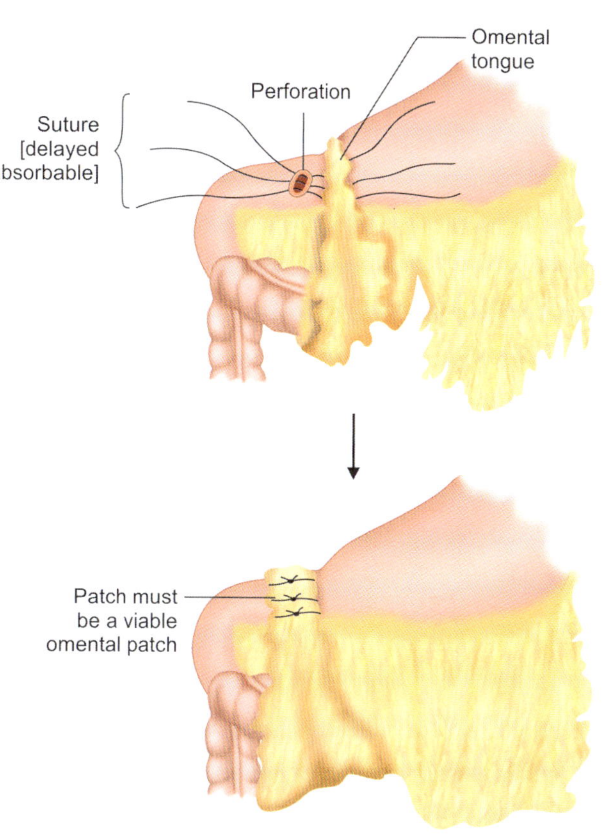

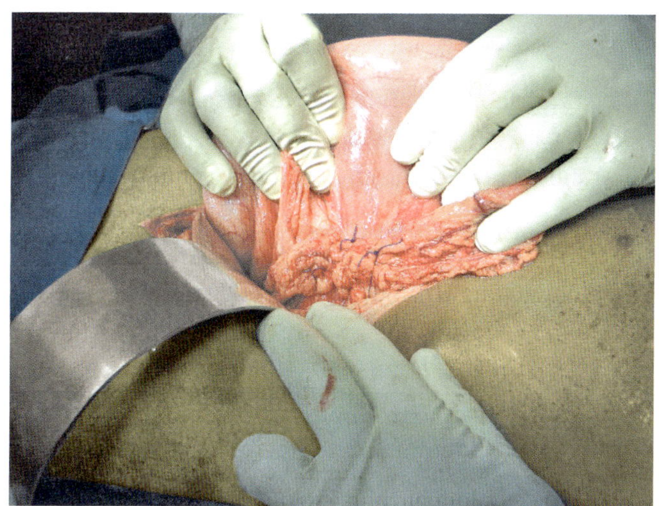

Operative picture showing repair of perforation with omental patch.

During Graham's omentopexy, care must be taken during introduction of the needle so that the posterior duodenal wall is not entrapped within the bite.

Sutures should be tied loosely enough so that blood supply to the omentum is not compromised.

Bleeding Peptic Ulcer

Risk Factors for Bleeding

Use of NSAIDs, *H. pylori* infection, smoking, alcohol consumption

Clinical Presentation

- Patients may present with hematemesis, melaena or hematochezia or together.
- Hypovolemic shock may develop in massive upper GI bleeding.
- Patient without any history of chronic liver disease or chronic alcoholism, bleeding peptic ulcer is the most likely cause of upper GI bleeding.

Diagnosis

In patients with suspected bleeding ulcer, endoscopy should be done as early as possible to get prognostic information based on endoscopic stigmata **(Forrest Classification)**.

Scoring System (for Risk Stratification, to Predict the Need for Surgery and Endoscopy)

(i) Glasgow-Blatchford score (GBS); (ii) Rockall score (Clinical Rockall score and Full Rockall score); and (iii) AIMS65

GBS score 0–1 denotes "very low risk", indicates no need for in-patient treatment and endoscopy. AIMS65 score ≥2 denotes risk of mortality is high. Rockall score ≤2 is associated with very low risk of mortality and bleeding and score 4–5 is associated with high risk of mortality.

Nonoperative Management of Bleeding Peptic Ulcer

(i) Airway control; (ii) Ventilation and oxygenation; (iii) Fluid resuscitation; (iv) PPI therapy; and (v) Diagnostic and therapeutic endoscopy or therapeutic embolization. In patients with bleeding peptic ulcer, PPI therapy for 6–8 weeks following successful endoscopic hemostasis is recommended. In recurrent bleeding, endoscopic hemostasis is the first-line treatment.

Endoscopic management (based on Blatchford score):

Very low-risk group: Outpatient endoscopy; *Low risk group:* Early in-patient endoscopy (≤24 hours of admission); *High risk group:* Urgent in-patient endoscopy (≤12 hours of admission)

Endoscopic management (based on Forrest classification):

- Spurting ulcer (Forrest Ia); Oozing ulcer (Forrest Ib); Ulcer with non-bleeding visible vessel (Forrest IIa)—Endoscopic hemostasis is recommended.
- Endoscopic therapy may be considered for adherent clot and should not be considered for flat pigmented spot or clean ulcer base.

Indications of Angioembolization in Bleeding Peptic Ulcer

(i) In hemodynamically stable patients, if failure of endoscopic hemostasis for two times and (ii) Endoscopic hemostasis not feasible.

Indications of surgery in bleeding peptic ulcer:

- Failure of repeated endoscopy
- Hemodynamic instability despite adequate resuscitation
- Ulcer larger than 2 cm at first endoscopy.

Gastroduodenal artery is the most common source of hemorrhage in bleeding duodenal ulcer.

Forrest classification	Stigmata of hemorrhage	Risk of rebleeding
Ia	Active spurting bleeding	High
Ib	Active oozing bleeding	High
IIa	Non-bleeding visible vessel	High
IIb	Adherent clot	Intermediate
IIc	Flat pigmented spot	Low
III	Clean base	Low

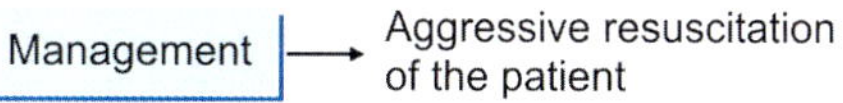

- Resuscitation with IV crystalloids via large bore IV lines (at least two)
- Rapid replacement of blood volume
- Catheterization to monitor urine output

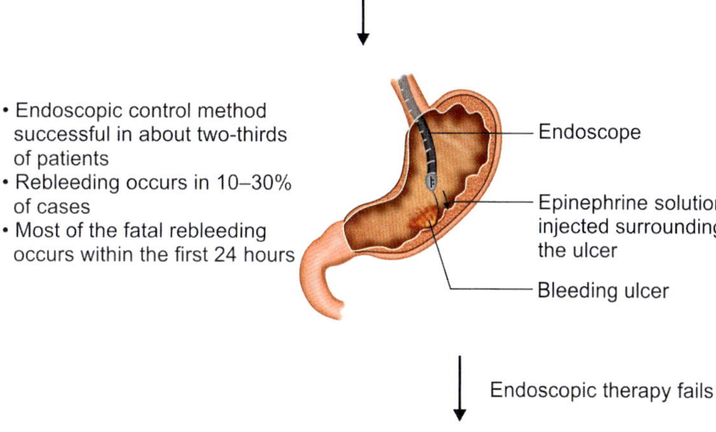

Emergency surgery of duodenal ulcer/gastric ulcer

Emergency surgery of duodenal ulcer

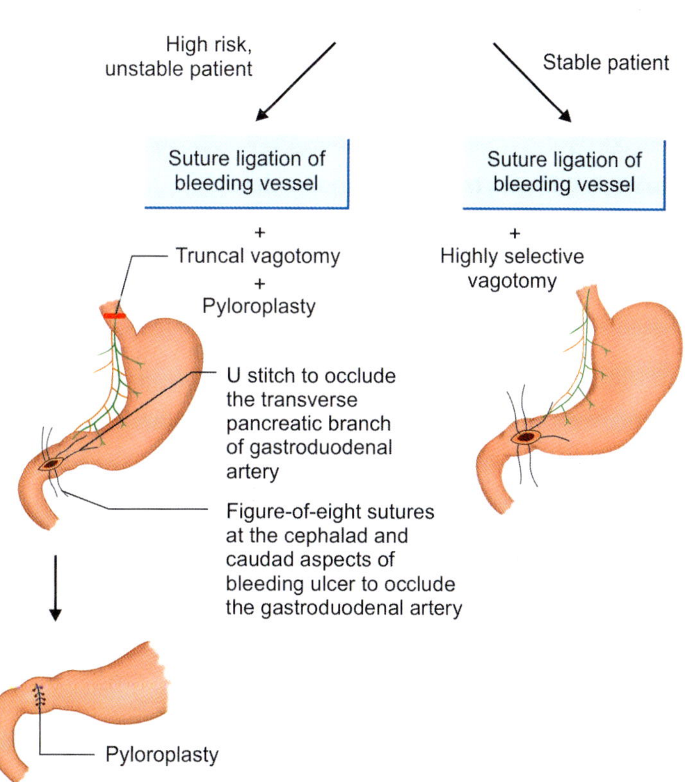

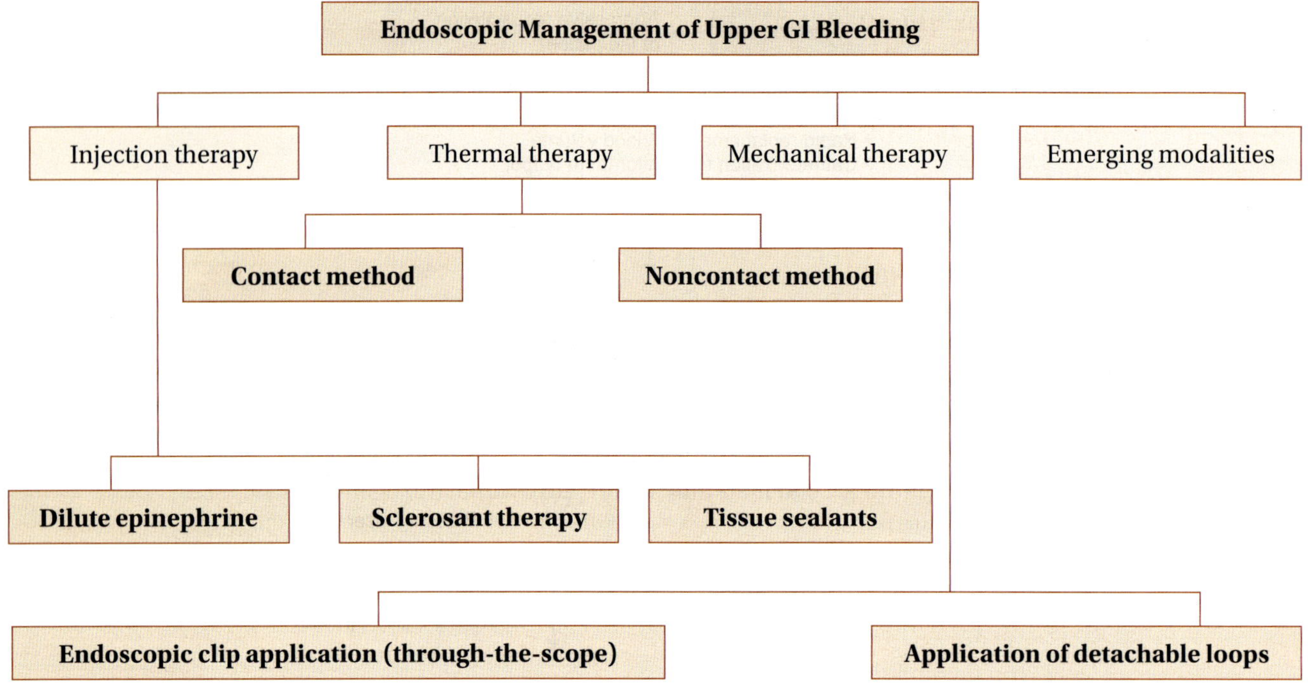

In Injection therapy, dilute epinephrine (1:10,000) is used but usually along with a second modality (cautery/clips). Except dilute epinephrine, injection therapy is not commonly used in non-variceal upper GI bleeding.

In sclerosant therapy, sclerosants used are: (i) Ethanol; (ii) Sodium morrhuate; (iii) Ethanolamine; and (iv) Polidocanol.

Tissue sealants are: (i) Thrombin; (ii) Fibrin; and (iii) Cyanoacrylate glue.

In Contact method of thermal therapy, either heater probe or monopolar or bipolar electrode are used.

In Noncontact method of thermal therapy, argon plasma coagulation is used.

Emerging endoscopic modalities for the management of non-variceal upper GI bleeding:

- **Over-the-Scope clip**—effective as first line and rescue management of non-variceal upper GI bleeding. OTSC is more effective in controlling bleeding from small, shallow, non-fibrotic ulcers.
- **Endoscopic suturing**—particularly effective for larger, deep, fibrotic ulcers.
- **Coagrasper**—a combination of thermal and mechanical hemostasis devices that delivers targeted monopolar coagulation energy at the site of bleeding.
- **Radiofrequency ablation**—particularly effective for the management of GAVE.
- **Endoscopic ultrasound guided angiotherapy**—acts by detecting vascular lesions by EUS and then injection of therapeutic agents into the lesion.
- **Topical hemostatic sprays:**
  - Hemospray—inorganic, absorbent powder rapidly concentrates clotting factors at the bleeding site and forms a coagulum.
  - Endoclot—starch-derived compound concentrates platelets, RBCs, and coagulation proteins at the bleeding site.
  - Ankaferd blood stopper—forms a protein mesh that acts as an anchor for RBC aggregation, resulting in formation of coagulum.

Emergency Surgery of Bleeding Gastric Ulcer

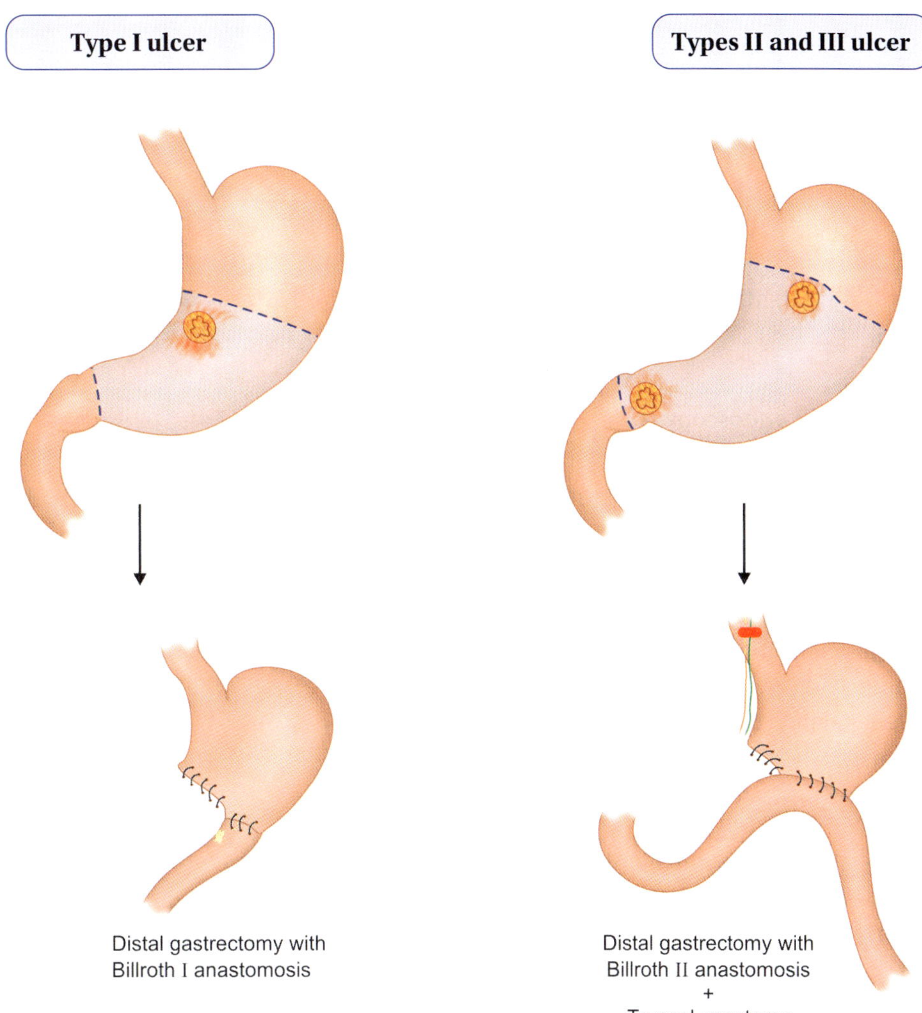

Distal gastrectomy with Billroth I anastomosis

Distal gastrectomy with Billroth II anastomosis
+
Truncal vagotomy

Causes of Non-variceal Upper Gastrointestinal Bleeding

Inflammation/ulcer	Neoplastic lesion	Vascular lesion	Procedure related	Others
Peptic ulcer disease	Gastric cancer	Dieulafoy's lesion	Endoscopic mucosal resection	Mallory–Weiss tear
Erosive esophagitis, gastritis, duodenitis	Esophageal cancer	Angiodysplasia	Endoscopic submucosal dissection	Cameron ulcer
Anastomotic ulcer	Gastrointestinal stromal tumor	Gastric antral vascular ectasia (GAVE)	Endoscopic sphincterotomy	
		Aortoenteric fistula		

Gastric Outlet Obstruction

Gastric outlet obstruction (GOO) is caused by benign or malignant mechanical obstruction or due to motility disorder. Among the benign causes, peptic ulcer disease is the most common.

Clinical Presentation

History of long-standing peptic ulcer disease, progressively worsening early satiety and vomiting, vomiting occurs later in the day, vomitus contains foul-smelling, nonbilious liquid and partially digested old food. Weight loss, cachexia, visible peristalsis, succussion splash, distended stomach outlined by ausculto-percussion.

Investigations

- For diagnosis, upper GI endoscopy is the investigation of choice.
- CT abdomen is indicated if obstruction is due to malignancy.
- Hypokalemic, hypochloremic metabolic acidosis is often present due to repeated vomiting.

Management

Conservative management includes: (i) Fluid resuscitation with normal saline and IV potassium supplementation; (ii) Nasogastric suction with Ryle's tube—to decompress the stomach and prevent aspiration; (iii) Nutritional support with total parenteral nutrition (if indicated); and (iv) *H. pylori* eradication therapy.

Definitive treatment options are: (i) Balloon dilation; (ii) Placement of self-expandable metal stent; and (iii) Surgery. Multiple dilations are often required for sustained response. Recurrent stricture after repeated dilations is the indication of surgical management. There is limited evidence support in favour of SEMS placement in benign GOO.

Surgery for GOO

Truncal vagotomy with gastrojejunostomy (open or laparoscopic approach). **Preoperative preparation includes:** (i) Decompression of stomach; (ii) Saline irrigation through Ryle's tube to remove the gastric contents; and (iii) Correction of dyselectrolytemia.

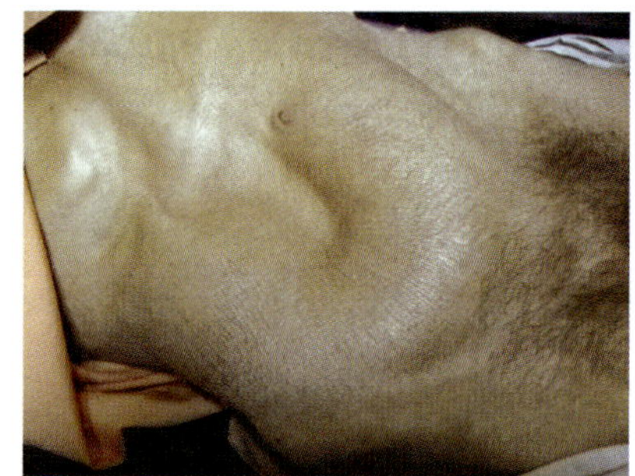

Distended stomach with visible peristalsis.

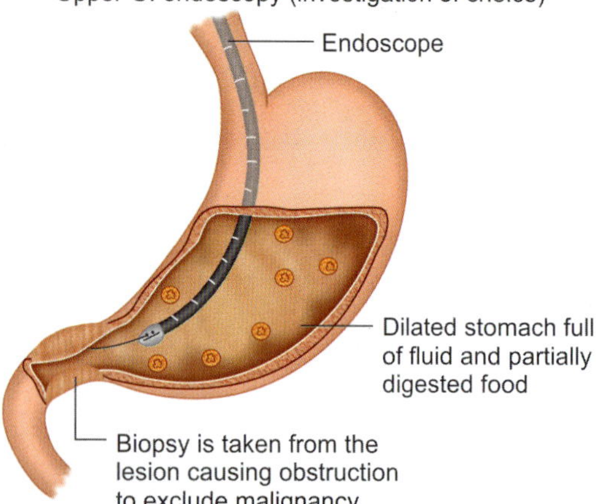

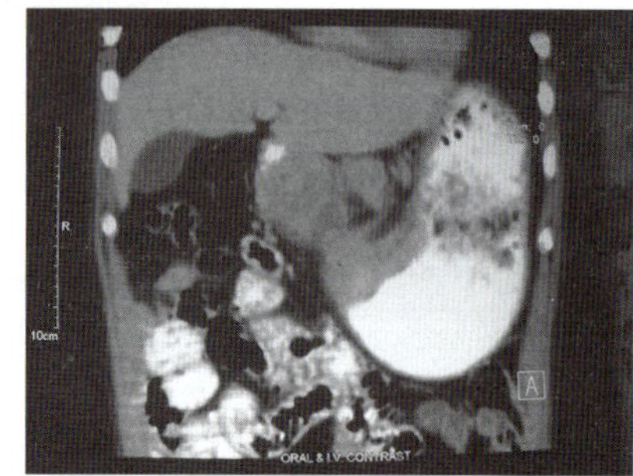

CECT showing contrast-filled distended stomach with food-debris.

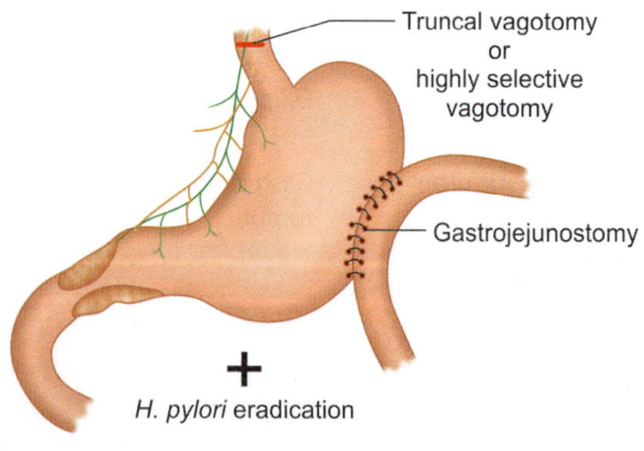

Balloon dilation is also effective in:

- Caustic stricture
- Stricture related to post-endoscopic submucosal dissection

Causes of Gastric Outlet Obstruction

Mechanical cause

Motility disorder

- Gastroparesis (due to long-standing diabetes)
- Post-surgical gastroparesis
- Medication-associated gastroparesis (narcotics, anticholinergics, calcium-channel blockers)
- Systemic disease-associated (amyloidosis, scleroderma)
- Paraneoplastic syndrome

Benign causes of GOO

- Peptic ulcer disease with secondary stricture
- NSAID-related stricture
- Anastomotic stricture
- Caustic-induced stricture
- Chronic pancreatitis
- Bouveret syndrome
- Bezoars

In pediatric population:

- Congenital hypertrophic pyloric stenosis
- Duodenal atresia
- Antral and duodenal webs

Malignant causes of GOO

- Carcinoma of gastric antrum
- Carcinoma at head of the pancreas
- Cystic neoplasm of pancreas
- GIST of stomach

Congenital Hypertrophic Pyloric Stenosis

A disease of the newborn characterized by **hypertrophy of the circular muscles of the pylorus**, resulting in gastric outlet obstruction. Gastric outlet obstruction leads to **hypokalemic, hypochloremic metabolic alkalosis.** This disorder is most commonly seen in **first-born male infants between the ages of 2 and 8 weeks of life**. Male infants are more affected (4:1) than females.

Etiology: Exact etiology is unknown. There is a higher risk for developing this disorder in offspring of parents with this condition.

Clinical presentation: Infants often present with frequent episodes of non-bilious projectile vomiting with or without significant weight loss and dehydration. On clinical examination, a mobile ovoid mass may be palpable (commonly referred as "**olive**") in the epigastrium or right upper quadrant. Visible gastric peristalsis may be seen from left upper quadrant to the epigastrium.

Diagnosis: USG is the preferred imaging modality. **Pyloric muscle thickness >3–4 mm and pyloric length >14 mm** is diagnostic.

Management: Treatment of choice is **Ramstedt pyloromyotomy**.

Gastritis

Classification of Gastritis (based on updated Sydney system)

Non-atrophic gastritis
- Superficial gastritis
- Diffuse antral gastritis
- Chronic antral gastritis
- Hypersecretory gastritis
- Type B gastritis

Atrophic gastritis

Autoimmune gastritis
- Type A gastritis
- Diffuse corporal gastritis
- Pernicious anemia-associated gastritis

Multifocal atrophic gastritis

Type B and AB gastritis

Special forms

Chemical

Bile reflux
NSAIDs

Radiation

Lymphocytic
- Celiac disease
- Varioliform (endoscopic)

Noninfectious granulomatous
- Sarcoidosis
- Crohn's disease

Eosinophilic

Other infectious gastritides

Phlegmonous gastritis

Type A Gastritis

- This autoimmune gastritis is characterized by presence of antibodies against parietal cells resulting in achlorhydria and decreased secretion of intrinsic factor (resulting in pernicious anemia). This gastritis mainly involves the body and fundic mucosa.
- There is hyperplasia of antral G cells resulting in hypergastrinemia.
- Autoimmune disease like Hashimoto's thyroiditis, Addison's disease may be associated.
- Patients with type A gastritis are at increased risk of gastric cancer.

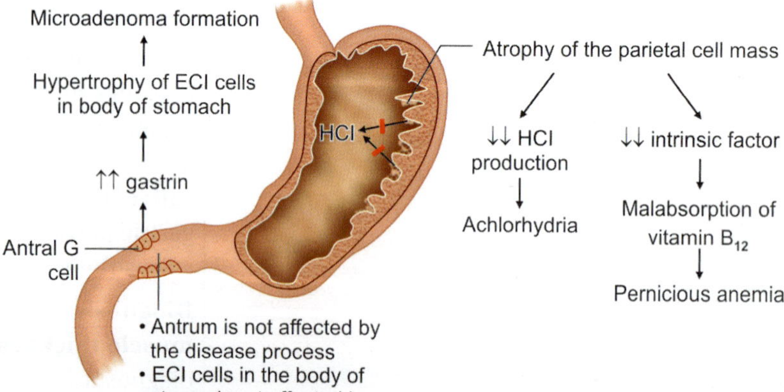

Type B Gastritis

- This gastritis is more common, involves mainly the antral mucosa, commonly associated with *H. pylori* infection.
- Patients are prone to develop peptic ulcer disease.
- This gastritis is also called hypersecretory gastritis due to oversecretion of HCl.
- Patients with pangastritis are at increased risk of intestinal type gastric cancer.

Erosive Gastritis

- The etiological factors of erosive gastritis are NSAIDs and alcohol.
- The endoscopic findings range from petechial hemorrhages to erosions and ulcers.

Granulomatous Gastritis

- This gastritis is characterized by presence of mucosal or submucosal granulomas.
- Based on etiology, granulomatous gastritis is classified into infectious, noninfectious, and idiopathic granulomatous gastritis.
- Crohn's disease and sarcoidosis are the common causes of noninfectious granulomatous gastritis and tuberculosis is one of the most common causes of infectious granulomatous gastritis.

Type AB Gastritis

- This gastritis involves mucosa of body and antrum.
- Multiple environmental factors are responsible for development of this type of gastritis.

Bile Reflux Gastritis

- This gastritis develops due to enterogastric reflux following postgastrectomy.
- Bile chelating or prokinetic agents are useful for relieving symptoms. Roux-en-Y diversion is the treatment of choice.

Lymphocytic Gastritis

- This gastritis is characterized by lymphocytic infiltration of surface and foveolar epithelium.
- Lymphocytic gastritis is associated with celiac disease and *H. pylori* infection.

Eosinophilic Gastritis

- This gastritis is characterized by eosinophilic infiltrate of the stomach, particularly gastric antrum.
- The etiology includes allergy to food (cow milk, soy protein) or drugs, connective tissue disorders or sometimes idiopathic.

Malignant Neoplasms of Stomach

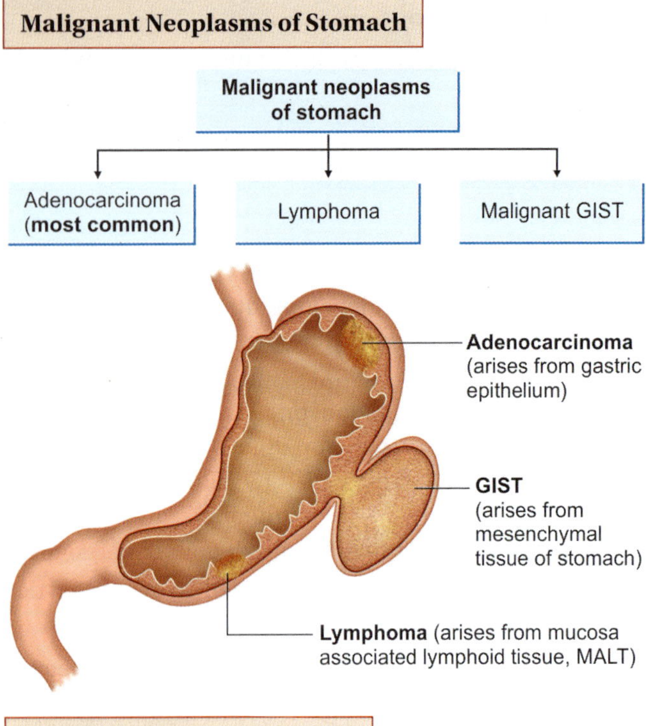

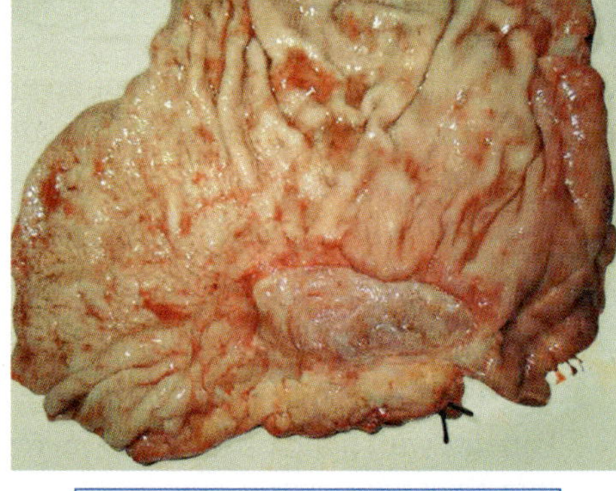

Adenocarcinoma of stomach.

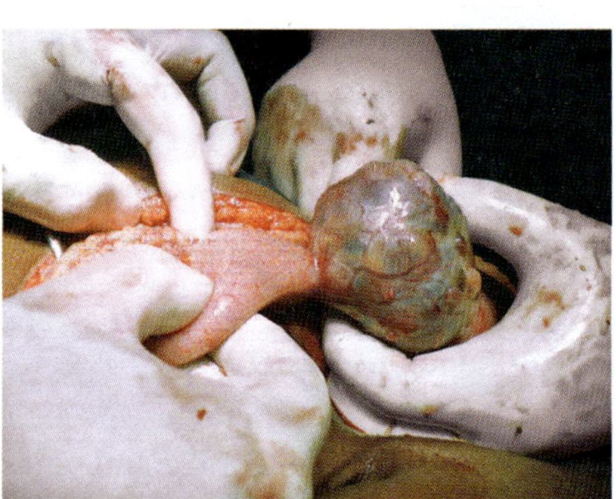

GIST of stomach.

Adenocarcinoma of Stomach

Risk Factors

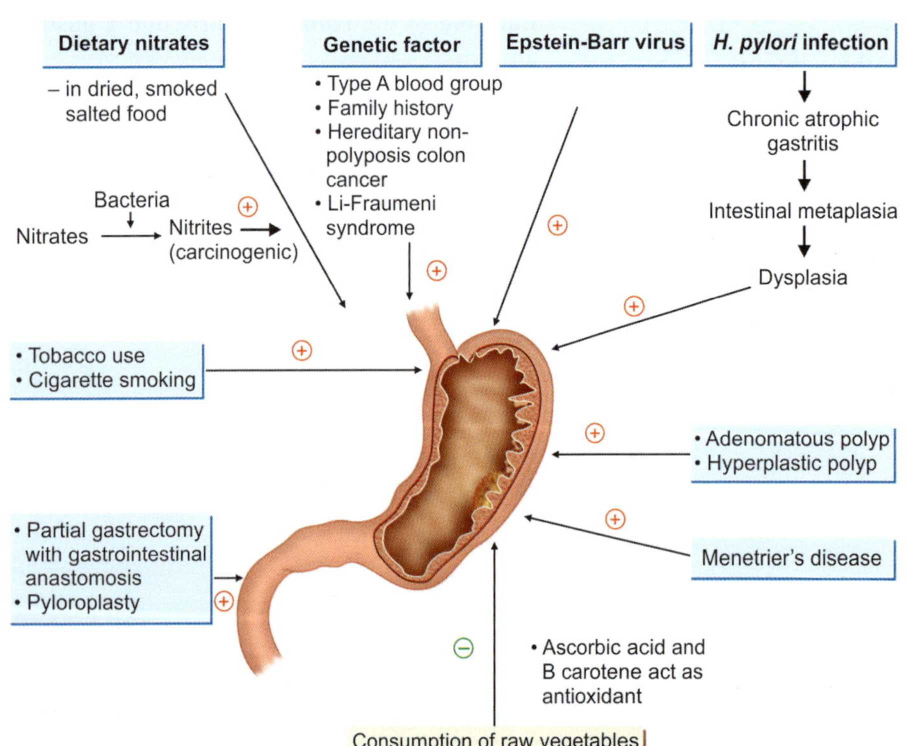

Risk factors associated with distal gastric cancer:

- *H. pylori* infection
- High-salt diet
- Intake of processed meat

Risk factors associated with cancer of gastroesophageal junction:

Barrett's esophagus

Hereditary Cancer Predisposition Syndromes Associated with Increased Risk for Gastric Cancer

- Hereditary Diffuse Gastric Cancer (mutation in the tumor suppressor gene *CDH1*)
- Lynch syndrome (mutation in any of DNA mismatch repair gene, *MLH1/MSH2/MSH6/PMS2*)
- Juvenile polyposis syndrome (mutation in *SMAD4/BMPR1A* genes)
- Peutz-Jeghers syndrome (mutations in *STK11* tumor suppressor genes)
- Familial Adenomatous Polyposis (mutation in *APC* gene).

Less Common Associated Syndromes

- Ataxia-telengiectasia
- Bloom syndrome
- Hereditary breast and ovarian cancer syndrome
- Li-Fraumeni syndrome
- Xeroderma pigmentosum
- Cowden syndrome.

Pathology

The 2010 WHO Classification of Gastric Cancer (Based on Histologic Pattern)

- Tubular adenocarcinoma
- Papillary adenocarcinoma
- Mucinous adenocarcinoma
- Poorly cohesive carcinoma, including signet-ring cell carcinoma
- Mixed carcinoma
- Others

Tubular Adenocarcinoma

Most common histologic type of early gastric carcinoma. This histologic type is characterized by irregular-shaped fused tumor cells of varying sizes with intraluminal mucus and debris.

Papillary Adenocarcinoma

This histologic type is commonly seen in early gastric carcinoma. This histologic variant usually found in cancer of proximal stomach and commonly associated with lymph node involvement and liver metastases.

Mucinous Adenocarcinoma

This histologic variant is characterized by clustered and scattered tumor cells in the extracellular mucin pools.

Poorly Cohesive Carcinomas, including Signet Ring Cell Carcinoma

These histologic variants are characterized by presence of signet ring cells and non-signet ring cells. These variants have propensity for lymphovascular invasion and lymph node metastases as well as duodenal invasion via submucosal and subserosal routes.

Lauren Classification System (1965) based on Histologic Pattern

- Intestinal type
- Diffuse type
- Indeterminate type

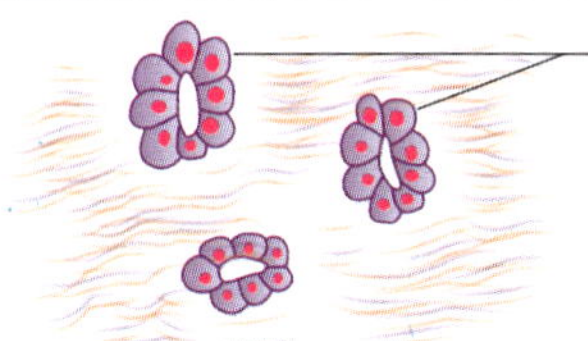

Intestinal Type

- Arises from precancerous lesion (e.g., gastric atrophy, intestinal metaplasia)
- More commonly in men
- More common in older age group
- More common in stomach cancer endemic zone
- Hematogenous spread
- Microsatellite instability

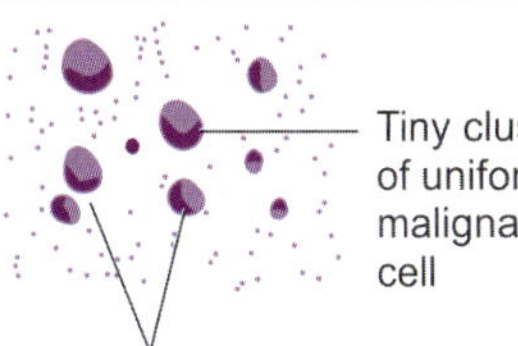

Diffuse Type

- Not arises from precancerous lesions
- More commonly in women and younger patients
- Higher familial occurrence (Blood group A)
- Transmural/lymphatic spread
- Tends to spread submucosally
- Early metastasis
- Prognosis less favorable
- Lack of expression of E-cadherin

Hereditary Diffuse Gastric Cancer

- An autosomal dominant syndrome characterized by development of diffuse gastric cancer at a young age.
- Truncating mutations in *CDH1* gene (gene encoding for E-cadherin) found in about half of the patients. Women with CDH1 mutations are at increased risk of developing lobular carcinoma of breast.
- Genetic testing for CDH1 mutations should be considered if any of the criteria are met: (i) Two gastric cancers in a family, one confirmed DGC diagnosed before 50 years; (ii) Three confirmed cases of DGC in first-or second-degree relatives independent of age; (iii) DGC diagnosed before age 40 years without a family history; and (iv) Personal or family history of DGC and lobular breast cancer, one diagnosed before age 50 years.
- Prophylactic total gastrectomy is recommended between age 18 and 40 years for CDH1 mutation carriers. CDH1 mutation carriers who are not willing for prophylactic gastrectomy, should be offered screening every 6–12 months by upper GI endoscopy with multiple random biopsies.

Borrmann's Classification System (based on macroscopic appearance of the tumor)

Type 1

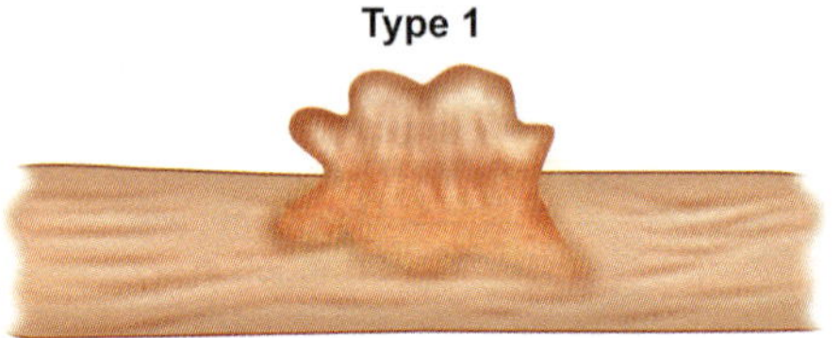

Polypoidal

Type 2

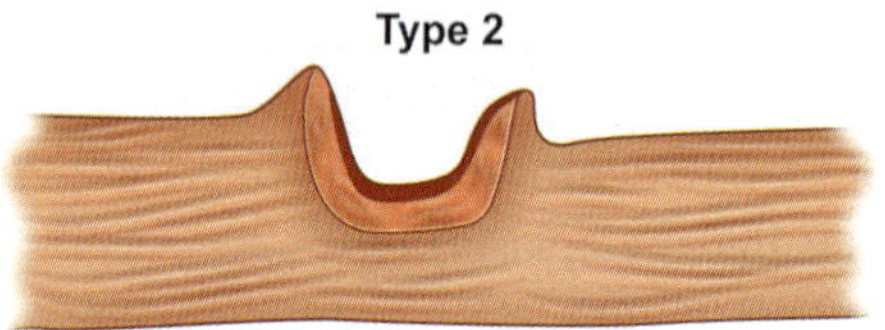

Ulcerating lesion with elevated border

Type 3

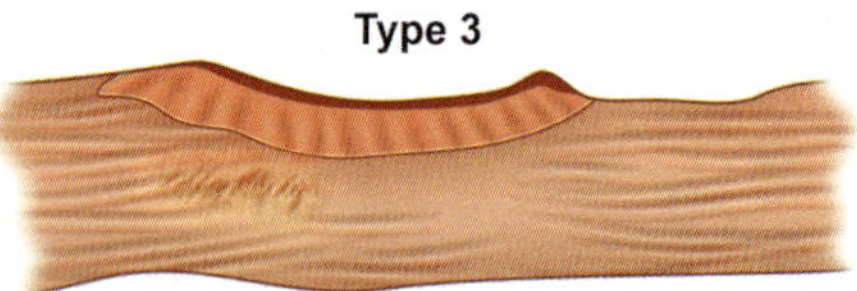

Ulcerating lesion with infiltration into the gastric wall

Type 4

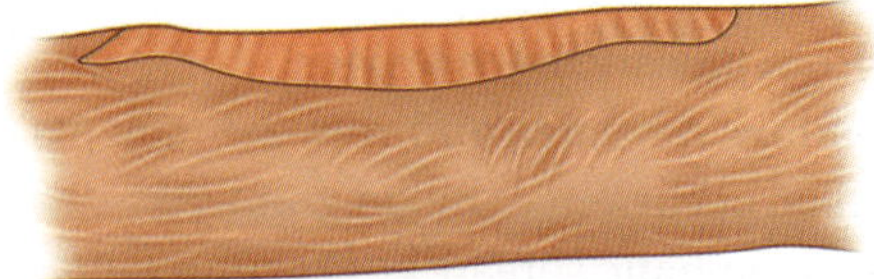

Diffusely infiltrating lesion

Type 5

Lesions that do not fit into any of the categories

Linitis plastica ('Leather bottle' Stomach)

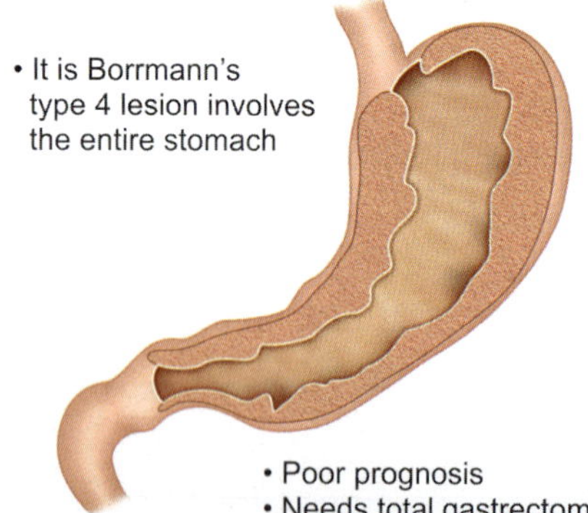

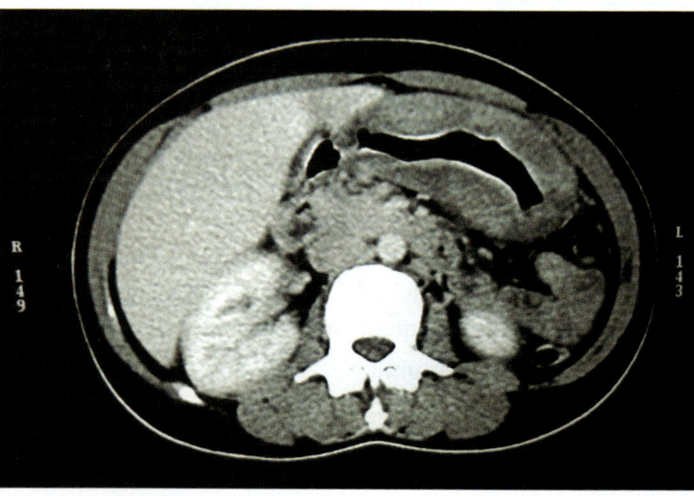

Linitis plastica is an aggressive and uncommon form of gastric carcinoma (infiltrating scirrhous type). Diagnosis is often delayed owing to absence of classic clinical presentation. **Endoscopic biopsy** is often negative due to mucosal sparing of the tumor. **CT abdomen** shows diffuse thickening of the stomach wall. **EUS** shows heterogeneous hyperechoic thickening as well as helpful for guided full thickness biopsy.

Early Gastric Cancer

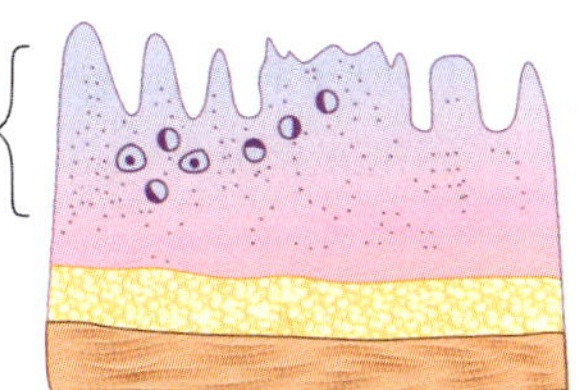

Classification of EGC (based on macroscopic appearance of the tumor): proposed by Japanese Endoscopic Society

Type I Protruded; Type II Superficial; Type III Excavated

Type II is subdivided into: IIa (Elevated); IIb (Flat); and IIc (Depressed)

Paris classification: Endoscopic classification of gastro-intestinal superficial neoplastic lesions

Type 0–I: Polypoid growth

Type 0–Ip (pedunculated growth); *Type 0–*Is (sessile growth)

Type 0–II: Nonpolypoid growth

Type 0–IIa (slightly elevated growth); *Type 0–IIb* (flat growth); *Type 0–IIc* (slightly depressed growth)

Type 0–III: Excavated growth.

Early Gastric Cancer (EGC)

EGC is defined as adenocarcinoma confined to the mucosa or submucosa irrespective of lymph node involvement.

EGC is more common in Japan than European countries due to mass screening of the asymptomatic population.

Conventional white light endoscopy is the diagnostic modality of choice. **Advanced endoscopic imaging modalities** and **endoscopic ultrasonography (EUS)** improve the diagnostic capabilities for early gastric cancer.

Treatment options for EGC are: (i) EMR (Endoscopic mucosal resection); (ii) ESD (Endoscopic submucosal dissection); and (iii) Gastrectomy (proximal, distal, or total).

EMR or ESD can be considered as adequate therapy in early-stage gastric cancer if: (i) Lesion ≤2 cm in diameter; (ii) Well or moderately well-differentiated; (iii) Does not penetrate beyond the superficial submucosa; (iv) Absence of lymphovascular invasion; and (v) Clear lateral and deep margins.

Advanced Endoscopic Imaging Techniques

Narrowed-spectrum endoscopy (Virtual chromoendoscopy): Using only a narrowed part of available spectral bandwidth ('blue light'). Types of virtual chromoendoscopy are: (i) Narrow band imaging (NBI); (ii) Flexible spectral imaging color enhancement (FICE); and (iii) I-SCAN.

I-SCAN are of: (a) I-SCAN1 (for detection of lesion); (b) I-SCAN2 (for lesion characterization); and (c) I-SCAN3 (for lesion demarcation).

Autofluorescence imaging (AFI): Based on real-time detection of fluorescence after excitation of natural fluorophores (e.g., collagen, flavins, NADPH) by short wavelength light.

Confocal laser endomicroscopy (CLE): Useful for cellular and subcellular imaging upto 250 micrometers below mucosa. Either IV (fluorescein) contrast agent or topical contrast agents (acriflavine,cresyl violet) are used. CLE are of two types: (i) Probe-based CLE and (ii) Integrated CLE.

Emerging technologies are: (i) Blue laser imaging (BLI) and (ii) Storz professional image enhancement system (SPIES).

Techniques of EMR: (i) Saline lift EMR and (ii) Cap-and-snare EMR.

Complications of EMR: (i) Bleeding; (ii) Perforation; (iii) Stricture formation; and (iv) Higher recurrence rate in comparison to ESD.

Advantages of ESD: (i) Margin status is well defined; (ii) More chance of en bloc resection; and (iii) Recurrence rate is less than EMR.

Limitations of ESD: (i) Greater skill and more instrumentation are required and (ii) Significant risk of complications (e.g., perforation)

Genetic Events in Gastric Cancer

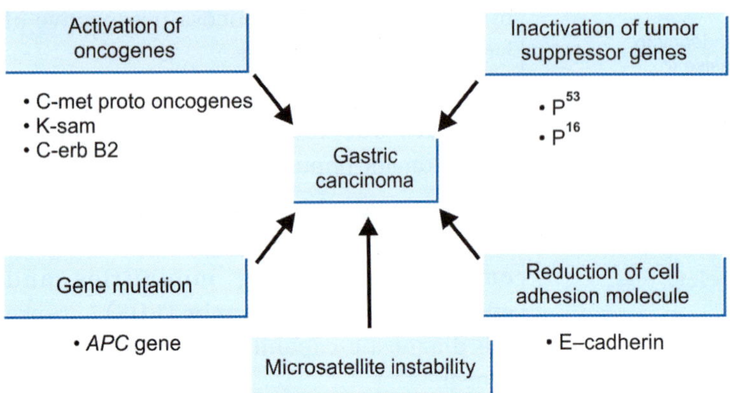

Correa Cascade

Inflammation—atrophy—metaplasia—dysplasia—carcinoma sequence is seen in development of intestinal-type gastric carcinoma. This is known as Correa cascade.

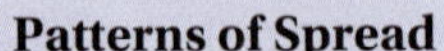

Patterns of Spread

Patterns of spread
- Local extension
- Lymphatic metastases
- Hematogenous metastases
- Transcelomic spread

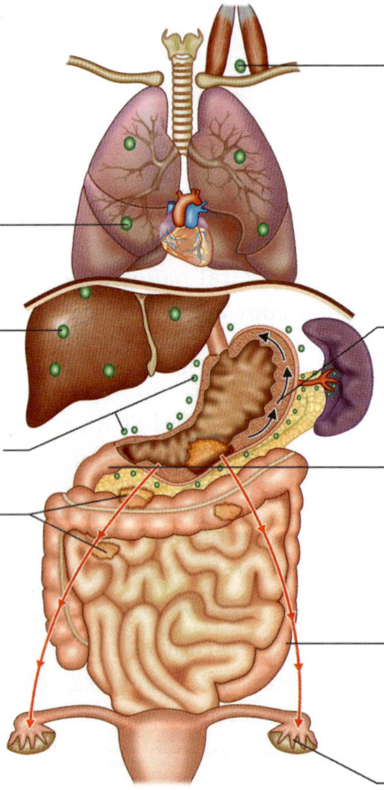

Involvement of left supraclavicular lymph node (Virchow's node)–Due to lymphatic spread of tumor via thoracic duct – **Troisier's sign**

Hematogenous spread to liver>lung>ovary>bone

Lymphatic metastases

Local extension to lesser and greater omentum, pancreas, liver, CBD, diaphragm spleen, and transverse colon

Submucosal spread into the esophagus due to continuity with esophagus through submucosal lymphatics

Submucosal spread occurs less commonly into the duodenum due to pyloric sphincter and submucosal Brunner's gland

Duodenal extension is mainly through muscular layer by direct extension and through subserosal lymphatics

[Duodenal extension carries poor prognosis]

Transcelomic spread causing ovarian mass (one or both sided) – **Krukenberg tumor**

Sixteen lymph node stations (1-16) have been mapped around the stomach as per **old classification of Japanese Research Society for Gastric cancer**.

1-6 stations—N1; 7-12 stations—N2; 13-16 stations—N3.

1 (Right cardiac nodes), 2 (Left cardiac nodes), 3 (Nodes along the lesser curvature), 4 (Nodes along the greater curvature), 5 (Suprapyloric nodes), 6 (Infrapyloric nodes).

7 (Nodes along the left gastric artery), 8 (Nodes along the common hepatic artery), 9 (Nodes around the celiac axis), 10 (Nodes at the splenic hilum), 11 (Nodes along the splenic artery), 12 (Nodes in the hepatoduodenal ligament).

13 (Nodes at the posterior aspect of the pancreatic head), 14 (Nodes at the root of the mesentery), 15 (Nodes in the mesocolon of the transverse colon), 16 (Para-aortic lymph nodes).

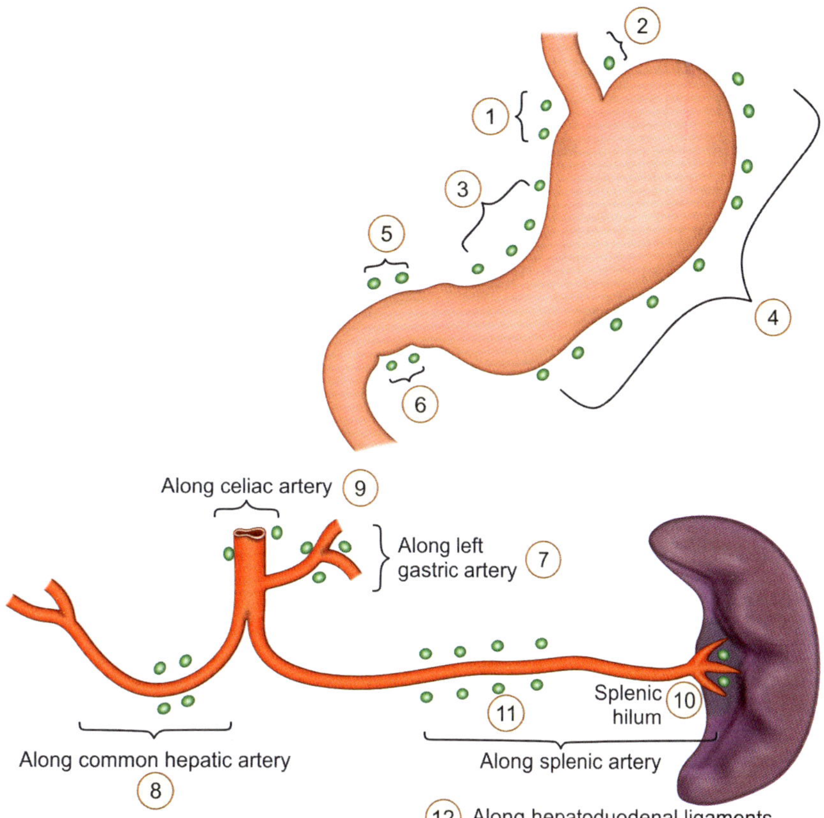

The Newer Classification (by Japanese Gastric Cancer Association) of Regional Lymph Nodes of Stomach

The regional lymph nodes of the stomach are classified into **station 1–20 and 110, 111, and 112**.

Station 1: Right paracardial LNs, including those along the first branch of the ascending limb of the left gastric artery.

Station 2: Left paracardial LNs including those along the esophagocardiac branch of the left subphrenic artery.

Station 3a: Lesser curvature LNs along the branches of the left gastric artery.

Station 3b: Lesser curvature LNs along the 2nd branch and the distal part of the right gastric artery.

Station 4sa: Left greater curvature LNs along the short gastric arteries (perigastric area).

Station 4sb: Left greater curvature LNs along the left gastroepiploic artery (perigastric area).

Station 4d: Right greater curvature LNs along the 2nd branch and distal part of right gastroepiploic artery.

Station 5: Suprapyloric lymph nodes along the 1st branch and proximal part of right gastric artery.

Station 6: Infrapyloric lymph nodes along the 1st branch and proximal part of the right gastroepiploic artery down to the confluence of the right gastroepiploic vein and the anterior superior pancreatoduodenal vein.

Station 7: LNs along the trunk of left gastric artery between its root and the origin of its ascending branch.

Station 8a: Anterosuperior LNs along the common hepatic artery.

Station 8p: Posterior LNs along the common hepatic artery.

Station 9: Celiac artery.

Station 10: Splenic hilar LNs including those adjacent to the splenic artery distal to the pancreatic tail, and those on the roots of the short gastric arteries and those along the left gastroepiploic artery proximal to its 1st gastric branch.

Station 11p: Proximal splenic artery LNs from its origin to halfway between its origin and the pancreatic tail end

Station 11d: Distal splenic artery LNs from halfway between its origin and the pancreatic tail end to the end of the pancreatic tail.

Station 12a: Hepatoduodenal ligament LNs along the proper hepatic artery, in the caudal half between the confluence of the right and left hepatic ducts and the upper border of the pancreas.

Station 12b: Hepatoduodenal ligament LNs along the bile duct, in the caudal half between the confluence of the right and left hepatic ducts and the upper border of the pancreas.

Station 12p: Hepatoduodenal ligament LNs along the portal vein, in the caudal half between the confluence of the right and left hepatic ducts and the upper border of the pancreas.

Station 13: Lymph nodes on the posterior surface of the pancreatic head cranial to the duodenal papilla.

Station 14v: LNs along the superior mesenteric vein.

Station 15: Lymph nodes along the middle colic vessels.

Station 16a1: Para-aortic LNs in the diaphragmatic aortic hiatus.

Station 16a2: Para-aortic LNs between the upper margin of the origin of the celiac artery and the lower border of the left renal vein.

Station 16b1: Para-aortic LNs between the lower border of the left renal vein and the upper border of the origin of the inferior mesenteric artery.

Station 16b2: Para-aortic LNs between the upper border of the origin of the inferior mesenteric artery and the aortic bifurcation.

Station 17: LNs on the anterior surface of the pancreatic head beneath the pancreatic sheath.

Station 18: LNs along the inferior border of the pancreatic body.

Station 19: Infradiaphragmatic LNs predominantly along the subphrenic artery.

Station 20: Paraesophageal LNs in the diaphragmatic esophageal hiatus.

Station 110: Paraesophageal LNs in the lower thorax.

Station 111: Supradiaphragmatic LNs separate from the esophagus.

Station 112: Posterior mediastinal LNs separate from the esophagus and esophageal hiatus.

Lymph node stations 1–12 and 14v are defined as **regional stations**.

Other lymph node stations are defined as **distant stations** and considered as M1 if metastases.

Lymph node stations 16, 19, 10, 110, and 111 are considered as regional stations if direct invasion of esophagus by the tumor.

Maruyama Index

Maruyama index is an independent prognostic factor of survival in gastric cancer. Maruyama index less than 5 has a better impact on survival. "Low Maruyama Index surgery" is now preferred over D-level surgery because it is associated with better disease-free survival and overall survival.

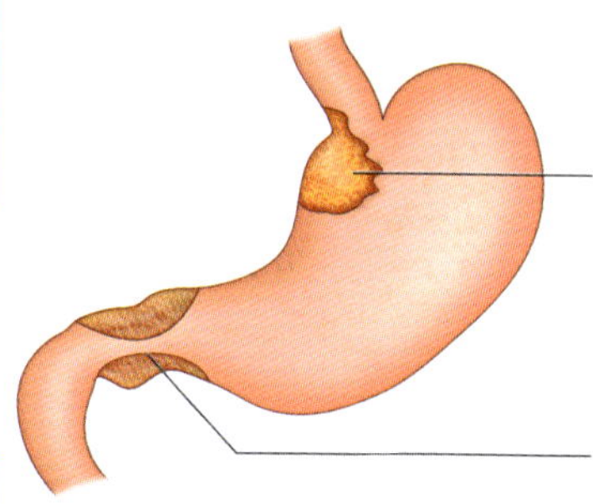

Clinical Presentation

Nonspecific symptoms: Epigastric discomfort or pain, loss of appetite, weight loss, early satiety.

Obstructive symptoms: Tumors in gastric antrum may cause gastric outlet obstruction whereas proximal tumor involving gastroesophageal junction may cause dysphagia.

Tumor bleeding may present as hematemesis or melaena or both. Melaena is more common in gastric cancer.

On clinical examination, visible peristalsis (if tumor in antral region), epigastric lump may be found. In advanced disease, jaundice, ascites, palpable left supraclavicular lymph node may present.

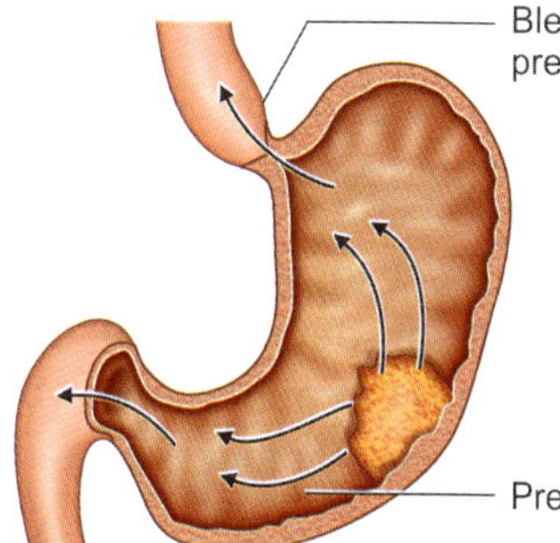

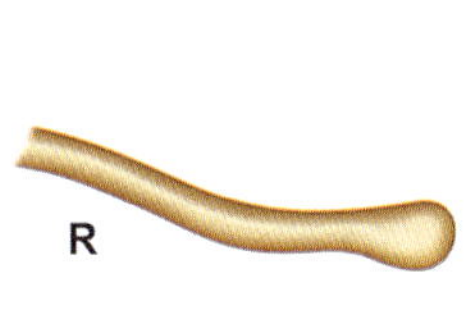

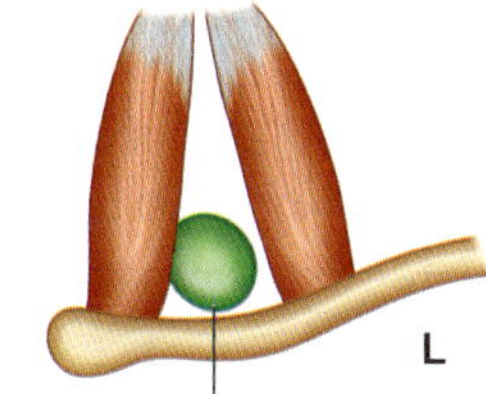

Uncommon Presentation

- Intestinal obstruction may develop due to diffuse peritoneal spread of tumor.
- Tumor involvement of transverse colon may cause fistula or obstruction.
- Secondary tumor deposit at the umbilicus (Sister Mary Joseph's nodule).

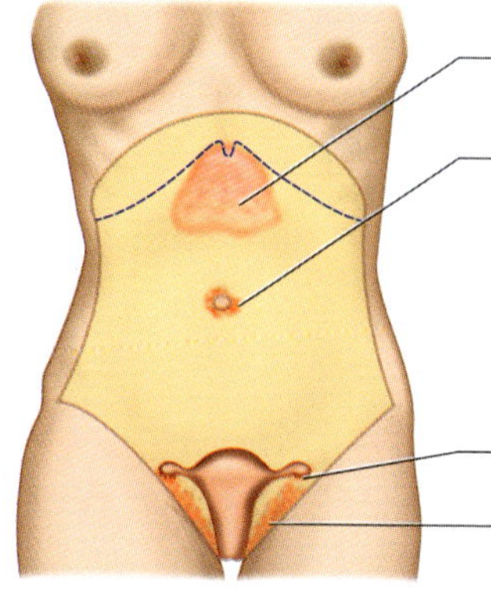

Investigations

Upper GI Endoscopy

Upper GI endoscopy with guided biopsy is the investigation of choice for diagnosis. The location of the tumor and its location relative to the esophagogastric junction must be assessed for proper treatment planning.

Multiple (6–8) biopsies should be performed to provide adequately sized material for histologic interpretation.

CT Abdomen

MDCT of abdomen and pelvis (with oral and IV contrast) is an useful imaging modality for preoperative staging. CT is useful for assessment of regional lymphadenopathy, liver metastases, and tumor penetration through the gastric wall.

Endoscopic Ultrasonography (EUS)

EUS is an important tool in the initial clinical staging of gastric cancer. This imaging modality can assess T and N status, but rarely M status. EUS is particularly important in patients who are being considered for EMR or ESD.

Staging Laparoscopy

Laparoscopy allows direct inspection of peritoneal and visceral surfaces for detection of CT-occult mestastases. Cytologic testing of peritoneal fluid can be done (positive peritoneal cytology is considered as M1 disease).

Advanced endoscopic imaging modalities (e.g., digital chromoendoscopy, confocal laser endomicroscopy) are particularly useful for diagnosis of early gastric cancer.

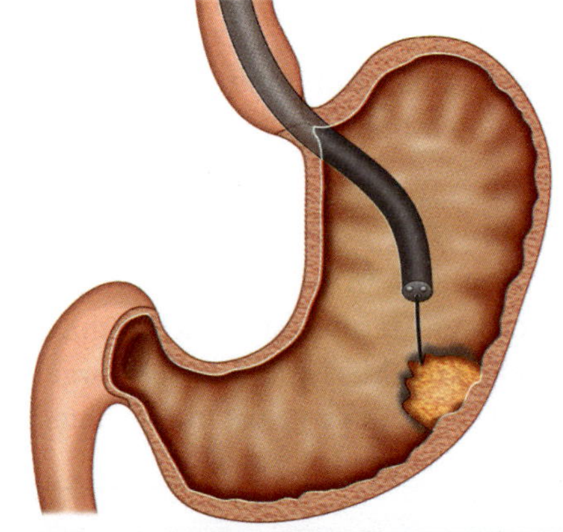

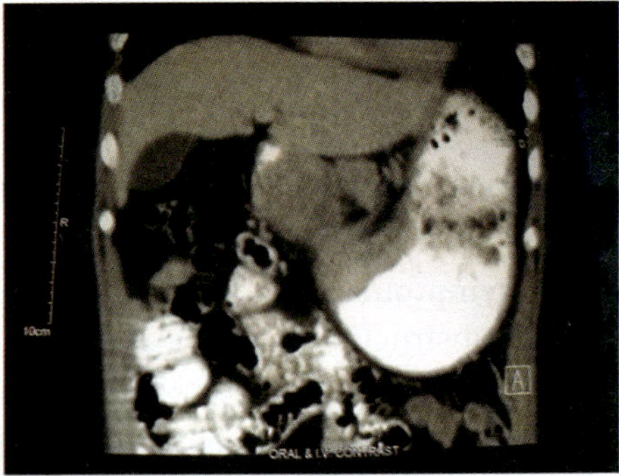

Assessment of HER2 overexpression should be considered in patients with locally advanced, recurrent, or metastatic tumors for whom trastuzumab therapy is being considered.

Microsatellite instability (MSI) or Mismatch repair (MMR) testing should be considered in all newly diagnosed gastric cancers. PD-L1 testing may be considered in patients with locally advanced, recurrent, or metastatic tumors who are potential candidates for treatment with PD-L1 inhibitors.

Treatment

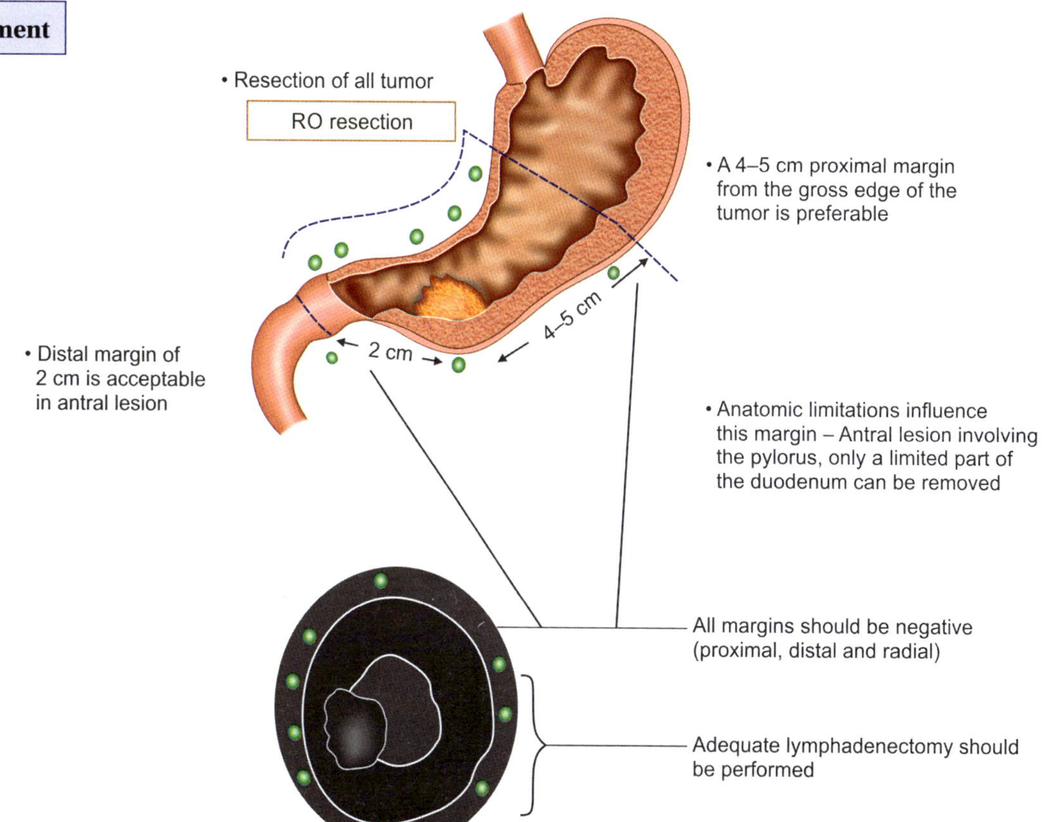

Surgery is the standard treatment for resectable gastric cancer. **Type of surgery (Gastrectomy/EMR or ESD)** depends on the T-stage of the tumor. **Types of gastrectomy** depends on the location of the tumor. **Extent of lymph node dissection** mainly depends on the expertise of the surgeon.

Types of Resection

Tis or T1a: EMR may be considered if expertise and facility is available.

T1b-T3: Distal gastrectomy/subtotal gastrectomy/total gastrectomy with ≥4 cm margin from gross tumor.

T4: Gastrectomy with en bloc resection of involved structures

Extent of Lymph Node Dissection

D1 lymph node dissection: D1 dissection entails gastrectomy and the resection of both the greater and lesser omentum (which would include the lymph nodes along right and left cardiac, lesser and greater curvature, suprapyloric along the right gastric artery, and infrapyloric area)

D2 lymph node dissection: D1 plus all the nodes along the left gastric artery, common hepatic artery, celiac artery, splenic hilum, and splenic artery.

Total gastrectomy with D2: D1 (nos 1–7) + Nos. 8a, 9, 10, 11p, 11d, 12a

Distal gastrectomy with D2: D1 (nos. 1, 3, 4sb, 4d, 5, 6, 7) + Nos. 8a, 9,11p, 12a

Proximal gastrectomy with D1+: D1 (1, 2, 3a, 4sa, 4sb, 7) + Nos. 8a, 9, 11p

Criteria of Unresectability

- Disease infiltration of the root of the mesentery or para-aortic lymph nodes highly suspicious on imaging or confirmed by biopsy
- Invasion or encasement of major vascular structures (excluding the splenic vessels)
- Distant metastasis or peritoneal seeding (including positive peritoneal cytology)

Limited gastric resection (R1 or R2 resection) may be considered in unresectable tumors with significant bleeding complications.

Tumor in Gastric Antrum

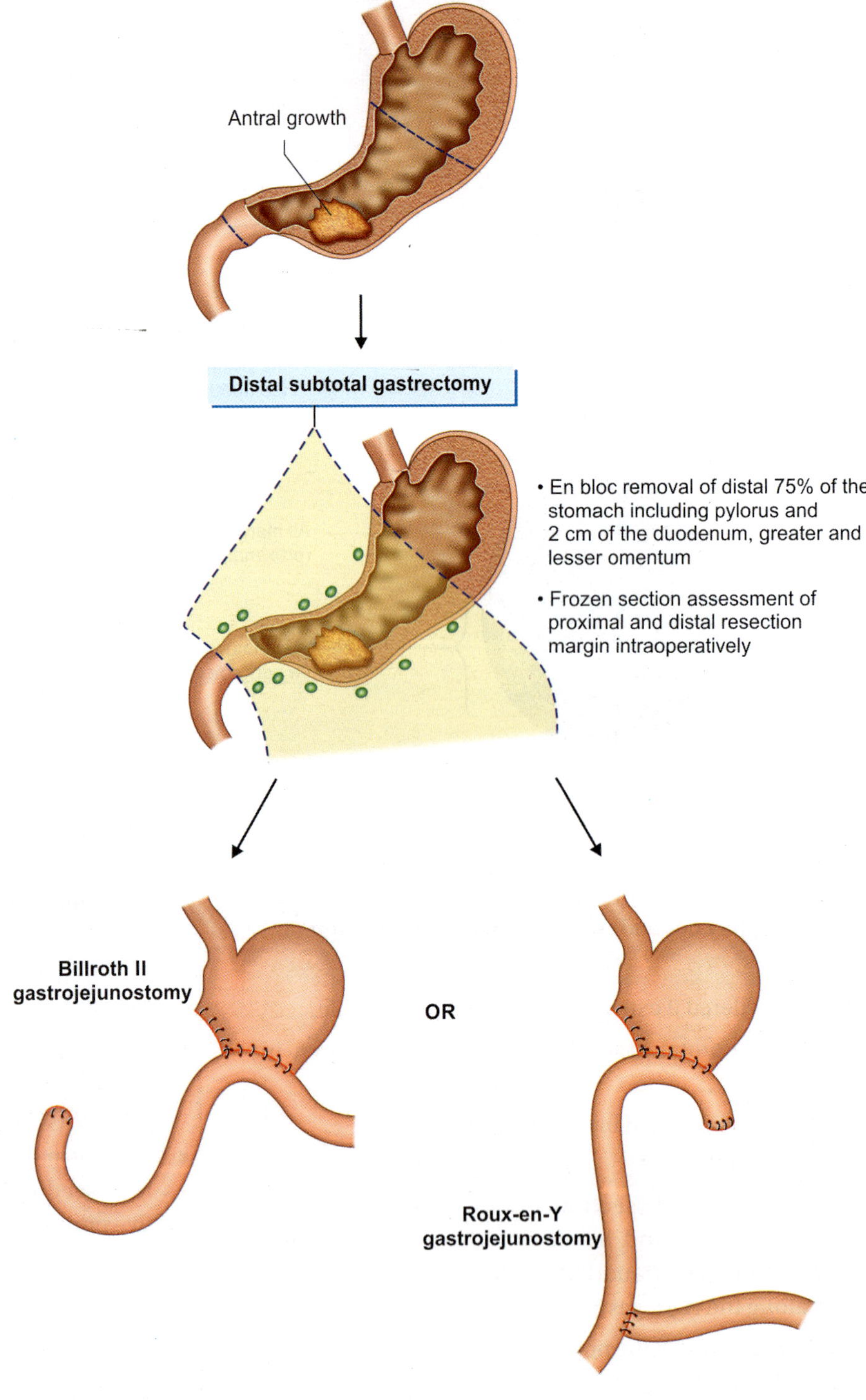

Tumor in Proximal Stomach or GE Junction

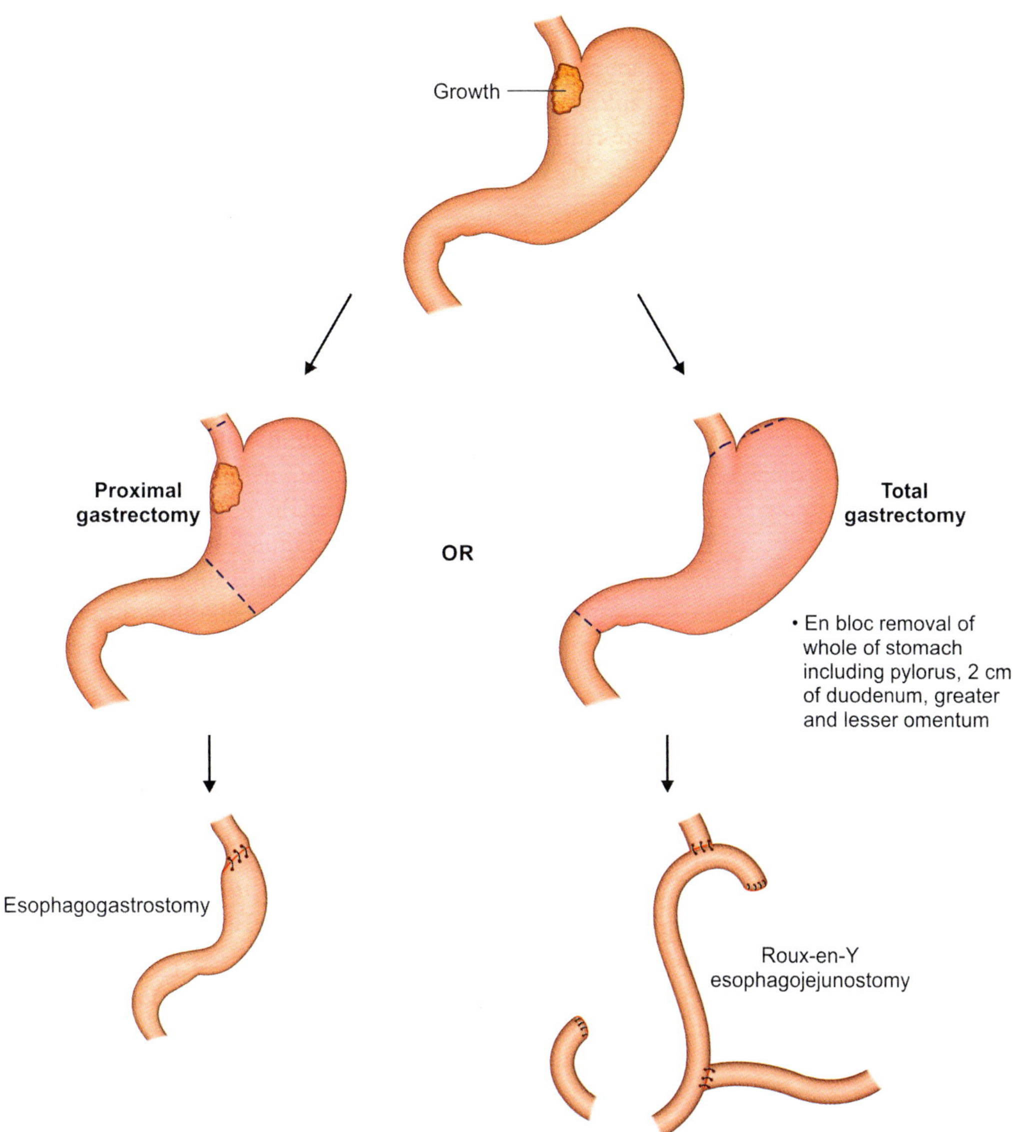

Tumor in Midbody or Fundus

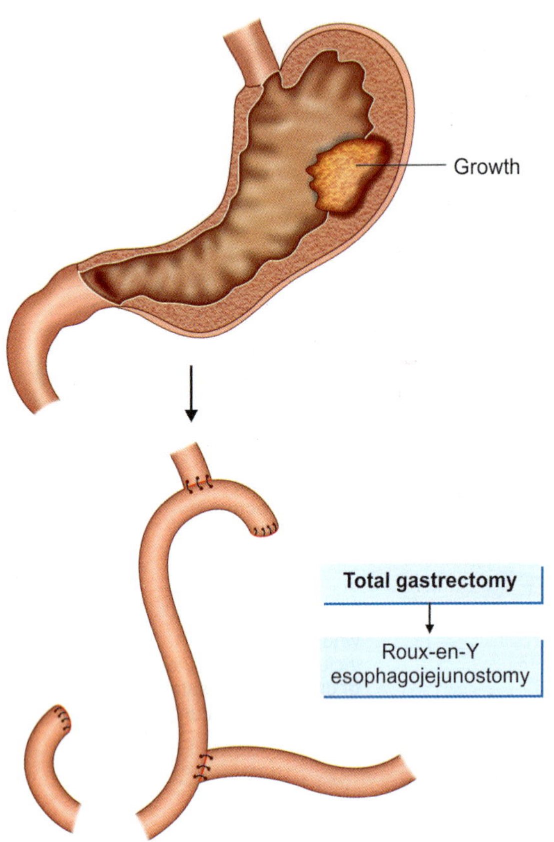

Types of Gastrectomy (Adapted from Japanese Gastric Cancer Treatment Guidelines 2014)

- *Total gastrectomy:* Total resection of the stomach including the cardia and pylorus.
- *Distal gastrectomy:* Resection of two-thirds of the stomach including the pylorus. The cardia is preserved.
- *Pylorus-preserving gastrectomy (PPG):* Resection of the stomach preserving the upper third of the stomach and the pylorus along with a portion of the antrum.
- *Proximal gastrectomy:* Resection of the stomach including the cardia (esophagogastric junction). The pylorus is preserved.

Pylorus Preserving Gastrectomy (PPG)

- Can be considered for middle-third early gastric cancers (cT1N0M0) but the distal tumor border must be atleast 4 cm proximal to the pylorus.
- Surgical principles of this gastrectomy is based on preservation of the infra-pyloric vessels and hepatic branch of the vagus nerve.
- Associated with lower incidence of dumping syndrome, bile reflux, gallstone formation and better nutritional advantages.
- Gastric stasis is typical complication of PPG.
- The short- and long-term oncological and survival outcomes are almost similar to distal gastrectomy.
- This type of gastrectomy can be performed by open or by laparoscopy-assisted (LAPPG) approach.

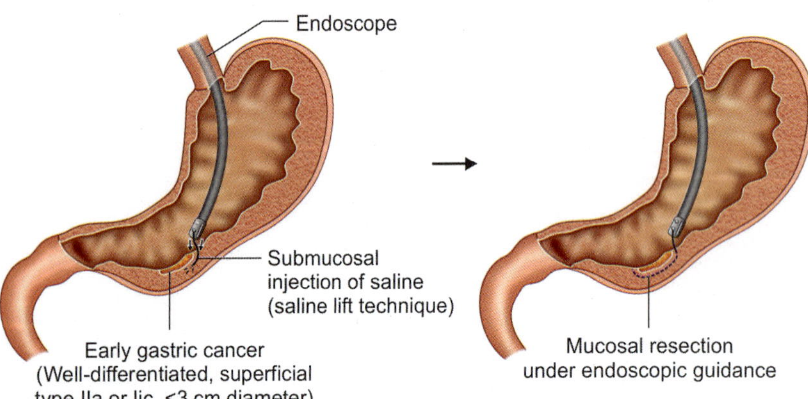

Endoscopic Mucosal Resection (EMR)

Endoscopic mucosal resection is an endoscopy-guided resection technique for treatment of various gastrointestinal lesions.

Indications: (i) Early gastric cancer; (ii) Barrett's high-grade dysplasia and mucosal cancer; and (iii) Colorectal adenoma.

Techniques: (i) Saline-lift EMR and (ii) Cap-and-snare EMR.

Complications: (i) Bleeding; (ii) Perforation; and (iii) Stricture.

Reconstruction Methods after Gastrectomy

Proximal gastrectomy	Distal gastrectomy	Total gastrectomy	Pylorus-preserving gastrectomy
Esophagogastrostomy	Billroth I gastroduodenostomy	Roux-en-Y esophagojejunostomy	Gastrogastrostomy
Jejunal interposition	Billroth II gastrojejunostomy	Jejunal interposition	
Double-tract method	Roux-en-Y gastrojejunostomy	Double tract method	
	Jejunal interposition		

Management of Unresectable Tumor

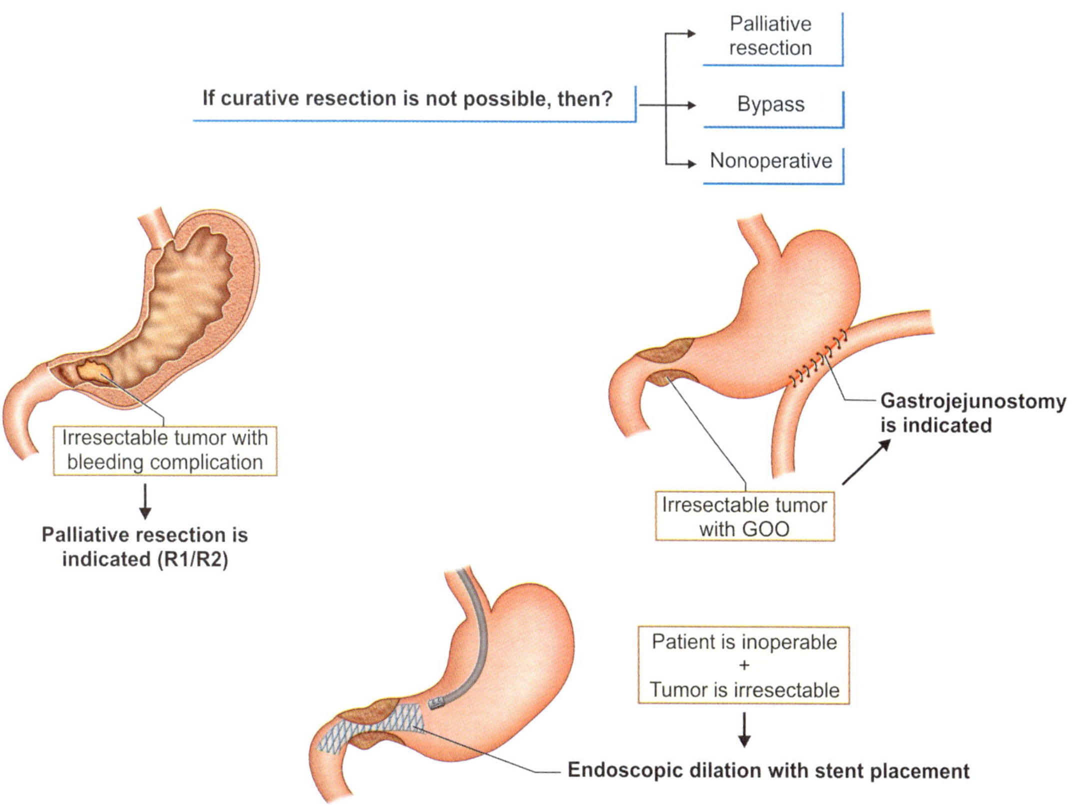

Management of acute bleeding in unresectable gastric cancer: (i) Endoscopic injection therapy or mechanical therapy (application of clips), ablative therapy; (ii) Angiographic embolization—if endoscopic therapy not successful; and (iii) Limited gastric resection (R1 or R2 resection). In case of chronic bleeding, external beam radiotherapy may be helpful.

Management of obstruction: (i) Placement of duodenal stent for gastric outlet obstruction or esophageal stent for esophagogastric junction/gastric cardia obstruction; (ii) Palliative gastrojejunostomy for GOO; (iii) Limited gastric resection; and (iv) Venting gastrostomy (if endoscopic therapy is unsuccessful).

Management of Long-term Subtotal Gastrectomy Survivors

Foods to be avoided—spicy foods, citrus juices (increase acid production) and caffeine, chocolate (decrease LES tone).

Monitoring of vitamin B_{12} level every 3 months for 3 years, every 6 months up to 5 years, then annually and supplementation of vitamin B_{12} (if clinically indicated).

Monitoring of iron level annually and supplementation of iron (if clinically indicated).

Gastrointestinal Stromal Tumor (GIST)

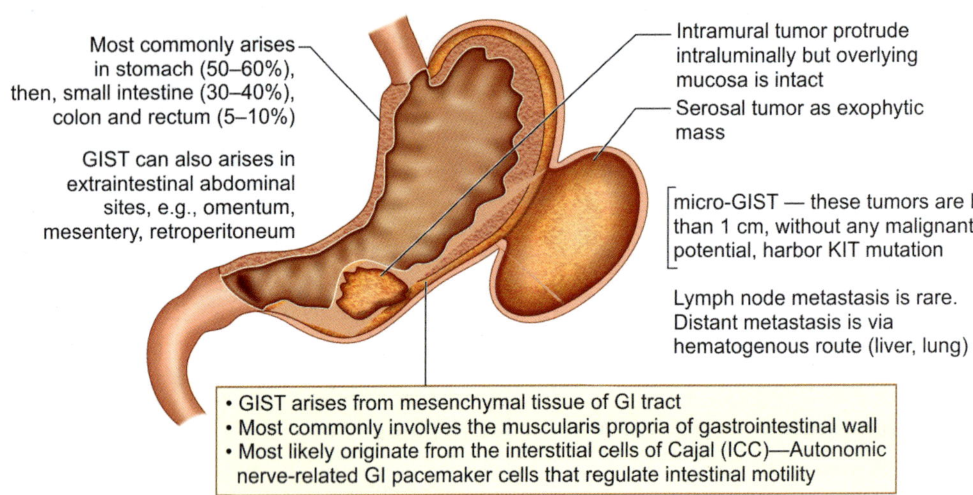

Interstitial cells of Cajal (ICC) are present in the myenteric plexus and regulate the gut peristalsis by coordinating the smooth muscle cells of the gut and the autonomic nervous system

GISTs are the most common soft tissue tumor of the GI tract. Stomach is the most common site, followed by small intestine. Uncommon sites are duodenum, rectum, esophagus, colon, and appendix.

Immunology

Most of the GISTs (80%) express KIT mutations. About 5% to 10% of GISTs have PDGFRA mutations. About 10–15% of GISTs have no detectable KIT or PDGFRA mutations, they are termed wild-type GIST. A majority of wild-type GISTs having loss of SDHB protein expression, termed as SDH-deficient GIST. A small group of patients with intestinal high-risk GIST lacking KIT/PDGFRA mutations having BRAF exon15 mutation (V600E). DOG1 is expressed independent of mutation type.

Most of the KIT mutations occur in exon 11, rarely in exon 13 and exon 17. Most of the PDGFRA mutations occur in exon 18, rarely in exon 12 and 14. KIT exon 11 mutations are most common in GISTs irrespective of tumor site. KIT exon9 mutations are specific for intestinal GIST. PDGFRA exon 18 mutations are common in gastric GIST. GIST with SDH mutations commonly arise in stomach, grow slowly, lymph node metastasis may present, commonly metastasize and usually resistant to imatinib.

Histopathology

Spindle cell type of GIST is most common (about 70%) followed by epithelioid or round cell type.

Clinical Presentation

Gastric GIST usually presented with abdominal pain, anorexia, weight loss or GI bleeding. Rarely, tumor may ulcerate and may cause significant intraperitoneal bleeding.

Diagnosis

Biopsy is indicated for confirmation of diagnosis if preoperative Tyrosine kinase therapy is planned. EUS-FNA biopsy is preferred over percutaneous biopsy because latter has more risk for hemorrhage and intra-abdominal tumor dissemination. Percutaneous image-guided biopsy is indicated for metastatic disease. Testing for mutations in KIT and PDGFRA is recommended, whereas in patients with wild-type GIST, germline mutation testing in *SDH* genes is to be considered who are SDH-deficient by immunohistochemistry. BRAF mutation analysis may be considered in GISTs that retain SDH expression.

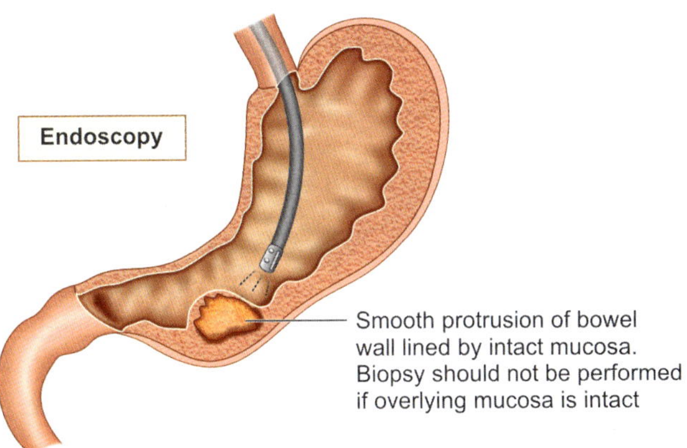

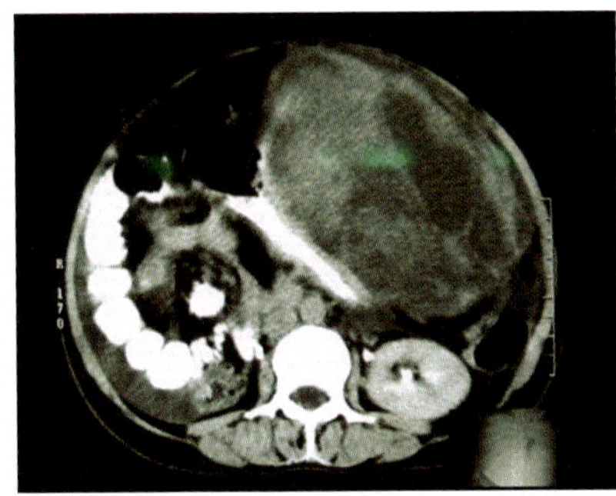

CECT shows characteristic peripheral enhancement pattern.

Role of Imaging

Imaging is indicated for diagnosis, initial staging, restaging, monitoring response to therapy and follow-up. **Contrast-enhanced CT** is the imaging modality of choice. If PET is selected for monitoring TKI therapy, a baseline PET should be done prior to initiation of therapy. In most of the cases, abdominal CT or MRI is used to assess response to TKI therapy using CT response criteria (Choi/RECIST/ WHO criteria).

Carney Triad

A triad of gastrointestinal stromal tumor, extra-adrenal paraganglioma and pulmonary chondromas.

Carney-Stratakis Syndrome

A dyad of gastrointestinal stromal tumor and familial paraganglioma.

GIST of the small intestine and colon have more aggressive biologic behavior than gastric GIST.

Risk Stratification

Gastric GIST: Guidelines for Assessing Malignant Potential

Tumor size	Mitotic rate	Predicted biologic behavior
≤2 cm	≤5 mitoses/50 HPFs >5 mitoses/50 HPFs	Metastasis rate 0% Metastasis rate 0%
>2 cm to ≤5 cm	≤5 mitoses/50 HPFs >5 mitoses/50 HPFs	Metastasis rate 1.9% Metastasis rate 16%
>5 cm to ≤10 cm	≤5 mitoses/50 HPFs >5 mitoses/50 HPFs	Metastasis rate 3.6% Metastasis rate 55%
>10 cm	≤5 mitoses/50 HPFs >5 mitoses/50 HPFs	Metastasis rate 12% Metastasis rate 86%

Non-gastric GIST: Guidelines for Assessing Malignant Potential

Tumor size	Mitotic rate	Predicted biologic behavior
Same	Same	Metastasis rate 0% Metastasis rate 50–54%
Same	Same	Metastasis rate 1.9–8.5% Metastasis rate 50–73%
Same	Same	Metastasis rate 24% Metastasis rate 85%
Same	Same	Metastasis rate 34–52% Metastasis rate 71–90%

Treatment

Surgery is the mainstay of therapy. Goal of surgery is R0 resection with pseudocapsule. Violation of the pseudocapsule and tumor spillage should be avoided to prevent dissemination of tumor cells into the peritoneal cavity. Elective lymphadenectomy is not indicated except in SDH-deficient GIST with significant lymph node enlargement. Laparoscopic resection may be considered if the tumor is in favorable anatomic sites (e.g., greater curvature of stomach, jejunum, ileum).

Tyrosine kinase therapy—Imatinib therapy is indicated for unresectable, metastatic, and recurrent GIST. GIST with KIT exon11 mutation responds to standard 400 mg Imatinib, whereas GIST with KIT exon9 mutation better responds to 800 mg Imatinib. GIST with PDGFRA mutations respond well to Imatinib therapy whereas SDH-deficient GIST or GIST with BRAF mutations are unlikely to respond. **Sunitinib** therapy is indicated in Imatinib-resistant/ Imatinib-intolerant GIST or SDH-deficient GIST. **Regorafenib** is indicated in locally advanced, unresectable or metastatic GIST resistant to imatinib and sunitinib.

GIST is resistant to chemotherapy and radiotherapy.

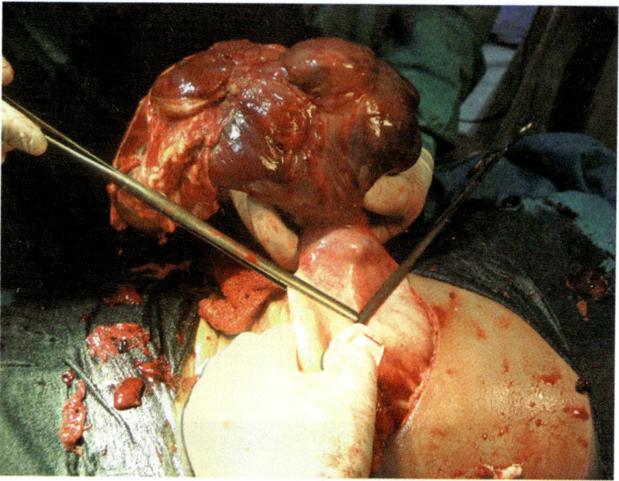

Operative picture showing resection of gastric GIST.

Other Uses of Imatinib Mesylate

- Newly diagnosed chronic myeloid leukemia in chronic phase
- Philadelphia chromosome-+ve acute lymphoblastic leukemia
- Locally advanced or metastatic dermatofibrosarcoma protuberans
- Chronic eosinophilic leukemia
- Systemic mastocytosis

Gastric Lymphoma

Stomach is the most common site of primary GI lymphoma (lymphoma arising in the gut without any evidence of systemic involvement at the time of presentation).

The most common gastric lymphoma is diffuse large B-cell lymphoma thought to arise in mucosa-associated lymphoid tissue (MALT). Low-grade MALT lymphoma arises in the setting of chronic gastritis associated with *H. pylori*. These low-grade lymphomas then transformed into high-grade lymphoma [t (11:18) translocation is a risk factor for high-grade lymphoma]

- Occurs in older patients with the peak incidence of sixth and seventh decades.
- More common in men (2 : 1).
- Most commonly involves the gastric antrum.
- Usually present with vague symptoms like epigastric pain, early satiety and fatigue. Systemic B symptoms (fever, weight loss, night sweat) may present in about 50% of patients.
- **Endoscopy** generally reveals nonspecific gastritis or gastric ulcerations. **EUS with EUS-guided biopsy** is diagnostic and can determine the depth of gastric wall invasion and nature of tumor. **CT chest and abdomen, bone marrow biopsy** should be done to exclude distant disease. ***H. pylori* testing** should be performed.
- Low-grade MALT lymphoma often disappears after *H. pylori* eradication therapy. If low-grade lymphoma persists after *H. pylori* eradication therapy, radiation therapy is the treatment for stage I disease. For advanced lesions, chemotherapy with or without radiation therapy is the treatment.

Primary treatment is chemotherapy: CHOP regimen (cyclophosphamide, doxorubicin, vincristine, and prednisone).
Subtotal gastrectomy is only indicated when there is bleeding or obstructive symptoms.

Menetrier's Disease

Menetrier's disease is a **protein-losing hypertrophic gastropathy** characterized by **massive gastric rugal folds** in the fundus and body with **antral sparing**, **increased mucus production** and **decreased acid secretion**.

Pathogenesis

The pathogenesis is not fully understood, but recent research suggests role of transforming growth factor alpha, epidermal growth factor receptor (EGFR) ligand, in developing this disease. This disease may be associated with cytomegalovirus infection (in children) or *H. pylori* infection.

Histopathology

Characteristic histologic feature is foveolar hyperplasia.

Clinical presentation

Usual clinical presentations include abdominal pain, vomiting, weight loss, anorexia, peripheral edema (due to hypoalbuminemia).

Diagnosis

Endoscopy reveals giant gastric rugal folds and biopsy should be performed to rule out carcinoma or lymphoma. Tests for CMV infection or *H. pylori* infection is also indicated.

Treatment

CMV-associated disease often spontaneously resolves within weeks to months. *H. pylori* eradication therapy is indicated for *H. pylori*-associated infection. Role of steroids, anticholinergics, octreotide is not well established. **Cetuximab**, an EGFR blocking monoclonal antibody is a highly effective therapeutic option.

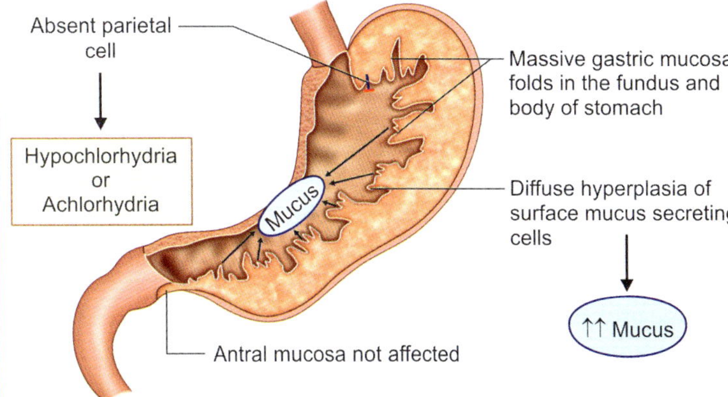

Differential Diagnosis

- Hyperplastic polyp
- Juvenile polyp
- Hypertrophic lymphocytic gastritis

Indications of Surgery (Subtotal or Total Gastrectomy)

- Intractable or debilitating disease
- Patients with increased risk of gastric carcinoma

Mallory-Weiss Tear

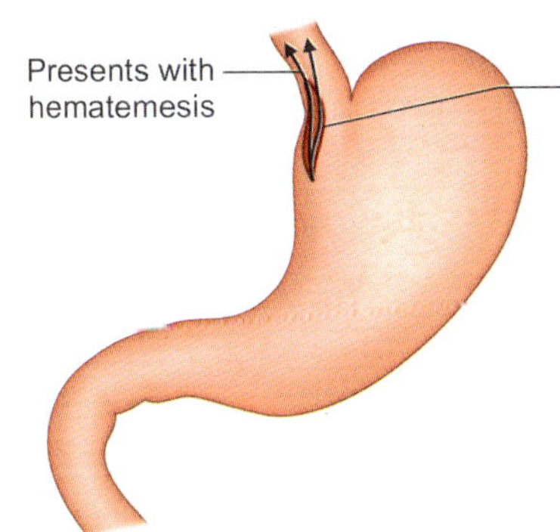

Forceful vomiting, retching or straining [commonly seen in alcoholics]

- Longitudinal tear in the mucosa of GE junction on the lesser curvature
- Endoscopy is diagnostic
- Managed by endoscopic methods (electric coagulation, epinephrine injection, band ligation, hemoclipping)
- Need for surgical intervention is rare If required, repair of mucosal tear with ligature through anterior gastrostomy approach

Differential Diagnosis

- Boerhaave syndrome
- Esophageal varices
- Bleeding peptic ulcer
- Arteriovenous malformations

Other Treatment Options

- Sengstaken-Blakemore tube application
- Angiographic embolization

Dieulafoy's Lesion

- A rare but life-threatening cause of acute upper GI bleeding.
- Dieulafoy's lesion is characterized by histologically normal, dilated tortuous submucosal artery.
- Most of the lesions are found in the proximal stomach on the lesser curvature, next common site is duodenum.
- Most of the patients are middle-aged or elderly male.
- Patients typically present with massive upper GI bleeding, often recurrent.
- Upper GI endoscopy is the diagnostic modality of choice.

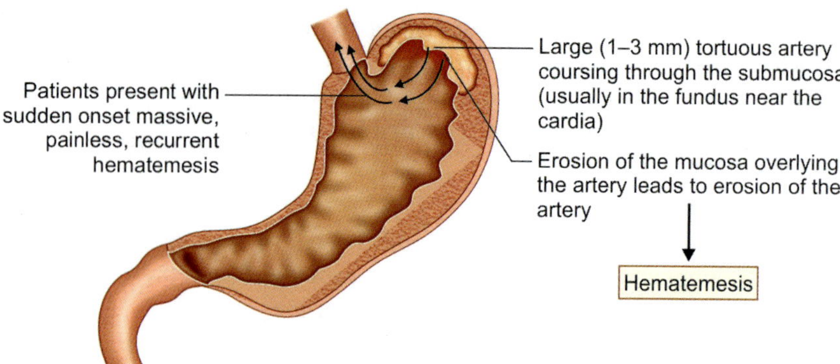

Treatment Options

- Endoscopic hemostatic procedures (multipolar electrocoagulation, laser photocoagulation, sclerotherapy, band ligation, hemoclip)
- Angiographic embolization (if failure of endoscopic therapy)
- Surgery is indicated if lesion is refractory to endoscopic or angiographic embolization methods. Surgical treatment includes under-running of the lesion or wedge resection of the involved part of the stomach.

Gastric Volvulus

Longitudinal axis of stomach

- Torsion along the stomach's longitudinal axis **(organoaxial)**
- Associated with diaphragmatic defect

Torsion along the vertical axis **(mesenteroaxial)**

Vertical axis of stomach

Organoaxial Volvulus

- Most common type of gastric volvulus (occurs in two-thirds of patients).
- Stomach is rotated (180°) around its long axis (along the cardiopyloric line), resulting in reversal of greater and lesser curvature.
- Usually associated with diaphragmatic defect.

Mesenteroaxial Volvulus

- Less common type of gastric volvulus, more common in children and young adults.
- Stomach is rotated around its short axis (from lesser curvature to greater curvature, perpendicular to cardiopyloric line).
- Stomach becomes upside-down, antrum is displaced above GE junction.
- Less commonly associated with diaphragmatic defect.

Clinical Presentation

The classical Borchardt triad of sudden onset severe epigastric pain, recurrent retching with production of little vomitus and inability to pass nasogastric tube, commonly present in acute gastric volvulus. Patient may present with vague abdominal pain. Mesenteroaxial volvulus usually presents as chronic volvulus (presents with intermittent epigastric pain, abdominal fullness after meals).

Diagnosis

Barium studies and CT abdomen are useful imaging modalities for diagnosis.

Management

Acute gastric volvulus is a surgical emergency due to complications including gangrene and perforation of stomach. Surgical management includes decompression of stomach, detorsion and gastropexy and repair of hiatal hernia (if present). Definitive surgical procedures include: (i) Fundoantral gastrostomy (Oozler's operation); (ii) Gastropexy with colonic displacement (Tanner's operation); and (iii) Partial gastrectomy. In asymptomatic patient, expectant nonoperative management may be considered.

Causes of Secondary Volvulus

- Paraesophageal hernia
- Wandering spleen
- Gastric ulcer
- Traumatic defects of diaphragm

X-ray Findings in Gastric Volvulus

Chest X-ray: Mediastinal or retrocardiac air-fluid level

Abdominal X-ray: (i) Unusual location of the gastric air bubble; (ii) Two air-fluid levels in the antrum and fundus; (iii) Large, distended stomach; and (iv) Collapsed small bowel

Bezoars

Bezoars are lump of hardened, undigested material accumulated in the GI tract.

Phytobezoars

Phytobezoars are the most common type of bezoar, composed of indigestible fruit and vegetable fibers (cellulose, hemicelluloses, lignin, etc.).

Predisposing factors are: (i) Following Billroth I or II gastrectomy, Roux-en-Y gastric bypass, sleeve gastrectomy; (ii) Diabetic gastroparesis; and (iii) Hypothyroidism.

Diagnosis is made by either contrast study or endoscopy.

Treatment includes: (i) Chemical dissolution (by cola, cellulose, papain, N-acetylcystein; (ii) Endoscopic retrieval; and (iii) Surgery—if both chemical therapy and endoscopic therapy fails.

Trichobezoars

Trichobezoars are made of hair, commonly associated with trichophagia (compulsive eating of one's hair). Patients usually present with gastric ulceration and obstructive symptoms.

Diagnosis is made by contrast study or endoscopy.

Endoscopic disruption is effective for small trichobezoars. Surgical intervention is indicated for large trichobezoars—a cast of stomach and duodenum is usually found. Psychiatric consultation is needed for trichophagia.

Diospyrobezoar

A special type of phytobezoar formed by persimmon fruit, difficult to treat, develop after massive ingestion of persimmons. Unripe persimmons contain large amount of phlobatannin which forms a tenacious glue that entraps fibers.

Rapunzel Syndrome

A special type of trichobezoar extending from the stomach to the small intestine or beyond.

Lactobezoars: Lactobezoars are pathological conglomeration of milk and mucus in stomach of milk-fed infants.

Pharmacobezoars: Pharmacobezoars are composed of medications, particularly enteric-coated preparations, psyllium preparations, aluminum hydroxide gel, sucralfate, guar gum.

Gastric Varices

Types of Gastric Varices (as per Sarin's Classification)

Gastroesophageal varices (GOV) type 1: Esophageal varices extending below the cardia into the lesser curvature.

Gastroesophageal varices (GOV) type 2: Esophageal varices extending into the fundus.

Isolated gastric varices (IGV) type 1: Varices located in the fundus.

Isolated Gastric varices (IGV) type 2: Varices located elsewhere in the stomach.

- GOV type 1 is the most common type of gastric varices. GOV2 and IGV1 are also termed as "cardiofundal varices".
- Risk of bleeding is highest in IGV1, followed by GOV2 and then GOV1.
- Isolated gastric varices commonly develop secondary to portal hypertension or secondary to splenic vein thrombosis.
- Patients commonly present with upper GI bleeding.
- Upper GI endoscopy can detect the location of varices. USG abdomen is indicated to exclude splenic vein thrombosis.

Prevention of first variceal hemorrhage: (i) In GOV2 and IGV1—Non-selective beta-blockers; (ii) In GOV1—same as esophageal varices

Treatment of variceal hemorrhage: (i) Restrictive transfusion, vasoactive drugs; (ii) TIPS (treatment of choice in cardiofundal varices); and (iii) Endoscopic therapy—endoscopic variceal ligation or cyanoacrylate glue injection.

Prevention of rebleeding: (i) GOV1—Non-selective beta-blockers and endoscopic therapy and (ii) In GOV2 or IGV1—TIPS or BRTO (Balloon-occluded Retrograde Transvenous Obliteration).

Postvagotomy Syndromes

Postvagotomy Diarrhea

- The incidence of diarrhea is highest after truncal vagotomy and almost negligible after selective or highly selective vagotomy.
- Vagotomy disrupts the integrity of gastric and duodenal pacemakers resulting in altered gut motility with bacterial overgrowth and impaired absorption of bile salts and bile acids—this is the **probable pathogenesis**.
- In most patients, diarrhea resolve within 3–4 months after vagotomy.
- Treatment is cholestyramine (anionic exchange resin). If not responding to cholestyramine, surgery is indicated.

Postvagotomy Gastric Atony

- After truncal or selective vagotomy, gastric emptying of solid is delayed.
- In contrast, emptying of liquids is accelerated, because of loss of receptive relaxation in the proximal stomach.
- Mechanical causes such as postoperative adhesions, afferent or efferent loop obstruction, internal hernia have to be ruled out.
- Patients with functional gastric outlet obstruction and documented gastroparesis, pharmacotherapy with metoclopramide or erythromycin is effective.

Incomplete Vagal Transection

- Sometimes truncal vagotomy procedure may be incomplete.
- Right vagus is more related with this problem than the left because of difficulty in identification during surgery.
- Patient may present with recurrent ulcer formation.
- Histologic confirmation of the transected specimen of nerve trunk is necessary.

Postgastrectomy Syndromes

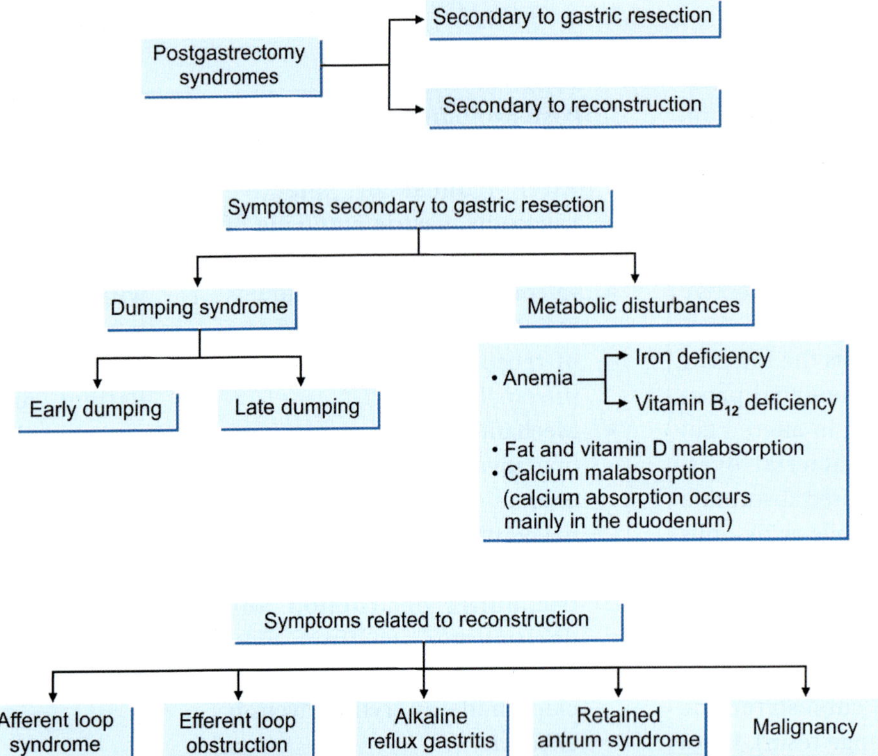

Early Dumping Syndrome

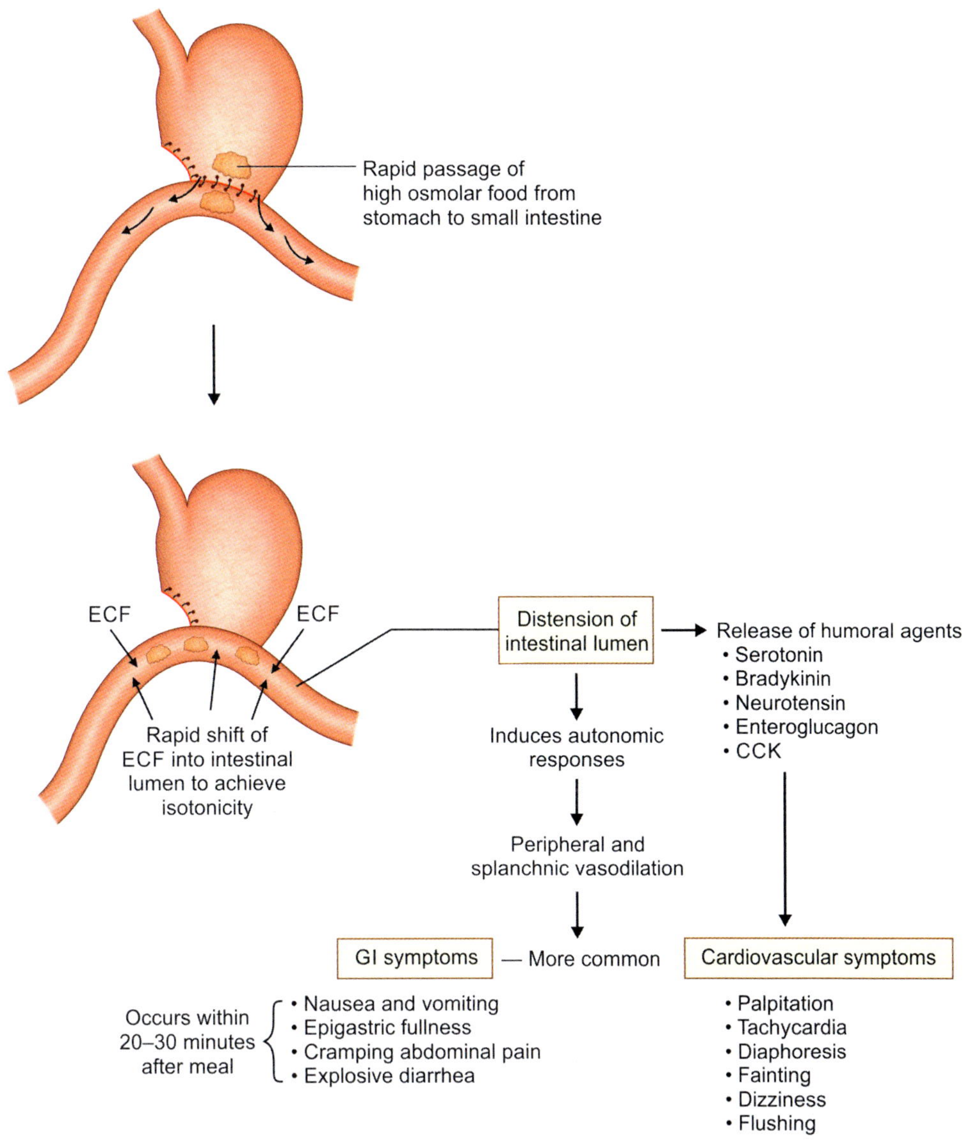

Medical Therapy

Modification of diet:

- Avoidance of liquid during meals
- Hyperosmolar liquid (e.g., milk-shake) have to be avoided.
- Addition of dietary fiber may be helpful.

Long-acting somatostatin analog—Octreotide

Surgical Management

- Surgery is indicated for patients not responding to medical therapy.
- Surgical options include: (i) Gastric bypass reversal and (ii) Gastric pouch restriction.

Late Dumping Syndrome

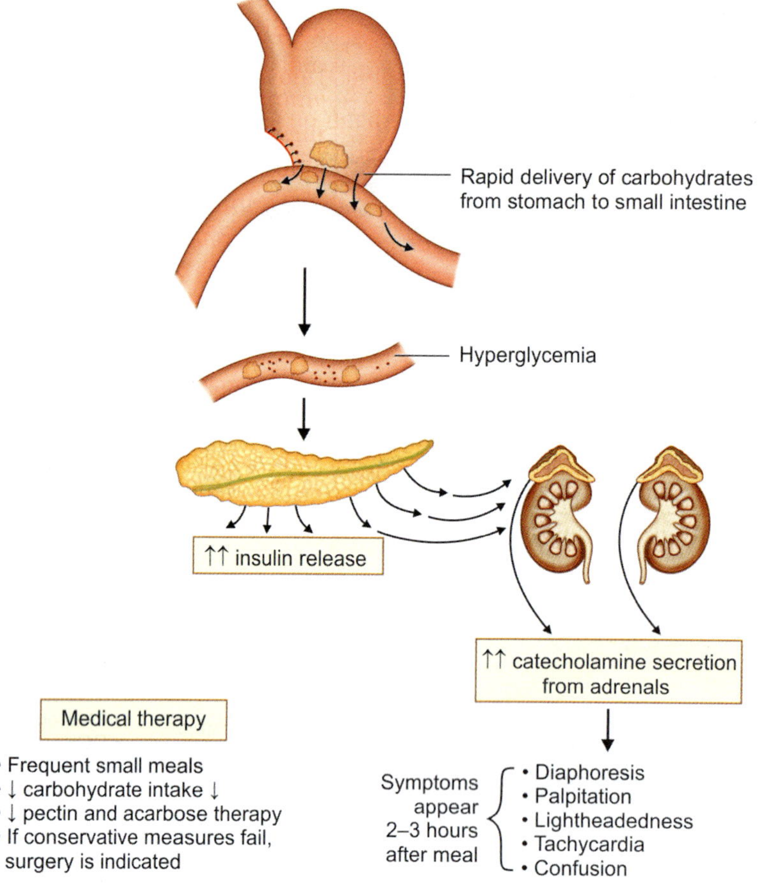

Afferent Loop Syndrome

Due to partial obstruction of the afferent limb resulting in partial emptying of its contents.

Pathology behind the syndrome:

- Kinking and angulation of the afferent limb
- Internal herniation behind the efferent limb
- Stenosis of gastrojejunal anastomosis
- Twisting of the afferent limb resulting volvulus
- Adhesion

If afferent limb is >30–40 cm and antecolic anastomosis, then chance of syndrome is more.

In both acute and chronic afferent loop syndrome, surgery is indicated.

Efferent Loop Obstruction

- Less common than afferent loop syndrome
- *Pathology behind the syndrome:* Herniation of the limb behind the anastomosis in a right to left fashion.
- Surgical intervention is almost always necessary.

Alkaline Reflux Gastritis

- Patients present with severe epigastric abdominal pain with bilious vomiting and weight loss.
- HIDA scan is diagnostic, endoscopy may be performed.
- In most of the patients, medical therapy is not beneficial. Surgery is indicated in these group.

Retained Antrum Syndrome

- It develops if residual antrum is left in the duodenal stump after Billroth II reconstruction.
- Retained antrum is exposed to alkaline secretions (duodenal, pancreatic, and biliary)

↓

↑↑Gastrin release

↓

↑↑HCl secretion

↓

Recurrent ulcer formation

- If medical therapy fails, surgery is indicated.

Roux Stasis Syndrome (Roux Syndrome)

- This syndrome may develop after distal gastrectomy with Roux-en-Y reconstruction. Gastric emptying (particularly for solid foods) is delayed.
- Clinical presentation includes abdominal pain and distension, postprandial bloating, vomiting (vomitus is nonbilious and contains solid food).
- Management includes dietary modification and prokinetic agents. If surgery is indicated, the type of surgery depends on the extent of gastrectomy, status of the Roux limb and condition of the patients.

Gallstone

The risk of gallstone formation increases after gastrectomy followed by reconstruction (particularly risk is more in Roux-en-Y reconstruction).

Marginal Ulcers

- A complication after gastrectomy followed by gastrojejunostomy. It is more common after Roux-en-Y reconstruction than after Billroth II reconstruction. Ulcers usually develop on the jejunal side of the anastomosis.
- Most of the marginal ulcers can be managed by PPI therapy, *H. pylori* eradication therapy and avoidance of NSAID use and smoking.

Gastric Cancer

- Gastrectomy or vagotomy (Truncal/selective) and drainage are risk factors for development of cancer (4 times risk than normal population).
- The time interval between the operation and development of malignancy is at least 10 years.

Case 1

History and Physical Examination

A 45-year-old male patient admitted in the surgical emergency ward with severe upper abdominal pain and vomiting for last 2 days. Patient was treated by local physician but pain not relieved. History of recurrent upper abdominal pain and intake of antacids and PPI for last 3 years. Patient is chronic alcoholic and smoker for last 15 years.

Physical Examination

Patient alert, conscious, cooperative

Pulse 116/min, BP 100/72 mm Hg, Respiratory rate 28/min

Examination of abdomen: Tenderness in epigastrium, card-board rigidity, liver dullness obliterated and IPS was absent

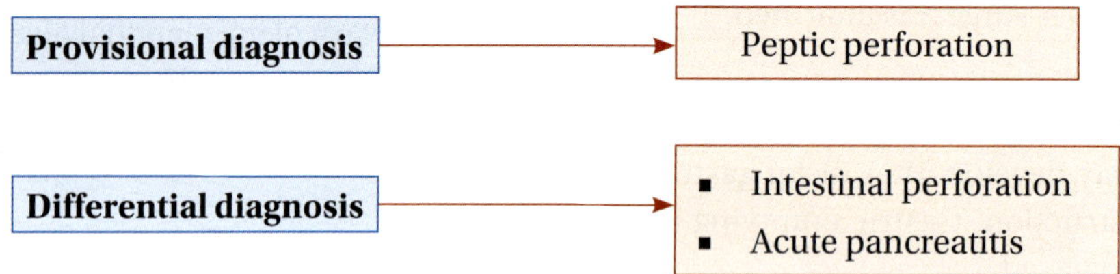

Investigations

X-ray of chest and abdomen (Erect/left lateral): Free gas under right dome of diaphragm. No need of any imaging for confirmation of diagnosis.

Discussion

History of recurrent upper abdominal pain with history of taking antacids highly suggestive of peptic ulcer disease. Chronic alcoholic and smoker male patient presented with acute onset severe upper abdominal pain along with epigastric tenderness, card-board rigidity, and obliterated liver dullness highly suggestive of peptic perforation. Chest X-ray confirmed the diagnosis by revealing free gas under right dome of diaphragm.

Management Algorithm

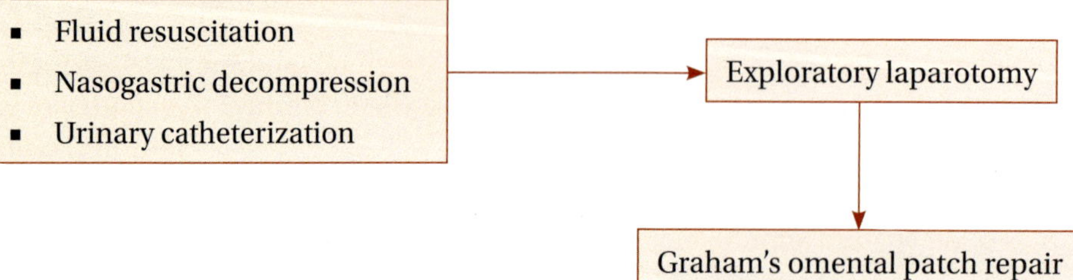

Case 2

History and Physical Examination

A 52-year-old male patient presented with recurrent vomiting for last 2 months. The vomitus contains old, undigested food particles. Patient also complained of vague upper abdominal pain and loss of appetite for last 3 months. No history of smoking or alcoholism.

Physical Examination

Anemia—present, Jaundice—absent, Nutritional status—poor, Neck nodes—not palpable

Abdominal examination: Epigastric fullness, visible peristalsis, and succussion splash present.

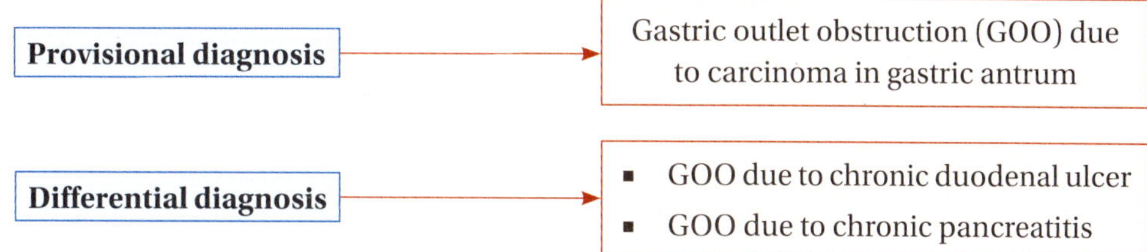

Investigations

Hb 8.2 gm%; Serum albumin 2.6 gm/dL; Na^+ 138 mEq/L, K^+ 2.6 mmol/L

Upper GI endoscopy: Ulceroproliferative lesion involving the gastric antrum, scope cannot be negotiated beyond the lesion.

Endoscopy-guided biopsy: Moderately differentiated adenocarcinoma

MDCT of abdomen and pelvis (with oral and IV contrast): Antral wall thickening and perigastric lymphadenopathy, mild ascites also present.

CT chest: No evidence of lung metastases.

Discussion

History and clinical examination findings suggestive of gastric outlet obstruction. Patient's age, no history suggestive of peptic ulcer disease, no history of smoking or alcoholism excludes the possibility of GOO due to peptic ulcer disease. The provisional diagnosis was also confirmed by UGI endoscopy and guided biopsy. Metastatic work-up (CT abdomen and CT chest) excluded distant metastases. Distal gastrectomy with D2 lymph node dissection planned.

Management Algorithm

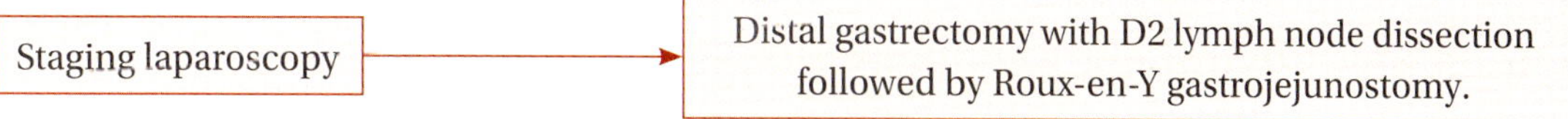

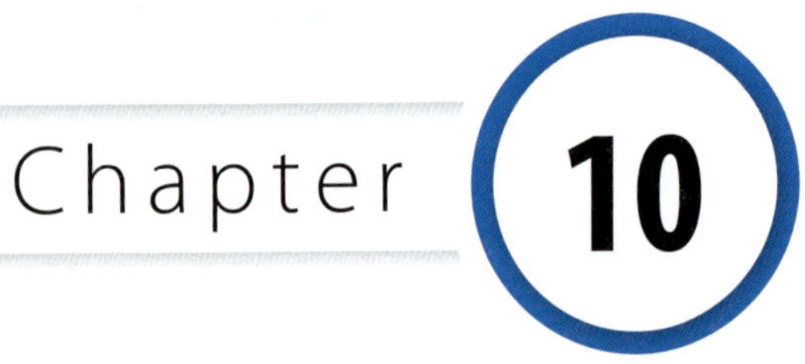

Intestine

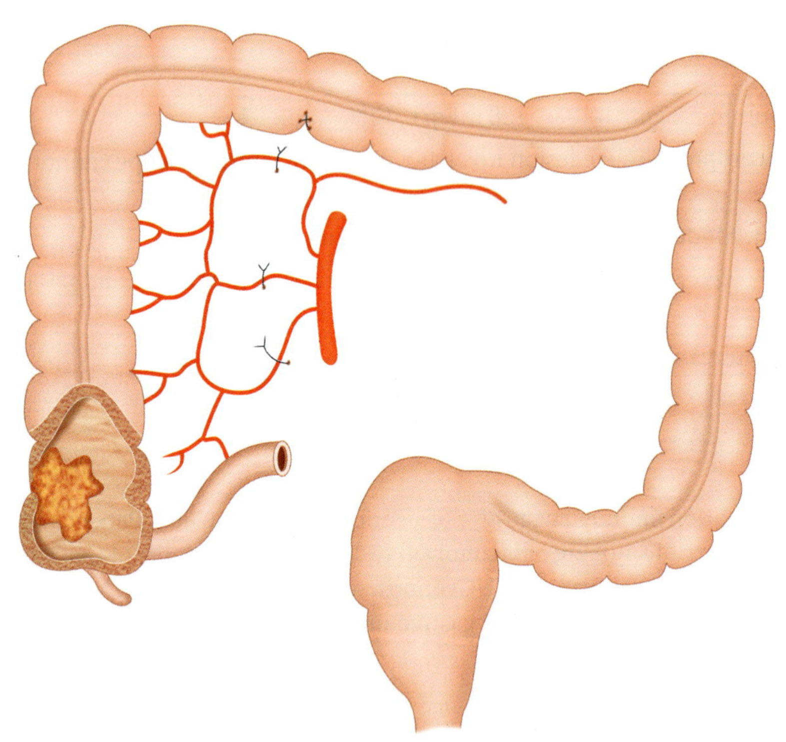

Important Topics

- Intestinal Obstruction
- Intussesception
- Crohn's Disease
- Intestinal Tuberculosis
- Meckel's Diverticulum
- Neoplasms of Small Intestine
- Short Bowel Syndrome
- Diverticular Disease of Colon
- Volvulus
- Ulcerative Colitis
- Colorectal Polyp
- Colorectal Cancer
- Stoma and its Management
- Enteroatmospheric Fistula
- Gastrointestinal Bleeding

'Medicine rests upon four pillars — philosophy, astronomy, alchemy, and ethics ………………., the fourth shows the physician those virtues which must stay with him up until his death, and it should support and complete the three other pillars.'

Paracelsus (C. 1493–1541)
Swiss Doctor and Chemist

Intestinal Obstruction

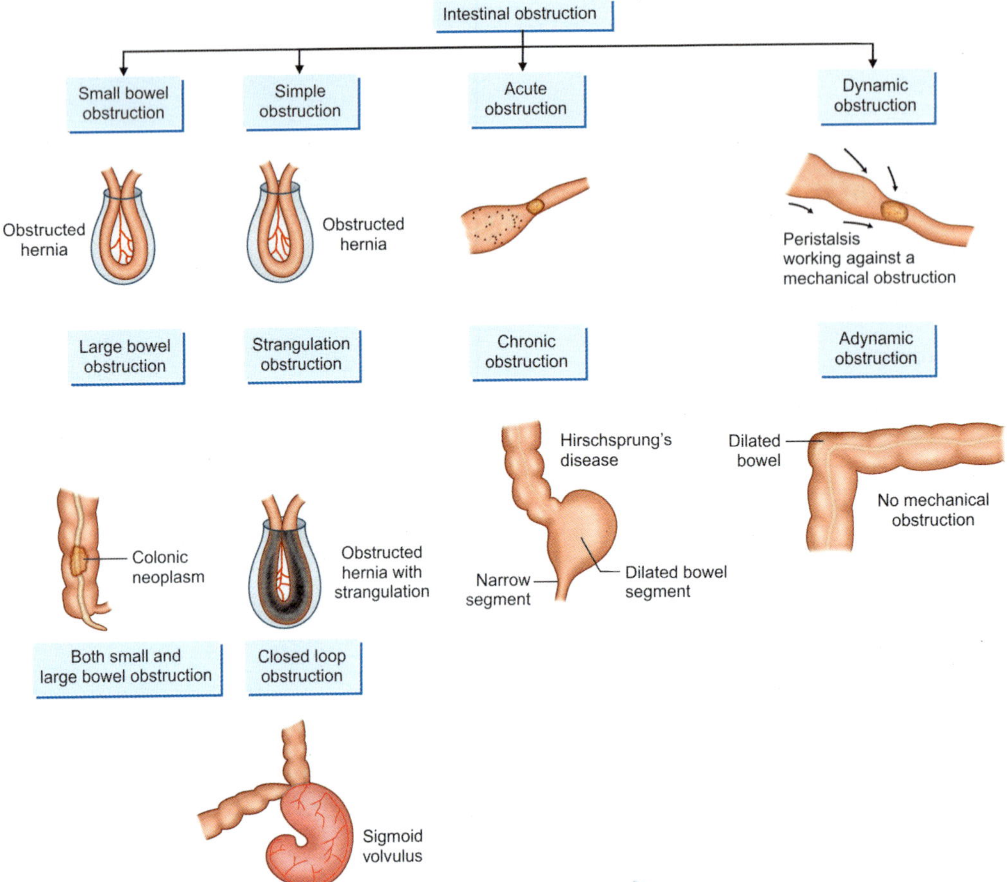

Small Intestinal Obstruction

- **Adhesions** secondary to surgery are the most common cause of small bowel obstruction.
- **Nonadhesive causes** of small bowel obstruction are obstructed hernias (inguinal, incisional, femoral hernias), congenital band, intussesception, worms, tuberculous stricture, Crohn's disease, etc.

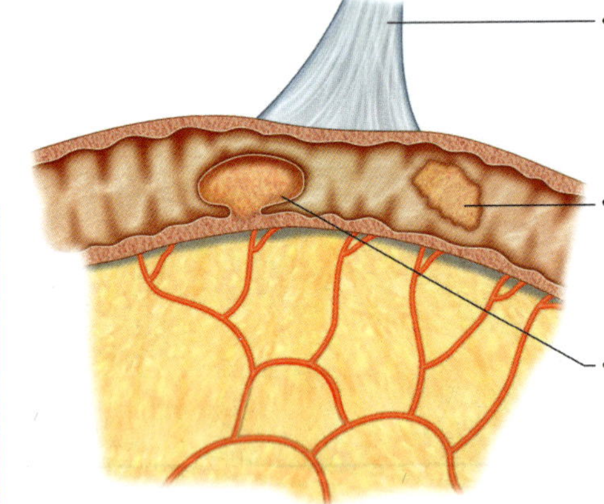

Causes of Small Intestinal Obstruction in Children

- Congenital atresia and stenosis (most common)
- Midgut volvulus
- Intussusception
- Meconium ileus
- Incarcerated inguinal hernia

'Adhesions' is defined as fibrous tissue that connects surfaces or organs within the peritoneal cavity that are normally separated. [Bologna guideline 2017 update]

Causes of peritoneal adhesion: (i) Abdominal surgery; (ii) Radiotherapy; (iii) Local response to neoplastic lesion; and (iv) Endometriosis.

Adhesions are most likely develop after gynecologic operations, appendectomy, colorectal operations.

Laparoscopic surgery reduces adhesion formation

- **Obstructed hernia** (inguinal, incisional, epigastric, femoral, internal hernia)
- **Neoplasm:** Peritoneal metastatic lesions secondary to ovarian, gastric, pancreatic, colonic carcinoma. Large intra-abdominal tumors may cause obstruction by extrinsic compression.
- **Intra-abdominal abscess:** Obstruction may develop due to local ileus adjacent to the abscess or intestine form a part of the wall of the abscess resulting in kinking of the intestine.

Pathophysiology of Obstruction

- Intestinal motility and contractile activity increases in an effort to propel the obstruction as well as luminal contents.
- Intestine becomes fatigued, contractions becoming less frequent and less intense. Intestine proximal to the obstruction gradually dilates.
- Fluid accumulates both intraluminally and in the bowel wall
- Mucosal absorption is decreased (absorptive flux) and intestinal secretion is increased (secretory flux).
- Microvascular perfusions of the intestine impaired resulting in ischemic changes in bowel followed by strangulation.

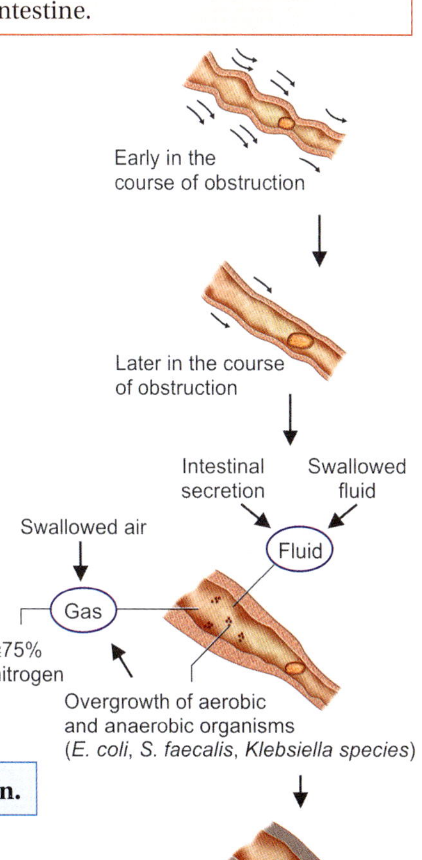

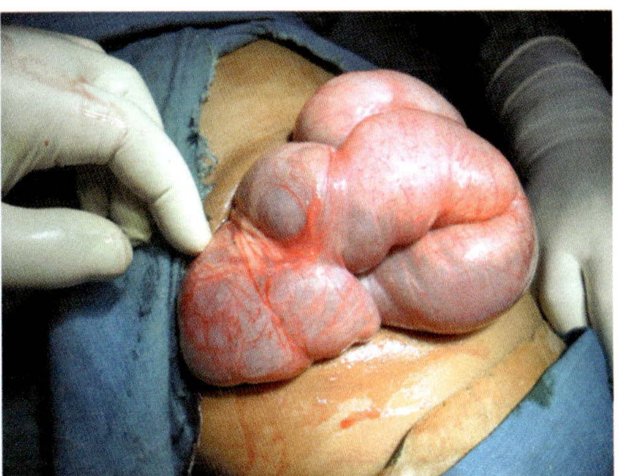

Adhesions causing obstruction.

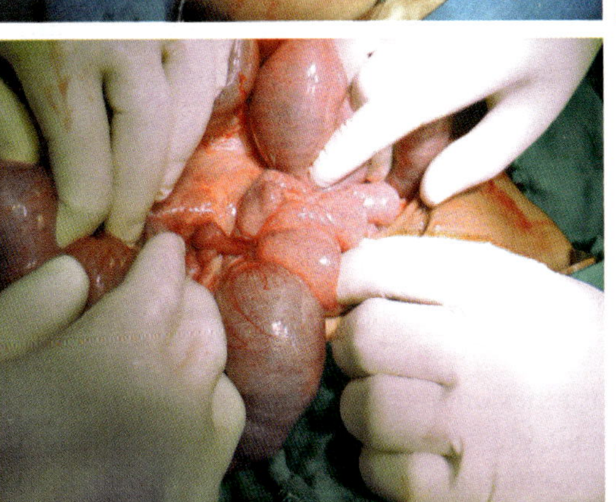

Bands causing obstruction.

Strangulation Obstruction

It is a consequence of obstruction where blood supply of the intestine is compromised resulting in ischemia and/or infarction of that obstructed bowel.

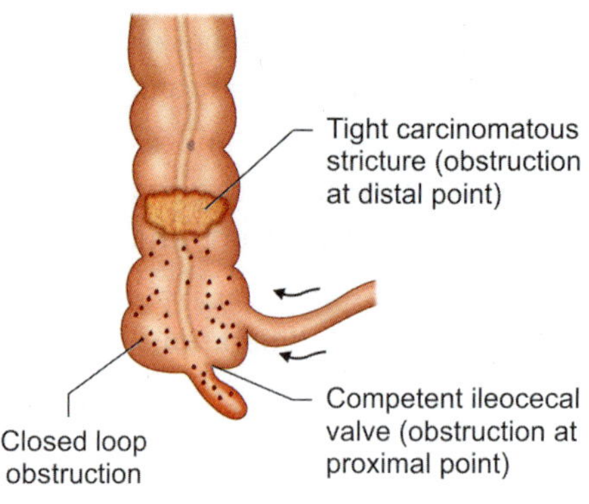

Closed Loop Obstruction

- A specific type of bowel obstruction where bowel is obstructed at both the proximal and distal point.
- Intestines are at higher risk of strangulation.
- This type of obstruction develops in sigmoid volvulus or a obstructing carcinomatous lesion in ascending colon with patent ileocecal valve.
- Urgent surgical intervention is indicated in closed loop obstruction.

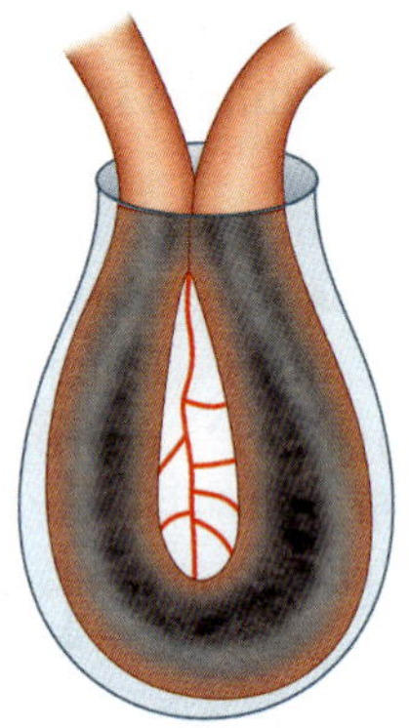

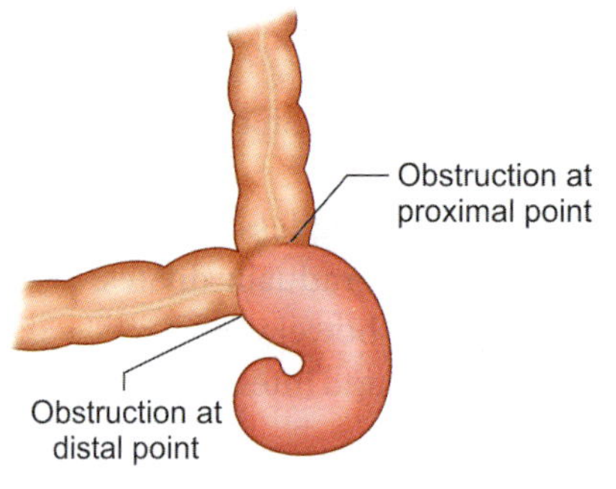

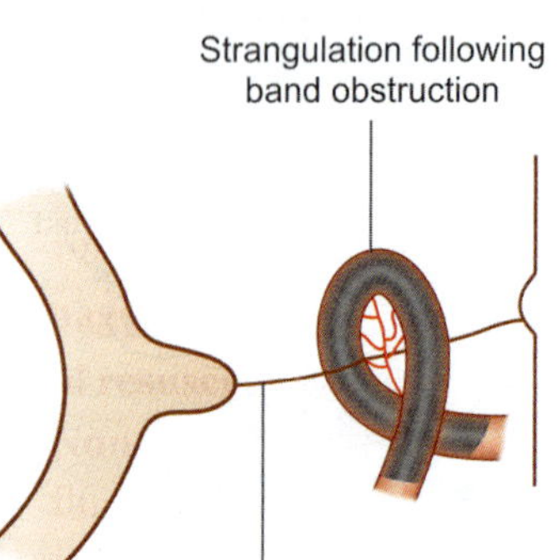

Pathophysiology of Strangulation Obstruction

Venous return is compromised before arterial supply
↓
↑↑ capillary pressure
↓
↑↑ capillary permeability leads to extravasation of fluid and RBC
↓
Then, arterial supply impaired
↓
Hemorrhagic infarction

Classification of Adhesion in General Surgery (Zuhlke et al.)

- **Grade 0:** No adhesions or insignificant adhesions
- **Grade 1:** Adhesions that are filmy and easy to separate by blunt dissection
- **Grade 2:** Adhesions where blunt dissection is possible but some sharp dissection necessary, beginning vascularization
- **Grade 3:** Lysis of adhesions possible by sharp dissection only, clear vascularization
- **Grade 4:** Lysis of adhesions possible by sharp dissection only, organs strongly attached with severe adhesions, damage of organs hardly preventable.

Clinical Presentation

Four Cardinal Features of Obstruction

1. Abdominal pain
2. Vomiting
3. Abdominal distension
4. Obstipation

Abdominal pain: Colicky pain due to hyperperistalsis against a fixed obstruction. Constant, severe pain is suggestive of strangulation/peritonitis.

Vomiting: The more distal the obstruction, the longer the interval between the onset of symptoms and the appearance of vomiting.

Abdominal distension: The more distal the obstruction, the more is the abdominal distension.

Obstipation: Cessation of flatus and bowel movement

History Taking

History of previous abdominal operations, radiation, malignancy, inflammatory bowel disease.

Physical Examination

- Any surgical scar over the abdomen (obstruction due to adhesion)
- Any palpable abdominal lump
- Signs of peritonitis
- Hernial orifices (to rule out obstructed hernia).

Digital Rectal Examination

- Any palpable rectal growth (responsible for large gut obstruction)
- Gross blood is suggestive of strangulation. Fecal impaction.

Features of hypovolemic shock: Oliguria, hypotension, tachycardia.

Features of strangulation: Fever, tachycardia, generalized tenderness, abdominal rigidity.

Clinical Presentations Depend on the Level of Obstruction

Proximal obstruction

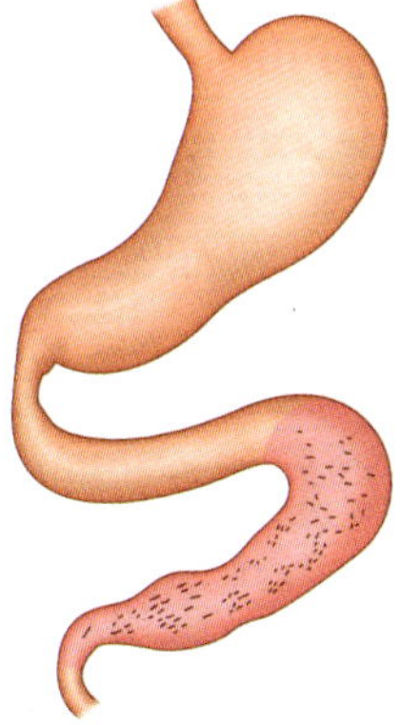

- Frequent vomiting
- Abdomen—not distended
- Intermittent pain—but not colicky

Mild intestinal obstruction

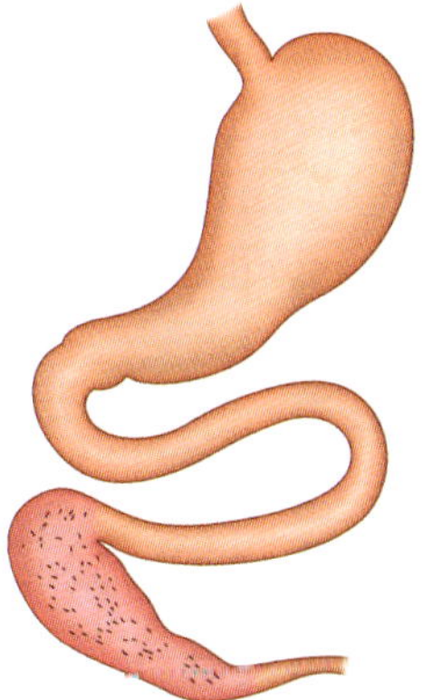

- Not so frequent vomiting
- Abdomen—moderately distended
- Intermittent colicky pain

Low intestinal obstruction

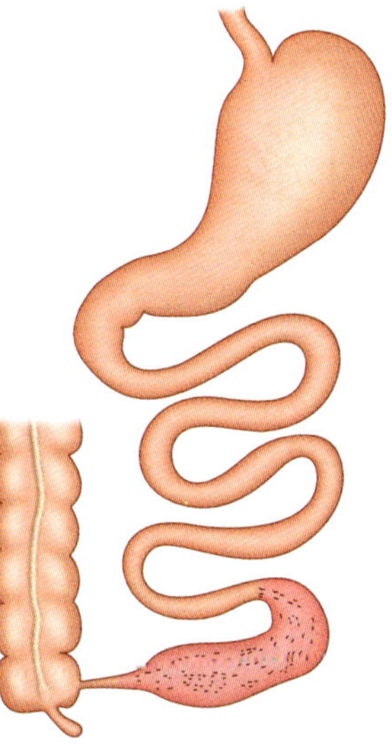

- Vomiting occurs late, if vomiting present, it will become feculent
- Marked abdominal distension
- Abdominal pain, not classic crescendo type

Diagnosis

Plain X-ray Abdomen

- Plain X-ray (in upright and supine position) should be the initial diagnostic modality. More the fluid levels, more severe and more distal the obstruction.
- X-rays do not detect early signs of strangulation or peritonitis. X-rays cannot provide anatomical details of obstruction.

CT Scan of Abdomen and Pelvis

- CT scan is superior to plain X-ray in diagnosis of small bowel obstruction. This imaging modality provides information about severity and etiology of obstruction. CT can be used for diagnosis of small bowel volvulus.
- **Multidetector CT and multiplanar reconstruction** helps to localize the level of obstruction.

Contrast Study

Contrast studies (water-soluble contrast agent) of the small bowel is particularly indicated for diagnosis of low-grade and partial small bowel obstruction. This imaging modality is more sensitive in the diagnosis of intraluminal and mural etiologies of obstruction.

USG Abdomen

USG abdomen has similar accuracy compared to plain X-ray. This imaging may be useful in pregnant patients with obstruction.

X-ray Findings Suggestive of Small Bowel Obstruction

Upright position

- Multiple air fluid levels
- Predominantly centrally located dilated bowel loops
- Air fluid levels in same loop of small bowel of unequal heights
- Valvulae conniventes are visible
- String of beads sign.

Supine position

- Dilated gas or fluid-filled small bowel (>3 cm)
- Small bowel dilated out of proportion to colon
- Stretch sign
- Absence of rectal gas

CT Findings Suggestive of Small Intestinal Obstruction

- A transition point with dilation of bowel proximally and distally.
- Decompressed colon
- Failure of contrast to pass beyond the transition point.
- Colon containing little gas or fluid.

CT Findings Suggestive of Bowel Ischemia

- Reduced bowel wall enhancement
- Thickening of bowel wall
- Mesenteric venous congestion
- Pneumatosis intestinalis
- Free fluid

CT Findings Suggestive of Small Bowel Volvulus

- Multiple transition points
- Posterior location of transition point
- Presence of 'Whirl sign'

Straight X-ray abdomen showing concertina appearance

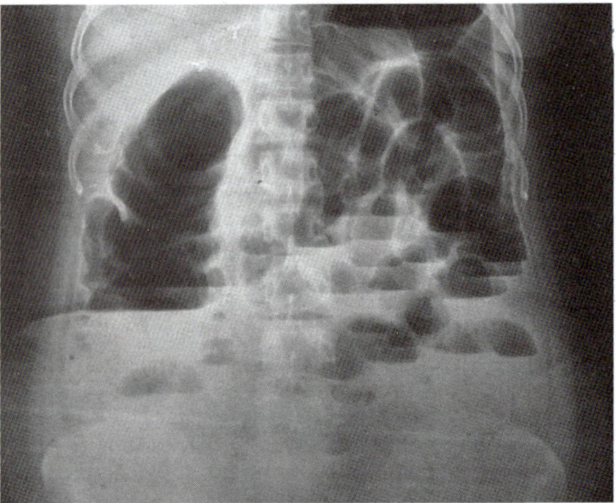

Straight X-ray abdomen showing multiple air-fluid level

Treatment

- **Fluid resuscitation:** Fluid resuscitation with isotonic fluid in IV route.
- **Decompression:** Decompression by nasogastric tube decreases abdominal distension, risk of aspiration.
- **Monitoring urine output:** Urine output should be monitored for assessing adequate fluid resuscitation.
- **Correction of electrolyte imbalance:** Hypokalemia must be corrected with IV supplement after satisfactory urine output is achieved.
- **Broad-spectrum antibiotics:** Antibiotics (coverage against gram-negative aerobes and anaerobes) are administered because of concerns that bacterial translocation may occur.
- **Operative or nonoperative management:** Patients with uncomplicated small bowel obstruction should ideally be considered for nonoperative management.

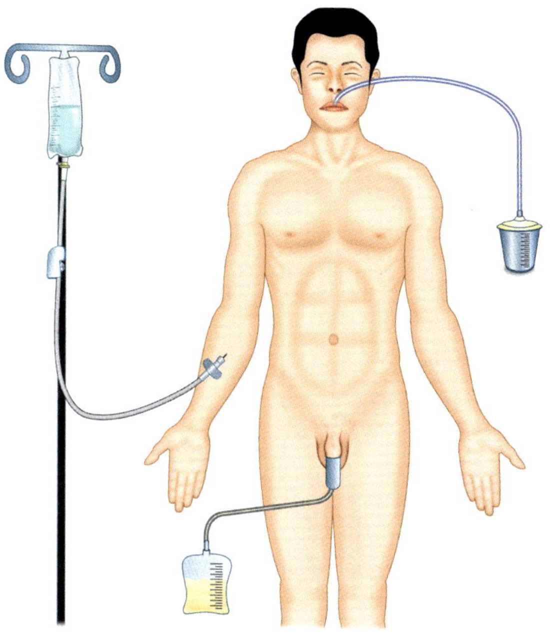

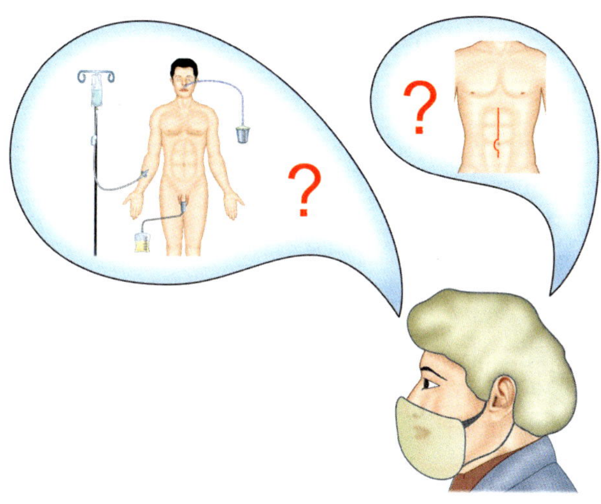

Early operative management is indicated if:

- Suspected bowel strangulation
- Signs of ischemia
- Closed loop obstruction
- Peritonitis

Nonoperative trial may be indicated in:

- Partial small bowel obstruction
- Adhesive small bowel obstruction without complications
- Obstruction in early postoperative period

Nonoperative to operative management if:

- Increasing or persistent symptoms after 72 hours trial of nonoperative management.
- Patient developing symptoms and signs of complications (continuous abdominal pain, localized tenderness, rebound tenderness, fever, tachycardia, leukocytosis).

Principles of Operative Management

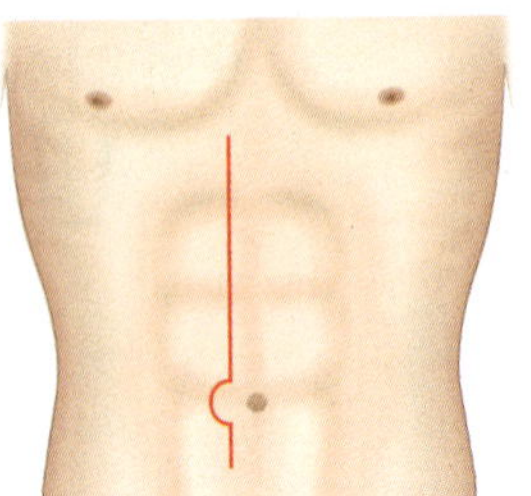

- If the site of obstruction is not known, **midline incision is the incision of choice.**
- If cecum is collapsed, obstruction is in the small intestine. If cecum is dilated, obstruction is in the large intestine.
- Regardless of etiology, affected intestine should be checked for viability. Viability is checked by **color of the intestine, peristalsis, marginal arterial pulsations.**

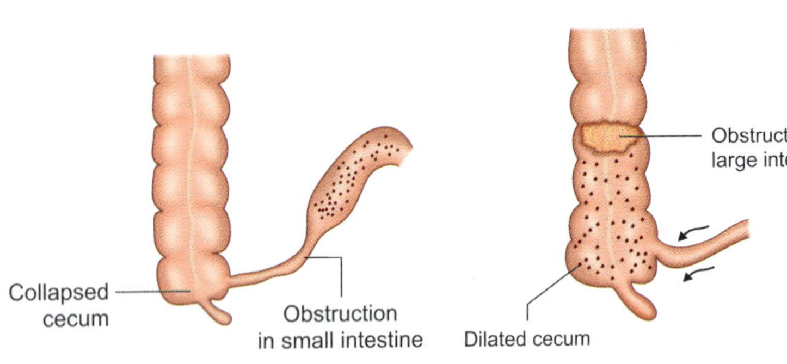

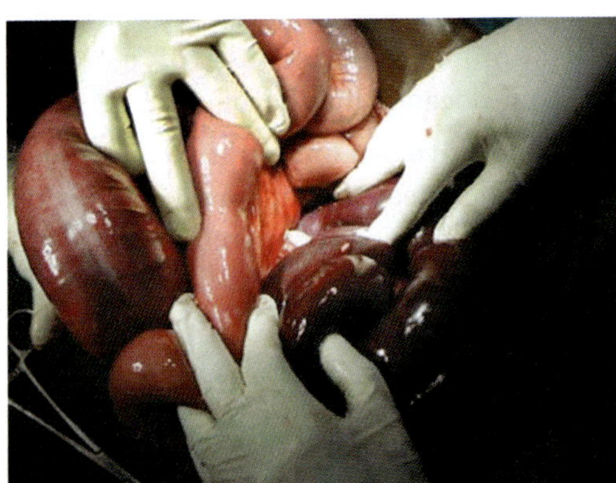

If a segment of intestine with questionable viability, then

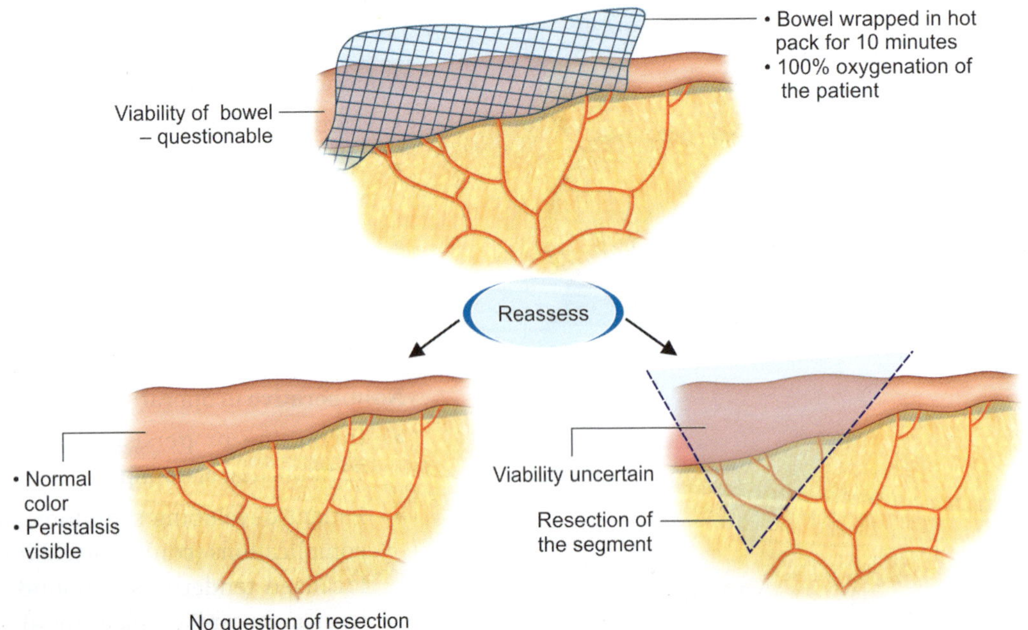

Types of Operative Procedures Depend on the Cause of Obstruction

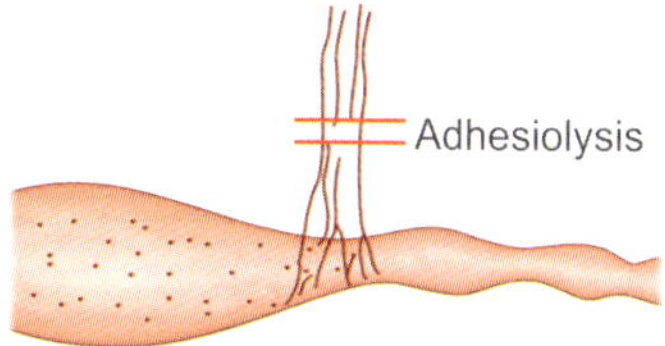

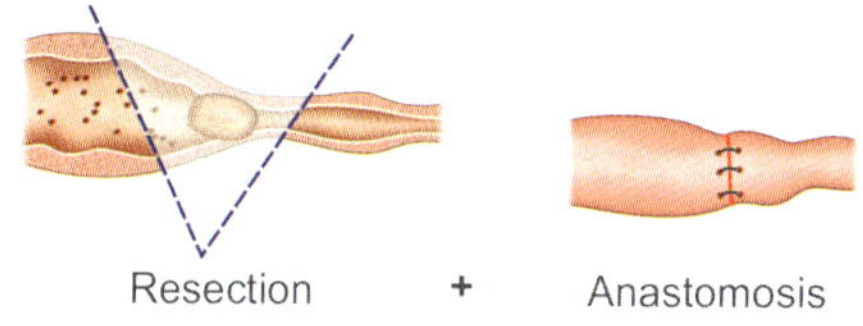

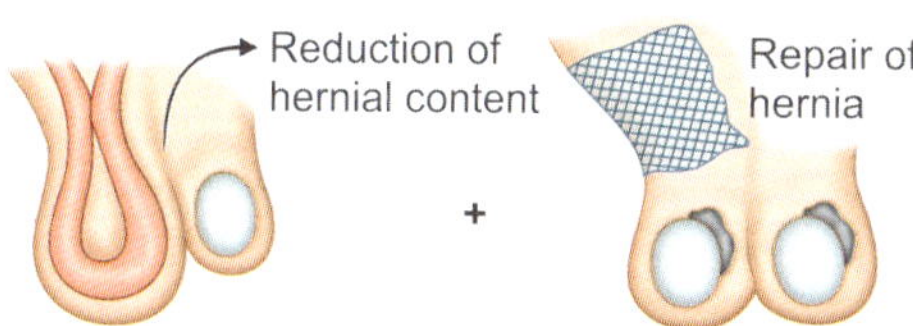

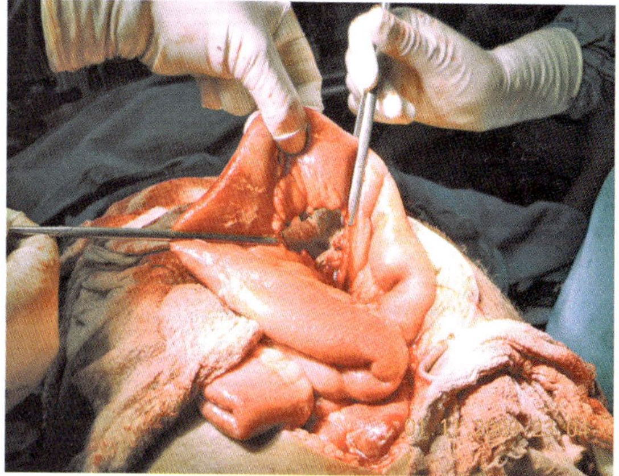

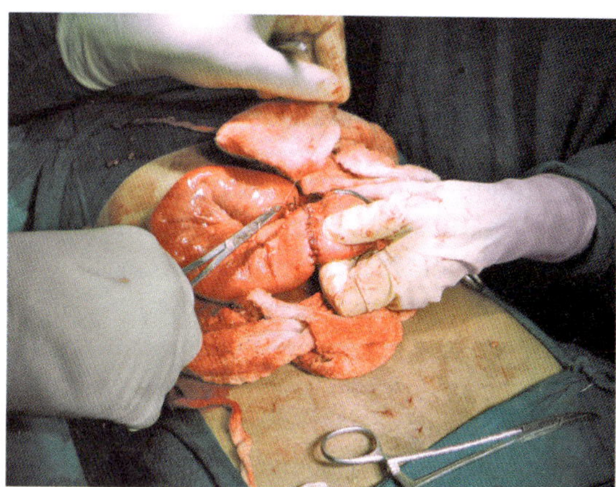

Different Types of Mechanical Small Bowel Obstruction

Operative picture of resection anastomosis.

Adhesive Small Bowel Obstruction

- Adhesions are the most common cause of small bowel obstruction.
- Risk of adhesive bowel obstruction is more after colorectal, oncologic gynecological and pediatric surgery. Laparoscopic surgery reduces adhesion formation.
- Patients with uncomplicated adhesive small bowel obstruction should be considered for nonoperative management.
- Operative management includes laparoscopic adhesiolysis and open adhesiolysis. Laparoscopic adhesiolysis is associated with more risk of bowel injuries.

Adhesiolysis invites further adhesions, so aggressive adhesiolysis should be avoided.

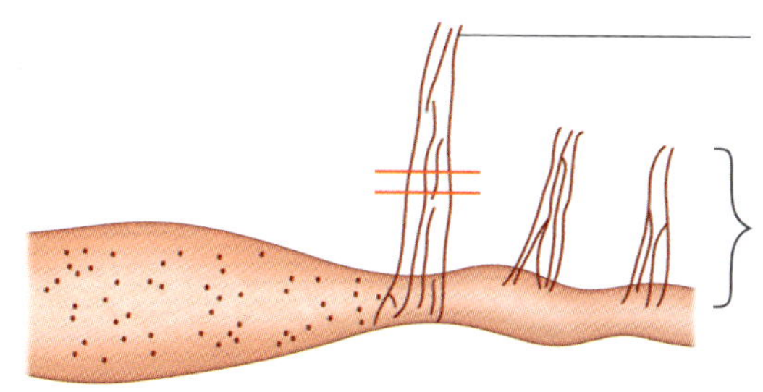

Obstruction from Enteric Strictures

- Small intestinal strictures are usually due to tuberculosis or Crohn's disease.
- Strictures due to lymphoma is more common than carcinomatous stricture.
- Surgical management is resection-anastomosis. Management of stricture due to Crohn's disease is somehow different.

Obstruction due to Worm Bolus

- A mass of roundworms *(Ascaris lumbricoides)* may obstruct the intestinal lumen, resulting in acute intestinal obstruction. Sometimes, the worm bolus act as lead point in intussusception or a pivot in small bowel volvulus.
- This condition commonly develops in children, usually following after antihelminthic therapy (antihelminthic drugs paralyze the worms and make them more likely to form a bolus).
- Patients with acute obstruction present with vomiting, severe colicky abdominal pain, constipation, abdominal distension. Vomitus may contain worms.
- Straight X-ray reveals multiple air-fluid levels with curvilinear soft-tissue-density cords. USG findings suggestive of roundworm obstruction are multiple pairs of curvilinear echogenic lines within an adynamic, fluid-filled small bowel.
- Most of the patients respond to conservative management. The aim of conservative management is "to starve the worms and hydrate the patient". Surgical intervention is indicated if patient is not responding to conservative management or in presence of complications (e.g., gangrene, perforation).

Obstruction due to Food Bolus

Patients at risk of food bolus obstruction are: (i) Elderly patient with no teeth or ill-fitting dentures and (ii) pt undergone partial gastrectomy. Food commonly responsible for bolus obstruction are—unchewed apple, coconut, brussel sprouts, dried fruits, orange pips. Intraluminal crushing of the bolus followed by milking through the ileocecal valve is effective in most of the patients. If this method is not successful, removal of bolus through enterotomy is indicated.

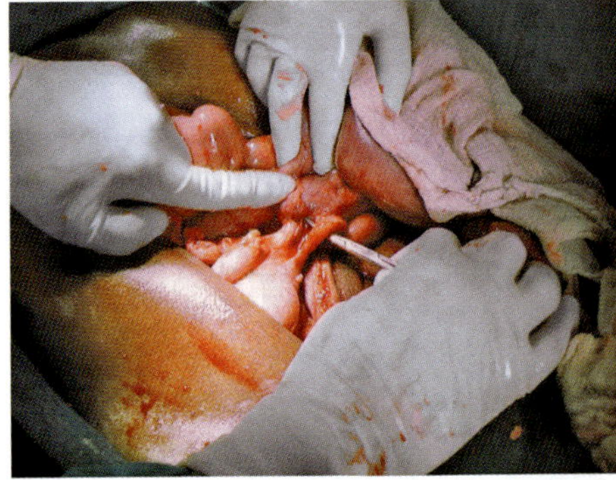

Stricture in the terminal ileum.

Other Causes of Bolus Obstruction

- Trichobezoars
- Gallstone
- Phytobezoars

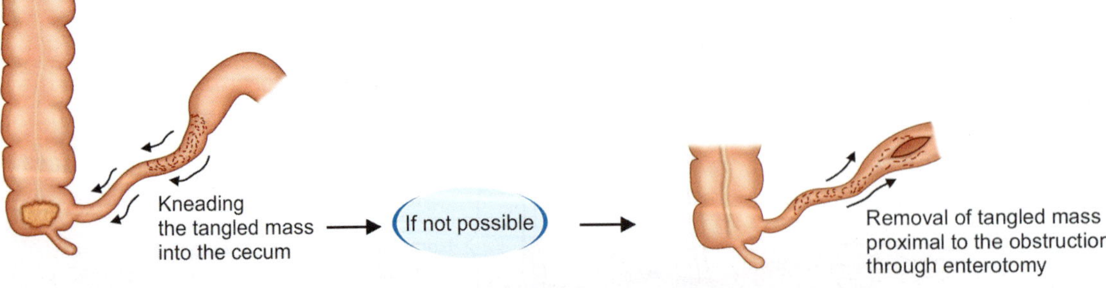

Operative technique of relieving worm bolus obstruction.

Intussusception

- **Intussusception** is defined as invagination of one segment of intestine into an immediately adjacent segment of the intestine.
- Intussusception is one of the most common causes of surgical emergencies in pediatric population.
- The **intussusceptum** is the proximal segment of intestine that invaginates into the distal segment **(intussuscipiens)**.

Pathophysiology

- The intussusception starts with a lead point. **In infants**, intussusception most commonly develops after weaning (due to hypertrophy of the Peyer's patches in lymphoid-rich terminal ileum following gastrointestinal infection or reaction to new food proteins)
- **In pediatric patients**, the lead point is usually hypertrophied Peyer's patch (secondary to adenovirus or rotavirus infection) or mesenteric lymphadenopathy. Pathological lead point is not so common.
- **In adult patients**, there is always a pathological lead point (polyp, submucosal lipoma, Meckel diverticulum, lymphoma).
- The lead point acts a focal area of traction that is responsible for telescoping of the proximal bowel segment into the distal segment.

Types of Intussusception

The Ileocolic type is the most common. Other types are-ileoileocolic, ileoileal, jejunojejunal and colocolic.

Retrograde intussusception (antiperistaltic or reverse intussusception) is defined as invagination of distal segment into proximal segment. Most common type of retrograde intussusception is jejuno-jejunal following Roux-en-Y gastrojejunostomy.

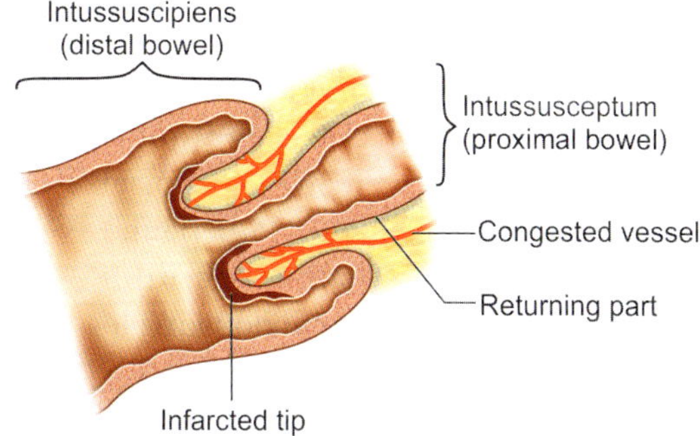

Pathological Lead Points in Pediatric Intussusception

- Meckel diverticulum
- Duplication cyst
- Aberrant tissue
- Intestinal polyp
- Lymphoma
- Henoch-Schönlein purpura.

Ileocolic type

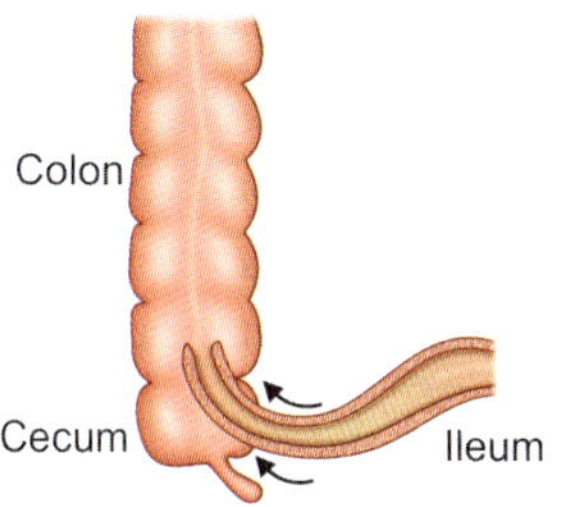

Ileoileocolic type

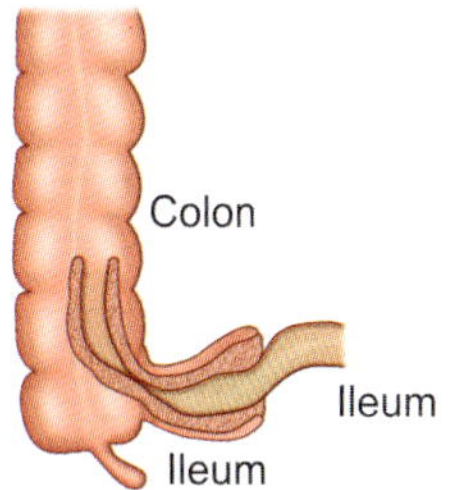

Ileoileal type

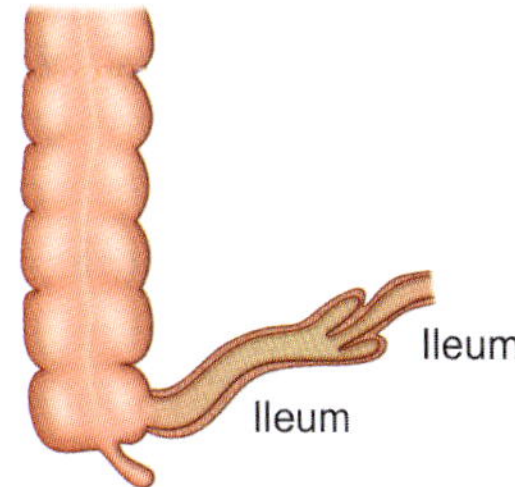

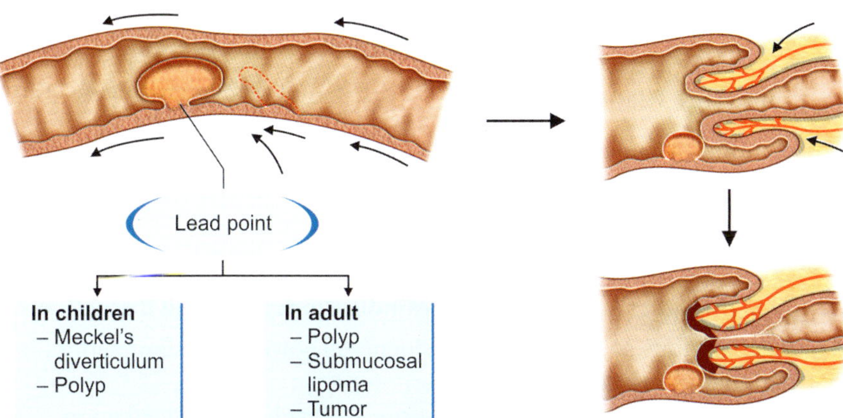

Clinical Presentation

- **Pediatric patients** present with intermittent and crampy abdominal pain, vomiting and bloody stool mixed with mucus ("red currant jelly" stool). This classic triad is present in only a few percentage of patients. Excessive irritability and crying are also common. On physical examination, a sausage-shaped mass is palpable in the right upper quadrant. "Dance sign" (emptiness of the ileocecal region) is rare and is not diagnostic.
- **Adult patients** commonly present with features of partial bowel obstruction—nausea, vomiting, constipation, change in bowel habits, lower GI bleeding.

Diagnosis

- **Plain X-ray of abdomen** may reveal features of intestinal obstruction or perforation but not a useful imaging modality for diagnosis of intussusception.
- **Ultrasonography** is the imaging modality of choice for screening intussusception in children. USG has nearly 100% sensitivity and specificity in diagnosing intussusceptions. This modality is also useful to detect pathological lead point. Color Doppler sonography is useful to detect degree of bowel ischemia.
- **CT abdomen** is not the first choice for diagnosis, but indicated if intussusception cannot be ruled out by other investigations (e.g., USG or contrast enema).
- **Contrast enema** is indicated if emergency USG facility is not available. Advantage of this modality is that it has a therapeutic role.

Management

Fluid resuscitation

- **Non-operative reduction:** Non-operative reduction by USG or fluoroscopy-guided pneumatic or hydrostatic enema is effective in most of the patients with acute idiopathic intussusception. Close observation after successful enema reduction is required because of increased chances of recurrence within the first 48 hours.
- **Surgical intervention:** Surgical intervention is indicated in following conditions: (i) Enema reduction is failed; (ii) Suspected or demonstrated pathological lead point; (iii) Features of peritonitis is present; (iv) Suspected bowel necrosis/perforation; and (v) Free air in abdominal X-ray.
- Bowel resection is indicated if—(i) Operatively irreducible intussusception; (ii) presence of pathological lead point; and (iii) perforation or necrosis of bowel.
- If preoperative imaging or peroperative findings strongly suggestive of malignancy or presence of gangrenous segment, operative reduction should be better avoided and resection of entire segment en bloc should be attempted.

Pathophysiology of Bloody Stool in Intussusception

Invagination of the intestine leads to dragging of the mesenteric vessels into the intussusceptum. These may lead to congestion and ischemia of that segment of intestine, resulting in mucosal edema and hemorrhage.

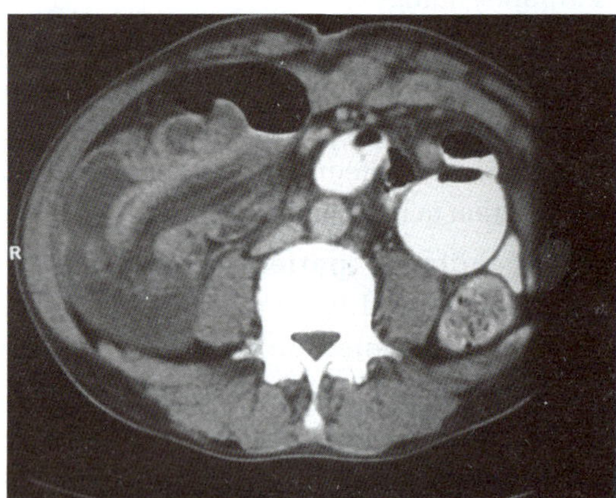

CT abdomen showing bowel-within-bowel configuration suggestive of intussusception.

Signs seen in USG

- "Target" or "doughnut" sign in transverse plane
- "Pseudokidney" sign in longitudinal plane

CT Findings Suggestive of Intussusception

- "Bulls-eye" appearance with concentric rings
- Gut-within-gut appearance

Contraindications of Enema Reduction

- Evidence of bowel necrosis or perforation
- Peritonitis
- Presence of pathological lead point

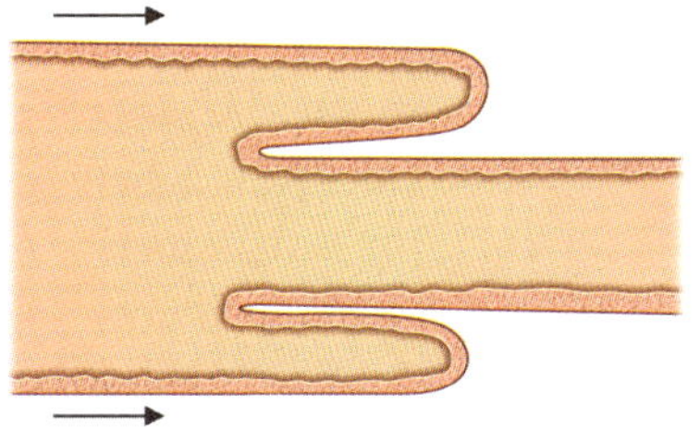

Squeezing the most distal part of the mass proximally—is the ideal technique.

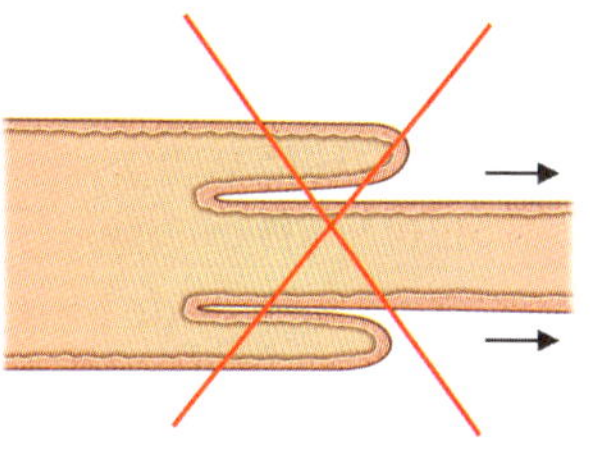

Do not pull.

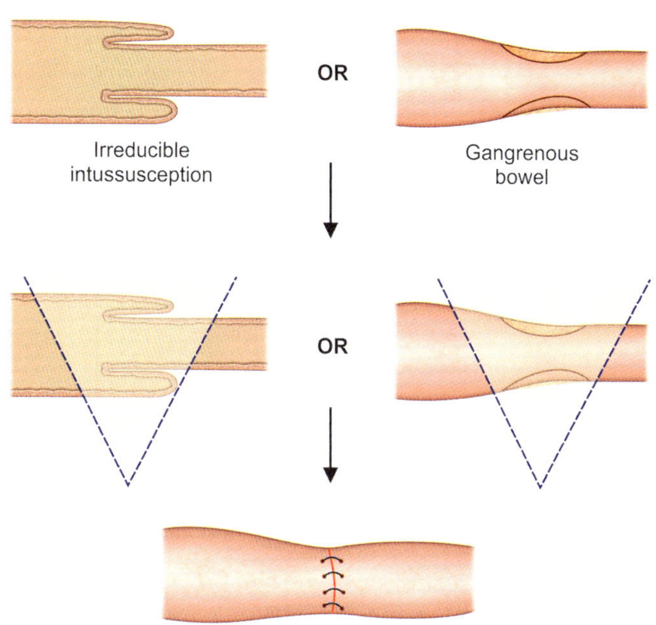

Crohn's Disease

A chronic idiopathic inflammatory disease of the alimentary tract characterized by **skip lesions** and **transmural inflammation.**

- **Bimodal age distribution:** First peak of incidence (15–30 years) and Second peak (55–60 years).
- **Genes associated with Crohn's disease:** *NOD2, IL23R, ATG16L1* genes.

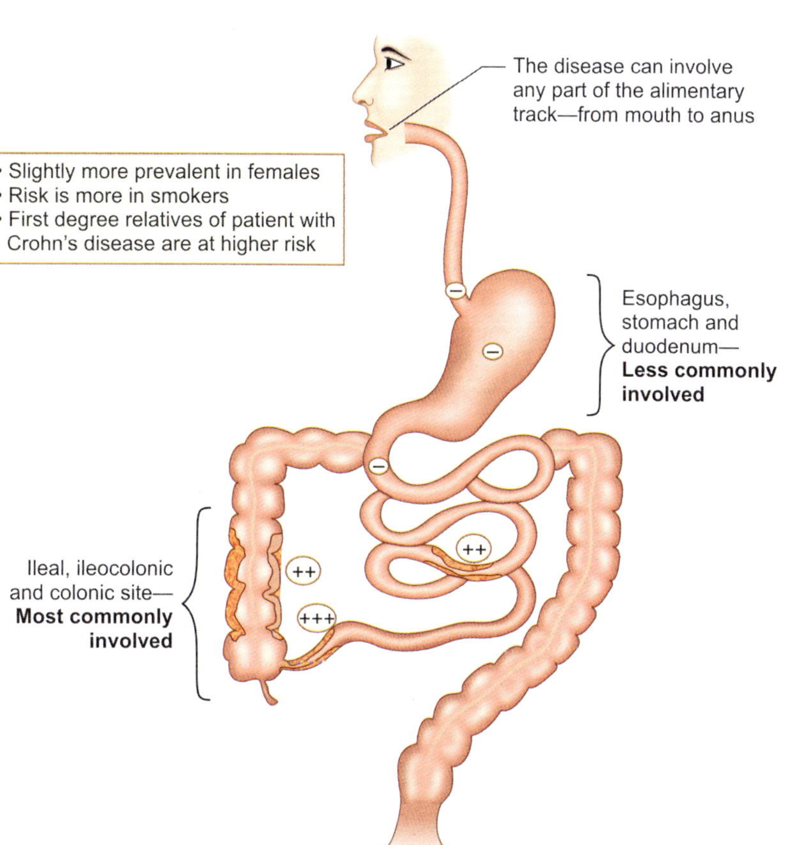

Pathophysiology

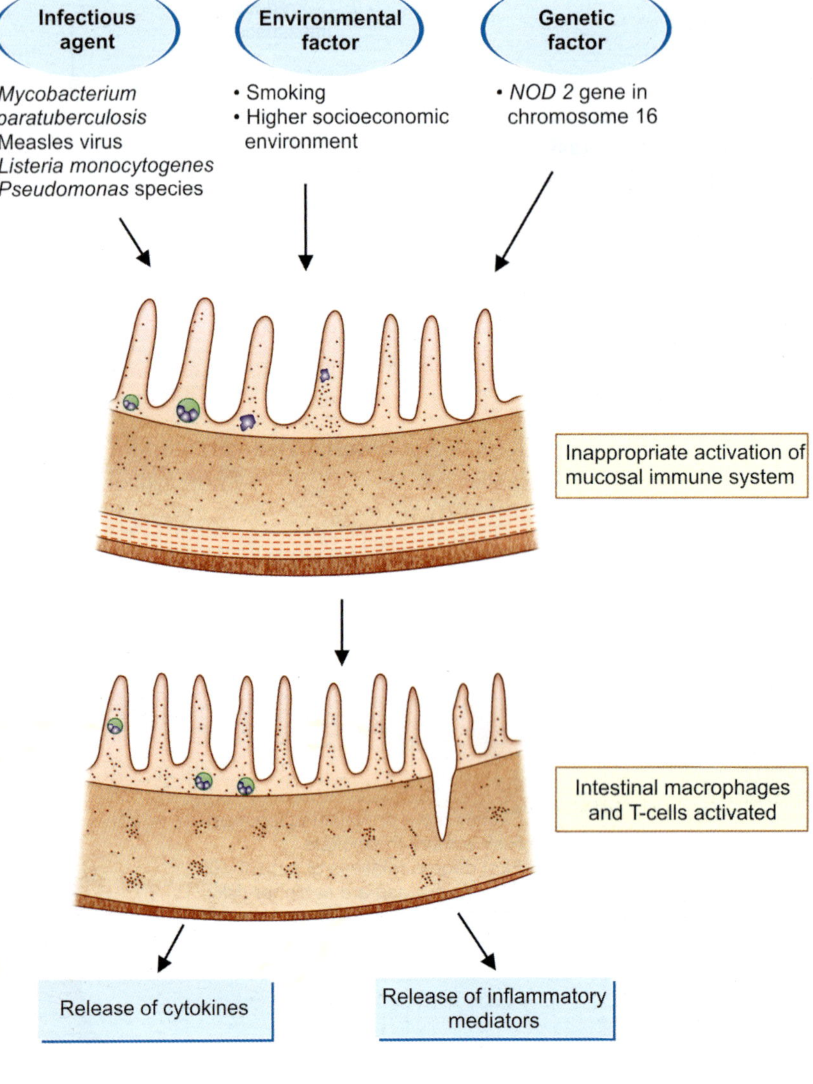

Macroscopic and Microscopic Features

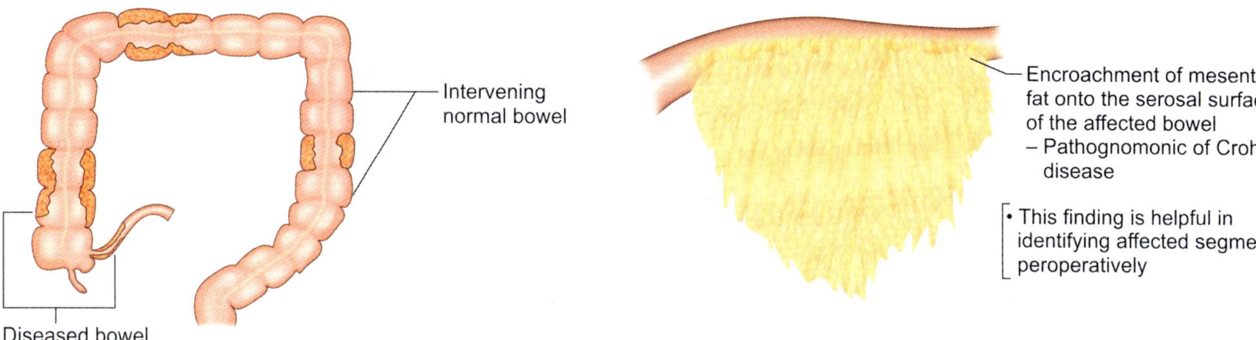

Characteristic Features of Crohn's Disease

- Skip lesions
- Creeping mesenteric fat
- Transmural involvement
- Sparing of the rectum
- Deep linear or serpiginous ulcers in the colon
- Presence of strictures and fistulas
- Presence of granuloma on biopsy.

Thickened mesentery
Enlarged lymph node
Thickened bowel with narrowed lumen
Characteristic findings in Crohn's disease

Aphthous ulcer (superficial ulcer with erythematous halo)

Linear or serpiginous ulcer (when multiple ulcers fuse in parallel to the long axis of the intestine)
Cobblestone appearance of mucosa
Ulcers coalescences transversely

Transmural involvement
Noncaseating granuloma with Langerhans giant cells
Deep fissuring ulcer

Distinguishing Features of Ulcerative Colitis

- In ulcerative colitis, the lesions are continuous.
- In ulcerative colitis, the inflammation is limited to the mucosa and submucosa.
- In ulcerative colitis, disease process is limited to the colon.

Clinical Presentation

Cardinal Symptoms of Crohn's Disease

- Abdominal pain (commonly at the right lower abdomen and increased after taking food)
- Chronic diarrhea (stool rarely contain mucus, pus or blood)
- Fatigue

Onset of symptoms is insidious. Severity of disease follows a waxing and waning course

Other Symptoms

- Weight loss
- Growth failure
- Anemia
- Recurrent fistulas
- Intestinal obstruction
- Extraintestinal manifestations

Classic Extraintestinal Manifestations

- Arthropathy (both axial and peripheral)
- Skin manifestations (e.g., erythema nodosum, pyoderma gangrenosum)
- Ocular manifestations (e.g., uveitis, scleritis, episcleritis)
- Hepatobiliary (e.g., primary sclerosing cholangitis)

Other Extraintestinal Manifestations

- Cholelithiasis
- Nephrolithiasis
- Osteonecrosis
- Thromboembolic (both venous and arterial)

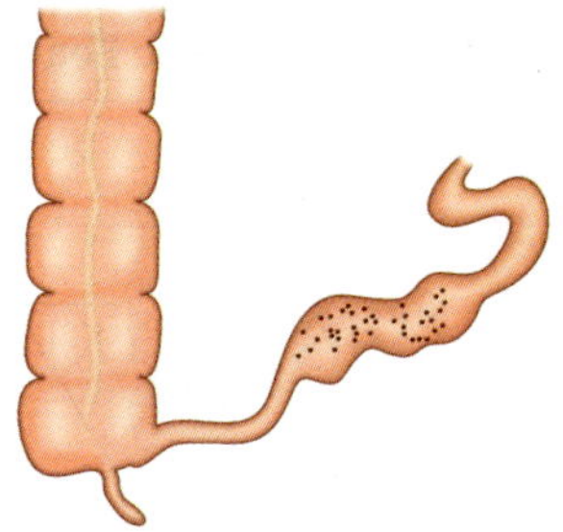

Intestinal obstruction due to stricture.

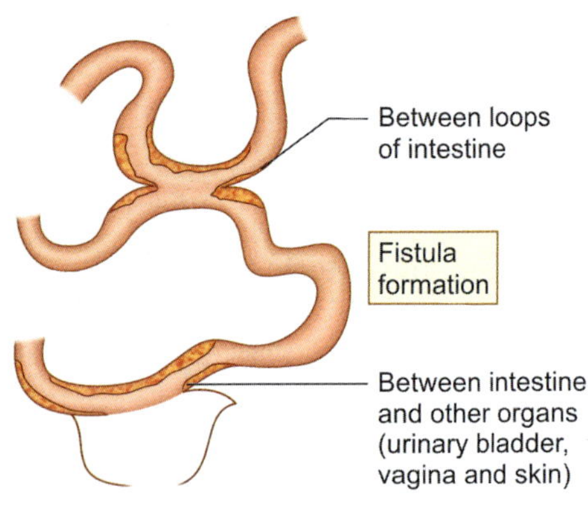

Fistulas in Crohn's Disease

- Enteroenteric
- Enterovesical
- Enterovaginal
- Enterocutaneous
- Perianal
- Perirectal

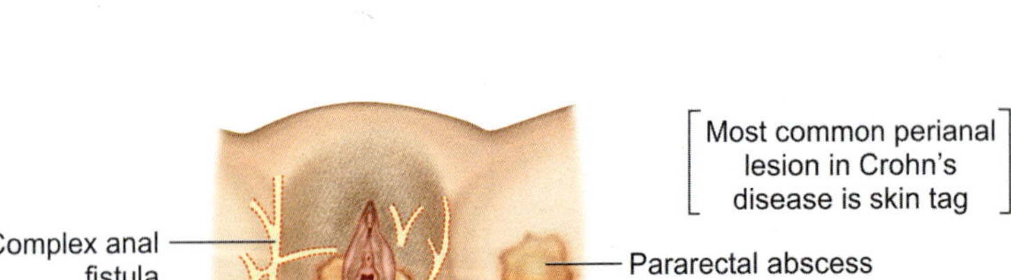

Anorectal Lesions in Crohn's Disease

Fistulizing lesions—abscess, perianal fistula, rectovaginal fistula.

Nonfistulizing lesions—fissures, deep ulcers, skin tags, anorectal strictures.

- Anorectal lesions may appear many years before the intestinal disease.
- Crohn's disease should be suspected in any patient with multiple, chronic perianal fistulas.

Oral Lesions in Crohn's Disease

- Lip swelling with or without fissures
- Oral mucosal swelling
- Deep linear ulceration
- Mucogingivitis
- Glossitis
- Palatal ulcerations.

- Crohn's disease affects the upper GI tract more commonly in children than adults.
- Esophageal involvement is rare in CD, but if occurs, always associated with extraintestinal manifestations.
- Patients with colonic involvement are at increased risk of colorectal cancer. **Risk factors are:** (i) Long duration of disease; (ii) Concomitant primary sclerosing cholangitis; and (iii) Family history of colorectal cancer.
- Patients with small bowel involvement are at increased risk of small bowel adenocarcinoma.

Immune-mediated Diseases Associated with Crohn's Disease

- Rheumatoid arthritis
- Multiple sclerosis
- Celiac disease
- Psoriasis
- Pericarditis
- Chronic bronchitis.

Investigations

- **Fecal calprotectin**—to differentiate the presence of inflammatory bowel disease from irritable bowel syndrome. Fecal calprotectin level <50 μg/g denotes that IBD is unlikely and level >200 μg/g denotes that the possible diagnosis is IBD. It is also used to evaluate response to therapy, and to predict relapse of the disease.
- **Anti-*Saccharomyces cerevisiae* antibodies (ASCAs)**—A serological marker with high specificity but considerably lower sensitivity.
- **Colonoscopy with intubation of the terminal ileum and biopsy**—is recommended as initial workup in patients with suspected IBD. Biopsies of uninvolved mucosa is recommended to assess the extent of histologic disease.
- **Small bowel imaging (Computed tomography enterography or Magnetic resonance enterography)**—as part of initial diagnostic workup. Due to absence of radiation exposure, MRE is preferred in young patients (<35 years) and in whom serial imaging may be required.
- **Endoscopic ultrasound or MRI of pelvis**—for characterization of perianal Crohn's disease, perirectal abscess.

Mucosal changes Suggestive of Crohn's Disease

- Mucosal nodularity
- Ulceration
- Mucosal edema
- Stenosis

Endoscopic Scoring Systems (To Quantify Distribution and Severity of Mucosal Involvement of Colon and Ileum)

- Simple Endoscopic Score for Crohn's disease (SES-CD)
- Crohn's Disease Endoscopic Index of Severity (CDEIS).

Disease Activity

- **Clinical disease activity is divided into:** (i) Remission; (ii) Mild; (iii) Moderate; and (iv) Severe.
- **Mild disease is characterized by**—(i) ambulatory patients, eating and drinking normally; (ii) <10% weight loss; and (iii) complications such as obstruction, abdominal mass, dehydration, fever are absent.
- **Severe disease is characterized by**—(i) significant weight loss; (ii) presence of complications such as obstruction, intra-abdominal abscess; and (iii) Persistence of symptoms despite aggressive therapy.

Risk Factors for Developing Intestinal Complications

- Ileal, ileocolonic and proximal GI tract involvement
- Extensive anatomic involvement
- Deep ulcerations

Phenotypic Classification (2005 Montreal Revision of the Vienna Classification)

Age at onset	A1	Disease onset at 16 years or younger
	A2	Disease onset 17–40 years age
	A3	Disease onset >40 years of age
Disease location	L1	Terminal ileum
	L2	Colon
	L3	Ileocolonic
	L4	Upper GI involvement
Disease behavior	B1	Nonstricturing, nonpenetrating
	B2	Stricturing
	B3	Penetrating

['p' is appended to the B subtype if presence of perianal fistulizing disease]

Management

Medical Therapy

Mild-to-moderately severe disease

- Sulfasalazine is effective for treating symptoms of colonic Crohn's disease.
- Controlled Ileal release budesonide is used for induction of symptomatic remission of ileocecal Crohn's disease.

Moderate-to-severe disease

- Oral corticosteroids are effective for relieving symptoms and signs of disease.
- Thiopurines (azathioprine, 6-mercaptopurine) are effective for steroid sparing in Crohn's disease.
- Methotrexate (up to 25 mg once weekly IM or SC) should be considered for alleviating signs and symptoms in steroid-dependent Crohn's disease and for maintaining remission.
- Anti-TNF agents (infliximab, adalimumab, certolizumab pegol) should be considered for Crohn's disease refractory to thiopurines or methotrexate or steroid-resistant Crohn's disease.
- Ustekinumab (anti-p40 antibody) should be considered for moderate-to-severe Crohn's disease who have failed previous treatment with corticosteroids, thiopurines, methotrexate, or anti-TNF inhibitors.
- Anti-integrin therapy (with Vedolizumab) or Natalizumab (anti-α4 integrin antibody) should be considered for induction of symptomatic remission in active Crohn's disease.

Severe disease

- IV corticosteroids and anti-TNF agents are considered for severely active Crohn's disease.

Disease Modifiers

- NSAIDs exacerbate disease activity.
- Cigarette smoking exacerbates disease activity and accelerates disease recurrence.
- Stress, depression, anxiety.

Surgical Management

Indications of surgery

Elective:

- Patient is unable to tolerate medical therapy due to side effects
- Disease activity not controlled with medical therapy
- Symptomatic small bowel strictures not amenable to medical therapy and/or dilation
- Enteric fistula with sepsis that persisting despite of medical therapy
- Patient with multifocal low-grade dysplasia, high-grade dysplasia, carcinoma of colon or rectum
- Colonic strictures that cannot be adequately surveyed endoscopically.

Emergency:

- Acute colitis with symptoms and signs of impending perforation
- Perforation of small or large intestine
- Fulminant colitis and toxic megacolon.
- Life-threatening lower GI bleeding or recurrent significant GI bleeding

Principles of surgery

- Surgery should be directed to the complications.
- Only the segment of bowel with complications should be managed ignoring other segments of diseased bowel.
- Stoma is preferred over primary anastomosis after resection in patients with sepsis, peritonitis or patient taking immunosuppressive therapy.

- **Surgical options for Crohn colitis:** (i) Total abdominal colectomy with ileo-rectal anastomosis (if disease is multifocal but rectum is disease-free); and (ii) Total proctocolectomy with permanent ileostomy.
- **The surgery of choice for emergency surgery in severe or fulminant colitis:** Subtotal or total colectomy with formation of end ileostomy and Hartmann closure of the distal bowel or creation of a mucous fistula.
- **The surgery of choice for multifocal low-grade dysplasia, high-grade dysplasia, nonadenoma-like DALM (Dysplasia-associated lesion or mass), carcinoma of colon or rectum:** Total proctocolectomy.

Management of Perianal Fistulizing Disease

- Infliximab is effective in treating perianal fistula, enterocutaneous fistula, and rectovaginal fistula.
- Adalimumab and certolizumab pegol are effective in treating perianal fistula in Crohn's disease.
- The combination of seton with infliximab has better overall fistula healing rate, longer duration of fistula closure, lower overall fistula recurrence rate.

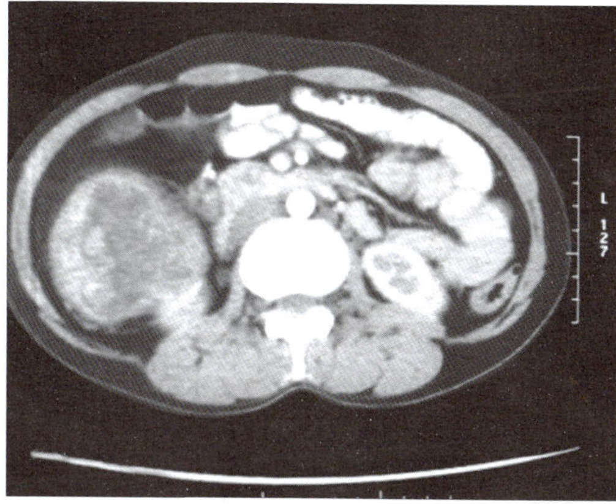

CT abdomen showing right colonic mass.

Management of Intestinal Obstruction

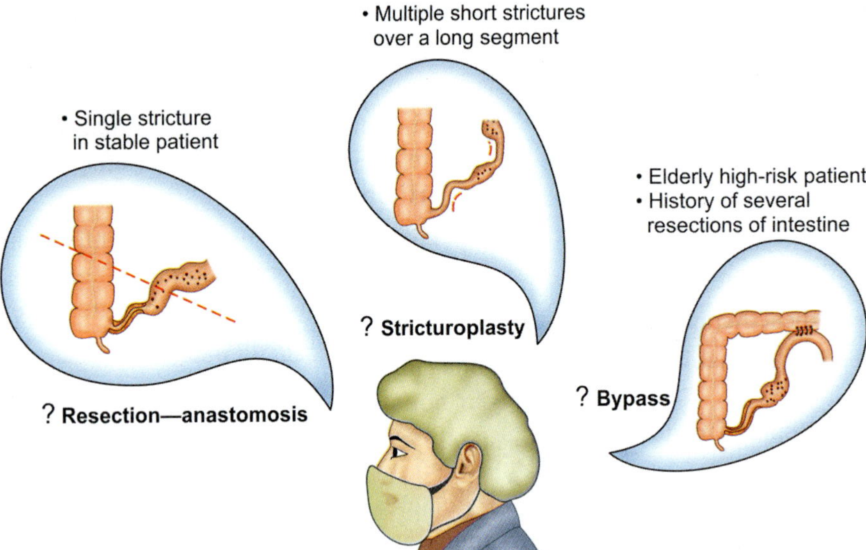

Indications of Stricturoplasty

- Multiple short strictures over a long segment.
- Previous extensive resections (>100 cm) of small bowel.
- Short bowel syndrome.
- Stricture at previous anastomotic site.

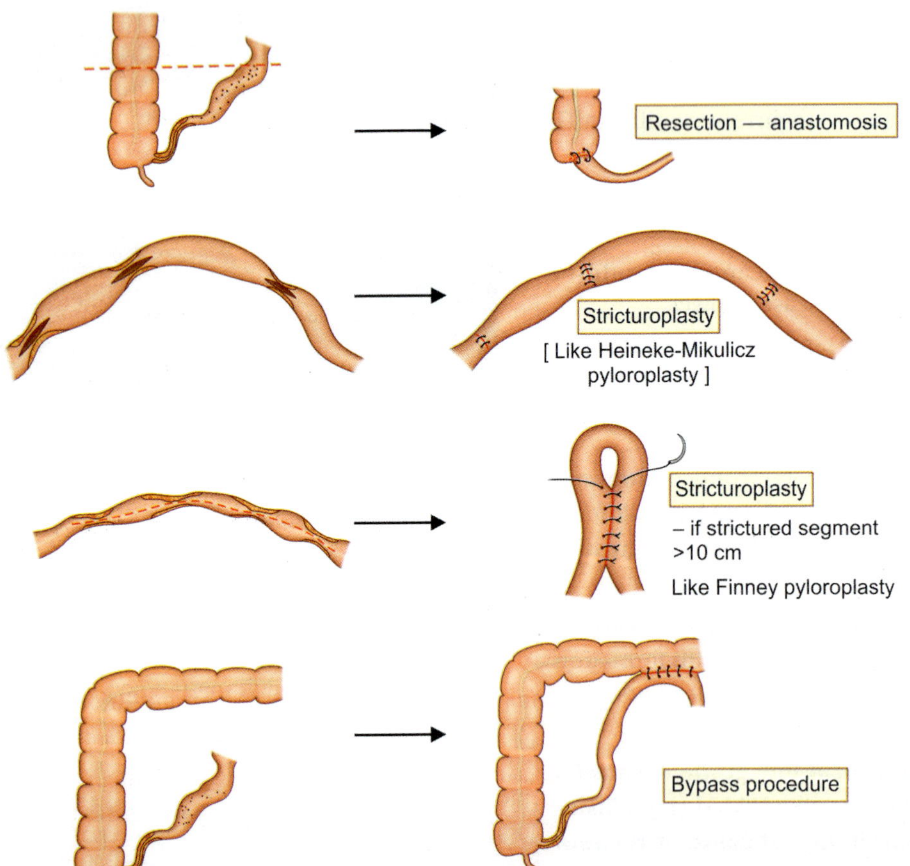

Contraindications to Stricturoplasty

- Fistula or abscess at the intended stricturoplasty site.
- Perforation of the small bowel.
- Intended stricturoplasty site close to bowel segment requiring resection.

Types of Stricturoplasty for Crohn's Disease

- Heineke-Mikulicz technique
- Finney technique
- Side-to-side isoperistaltic stricturoplasty (Michelassi stricturoplasty).
- Michelassi stricturoplasty is the preferred technique for long stenotic segments or multiple and close strictures.

Management of Fistula	Infliximab, thiopurines, tacrolimus are effective for treatment of fistulizing Crohn's disease.

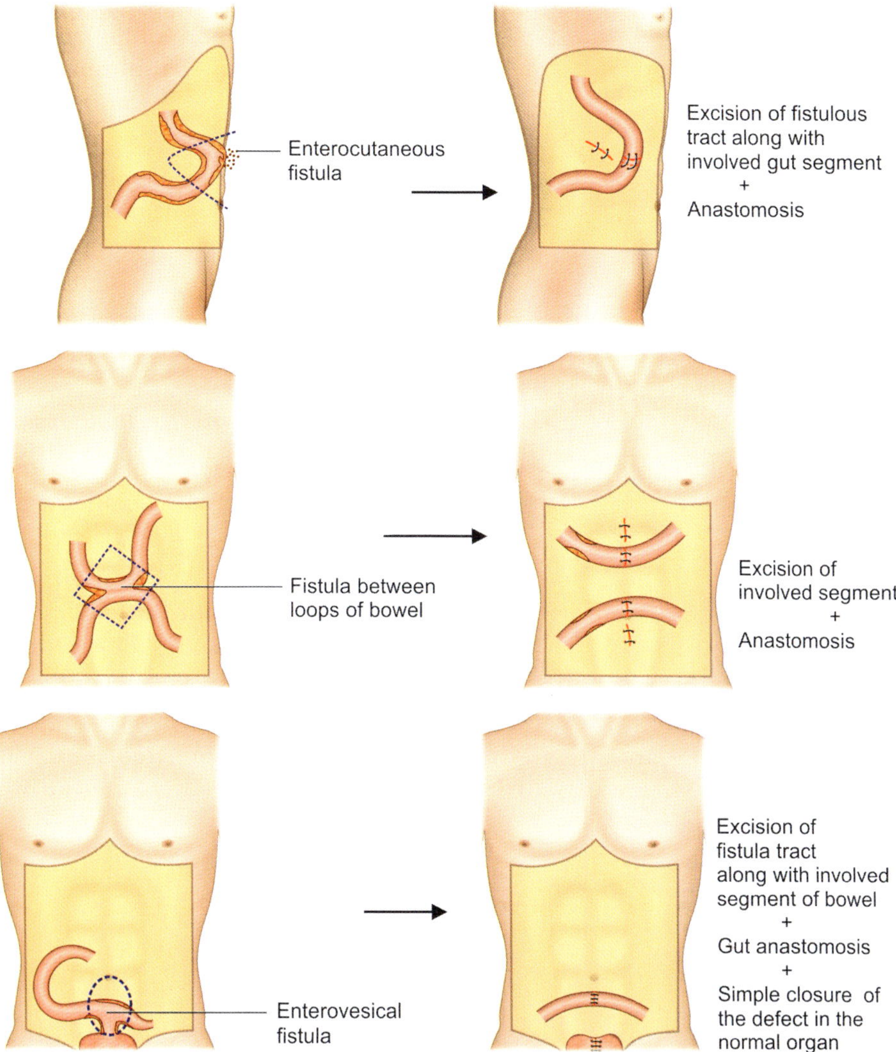

Management of Anorectal Lesions in Crohn's Disease

- Fistulotomy is indicated in superficial, low trans-sphincteric and low intersphincteric fistulas.
- High trans-sphincteric, suprasphincteric fistulas are treated with seton. The combination of seton with infliximab has better overall fistula healing rate, longer duration of fistula closure, lower overall fistula recurrence rate.
- Conservative management is sufficient for anal fissure. Perianal abscess should be drained but liberal excision of tissues should be avoided.
- Skin tags and hemorrhoids should not be excised unless they cause symptoms.

Risk Factors for Postoperative Recurrence

- Patients with penetrating disease (i.e., fistula, abscess, perforation)
- Two or more prior surgeries
- Disease in the ileum and colon (rather than ileum alone)
- Shorter time interval between time of diagnosis and surgery (<10 years)
- Perianal fistula
- Longer segment of bowel requiring resection
- Active tobacco smoking after surgery

Typhoid Enteritis

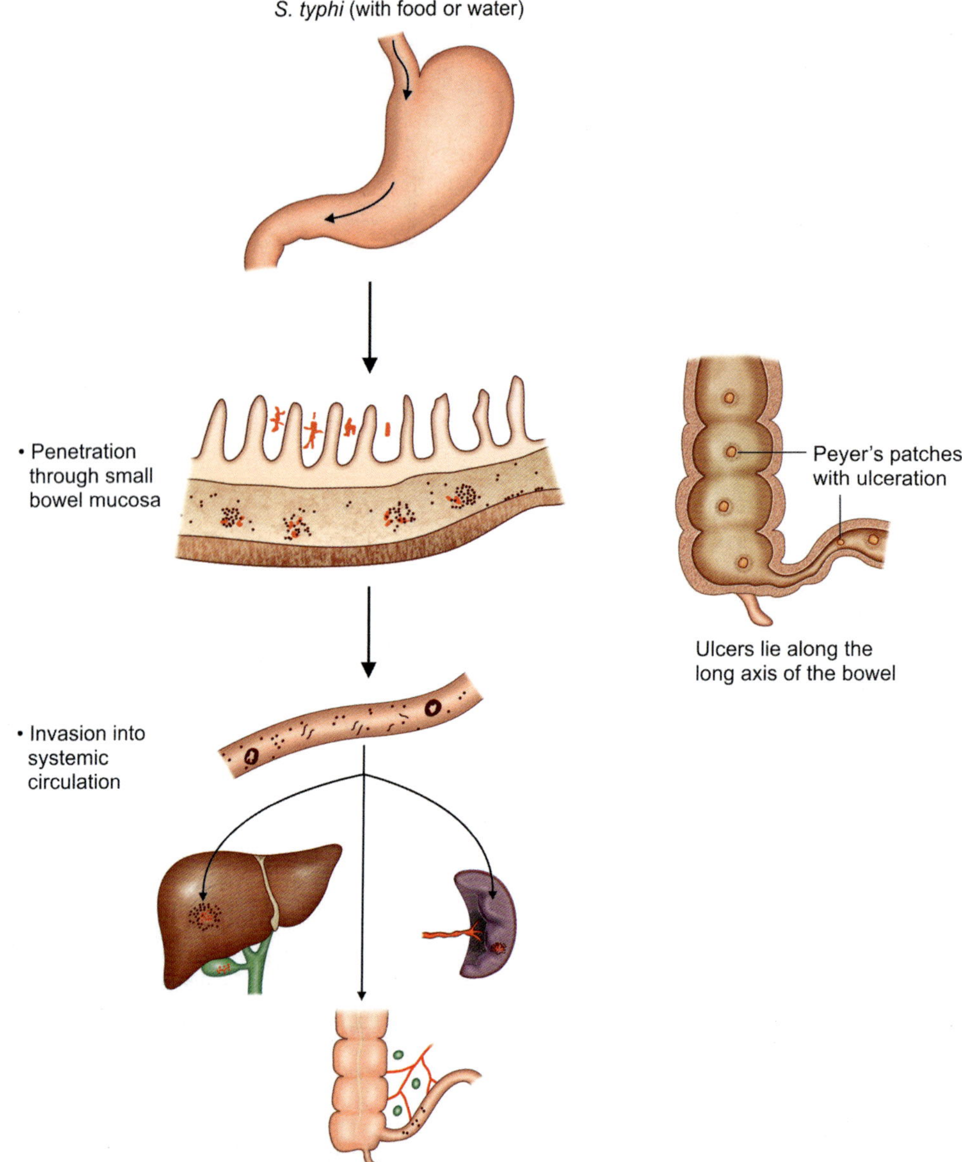

- A systemic illness caused by ***Salmonella typhi***. The organisms enter through Peyer's patches and then proliferate in the mucosal macrophages. **Typhoid ulcers lie along the longitudinal axis of the intestine (mostly ileum) on the antimesenteric border**.
- Typhoid intestinal perforation is the most serious complication of typhoid fever. **Classically a single perforation occurs through the Peyer's patch**. Multiple perforations are not common. Mostly perforation develops at the **3rd week of typhoid fever**.
- Surgery is indicated for perforation. **Primary repair** is sufficient for single perforation. **Segmental resection and anastomosis** is indicated for large solitary perforation and for adjacent multiple perforations. **Ileostomy** may be considered if patient's condition is unstable, delayed presentation or heavily contaminated abdomen.

Intestinal Tuberculosis

Intestinal tuberculosis is one of the forms of **abdominal tuberculosis.**

Other Forms of Abdominal Tuberculosis

- Tuberculous lymphadenopathy
- Peritoneal tuberculosis (wet—ascitic, fixed—fibrotic and dry—plastic type)
- Visceral tuberculosis

Pathophysiology

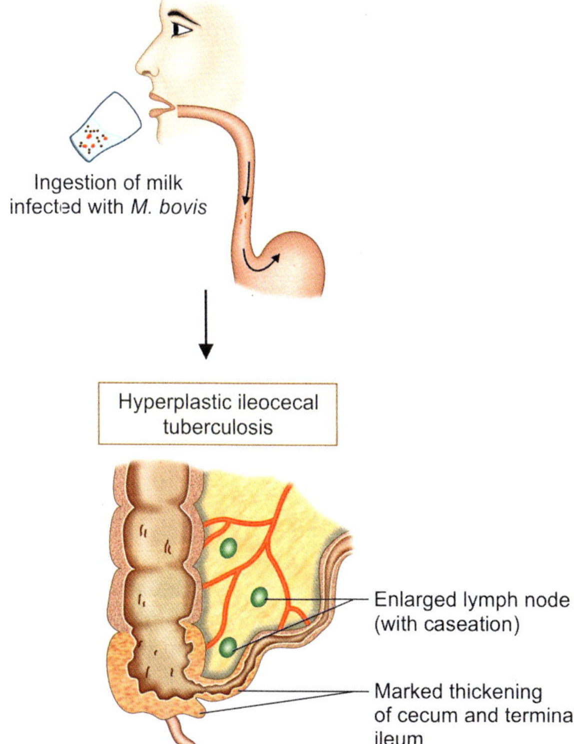

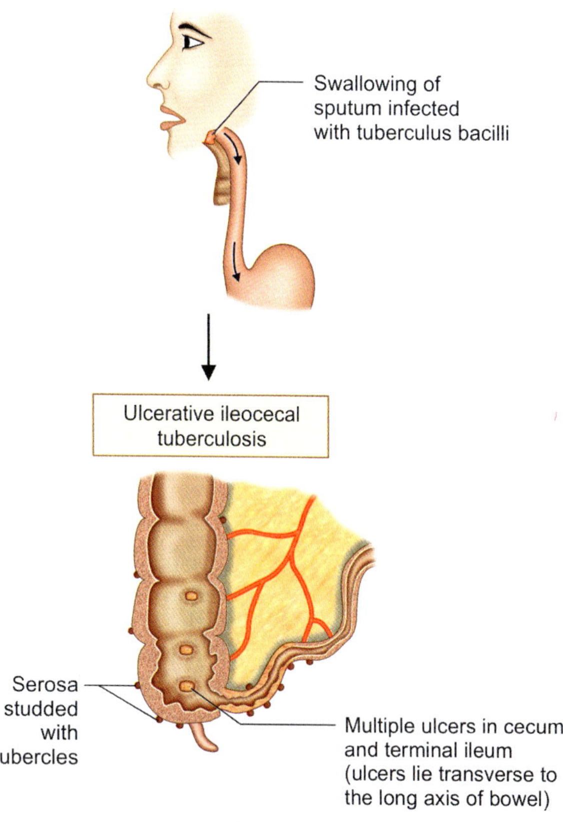

- **Caseating and noncaseating granulomas, caseation necrosis** are characteristic histological findings in intestinal tuberculosis.
- The **ileocecal region** is most commonly involved in intestinal tuberculosis.

Granulomatous Diseases

Tuberculosis

- Leprosy
- Histoplasmosis
- Sarcoidosis
- Schistosomiasis

Crohn's disease

Characteristic Features of Granuloma in Intestinal Tuberculosis (Can be Differentiated from Granulomas of Crohn's Disease)

- Larger (>400 μm) granulomas
- Confluent granulomas
- Submucosal location
- >4 locations of granuloma
- Multiple granulomas and cecal location.

Clinical Presentation

- Colicky abdominal pain, episodes of subacute intestinal obstruction, diarrhea, loss of appetite, weight loss are common clinical presentations. Patient may develop acute episode of intestinal obstruction.
- In **predominant ulcerative form**, diarrhea is commonly present whereas in **predominant hypertrophic form**, abdominal pain and episodes of intestinal obstruction are typically present. Patient may also present with right iliac fossa mass (firm, tender and ill-defined).
- **Perforation of the tuberculous ulcer** is not so common.

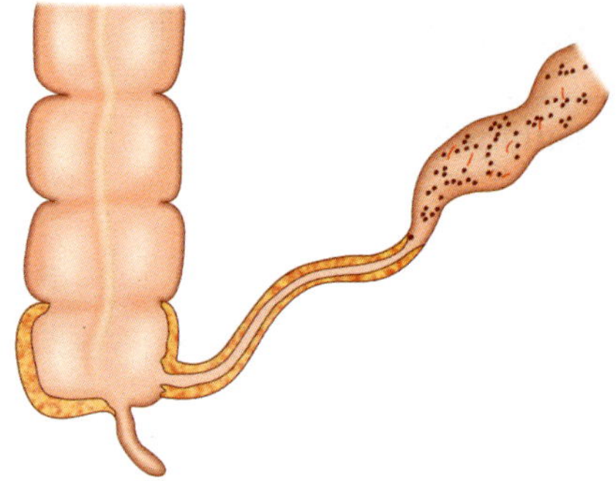

Recurrent episodes of subacute intestinal obstruction

Diagnosis

- **Straight X-ray abdomen:** Dilated bowel loops with multiple air-fluid levels if patient presents with acute intestinal obstruction.
- **Barium meal follow through:** Narrowed terminal ileum, widening of ileocecal angle, and pulled up cecum are characteristic findings in ileocecal tuberculosis.
- **CT abdomen:** Circumferential wall thickening of cecum and terminal ileum associated with mesenteric lymphadenopathy are suggestive of ileocecal tuberculosis.
- **Colonoscopy:** Classic colonoscopy findings in ileocecal tuberculosis are nodular or ulcerative lesions with surrounding erythematous mucosa, thickened edematous ileocecal valve.

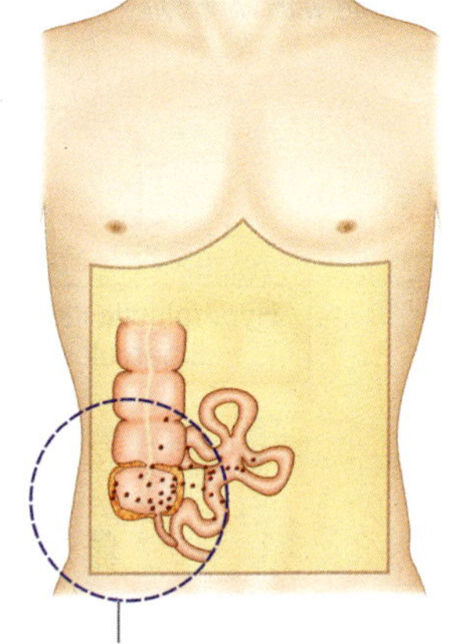

Mass in the right iliac fossa–The mass is firm, tender and very ill-defined

Management

- Most of the patients with intestinal tuberculosis respond to antituberculous therapy if early diagnosis and treatment is started. Surgery is indicated for acute intestinal obstruction, recurrent subacute intestinal obstruction even after completion of ATD therapy, for perforation or fistula.
- If patient with ileocecal tuberculosis presents with acute intestinal obstruction, ileotransverse anastomosis to bypass the diseased segment is the preferred option in poor surgical candidates. Right hemicolectomy is another surgical option if patient is well-nourished or on ATD therapy.
- Tubercular perforation is managed by resection of involved segment followed by primary anastomosis.

Radiological signs (Barium Studies) in Ileocecal Tuberculosis

String sign—persistent narrow stream of barium of diseased segment suggestive of stenosis.

Stierlin sign—lack of barium retention in the diseased segment with normal configured barium column on either side, suggestive of acute inflammation of the diseased segment.

"inverted umbrella" sign—thickening of the lips of the ileocecal valve and wide gaping of the valve with narrowing of the terminal ileum.

"Goose neck deformity"—loss of normal ileocecal angle, dilated terminal ileum appearing hanging from the retracted and fibrosed cecum.

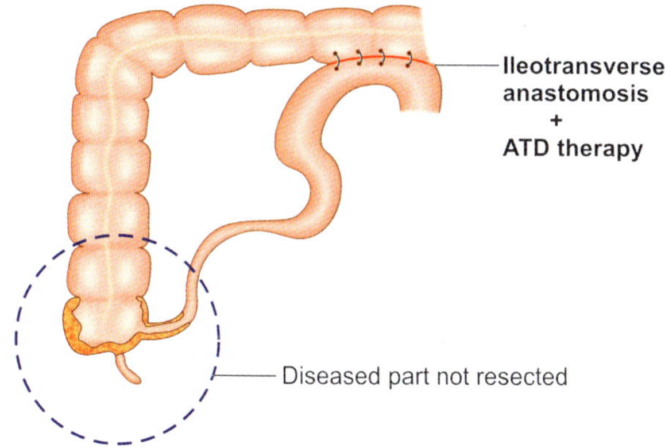

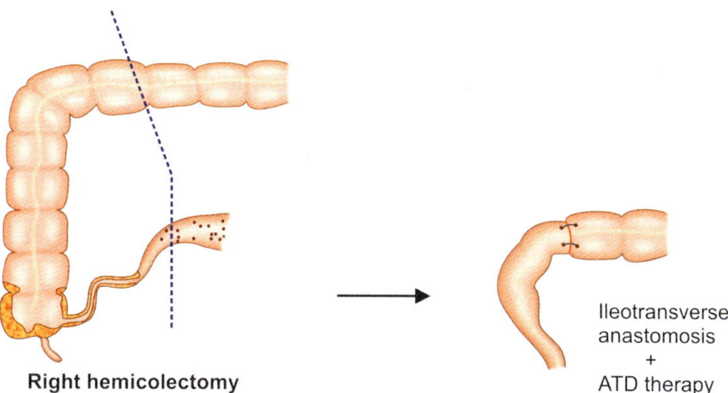

Complications of Bypass Procedure in Ileocecal Tuberculosis

- Blind loop syndrome
- Fistula formation
- Chance of recurrence in the involved segment

Characteristic Appearance to Differentiate between Jejunum and Ileum

Jejunum	Ileum
Larger luminal diameter	Smaller luminal diameter
The mesentery of jejunum contains single arterial arcade	The mesentery of ileum contains two or three sets of arterial arcade.
Mesenteric fat not encroaching the gut wall.	Mesenteric fat encroaching the gut wall.

Plica Circulares (Valvulae Conniventes or Folds of Kerckring)

- Plica circulares are the circular mucosal folds of the small intestine. These folds are thicker and closely spaced in the distal duodenum and jejunum and thinner and widely spaced in the ileum.
- In small bowel obstruction, valvulae conniventes may become prominent.

Ligament of Treitz

- The ligament of Treitz is also known as suspensory ligament of duodenum.
- This ligament is composed by two components: (i) Suspensory muscle of the duodenum and (ii) Accessory muscle (Hilfsmuskel).
- This ligament suspends the duodenojejunal flexure.
- **Clinical importance:** (i) This ligament is landmark to discriminate between upper GI and lower GI bleeding; (ii) Serve as a landmark to the Surgeons to identify the duodenojejunal flexure; and (iii) Landmark for the radiological diagnosis of intestinal malrotation.

Jejunal and Ileal Diverticula

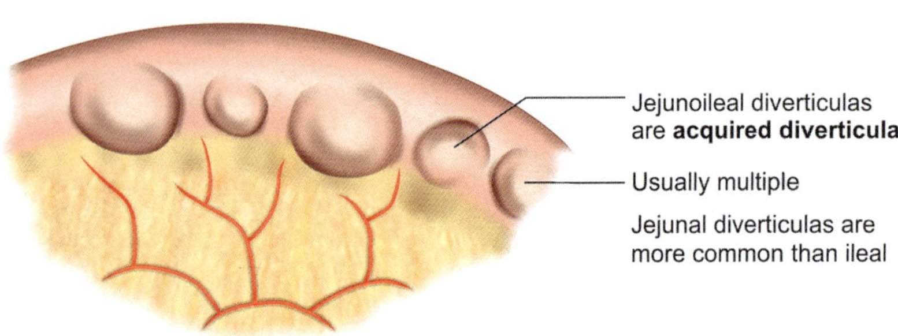

- Jejunoileal diverticulas are **false diverticula of pulsion type**.
- More common in the proximal jejunum followed by distal jejunum and then ileum.
- These diverticulas involve **only the mucosal and submucosal layers**.
- The herniation occurs through the **weakest part of the intestine (mesenteric side)**.
- Most of the patients are **asymptomatic**. Symptoms are usually nonspecific like vague abdominal pain, constipation, diarrhea. Some patients may present with intestinal obstruction or diverticulitis or perforation.
- USG can detect jejunoileal diverticula but **CT abdomen is the imaging modality of choice**.
- **No need of active management** for asymptomatic diverticulas. Complicated diverticulas are managed by **resection of involved segment followed by anastomosis**.

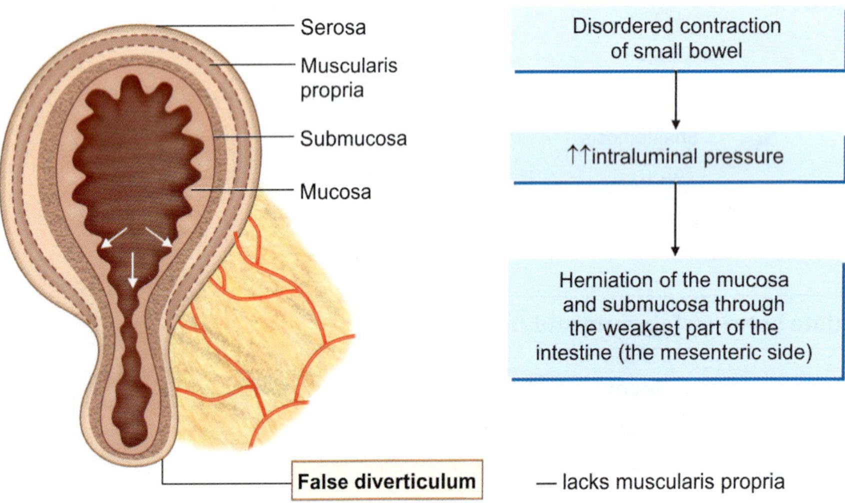

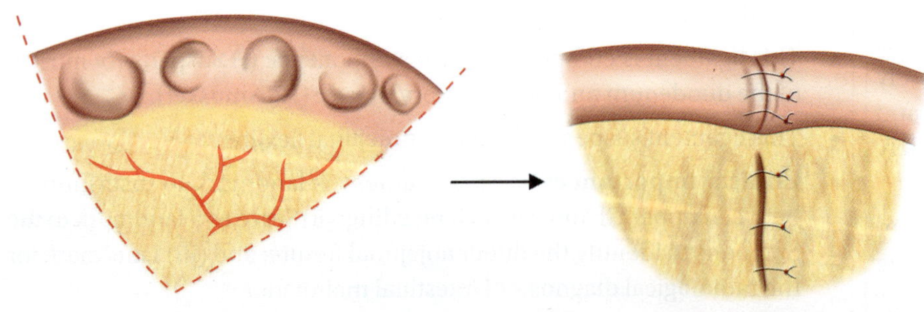

Duodenal Diverticula

Duodenum is the most common site for diverticula after the colon. Duodenal diverticula is the **most common acquired diverticula of the small intestine**. Most of the duodenal diverticula arise in the periampullary region and project from the medial wall of the duodenum.

Clinical Presentation

Most of the patients are asymptomatic. Patients may present with complications like cholangitis, pancreatitis, cholelithiasis (diverticula causes distortion of ampulla of Vater that leads to obstruction of the CBD). Diverticulitis, hemorrhage, perforation rarely develop in few percentage of patients. Blind loop syndrome may develop resulting in steatorrhea, Vitamin B_{12} deficiency anemia.

Diagnosis

Most of the diverticulas are discovered incidentally during endoscopy, imaging or peroperatively. Barium meal follow through study is the best diagnostic modality. Upper GI endoscopy may miss the diagnosis unless a side-viewing endoscope is used. CT is another imaging modality for diagnosis but with lower sensitivity.

Treatment

Surgery is not considered for asymptomatic and incidental diverticula. Surgery is indicated for symptomatic and complicated diverticula. Different surgical options are: (i) Diverticulectomy; (ii) Diverticulum inversion; and (iii) Duodenal resection.

Types of Duodenal Diverticula

Extraluminal (acquired diverticula)—most common type.

- Periampullary (located adjacent to or in the ampulla of Vater)
- Juxtapapillary (located about 2 cm from the ampulla of Vater)

Intraluminal (congenital)—develops due to incomplete recanalization of the intestinal lumen.

"Windsock" sign—a barium-filled sac within the duodenum and surrounded by a narrow radiolucent line.

Classic sign in upper gastrointestinal contrast series found in intraluminal duodenal diverticula.

Careful detection of the ampulla is important during surgical dissection to avoid injury to the CBD and main pancreatic duct.

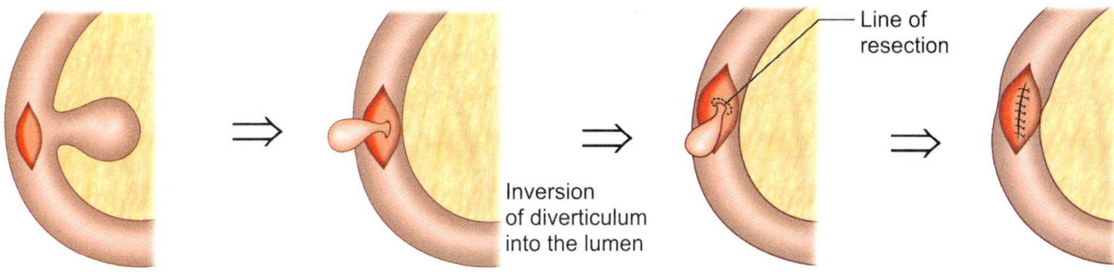

Meckel's Diverticulum

- Meckel's diverticulum is the most common congenital anomaly of the gastrointestinal tract.
- It is the **vestigial remnant of the omphalomesenteric duct**.
- It is a **congenital and true diverticulum** of the small intestine arises from the antimesenteric border. This diverticulum derives its blood supply from right vitelline artery which becomes the superior mesenteric artery.

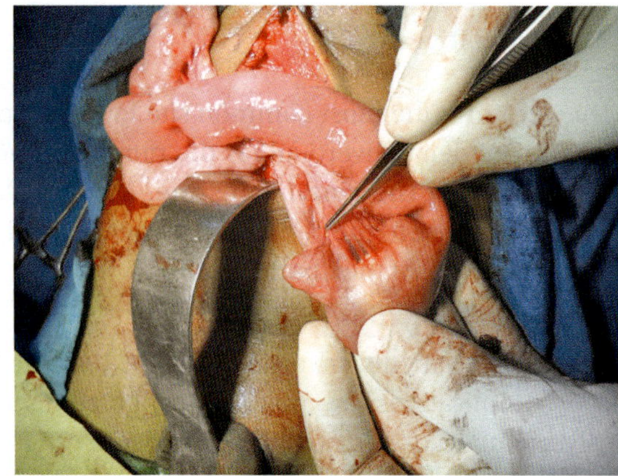

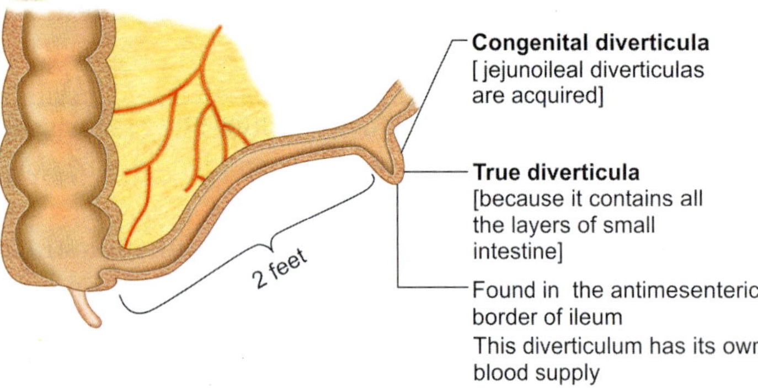

- **The omphalomesenteric duct (Vitelline duct)** acts as communicating tract between the embryonic sac and the primitive midgut during the early part of development. The vitelline duct normally obliterates during the eighth week of gestation.
- **The cell lining of the vitelline duct is pluripotent**, so heterotopic mucosa may be found in Meckel's diverticulum.

Rule of 2s

– Found in about 2% of general population
– (2:1) male predominance
– 2 ft proximal to the ileocecal valve (in adults)
– 2 inches in length

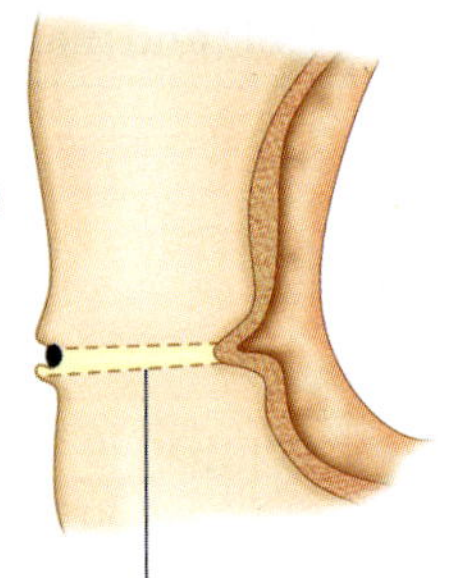

Result of incomplete obliteration of vitelline (omphalomesenteric) duct

Gastric mucosa
Pancreatic acini
Colonic mucosa
Heterotopic mucosa

- About 60% of Meckel's diverticula contain heterotopic mucosa.
- Gastric mucosa is the **most common heterotopic mucosa** (found in about 50% of all Meckel's diverticula).
- Pancreatic acini is the **second most common heterotopic mucosa**.

Clinical Presentation

Most of the Meckel's diverticulum are asymptomatic.

GI bleeding

- This diverticulum is the most common cause of painless significant lower GI bleeding in previously healthy infant. GI bleeding is the most common presentation in children with Meckel's diverticulum.
- Bleeding is related to presence of ectopic gastric mucosa in the diverticulum that secretes acid causing ulceration of mucosa of diverticulum and adjacent ileum

Long diverticula: Height-to-diameter ratio >2. Ectopic mucosa mostly found in the tip and body of the diverticulum.

Short diverticula: Height-to-diameter ratio ≤2. Ectopic mucosa has wide distribution including the base.

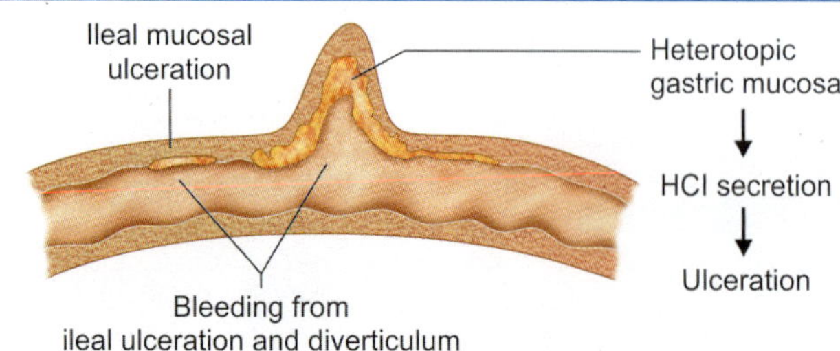

Obstruction

Meckel's diverticulum may cause intestinal obstruction by: (i) ileoileal and ileocolic intussusception; (ii) volvulus of small intestine around the fibrous band extending from diverticulum to the umbilicus; (iii) entrapment of small bowel beneath the mesodiverticular band; and (iv) incarceration of Meckel's diverticulum in an inguinal hernia (Littre's hernia).

Intestinal obstruction is the most common presentation in adults with Meckel's diverticula.

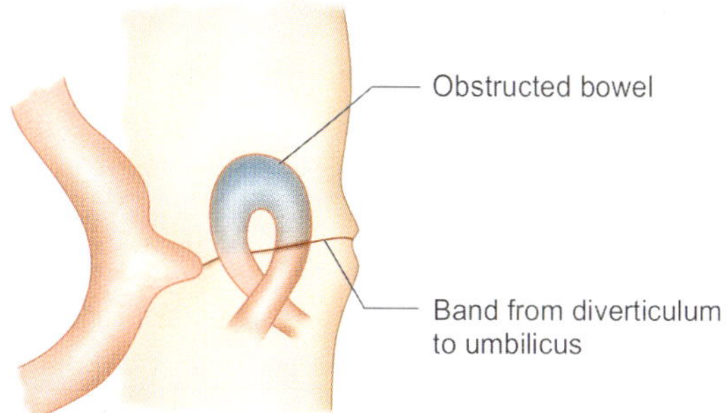

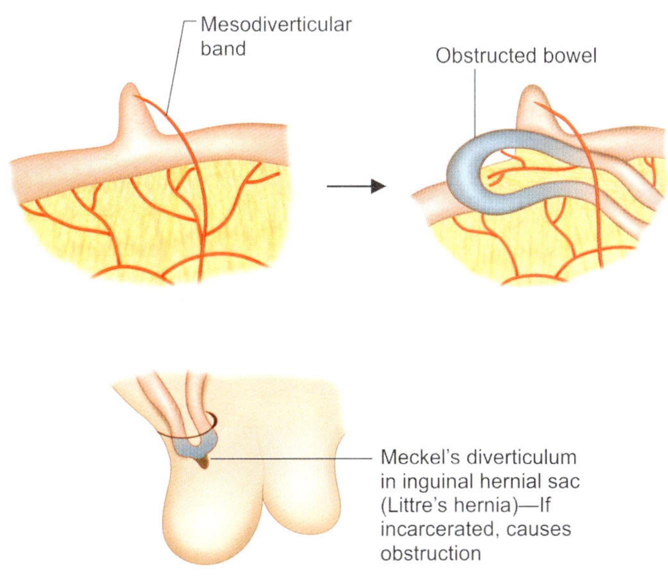

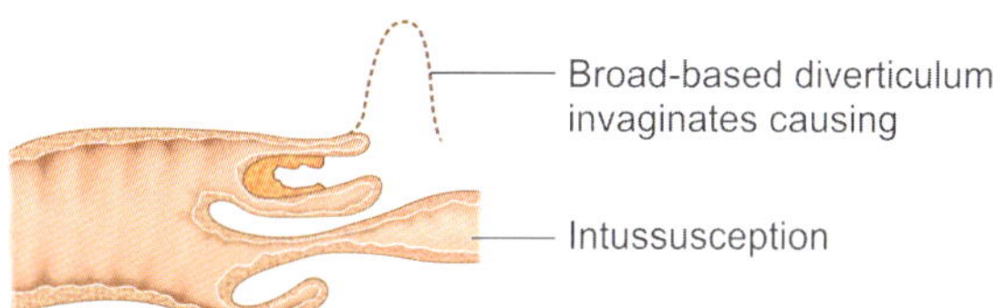

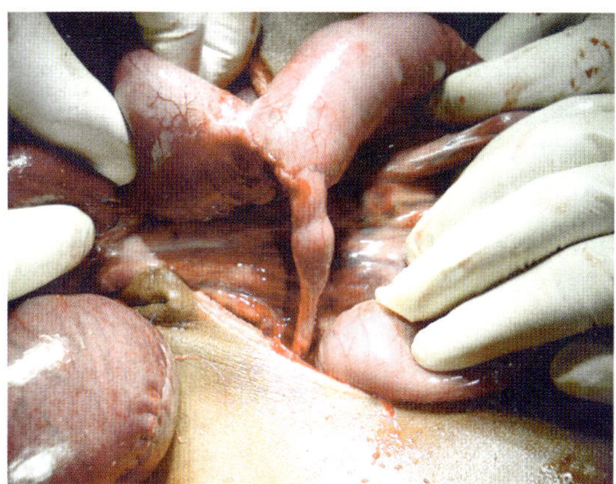

Operative picture—Meckel's diverticulum with band from the tip of the diverticulum.

Diverticulitis

This diverticulitis is caused by obstruction of the diverticular opening by enterolith, inflammatory tissues, parasites. Meckel's diverticulitis may mimic acute appendicitis. So, Meckel's diverticulitis should always be considered as a differential diagnosis in a patient with right iliac fossa pain.

On surgical exploration in a patient with a clinical diagnosis of acute appendicitis, if appendix is found to be normal, always search for a inflamed Meckel's diverticulum.

Neoplasm

Neoplasm of Meckel's diverticulum is extremely rare. Among the neoplastic lesions, carcinoid tumor is the most common.

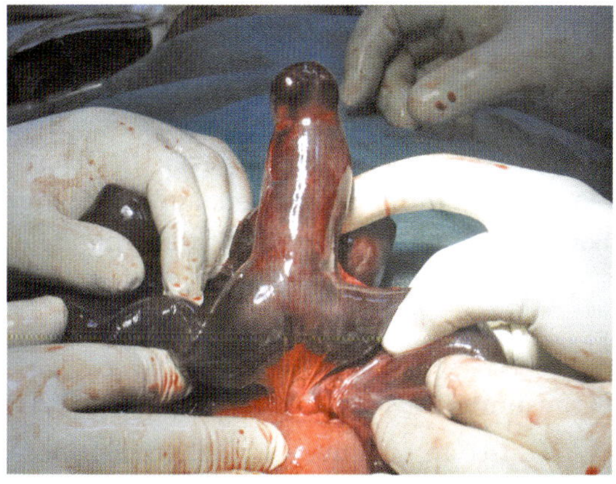

Operative picture showing Meckel's diverticulum with gangrenous changes.

Diagnosis

- In most of the patients, Meckel's diverticulum is detected as an incidental finding during intraoperative period.
- **Meckel scintigraphy:** Scintigraphy with 99mTc-pertechnetate detects the ectopic gastric mucosa in Meckel's diverticulum. This radiotracer is selectively taken up by the mucin-producing cells of the gastric mucosa. This modality should be used when no active GI bleeding is present. In children, this scan has high sensitivity and specificity but not in adults. The accuracy of this scan may be increased by using pentagastrin (to stimulate the uptake of the radioisotope), histamine blockers (to inhibit the secretion of the radioisotope once it is taken up) and glucagon (to decrease the "wash-out" of the radioisotope).

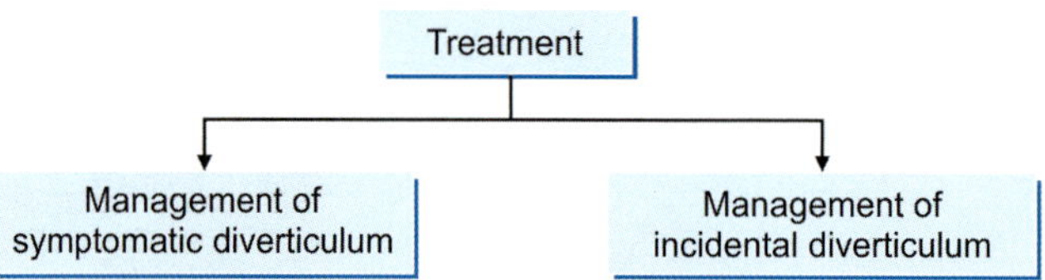

Surgery is indicated for following complications: (i) GI bleeding; (ii) Diverticulitis; (iii) Diverticulitis with perforation; and (iv) Intestinal obstruction.

The surgical options (open or laparoscopic approach) are: (i) Diverticulectomy; (ii) Wedge resection; and (iii) Segmental resection.

Diverticulitis of a long Meckel's diverticulum: Diverticulectomy.

Diverticulitis of a short diverticulum: Wedge resection.

Diverticulitis complicated by perforation of base or complicated intestinal obstruction: Wedge or segmental resection.

Bleeding from a short diverticulum: Wedge resection or segmental resection. Diverticulectomy may be considered in a long diverticulum.

Laparoscopic approaches are: (i) Diverticulectomy with endostaplers and (ii) Wedge or segmental resection with intracorporeal or extracorporeal anastomosis.

LATUM (Laporoscopic-assisted Transumbilical Meckel's Diverticulectomy)

LATUM is an effective surgical procedure for management of Meckel's diverticulum. This procedure allows palpation of the diverticulum and avoid use of staplers.

Incidental diverticulum with following factors are associated with increased risk of complications: (i) Male patient; (ii) Patient's age is less than 45 years; (iii) Diverticula longer than 2 cm; and (iv) Abnormal features within the diverticulum.

Incidental diverticulum with any of these risk factors may be considered for surgery (diverticulectomy for long diverticula and wedge or segmental resection for short diverticula).

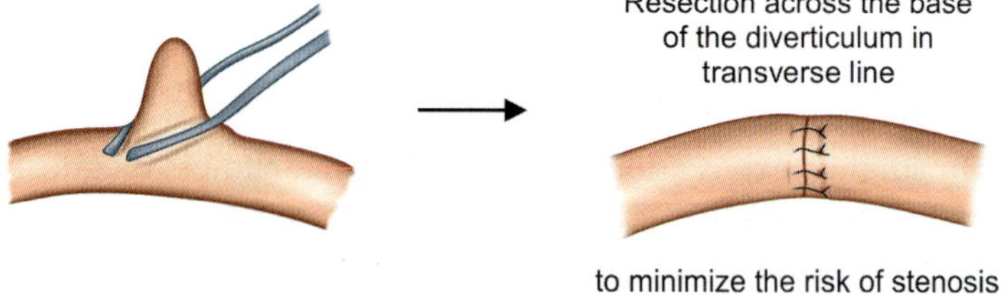

Diverticulectomy

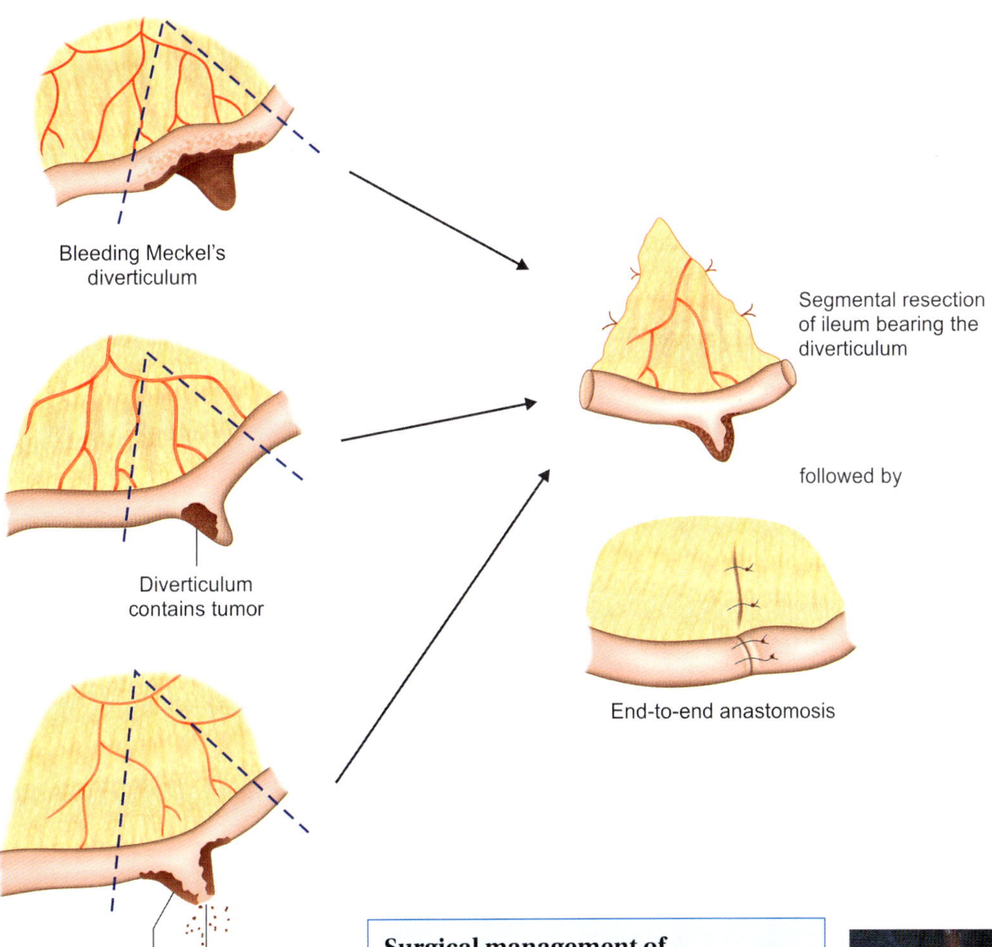

Surgical management of symptomatic Meckel's diverticulum.

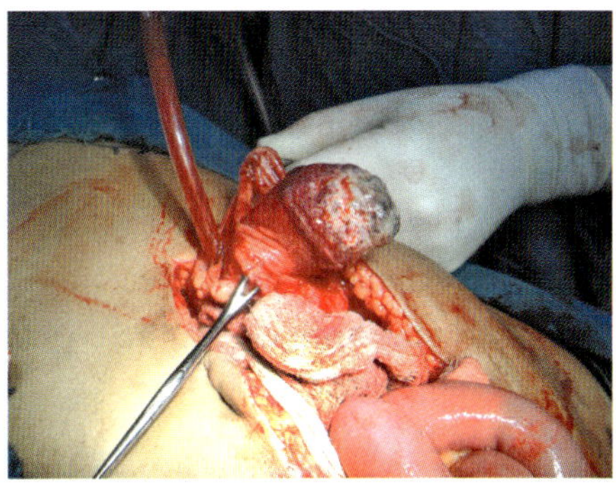

Lipoma of the small intestine.

Neoplasms of Small Intestine

Common benign neoplasms of small intestine are—lipoma, benign GIST, adenoma.

Common malignant neoplasms are—adenocarcinoma, carcinoid tumor, lymphoma, sarcoma, metastatic tumors.

Risk Factors Associated with Small Bowel Neoplasm

Hereditary syndromes

Peutz-Jeghers syndrome (hamartomatous polyps in the jejunum and ileum), Familial adenomatous polyposis (adenoma and adenocarcinoma), Gardner syndrome (multiple desmoid tumors)

Celiac disease (lymphoma and carcinoma)

Crohn's disease (adenocarcinoma)

Dietary habits (saturated fat intake associated with increased risk)

Small Intestine

- 70% of the total length of the GI tract.
- 90% of total mucosal surface of the GI tract.
- Small intestinal neoplasms accounting for about 3–6% of all GI neoplasms.

Clinical Presentation

Patients commonly present with nonspecific symptoms, e.g., dyspepsia, anorexia, malaise, vague abdominal pain. Patient may present with GI bleeding, intestinal obstruction, perforation.

Clinical presentations may depend on the type of tumor (e.g., symptoms of carcinoid syndrome may be present in carcinoid tumor).

Diagnosis

Barium enteroclysis: It is one of the useful imaging modalities for the diagnosis of small bowel neoplasms. The drawbacks of this modality are-time consuming, poorly tolerated by the patients and not sensitive for detection of small and/flat lesions.

MDCT and MRI enteroclysis: Both these imaging modalities can detect the exact location, appearance, mesenteric involvement of the tumor along with remote metastatic spread.

Balloon enteroscopy: Allows complete visualization of the small intestine with diagnostic and therapeutic potential.

Wireless video capsule endoscopy: Allows complete visualization of the small intestine without any diagnostic potential.

Management

Adenocarcinoma: Wide segmental resection with regional lymphadenectomy followed by adjuvant chemotherapy.

Carcinoid tumor: Wide segmental resection with regional lymphadenectomy.

Lymphoma: Surgical resection followed by adjuvant chemotherapy.

GIST: Wide segmental resection followed by KIT inhibitor therapy (if indicated). Regional lymphadenectomy is not required.

Adenocarcinoma

Adenocarcinoma is the most common primary malignant tumor of the small intestine. Tumors most commonly develop in the duodenum and proximal jejunum (adenocarcinoma associated with Crohn's disease mostly located in the ileum). Risk factors associated with small bowel adenocarcinoma are—Crohn's disease, Celiac disease, Peutz-Jegher's syndrome, Familial adenomatous polyposis.

Carcinoid Tumors

Carcinoid tumors are the second most common primary malignancy of the small intestine. These tumors are commonly found in the ileum (within 60 cm of the ileocecal valve). Small bowel carcinoids are likely to be associated with MEN1 syndrome.

Lymphoma

Lymphoma of the small intestine may present as a primary neoplasm of the small intestine or as a component of systemic disease. Stomach and small intestine are the most common sites of primary gastrointestinal lymphoma. Small-bowel lymphomas are commonly associated with Celiac disease, Crohn's disease, AIDS, long-term immunosuppressive therapy.

Gastrointestinal Stromal Tumor (GIST)

GIST can occur anywhere in the small intestine. Malignant GIST most commonly develop in the distal ileum.

Metastatic Tumor

Adenocarcinoma, carcinoid tumors are common intra-abdominal causes of metastasis, most common extra-abdominal cause is cutaneous melanoma.

Factors Responsible for Rarity of Tumors in the Small Intestine

- Rapid transit time—allowing minimal contact time between the carcinogens and the intestinal mucosa.
- High concentration of lymphoid tissue.
- Increased secretion of IgA.
- Increased liquidity and alkaline pH of the small intestinal contents—decrease the mechanical and chemical inflammation of the mucosa.
- Low bacterial load (particularly anaerobic bacteria)—less chance of carcinogen production.
- Rapid turnover of intestinal epithelial cells.

Enteroclysis

Enteroclysis is a radiological study of small intestine by intubation of the duodenum or jejunum and instillation of the contrast agent through that tube (Bilbao Dotter tube).

Different types of enteroclysis are:

- Single-contrast enteroclysis (low density barium)
- Air-contrast enteroclysis (medium density barium and air)
- Methylcellulose enteroclysis (high density barium and methylcellulose).

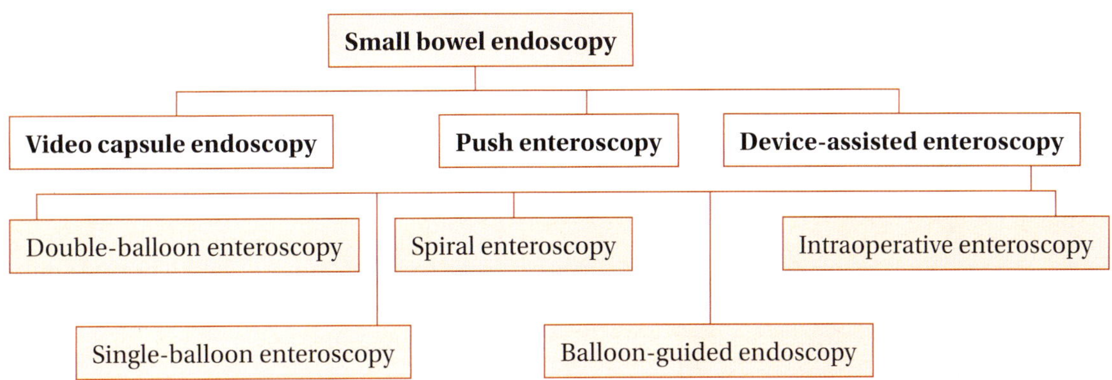

Video Capsule Endoscopy (VCE)

VCE consists of three components: (i) a capsule endoscope; (ii) a sensing system with data recorder; and (iii) computer workstation for image review and interpretation. This imaging system allows real-time review of images of small bowel.

It is the first-line investigation in patients with obscure gastrointestinal bleeding (OGIB).

Limitations: (i) unable to obtain biopsy specimens or perform therapeutic interventions; (ii) unable to cross altered anatomy; (iii) inability to control its movement through GI tract; (iv) Difficulty in localizing the lesion; and (v) may miss clinically important duodenal and proximal jejunal lesions (due to rapid transit through the duodenal loop).

Contraindications: (i) Pregnancy; (ii) History of small bowel resection; (iii) prior abdominopelvic radiation; and (iv) established diagnosis of Crohn's disease.

Complications: Capsule retention (particularly in Crohn's patients).

Push Enteroscopy

- An endoscopic evaluation technique for visualization of proximal jejunum.
- A dedicated push enteroscope is used in this procedure.

Limitations: Diagnostic and therapeutic procedures in the distal part of the small intestine are not feasible by this procedure.

Device-assisted enteroscopy (DAE) should be considered as first line investigation in patients with OGIB when small bowel video capsule endoscopy is contraindicated or unavailable.

Types of DAE are—Double-balloon enteroscopy (DBE), Single-balloon enteroscopy (SBE), Spiral enteroscopy (SE), Balloon-guided endoscopy, Intraoperative enteroscopy.

Double-balloon Enteroscopy (DBE)

DBE consists of three components: (i) an enteroscope; (ii) an overtube; and (iii) balloon-pump system (balloon is made of latex, balloon is fitted at enteroscope).

Three types of double-balloon enteroscopes: (i) Diagnostic; (ii) Therapeutic; and (iii) Short model.

Advancement of enteroscope and accompanying overtube through the small bowel is achieved by alternating inflation and deflation of the two balloons along with instrument insertion and retraction—**"push and pull" technique**.

DBE can be performed as—(i) Antegrade approach (oral) or (ii) Retrograde approach (anal). Complete small-bowel visualization can be achieved by a combined approach.

Procedures that can be done: (i) obtain biopsy specimens; (ii) polypectomy; (iii) stricture dilation; and (iv) retrieval of foreign bodies.

Adverse events—(i) perforation; (ii) bleeding; (iii) pancreatitis; and (iv) aspiration pneumonia.

Spiral Enteroscopy (SE)

SE consists of two components: (i) an enteroscope and (ii) a specialized overtube (made of polyvinyl chloride) with a spiral raised element at its distal end.

This enteroscopy is performed by rotational endoscopy technique.

Advantage: Less procedure time.

Limitation: Complete small bowel visualization rate is very low.

Adverse events: (i) Perforation and (ii) Mucosal tear.

Single-balloon Enteroscopy (SBE)

SBE consists of three components—(i) an enteroscope and (ii) an overtube (iii) balloon-pump system (balloon made of silicone, balloon is fitted at overtube).

This enteroscopy is performed by **"push and pull"** technique.

Procedures that can be done—same as DBE.

Adverse events—same as DBE.

Balloon-guided Endoscopy

This system consists of: (i) balloon inflation-deflation system and (ii) single-use latex-free balloon catheter.

Balloon catheter is inserted through the 3.7 mm working channel of a standard colonoscope, enteroscopy is performed by push-pull technique.

Intraoperative Enteroscopy

- Enteroscopy is done by a flexible endoscope via oral route or via an enterotomy during the surgical procedure.
- Intraoperative enteroscopy is indicated in massive mid-gut bleeding, lesions not accessible or difficult to treat by balloon enteroscopy.

Short Bowel Syndrome

Short bowel syndrome develops when remaining small bowel length is less than 200 cm. Life-long dependency on TPN can be avoided if small bowel length is 60 cm with completely functioning colon or small bowel length is 100 cm in absence of colon. Ultrashort bowel syndrome develops when length of small bowel is less than 10 cm or 10% of expected for the age.

Etiology

- Congenital—intestinal atresia
- *Related to resection (massive or multiple):*
  - Necrotizing enterocolitis
  - Gastroschisis
  - Mesenteric arterial embolism or venous thrombosis
  - Crohn's disease
  - Malignancy
- *Functional (due to physiological loss of function):*
  - Radiation enteritis
  - Refractory sprue
  - Congenital villous atrophy

Anatomic Subtypes

- Type I—resection includes most of the jejunum, remains at least 10 cm terminal ileum, ileocecal valve, colon; jejunoileal anastomosis
- Type II—resection includes most of the ileum, ileocecal valve, proximal colon; jejunocolic anastomosis
- Type III—resection includes all of the ileum and colon, part of the jejunum; output via end jejunostomy

Phases of Intestinal Adaptation

(i) Acute phase (up to 4 weeks of resection, characterized by dysmotility, malabsorption, diarrhea, gastric hypersecretion); (ii) Adaptive phase (duration 1–2 years, most of the adaptive changes happen in this phase); and (iii) Maintanence phase.

Clinical Manifestations

In type I: Dehydration in initial phase and symptoms due to hypersecretion of HCl.

In type II: Vitamin A, D, K and B_{12} deficiency, steatorrhea

In type III: Dehydration, nutritional deficiency.

Medical Management

In acute phase: (i) Management of fluid and electrolyte imbalance; (ii) Replacement of water-soluble vitamins; (iii) Loperamide (for diarrhea); (iv) PPI or H_2 blocker therapy; (v) Cholestyramine (to increase bile salt retention); and (vi) Enteral nutrition.

In adaptive phase: (i) Enteral nutrition and (ii) Calcium and magnesium supplementation.

In maintenance phase: (i) Enteral nutrition; (ii) Supplementation of vitamin A, D, E and B_{12}; (iii) Supplementation of calcium, iron, zinc, magnesium; and (iv) Teduglutide (in parenteral nutrition-dependent patients).

Intestinal Rehabilitation

(i) Educational counseling; (ii) Nutritional assessment; (iii) Monitoring of complications; and (iv) Stoma care (if indicated).

Surgical Management

- Colonic interposition
- Tapering enteroplasty
- Longitudinal intestinal lengthening and tailoring (LILT)
- Serial transverse enteroplasty (STEP)
- Spiral intestinal lengthening and tailoring (SILT)
- Intestinal transplantation.

Teduglutide is a recombinant human analog of glucagon-like peptide-2 (GLP-2). It promotes crypt cell growth and increase villous height, increases intestinal barrier function and absorption. Teduglutide may decrease requirement of parenteral nutrition in parenteral nutrition-dependent patients. Since 2012, teduglutide is approved by FDA and EMA for the treatment of parenteral nutrition-dependent adult patients with short bowel syndrome.

Etiologies of Short Bowel Syndrome

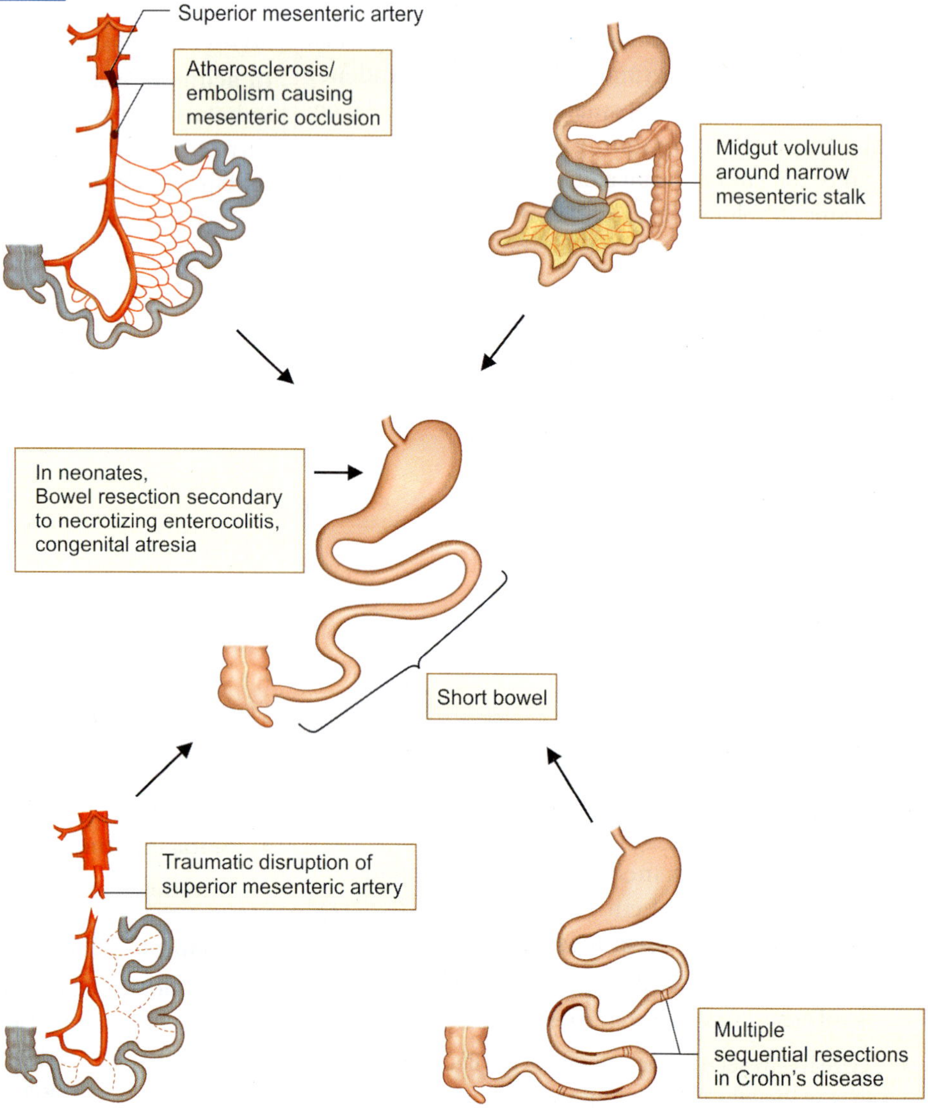

Superior mesenteric artery

Atherosclerosis/ embolism causing mesenteric occlusion

Midgut volvulus around narrow mesenteric stalk

In neonates, Bowel resection secondary to necrotizing enterocolitis, congenital atresia

Short bowel

Traumatic disruption of superior mesenteric artery

Multiple sequential resections in Crohn's disease

Outcome of SBS Depends on the following Factors

- Remaining intestine (length and location)
- Presence of functioning colon
- Presence or absence of Ileocecal valve
- Underlying disease (e.g., malignancy, Crohn's disease, radiation enteritis)
- Intestinal adaptation
- Patient related (age, BMI)

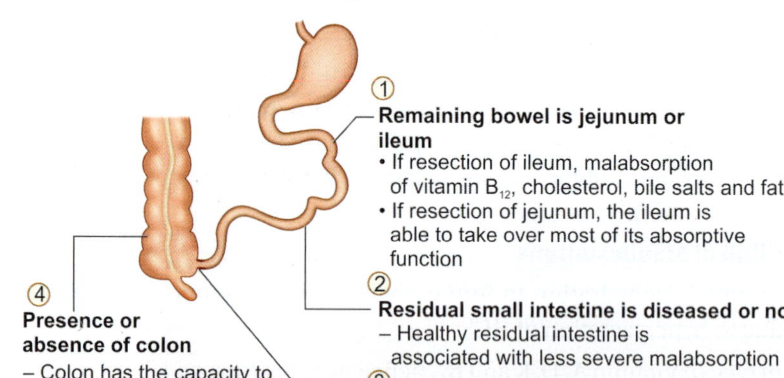

Colonic Interposition

A surgical method to slow transit time in patients with short bowel syndrome. This technique is indicated when sufficient length of intestine is not available for conventional bowel lengthening procedures.

In this procedure, a segment of colon is relocated to the small intestines while maintaining peristaltic directionality.

Complications: (i) Colonic dilatation and (ii) Enterocolitis

Longitudinal Intestinal Lengthening and Tailoring (LILT) Procedure

- A surgical technique of bowel lengthening for short bowel syndrome, first described by Adrian Bianchi.
- **Criterias ideal for LILT procedure are:** (i) Intestinal diameter >3 cm; (ii) Length of residual small bowel >40 cm; and (iii) Length of dilated bowel >20 cm.
- **This technique includes:** (i) Creation of an avascular space along the mesenteric border of a dilated loop of bowel; (ii) Splitting of the bowel lengthwise, taking care to allocate alternating blood vessels each side; and (iii) 2 "hemi-loops" are created and then anastomosing end-to-end in a isoperistaltic fashion.
- This technique creates a loop of intestine that is twice the length and half the original diameter of the original bowel.
- **Complications:** (i) Anastomotic stenosis; (ii) Staple line leakage; (iii) Interloop abscess; and (iv) Fistula formation.

Spiral Intestinal Lengthening and Tailoring (SILT)

- SILT is a emerging surgical technique of intestinal lengthening for short bowel syndrome.
- This technique requires less mesenteric dissection than Bianchi procedure and more physiological than STEP procedure.

Tapering Enteroplasty

This surgical procedure is indicated in: (i) Jejunal atresia with dilated bowel and (ii) Vascular anatomy of the dilated bowel does not permit bowel division for a lengthening procedure.

This technique includes: (i) Excision of a wedge of the antimesenteric border of the dilated bowel using a stapling device and (ii) Suturing the remnant bowel into a tube.

Complication: Anatomotic leakage.

Serial Transverse Enteroplasty (STEP)

A simpler surgical technique of bowel lengthening for short bowel syndrome.

This procedure is indicated if: (i) Patient develops redilatation of the bowel after a LILT procedure and (ii) Patients have foreshortened mesentery or previous surgeries without intact both leaves of mesentery.

This technique includes narrowing of the luminal channel by firing a series of staples perpendicular to the long axis of the bowel in a zig-zag pattern, resulting in tapering without loss of surface area.

Advantages of this technique: (i) No need of anastomosis; (ii) Minimal mesenteric dissection; and (iii) Can be performed for redilation of bowel after a LILT or STEP procedure.

Intestinal Transplantation

Indications: (i) Patients with short bowel syndrome who experience parenteral nutrition failure and (ii) Ultra-short bowel syndrome.

In the absence of liver disease, isolated intestinal transplantation (SBTx) is the procedure of choice.

In children, combined liver-intestinal transplantation (SB-LTx) is most commonly performed. In adults, isolated intestinal transplantation is most commonly performed.

Contraindications: Active infection, malignancy.

Diverticular Disease of Colon

Diverticular disease covers the spectrum from diverticulosis to diverticulitis.

Diverticulosis: A clinical condition in which multiple diverticulas develop anywhere in the intestine (most commonly in the sigmoid colon). Diverticulosis is characterized by false diverticula, muscular thickening, and redundant folds of mucosa.

Symptomatic uncomplicated diverticular disease (SUDD): Diverticulosis with associated chronic abdominal pain in the absence of clinically overt colitis.

Complicated diverticulitis: Diverticulitis associated with uncontained free, perforation with a systemic inflammatory response, fistula, abscess, stricture, or obstruction.

Uncomplicated diverticulitis: Diverticulitis not associated with any of these complications.

Right-sided diverticulosis is more common in Asian countries and left-sided diverticulosis is more common in Western population.

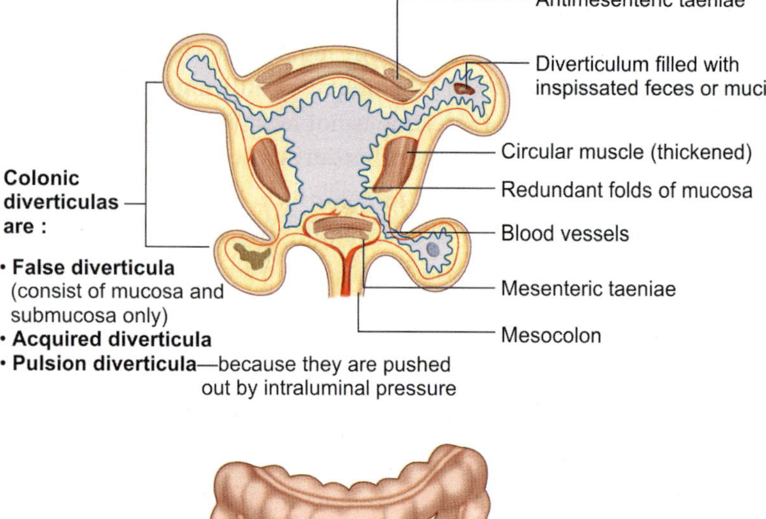

Myochosis coli

Thickening of colonic smooth muscles before the appearance of diverticula.

Pathophysiology

Predisposing factors related to diverticulosis: (i) Low fiber diet; (ii) abnormal colonic motility; and (iii) colonic wall resistance.

Abnormal colonic motility results in exaggerated segmental muscle contractions in colonic segment. This lead to maximal intraluminal pressure in sigmoid colon (this colonic segment is the narrowest part of the colon) resulting in outpouching of mucosa and submucosa through the weakest part of the colonic wall.

Diverticula tend to occur at 4 weak points where the vas rectae penetrate the circular muscle (each side of the mesenteric taenia and mesenteric border of the two antimesenteric taenia).

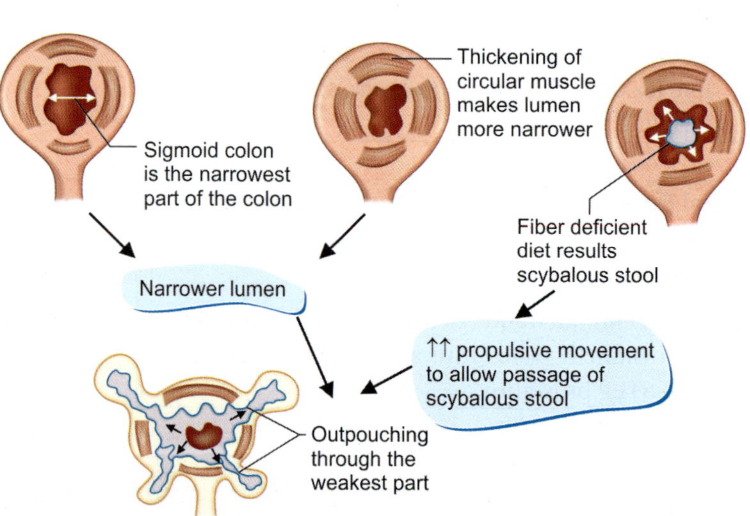

Diverticulosis occur at younger age in patients with **Ehlers-Danlos syndrome and Marfan syndrome.**

Clinical Presentation of Diverticulitis

Classic presentation of sigmoid diverticulitis—pain in the left lower quadrant, fever, leukocytosis.

Patients of complicated diverticulitis with free perforation and generalized peritonitis present with rigidity and diffuse guarding. Presence of fecaluria, pneumaturia, or pyuria are suggestive of colovesical fistula. Passage of stool per vagina is suggestive of colovaginal fistula.

Patient may present with features of intestinal obstruction due to stricture (as result of recurrent episodes of diverticulitis) or due to abscess formation.

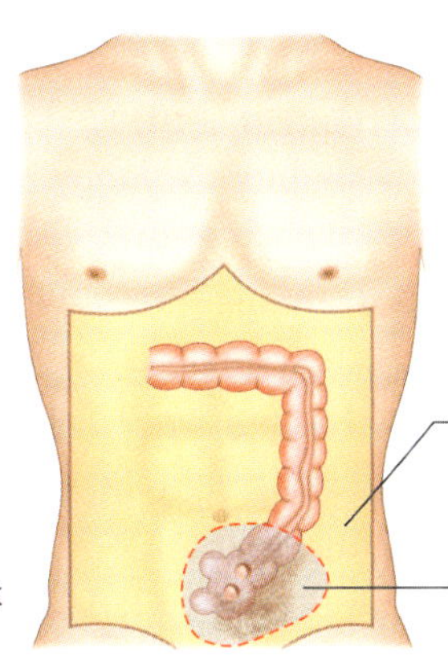

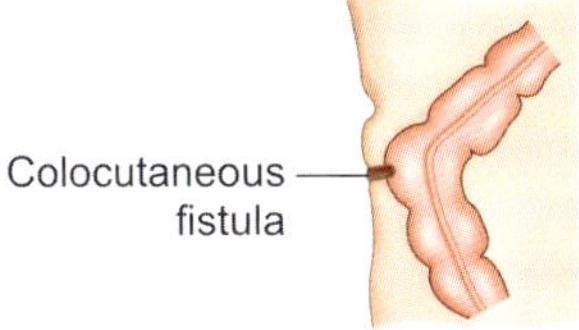

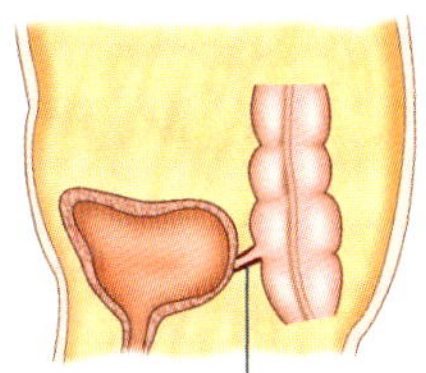

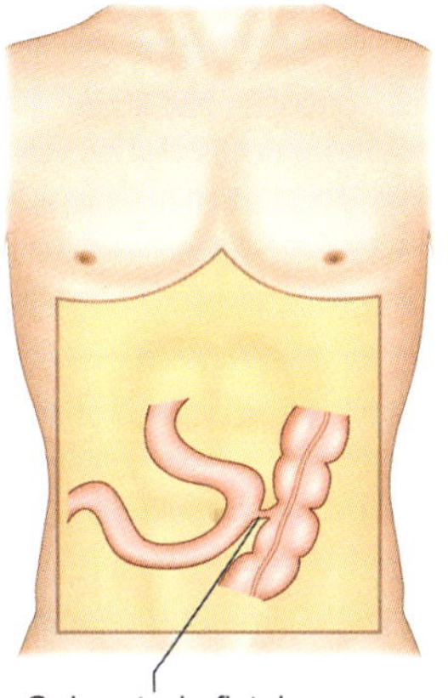

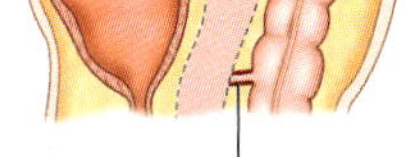

Saint's Triad

- Cholelithiasis
- Hiatal hernia
- Diverticulosis of the colon

Differential Diagnosis

- Inflammatory bowel disease
- Irritable bowel syndrome
- Urinary tract infection
- Kidney stone
- Pelvic inflammatory disease

Diagnosis

MDCT abdomen and pelvis with IV and intaluminal contrast: The most appropriate initial imaging modality. This imaging accurately reveals the location of the infection, extent of the inflammatory process, location of an abscess.

Abdominal USG: Another imaging modality that can be used for initial evaluation in a patient with suspected diverticulitis where CT scan is not available or contraindicated (pregnant patient, contrast allergy). USG may miss complicated diverticulitis.

MRI abdomen: Another imaging modality with high sensitivity and specificity and can be used where CT scan is contraindicated. MRI may be better in differentiating diverticulitis from colorectal neoplasia.

CT Findings in Uncomplicated Diverticulitis

- Inflamed diverticulum
- Colonic wall thickening (wall thickness >3 mm on the short axis of the lumen)
- Pericolic fat stranding

CT Findings in Complicated Diverticulitis

- Fluid-containing mass with or without air and enhancing wall
- Contained or free extraluminal air pockets
- Fistula

Management

Nonoperative management: Antibiotic therapy is not beneficial in uncomplicated early-stage disease (Hinchey I and Ia). All other stages of diseases are treated with oral or IV antibiotics.

Image-guided percutaneous drainage—in stable patients with abscesses more than 3 cm.

Laparoscopic or open drainage of abscess—(i) if patient not responding to percutaneous drainage or antibiotic therapy and (ii) percutaneous drainage is not technically feasible.

Elective sigmoid colectomy—in all patients recovered from complicated diverticulitis and selected patients recovered from uncomplicated diverticulitis.

Urgent sigmoid colectomy—in patients with generalized peritonitis, purulent or feculent peritonitis with features of overwhelming systemic inflammatory response.

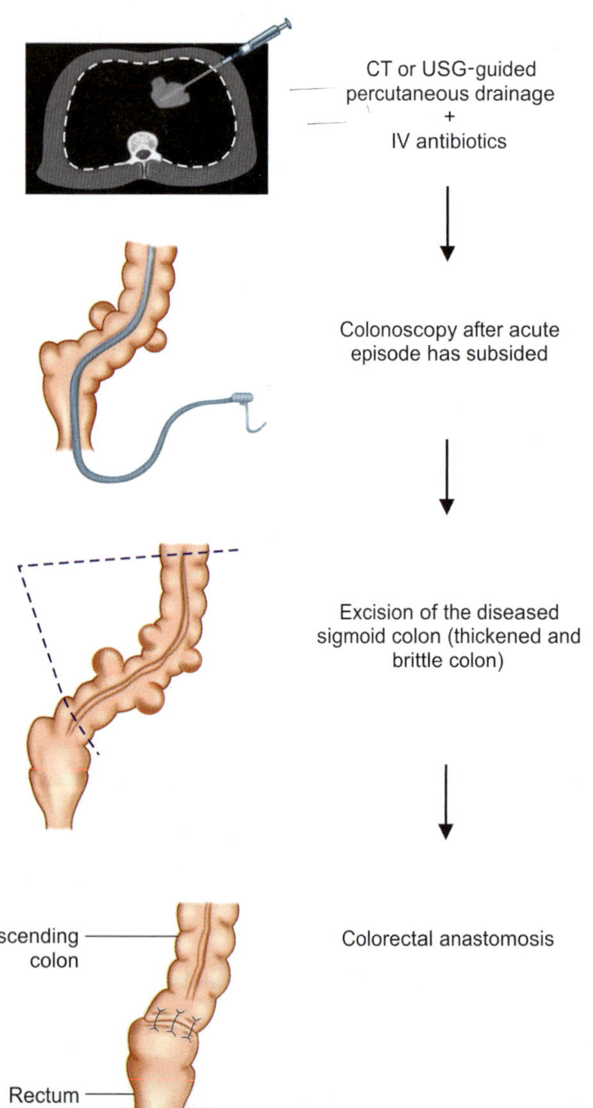

Measures to Reduce the Risk of Diverticulitis

- High-fiber diet
- Reduced intake of red meat
- Cessation of smoking
- Physical activity
- Weight loss

Principles of Elective Sigmoid Colectomy

- All diseased segments of the colon should be resected.
- The distal resection margin should be in a healthy rectum.
- Laparoscopic approach is preferred if expertise is available.

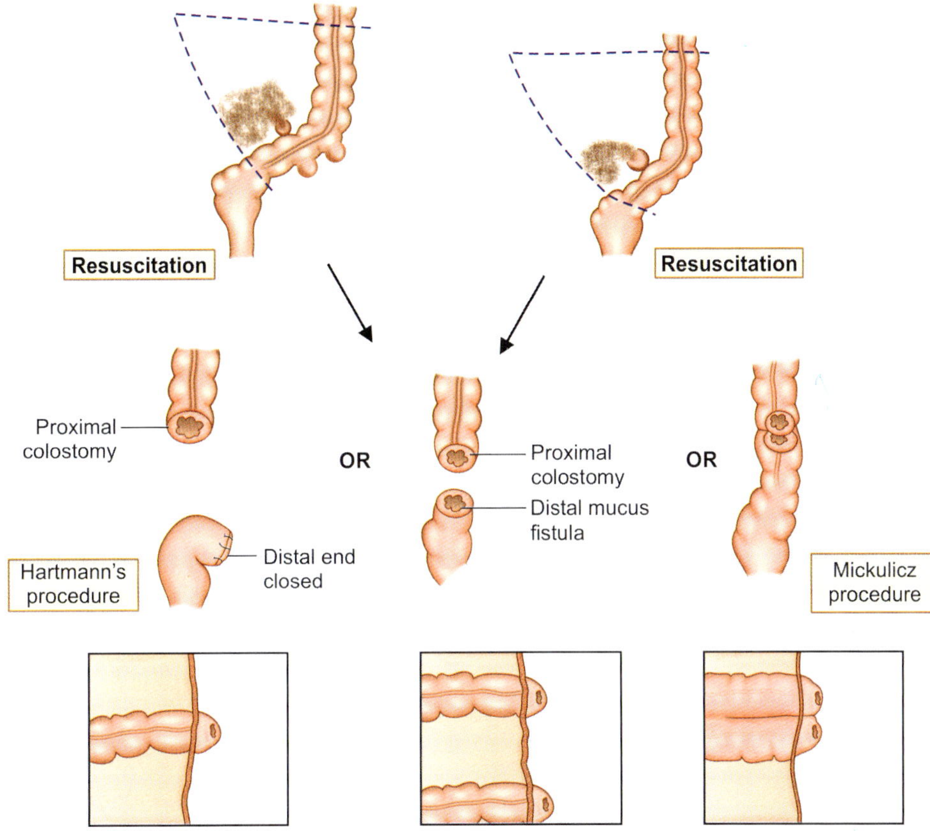

Following urgent sigmoid colectomy, the type of bowel continuity restoration depends on patient factors, intraoperative factors and surgeon's choice.

Options are: (i) Primary colorectal anastomosis; (ii) Primary colorectal anastomosis with a diverting stoma (colostomy or ileostomy); (iii) Hartmann procedure; and (iv) Mickulicz procedure.

Management of Fistula

- Imaging should be done to delineate the site and complexity of the fistula tract.
- Other causes of fistula (e.g., Crohn's disease, malignancy) should be ruled out.
- The basic principle of surgical management is to excise the diverticular segment of the bowel and to repair the defect of the involved organ.

Management of Obstruction

- Resection of diseased segment followed by primary anastomosis
- Hartmann procedure
- Stenting (if patient is inoperable).

Sigmoid Volvulus

Sigmoid volvulus is the most common volvulus of the colon. It is a common cause of large bowel obstruction in adults and exceedingly rare in pediatric age group. Sigmoid volvulus is more common in male population.

Anatomical Predisposing Factors

(i) Redundant sigmoid colon; (ii) Dolichomesentery (mesentery that is wider than long); and (iii) Narrowing of the base of the sigmoid mesentery.

Other predisposing factors: (i) High residue diet; (ii) Habitual constipation; (iii) Colonic motility disorders; (iv) Postoperative adhesions; (v) Internal herniation; and (vi) Pregnancy (gravid uterus displaces the redundant)

Pathophysiology

Types of Obstruction in Sigmoid Volvulus

- Closed loop obstruction in the twisted segment.
- Simple obstruction in colonic segment proximal to the proximal point of torsion.
- Double closed loop obstruction in protracted volvulus with competent ileocecal valve.

Morphological changes in Sigmoid Volvulus

- Grossly enlarged sigmoid colon
- Hypertrophied colonic wall
- Thickened sigmoid mesocolon with prominent vessels
- Obliteration of haustrations
- Splayed out taeniae.

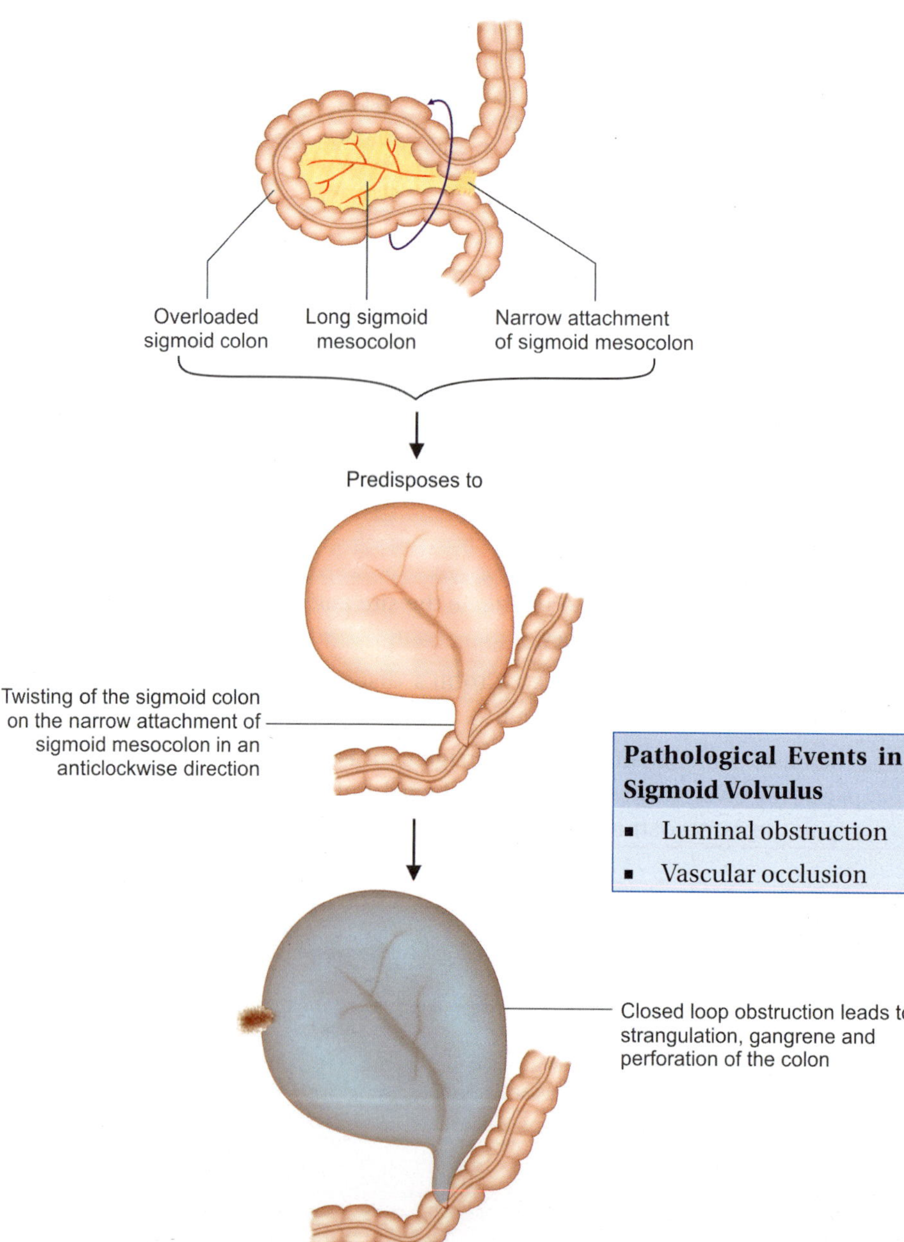

Pathological Events in Sigmoid Volvulus

- Luminal obstruction
- Vascular occlusion

Clinical Presentation

- Common presentations are abdominal pain, vomiting, obstipation.
- On clinical examination, asymmetric abdominal distension, varying degrees of tenderness, diminished or increased bowel sounds are common findings.
- Rebound tenderness and features of shock are suggestive of colon ischemia or perforation.

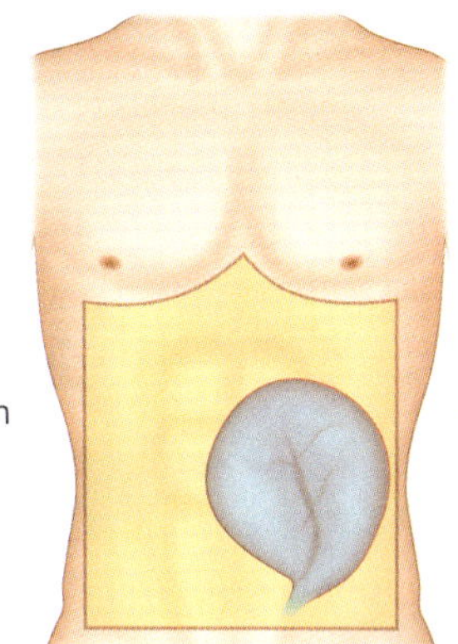

Diagnosis

Plain abdominal radiograph—the initial imaging modality in a patient with suspected sigmoid volvulus. "coffee bean" sign or "bent inner tube" sign are characteristic of sigmoid volvulus. Plain X-ray may also detect other conditions that are included in differential diagnosis. Associated complications like pneumoperitoneum or pneumatosis may also be revealed, if present.

Contrast enema—is indicated if plain abdominal radiograph is not diagnostic. Contrast enema (water-soluble contrast or barium) usually shows the point of colon torsion as a "bird's beak" like termination. Barium enema can only be used in absence of bowel ischemia or perforation.

Contrast-enhanced CT—is now the preferred imaging modality for confirmation of diagnosis of sigmoid volvulus. CT can also detect any ischemic changes in involved colonic segment. Other conditions that are included in the differential diagnosis, may also be detected.

Differential Diagnosis

- Colonic pseudo-obstruction
- Toxic megacolon
- Ileosigmoid knotting
- Cecal volvulus.

X-ray Signs in Sigmoid Volvulus

- "coffee bean" sign
- Frimann-Dahl sign
- "bent inner tube" sign
- "northern exposure" sign
- "ace of spades" sign

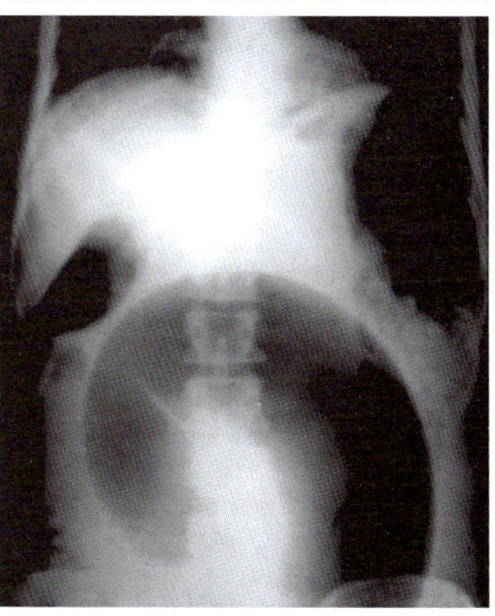

"Coffee bean" sign

CT Signs in Sigmoid Volvulus

- Whirl sign
- "X-marks-the-spot" sign
- "split-wall" sign.

Management

In the absence of colonic ischemia or perforation, the initial treatment of sigmoid volvulus is endoscopic detorsion (by rigid or flexible sigmoidoscopy or colonoscopy) followed by placement of a decompression tube for 48–72 hours.

Sigmoid colectomy with colorectal anastomosis should be considered during the index admission. Chance of recurrence is more after nonresectional surgical options (e.g., intraperitoneal or extraperitoneal sigmoidoplasty, mesosigmoidoplasty).

Emergency surgical intervention is indicated if endoscopic detorsion is unsuccessful or clinical features of ischemia, perforation or peritonitis are present. Resection of the gangrenous sigmoid colon should be done without detorsion and minimal handling (to minimize release of colonized microorganisms and endotoxins), followed by primary colorectal anastomosis (with or without proximal defunctioning stoma) or Hartmann procedure.

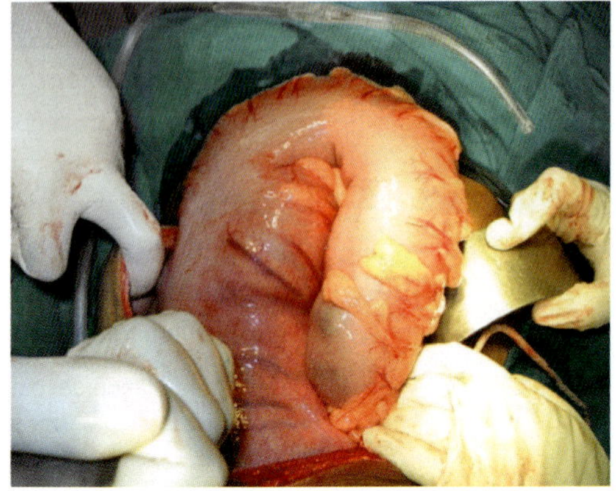
Intraoperative picture of sigmoid volvulus.

Rigid sigmoidoscopy and insertion of flatus tube to derotate the gut and deflate the colon
↓
Flatus tube remains for at least 48 hours
↓
Resuscitation and bowel preparation
↓
Elective procedure (Should be done because recurrence rate after decompression only is about 50%)
↓
Resective procedures | Nonresective procedures

Resection of sigmoid colon followed by colorectal anastomosis.

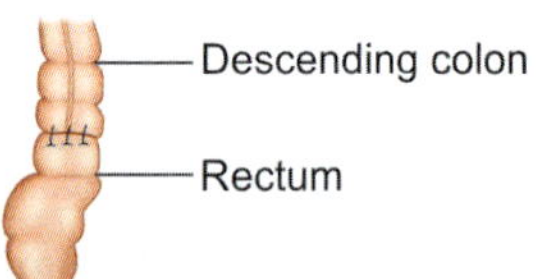

Resection of sigmoid colon followed by Hartmann procedure.

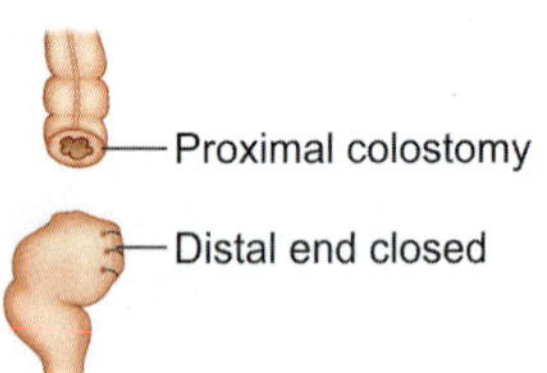

Resection of sigmoid colon followed by Mikulicz's procedure.

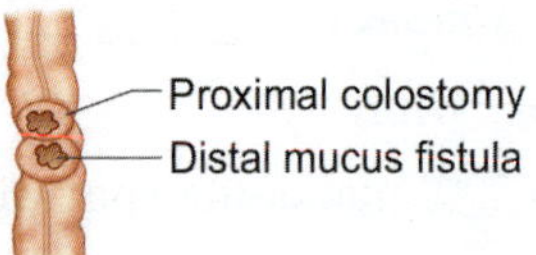

Mesosigmoidoplasty

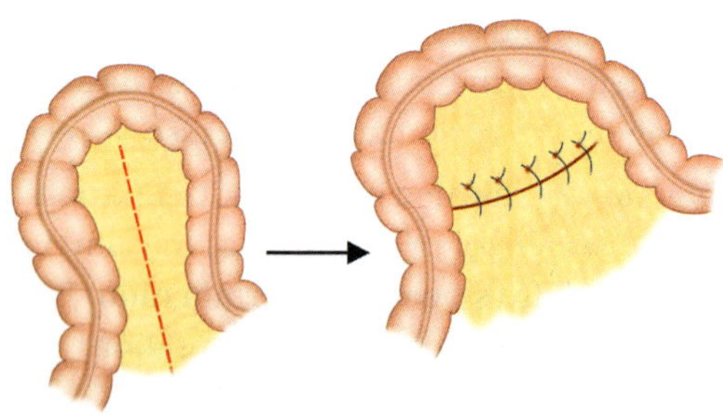

Sigmoidopexy

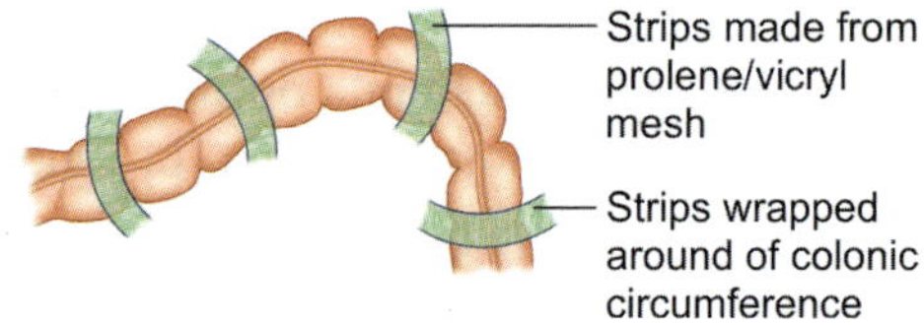

Endoscopic Fixation of the Sigmoid Colon

- This procedure is indicated if patient is not fit for any abdominal operations.
- The percutaneous endoscopic colostomy (PEC) technique is used to fix the sigmoid colon to the anterior abdominal wall by using T fasteners or by percutaneous tube colostomy placement.

Cecal Volvulus

Cecal volvulus is a uncommon cause of intestinal obstruction. This volvulus most commonly develops in 2nd and 3rd decades of life, compared to sigmoid volvulus that occurs in 6th to 8th decade of life. Cecal volvulus is more common in women.

Types of Cecal Volvulus

Most common type of cecal volvulus is **organoaxial type**, where clockwise axial twisting occurs involving the cecum, terminal ileum, and the ascending colon. **Cecal bascule** is another variant, not so common. In cecal bascule, anterior and superior folding of the mobile cecum over the fixed ascending colon without any torsion.

Predisposing Factors

Mobile cecum, previous abdominal surgery, postoperative adhesions, chronic constipation, high-residue diet are important contributing factors for the development of volvulus.

Clinical Presentation

Most of the patients with cecal volvulus present with features of acute intestinal obstruction. Patients with mobile cecum syndrome usually present with recurrent attacks of right lower quadrant pain, abdominal distension and relief of pain after passage of flatus, before the onset of acute volvulus. Features of peritonitis and shock are usually present in patients with gangrene or perforation.

Diagnosis

Plain abdominal radiograph may show cecal dilatation, single air-fluid level, left upper quadrant cecum.

Contrast-enhanced CT is now the preferred diagnostic imaging modality for cecal volvulus. CT can distinguish between organoaxial cecal volvulus from cecal bascule.

Management

Endoscopic reduction is not recommended due to high rate of failure and increased risk of perforation.

Resectional operative procedures are indicated for nonviable or perforated bowel. Resection followed by primary anastomosis or resction followed by ileostomy or mucus fistula are different options.

For patients with viable bowel, both resection and **nonresectional operative procedures** (detorsion alone, detorsion followed by cecopexy, cecostomy) are the options. Resectional procedure is preferred in good surgical candidates.

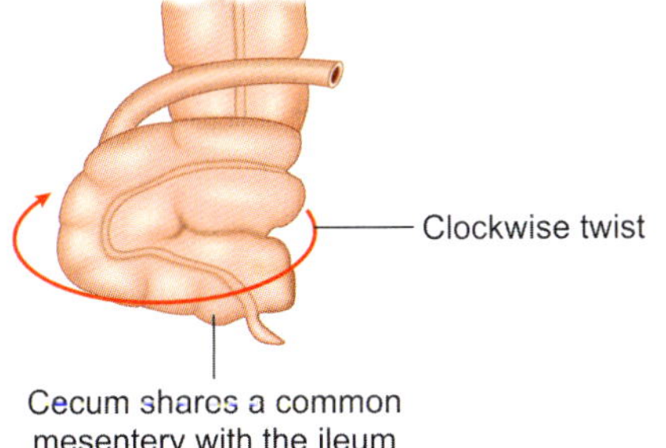

Organoaxial cecal volvulus

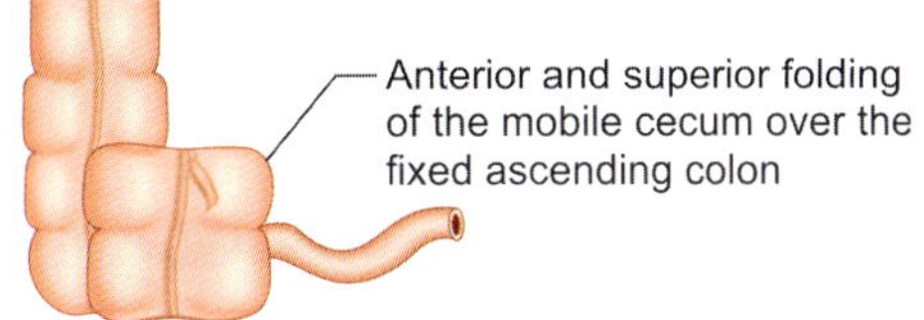

Cecal bascule

CT Findings in Cecal Volvulus

- "Whirl" sign
- "Coffee-bean" sign
- "Bird beak" sign.

Ileosigmoid Knotting

Ileosigmoid knotting is also known as **compound volvulus or double volvulus**. Ileosigmoid knotting is a rare cause of **double closed loop obstruction**, characterized by twisting of the ileum around the base of the sigmoid colon or vice-versa. This condition is more common in males in 3rd to 5th decades.

Predisposing Factors

Hypermobile ileum and sigmoid colon with elongated mesentery and a narrow base and intake of bulky diet after fasting are the main predisposing factors. Relaxed anterior abdominal wall, postoperative adhesions, internal herniation are other contributing factors.

Classification

Ileosigmoid knotting is classified into three types:

Type I: The ileum (active component) wraps itself around the sigmoid colon (passive component) in a clockwise or anticlockwise direction (type A when clockwise and type B when anticlockwise);

Type II: The sigmoid colon (active component) wraps itself around a loop of ileum (passive component) in a clockwise or anticlockwise direction;

Type III: The ileocecal segment (active component) wraps itself around the sigmoid colon (passive component); Undetermined type it is impossible to determine the revolved segment. Type I is most common, followed by type II and type III.

Clinical Presentation

Common presentations are abdominal pain, vomiting, obstipation, asymmetric abdominal distension, hypokinetic, hyperkinetic or absent peristaltic sound. In presence of bowel ischemia or perforation, rebound tenderness and features of shock may be present.

Diagnosis

Plain abdominal radiograph reveals distended ileal loops with a dilated sigmoid colon. CT reveals the findings of sigmoid volvulus along with twisted and dilated small intestine, medial deviation of the cecum and descending colon.

Management

Emergency surgical intervention is indicated. If both sigmoid colon and loops of small intestine are viable, untwisting of the knot may be attempted (but untwisting is technically difficult and increased risk of perforation) followed by appropriate measures depending on the viability of the active and passive components. If both intestine are gangrenous, resection followed by primary anastomosis or stoma formation is the surgical procedure of choice.

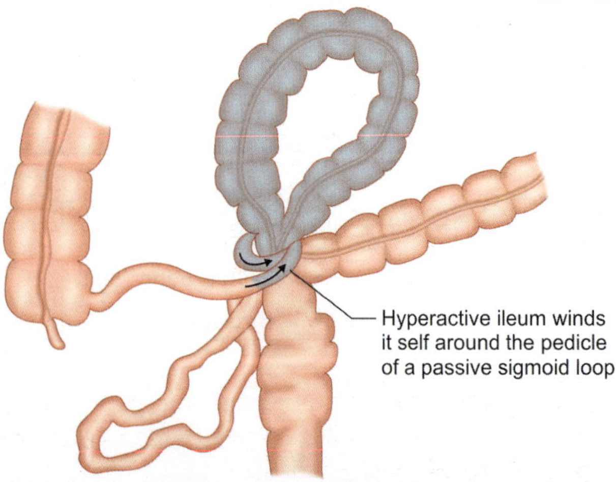

Type I ileosigmoid knotting

Characteristic Features of Ileosigmoid Knotting

- A double closed loop obstruction.
- Both small and large intestine are involved.
- Preoperative accurate diagnosis is difficult.
- Early gangrenous changes of bowel.
- High morbidity and mortality if delay in diagnosis and surgical intervention.

Acute Colonic Pseudo-obstruction

Acute colonic pseudo-obstruction (Ogilvie syndrome) is characterized by acute colonic distension in the absence of mechanical obstruction. This condition commonly occurs in older, hospitalized patients with severe comorbid illnesses, or recovering from surgery or traumatic injuries.

Pathophysiology

Exact pathogenesis is not known. An imbalance in colonic motor activity as a result of acute illness in a setting of chronic disease is most likely responsible.

Risk Factors Associated with ACPO

Surgical (cardiac surgery, solid organ transplantation, major orthopedic surgery, spine surgery); **Cardiorespiratory diseases** (myocardial infarction, congestive heart failure, chronic obstructive pulmonary disease); **Neurological** (dementia, Parkinson's disease, stroke, spinal cord injury); **Metabolic** (dyselectolytemia, diabetes, renal failure); **Medications** (opioids, anticholinergics, anti-Parkinson agents, clonidine); **Obstetric** (Cesarean section, normal vaginal delivery, normal pregnancy); **Infections** (Varicella-zoster virus, herpes virus, cytomegalovirus); **Miscellaneous** (major burn or trauma, severe sepsis).

Clinical Presentation

Abdominal pain, vomiting, constipation or obstipation, significant abdominal distension (with tympanic note on percussion) are common. On auscultation, high-pitched bowel sound are often present. Increasing abdominal pain, fever, abdominal tenderness are highly suggestive of colon ischemia or perforation.

Diagnosis

Diagnostic imaging is indicated to confirm large bowel obstruction and to rule out mechanical cause of obstruction. **Plain abdominal radiograph** is often helpful to detect mechanical cause of obstruction, such as sigmoid volvulus as well as complications (e.g., perforation). Pancolonic distension (in pseudo-obstruction) and paucity of gas in rectum or sigmoid colon (suggestive of mechanical obstruction) are X-ray findings that are helpful to differentiate between pseudo-obstruction and mechanical obstruction.

Contrast-enhanced abdominal CT or water-soluble contrast enema is essential to exclude mechanical cause of obstruction.

Management

Treatment options: (i) Conservative management; (ii) Neostigmine therapy; (iii) Endoscopic decompression; and (iv) Surgical intervention.

Conservative management is appropriate if patient without any clinical and radiological evidences of colon ischemia or perforation and cecal diameter is less than 12 cm. Management includes—(i) Fluid resuscitation; (ii) Correction of any dyselectrolytemia; (iii) Introduction of nasogastric and rectal tubes; (iv) Avoidance of opiods and anticholinergic drugs; and (v) Knee-chest or prone positioning. Conservative management can be continued up to 72 hours if no features of peritonitis or cecal diameter <12 cm.

Neostigmine therapy (2 mg IV over 2–5 minutes in cardiac-monitored setting) is indicated if conservative management fails. Neostigmine is contraindicated in pregnancy, uncontrolled arrhythmia or severe bronchospasm. Neostigmine therapy may be used with caution in patients with bradycardia, recent myocardial infarction, COPD, renal insufficiency.

Endoscopic decompression of the colon may be considered if patient not responding to neostigmine therapy or contraindicated.

Surgical intervention is indicated if colon ischemia or perforation is present or failure of neostigmine and endoscopic therapy. Tube cecostomy or cecostomy is an option if colon is viable. In presence of ischemia or perforation, either resection-anastomosis or resection with end ostomy are the surgical options.

Features suggestive of colon ischemia or perforation: (i) Fever; (ii) Abdominal tenderness; (iii) Leukocytosis; and (iv) Cecum dilation.

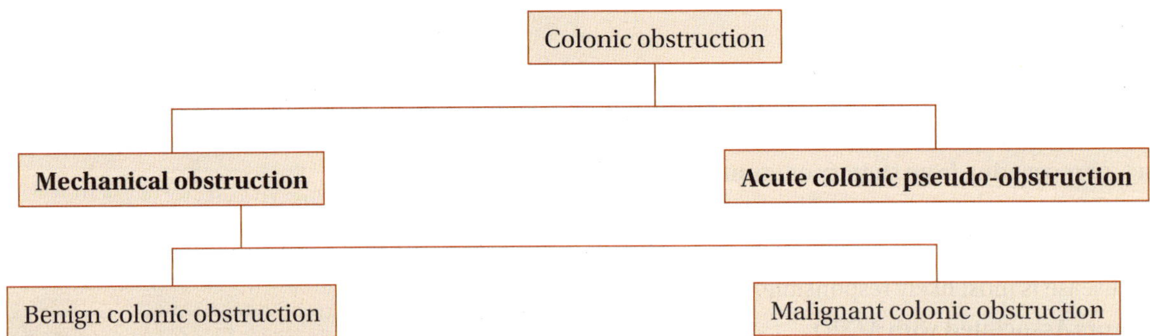

Causes of Benign Colonic Obstruction

- Volvulus
- Inflammatory bowel disease
- Anastomotic stricture
- Radiation injury
- Intussusception
- Diverticulitis
- Ischemic colitis

Treatment Options

- **Endoscopic detorsion followed by surgery**—in sigmoid volvulus without any clinical evidences of gangrene or perforation.
- **Emergent surgery**—in sigmoid volvulus or cecal volvulus with gangrenous changes or perforation.
- **Endoscopic balloon dilation**—in anastomotic strictures and strictures related to inflammatory bowel disease.
- **Colonic SEMS**—as a bridge therapy in patients with strictures waiting for surgery.

Causes of Malignant Colonic Obstruction

- Adenocarcinoma of colon (mostly left colon)
- Metastatic tumor of colon
- Pelvic tumors causing extrinsic compression

Treatment Options

- **Emergent surgery**—in good surgical candidates.
- **Colonic SEMS**—(i) as a bridge therapy to surgical resection and (ii) as palliative therapy in patients with poor performance status.
- **Transanal colonoscopic decompression tube placement**
- **Tumor debulking**—by endoscopic laser therapy, argon plasma coagulation, snare polypectomy

Useful Facts Related to Colonic Stenting

Uncovered stents have better outcome than covered stents (chance of stent migration is lower).

Absolute contraindication of colonic stenting is perforation.

- Colonic SEMS placement is performed by either TTS (through-the-scope) technique or OTW (over-the-guidewire) technique.
- Stricture dilation either just before or after colonic stent placement should be avoided (risk of colonic perforation is high).

Adverse events related to colonic stenting: (i) Early-perforation, stent failure, re-obstruction, bleeding and (ii) Late-re-obstruction, stent migration.

Factors associated with increased risk of stent-related perforation—Diverticular strictures, stricture dilation just before or after stenting, concurrent bevacizumab therapy.

Ulcerative Colitis

Ulcerative colitis is **chronic immune-mediated inflammatory bowel disease** of **unknown etiology**, affecting **the large intestine**.

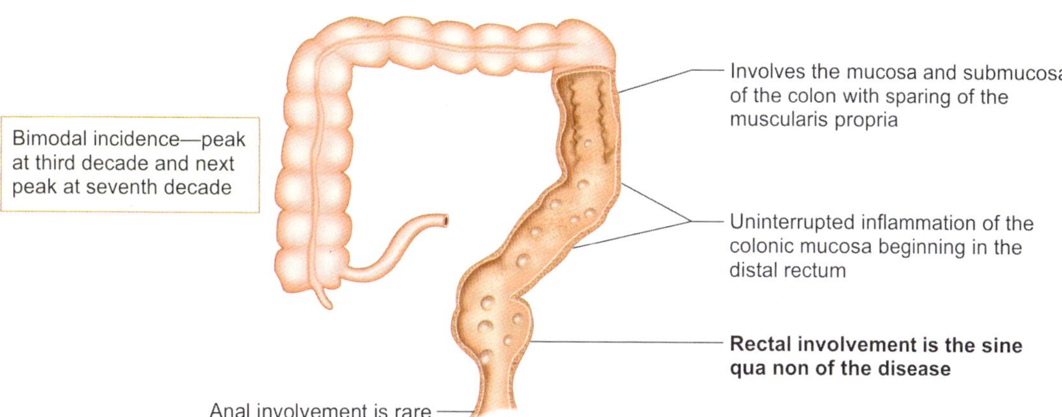

Pathophysiology

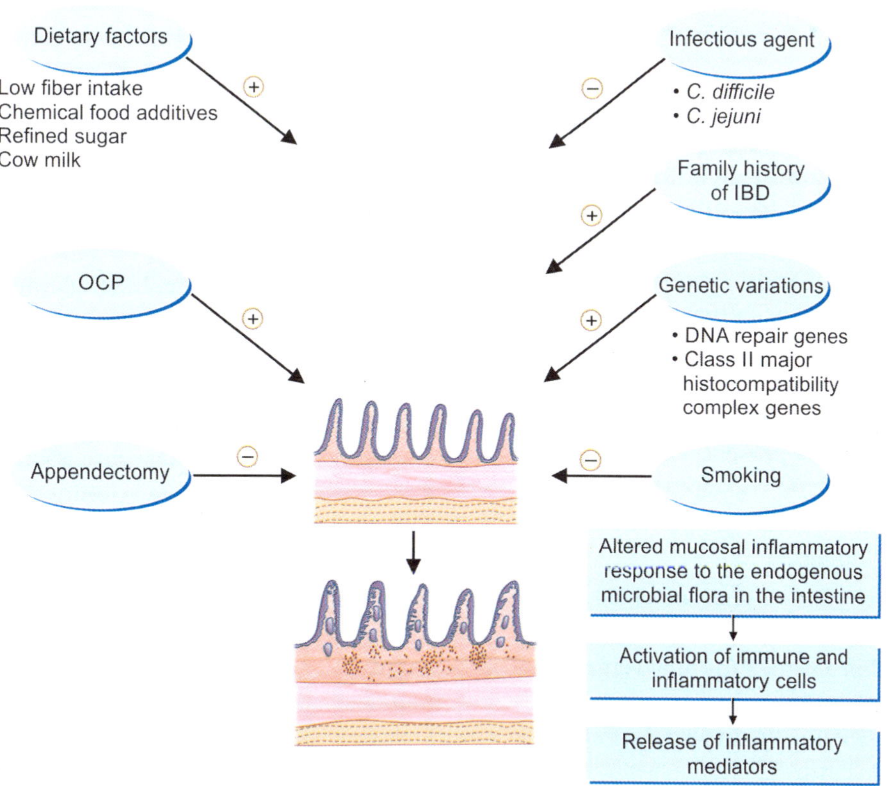

Macroscopic and Microscopic Appearance

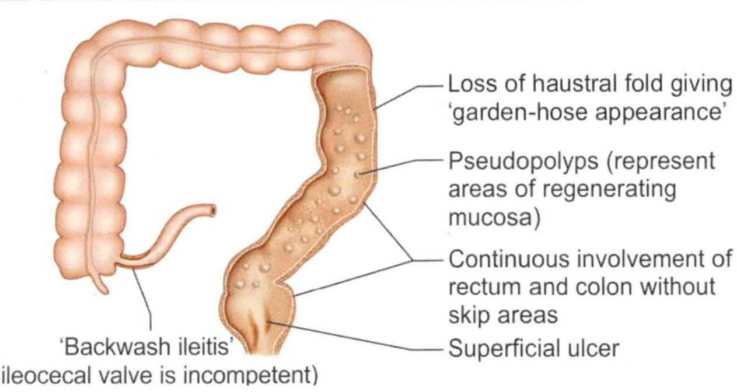

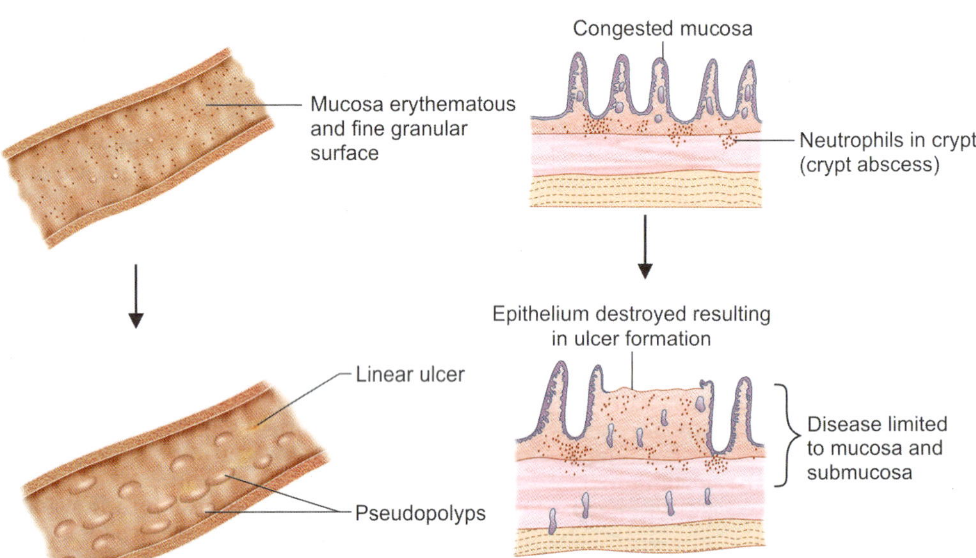

Clinical Presentation

The initial presentation of ulcerative colitis are the symptoms of proctitis, namely, rectal bleeding, urgency, and tenesmus. Other symptoms are increased frequency of bowel movements, watery stool mixed with blood and mucus, abdominal discomfort. **There is symptoms of active disease alternating with periods of remission.** Clinical presentation mostly depends on the extent of disease involvement. **Patients with proctitis** commonly present with urgency and tenesmus (sensation of incomplete evacuation of bowel), while, **patients with pancolitis** present with abdominal cramping pain and bloody diarrhea.

Abdominal tenderness, blood with mucus in per rectal examination are common clinical findings.

Extent of ulcerative colitis is characterized by Montreal Classification system:

E1—Proctitis (within 18 cm of the anal verge, distal to the rectosigmoid junction); E2—Left-sided colitis (extending from the rectosigmoid junction to the splenic flexure); E3—Extensive colitis (extension proximal to splenic flexure).

Severity of Ulcerative Colitis (According to Truelove and Witt's Criteria)

- **Mild colitis—**<4 bowel movements daily, normal temperature and heart rate, hemoglobin >11 g/dL, ESR <30 mm/hour
- **Severe colitis—**>6 bloody stools/day along with any of the following: fever (temperature >37.5°C), tachycardia (heart rate >90 beats/min), anemia (hemoglobin <75% of normal), ESR >30 mm/hour.
- **Moderately severe colitis—**Intermediate between mild and severe.

Toxic or Fulminant Colitis

>10 bloody stools/day, fever (temperature >37.5°C), tachycardia (>90 beats per minute), anemia requiring transfusion.

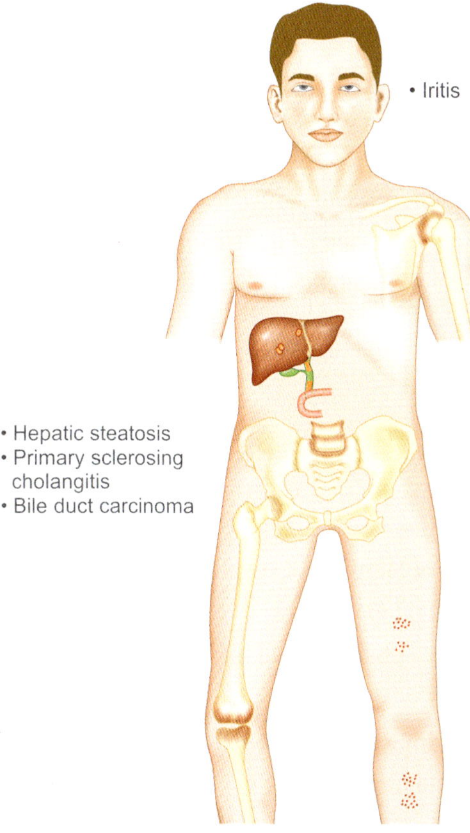

Extraintestinal Manifestations

Extraintestinal manifestations may develop about one-third of patients with ulcerative colitis.

Peripheral arthritis is the most common extraintestinal manifestation.

Other common extraintestinal manifestations are primary sclerosing cholangitis, pyoderma gangrenosum.

Toxic Megacolon

- Toxic megacolon is a rare, life-threatening complication of ulcerative colitis.
- It is characterized by **nonobstructive complete or segmental dilatation of colon exceeds 6 cm with systemic toxicity. The dilatation is typically most prominent in the transverse colon.**
- For diagnosis, proper history and clinical examination, plain radiograph of abdomen and awareness of this complication, are essential.
- **Medical therapy** is the first-line of treatment. Medical therapy consists of fluid resuscitation, correction of dyselectrolytemia, intravenous steroid therapy. Infliximab is the preferred second-line treatment.
- **Surgery is indicated** if no significant clinical improvement after 24–36 hours of aggressive medical therapy or any signs of perforation.
- Total abdominal colectomy with ileostomy and preservation of rectum is the **preferred surgical option**.

Other Causes of Toxic Megacolon

- Crohn's colitis
- *Clostridium difficile* colitis
- Infectious colitides (*Salmonella*, *Shigella*, Cytomegalovirus)

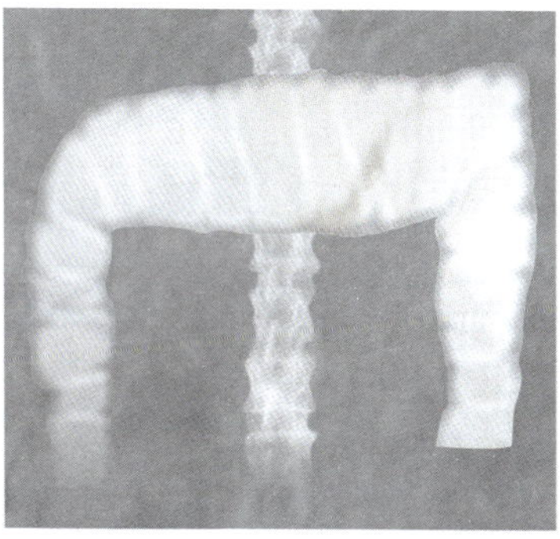

In plain radiograph, segmental or complete colonic dilatation >6 cm.

Diagnosis

Lower GI Endoscopy with Biopsy

Complete colonoscopy with examination of the ileum with biopsy is ideal for diagnosis but often associated with increased risk of perforation in severe disease. In severe disease, sigmoidoscopy with biopsy is sufficient.

Biopsy should be taken from diseased segment as well as from endoscopically normal-appearing proximal colon and distal rectum.

Upper GI Endoscopy

Upper GI endoscopy is indicated only in patients with symptoms of upper GI involvement.

CT Enterography or MR Enterography

Routinely not indicated in ulcerative colitis, but indicated for small bowel assessment where Crohn's disease is suspected. These imagings are also used to exclude other diagnosis based on symptoms and extraintestinal manifestations. CT abdomen is also indicated in suspected disease complications (e.g., colonic perforation).

Barium Enema

Role of barium enema is limited in the era of endoscopy. This imaging is particularly helpful to assess the colonic segment proximal to a colonic stricture. Barium enema should not be used in severe colitis.

Plain Radiograph of Abdomen

Abdominal X-ray is indicated if there is suspicion of colonic perforation or toxic megacolon.

Serologic Markers

Perinuclear antineutrophil cytoplasmic antibodies (pANCAs) may be found in about 70% of patients with ulcerative colitis, but cannot be used for establishing the diagnosis.

Endoscopic Findings in Ulcerative Colitis

- Continuously inflamed colonic segment involving the distal rectum
- Loss of vascular markings
- Friable mucosa
- Erosions, deep ulcerations, spontaneous bleeding.

CT Features Suggestive of Ulcerative Colitis

- Colonic mural thickening and enhancement
- Pericolonic fat stranding
- Rectal narrowing
- Widening of presacral space.

Radiological Evaluation of Ileoanal Pouch

- Pouchogram
- Pouch endoscopy
- Abdominal/pelvic MRI
- CT enterography

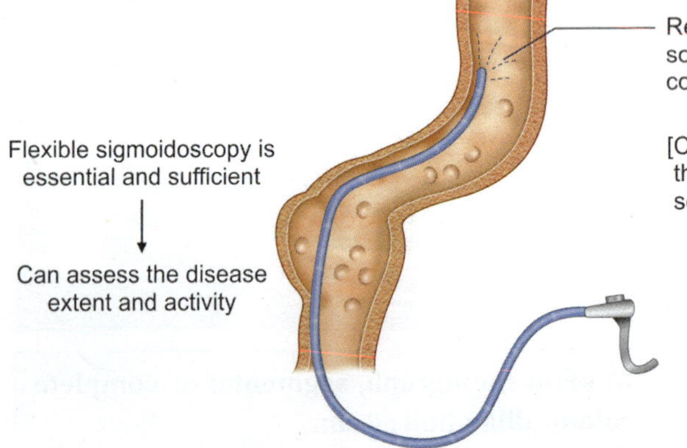

Assessment of Severity

Laboratory Investigations

- C-reactive protein (CRP), Erythrocyte sedimentation rate (ESR), Hemoglobin level, Serum albumin.
- Fecal calprotectin.

Quantitative Disease Activity Score

- Mayo score
- Simple Clinical Colitis Activity Index (SCCAI)
- Pediatric UC Activity Index (PUCAI).

Endoscopic Severity Score

Ulcerative Colitis Endoscopic Index of Severity (UCEIS) score

Mayo Score

Mayo score is based on: (i) stool frequency (Score 0–3); (ii) Rectal bleeding (Score 0–3); and (iii) Findings on endoscopy (Score 0–3).

Score 0: Normal; **Score 1:** Mild disease; **Score 2:** Moderate disease; **Score 3:** Severe disease.

Poor Prognostic Factors

- Age <40 years at diagnosis
- Extensive colitis (E3)
- Severe endoscopic disease (Mayo score 3, UCEIS score ≥7)
- Hospitalization for colitis
- Elevated CRP
- Low serum albumin

Calprotectin

- Calprotectin is a calcium- and zinc-binding protein, accounts for about 60% of soluble proteins in the cytosol fraction of neutrophils.
- **Fecal calprotectin (FC)** level is related to endoscopic and histologic severity of inflammation in ulcerative colitis.
- FC level may be used as marker of disease activity to guide treatment.

UCEIS score	Mayo endoscopic subscore	Endoscopic features
0	0	Normal
1–3	1	Erythema, decreased vascular pattern, mild friability.
4–6	2	Marked erythema, absent vascular pattern, friability, erosions.
7–8	3	Spontaneous bleeding, ulceration

Management

Medical Management

Induction of remission in mildly active ulcerative colitis

- **Mildly active ulcerative proctitis:** Rectal 5-aminosalicylate enema (1 g/day).
- **Mildly active left-sided ulcerative colitis:** Rectal 5-aminosalicylate enema (at least 1 g/day). Oral 5-ASA (at least 2 g/day) may be given along with rectal 5-ASA enema (at least 1 g/day).
- **Mildly active extensive colitis:** Oral 5-ASA (at least 2 g/day). Patients who are intolerant or nonresponsive to rectal and oral 5-ASA, budesonide multimatrix (9 mg/day) with a colonic deliver technology, is recommended for left-sided and extensive colitis.

Patients not responding to budesonide MMX, oral systemic corticosteroid (0.75–1 mg/kg oral prednisone-equivalent, not more than 60 mg/day) is recommended.

Maintenance of remission in mildly active ulcerative colitis

- **Mildly active ulcerative proctitis:** Rectal ASA (1 g/day)
- **Mildly active left-sided or extensive colitis:** Oral 5-ASA (at least 2g/d)

Induction of remission in moderately to severely active ulcerative colitis

- Budesonide MMX
- Oral systemic corticosteroids
- Anti-TNF therapy (infliximab, adalimumab).

Maintenance of remission in moderately to severely active ulcerative colitis

- Thiopurines
- Anti-TNF therapy
- Vedolizumab
- Tofacitinib

Systemic corticosteroid should not be used for maintenance of remission.

Rectal 5-ASA Agent

Mesalamine

Oral 5-ASA Agents

- Mesalamine
- Olsalazine
- Sulfasalazine

Budesonide

A second-generation corticosteroid with high first-pass metabolism and minimal systemic side effects. Oral formulations of budesonide release the drug only in the distal ileum and proximal colon.

Budesonide Multimatrix

Budesonide-MMX is a once-daily novel oral formulation for topical release throughout the colon by using Multimatrix technology.

Mesalamine multimatrix preparation is also available.

Opioids and **anticholinergics** should be avoided in acute severe ulcerative colitis as they may precipitate colonic dilation and toxicity.

Management of Acute Severe Ulcerative Colitis

- Patient should be admitted to the hospital.
- Fluid resuscitation with correction of dyselectrolytemia, intravenous corticosteroid therapy (methylprednisolone 60 mg/d or hydrocortisone 100 mg 3–4 times per day) should be initiated immediately. If patient not responding to IV corticosteroid therapy within 3–5 days, then medical rescue therapy with infliximab or cyclosporine should be considered.
- All patients need close monitoring to detect any symptoms of complications that need surgical rescue therapy (e.g., colonic perforation, toxic megacolon, massive hemorrhage).
- Stool testing for *C.difficile* infection is recommended for all patients.

Surgical Management

Emergency indications

- Acute severe ulcerative colitis, not responding to medical rescue therapy
- Acute fulminant colitis, not responding to medical therapy
- Toxic megacolon, not responding to medical therapy or with any signs of perforation
- Colonic perforation
- Severe colorectal bleeding
- Acute obstruction from colonic stricture

Elective indications

- Chronic refractory ulcerative colitis
- Dysplasia-associated lesion or mass (DALM) detected by colonoscopy
- Colorectal carcinoma
- Presence of extraintestinal manifestations
- Failure of medical therapy

Surgical options for Ulcerative colitis

- Total proctocolectomy with IPAA (ileal-pouch anal anastomosis)—**surgical procedure of choice.**
- Total proctocolectomy with Brooke ileostomy
- Total proctocolectomy with continent ileostomy (Kock pouch)
- Total abdominal colectomy with ileorectal anastomosis

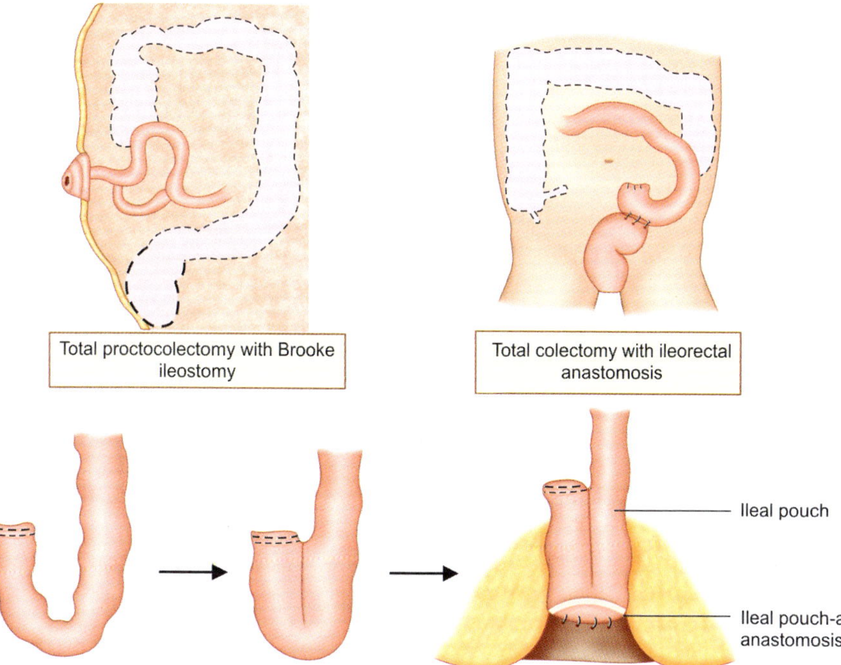

Total proctocolectomy with Brooke ileostomy

Total colectomy with ileorectal anastomosis

Total proctocolectomy with Ileal pouch-anal anastomosis (IPAA) — **most preferred procedure**

Extraintestinal Manifestations not Improved after Surgery

- Ankylosing spondylitis
- Primary sclerosing cholangitis
- Pyoderma gangrenosum.

Chronic Refractory Ulcerative Colitis

Patients who are refractory to induction of remission with biologics, corticosteroids, or small molecule therapies or Patients who are corticosteroid dependent.

Complications of Total Proctocolectomy with IPAA

- Related to pelvic dissection—sexual and bladder dysfunction, infertility
- Related to anastomosis—anastomotic leak, pelvic abscess, fistula, stricture
- Related to pouch—pouch failure, pouchitis, pouch leakage
- Prepouch ileitis (nonspecific inflammation proximal to the pouch in the neoterminal ileum).

Types of Ileal Pouch

- S-pouch (Parks, 1978)
- J-pouch (Utsonomiya, 1980)
- W-pouch (Nicholls, 1984)

The J-pouch is the most preferred ileal pouch design.

Total Proctocolectomy with IPAA (Ileal Pouch-anal Anastomosis)

This operative procedure involves total colectomy, proctectomy, formation of an ileal pouch, and ileal pouch-anal anastomosis. This is the surgical procedure of choice in ulcerative colitis.

Advantages: (i) Complete disease removal with preservation of intestinal continuity; (ii) Acceptable stool frequency; (iii) Good fecal continence; and (iv) Quality of life (QoL) is better than Brooke ileostomy, Kock pouch.

Total Proctocolectomy with Brooke Ileostomy

This operative procedure involves total colectomy, resection of rectum and anal canal (intersphincteric) and creation of a permanent Brooke ileostomy. **This procedure may be considered** in elderly patients not suitable for total proctocolectomy with IPAA and in patients with poor sphincter function. **The main drawback** of this procedure is a permanent stoma, which causes altered body image.

Total Proctocolectomy with Continent Ileostomy (Kock Pouch)

This procedure involves proctocolectomy with creation of an ileal pouch with a valve mechanism, to make the ileostomy continent. No external appliance is required. **The indications are:** (i) Pouch failure after IPAA and redo IPAA is not feasible and (ii) Patient wants conversion after Brooke ileostomy due to dissatisfaction with ileostomy.

Total Abdominal Colectomy with Ileorectal Anastomosis

This operative procedure involves total colectomy with restoration of intestinal continuity by ileorectal anastomosis. **The indications are:** (i) Patient with indeterminate colitis and (ii) Patient wants to avoid IPAA or a permanent stoma. **Absolute contraindications are:** (i) Active rectal disease; (ii) Associated rectal dysplasia or carcinoma; and (iii) Incompetence of anal sphincters.

Complications of Kock Pouch

- Sepsis
- Incontinence
- Valve prolapse
- Dysfunction of valve
- Pouchitis.

Complications of Total Proctocolectomy with Brooke Ileostomy

- Related to pelvic dissection—sexual and bladder dysfunction.
- Related to stoma—peristomal skin changes, retraction, parastomal herniation, prolapse.
- Delayed perineal wound healing.

Complications of Total Abdominal Colectomy with Ileorectal Anastomosis

- Anastomotic leakage
- Pelvic sepsis
- Late carcinogenesis in rectum
- Proctitis.

Surveillance Colonoscopy to Detect Dysplasia or Colorectal Carcinoma in Ulcerative Colitis

- Annual surveillance colonoscopy (standard or high-definition white-light endoscopy) should be started 8 years after diagnosis in patients with pancolitis and left-sided colitis. If no dysplasia is detected, subsequent surveillance colonoscopy should be performed every 3 years for 10 years, biennially for the next 10 years and then annually. Patients with primary sclerosing cholangitis should undergo annual surveillance colonoscopy from the time of diagnosis.
- Two to four random biopsies should be taken at 10 cm intervals along with targeted biopsies from suspicious lesions (e.g., raised lesions, abnormal pit patterns, irregular plaques). Dye spray chromoendoscopy with methylene blue or indigo carmine are recommended for better identification of dysplasia.

Factors Associated with Increased Risk of Malignancy

- Risk is more in pancolitis (proximal to the splenic flexure) than left-sided colitis
- Duration of disease (>8 years with pancolitis)
- Diagnosis of ulcerative colitis at a young age
- Family history of inflammatory bowel disease
- Comcomitant primary sclerosing cholangitis.

Colorectal Polyp

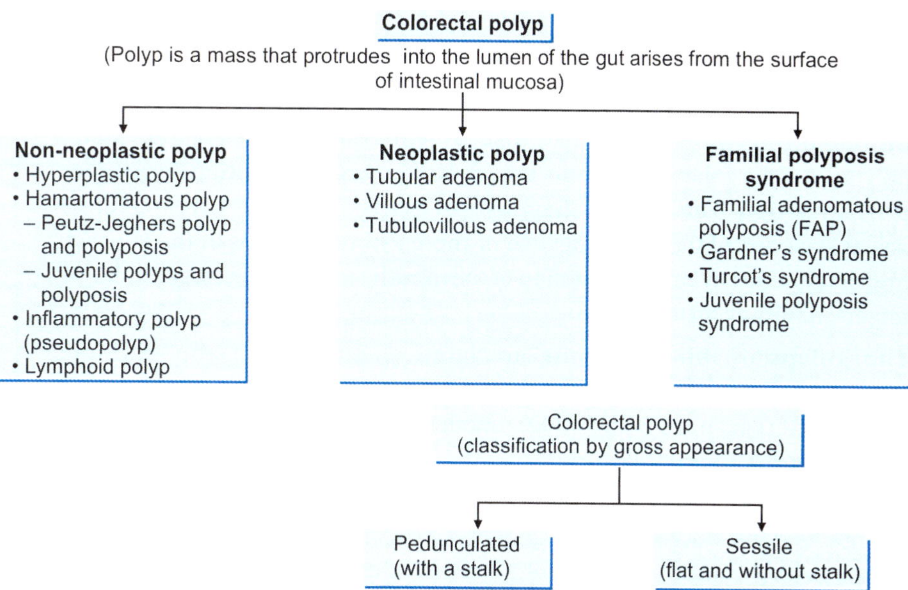

Hyperplastic Polyp

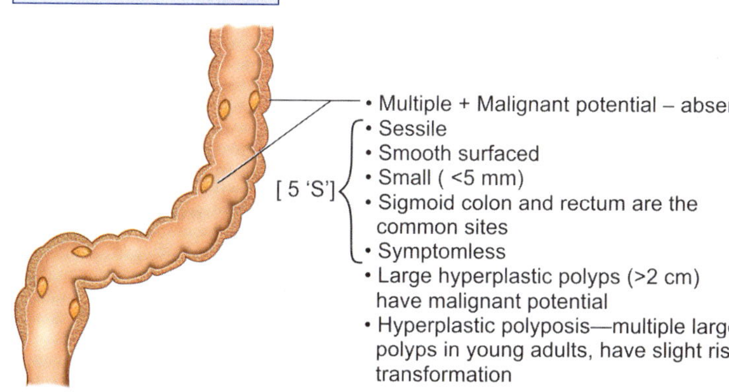

- Hyperplastic polyps are the **most common type of colorectal polyps.**
- These polyps are **usually less than 5 cm** (diminutive polyps).
- These polyps are sometimes cannot be distinguished from adenomatous polyps on colonoscopy.
- **"Resect and discard" strategy** may be considered for diminutive colonic polyps. **"Diagnose and leave behind" strategy** is appropriate for rectosigmoid diminutive hyperplastic polyps.

Hamartomatous Polyp

Hamartomatous polyps consist of connective tissue and smooth muscle covered by hypertrophic epithelium. These polyps appear as pedunculated, smooth polyps. These polyps may present as sporadic hamartomatous polyp (juvenile polyp) or as part of polyposis syndrome (Peutz-Jeghers syndrome, Juvenile polyposis syndrome).

Sporadic Hamartomatous Polyp (Juvenile Polyp)

Characteristic features of sporadic hamartomatous polyp: (i) Solitary; (ii) Smooth surfaced; (iii) Slightly lobulated; (iv) Stalk present; (v) Presents at an early age, usually below 5 years of age ('juvenile' polyp); (vi) No malignant potential; and (vii) Highly vascularized.

Patients commonly present with rectal bleeding. Sometimes, polyp with long pedicle may prolapse through anus.

Treatment is polypectomy.

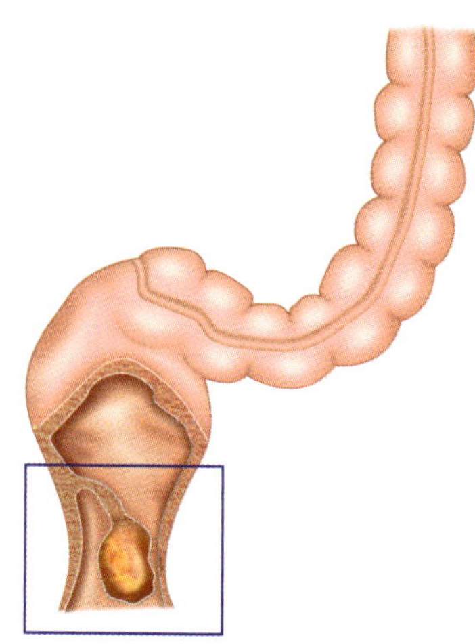

Juvenile rectal polyp.

Peutz-Jeghers Syndrome (PJS)

An autosomal dominant polyposis syndrome (due to germline mutations in the *STK11* gene on chromosome 19p13.3) characterized by **polyposis of the small intestine** (mostly the proximal jejunum) and, to a lesser extent, polyposis of the colon and rectum, **mucocutaneous pigmentation** and **cancer predisposition**. **The clinical diagnosis of PJS** is made when an individual has at least two of the following: two or more PJS-type polyps of the GI tract, mucocutaneous hyperpigmentation of the mouth, lips, nose, eyes, genitalia, or fingers; or family history of PJS.

The polyps of this syndrome are large, pedunculated and multiple hamartomatous polyps throughout the GI tract. Histologically, these polyps are characterized by interdigitating smooth muscle bundles in a characteristic branching tree appearance throughout the lamina propria.

Mucocutaneous hyperpigmentation presents as dark bluish macules in perioral regions, buccal mucosa, genital region, hands and feet. The macules appear at birth and may fade in puberty and childhood.

Patients are at increased risk of wide variety of epithelial malignancies (colorectal, stomach, pancreas, breast, ovary). Risk of colorectal cancer is highest among different malignancies, followed by breast and the stomach. Females are also at risk of sex cord tumors with annular tubules (SCTAT), a benign tumor of ovaries and males are at risk of Sertoli cell tumor of testes.

Clinical presentation of GI polyps are GI bleeding, intussusception, intestinal obstruction. **Small bowel polypectomy** is indicated for all polyps causing symptoms and polyps more than 1 cm.

Recommended screening program for patients known to have PJS are: (i) Colonoscopy every 2–3 years, beginning at age 20 years; (ii) Mammography and breast MRI annually and clinical breast examination every 6 months, beginning at age 25 years; (iii) Upper GI endoscopy (for screening of gastric cancer) every 2–3 years, beginning at age 20 years; (iv) CT or MR enterography or video capsule endoscopy (for screening of small intestinal cancer), beginning at age 8–10 years; (v) MRCP with contrast or EUS every 1–2 years, beginning at age 30 years; (vi) Pap smear and pelvic examination annually, beginning at age 18–20 years; and (vii) Testicular examination and observation for feminizing changes annually, beginning at age 10 years.

Juvenile Polyposis Syndrome (JPS)

An autosomal dominant polyposis syndrome characterized by multiple hamartomatous polyps in the colon (mostly right-sided colon) and rectum, present during childhood. **The clinical diagnosis of Juvenile polyposis syndrome** is met if an individual fulfills any of the three criterias: (i) At least five juvenile polyps in the colon; (ii) multiple juvenile polyps throughout the GI tract; and (iii) at least one juvenile polyp in an individual with a family history of JPS.

Polyps may be transformed into adenoma and eventually carcinoma. Treatment is prophylactic surgery. Total abdominal colectomy with ileorectal anastomosis is preferred if rectum is not involved. If rectum is involved, surgery of choice is total proctocolectomy with ileal pouch-anal anastomosis.

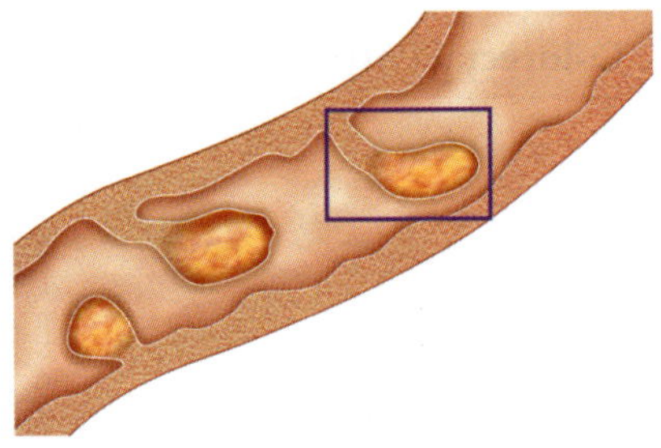

Multiple, pedunculated hamartomatous polyps in Peutz-Jeghers syndrome.

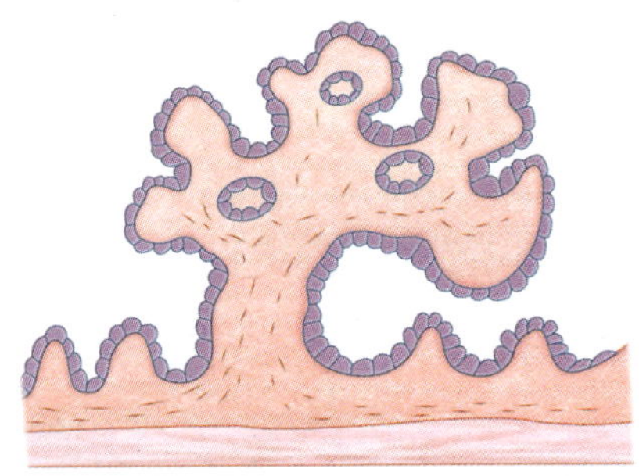

Characteristic histologic appearance (branching tree) of Peutz-Jeghers polyps.

Extraintestinal Sites of Polyps in Peutz-Jeghers Syndrome

- Renal pelvis
- Bronchus
- Gallbladder
- Nasal passages
- Urinary bladder
- Ureter

Genetic Events Associated with Juvenile Polyposis Syndrome

- Mutations in *SMAD4* gene
- Mutations in *BMPR1A* gene

Inflammatory Polyp (Pseudopolyp)

- Inflammatory polyps develop due to re-epithelialization on the undermined ulcers in inflammatory bowel disease, mostly in **Ulcerative colitis and rarely in Crohn's disease**. This type of polyp also may develop after **amebic colitis, ischemic colitis**.
- **These are not true polyps.** These polyps have no malignant potential, but these polyps cannot be differentiated from adenomatous polyps in colonoscopy.
- **Treatment** is polypectomy.

Adenomatous Polyp

Adenomatous polyps are benign neoplastic colorectal polyps originating from the mucus-secreting colonic epithelium. **Adenomatous polyps are histologically classified into:** (i) Tubular adenoma; (ii) Villous adenoma; and (iii) Tubulovillous adenoma.

Tubular Adenoma

Tubular adenoma is the most common type (65–80% of adenomatous polyp). These polyps have histological appearance of branched tubular glands (glandular elements more than 75%). Most commonly found in the distal colon and rectum. Polyps may be single or multiple, pedunculated or sessile. Tubular adenomas are usually pedunculated. The malignant potential of an adenoma depends on size (>5 mm), growth pattern and degree of epithelial atypia.

Villous Adenoma

These polyps are most commonly found in the rectosigmoid area, but may be located anywhere in the colon. Villous adenomas have histological appearance of long, finger-like projections (villous fronds). These polyps are more commonly sessile and likely to have severe atypia or dysplasia.

Tubulovillous Adenoma

These adenomatous polyps have both tubular and villous components. About 10–25% of adenomatous polyps are tubulovillous type.

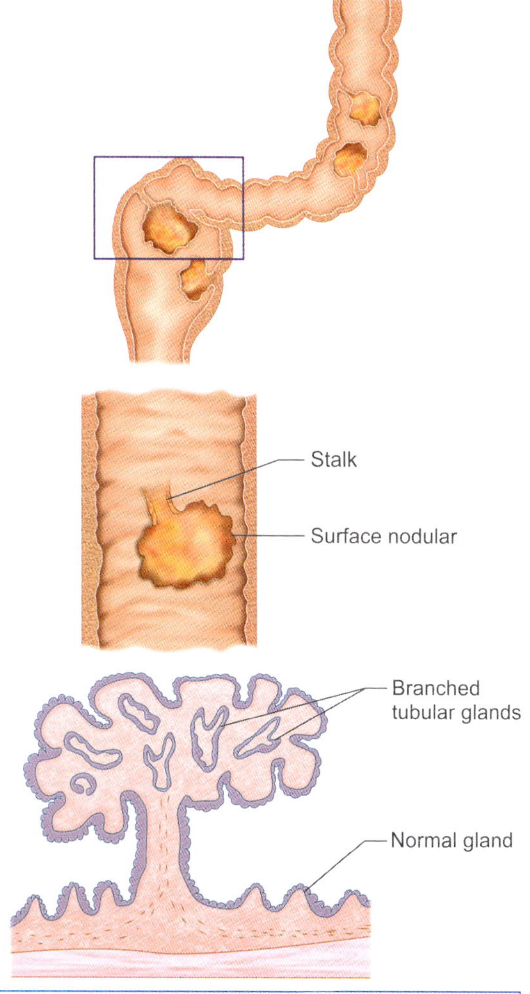

Macroscopic and microscopic appearance of tubular adenoma.

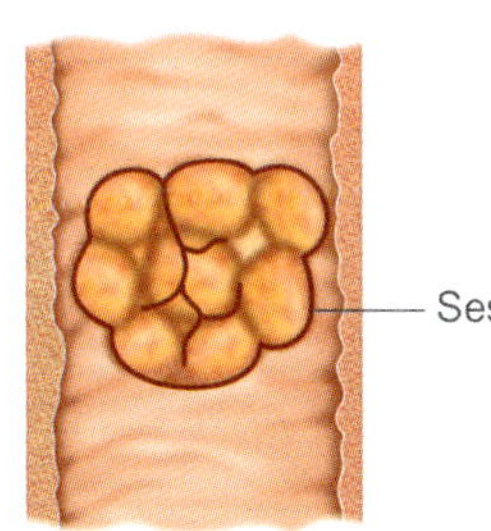

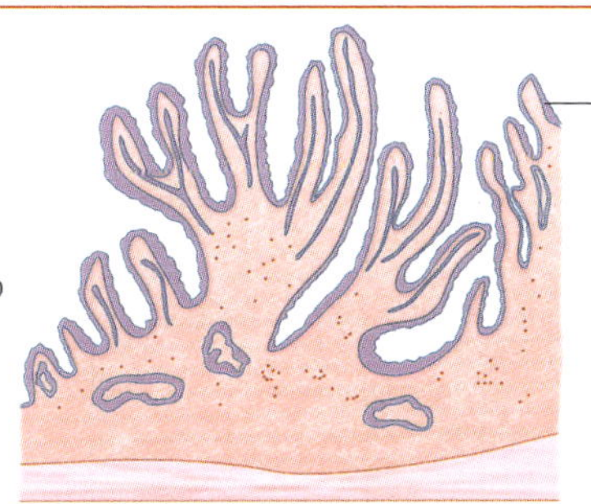

Macroscopic and microscopic appearance of villous adenoma.

Clinical Presentation

Most of the adenomatous polyps are asymptomatic and only detected during screening colonoscopy. Larger polyps may present with lower GI bleeding, obstruction. Secretory diarrhea associated with hypokalemia (Mckittrick-Wheelock syndrome) is a rare presentation of villous adenoma.

Management

Cold snare polypectomy is the preferred technique for resection of diminutive polyps (≤ 5 mm). This technique is also preferred for resection of sessile polyps 6–9 mm in size.

Hot snare polypectomy (with or without submucosal injection of normal saline or hyaluronic acid) is the most commonly used technique for resection of sessile polyps 10 mm or more. HSP is also the preferred technique for resection of pedunculated polyps. For resection of large pedunculated polyps, pretreatment of the stalk with mechanical hemostasis (with endoloops or clips) or injection of dilute adrenaline is recommended to decrease the risk of postpolypectomy bleeding.

Endoscopic mucosal resection (EMR) is recommended for large, laterally spreading and sessile polyps ≥20 mm in size.

Surgery is indicated for (i) resection of colonic and rectal lesions with high suspicion of submucosal invasive carcinoma; (ii) Pedunculated polyp with Haggitt's criteria level 4; and (iii) Multiple polyps.

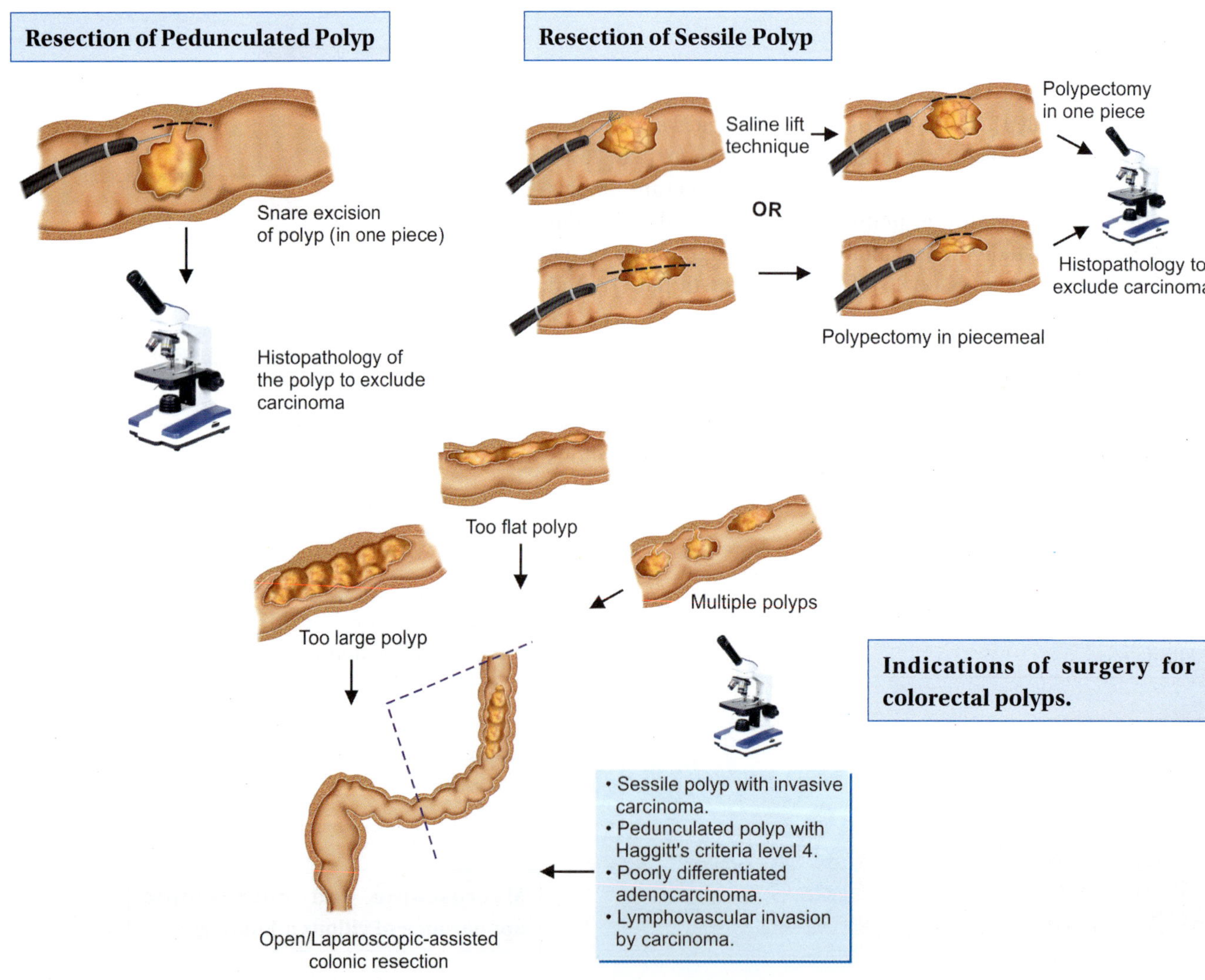

Indications of surgery for colorectal polyps.

Familial Adenomatous Polyposis (FAP)

FAP is an **autosomal dominant polyposis syndrome** characterized by **germline mutation in the *APC* gene** (chromosome 5q21), presence of **multiple adenomatous polyps (>100) in the large intestine** and **extracolonic polyps, presence of extraintestinal manifestations** and **cancer predisposition.**

Colonic mucosa is studded with hundred to thousands of adenomatous polyps. Gastric, duodenal and periampullary polyps (adenomatous polyps) may also found. Most of the gastric polyps are basically fundic gland hyperplasia.

Extraintestinal manifestations include congenital hypertrophy of the retinal pigmented epithelium (CHRPE), desmoid tumors, osteoma of the skull, mandible, supernumerary teeth.

The lifetime for colorectal cancer in FAP patients approaches 100% by the age 50 if colon is not surgically removed. Most of the cancers develop in the left colon. Patients with FAP are also at increased risk of other malignancies, including duodenal cancer, hepatoblastoma, thyroid cancer, and gastric cancer.

Variants of FAP

The variants of FAP are: (i) Attenuated FAP; (ii) Gardner's syndrome; and (iii) Turcot's syndrome.

Patients with attenuated FAP present with fewer polyps (10-100) later in life. These polyps are mostly diminutive sessile adenomatous polyps, commonly develop in the right colon. APC gene mutation found in only about 30% of patients. The onset of colorectal carcinoma is delayed compared to classical FAP. Risks of other cancers are same as classical FAP.

Gardner's syndrome includes colonic polyps, epidermal inclusion cyst, osteomas, desmoid tumor. **Turcot's syndrome** includes colonic polyps, brain tumors (glioblastoma multiforme and medulloblastoma).

Genetic testing

When a patient clinically diagnosed as FAP, genetic testing should be done to detect *APC* gene mutations. Screening of first-degree relatives in patients with FAP (patient is positive for *APC* gene mutation or no mutation is found or genetic testing is not done): Sigmoidoscopy at age 10–12 years, then annually up to age 35, then every 3 years. Upper GI endoscopy every 1–3 years, starting when colorectal polyp is first detected.

Management

Treatment is prophylactic surgery. Three different surgical options available for classical FAP and attenuated FAP: (i) Total proctocolectomy with ileal pouch anal anastomosis (most preferred procedure); (ii) Total abdominal colectomy with ileorectal anastomosis; and (iii) Total proctocolectomy with permanent end ileostomy.

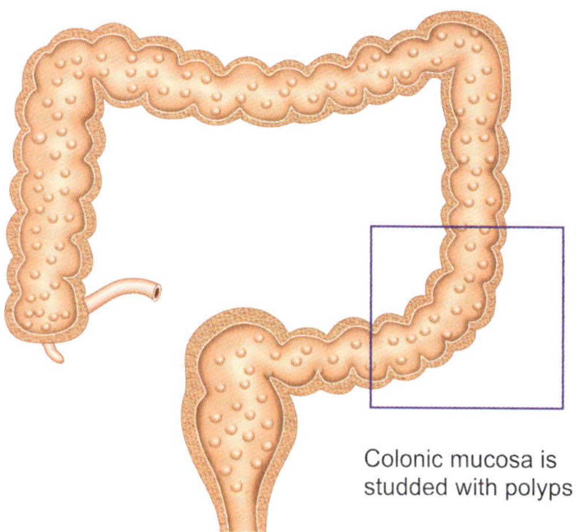

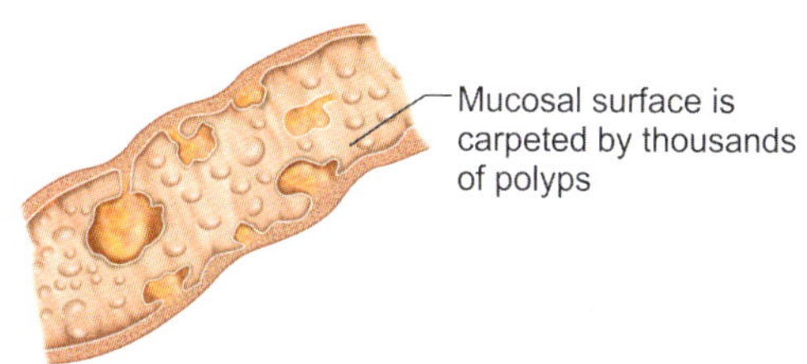

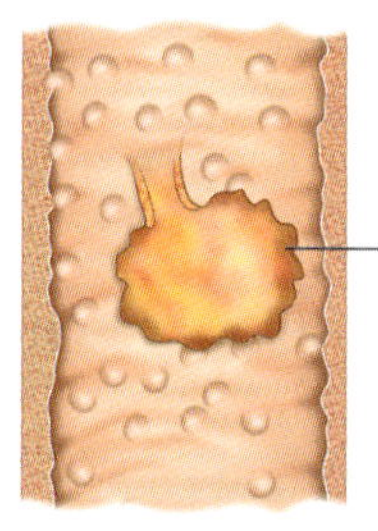

Congenital Hypertrophy of the Retinal Pigmented Epithelium (CHRPE)

- CHRPE is present as early as at 3 months of age in affected persons (with APC mutation).
- This abnormality predicts FAP with 97% sensitivity. This abnormality can be detected in about two-third of patients of FAP by indirect ophthalmoscopy.
- This is the most common and earliest extracolonic manifestation in FAP patients.
- CHRPE occurs in patients with mutations in the central portion of the gene.

Colon Cancer

Most common malignancy of the GI tract.

Types of Colon Cancer

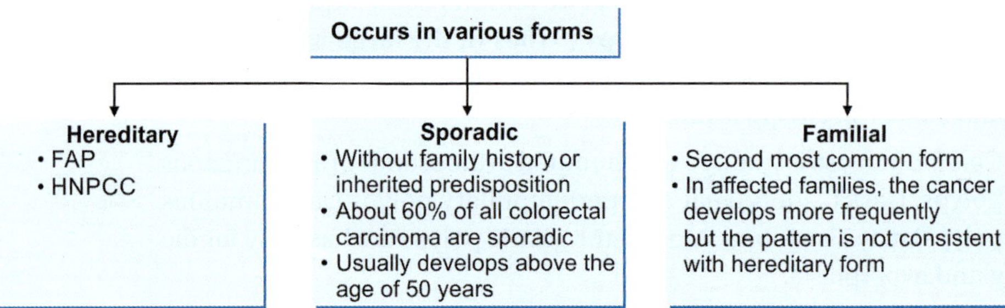

Other high-risk inherited syndromes

- MutY human homolog (MUTYH)-associated polyposis (MAP)
- Peutz-Jeghers syndrome
- Juvenile polyposis syndrome
- Serrated polyposis syndrome
- Turcot syndrome
- Gardner syndrome.

Characteristic Phenotypic Features of Lynch Syndrome

- Presence of less than 100 polyps (diminutive and flat)
- Preferential right-sided colonic tumor location
- Multiple synchronous and colorectal cancers
- Poorly differentiated tumors
- Crohn's like lymphoid reaction (peri-tumoral lymphocyte aggregates).

In Women with Lynch Syndrome

- Colon cancer is most common
- Endometrial cancer is second most common.

Lynch Syndrome (Hereditary Nonpolyposis Colorectal Cancer, HNPCC)

- Lynch syndrome is the most common inherited syndrome responsible for colon cancer predisposition. About 2–5% colorectal cancers arise from this inherited cancer syndrome. Patients with Lynch syndrome have up to 80% lifetime risk for developing colorectal carcinoma.
- This syndrome is caused by germline mutations in one of the four DNA mismatch repair genes *(MLH1, MSH2, MSH6, or PMS2)*. Deletions in the *EPCAM* (Epithelial cell adhesion molecule) gene may also cause Lynch syndrome.
- This syndrome predisposes to extracolonic malignancies involving the endometrium (up to 60% life time risk), stomach, ovary, pancreas, ureter and renal pelvis, biliary tract, brain, and small intestine, as well as keratoacanthoma and sebaceous gland adenoma.

Diagnosis

Initially, the diagnosis of Lynch syndrome was based on Amsterdam criteria II. Germline sequencing of the mismatch repair genes now the gold standard for diagnosis of this syndrome. Bethesda guideline was developed and later updated to identify patients who should be tested for microsatellite instability.

Cancer Surveillance in Patients with Lynch Syndrome

- Colon cancer surveillance: Colonoscopy should be started between 20 and 25 or 2 and 5 years younger than the youngest diagnosis age in the family, which one is earlier and should be repeated every 1–2 years.
- There is no clear evidence to recommend screening for cancer of endometrium, ovary, stomach, duodenum, small bowel, pancreas, and brain.

Management

Total colectomy with ileorectal anastomosis is treatment of choice in patients with Lynch syndrome with colon cancer or endoscopic resection of polyps not feasible. Less-extensive surgical procedures should be considered for patients older than 60–65 years or those with underlying sphincter dysfunction.

Risk Factors

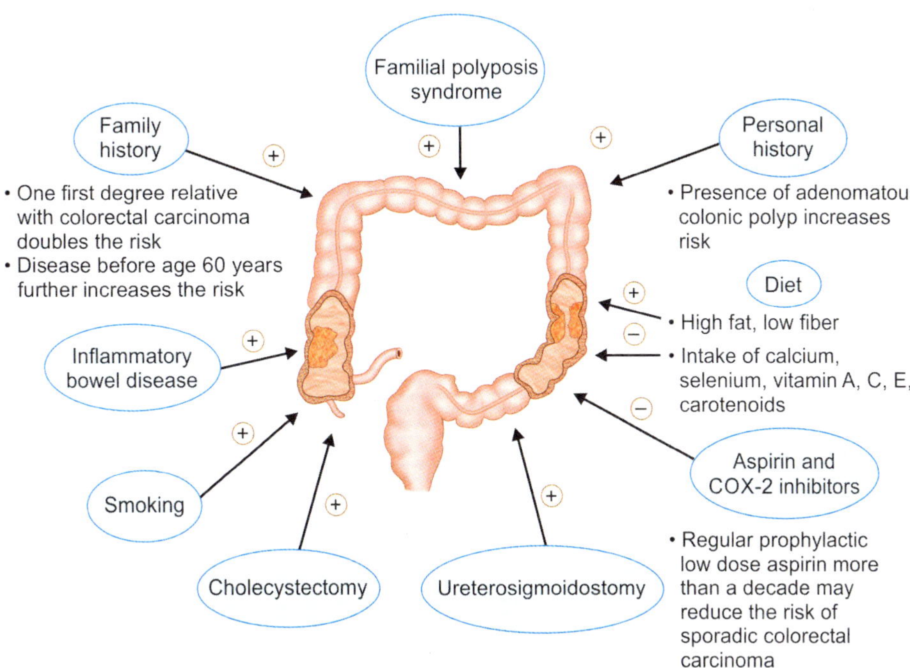

Molecular Pathways of Colorectal Cancer

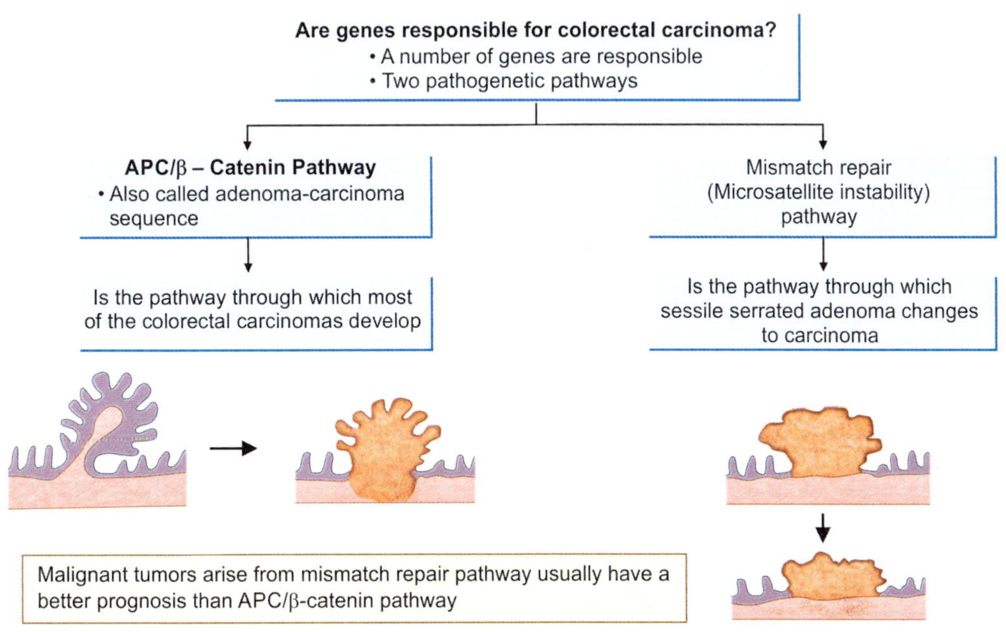

Adenoma-carcinoma Sequence

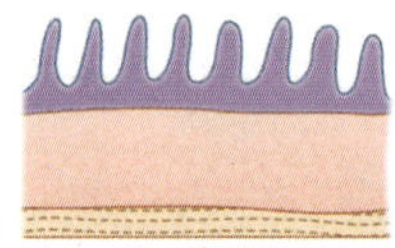

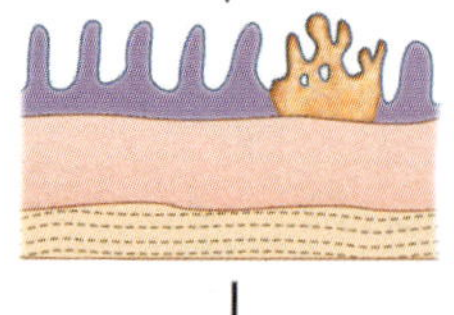

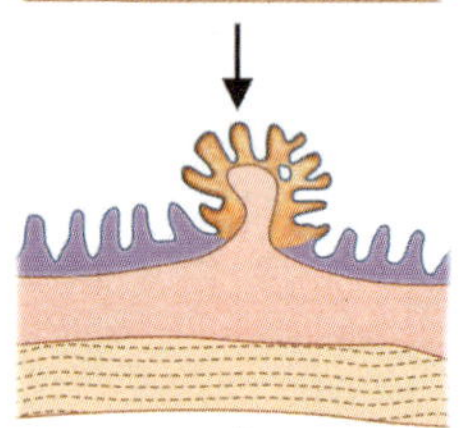

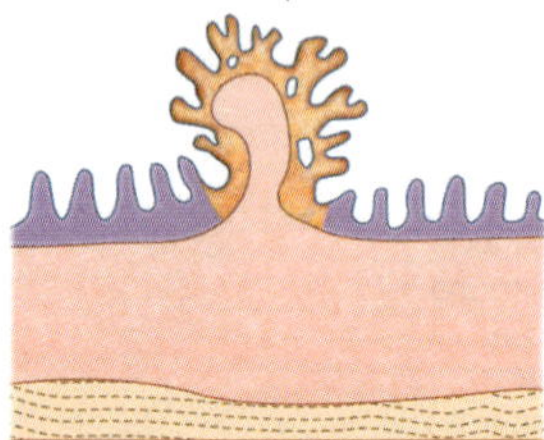

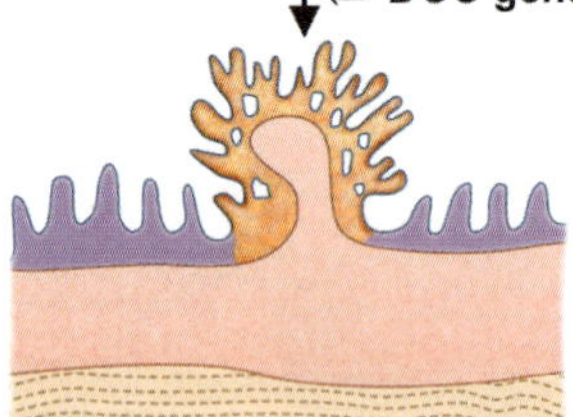

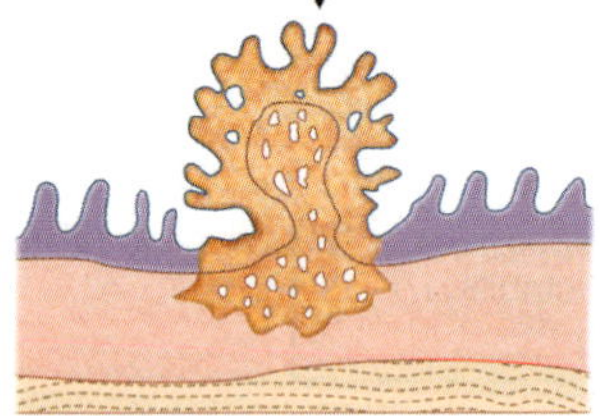

Genetic Events Associated with Colon Carcinoma

- *APC* gene mutation
- *KRAS* gene mutation
- *NRAS* gene mutation
- *BRAF* gene mutation
- *P53* gene mutation
- *PIK3CA* gene mutation
- *DCC* gene deletion
- Microsatellite instability-high (MSI-H).

Characteristic Features of MSI-H Colorectal Tumors

- Tumors are commonly right-sided and high grade.
- Tumors are larger at the time of diagnosis but not commonly associated with lymph node metastasis.
- Commonly associated with increased peritumoral lymphocytic infiltration.
- Better long-term prognosis than microsatellite-stable (MSS) tumors.

Macroscopic and Microscopic Appearance

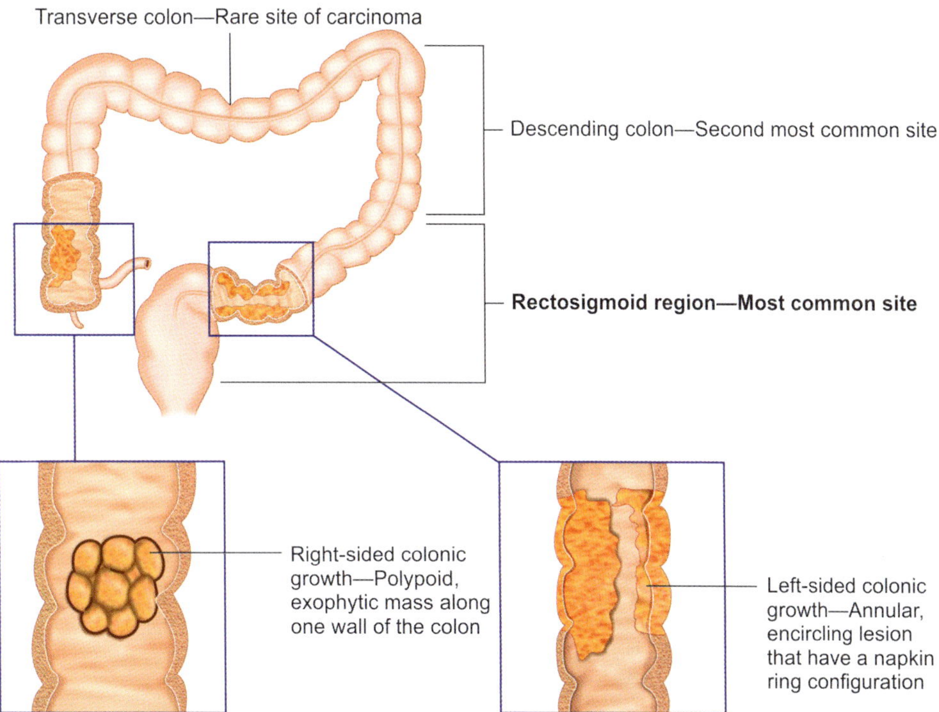

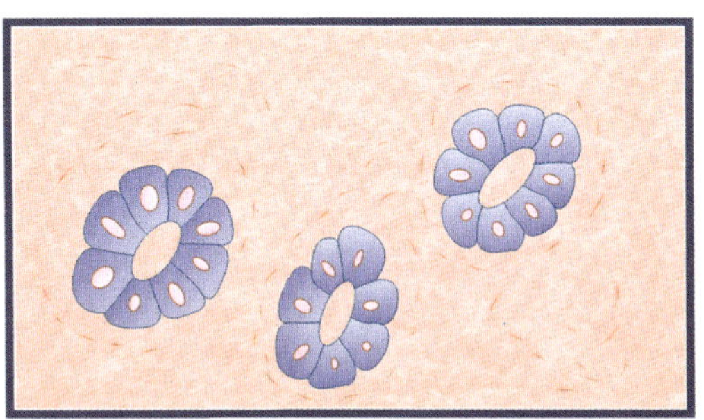

Histologic appearance of adenocarcinoma.

- **Signet ring cell adenocarcinoma** carries adverse prognosis.
- **Small cell carcinoma** carries adverse prognosis.
- Prognosis of **mucinous adenocarcinoma** is controversial.
- **Medullary carcinoma** is associated with MSI-H.

Most of the colonic carcinomas are adenocarcinomas (well differentiated, moderately differentiated, and poorly differentiated).

Other uncommon histologic types are:

- Neuroendocrine carcinoma
- Small cell carcinoma (high grade neuroendocrine tumor)
- Squamous cell carcinoma
- Adenosquamous carcinoma
- Spindle cell carcinoma
- Medullary carcinoma
- Undifferentiated carcinoma.

Histologic variants of adenocarcinoma:

- Mucinous adenocarcinoma
- Signet ring cell adenocarcinoma (more than 50% cells showing "signet ring" morphology).

Spread of Colon Cancer

Spread of colonic carcinoma
- Local spread
- Lymphatic spread
- Hematogenous spread

Local Spread

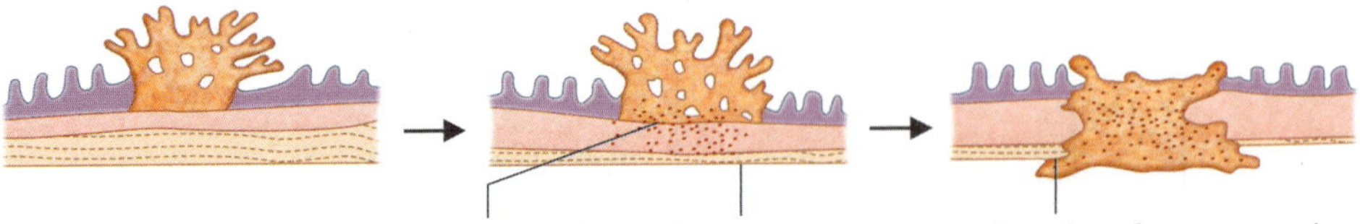

Lymphatic Spread

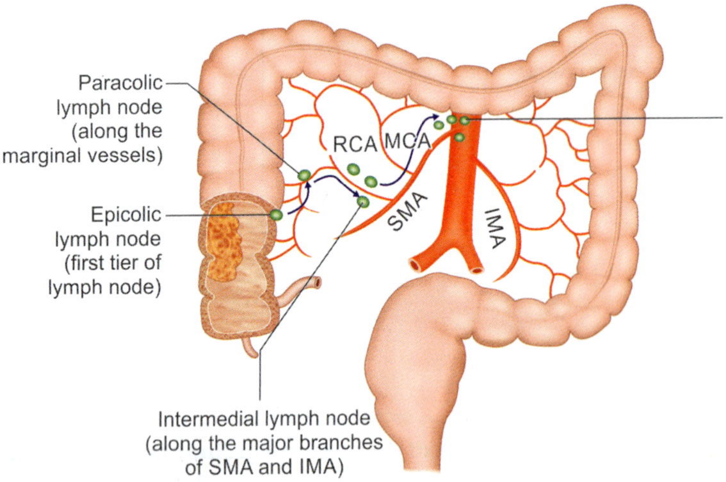

Submucosal lymphatics
↓
Epicolic lymph nodes
↓
Paracolic lymph nodes
↓
Intermediate lymph nodes
↓
Principal lymph nodes

Types of Regional Lymph Nodes of Colon

- **Epicolic lymph nodes:** Lymph nodes that are located in the colonic wall under the peritoneum.
- **Paracolic lymph nodes:** Lymph nodes that are present along the marginal vessels.
- **Intermediate lymph nodes:** Lymph nodes that are present along the major branches of superior or inferior mesenteric artery.
- **Apical (Principal) lymph nodes:** Lymph nodes that are present around the origin of SMA/IMA.

Hematogenous Spread

- **Liver** and **peritoneum** are the two most common sites of metastases. Liver is the most common site of visceral metastases. Colorectal liver metastases (CRLM) either present as synchronous mestastases or metachronous metastases. About 20% of patients present with **synchronous metastases**. About half of the patients eventually develop **metachronous liver metastases**. The metastatic spread to the liver is through the portal venous system.
- **Peritoneal metastasis** is associated with poor prognosis compared to other metastatic sites.
- **Other sites of metastases** are lungs, brain, bones, ovaries.

Clinical Presentation

Growth in right colon

Palpable lump in upper abdomen with anemia

- Closed loop obstruction (in the setting of patent ileocecal valve and occlusive growth in right colon)
- Anemia (due to occult blood loss)
- Mass in right iliac fossa
- Symptoms and signs of appendicitis

⊙ Wide lumen and liquid feces in right colon—Decreased chance of obstruction

Growth in left colon

- Change in bowel habit
  - Alternate constipation and diarrhea
- Passage of blood and mucus in stool
- Narrow lumen and solid feces with stenosing growth
  - Increased chance of obstruction
- Lump in left iliac fossa

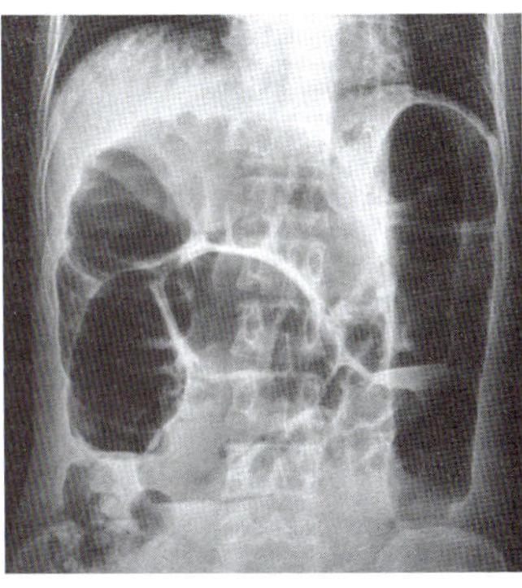

Straight X-ray abdomen findings suggestive of large gut obstruction.

- Careful history taking, particularly family history of colon polyps and colon cancer is important to suspect high-risk inherited syndromes.
- The clinical presentations of right-sided colon cancer and left-sided colon cancer are characteristically different. Advanced cancer may present with features of large gut obstruction or perforation or bleeding from tumor.

A middle aged or older patient recently presents with **alteration of bowel habit, colon cancer** should be in differential diagnosis.

Investigations

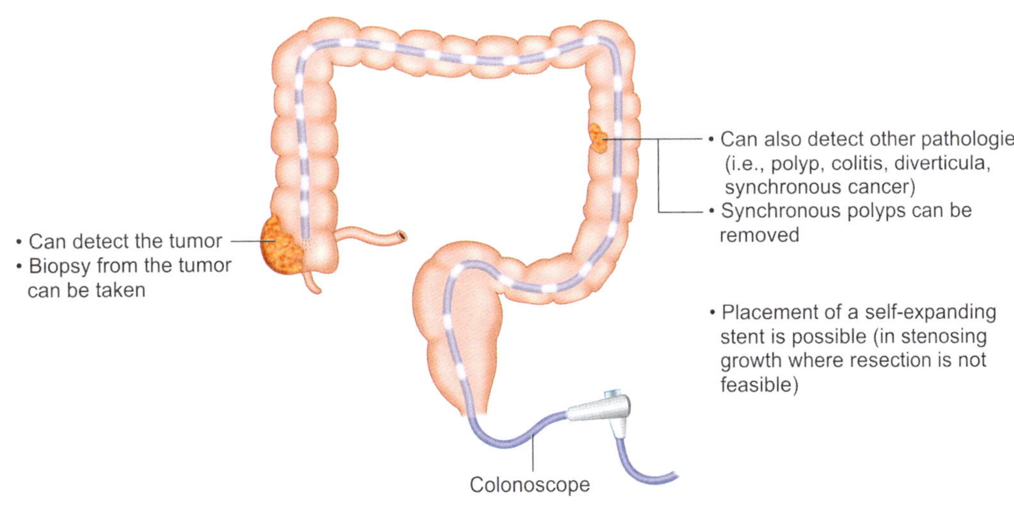

Colonoscopy

Colonoscopy is indicated to detect the location of the tumor as well as guided biopsy from the tumor for histologic diagnosis. Colonoscopy can also detect associated pathologies (i.e., synchronous adenoma, diverticula, synchronous cancer). Complete evaluation of the colorectal mucosa is essential to detect any synchronous cancer or adenoma.

CT Scan of Chest, Abdomen and Pelvis

- CT abdomen and pelvis with oral and IV contrast is indicated to detect distant metastases to abdominal organs (particularly liver), abdominal lymph nodes. CT abdomen can also detect adjacent organ involvement, that may the change the operative plan. CT chest is helpful to detect lung metastases.
- If CT with IV contrast is contraindicated, noncontrast chest CT with MRI of abdomen and pelvis with IV gadolinium-based contrast agent may be considered. If both iodinated contrast agent and gadolinium contrast are contraindicated, MRI abdomen and pelvis without contrast or PET/CT imaging may be considered.
- If there is difficulty to differentiate a proximal rectal cancer and a low-lying sigmoid cancer, MRI of abdomen and pelvis is particularly helpful.

CEA (Carcinoembryonic Antigen) Estimation

Preoperative CEA level estimation is indicated to establish a baseline value. During surveillance period, elevation of CEA level is indicative of recurrence.

Mismatch repair (MMR) or **Microsatellite instability (MSI)** testing is recommended in all newly diagnosed patients with colon cancer. All patients with metastatic colorectal cancer should be tested for **KRAS, NRAS and BRAF mutations.**

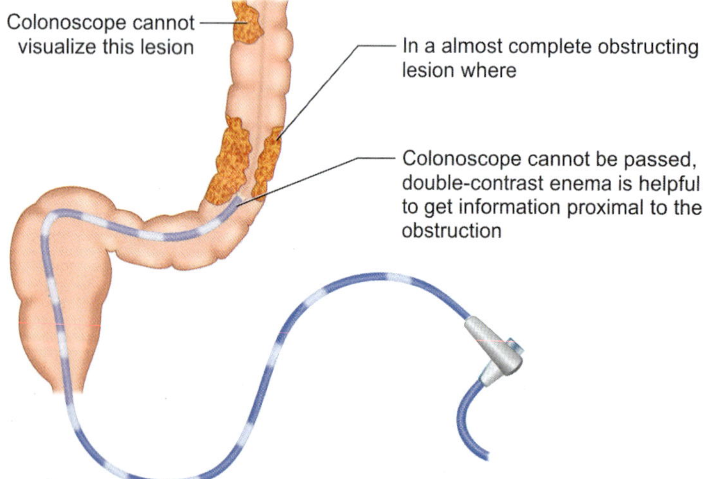

Complete Preoperative Colonic Evaluation in Presence of Endoscopically Obstructing Lesion

- CT colonography
- Colon capsule endoscopy
- Double-contrast enema (if no other options are available)

Management

In resectable colon cancer without widespread distant metastases, the treatment of choice is colectomy with en bloc removal of lymph nodes. The extent of colectomy depends on the location of the tumor and its lymphovascular drainage. In the absence of synchronous lesion, the 5–7 cm of proximal and distal margin must be maintained. The lymphadenectomy should include intermediate and central (pericolic) lymph nodes. Any suspicious nodes at the origin of the tumor feeding vessels (i.e., apical lymph node) and outside the field of dissection should be removed. Grossly involved adjacent organ should be removed en bloc.

Management of synchronous cancer: Synchronous cancers in the same segment of the colon are treated by segmental colectomy whereas synchronous cancers in the separate segments are treated by extended resection or two separate resections.

Management of colon cancer with underlying colonic disease (e.g., Lynch syndrome, ulcerative colitis): Colon cancer in a patient with Lynch syndrome is treated with total colectomy or segmental colectomy. Colon cancer in a patient with ulcerative colitis, proctocolectomy is the ideal surgical option.

Minimally invasive colectomy is a surgical option for colon cancer. Minimally invasive colectomy have demonstrated equivalent oncologic outcomes including overall and recurrence-free survival rates compared to open colectomy.

Management of liver and lung metastases: Presence of resectable synchronous liver or lung metastases can be treated by staged or simultaneous resection.

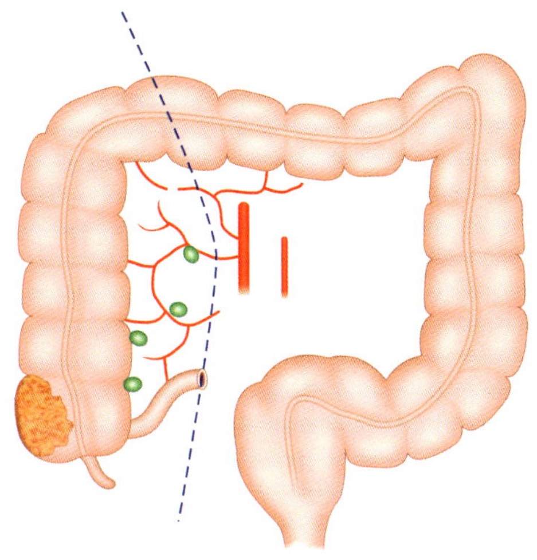

Resection of primary tumor

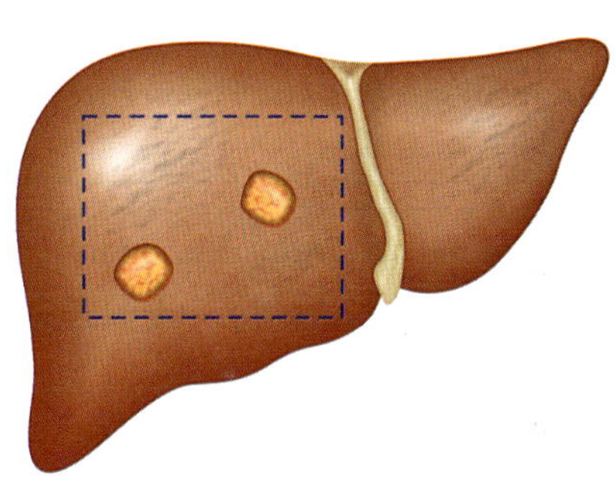

Resection of metastases

Complete Mesocolic Excision (CME) with Central Vascular Ligation

A newly evolving concept in colon cancer surgery. It involves:

- Sharp dissection of the visceral plane from the parietal one along the Toldt fascia with complete mobilization of the entire mesocolon up to the mesenteric root (resulting specimen is composed of tumor and its lymphatic drainage with no tears in the fascial layers on each side of the mesocolon)
- Central division of the feeding arteries at their origin (for right colon cancers, division is done at the level of superior mesenteric artery and for left colon cancers, at the level of inferior mesenteric artery or aorta). Various prospective studies showed better lymph node harvest and better survival compared to non-CME colectomy.

Principles of Pathologic Review

Parameters should be assessed—(i) Grade of the tumor; (ii) Depth of penetration; (iii) Number of lymph nodes evaluated and number of positive lymph nodes; (iv) Status of proximal, distal, radial and mesenteric margins; (v) Lymphovascular invasion (LVI); (vi) Perineural invasion; (vii) Tumor deposits; and (viii) Tumor budding.

A minimum of 12 lymph nodes should be examined for accurate staging.

The **radial margins (circumferential resection margin)** should be assessed in all colonic segments with non-peritonealized surfaces. Segments of colon that are completely encased by peritoneum (transverse colon), the mesenteric resection margin is the only relevant radial margin.

Tumor in the Cecum or Ascending Colon

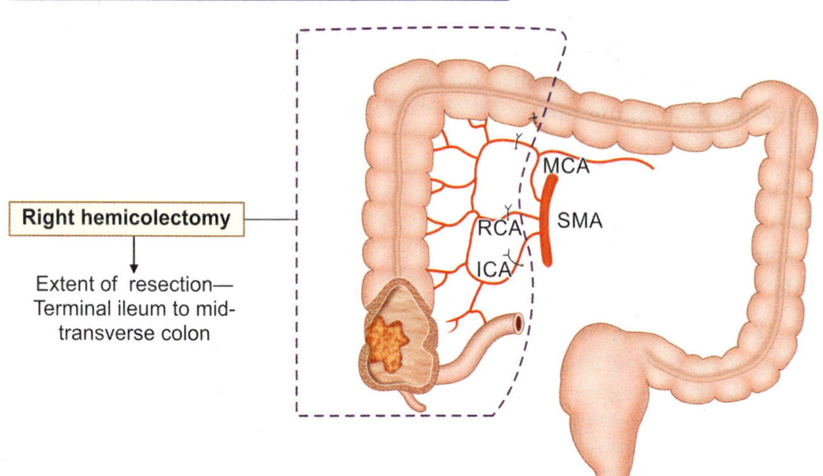

Type of colectomy

Right hemicolectomy.

Division of the following vessels

- Ileocolic artery
- Right colic artery
- Right branch of middle colic artery.

Extent of resection

5–10 cm of terminal ileum to right part of transverse colon.

Anatomical structures at risk

- Right ureter
- Duodenum
- Gonadal vessels.

Tumor in the Hepatic Flexure or Right Part of the Transverse Colon

- **Type of colectomy:** Extended right colectomy.
- **Division of the following vessels:**
  - Ileocolic artery
  - Right colic artery
  - Middle colic artery at its origin.
- **Extent of resection:** Terminal ileum to left part of transverse colon.
- **Anatomical structures at risk:** Right ureter, duodenum, gonadal vessels.

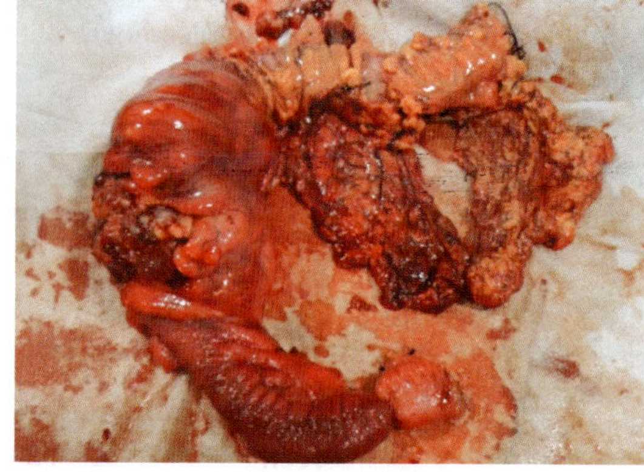

Operated specimen of extended right hemicolectomy.

Tumors in the Mid Part of Transverse Colon

- **Type of colectomy:** Extended right colectomy or transverse colectomy.
- **Division of the following vessels:**
  - Middle colic artery (in transverse colectomy)
  - Ileocolic, right colic and middle colic artery (in extended right colectomy).
- **Extent of resection:** Transverse colon (both hepatic flexure and splenic flexure are often mobilized for a tension-free anastomosis).
- **Anatomical structures at risk:** Right ureter, duodenum, gonadal vessels, and spleen (in transverse colectomy).

Tumor in the Distal Transverse Colon and Splenic Flexure

- **Type of colectomy:** Right colectomy extended to the splenic flexure.
- **Division of the following vessels:** Ileocolic, right colic and middle colic artery.
- **Extent of resection:** Terminal ileum to proximal descending colon
- **Anatomical structures at risk:** Right ureter, duodenum, gonadal vessels, spleen

Tumor in the Distal Transverse Colon, Splenic Flexure and Descending Colon

- **Type of colectomy:** Left hemicolectomy
- **Division of the following vessels:** Left branch of the middle colic artery, inferior mesenteric vein and left colic vessels
- **Extent of resection:** Splenic flexure to sigmoid colon
- **Anatomical structures at risk:** Left ureter, spleen, left kidney

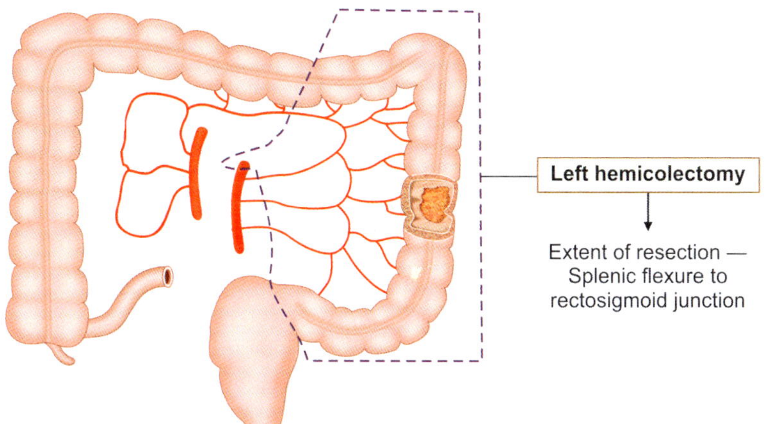

Tumor in the Sigmoid Colon

- **Type of colectomy:** Sigmoid colectomy
- **Division of the following vessels:** Inferior mesenteric artery at its origin
- **Extent of resection:** Sigmoid colon
- **Anatomical structures at risk:** Left ureter, left kidney, gonadal vessels

Minimally Invasive Approaches to Colectomy

Minimally invasive approaches are now preferred surgical options for elective colectomy among many surgeons.

Several large multi-institutional RCTs (e.g., COLOR trial, COST trial, CLASICC trial) showed equivalent outcomes including DFS (Disease-free survival), OS (Overall survival), and recurrence between **open and laparoscopic colectomy**.

RCTs showed similar long-term oncologic outcomes between **hand-assisted laparoscopic colectomy and conventional laparoscopic or open colectomy** but hand-assisted laparoscopic colectomy was associated with less pain and shorter recovery.

Different studies demonstrated no differences in postoperative morbidity or short-term cancer-related outcomes between **robotic colectomy and laparoscopic colectomy** but robotic colectomy was associated with increased operative time, increased cost and less blood loss, shorter hospital stays.

The two approaches for laparoscopic colectomy are: (i) Lateral-to-medial (L-M) approach and (ii) Medial-to-lateral (M-L) approach. The European Association of Endoscopic Surgeons (EAES) consensus statement 2004 recommended medial-to-lateral approach for laparoscopic colectomy.

Minimally invasive colectomy in colon cancer is not recommended in:

- T4 colon cancer
- Tumor with acute obstruction or perforation
- Patients with high risk of prohibitive abdominal adhesions.

Management of Colorectal Emergencies

Management of acute bleeding from tumor: (i) Resuscitation; (ii) Localization of bleeding (by urgent colonoscopy or CT angiography or radionuclide imaging); and (iii) Surgical resection (if previous options fail).

Management of obstructing right colon cancer:

(i) Right colectomy with primary anastomosis with or without diverting stoma—preferred option if patient is stable

(ii) Right colectomy with terminal ileostomy and colonic fistula—preferred option in resectable tumor in unstable patients

(iii) Ileotransverse anastomosis (side-to-side anastomosis between terminal ileum and transverse colon)—if tumor is unresectable.

(iv) SEMS placement—as palliative option only, as bridge to elective surgery is not recommended.

Management of obstructing left-sided colon cancer:

(i) Initial stenting (self-expanding metal stent) followed by interval colectomy—if endoscopic stenting facility is available and Bevacizumab therapy is not planned.

(ii) Resection and primary anastomosis—for resectable tumor in stable patients.

(iii) Hartmann's procedure—preferred in resectable tumor in unstable patients.

(iv) Loop colostomy—preferred in unresectable tumor in unstable patients.

(v) Transanal tube decompression—in high-risk patients as bridge to surgery (BTS) option

Management of perforation: In most of the cases of colorectal carcinoma, perforation occurs at the tumor site (about 70%). If perforation develops proximal to the obstructing tumor in uninvolved colonic segment, the tumor is treated by colon resection and perforation is treated by repair or resection. If perforation at the tumor site, treatment is formal resection with or without anastomosis, with or without stoma.

Self-expanding metal stenting is contraindicated in perforated colon cancer.

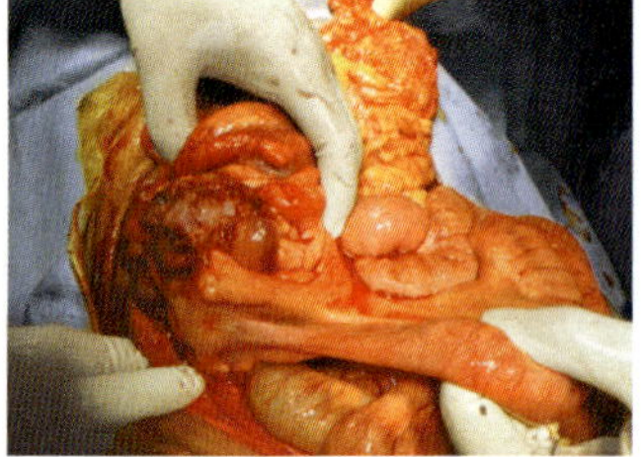

Carcinoma of right colon.

Management of Obstruction from Resectable Tumor

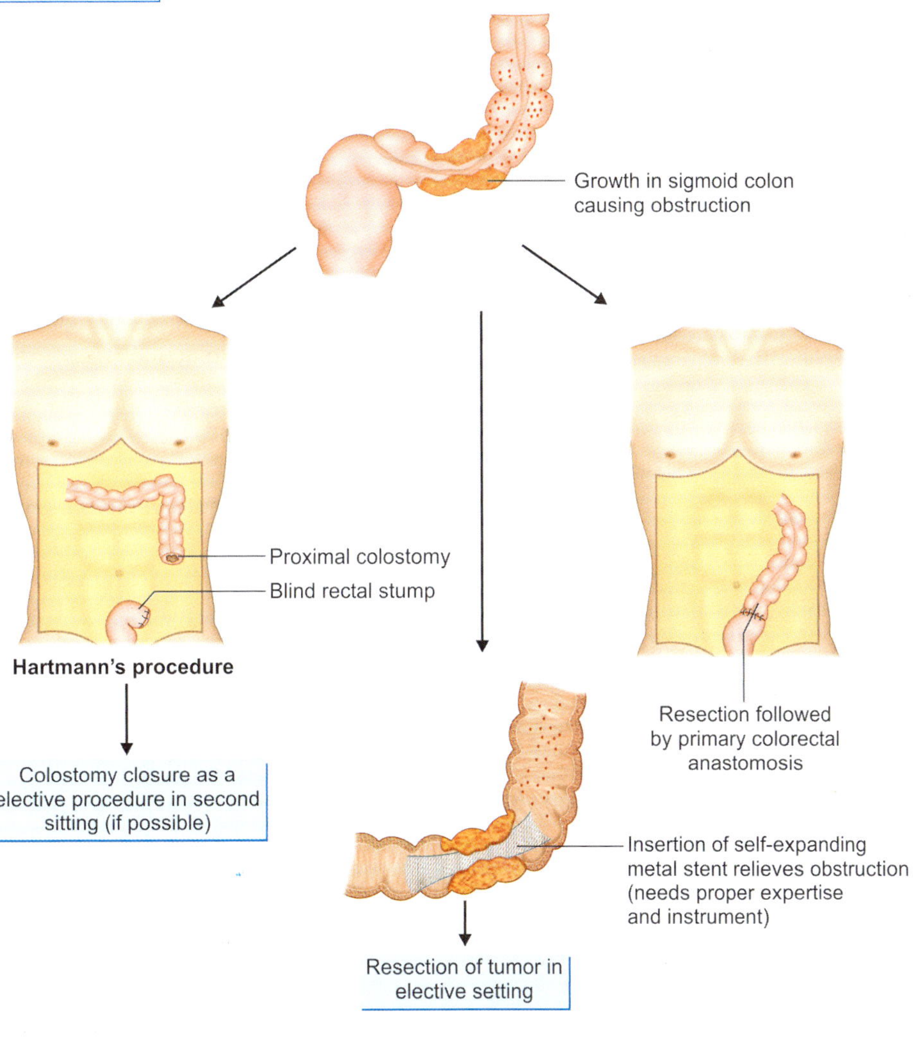

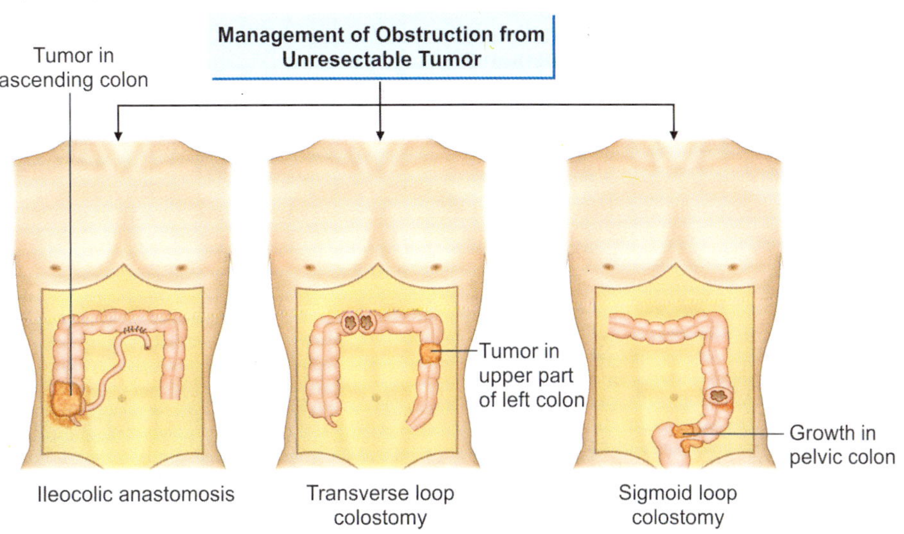

Stoma and its Management

Types of Ostomy

- Ileostomy (created from small intestine) or colostomy (created from large intestine).
- Temporary or Permanent
- Defunctioning or Decompressing
- End stoma (End ileostomy, End colostomy); Loop stoma (Loop ileostomy, Loop colostomy); End loop stoma (End loop ileostomy, End loop colostomy, End loop ileocolostomy)
- *Types of colostomy:* Loop transverse colostomy, Double-barrel transverse colostomy, Loop sigmoid colostomy, Double-barrel sigmoid colostomy, Ascending loop colostomy, Hartmann procedure.

Indications

- Defunctioning loop ileostomy—to protect a distal anastomosis (following colocolic anastomosis after segmental colon resections).
- Decompressing loop ileostomy—in colonic obstruction where ileocecal valve is incompetent.
- Permanent ileostomy—After proctocolectomy in ulcerative colitis, Crohn's disease, Familial Adenomatous Polyposis.
- Defunctioning loop colostomy—usually transverse loop colostomy, after colorectal anastomosis, in high anal fistula, after repair of rectal injury.
- Decompressing loop colostomy—large bowel obstruction due to colon cancer, where curative resection is not feasible or distant metastases present; Sigmoid loop colostomy for high anorectal malformation and Hirschsprung's disease.
- Permanent colostomy—after abdomino-perineal resection (APR), in unresectable rectal cancer, sphincter complex is damaged beyond repairable.
- End loop ileostomy and end loop colostomy—Same indications of standard loop ileostomy or loop colostomy.
- End loop ileocolostomy—following intestinal resection where primary anastomosis is not justified.
- Hartmann procedure—in gangrenous sigmoid volvulus, following sigmoidectomy, where primary anastomosis is not justified.

Diseases or Conditions Commonly Associated with Stoma Formation

(i) GI malignancy; (ii) Malignant bowel obstruction; (iii) Traumatic bowel injury; (iv) Inflammatory bowel disease; (v) Sigmoid volvulus; and (vi) Diverticulitis.

Complications

Early complications (within 1 month of surgery): (i) Peristomal skin complications (e.g., allergic dermatitis, pseudoverrucous lesions, cellulitis, peristomal varices, mucosal transplantation, pyoderma gangrenosum); (ii) Leakage; (iii) Ischemia; (iv) Peristomal breakdown; (v) Mucocutaneous separation; (vi) Cutaneous infection; and (vii) Retraction.

Late complications (>1 month of surgery): (i) Prolapse; (ii) Parastomal hernia; (iii) Obstruction; and (iv) Stenosis.

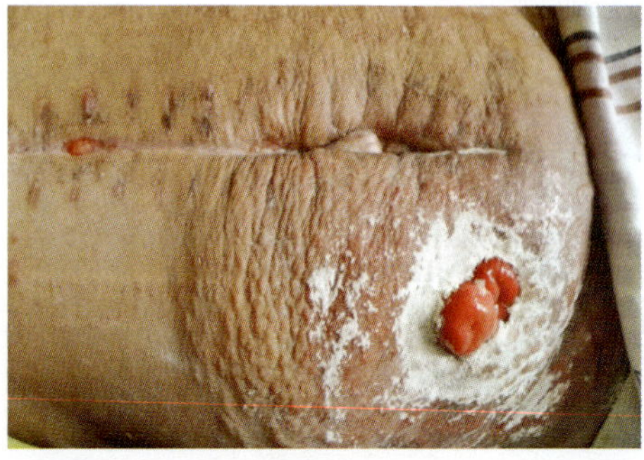

Loop ileostomy with barrier cream (to protect the peristomal skin from the effluent).

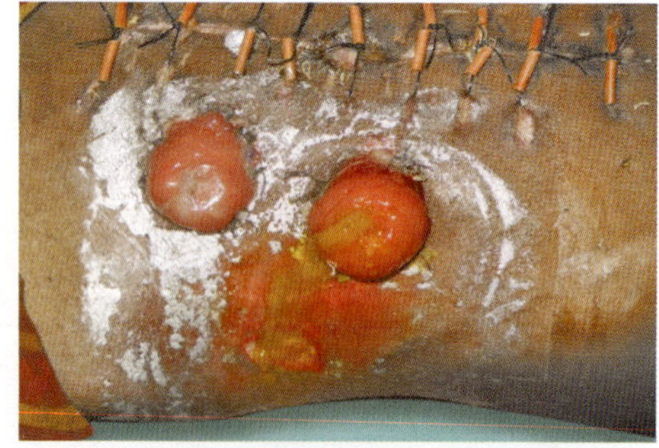

Proximal end as stoma, distal end as mucous fistula.

Stoma site marking: During marking of stoma site, following points have to be considered:

- Type of ostomy (ileostomy or colostomy, loop or end)
- Body habitus
- History of radiation, occupation
- Indication of stoma
- Stoma should be within the 'Ostomy triangle' (formed by anterior superior iliac spine, pubic tubercle and umbilicus) overlying the rectus muscle
- Marking should be evaluated in multiple positions (supine, seated and standing position) and site must be visible to the patient
- *Sites to be avoided:* Skin fold, the umbilicus, bony prominences, expected incision site, previous surgical sites, belt line.

Following features related to stoma should be checked in postoperative period:

- Color of the stoma (healthy stoma is pink to bright red)
- Output
- Rod (if given) is secured in place or not
- Skin condition
- Stoma spout and size
- Sutures surrounding the stoma.

Facts Related to Ostomy

- Loop ileostomy is preferred over transverse loop colostomy for temporary fecal diversion.
- Loop ileostomy is associated with less risk of prolapse, infectious complications, less odor, easier ostomy care.
- Loop ileostomy is associated with more dehydration, greater need for dietary alterations.
- Obstructive complications after ostomy reversal is more common in ileostomy.
- Ileostomies should protrude at least 2 cm over the skin surface, colostomies should protrude at least 1 cm.
- Placement of lightweight polypropylene mesh at the time of permanent ostomy creation can decrease parastomal hernia rates.
- Different techniques of ostomy creation: (i) Open ostomy creation; (ii) Laparoscopic ostomy creation; and (iii) Trephine ostomy creation.

Personal Issues Related to Ostomy

- Clothing adjustment
- **Modification of dietary habits:** (i) Slow and thorough chewing of solid foods and (ii) Ostomates have to be oriented about the foods causing odor, gas, constipation, diarrhea, altered color of output.
- Management of stoma and pouch bag
- Returning to work—Ostomates must be open about the stoma to other colleagues in workplace.
- Sexual relationship—in the initial period, sexual function usually impaired, that improves with time. No contraindication regarding pregnancy.
- Participation in sports—contact sports are better avoided.

Odor Producing
Cabbage, broccoli, garlic, cod liver oil, onion, peanut butter, egg, fish.
Odor Control
Orange juice, cranberry juice, tomato juice, yogurt, butter milk.
Gas Producing
Alcoholic beverages, carbonated beverages, cabbage, cauliflower, cucumber, dairy products, milk, nuts, radishes.
Color Changing
Beets, iron pills, strawberries, tomato sauces.

Increased Stool Forming
Alcoholic beverages, raw vegetables, fresh fruits, whole grain, cooked cabbage, milk.
Diarrhea Controlling
Banana, boiled rice, peanut butter, toast.
Stoma Obstructing
Apple peels, raw cabbage, corn, whole kernel, coconut, dried fruit, mushroom, orange, pineapple.
Constipation Relieving
Water, warm or hot beverages, fruit juice, coffee, cooked vegetables, cooked fruits.

Enteroatmospheric Fistula (EAF)

The opening of fistula onto open abdomen, exposing and communicating the bowel and its effluent to the atmosphere.

Risk factors: (i) Delayed abdominal closure; (ii) Anastomotic disruption; (iii) Bowel injury during dissection; (iv) Use of polypropylene mesh directly over the bowel; (v) Presence of intra-abdominal abscess; (vi) Development of abdominal compartment syndrome; (vii) Multiple re-exploration; and (viii) Large amount of fluid resuscitation (>5L/24 hr).

Measures to prevent EAF: (i) Early abdominal wall closure; (ii) No direct application of NPWT on the bowel; (iii) Bowel coverage with omentum or skin; and (iv) No direct application of polypropylene mesh on bowel.

Classification:

- Based on fistula effluent output: Low (<200 mL/day); Moderate (200–500 mL/day); High (>500 mL/day).
- Based on anatomic location: Proximal and Distal.
- Based on location in the open abdomen: Superficial and Deep.

Management:

Early recognition and control of sepsis.

Source control: Any intra-abdominal abscess or infected collections have to be drained by image-guided drainage method.

Nutritional support: Early enteral nutrition should be started as early as possible, if no other contraindication. Significant nitrogen and protein loss must be replaced. Vitamin and trace element loss must be replaced.

Isolation of fistula effluent: Isolation helps to (i) maintain the peritoneal cavity clean; (ii) accurate measurement of fistula effluent; (iii) ensure skin protection; (iv) better nursing care of the patients; and (v) allow better mobility of the patient. Negative pressure wound therapy, with specific variants (e.g., Nipple VAC, Fistula VAC, Tube VAC, Ring and silo VAC) are preferred techniques of EAF isolation.

Definitive treatment: Fistula closure and reconstruction of the abdominal wall defect. Treatment should be postponed at least 6 months and only after the patient and the wound healed completely.

Gastrointestinal Bleeding

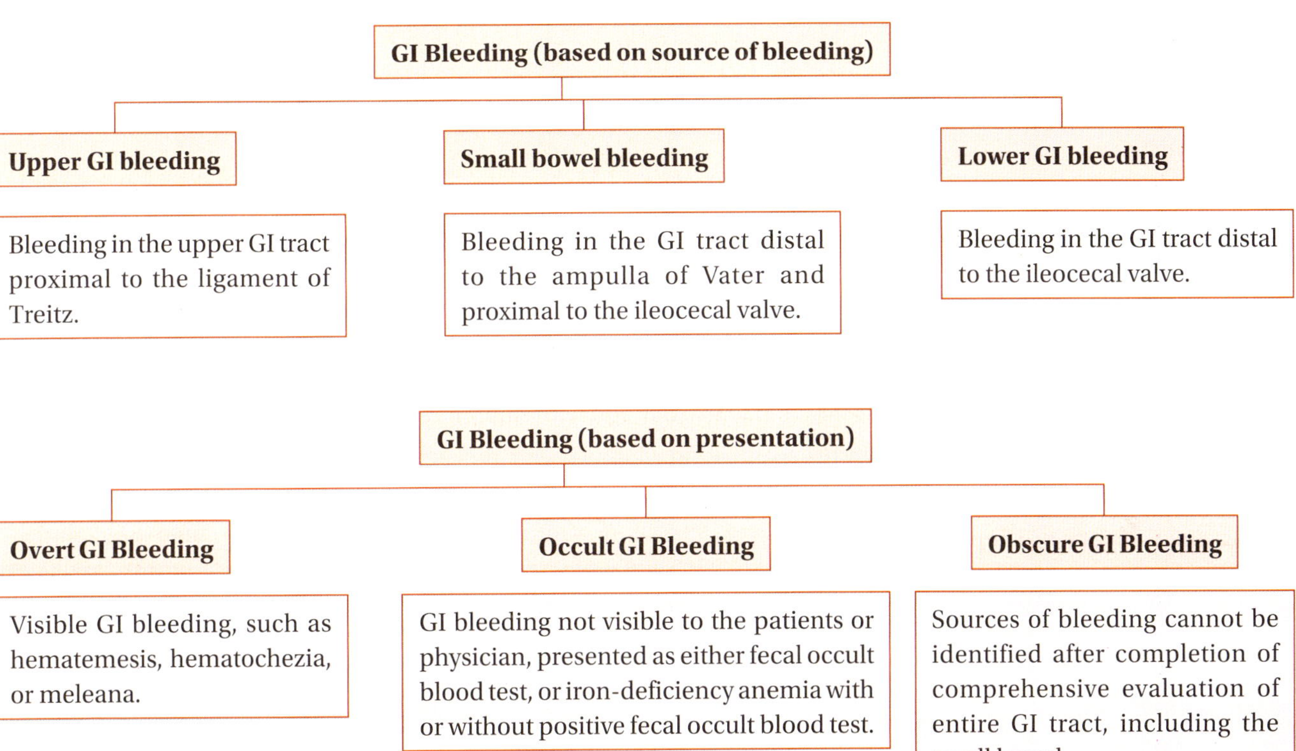

Causes of GI Bleeding

Upper GI bleeding	Small bowel bleeding	Lower GI bleeding
Peptic ulcer	Angiectasias of small bowel	Diverticulosis
Gastroduodenitis	Small bowel tumors (e.g., GIST, carcinoid, lymphomas)	Ischemic colitis
Varices/portal hypertensive gastropathy	Inflammatory bowel disease	Hemorrhoids
Esophagitis	Dieulafoy's lesions	Angiectasias
Erosive duodenitis	NSAID ulcers	Inflammatory bowel disease
Malignancy	Meckel diverticulum	Colorectal tumors
Vascular ectasia	Polyposis syndrome	Radiation proctopathy
Mallory-Weiss tear		Rectal varices
		Postpolypectomy

Treatment Options for Small Bowel Bleeding [Adapted from ACG Guideline]
Medical treatment: PRBC transfusion, Iron (oral or IV)
Endoscopic therapy: Endoscopic hemostasis therapy
Somatostatin analogs (acts by inhibition of angiogenesis, decreasing splanchnic blood flow)—may be considered in angiectasia patients who are not candidates for endoscopic therapy.
Thalidomide (acts as antiangiogenic agent by inhibiting VEGF) may be considered in angiectasia patients who are not candidates for endoscopic therapy or after failure of endoscopic therapy.
Transarterial embolization: Selective mesenteric embolization.
Surgical intervention: Indicated for lysis of adhesions to perform successful DAE.

Treatment Options for Lower GI Bleeding
Endoscopic hemostasis therapy
a. Epinephrine injection therapy (1:10,000 or 1:20,000 dilution with saline) b. Contact thermal therapy (Bipolar electrocoagulation, Unipolar electrocoagulation, Heat probe) c. Noncontact thermal therapy (Argon plasma coagulation) d. Through-the-scope clipping devices e. Band ligation f. Hemostatic topical powder/sprays (Hemospray, EndoClot, Ankaferd Bloodstopper) g. Over-the-scope clip (OTSC).
Angioembolization
Angioembolization is indicated in patients with high risk clinical features and ongoing bleeding, not responding to resuscitation, negative upper GI endoscopy, and unlikely to tolerate urgent bowel preparation and colonoscopy. Superselective embolization is done with microcoils, polyvinyl alcohol particles, gelfoam.
Surgical intervention
Surgical intervention is indicated for colorectal tumors, ischemic colitis, ulcerative colitis, Crohn's colitis.

Management of Diverticular Bleeding
Through-the-scope endoscopic clips, endoscopic epinephrine injection therapy, thermal coagulation
Management of Angiectasia Bleeding
Argon-plasma coagulation
Management of Postpolypectomy Bleeding
Endoscopic clip, contact thermal therapy, band ligation, over-the-scope clip, hemostatic topical powder/spray

Hemostatic Topical Powder/Spray

Hemostatic topical powders/sprays are the newly emerging endoscopic hemostatic agents. The available agents are—(i) Hemospray (TC-325); (ii) EndoClot; and (iii) Ankaferd Blood Stopper (ABS).

These hemostatic agents are particularly effective for control of postpolypectomy bleeding, bleeding from solitary rectal ulcer, radiation proctitis and colorectal tumors.

Hemospray: A mineral-based powder, delivered via an endoscopic catheter using pressurized carbon dioxide as delivery system. Hemospray acts by (i) Creating a barrier layer over the bleeding site and acts as tamponade; (ii) Concentrate the clotting factors and blood elements by absorbing the fluid elements of blood; and (iii) Initiates fibrin plug by platelet aggregation and activation of clotting cascade.

EndoClot: Absorbable polysaccharide elements derived from plant starch. EndoClot acts by absorbing the fluid component of the blood, forming a gel composed of concentrated RBCs, platelets, and coagulation factors.

Ankaferd Blood Stopper: A combination of plant extracts. ABS rapidly (<1 s) forms a encapsulated protein network that act as an anchor for RBC aggregation ('ABS web') without involving platelets and coagulation factors.

Case 1

History and Physical Examination

A 36-year-old male patient admitted in the surgical emergency ward with acute onset abdominal pain, absolute constipation and vomiting for last 2 days. Patient had a history of exploratory laparotomy 2 years back. No history of hematemesis or melena. Patient is chronic alcoholic for last 8 years.

Physical examination

Patient dehydrated; Pulse—100/min, BP—100/70 mm Hg, Respiratory rate—20/min

Abdomen—distended, diffuse tenderness all over the abdomen, no rebound tenderness, IPS—sluggish Per rectal examination—Rectum empty, no ballooning, no growth palpable.

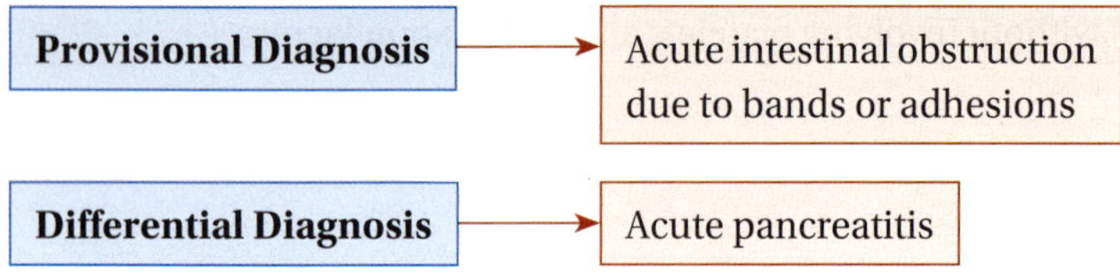

Investigations

Straight X-ray abdomen—Predominantly centrally located multiple air-fluid levels, valvulae conniventes

Hb—11.7 gm%, Total WBC count—10,000/cumm, Na^+—130 mEq/L, K^+—2.8 mmol/L, Fasting blood sugar—89 mg/dL, Serum urea—80 mg/dL, Creatinine—1.6 mg/dL.

Discussion

History of abdominal pain, vomiting, absolute constipation, all suggestive of acute intestinal obstruction. History of exploratory laparotomy also indicated that band-adhesion as the most likely cause of obstruction. All clinical findings were also suggestive of acute intestinal obstruction. Straight X-ray findings confirmed the clinical diagnosis. As clinical features suggestive of acute intestinal obstruction without any complications (without any features of peritonitis) and X-ray findings also suggestive of small intestinal obstruction, nonoperative trial was planned.

Management Algorithm

- Fluid resuscitation
- Nasogastric decompression
- Monitoring of urine output
- Correction of dyselectrolytemia
- IV antibiotics

→

- Monitoring of symptoms and clinical findings (particularly clinical features of peritonitis)
- Laboratory investigations
- Straight X-ray of abdomen

↓

- Patient became toxic, rebound tenderness appeared
- Leukocytosis
- Air-fluid level increased in X-ray

→

Decision of nonoperative to operative management (Exploratory laparotomy) was taken.

Case 2

History and Physical Examination

A 58-old-year male patient presented in the surgical OPD with history of alternate constipation and diarrhea for last 3 months. Patient also complained passage of mucus with stool for same duration. History of significant weight loss was present. Patient was treated by local physician but symptoms not relieved. No history of melena or hematochezia. Patient is chronic smoker for last 15 years.

Physical examination

Anemia—present, jaundice—absent, cervical lymph nodes—not palpable.

Examination of abdomen—Abdomen soft, no specific point of tenderness, no lump palpable.

Per rectal examination—No growth palpable.

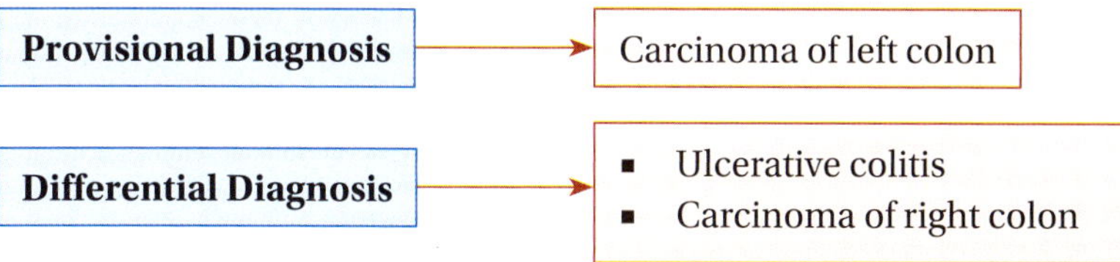

Investigations

Colonoscopy: A ulceroproliferative lesion in the sigmoid colon almost obliterating the lumen. Scope could not be negotiated proximal to the lesion.

Colonoscopy-guided biopsy revealed moderately differentiated adenocarcinoma.

CT abdomen and pelvis with oral and IV contrast: Irregular wall thickening at the sigmoid colon region, pericolic lymphadenopathy, no liver metastases.

CT chest: No lung mestastases.

CT colonography: No lesion detected proximal to the sigmoid growth.

CEA: 15 ng/mL

Discussion

Recent history of alteration of bowel habit along with passage of mucus with stool and history of significant weight loss highly suggestive of colon cancer, particularly left-sided colon cancer. Colonoscopy and colonoscopy guided-biopsy confirmed the diagnosis of left-sided colon cancer (sigmoid colon cancer). Raised CEA level also suggestive of colon cancer. CT colonography performed to exclude synchronous lesion as colonoscope could not be negotiated proximal to the lesion. No distant metastases found in CT abdomen and chest. Curative resection (sigmoid colectomy) was planned.

Management Algorithm

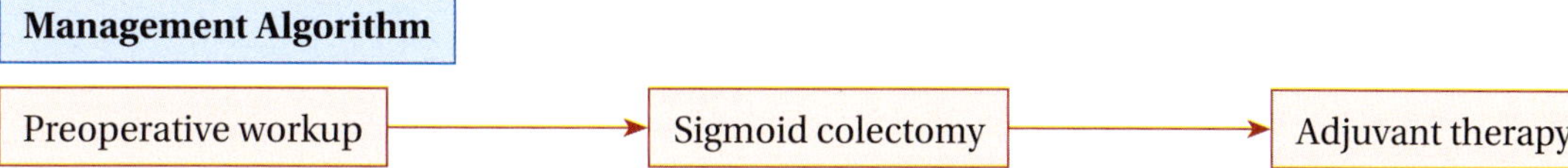

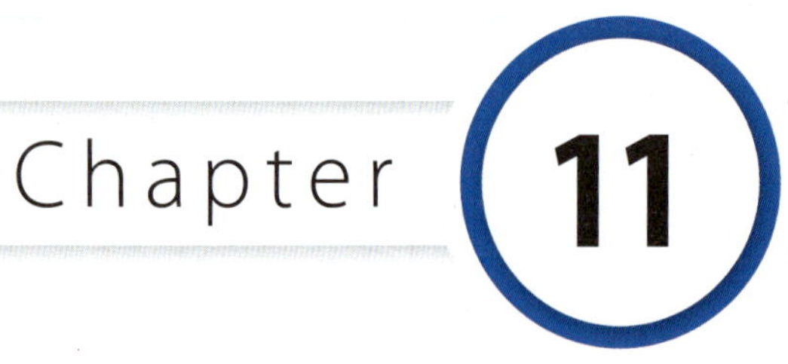

Chapter 11

Appendix

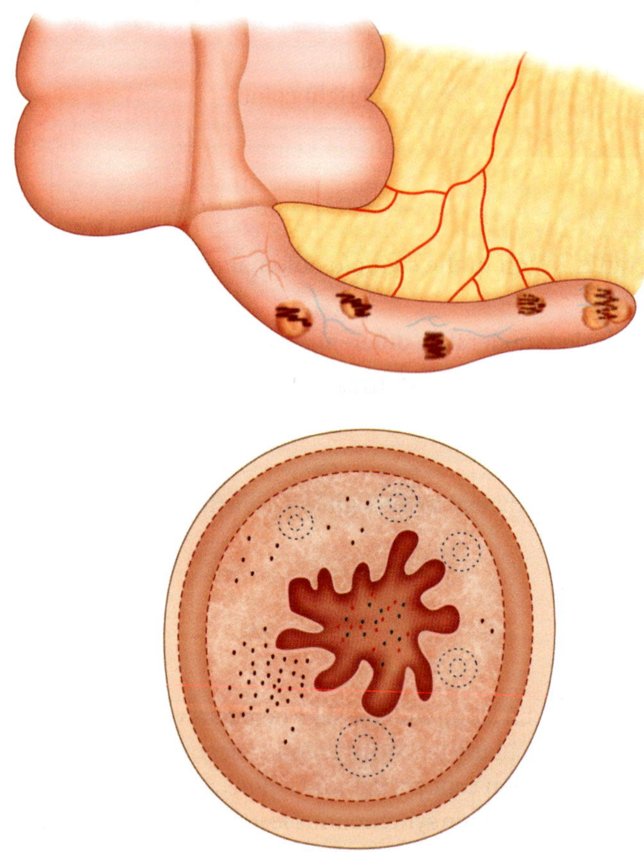

Important Topics

- Acute Appendicitis
- Appendicular Lump
- Carcinoids of the Appendix

'An organism is a molecular society, and biological order is a kind of social order. Social order is opposed to revolution, which is an abrupt change of order and to anarchy, which is the absence of order.'

André Lwoff (1902–1994)
French Microbiologist

Acute Appendicitis

Acute appendicitis is one of the common causes of acute lower abdominal pain in young adults, most common surgical pathology in children, and most common cause of nongynecological or obstetric-related emergency surgery in pregnant women.

Pathophysiology

Obstruction of the appendicular lumen is the major causative factor of acute appendicitis.

Causes of Obstruction

- Fecalith (composed of inspissated fecal material, calcium phosphates, bacteria, epithelial debris)
- Hyperplastic lymphoid follicles
- Intestinal parasites particularly *Oxyuris vermicularis* (pinworm)
- Carcinoma of cecum

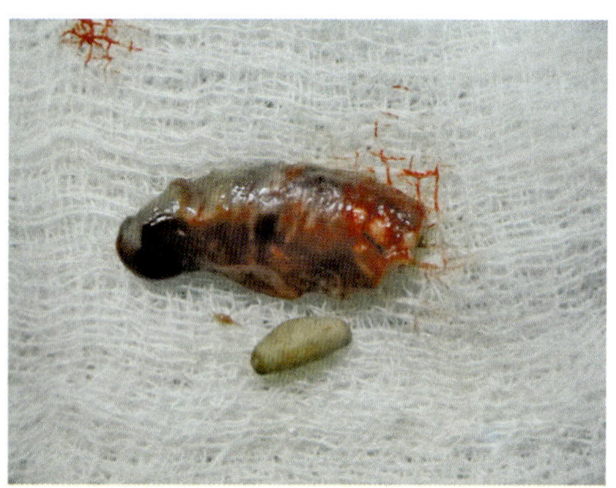

What Happens after Obstruction?

Closed loop obstruction by fecalith/hyperplastic lymphoid follicles/worms/cecal growth

↓

Appendiceal mucosa secretes fluid against obstruction

↓

↑ intraluminal pressure (this increased intraluminal pressure causes visceral pain, manifested as periumbilical pain)

↓

Increased pressure in the appendiceal wall exceeds capillary pressure

↓

Mucosal ischemia

↓

Luminal bacterial overgrowth and translocation of bacteria across the appendiceal wall

Commonly isolated organisms in inflamed appendix: *E. coli, Streptococcus viridans, Pseudomonas, Bacteroides*

↓

Inflammation, edema and necrotic change

↓

Perforation resulting in abscess [Perforation develops at least 48 hours from the onset of symptoms]

[*Pepto-Streptococcus, Lactobocillus, Fusobacterium Nucleatum*—found in a few percentage of patients]

OR

Phlegmonous mass (appendicular lump)—Formed by greater omentum, loops of small intestine and inflamed appendix

[Inflammation of the adjacent peritoneum causes localized pain in right iliac fossa]

Clinical Presentation

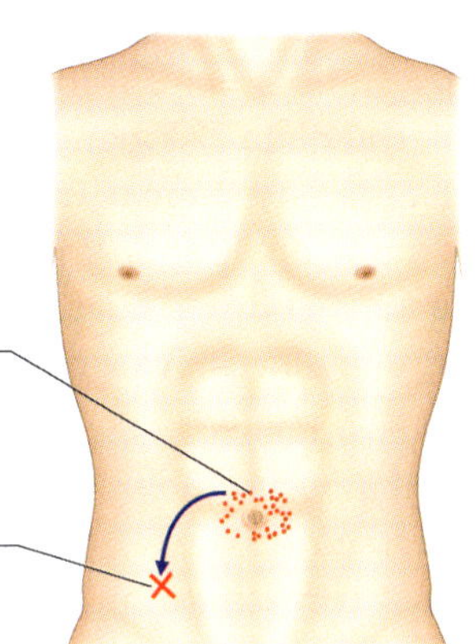

Tenderness at McBurney's point is minimal or absent in:

- Appendicitis in retrocecal, pelvic or postileal type
- Appendicitis in 2nd and 3rd trimester of pregnancy
- In high up cecum with appendicitis
- Extremely obese patients

Risk Factors for Perforation

- Extremes of age (Pediatric and geriatric population)
- Presence of appendicolith
- Immunosuppressive state
- Diabetes mellitus
- Previous abdominal surgery (due to restricted spread of greater omentum)

Different Positions of the Appendix

- Retrocecal
- Pelvic
- Postileal
- Subcecal
- Preileal
- Paracecal

McBurney's Point

A point that lies one-third of the distance laterally on a line drawn between right anterior superior iliac spine and the umbilicus.

- Pain in right iliac fossa
- Loss of appetite
- Nausea or vomiting
- Rise of temperature
- Discomfort on moving, walking or coughing
- Tenderness at **McBurney's point**
- Rebound tenderness at RIF
- Percussion tenderness
- Muscle guarding
- Urinary frequency and diarrhea (Appendicitis in **subcecal and pelvic type**)
- **Diagnosis of acute appendicitis is difficult in children and elderly person**

Clinical Signs in Acute Appendicitis

- **Rovsing sign:** Palpation of the left lower quadrant may elicit pain in the right lower quadrant.
- **Dunphy sign:** Coughing causes increased abdominal pain in the right lower quadrant.
- **Psoas sign (Obraztsova's sign):** On left lateral decubitus position, passive extension of the right hip causes pain in right lower quadrant. This sign is typically found in retrocecal appendicitis.
- **Obturator sign:** On right knee in flexed position, passive internal rotation of the right hip causes pain in the right lower quadrant. This sign is typically found in inflammation of the pelvic appendix.

Diagnosis

Clinical scoring system: This system is helpful to exclude acute appendicitis and to identify intermediate-risk patients needing of imaging for diagnosis. Among different clinical scoring systems, Alvarado score, Appendicitis Inflammatory Response (AIR) score, and new Adult Appendicitis Score are sufficiently sensitive. AIR score is the most sensitive and specific among different clinical prediction models.

Alvarado score (cutoff score <5) is sufficiently sensitive to exclude acute appendicitis but not sufficiently specific in diagnosing acute appendicitis in adults. Alvarado score is less accurate in acute appendicitis in pregnancy (in first trimester of pregnancy, nausea and vomiting are common and WBC count becomes higher). This scoring system is also unreliable in differentiating complicated from uncomplicated appendicitis in elderly patients.

Imaging: Diagnostic imaging is indicated for intermediate-risk adult patients according to the AIR/Alvarado score.

Point-of-care ultrasound (POCUS) is a useful diagnostic modality with satisfactory sensitivity and specificity for acute appendicitis in adult and pediatric patients.

Contrast enhanced CT scan is particularly indicated after the negative USG and to differentiate complicated appendicitis from uncomplicated appendicitis. Contrast-enhanced low-dose CT scan is preferred over contrast-enhanced standard-dose CT. In children, MRI is preferred over CT to avoid radiation when US findings are inconclusive.

Graded compression transabdominal grayscale US is the preferred first-line imaging modality in pregnant women with suspected acute appendicitis. MRI is indicated when USG is inconclusive. MRI has almost similar sensitivity and specificity as CT.

Diagnostic laparoscopy is indicated to establish or rule out acute appendicitis or other diagnoses if cross-sectional imaging is negative but right iliac fossa pain is not resolving.

Clinical Scoring Systems for Acute Appendicitis

- Alvarado score (also known as the MANTRELS score)
- Appendicitis inflammatory response (AIR) score
- Pediatric appendicitis score (PAS)
- The Raja Isteri Pengiran Anak Saleha Appendicitis (RIPASA) score
- The new Adult Appendicitis Score (AAS)

Among them, **Alvarado and Appendicitis Inflammatory Response score** are most often used scoring systems in clinical settings.

Clinical Scoring Systems for Pediatric Patients

- Pediatric appendicitis score (PAS)
- Alvarado score
- Appendicitis inflammatory response (AIR) score
- Pediatric Appendicitis Laboratory Score (PALabS)
- Appendicitis-PEdiatric score (APPE).

Among them, **PAS and Alvarado score** are commonly used to exclude acute appendicitis.

USG Findings Suggestive of Acute Appendicitis

- Noncompressible appendix with diameter more than 6 mm
- Thickened wall
- Absence of gas in the lumen
- Appendicoliths
- Hypoperistalsis
- Hyperechogenic periappendicular fat

Based on CT findings, acute appendicitis is classified into:

- Uncomplicated appendicitis
- Complicated appendicitis

Complicated appendicitis includes:

- Perforation of appendix
- Gangrenous appendix
- Appendicular abscess or phlegmon

CT Findings Suggestive of Acute Appendicitis

- Appendiceal dilatation (>6 mm in diameter)
- Thickened appendiceal wall >2 mm ('target sign')
- Periappendiceal inflammation (fat stranding, thickening of mesoappendix)
- Thickening of the cecal apex ('arrowhead sign')
- Presence of fecalith

Alvarado Score

Migratory right iliac fossa pain	1
Anorexia	1
Nausea or vomiting	1
Tenderness	2
Rebound tenderness	1
Elevated temperature	1
Leukocytosis ≥10 × 10^9/L	2
Shift to the left	1
	10

Score <3: Low possibility of appendicitis
Score 4–6: Diagnostic imaging needed
Score ≥7: High possibility of appendicitis.

Appendicitis Inflammatory Response (AIR) Score

Vomiting	1
Pain in right lower quadrant	1
Rebound tenderness:	
Light	1
Medium	2
Strong	3
Body temperature >38.5°C	1
Polymorphonuclear leukocytes:	
70–84%	1
≥85%	2
WBC count:	
10.0– 14.9 × 10^9/L	1
≥15.0 × 10^9/L	2
CRP concentration:	
10-49 g/L	1
≥50 g/L	2
Total score	**12**

Score 0–4: Low probability; **Score 5-8:** Indeterminate group; **Score 9-12:** High probability

CT Findings Suggestive of Complicated Appendicitis

- Extraluminal appendicolith
- Extraluminal air
- Periappendiceal abscess
- Appendiceal wall enhancement defect
- Periappendiceal fat stranding.

Pediatric Appendicitis Score (PAS)

Migration of pain	1
Anorexia	1
Nausea/vomiting	1
Tenderness	2
Cough/hopping/percussion tenderness	2
Increase in temperature	1
Leukocytes >10,000/μL	1
Polymorphonuclear neutrophilia >75%	1
Total score	**10**

Score <4 (Low risk): No need of imaging, consider other causes of pain.

Score 4–6 (Equivocal): Imaging is indicated.

Score >6 (High risk): Surgical consultation is warranted.

Role of Serum Biomarkers in Acute Appendicitis

Serum biomarkers are emerging as reliable diagnostic tools in acute appendicitis but still not recommended.

Promising biomarkers in adult patients:
- C-reactive protein (CRP)
- Ischemia modified albumin (IMA)

Promising biomarkers in pediatric patients:
- CRP
- Calprotectin
- Appendicitis Urinary Biomarker (AuB-leucine-rich α-2-glycoprotein)

Differential Diagnosis

In Preschool Aged Children

- Intussusception
- Meckel's diverticulitis
- Gastroenteritis

In School Aged Children

- Mesenteric lymphadenitis
- Gastroenteritis

In Adults

- Colitis
- Diverticulitis
- Pyelonephritis

In Women of Childbearing Age

- Ectopic pregnancy
- Twisted ovarian cyst
- PID

Valentino Syndrome

Patient with perforated peptic ulcer presents with pain in right lower quadrant or right iliac fossa mimicking acute appendicitis due to gastrointestinal contents leaking from perforated peptic ulcer and passage of that contents through the right paracolic gutter into right iliac fossa.

Management

Nonoperative management with antibiotics: NOM with antibiotics is a treatment approach in uncomplicated acute appendicitis without appendicoliths in adult and pediatric patients, but not in pregnant patients. The drawback of this approach are: (i) Chance of NOM failure and (ii) Misdiagnosing complicated appendicitis. Appendicolith is an independent predictive factor for perforation and failure of NOM in uncomplicated acute appendicitis.

Appendectomy: Laparoscopic appendectomy should be the first choice in both uncomplicated and complicated acute appendicitis in adults and children where equipment and expertise are available. In uncomplicated appendicitis, emergency surgery is not always indicated but delay should not be more than 24 hours. In complicated appendicitis, early appendectomy within 8 hours should be performed.

Treatment options for acute appendicitis with phlegmon or abscess are appendectomy (laparoscopic or open) or percutaneous drainage with antibiotics. Interval appendectomy is not routinely recommended in children and young adults (<40 years) after NOM for appendicitis with phlegmon or abscess. Interval appendectomy is indicated in patients with recurrent symptoms. Colonic screening with colonoscopy and interval full-dose contrast-enhanced CT scan is indicated after nonoperative management of acute appendicitis in patients older than 40 years to exclude colonic neoplasms.

Different Laparoscopic Approaches of Appendectomy in Adult Patients

- Conventional three-port laparoscopic appendectomy (CLA)
- Single-incision laparoscopic appendectomy (SILA)

Different Laparoscopic Approaches of Appendectomy in Pediatric Patients

- Conventional three-port laparoscopic appendectomy (CLA)
- Single-incision laparoscopic appendectomy (SILA)
- Transumbilical laparoscopically assisted appendectomy (TULAA)

Open Appendectomy

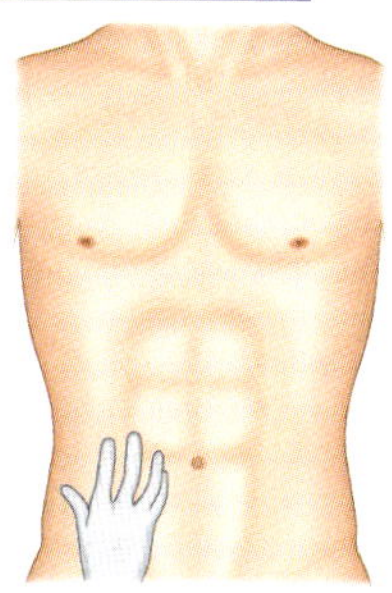

- Preoperative single dose of broad-spectrum antibiotic significantly reduces the chance of postoperative wound infection and intra-abdominal abscess. Postoperative antibiotic is not recommended in uncomplicated appendicitis.
- Regional anesthesia is preferred over general anesthesia for open appendectomy.
- After anesthesia and prior to incision, right lower quadrant should be palpated to rule out appendicular lump.

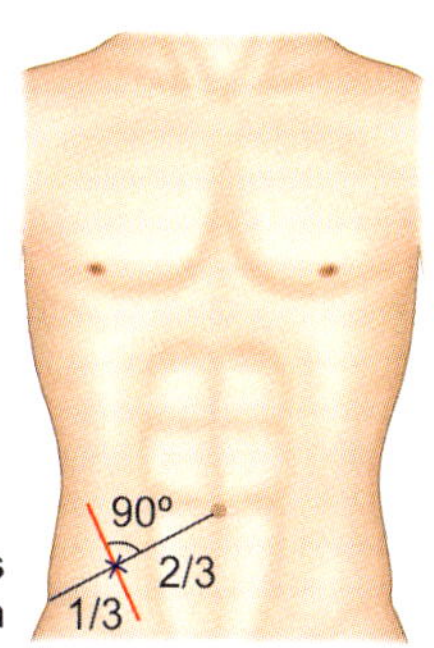

[In acute condition, McBurney's Gridiron incision is preferred]

OR

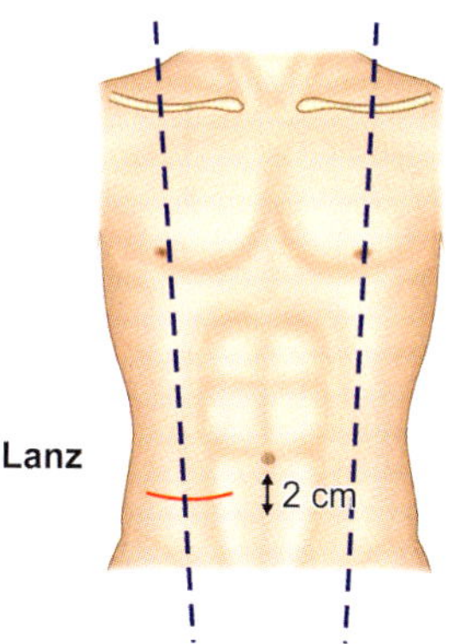

Incisions for Appendectomy

- McBurney's gridiron incision (most preferred for emergency appendectomy)
- Rutherford Morrison incision
- Lanz incision

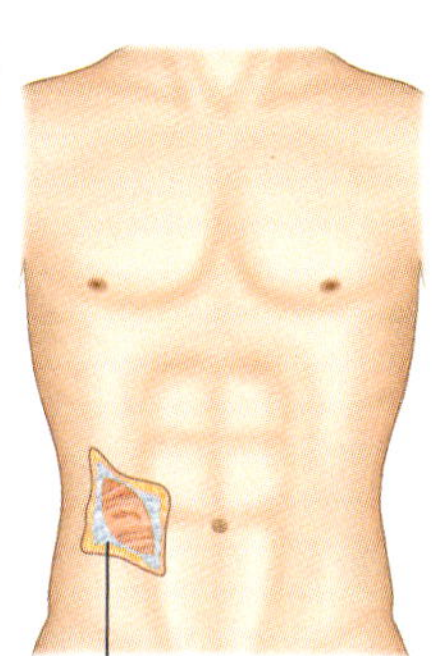

Division of external oblique aponeurosis along the direction of fibers

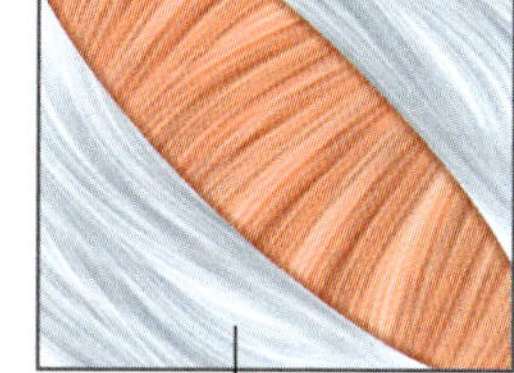

Fibers of external oblique aponeurosis

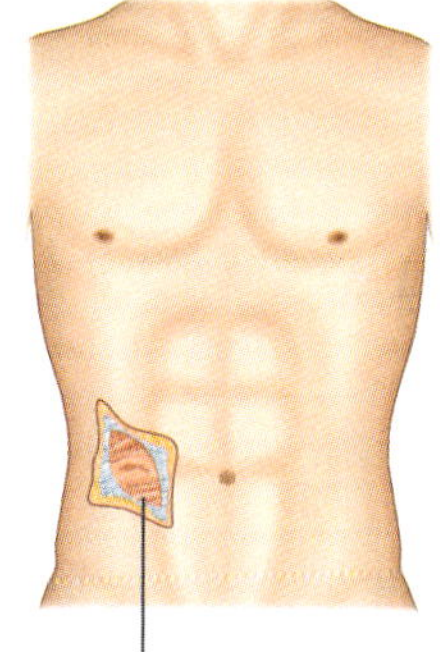

Internal oblique and transversus abdominis are splitted along the direction of muscle fibers

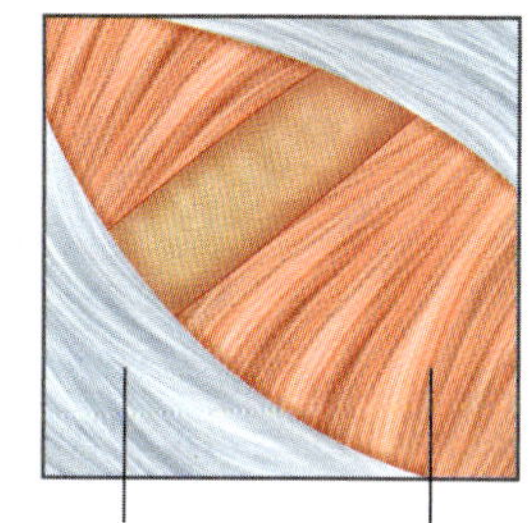

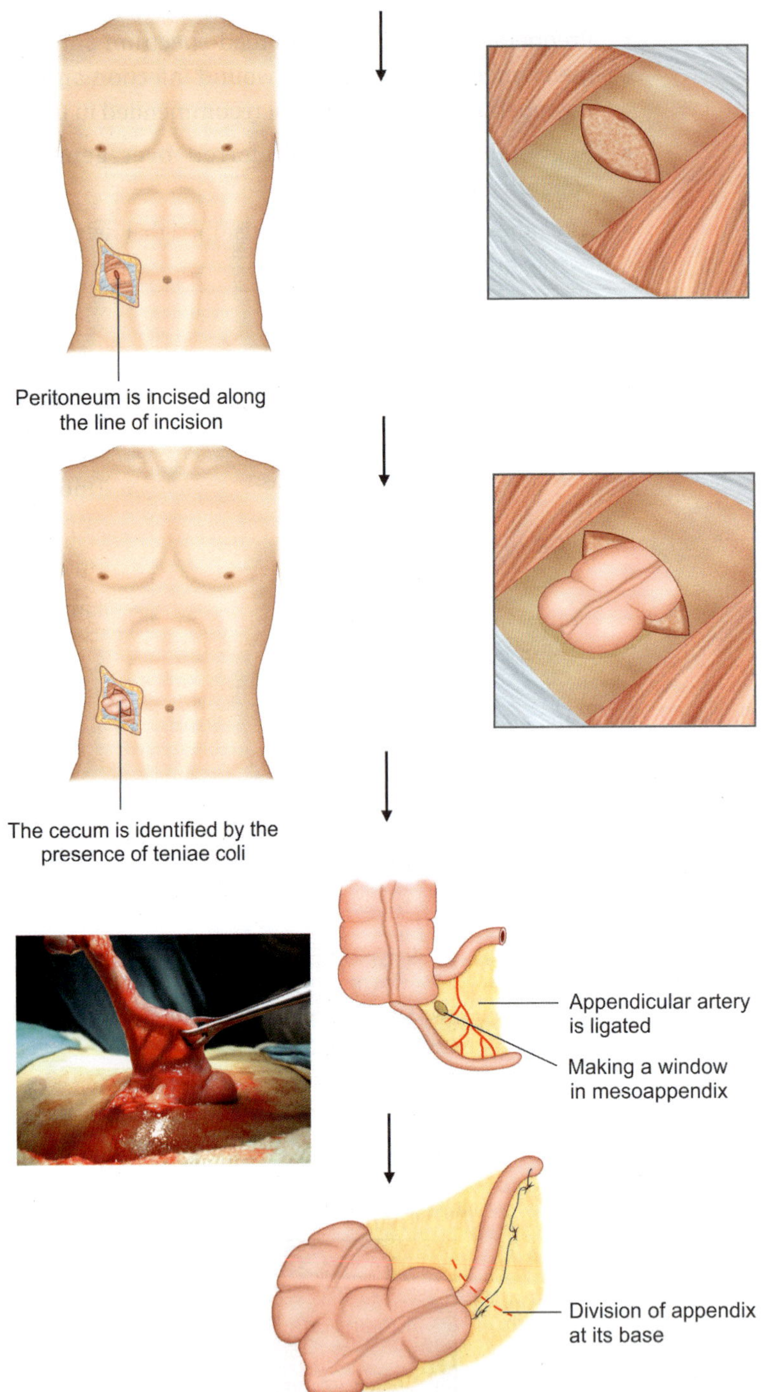

Intraoperative peritoneal irrigation does not have any advantage of preventing development of postoperative intraabdominal abscess in complicated appendicitis.

Drain after appendectomy for perforated appendicitis and abscess/peritonitis is not effective for prevention of intraabdominal abscess formation.

Most of the international guidelines suggest appendectomy in a case of normal appearing appendix during surgery for suspected acute appendicitis.

Laparoscopic Appendectomy

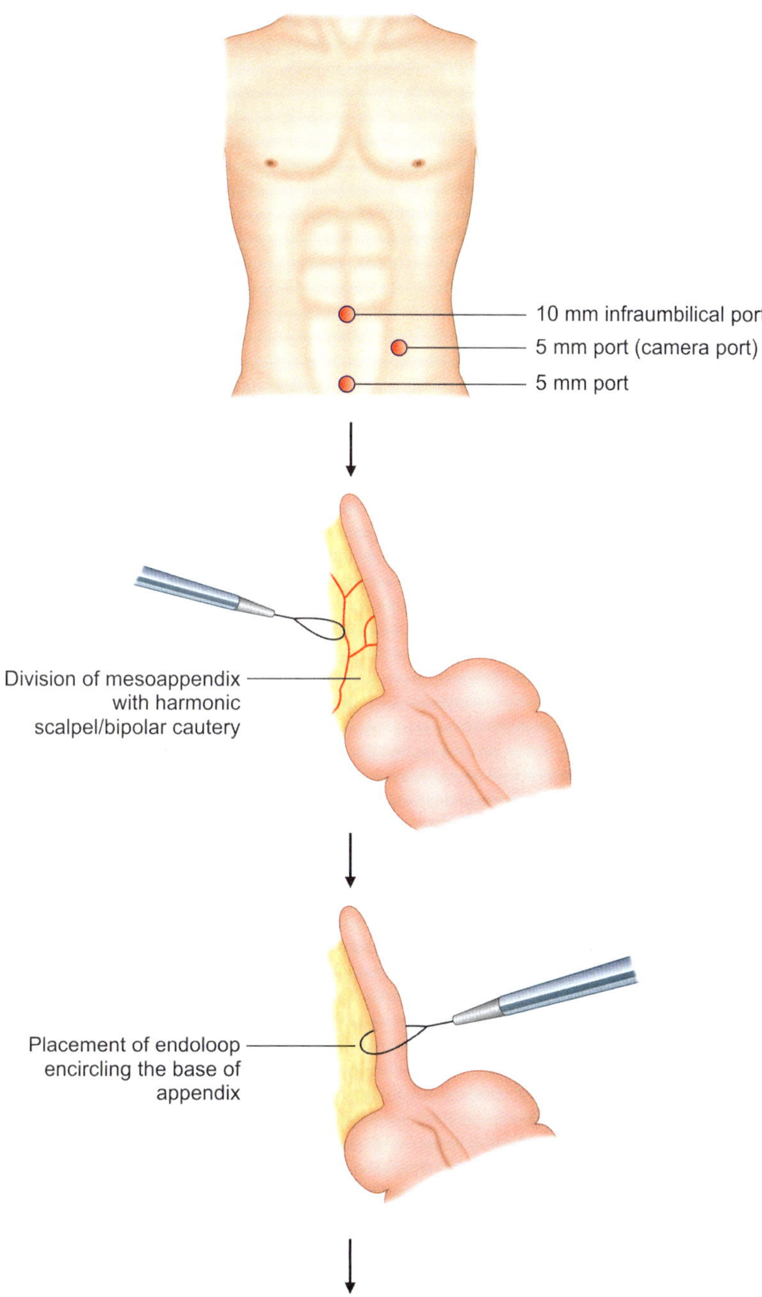

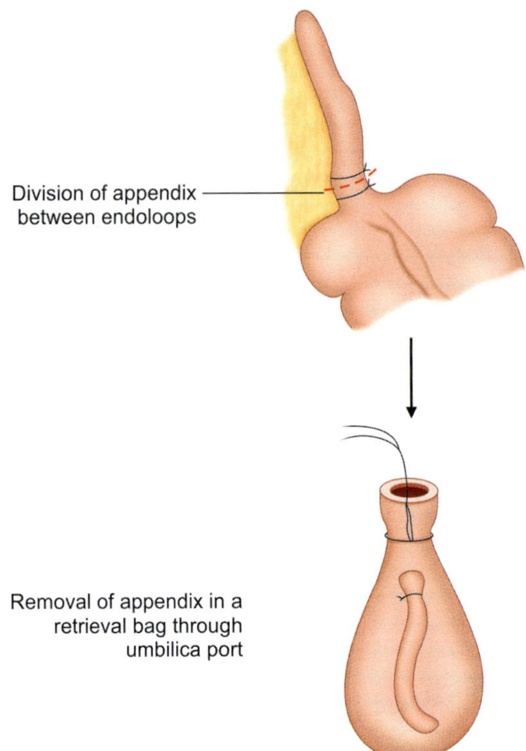

Techniques of mesoappendix dissection in laparoscopic appendectomy:

- Bipolar energy
- Unipolar electrosurgery-Endoloops
- Metal clips
- LigaSure
- Harmonic scalpel

Methods of appendicular stump closure in laparoscopic appendectomy:

- Simple ligation
- Endoloop
- Polymeric clip
- Endostapler

Stump Appendicitis

A uncommon, late complication of appendectomy (open or laparoscopic), where inflammation occurs in the remaining appendicular stump.

To prevent stump appendicitis, surgeon must follow the following principles during appendectomy:

(i) Complete exposure of mesoappendix, taenia coli of the cecum, and appendico-cecal junction
(ii) Ligation of recurrent or accessory branch of appendicular artery (artery of Seshachalam)
(iii) Remaining stump length should be less than 0.5 cm.

Stump appendicitis presents with similar symptoms and signs of acute appendicitis. A high index of suspicion along with imaging (USG or CT) can detect stump appendicitis early and can avoid complications (e.g., stump gangrene, cecal perforation, peritonitis).

Completion appendectomy (open or laparoscopic) with or without invagination is the treatment of choice.

Acute Appendicitis in the Elderly

In elderly patients, classic symptoms, and signs of acute appendicitis are not always present. Incidence of complicated appendicitis is also more in this population.

CT abdomen is helpful for diagnosis and also to differentiate between uncomplicated and complicated appendicitis.

If equipments and expertise are available, laparoscopic appendectomy is the preferred surgical option. If preoperative imaging shows periappendiceal abscess, percutaneous drainage is the treatment. Colonic screening should be done both after nonoperative and operative management to rule out any colonic neoplasm.

Acute Appendicitis in Children

Diagnosis is often difficult particularly in younger children due to lack of communication, inadequate clinical examination, overlap of symptoms with other common pediatric illnesses. Often, acute appendicitis present with complications like perforation or abscess due to:

(i) Delayed diagnosis
(ii) Thin-walled appendix
(iii) Short omentum.

The combination of Pediatric Appendicitis Score and USG is highly accurate for diagnosis. MRI should be preferred over CT (same sensitivity and specificity as CT) as second-line imaging modality to avoid CT radiation dose.

Treatment is emergency appendectomy (laparoscopic or open).

Acute Appendicitis in Pregnancy

Acute appendicitis is the most common cause of nongynecological or obstetric-related emergency surgeries in pregnant women. Symptoms and signs of appendicitis are same but localization of tenderness is shifted (more laterally and superiorly) due to gravid uterus.

For diagnosis, imaging should be either USG or MRI. MRI is particularly indicated if USG is inconclusive.

If acute appendicitis is highly suspected, emergency appendectomy (open or laparoscopic) should be done because delay in surgery may lead to perforation or abscess resulting in increased risk of fetal loss.

Appendicular Lump (Appendiceal Mass)

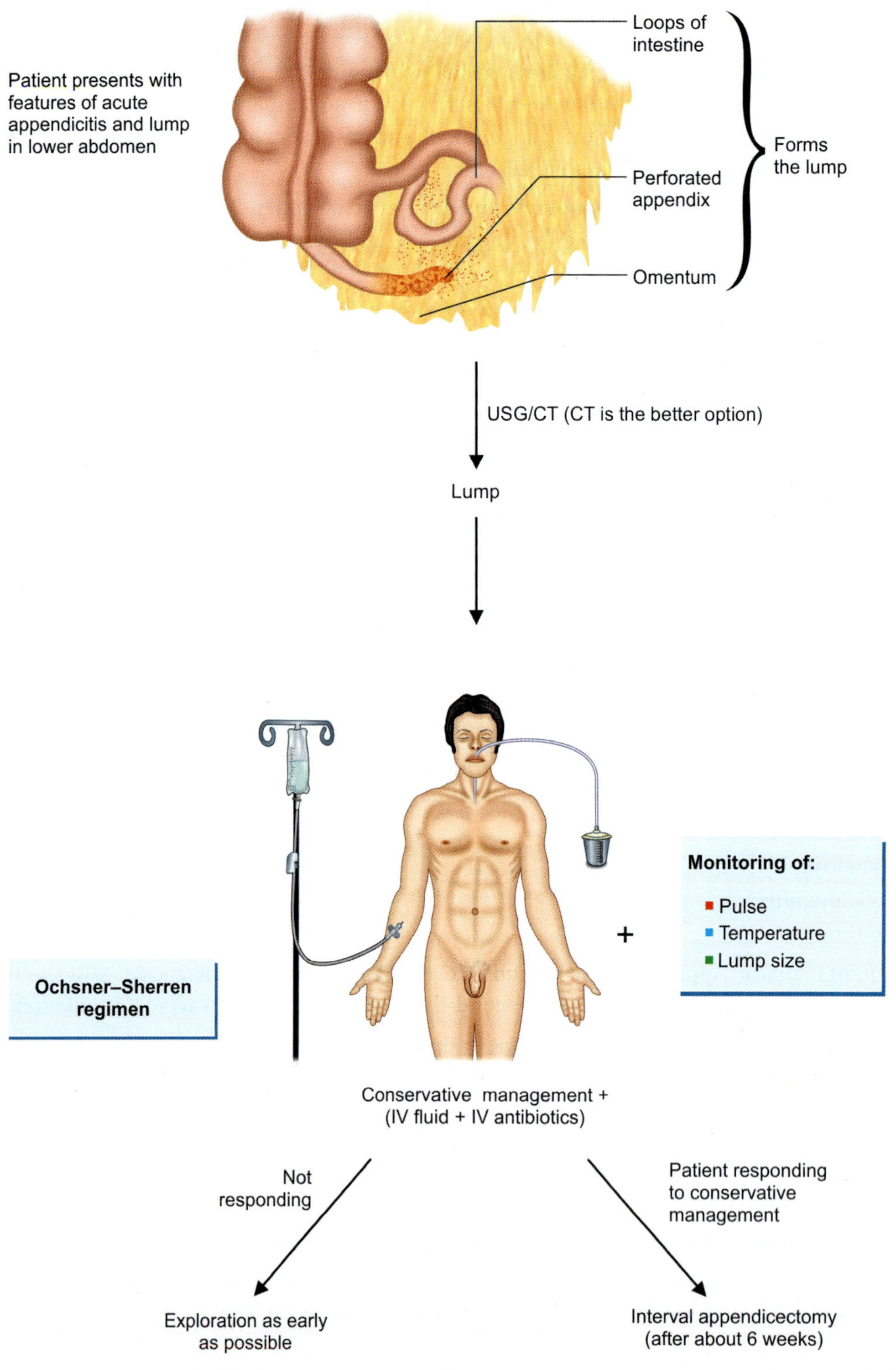

In patients with recurrent symptoms.

Carcinoids of the Appendix

- Carcinoid tumors are **neuroendocrine tumors that arise from Kulchitsky cells of the crypts of Lieberkühn**.
- Carcinoid tumor is the **most common neoplasm of the appendix**.
- Most of the appendiceal carcinoids are located at the tip of appendix.
- Most of the carcinoids present as recurrent appendicitis.
- Unlike carcinoids of other sites, appendiceal carcinoid rarely gives rise to metastases.
- **Appendicectomy** is indicated for tumor <2 cm. For tumor >2 cm, involving the base of appendix or mesoappendix, **right hemicolectomy** is recommended.
- Patient with appendiceal carcinoids may present with **second primary tumors** (specially tumors in GI and genitourinary tract), screening investigations (e.g., colonoscopy) are necessary to detect the second malignancy.

Case 1

History and Physical Examination

A 32-year-old female patient presented with pain in the right lower abdomen for last 2 days. Patient also complained 1–2 episodes of vomiting during this period. No history of dysuria or increased frequency of urination. No history of similar type of pain in the past. No history of constipation or diarrhea. No significant abnormality in menstrual and obstetric history.

Physical Examination:

Patient alert, conscious, cooperative

Anemia, jaundice: absent, pulse: 100/min, Temperature: 101°F

Examination of abdomen: Abdomen soft, tenderness in right iliac fossa, rebound tenderness present, no lump palpable in RIF

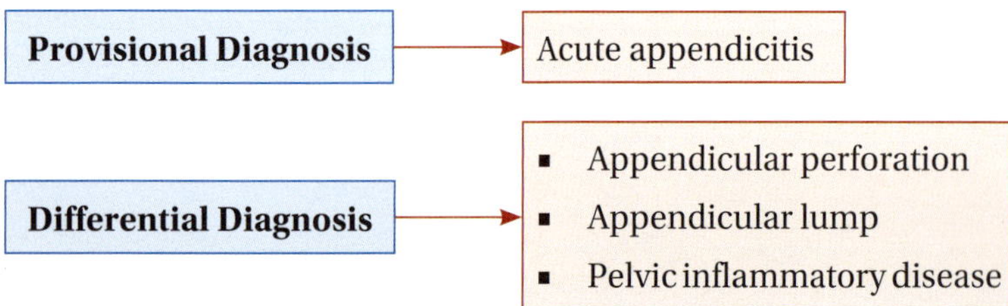

Investigations

USG abdomen: Noncompressible appendix with 7 mm diameter and presence of fecalith.
Hb: 11.2 gm%, Total leucocyte count: 12,000/cumm.

Discussion

History of acute onset right lower abdominal pain with clinical findings of tenderness and rebound tenderness in RIF almost suggestive of acute appendicitis. USG abdomen confirmed the clinical diagnosis. Emergency appendectomy was planned.

Management Algorithm

Palpation of the RIF after anesthesia to exclude appendicular lump → If no lump is palpable, then appendectomy

Case 2

History and Physical Examination

A 35-year-old female patient presented in the emergency department with acute onset pain in the right lower abdomen. Patient had a history of recurrent attack of pain in the same region in last 2 years. No history of dysuria. Menstrual and obstetric history were normal.

Physical Examination:

Temperature: 100.2°F, pulse: 96/min, BP: 110/78 mm Hg

Examination of abdomen: Tenderness in the right iliac fossa, no rebound tenderness, no lump palpable in RIF

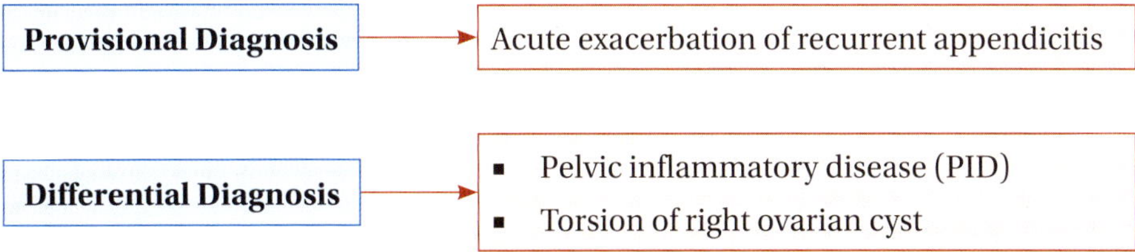

Investigations

Hb: 12.8 gm%, Total WBC count: 8000/cumm, Blood sugar (F): 88 mg/dL
CT abdomen revealed appendiceal inflammation

Discussion

Acute onset pain in the right lower abdomen along with recurrent pain in the same region consistent with acute exacerbation of recurrent appendicitis. CT abdomen also confirmed the diagnosis of appendiceal inflammation and excluded tubo-ovarian pathology. Therefore, appendectomy was planned.

Management Algorithm

Appendectomy → Histopathology revealed well-differentiated neuroendocrine tumor measuring 1 cm at the maximum dimension at the tip of the appendix, infiltrated few areas of the muscular layer. The diagnosis of carcinoid tumor was confirmed by immunohistochemistry (positive for chromogranin A and synaptophysin).

↓

As the tumor size was less than 2 cm and at the tip of the appendix, there was no need of further treatment.

Diseases of Rectum and Anal Canal

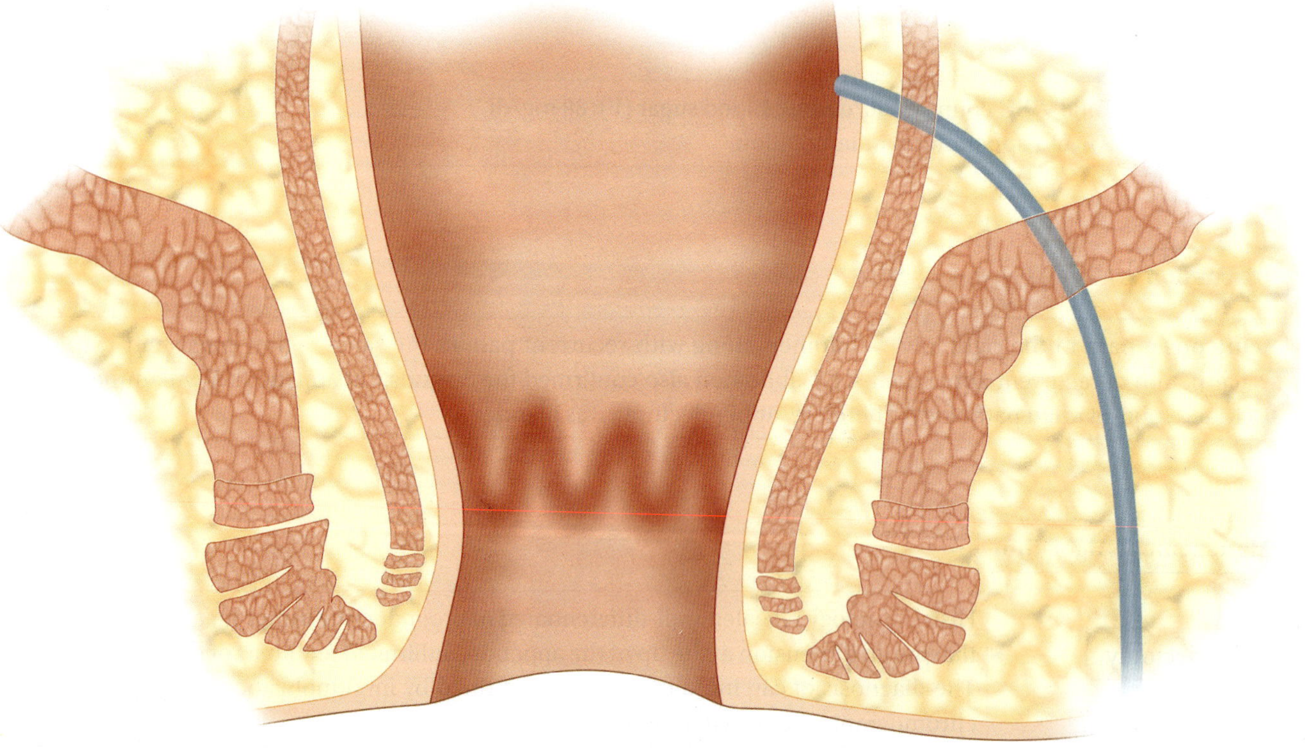

Important Topics

- Rectal Prolapse
- Anal Fissure
- Anorectal Abscess
- Hemorrhoids
- Pilonidal Disease
- Fecal Incontinence
- Rectal Cancer
- Anal Carcinoma
- Surgical Staplers

'[F]rom the simplicity Nature employs in all her works. We may conclude …… From these considerations it is highly probable that the question about the mutual union and anastomosis of the vessels can be solved; for if Nature once circulates the blood within vessels and combines their ends in a network, it is probable that they are joined by anastomosis at other times too.'

Marcello Malpighi (1628–1694)
Italian Physician, Physiologist and Microscopist

Rectal Prolapse

Rectal prolapse (Procidentia) is **intussusception of the rectum** with external protrusion through the anus. **Complete rectal prolapse** is circumferential protrusion of full thickness of rectum. **Mucosal prolapse** is circumferential protrusion of the rectal mucosa.

Types of Rectal Prolapse

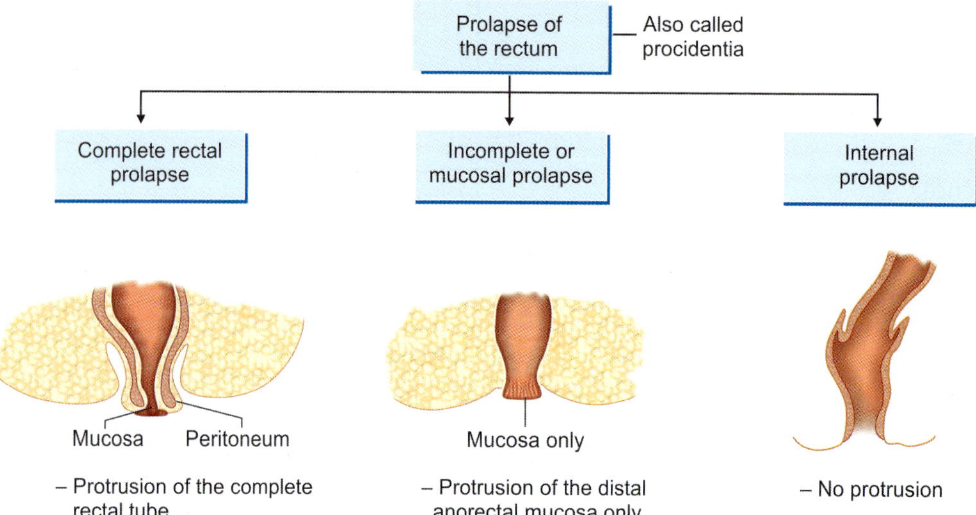

Pathophysiology

Exact pathophysiology is not known. Rectal prolapse is commonly associated with **some anatomical abnormalities**.

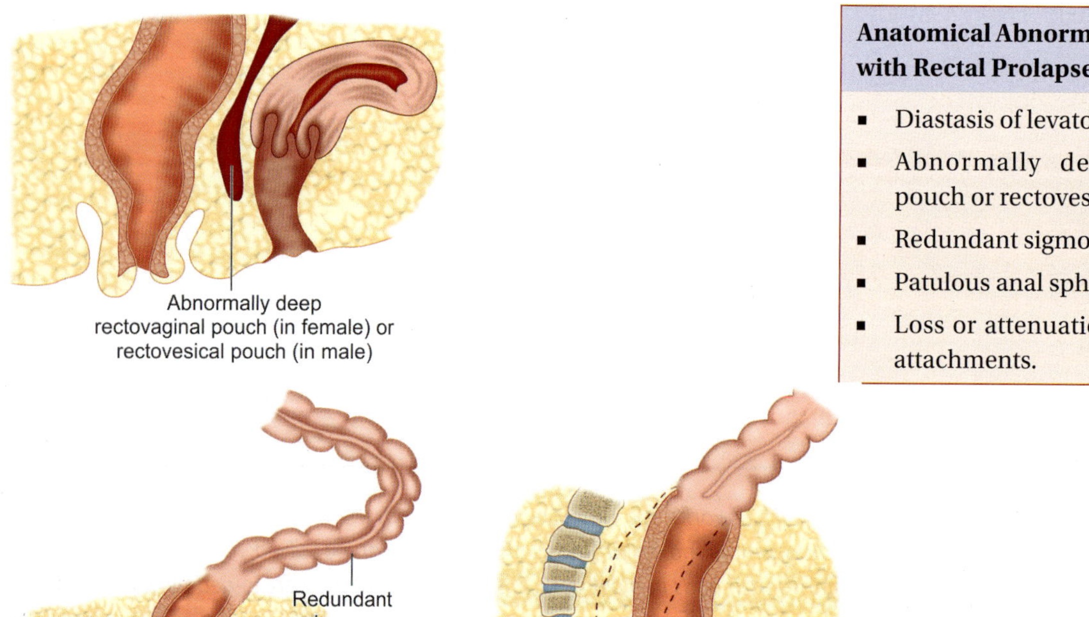

Anatomical Abnormalities Associated with Rectal Prolapse

- Diastasis of levator ani
- Abnormally deep rectovaginal pouch or rectovesical pouch
- Redundant sigmoid colon
- Patulous anal sphincter
- Loss or attenuation of rectal sacral attachments.

Clinical Presentation

Mucosal Prolapse

Children presents **after a diarrheal episode** or **acute illness** causing loss of body weight. This prolapse only apparent during defecation.

Complete Rectal Prolapse

More common in **elderly women**. Peak age of incidence in women is seventh decade. Age of incidence in men is usually **≤40 years**. **Rectal prolapse in younger patients is** usually associated with autism, syndromes associated with developmental delay, psychiatric comorbidities.

Initially the prolapse apparent during defecation. Later, patient presents with soiling of underclothes with blood and mucus. Constipation commonly present in these patients. Incontinence of feces and flatus also may be present. In long standing cases, ulceration over the prolapsed mucosa may be found. Symptoms of associated urinary incontinence, vaginal/uterine prolapse may present.

Differential Diagnosis of Mucosal Prolapse

- Prolapsed juvenile rectal polyp
- Apex of intussusception.

Differential Diagnosis of Complete Rectal Prolapse

- Prolapsed internal hemorrhoids
- Mucosal prolapse.

Coexisting Pathologies that May Present

- Cystocele
- Vaginal vault prolapse
- Enterocele
- Anterior solitary rectal ulcer.

Clinical Evaluation

No prolapse on physical examination: Patient has to be asked to reproduce the prolapse by straining in sitting or squatting position.

Full inspection of the perineum: Concentric folds of prolapsed tissue (in complete rectal prolapse) or radial folds of mucosa around the anus (in mucosal prolapse) can be seen. Sometimes, associated vaginal or uterine prolapse may be apparent.

Digital rectal examination: Palpation reveals double thickness of tissue in complete rectal prolapse and mucosa only in mucosal prolapse. Patulous anus with diminished sphincter tone is commonly revealed in digital rectal examination.

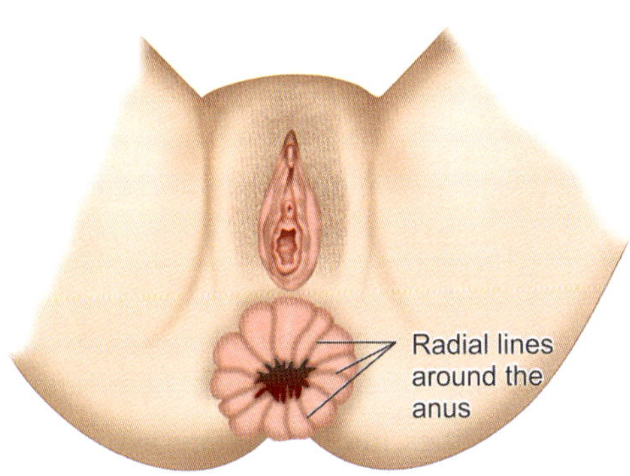

Mucosal Rectal Prolapse

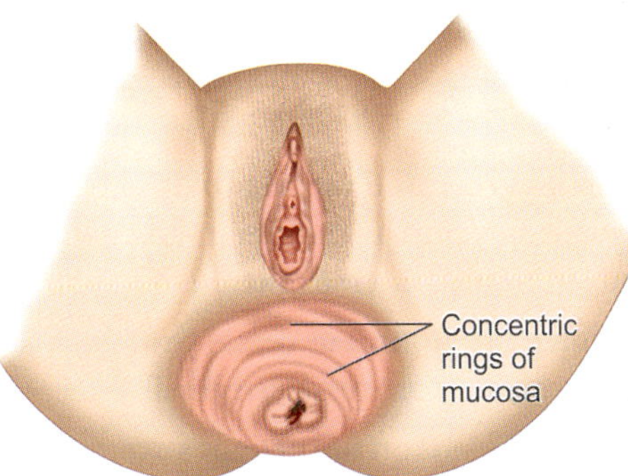

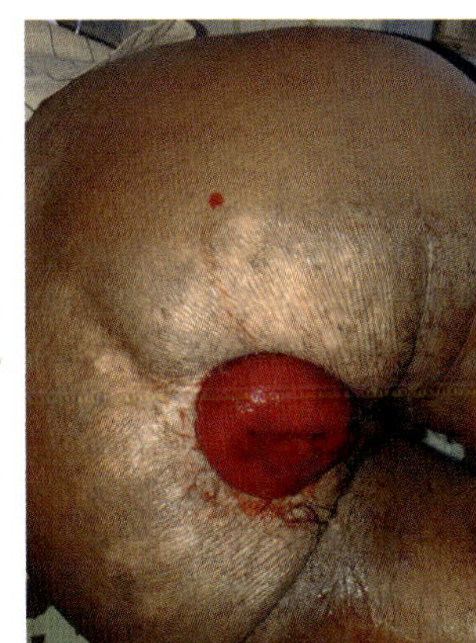

Complete Rectal Prolapse

Oxford Rectal Prolapse Grading System

Internal Rectal Prolapse

I (Low grade): Descends no lower than proximal limit of the rectocele

II (Low grade): Descends into the level of the rectocele, but not onto sphincter/anal canal

III (High grade): Descends onto sphincter/anal canal

IV (High grade): Descends into sphincter/anal canal

External Rectal Prolapse

V (Overt rectal prolapse) Protrudes from anus

Rectocele

Protrusion of the rectum into the posterior wall of the vagina due to defect in the integrity of rectovaginal septum.

Cystocele

Pathologic descent of the anterior vaginal wall and overlying bladder base due to defect in pubocervical fascia.

Enterocele

Herniation of the pelvic peritoneum into the rectovaginal space containing the small intestine due to defect of the rectovaginal fascia.

Investigations

Defecography: If prolapse cannot be seen during physical examination, then fluoroscopic defecography or MRI defecography is indicated. Defecography can also detect cystocele, enterocele, and vaginal vault prolapse.

Colonoscopy: It is indicated to rule out any polyp or neoplastic lesion. Plan of management may be changed if significant colonoscopic findings.

Urodynamic study: It is indicated in patients with associated urinary incontinence.

Anorectal manometry: It is indicated in patients of rectal prolapse with associated constipation to assess pelvis dyssynergia. Patients with pelvic dyssynergia are not the ideal candidates for surgical procedures that exacerbate constipation.

Management

Mucosal prolapse in children is a self-limiting condition. Most of the patients respond to conservative measures. Digital repositioning (parents are taught the technique), correction of bowel habit, judicious use of laxatives and improvement of general health are sufficient for definitive management. Prolapse associated with underlying congenital conditions (e.g., myelomeningocele, spina bifida, Hirschsprung disease, congenital hypothyroidism) may need surgical intervention.

The immediate management of incarcerated rectal prolapse is reduction if no evidence of full-thickness ischemia. Reduction is done by continuous steady pressure under intravenous sedation or general anesthesia in the emergency setup. Topical application of sugar reduces edema and aid in reduction of incarcerated prolapsed rectum.

Surgery is the treatment of choice for complete rectal prolapse. Decision of surgery should be taken as early as possible as delay may lead to incarcerated prolapse, irreversible fecal incontinence and increased risk of recurrence.

Abdominal or perineal approach depends on the patient's age, associated comorbidities, life expectancy, associated pelvic floor defects and surgeon's preference. **Abdominal approach is the procedure of choice unless specific indications for perineal approach are present.**

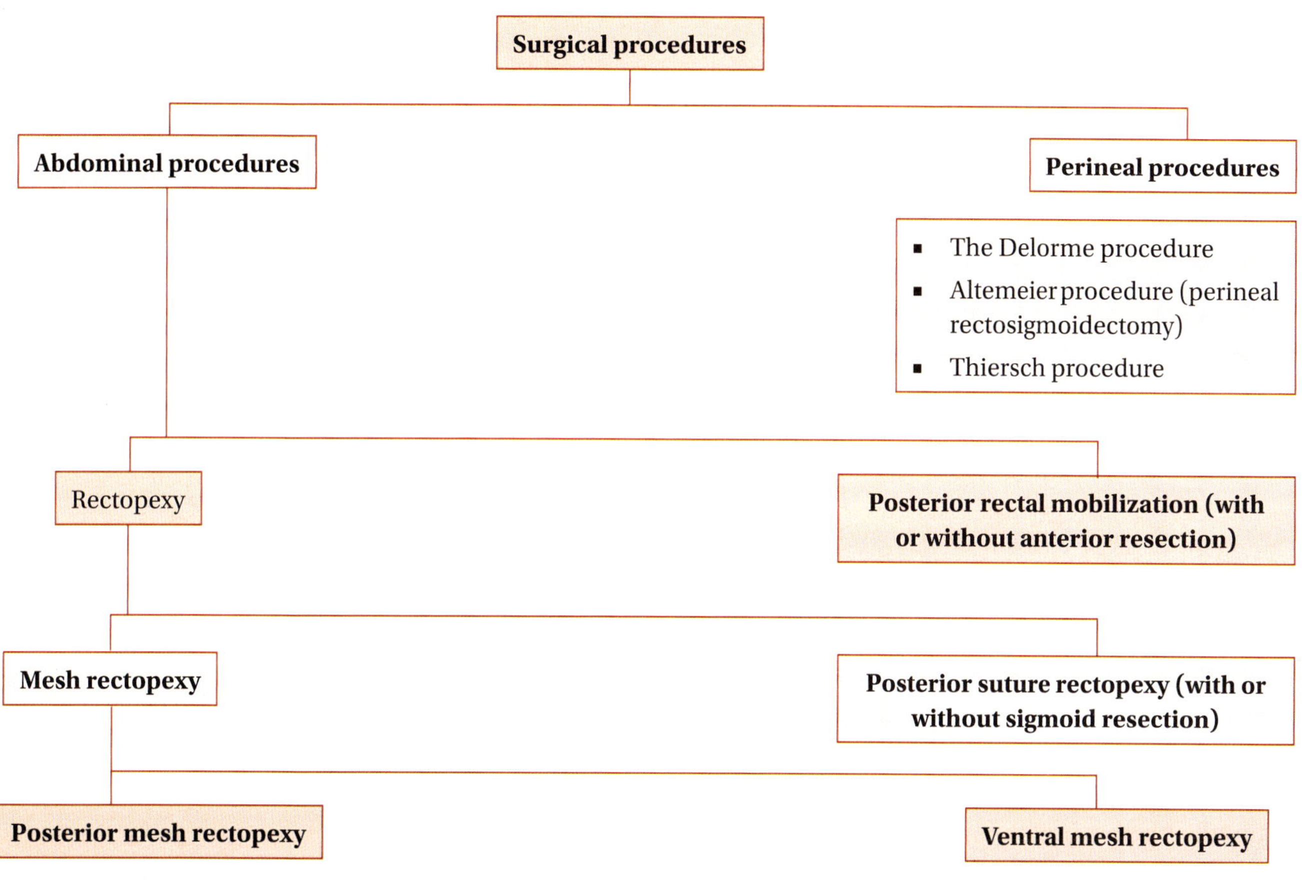

Advantages of Abdominal Procedures

- Less chance of recurrence
- Better functional outcomes
- Can address the associated constipation or incontinence.

Disadvantages of Abdominal Procedures

- More postoperative morbidity and mortality
- Risk of injury to the pelvic nerves.

Surgical Procedures for Rectal Prolapse that Exacerbate Constipation

- Posterior rectal mobilization
- Transection of lateral ligaments during posterior suture rectopexy
- Levatorplasty during perineal proctosigmoidectomy.

Indications of Perineal Procedures

- Elderly, frail patients
- Patient with extensive comorbid illness
- Decreased life expectancy
- Prior pelvic surgery or radiation.

Advantages of Perineal Procedures

- Less postoperative morbidity and mortality
- Less invasive procedure
- Lower risk of injury to the pelvic nerves
- Shorter length of hospital stay
- Concomitant anorectal pathologies (e.g., hemorrhoids, rectocele, cystocele etc.) can be treated.

Disadvantages of Perineal Procedure

- Higher recurrence rate
- Less improvement of fecal incontinence.

Posterior rectal mobilization (with or without concomitant anterior resection): Rectum is mobilized from sacral promontory to the levators in the plane between mesorectal fascia and the presacral fascia. This procedure with or without anterior resection has high recurrence and complication rate.

Posterior suture rectopexy (with or without sigmoid resection): Suturing the rectum to the sacral promontory with nonabsorbable suture to prevent the telescoping of the redundant bowel. Posterior suture rectopexy with sigmoid resection is known as **Frykman-Goldberg procedure**. Addition of sigmoidectomy to the suture rectopexy decreases the recurrence rate, improves functional outcome.

Posterior mesh rectopexy: In posterior mesh rectopexy **(Modified Ripstein and McMahan procedure)**, posterior fixation of the mesh to the sacrum with attachment of the ends of the mesh to the rectum laterally.

In original Ripstein procedure, a band of rectangular mesh is placed around the anterior aspect of the rectum at the level of peritoneal reflection, mesh is secured to the anterior surface of the rectum, sides of the mesh were sutured to the presacral fascia.

Modified Wells procedure: In this procedure, polypropylene or polyester or biological mesh is used for posterior fixation of the rectum. This procedure is popular for laparoscopic approach. **Original Wells procedure** includes fixation of the rectum using polyvinyl alcohol sponge and transection of the lateral ligaments.

Ventral rectopexy: In this procedure, anteriorly, the rectum is mobilized from the vagina (or prostate) down to the perineal body, posteriorly, a small area of sacrum and without lateral dissection. The synthetic or biological mesh buttresses the anterior wall of the rectum at the point of intussusception and resuspends the rectum to the sacral promontory.

Complications of rectopexy: (i) Presacral bleeding; (ii) Fecal impaction; (iii) Stricture; (iv) Pelvic abscess; (v) Rectal erosion; (vi) Recurrence; and (vii) Constipation. Division of lateral ligaments (containing parasympathetic innervations) during rectopexy increases the severity of constipation.

Laparoscopic mesh rectopexy has similar recurrence rate and morbidity compared to open mesh rectopexy and also associated with less postoperative pain, early return of bowel function, and shorter hospital stay.

The Delorme procedure: This procedure involves a circumferential mucosal sleeve resection and imbrication of the muscularis layer with serial vertical sutures. Complications include: infection, urinary retention, bleeding, fecal impaction.

The Altemeier procedure: This procedure involves a transanal full-thickness resection of the prolapsed rectum and a coloanal anastomosis. Concomitant levatorplasty may decrease the recurrence rate of this procedure. Complications include: bleeding from the suture staple line, pelvic abscess, anastomotic leak.

The Thiersch procedure: This procedure involves placing a nonabsorbable suture (e.g., polypropylene, nylon) encircling the anal canal under the skin. The suture is tightened to a point that allows passage of one finger only. This procedure may be indicated in patients with significant comorbidities with short life expectancy. Complications include: anal stenosis, fecal impaction, high recurrence rate.

Operations for internal rectal prolapse: (i) STARR (Stapled Transanal Rectal Resection) procedure and (ii) EXPRESS (External Pelvic Rectal Suspension) procedure.

Posterior Mesh Rectopexy

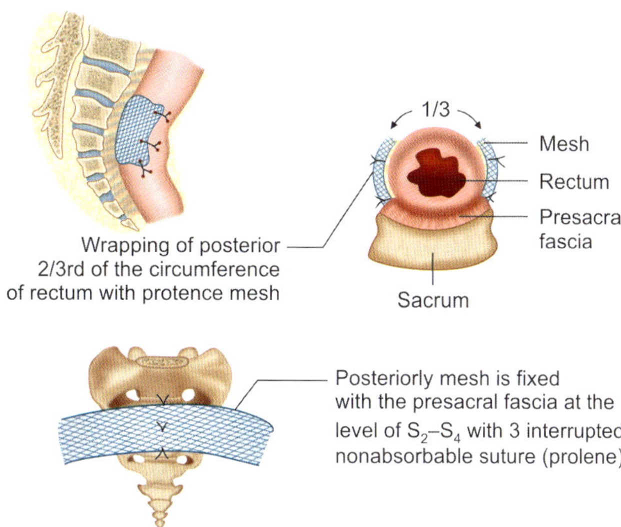

Ventral Mesh Rectopexy

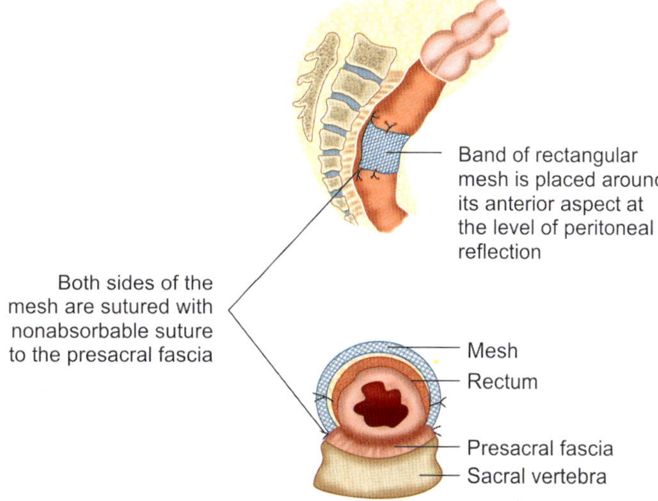

Posterior Suture Rectopexy with Sigmoid Resection

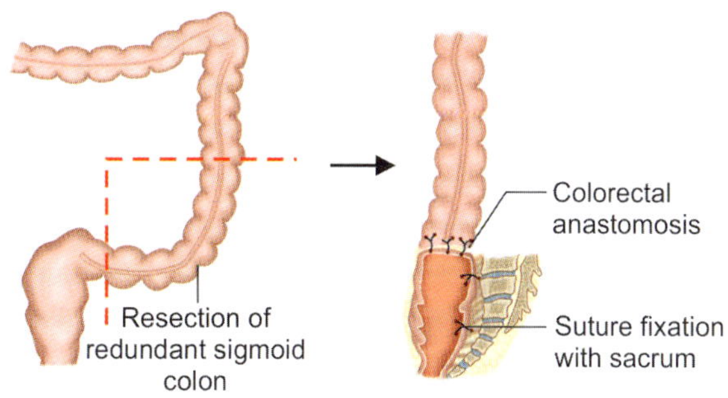

Anal Fissure

Anal fissure (Fissure-in-ano) is a **longitudinal tear** within the anal canal that **extends from the dentate line toward the anal verge**.

Acute fissure: Symptoms persisting for less than 8 weeks. In acute fissure, a linear tear or laceration is visible.

Chronic fissure: Symptoms persisting for more than 8 weeks.

Classic Findings in Chronic Fissure

- Hypertrophied anal papilla at the proximal aspect of the fissure
- Edematous skin tag **(sentinel piles)** at the distal aspect of the fissure
- Exposed internal sphincter at the base of the fissure.

Posterior midline: Most common location.

Anterior midline: Common in females.

Both anterior and posterior: About 3% of patients.

Fissure at lateral location and multiple fissures: Crohn's disease, tuberculosis, HIV, syphilis, hidradenitis suppurativa.

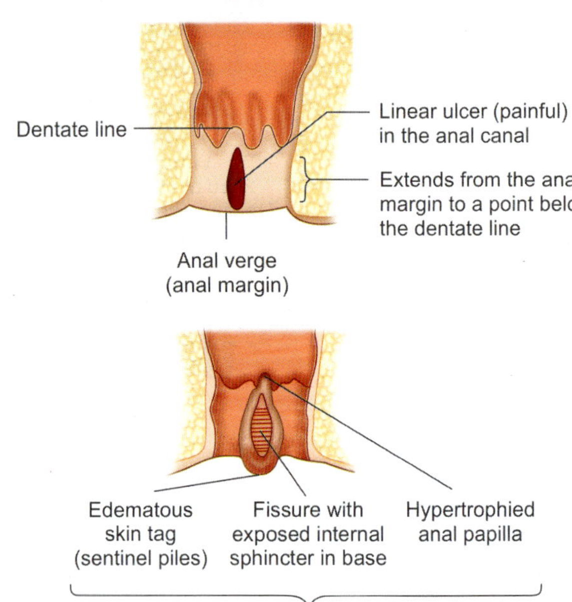

Classic findings in fissure-in-ano

Pathophysiology

Predisposing Factors

- Local trauma due to constipation
- Scarring from previous anal surgery
- High resting anal canal pressure

Why posterior midline is the most common site?

In the posterior part of anal canal, there is lack of anatomical support due to elliptical arrangement of external sphincter fibers, that favors early tearing of anoderm.

Decreased mucosal perfusion of the posterior midline due to characteristic pattern of blood supply.

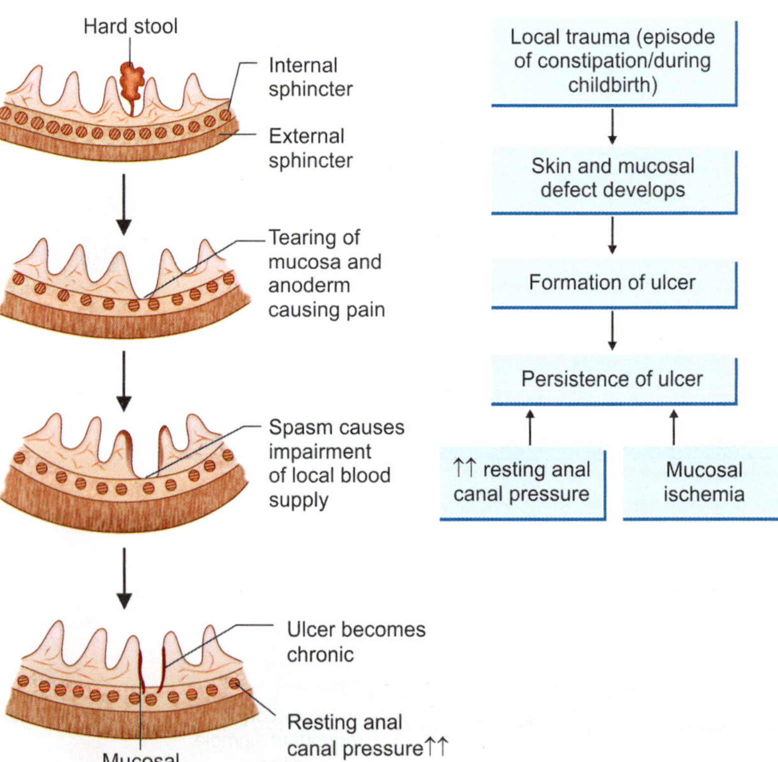

Diagnosis

Most common presentation is sharp and agonizing pain, starts during defecation and lasts for a few hours. Patient often describes a tearing sensation during defecation. Patient tends to become constipated due to pain. Fecal impaction commonly found in children and elderly patients. Bleeding is slight and usually streaks on the stool or toilet paper.

Typical history, tightly closed puckered anus, inspection of the lower end of fissure are sufficient to diagnose acute fissure. In chronic fissure, classic findings (e.g., sentinel piles, hypertrophied anal papilla) are present.

Digital rectal examination and proctoscopy should be avoided in acute fissure. DRE and proctoscopy should be delayed for 4–6 weeks when acute pain resolves.

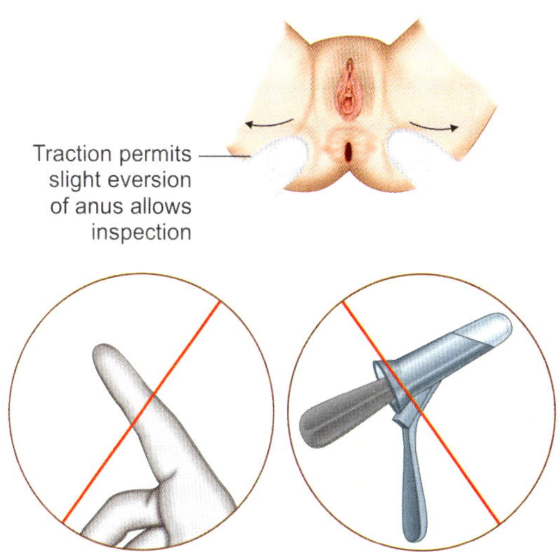

Management

Acute Anal Fissure

First-line treatment is warm-water sitz bath (relieves discomfort by decreasing muscle spasm) and bulk laxatives (changes the consistency of stool).

Chronic Anal Fissure

Chronic fissure is managed by medications **("chemical sphincterotomy")** or by surgical intervention.

Topical nitroglycerine: It is a nitric oxide donor. Nitric oxide is a potent smooth muscle relaxant and vasodilator. Topical application of nitroglycerine 0.2% ointment causes healing of anal fissure by reducing tone of internal anal sphincter and increasing mucosal blood flow. Headache is a significant side effect. Other side effects are orthostatic hypotension, syncopal attack, tachyphylaxis.

Topical calcium channel blockers (Nifedipine 0.3%, Diltiazem 2%): Calcium channel blockers cause healing of fissure by reducing the resting anal sphincter tone. Headache is less frequent than topical nitrates. Oral calcium channel blockers are not preferred due to higher incidence of systemic side effects.

Botulinum toxin: Injection of botulinum toxin A (20–60 units) is preferred as second-line therapy following treatment with topical therapy. Botulinum toxin helps in healing of fissure by temporary paralysis of sphincter muscles by preventing the presynaptic release of acetylcholine. The toxin can be injected into internal sphincter, intersphincteric plane or external sphincter at 3 and 9 o'clock position. Side effects are transient incontinence to flatus and stool, perianal hematoma.

Surgical management: Surgical management with Lateral internal sphincterotomy (LIS) can be selected as first-line therapy for chronic fissure in patients with no underlying fecal incontinence. LIS is also the surgery of choice in refractory anal fissure. Other surgical options are fissurectomy (excision of the fissure with or without advancement flap), manual anal dilation with four finger insertion technique (associated with high risk of postoperative incontinence).

Newer surgical approaches are tailored sphincterotomy, calibrated sphincterotomy, V-Y advancement flap. These newer procedures are associated with low risk of fecal incontinence.

Management of low-pressure anal fissure: This type of fissure typically found in postpartum patients. If conservative management fails, fissurectomy with skin advancement flap is the preferred treatment option.

Lateral Internal Sphincterotomy (Open/Closed Approach)

In this surgical procedure, division of a portion of internal sphincter (as far as proximally as the dentate line) is done by open or closed approach to reduce anal canal pressure and facilitate healing of the fissure. No significant difference in postoperative pain, incontinence and overall outcomes between open and closed surgical sphincterotomies.

Contraindications of lateral sphincterotomy: (i) Pre-existing fecal incontinence; (ii) History of fistulotomy or fistulectomy; and (iii) Prior obstetric injury to the anal sphincter.

Complications of lateral sphincterotomy: (i) Transient incontinence; (ii) Anorectal seepage; and (iii) Relapse.

Closed Sphincterotomy

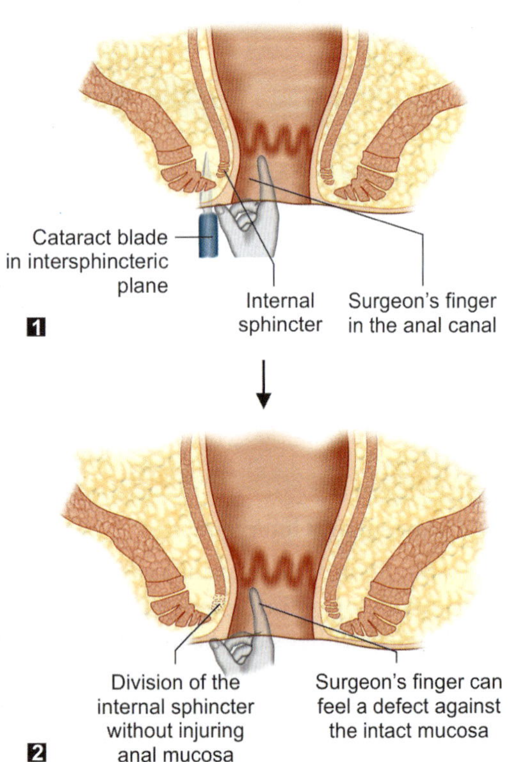

Tailored sphincterotomy: Sphincterotomy limited to the length of the fissure.

Calibrated sphincterotomy: Division of the internal sphincter according to the degree of hypertonia and to the sphincter length (based on the anal manometric findings).

Open Sphincterotomy

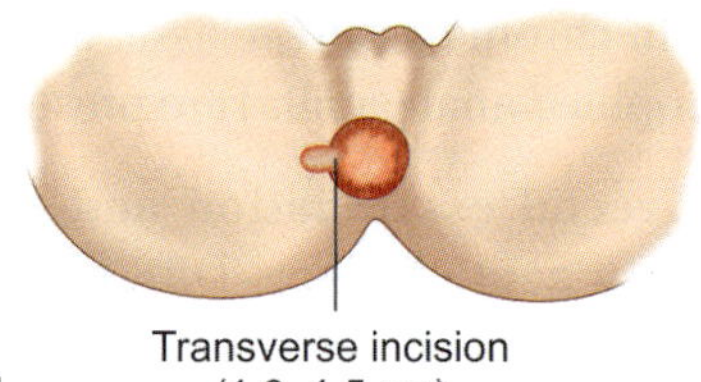

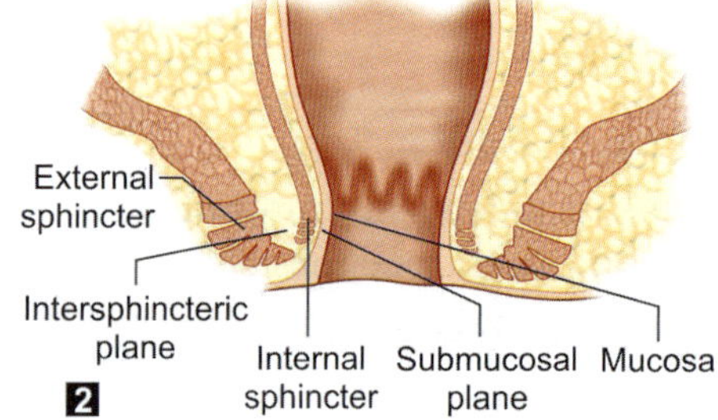

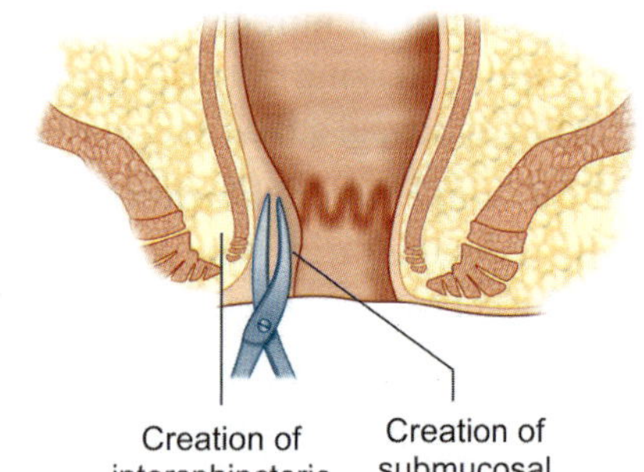
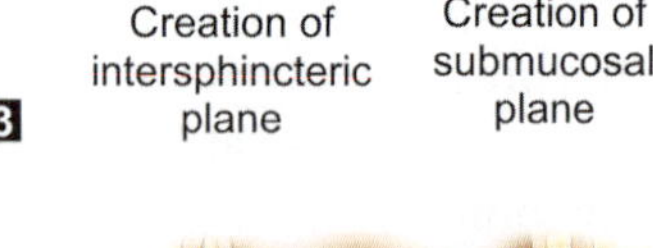

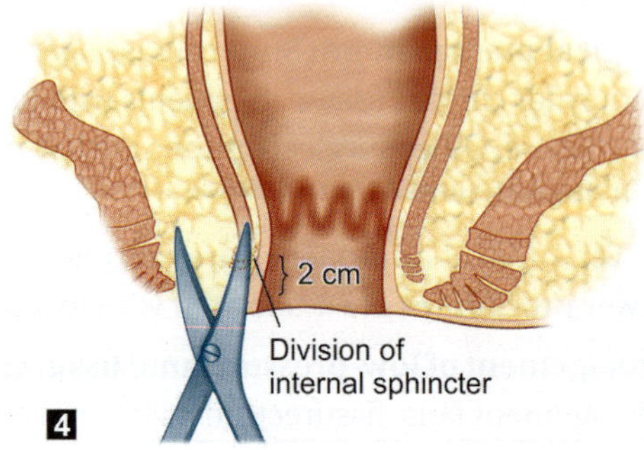

Anorectal Abscess

Infection of the secretion of the anal glands related to **anal crypts** is primarily responsible for development of anorectal abscess **(Cryptoglandular theory)**.

Types of anorectal abscess (based on location)

- Perianal abscess **(most common)**
- Ischiorectal abscess
- Intersphincteric abscess
- Supralevator abscess
- Submucosal abscess.

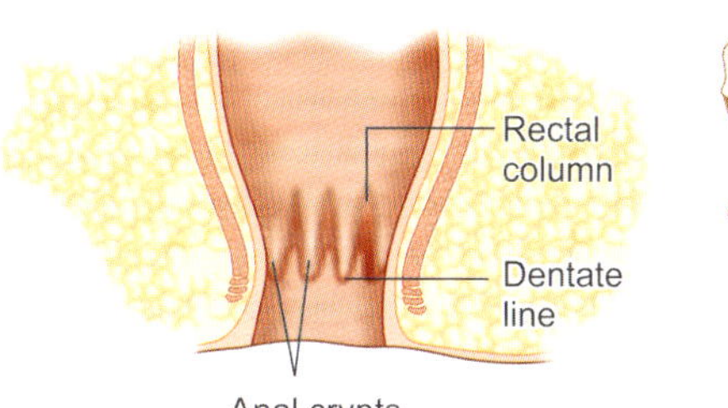

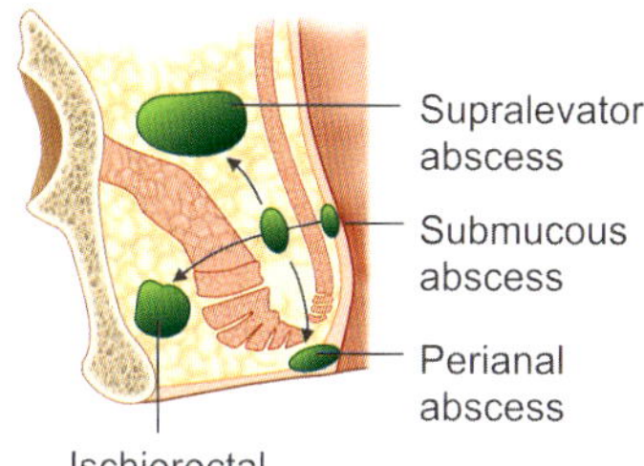

Superficial Abscesses

- Perianal abscess
- Ischiorectal abscess
- Submucosal abscess.

Deeper Abscesses

- Intersphincteric abscess
- Supralevator abscess.

Clinical Presentation

Perianal pain and swelling are common clinical presentations of superficial abscess. Erythematous, fluctuant, defined subcutaneous mass near the anal orifice is suggestive of **perianal abscess**.

Deeper abscesses may present with pain in the perineum, low back or buttock. **It is difficult to diagnose deeper abscesses by clinical examination alone**.

Thirty to seventy percent of patients with anorectal abscess present with concomitant fistula-in-ano.

Diagnosis

For superficial abscess, no need of imaging for diagnosis. Clinical diagnosis is sufficient for management.

For diagnosis of occult anorectal abscesses, imaging with MRI, CT, or Endoanal ultrasound is indicated.

MRI is the imaging modality of choice for complex anorectal sepsis.

Differential Diagnosis

- Pilonidal disease
- Hidradenitis suppurativa
- Perianal Crohn's disease
- Sexually transmitted infections
- Anal cancer.

Management

Primary treatment is early incision and drainage of abscess. Delay in drainage may result in chronic infection and destruction of tissues. Drainage should be done under regional or general anesthesia. Whether external or internal drainage, depends on the location of the abscess.

The incision should be as close as possible to anal verge to minimize the length of potential fistula tract.

Pus must be sent for culture and sensitivity.

Risk Factors for Recurrence after Surgical Drainage

- Inadequate drainage
- Multiloculated abscess
- Horse-shoe type abscess.

Drainage of Perianal Abscess

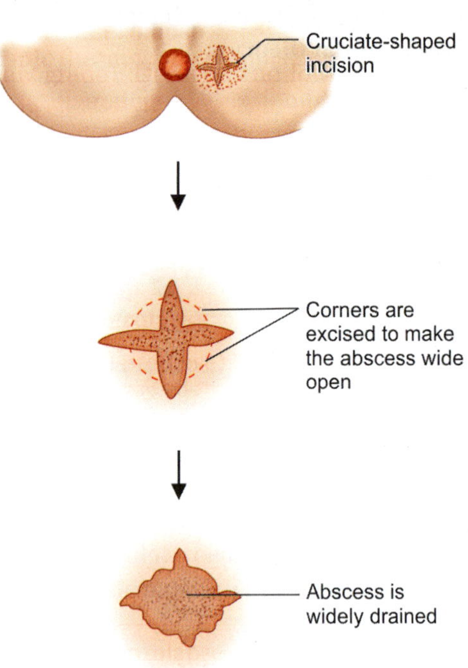

Drainage of Submucosal Abscess

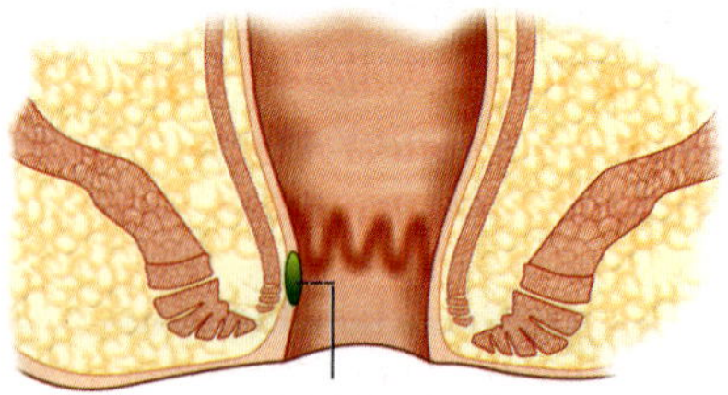

Drainage of Ischiorectal Abscess

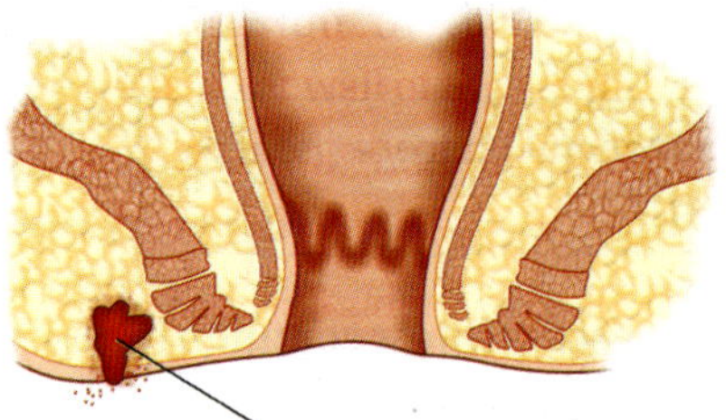

Drainage of Intersphincteric Abscess

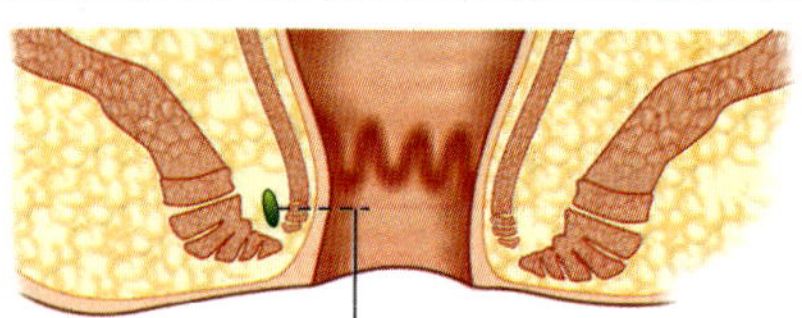

Drainage of Supralevator Abscess

It is essential to detect the origin of supralevator abscess before drainage. If the abscess is due to upward extension of intersphincteric abscess, it **should be drained transrectally**. If the abscess is due to upward extension of ischiorectal abscess, then it **should be drained transperineally through the ischioanal fossa.**

Horseshoe-type Anorectal Abscess

Abscess originating in the deep posterior anal space or deep anterior anal space. Then unilateral or bilateral extension into ischiorectal space.

Drainage is done by **Hanley procedure** (drainage of deep posterior anal space via fistulotomy and additional incisions into the ischiorectal space) or **modified Hanley technique** (partial sphincterotomy with seton placement).

External Drainage Through Perianal Skin

- Perianal abscess
- Ischiorectal abscess
- Supralevator abscess (due to upward extension of ischiorectal abscess).

Internal Drainage Through Anal Canal

- Intersphincteric abscess (via internal sphinctero-tomy)
- Submucosal abscess
- Supralevator abscess (due to upward extension of intersphincteric abscess).

Fistula-in-ano

Fistula-in-ano (Anal fistula) is a tract that connects the perineal skin to the anal canal. Anal fistula is the **chronic form of anorectal suppurative process** and develops due to **epithelialization of the anorectal abscess drainage tract**.

Classification of Fistula-in-ano

Based on Relationship of Fistula to the External Sphincter

- Intersphincteric (most common)
- Transsphincteric
- Suprasphincteric
- Extrasphincteric

Simple Anal Fistula

Intersphincteric and low transsphincteric fistulas that involve less than 30% of the sphincter complex.

Complex Anal Fistula

- Transsphincteric fistulas that involve greater than 30% of the external sphincter
- Suprasphincteric fistula
- Extrasphincteric fistula
- Horseshoe fistula
- Fistulas associated with inflammatory bowel disease, radiation, malignancy, preexisting fecal incontinence
- Anterior fistula in female.

Fistula-in-ano may be Associated with Specific Diseases

- Crohn's disease
- Tuberculosis
- Lymphogranuloma venereum
- Malignancy
- Actinomycosis infection.

Intersphincteric Fistula

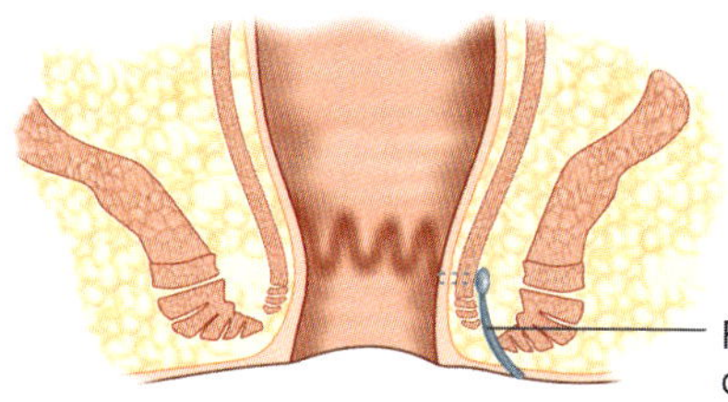

Transsphincteric Fistula

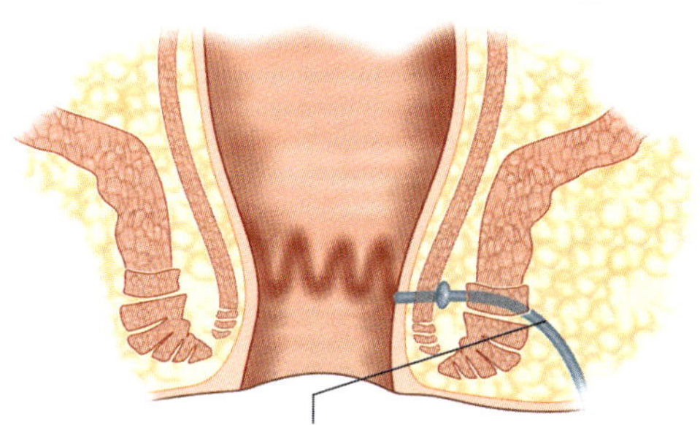

Suprasphincteric Fistula

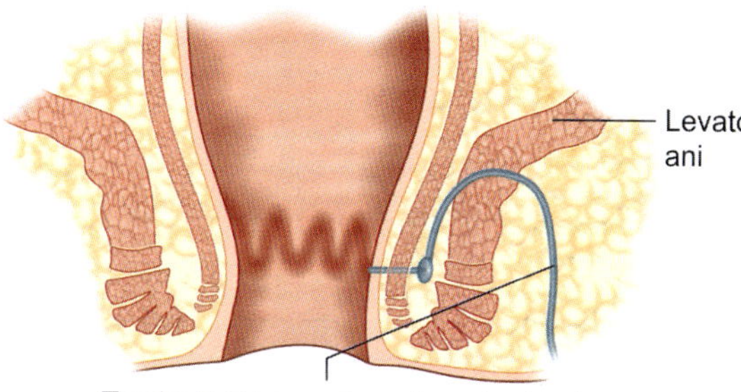

Extrasphincteric Fistula

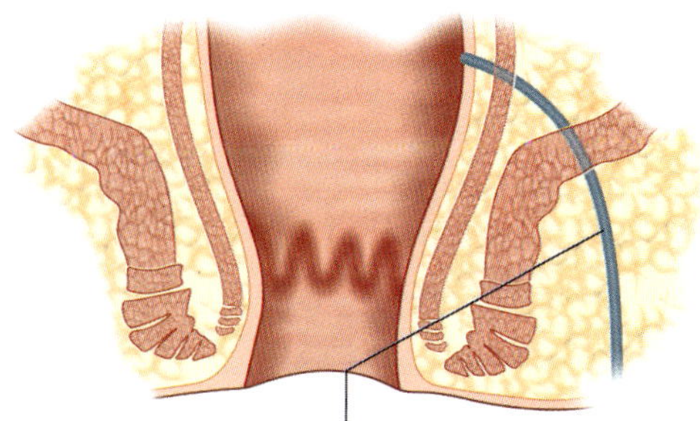

Clinical Manifestation

- **Classic presentation:** Pain and swelling in the perianal region, gradually increasing, then mucopurulent discharge from the swelling and pain relieves. This history often repeats few months interval.
- Serosanguineous discharge from the perianal region or from the anal canal.
- History of surgical intervention for fistula, same symptoms after few months of operation **(Recurrent fistula)**.

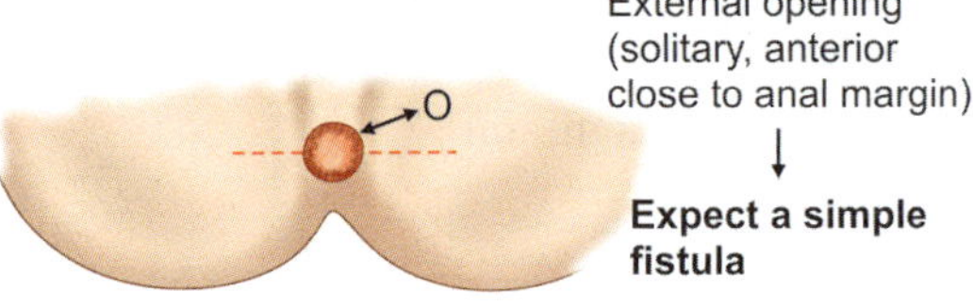

Clinical Evaluation

Inspection of Perianal Region and Perineum

Following points should be noted during inspection:

- *External opening:* Single or multiple, anterior or posterior, distance from the anal margin, presence of any active seropurulent discharge.
- Presence of any surgical scar.

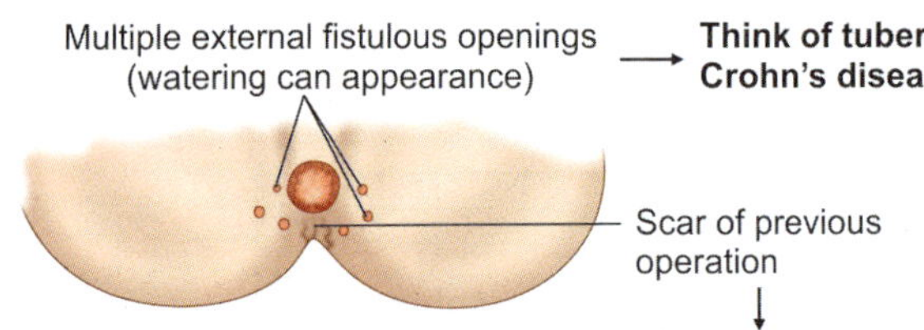

Causes of "Watering can Perineum"

- Multiple urethrocutaneous fistula
- Perianal fistulizing Crohn's disease
- Tuberculosis
- Actinomycosis
- Schistosomiasis.

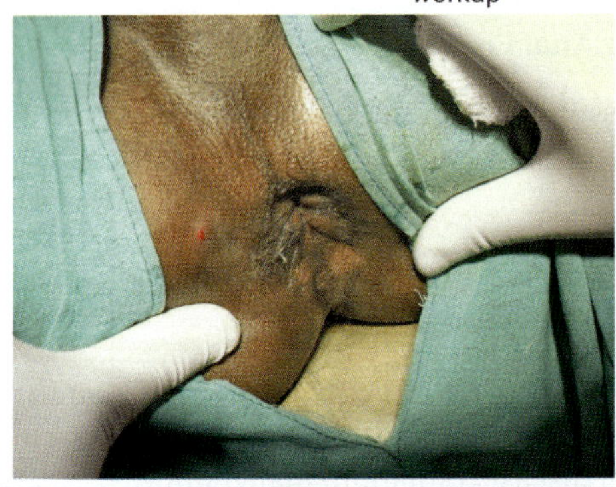

Palpation of the Perianal Region and Anal Canal

It is important to find out the internal opening because chance of recurrence after surgery is high if internal opening cannot be located.

In most of the patients, internal opening can be felt at the dentate line as an indurated nodule.

External Opening is Single and Anteriorly Placed Without any Active Seropurulent Discharge

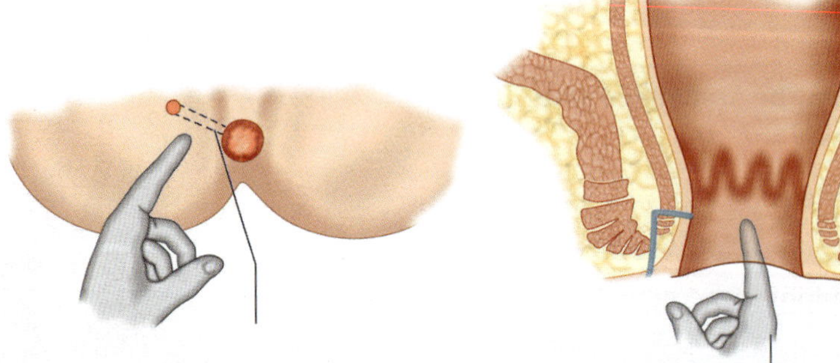

Proctoscopy

Proctoscopy is done to identify the internal opening and to detect other associated pathologies.

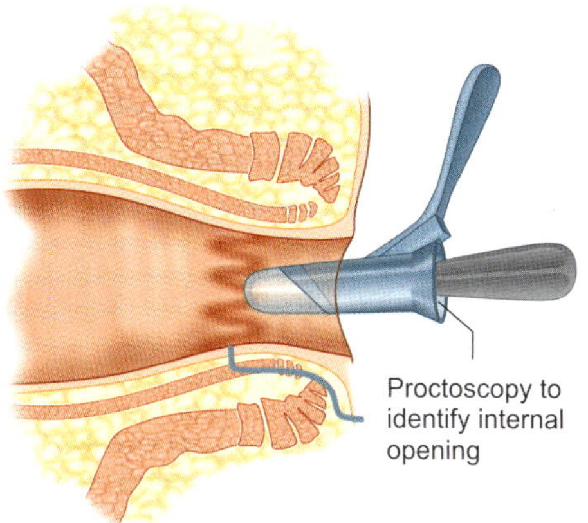

Probing of the Fistula Tract

- Gentle probing of the external opening is helpful to confirm the presence of fistula track and identification of the internal opening.
- Care must be taken to avoid creating any false tract.
- If internal opening cannot be identified by probing, methylene blue is injected into the external opening with pediatric feeding tube.

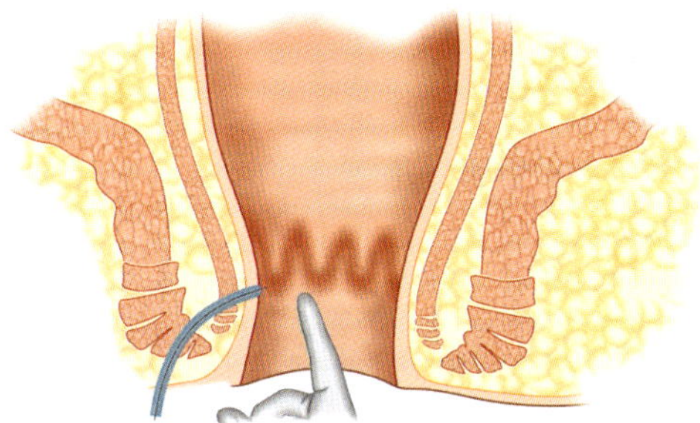

Goodsall's Rule

- This rule is helpful to locate the internal opening in fistula-in-ano.
- This rule states that if an external opening is anterior to an imaginary transverse anal line, straight radial tract runs directly into the anal canal. If the external opening is posterior to the imaginary line, curvilinear tract runs into the posterior midline.
- Exception to this rule: (i) Anterior openings more than 3 cm from the anal verge; and (ii) Multiple external openings.

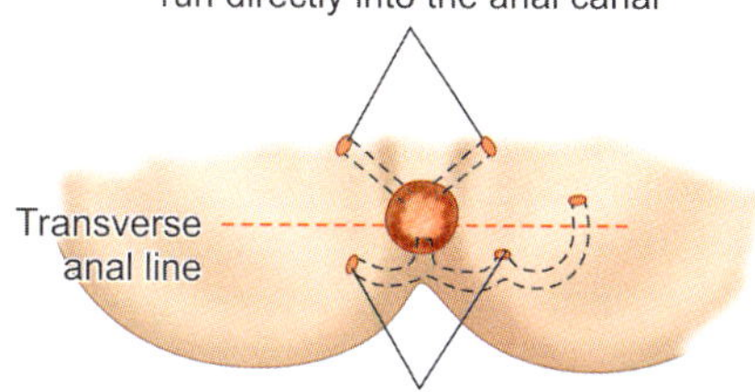

Investigation

In simple fistula: No imaging is indicated.

In complex fistula and recurrent fistula-in-ano: MRI, endoanal ultrasound (EUS), CT or fistulography is indicated.

MRI is particularly helpful to delineate primary fistula tract and its extensions, internal opening, and associated anorectal abscesses.

Two-dimensional or three-dimensional EUS with or without hydrogen peroxide enhancement is also a useful imaging modality for diagnosis and classification of fistula-in-ano.

The role of CT and fistulography is limited for assessment of complex fistulas and recurrent fistula.

Treatment

The treatment of choice for fistula-in-ano is surgery.

The goals of surgical management are:

- Obliteration of the internal opening and associated epithelialized tracts
- Preservation of anal sphincter function
- Prevention of recurrence.

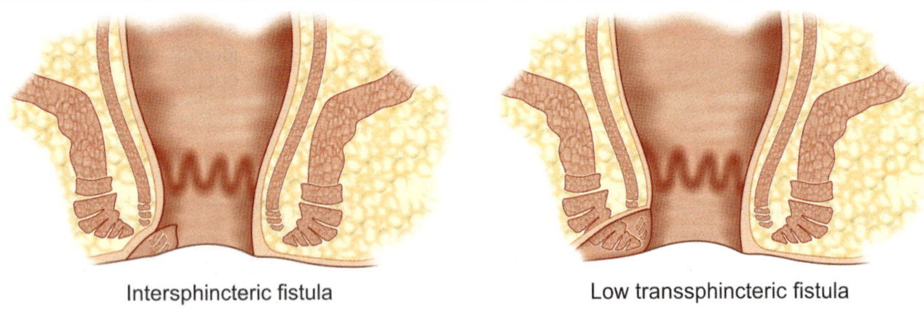

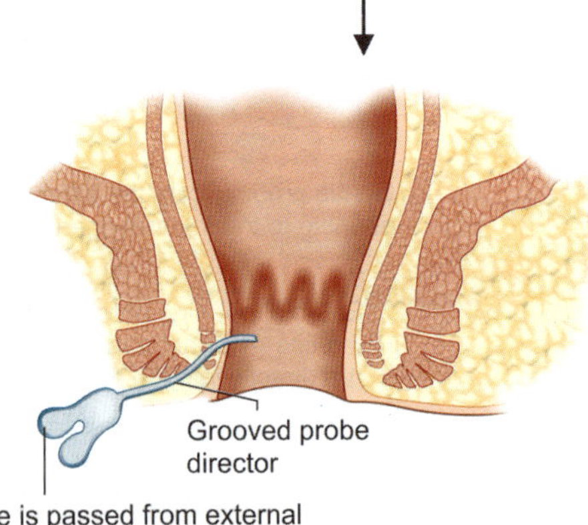

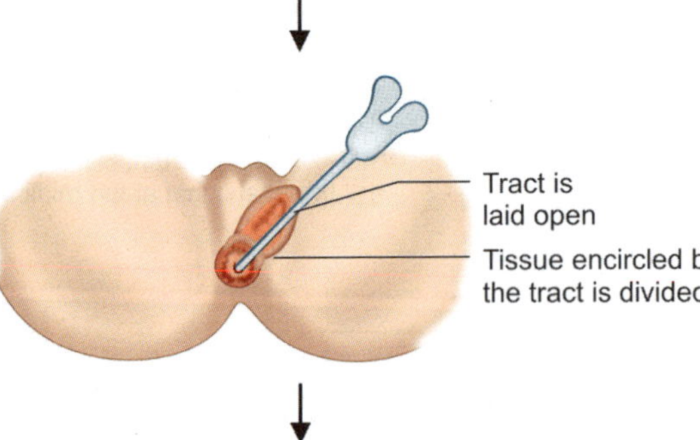

All secondary tracts should be drained through the fistulotomy incision.

All tracts must be curetted and curetted tissue should be sent for biopsy.

Marsupialization of the wound edges with running absorbable suture is associated with faster wound healing, less postoperative bleeding.

Different surgical options are:

Sphincter sacrificing procedures

- Fistulotomy
- Fistulectomy
- Cutting seton

Sphincter-preserving procedures

- Endoanal advancement flap
- LIFT (Ligation of intersphincteric fistula tract)
- Modified LIFT
- VAAFT (Video-assisted anal fistula treatment)
- Fistula plug
- Fibrin glue

Fistulotomy

Fistulotomy is an effective treatment for simple anal fistula where whole of the fistula tract is cut to lay it open.

Risk factors for recurrence after fistulotomy:

(i) Complex fistula
(ii) Internal opening cannot be identified preoperatively.

Risk factors for fecal incontinence after fistulotomy: (i) Recurrent fistula; (ii) Complex fistula; and (iii) Previous anorectal surgery.

Fistulectomy

- Fistulectomy is also a treatment option for simple fistula where fistula tract is resected.
- This procedure is associated with more healing time, increased risk of incontinence but almost equal recurrence rate compared with fistulotomy.

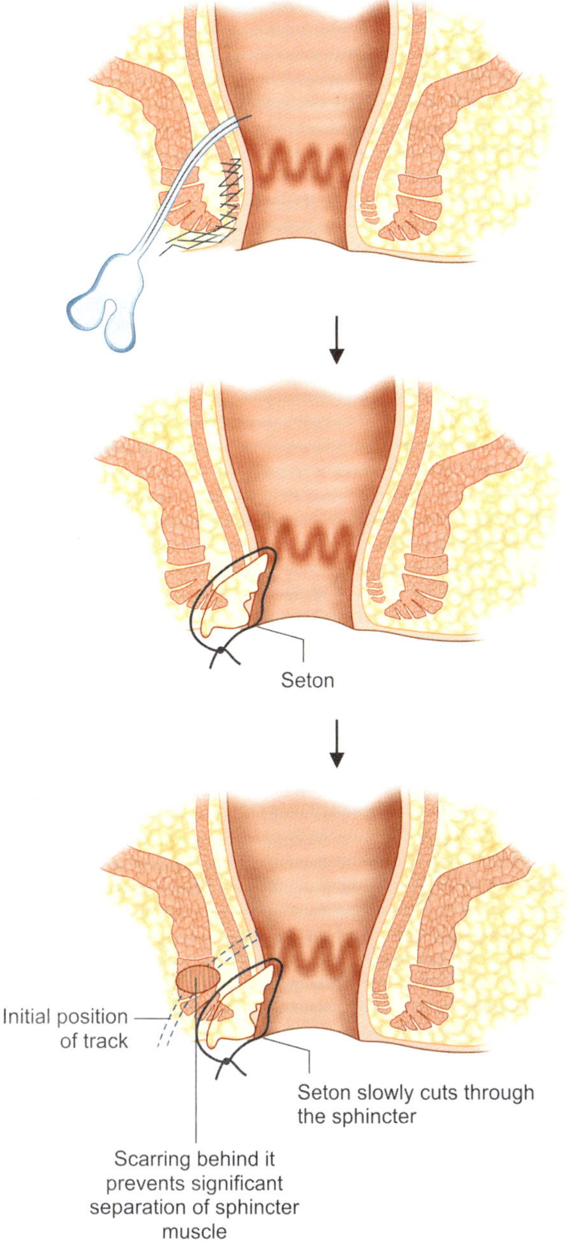

Cutting Seton Technique

Cutting Seton

Cutting seton is an effective treatment option for complex cryptoglandular anal fistulas. This technique involves threading of a nonabsorbable suture (e.g., silk, nylon) through the fistula tract and backout through the anus and loosely tied. This is periodically (2-week interval) tightened so that tract is slowly lay open (sphincter muscle is divided by the process of ischemic necrosis) with minimal risk of fecal incontinence (fibrosis develops and replace the defect of sphincter muscle).

Draining Seton

Draining seton is used for long-term drainage of infective process. This seton is particularly indicated in complex fistulas associated with Crohn's disease.

'Seton' term is derived from a Latin word 'Seta' which means bristle.

Types of seton

- Cutting seton
- Draining seton

Materials used as seton

- Sutures (nylon, polypropylene)
- Stainless-steel wires
- Medicated Kshar Sutra
- Silicone
- Rubber band
- Silastic vessel loop.

Endoanal Advancement Flap

This method is based on curettage of the fistula tract; suture closure of the internal opening; mobilization of a segment of proximal healthy anorectal mucosa, submucosa, and muscle to cover the internal defect.

Advantages: (i) Minimal impairment of sphincter function; (ii) Rapid healing; and (iii) Less risk of anal canal deformity.

Factors associated with increased risk of flap failure: (i) Underlying Crohn's disease; (ii) Prior radiation; and (iii) Multiple attempted repair.

LIFT (Ligation of Intersphincteric Fistula Tract)

- This technique is based on incision at the intersphincteric groove; identification of the intersphincteric tract; ligation of the intersphincteric tract close to the internal opening and removal of the intersphincteric tract; scraping out all granulation tissue of rest of fistulous tract; suturing of the defect at external sphincter muscle.
- LIFT is used for both simple and complex transsphincteric fistula.

Modified LIFT Procedure

This technique involves omission of the fistula tract division; excision of the lateral aspect of the tract; combined use of a seton, fistula plug (LIFT-plug), or biological mesh interposition (Bio-LIFT).

Fibrin Glue

Fibrin glue is a biological glue made of fibrinogen, thrombin along with Aprotinin, factor XIII and calcium. This technique is associated with high recurrence rate in long-term follow up.

VAAFT (Video-assisted Anal Fistula Treatment)

- This technique allows surgeon to visualize inside the fistula tract and locate the internal opening by using fistuloscope.
- This technique is based on insertion of video telescope (fistuloscope) into the fistula tract to locate internal opening, any secondary tracts; cleaning of the fistula tract using unipolar electrosurgery, fistula brush and forceps and continuous irrigation; closure of the internal opening by stitches and staples from inside the anal canal.

Fistula Plug

This treatment option involves use of acellular collagen matrix to close the primary internal opening and to provide a scaffold for tissue-in-growth that will obliterate the fistula tract.

Commercially available fistula plug are:

Lyophilized porcine intestinal submucosa and synthetic absorbable biomaterial.

Management of Fistula-in-ano Associated with Crohn's Disease

- **Fistulotomy** is indicated for symptomatic, simple, low anal fistulas and **draining seton** is indicated for symptomatic, complex fistulas. **The combination of seton with infliximab** has better overall fistula healing rate, longer duration of fistula closure, lower overall fistula recurrence rate.
- Adalimumab and certolizumab pegol are also effective in treating perianal fistula in Crohn's disease.
- Complex anal fistula associated with Crohn's disease may be treated with **Endoanal advancement flap, LIFT or fistula plug** with good functional outcome. **Fecal diversion or proctectomy** may be indicated in patients with intractable perianal disease.

Hemorrhoids

Hemorrhoids are **prolapse of the anal cushions** causing symptoms.

Anal Cushion

Anal cushions are composed of **tufts of anastomosing arterioles and venules** in the anorectal submucosa embedded within smooth muscle (Treitz muscle) and elastic connective tissue and covered by anorectal mucosa.

Location of the Major Anal Cushions

- Right anterior (11 o'clock)
- Right posterior (7 o'clock)
- Left lateral (3 o'clock).

Blood Supply of the Anal Cushions

- Superior rectal artery arising from the inferior mesenteric artery
- Middle rectal arteries arising from the internal iliac arteries
- Inferior rectal arteries arising from the pudendal arteries.
- **The venous drainage** is to the portal venous system above the level of the dentate line and to the systemic venous system below the dentate line.

Pathological Changes in Anal Cushions in Hemorrhoids

- Abnormal venous dilatation
- Vascular thrombosis
- Rupture of anal subepithelial muscles.

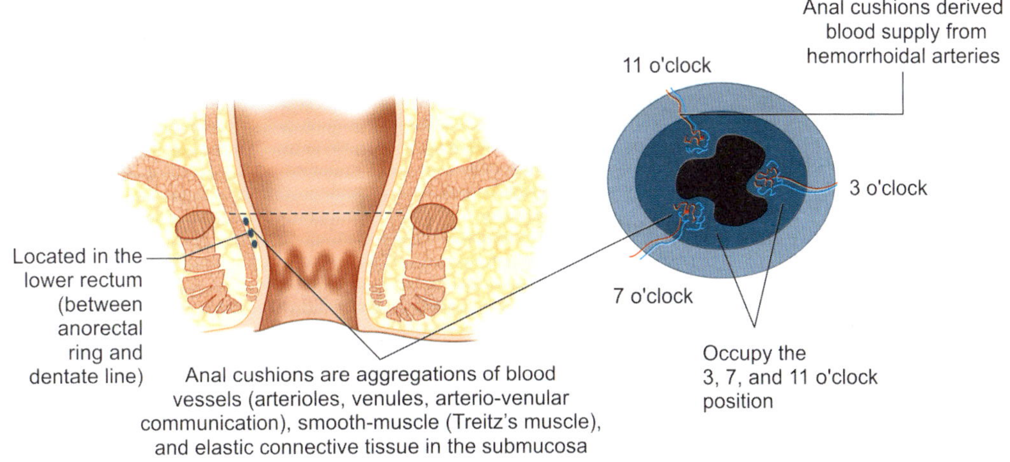

Predisposing Factors

- Chronic constipation
- Excessive straining
- Prolonged sitting in toilet
- Advanced age.

Causes of Secondary Hemorrhoids

- Pregnancy
- Ascites
- Portal hypertension
- Large rectosigmoid growth.

Pathophysiology

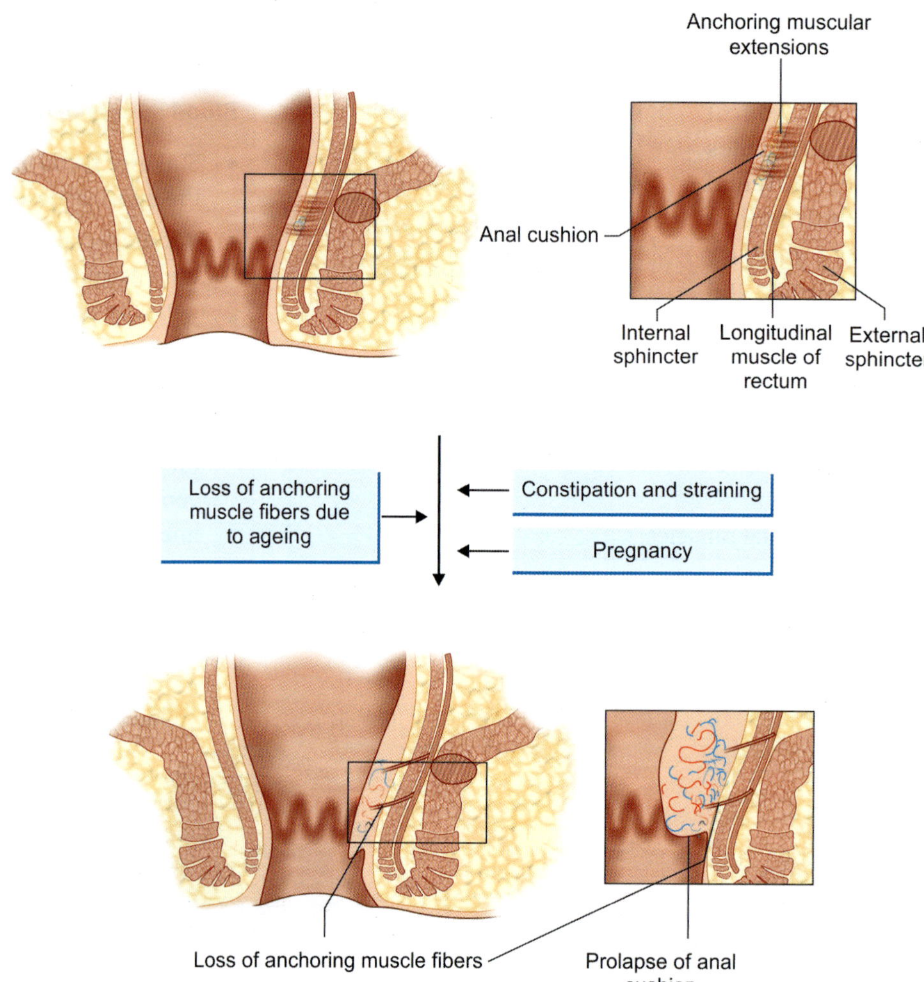

Types of Hemorrhoids

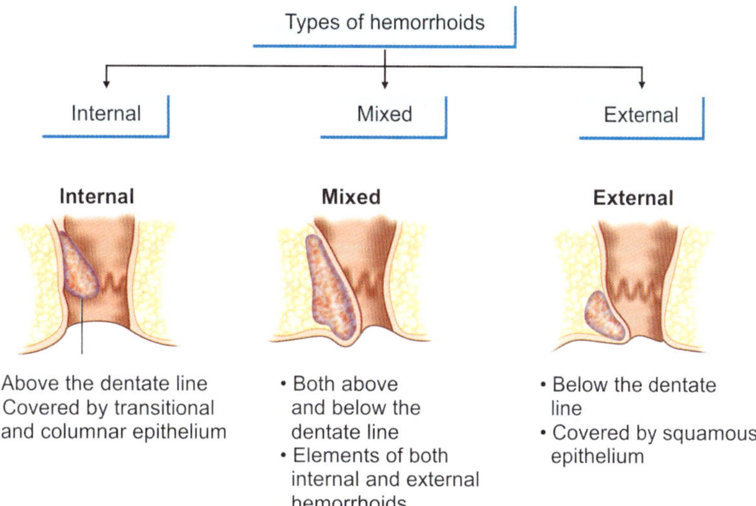

Types of Internal Hemorrhoids

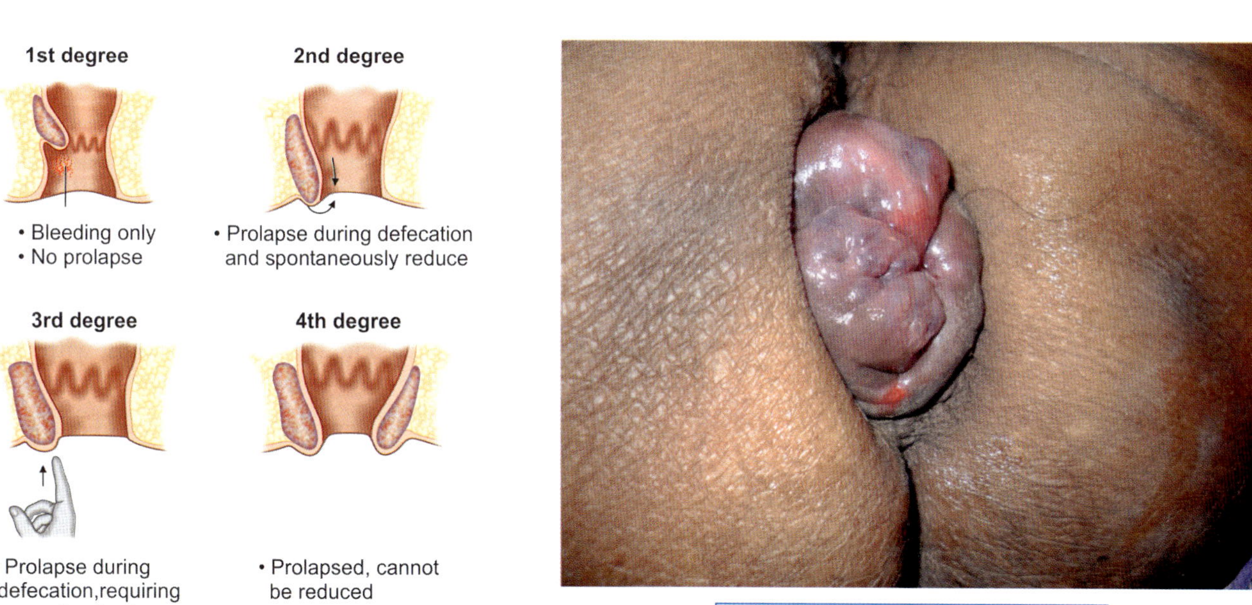

4th Degree Hemorrhoids.

Clinical Presentation

- **Painless bleeding** with bowel movements, bright red in color, usually drip into the toilet after defecation.
- **Prolapse** depending on the degree of internal hemorrhoids.
- **Pain** only in thrombosed external hemorrhoids (external hemorrhoids are covered by squamous epithelium and innervated by somatic pain fibers).
- **Mucoid discharge** may be associated in 4th degree hemorrhoids.

Differential Diagnosis

- Rectal prolapse
- Colorectal cancer
- Diverticulitis.

Clinical Evaluation

Visual inspection of the anus

Visual inspection is commonly done in lateral decubitus or knee-chest or prone position. In first-degree hemorrhoids, no abnormality is seen. After straining, second-degree hemorrhoids become apparent. Third-degree and fourth degree hemorrhoids are readily recognized. Other associated pathologies (e.g., fissure, fistula), if present, may be detected.

Digital rectal examination (DRE)

DRE should be done at rest and after straining to assess associated anal pathologies and sphincter tone.

Proctoscopy

Proctoscopy is done to confirm the findings during inspection and DRE.

Complete colonoscopic evaluation is indicated in selected patients.

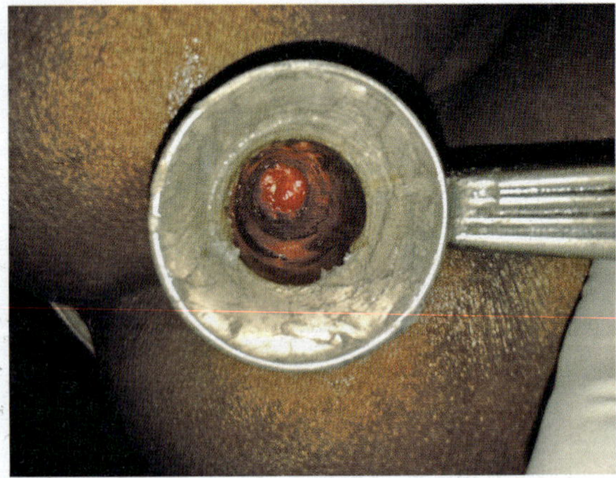

Indications for Complete Colon Evaluation in Symptomatic Hemorrhoids and Rectal Bleeding

As per guidelines by US Multi-Society Task Force on Colorectal Cancers:

- Age ≥50 years if no complete examination within 10 years.
- Age ≥40 years or 10 years younger than age at diagnosis with history positive for a single, first-degree relative with colorectal cancer or advanced adenoma diagnosed at age <60
- Age ≥40 years or 10 years younger than age at diagnosis with history positive for two first-degree relatives with advanced adenomas or colorectal cancer
- Positive fecal immunochemical testing (FIT)
- Positive FIT-fecal DNA test.

Treatment

Conservative Management

- Dietary modification (adequate fluid and fiber intake)
- Maintenance of proper bowel habit (avoidance of straining and limiting time on commode)
- Use of phlebotonics.

Office-based Procedures

Rubber band ligation, Sclerotherapy and infrared coagulation are office-based procedures, indicated in Grade I and II hemorrhoids where medical treatment fails.

Flavonoids (diosmin, micronized purified flavonoid fraction, rutosides) and **Calcium dobesilate** (synthetic compound) are phlebotonics. Flavonoids are derived from plant extracts.

Phlebotonics act by following mechanisms:

- Strengthening of vessel wall
- Increasing venous tone
- Normalizing capillary permeability.

Rubber Band Ligation

Most effective office-based procedure.

Mechanism of action: Ligation of hemorrhoidal tissue by rubber band resulting in ischemia and necrosis of the tissue followed by scar fixation to the rectal wall.

Banding can be performed in a single session or multiple sessions.

Contraindications: (i) Coagulation disorders; and (ii) Patient on anticoagulant therapy.

Complications: (i) Anorectal pain; (ii) Bleeding; (iii) Thrombosis of external hemorrhoids; (iv) Vasovagal symptoms; (v) Misplacement of band near or below the dentate line; and (vi) Pelvic sepsis.

Rubber band should be placed well above the dentate line to avoid postprocedure severe anorectal pain (above the dentate line, somatic sensitivity is absent).

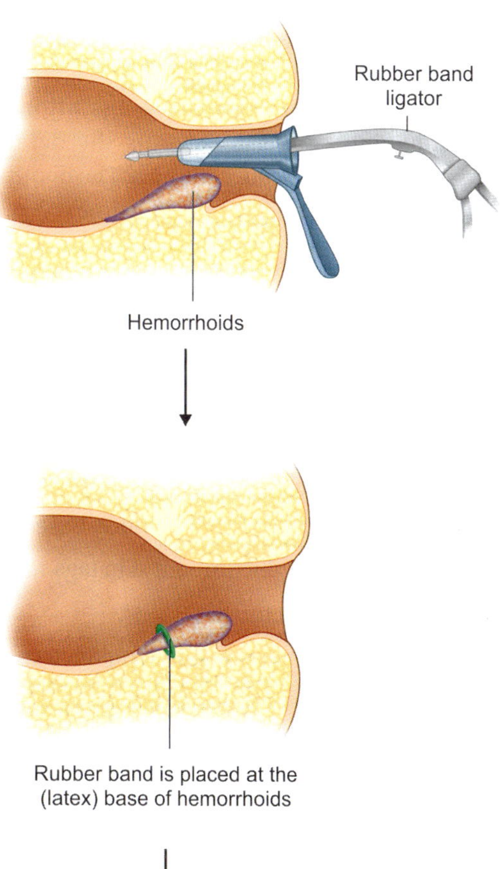

Sclerotherapy

Mechanism of action: The sclerosant is injected into the submucosa at the apex of a hemorrhoidal bundle resulting in fibrosis of the submucosa followed by fixation of the hemorrhoidal tissue.

Sclerosants are: (i) 5% phenol (1–3 mL) in almond or vegetable oil; (ii) Sodium tetradecyl sulfate (0.5–2.0 mL of 1%); and (iii) Sodium morrhuate.

Complications: (i) Mucosal ulceration or necrosis; (ii) Prostatic abscess; (iii) Retroperitoneal sepsis; (iv) Hematuria; (v) Hematospermia; (vi) Recto-urethral fistula; and (vii) Transient bacteremia.

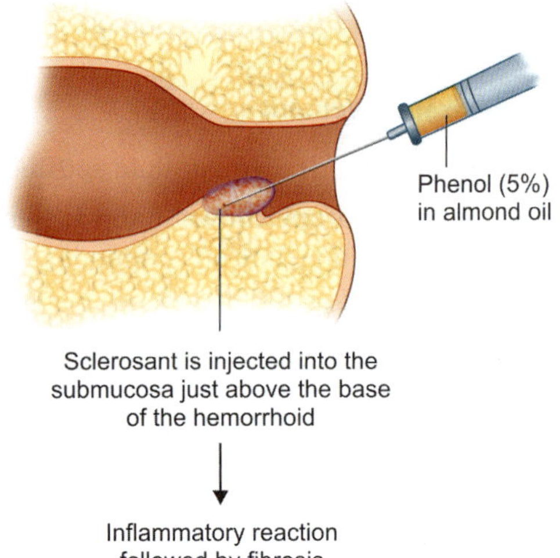

Infrared Coagulation

Application of infrared wave causes coagulation of tissue protein, resulting in coagulation of hemorrhoids. The mucosa covering the hemorrhoids is exposed to the infrared wave. The depth of coagulation depends on the exposure time.

Hemorrhoidectomy

Indications of hemorrhoidectomy:

- In grade III and IV hemorrhoids
- Failure of office-based procedures
- In patients who cannot tolerate office-based procedures
- Hemorrhoids with concomitant skin tags

Types of hemorrhoidectomy:

- Milligan-Morgan or open hemorrhoidectomy
- Ferguson or closed hemorrhoidectomy

Complications of hemorrhoidectomy:

(i) Reactionary hemorrhage; (ii) Acute retention of urine; (iii) Postoperative pain; (iv) Secondary hemorrhage; (v) Flatus incontinence; and (vi) Anal stenosis

Closed hemorrhoidectomy is associated with less postoperative pain, hemorrhage, more rapid wound healing but similar recurrence rate compared to open hemorrhoidectomy.

Hemorrhoidectomy can be performed by:

- Conventional surgical devices (e.g., scissors, etc.)
- Bipolar energy device
- Ultrasonic shears

Causes of Anal Stenosis

- Over-aggressive hemorrhoidectomy
- Crohn's disease
- Trauma
- Radiation therapy

Open Hemorrhoidectomy

Application of artery forceps to the skin covering the component of piles

Application of artery forceps to the mucosal covered component of piles

V-shaped incision in the perianal skin

Sphincter is swept away from hemorrhoids

Ligature (absorbable suture) is applied

Bridge of skin and mucous membrane must remain between each wound

['Clover leaf' appearance]

Closed Hemorrhoidectomy

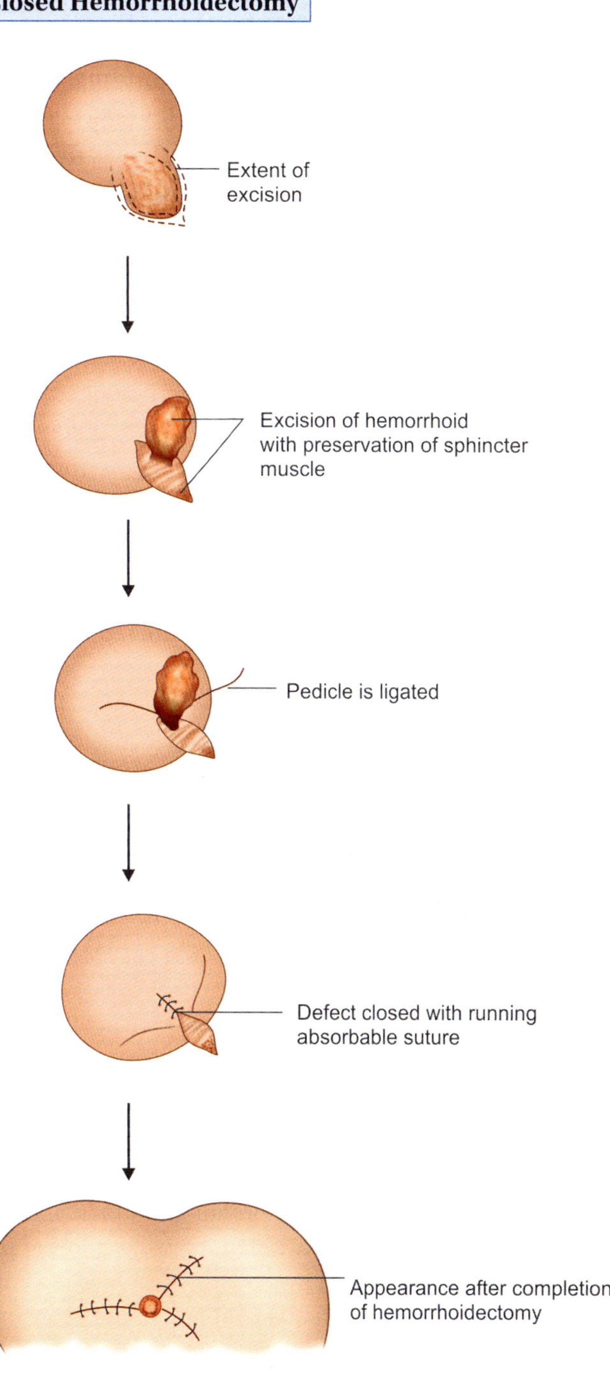

Stapled Hemorrhoidopexy

This procedure is based on creating a mucosa-to-mucosa anastomosis by excising the submucosa proximal to the dentate line, resulting in cephalad relocation of the anal cushions.

Limitation: It is not effective for external hemorrhoids.

Complications: (i) Rectovaginal fistula; (ii) Staple line bleeding; (iii) Stricture at staple line; (iv) Rectal perforation; and (v) Recurrence.

Stapled hemorrhoidopexy is associated with more recurrence rate than conventional hemorrhoidectomy.

Doppler-guided/Assisted Hemorrhoid Artery Ligation (DGHAL) or Transanal Hemorrhoidal Dearterialization

In this method, each hemorrhoid artery is ligated by using an anoscope fashioned with Doppler probe.

Advantages: (i) Less postprocedural pain and (ii) No need of tissue excision.

Thrombosed External Hemorrhoids

Patients present with painful perianal mass with throbbing pain.

Treatment is aimed to relief severe pain, prevention of recurrent thromboses, and management of residual skin tag.

Treatment options for thrombosed external hemorrhoids: (i) Topical application of 0.2% nitroglycerine; (ii) Incision and evacuation of thrombus; and (iii) Excision of hemorrhoids (using an elliptical incision).

Excision of hemorrhoids may cause more rapid symptom resolution.

Pilonidal Disease

Pilonidal disease is an acquired condition related to trauma of the hair shafts and characterized by chronic sinus form (sinus tract containing hair shafts) or acute form as abscess.

Classic site is the natal cleft or gluteal cleft.

Risk factors: (i) Obesity; (ii) Repeated trauma or irritation to the gluteal cleft skin; (iii) Hirsute body habitus; and (iv) Family history of pilonidal disease.

Spectrum of pilonidal disease: (i) Acute form as abscess and (ii) Chronic form as single or multiple subcutaneous branching sinus tracts with a characteristic midline pit (opening of a sinus tract) in the gluteal cleft. The sinus tracts from the midline pit often courses in the cephalad direction, sometimes in a caudal direction.

The sinus tract characteristically contain hair debris.

Unusual Sites of Pilonidal Sinus

- Finger web (barber's pilonidal sinus)
- Umbilicus
- Perineum
- Breast (women engaged in sheep shearing, dog beauticians).

Follicular Occlusion Tetrad

A symptom complex consisting of four diseases having similar pathophysiology (follicular occlusion in apocrine gland bearing areas).

This tetrad consists of Hidradenitis suppurativa, acne conglobata, dissecting cellulitis of the scalp and **pilonidal sinus**. Commonly, each condition presents singly.

Etiological Theories

Bascom's Theory

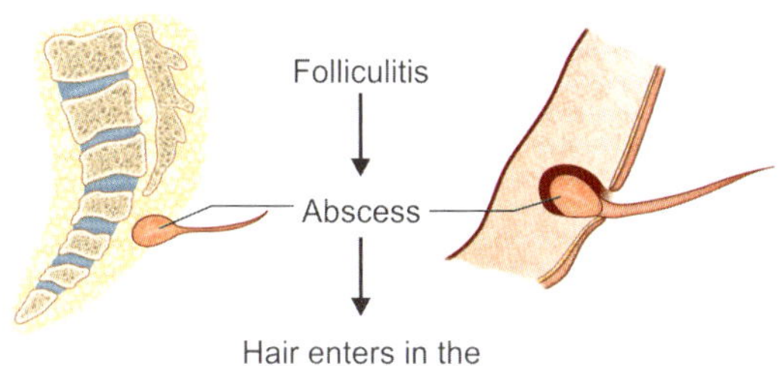

Hair enters in the abscess cavity due to suction

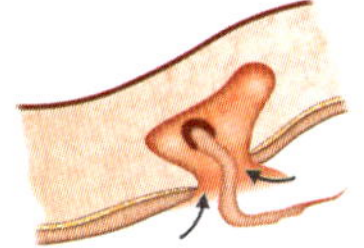

Movement of gluteal crease creates suction, hair enters in the abscess cavity

Karydaki's Theory

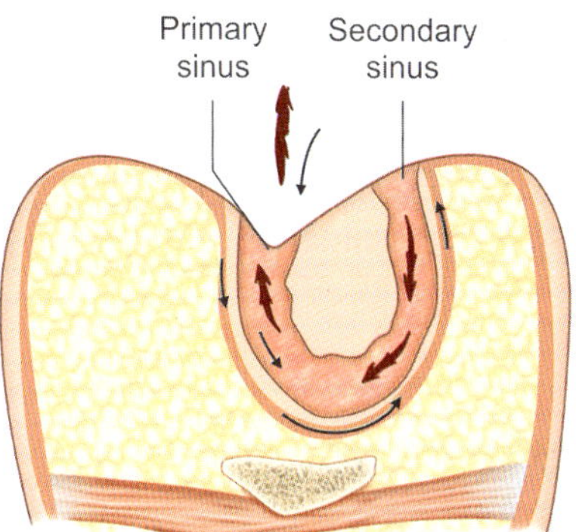

Shafts of loose hair inserts into the depth of the natal cleft, resulting in foreign body reaction.

Secondary opening develops due to self-propelling ability of the hair or spontaneous rupture of abscess.

Clinical Presentation

- Most of the patients are **hirsute and obese. Males** are more commonly affected.
- **Characteristic presentation is midline pits (fistulous opening) in the gluteal cleft.**
- **Pilonidal abscess** often presenting as tender, fluctuant mass with cellulitis. Continuous or intermittent serous or purulent discharge from the secondary openings or pits.
- **Malignant degeneration** (predominatly squamous cell carcinoma) is rarely reported in long-standing pilonidal disease.

Differential Diagnosis

- Perianal fistula in Crohn's disease
- Hidradenitis suppurativa
- Actinomycosis
- Sacral osteomyelitis.

Treatment

Treatment of Acute Pilonidal Abscess

Incision and drainage of abscess is the treatment. Incision should be paramedian next to the natal cleft. Elimination of hair in the gluteal cleft and surrounding region by surgeon-performed shaving or laser epilation promotes healing and decreases the chance of recurrence. Hair removal should be repeated every 1–2 weeks until healing of acute disease.

Treatment Options for Chronic Pilonidal Disease

- Phenol application (hair removal, curettage of the cyst, application of 1–3 mL of crystallized phenol into the cyst and tracts)
- Surgical excision (Excision of diseased tissue with off-midline primary closure/Excision with healing by secondary intention/Excision with marsupialization)
- Flap-based procedures
- Video-assisted ablation of pilonidal sinus (VAAPS)
- Endoscopic pilonidal sinus treatment (EPSiT).

Karydaki's Procedure

The Karydakis procedure is an **off-midline excisional procedure**.

Midline follicle excision and lateral drainage (described by Bascom)

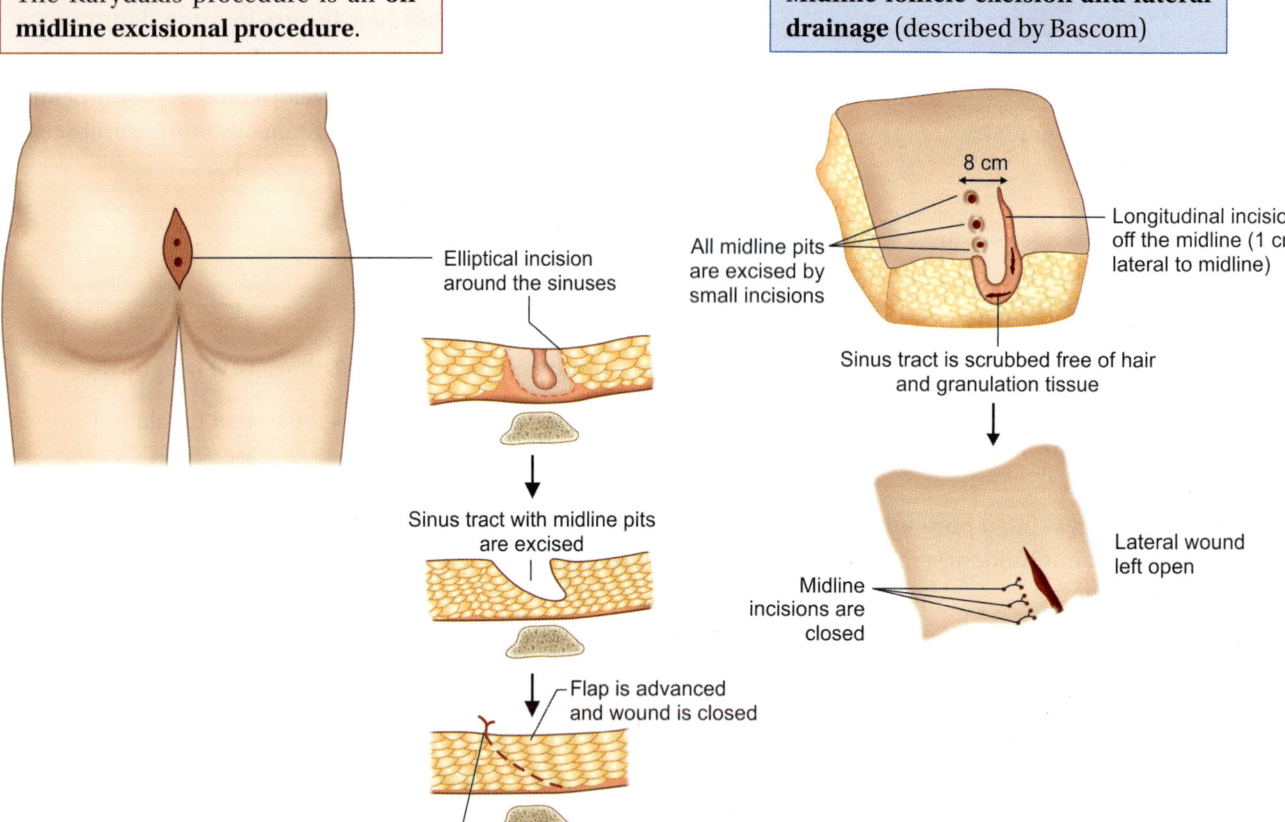

Off-midline closure is associated with faster healing, lower rates of infection, lower rates of recurrence.

Flap-based Procedures

Indications: (i) Complex chronic pilonidal disease and (ii) Recurrent pilonidal disease.

Different techniques are: (i) Rhomboid or Limberg flap; (ii) Karydakis flap; (iii) Cleft-lift technique (Bascom's technique); (iv) Z-plasty; and (v) V-Y advancement flap.

Limberg or Rhomboid flap: This is the most common flap-based procedure for pilonidal disease. This procedure involves excision of diseased tissue in rhomboid shape followed by coverage of the defect by rhomboid flap.

Modified Limberg flap: In this modification, lower end of the flap is completely outside the natal cleft.

Z-plasty

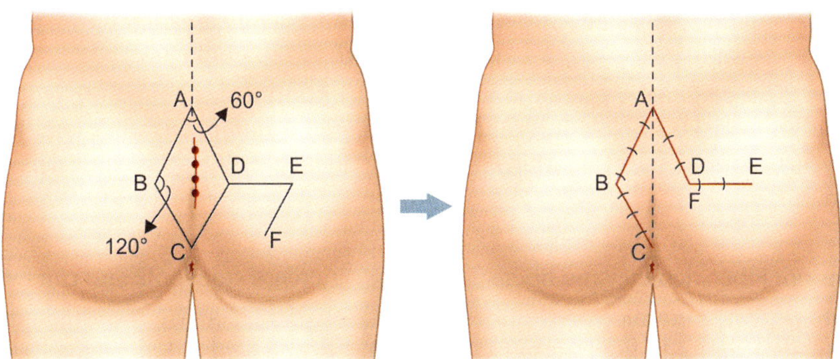

VAAPS and EPSiT

The basic steps of VAAPS and EPSiT are almost same. **These procedures involve:** (i) Insertion of fistuloscope (the same fistuloscope for VAAFT) through the external opening of pilonidal sinus; (ii) Identification of the anatomy of sinus tract and any secondary tracts or abscess cavity; (iii) Removal of hair, infected tissue, any debris from the sinus tract using forceps; (iv) Ablation of main sinus tract and any secondary tract or abscess cavity using monopolar electrosurgery; and (v) Necrotic material is removed using endobrush and sinus tract is cleaned using irrigation solution.

Advantages of VAAPS and EPSiT: (i) Less postoperative pain; (ii) Quicker healing; (iii) Shorter length of hospital stay; and (iv) Also effective for recurrent disease.

Drawbacks: (i) Needs specialized instrumentation and proper training and (ii) Long-term outcome is still unclear.

Fecal Incontinence

Fecal incontinence is the uncontrolled passage of feces or gas over atleast 1 month duration, in an individual of atleast 4 years of age, who had previously achieved control. [ASCRS guideline 2015].

Types: (i) Urge incontinence (patient experiences the urge to defecate, but cannot reach the toilet in time); (ii) Passive incontinence (patient not aware of the need to defecate before the incontinent episode); and (iii) Nocturnal incontinence (associated with diabetes mellitus and scleroderma).

Causes: (i) Obstetric causes (vaginal delivery, forceps delivery, prolonged labor); (ii) Anorectal procedures (e.g., fistulectomy, hemorrhoidectomy, internal anal shincterotomy, fistulotomy); (iii) Neurological disorders (e.g., dementia, stroke, multiple sclerosis, spinal cord lesions); (iv) Diabetes mellitus; (v) Scleroderma; and (vi) Rectal prolapse.

Scoring systems (to assess the nature, severity and impact of incontinence on quality of life): (i) Fecal incontinence severity index; (ii) St. Marks incontinence score; (iii) Cleveland clinic Florida fecal incontinence score; and (iv) Park's incontinence score.

Clinical examination includes: (i) Inspection of anus and perianal areas (any scar of anorectal procedures, rectal prolapse if any, skin excoriation); (ii) Elicitation of pinprick sensation in perianal area and anal wink reflex; (iii) Digital anorectal examination (to exclude any palpable rectal mass, clinical estimation of anal resting and squeeze pressures); and (iv) Anoscopy and proctoscopy—to detect any possible pathologies.

Diagnostic evaluation: The diagnostic evaluation includes: (i) Anorectal manometry; (ii) Rectal sensation; and (iii) Rectal compliance. Endoanal USG or MRI should be considered if patient has weak anal sphincter pressure and surgery is being planned. Colonoscopic evaluation is needed if patient presents with clinical presentations suggestive of colorectal carcinoma.

Management:

- **Dietary modification:** Fiber-rich diet and fiber supplements increase stool bulk and can reduce watery stools.
- **Pharmacologic therapy:** Loperamide and diphenoxylate-atropine (decreases intestinal motility and increases internal anal sphincter tone), Cholestyramine (binds cathartic bile acids), Kaopectate (absorbs excess fluid in stool), Opioids (decreases intestinal motility, intestinal secretion, and increases absorption) are recommended as first-line therapy.
- **Biofeedback training or pelvic floor rehabilitation:** Indicated if patient not responding to dietary modifications and pharmacologic therapy.
- **Treatment of associated anorectal disorders:** If patient having rectovaginal fistula, rectal prolapse; these should be treated first because most of the patients improves after treatment of the these disorders.
- **Sphincteroplasty:** An effective treatment in patients with defined defect in external anal sphincter.
- **Dynamic graciloplasty:** This technique utilizes continuous electrical stimulation of gracilis muscle, thereby converting type II (fast-twitch, fatigue-prone) to type I (slow-twitch, fatigue-resistant) muscle fibers.
- Injection of biocompatible bulking agents (Nonanimal stabilized hyaluronic acid dextranomer gel)
- **Sacral neuromodulation:** Acts by modulating rectal sensation and changing brain activity related to continence mechanism.
- **Artificial bowel sphincter** is indicated in following conditions: (i) Extensive sphincter destruction (>180°); (ii) Neurogenic incontinence from spinal cord injury; and (iii) Patient with congenital malformation having incontinence. Complications of this procedure are—(i) Infection; (ii) Anorectal ulceration; (iii) Device malfunction; and (iv) Device migration.
- **Colostomy:** Colostomy (particularly an end sigmoid colostomy) is indicated in severe fecal incontinence when all other treatment options fail.
- **Newer techniques:** Percutaneous tibial nerve stimulation and Magnetic sphincter are emerging techniques but still not recommended for clinical use presently.
- **Supportive treatment:** Proper perianal skin care, use of zinc-oxide based protective ointments.

Rectal Cancer

Rectum is devoid of cardinal features of large intestine—teniae coli, appendices epiploicae, sacculations, and well-defined mesentery.

The upper limit of the rectum is defined by sacral promontory, the splaying of the teniae coli, the proximal valve of Houston, the level of the peritoneal reflection or the junction of sigmoid mesocolon and mesorectum.

The lower limit of rectum is anorectal ring (surgical landmark) or dentate line (anatomical landmark) or upper border of the anal sphincter and puborectalis muscles (radiological landmark).

Length of rectum is 12–15 cm. After mobilization during surgery, the length is increased up to 15–20 cm.

Upper third of rectum (from the anal verge 12–15 cm)—completely covered by peritoneum except a small posterior segment.

Middle third of rectum (7–11 cm)—covered by peritoneum anteriorly.

Lower third of rectum (0–6 cm)—no peritoneal coverings.

Tumor within 15 cm from the anal verge are classified as rectal cancer.

Rectal cancer shares most of the risk factors, genetic and morphologic characteristics of colon cancer. **Anatomically**, rectal cancer is different from colon cancer in many aspects. **From surgical aspect**, rectal cancer surgery is also different from colon cancer surgery.

Rectal Cancer Surgery is Different from Colon Cancer Surgery

- Rectum is located within the narrow pelvis, so surgery is technically difficult.
- Increased risk of complications due to close proximity of urogenital organs and autonomic nerves.
- Principles of total mesorectal excision (TME) is followed during rectal cancer surgery.
- Higher risk of local recurrence after rectal cancer surgery.

Spread of Rectal Cancer

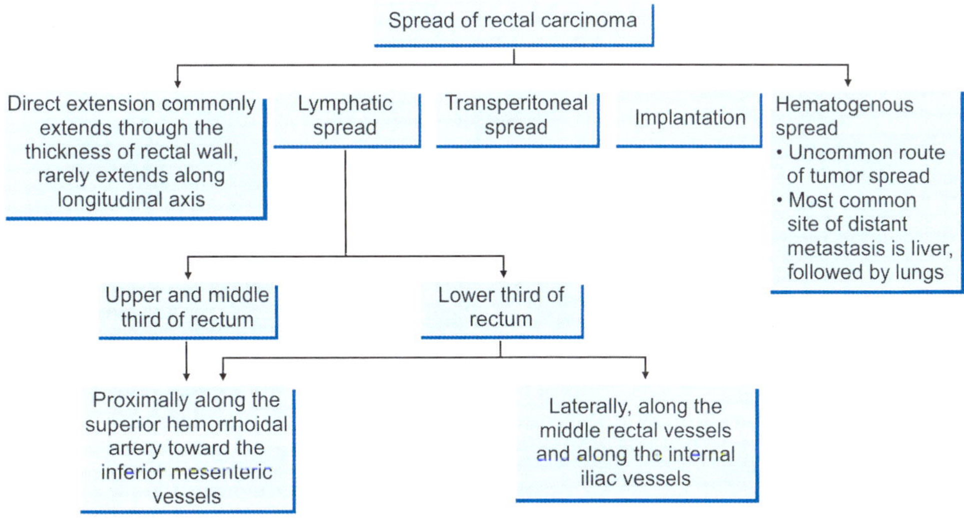

Clinical Presentation

- Rectal bleeding is the most common symptom of rectal cancer. **[Rectal carcinoma must be ruled out in any adult patient presents with rectal bleeding]**.
- Alteration of bowel habit.
- Passage of mucus with stool.
- Sense of incomplete evacuation.
- Sense of rectal 'fullness'.
- Subacute intestinal obstruction (complete obstruction rarely develops in carcinoma rectum).
- Weight loss, anorexia.
- Rectal pain or low back pain (if there is extensive local invasion).
- Family history of rectal cancer, FAP, HNPCC, and IBD may be present.

Diagnosis

- **Histological diagnosis is essential for elective treatment.**
- **If the growth is palpable during digital rectal examination,** tissue must be retrieved by the punch biopsy for histological assessment.
- **If tumor is detected in colonoscopy,** colonoscopy guided biopsy is indicated for histological diagnosis.

Assessment of Tumor

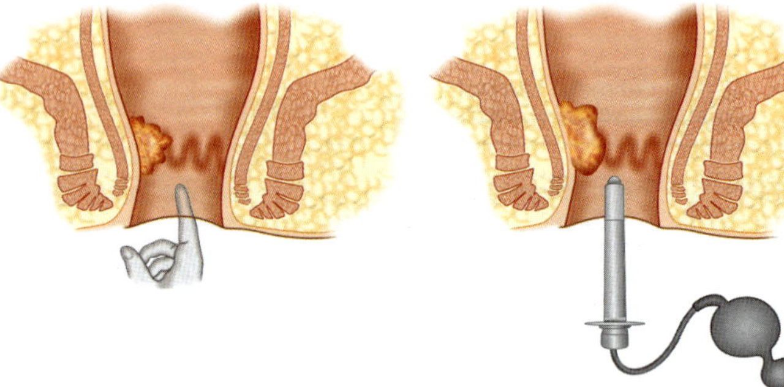

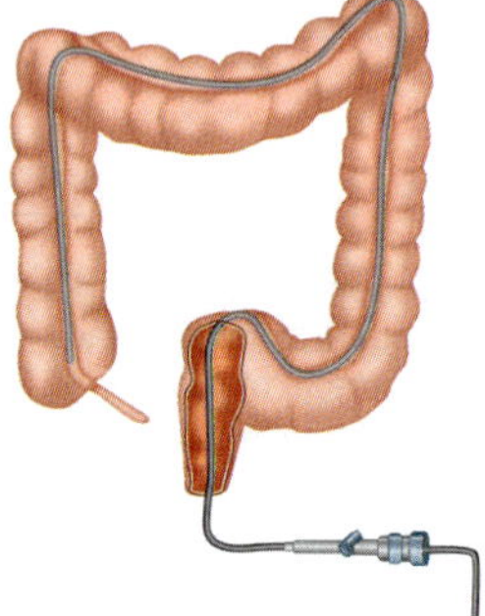

Digital rectal examination (DRE)

Assess –
- Tumor size, position, mobility and fixation
- Distance from anal verge or dentate line
- Relationship to the sphincter mechanism
- Relationship to adjacent organs and sacrum

Rigid sigmoidoscopy

Assess –
- Proximal and distal levels of the tumor from the dentate line
- Circumferential involvement
- Relationship with vagina and posterior peritoneal reflection

Full length colonoscopy

Assess –
- Presence of any synchronous lesions or polyp syndromes

Pelvic examination is indicated to assess vaginal involvement.

If full colonic evaluation is not feasible by colonoscopy, then

Evaluation is done by:

- Second attempt by conventional colonoscopy
- CT colonography
- Colon capsule endoscopy
- Contrast enema (if other options are not available).

Full colonic evaluation is essential because if synchronous polyp or tumor or polyposis syndrome is detected, the plan of management will be different.

In emergency setting (presenting with acute obstruction or perforation), **colonoscopy should be done in postoperative period**.

- Incidence of **synchronous adenoma or other polyps**–up to 30%
- Incidence of **synchronous colorectal cancer**–1-3%.

Staging

Clinical staging is important for treatment decisions (surgery/neoadjuvant therapy).

Rectal cancer protocol MRI is the imaging modality of choice for **locoregional staging**. EUS is indicated to evaluate pelvis only when MRI is contraindicated.

Metastatic workup includes: Contrast-enhanced CT scan of abdomen and pelvis, CT chest.

Role of Carcinoembryonic antigen (CEA):

- Baseline CEA level is prognostic of long-term survival
- Baseline CEA acts as a reference during post-therapy surveillance and also correlates with treatment response.

Staging protocol after neoadjuvant therapy includes: (i) Clinical assessment; (ii) Colonoscopy; (iii) Pelvic MRI; and (iv) Contrast enhanced CT abdomen and pelvis. **Functional MRI and/or PET/CT scan** is better imaging modality for assessing treatment response.

Pelvic MRI with contrast can assess:

- Depth of tumor penetration
- Distance from the anal verge to the lower end of tumor
- Tumor length
- Involvement of mesorectal fascia
- Assessment of **circumferential resection margin (CRM),** N stage, presence/absence of suspicious extramesorectal lymph nodes.

Circumferential Resection Margin (CRM) in Rectal Cancer

The CRM by MRI is measured at the closest distance of the tumor to the mesorectal fascia. **Clear CRM** is tumor >1 mm from mesorectal fascia and levator muscles and not invading into the intersphincteric plane. **Involved CRM** is tumor within 1 mm of mesorectal fascia or within 1 mm from levator muscle (for lower third rectal tumors).

Positive CRM is associated with increased risk for local recurrence and decreased survival.

Pelvic MRI Requirements

- Minimum magnet strength—1.5 Tesla
- External surface body coil or endorectal coil
- Slice thickness 1-3 mm
- 2D T2-weighted sequences for T staging and lymph node assessment
- T1-weighted sequences for assessment of other pelvic organs.

Role of EUS in Rectal Cancer

- For clinical staging when MRI is contraindicated
- To differentiate between early T stages (T1 or T2).

Treatment

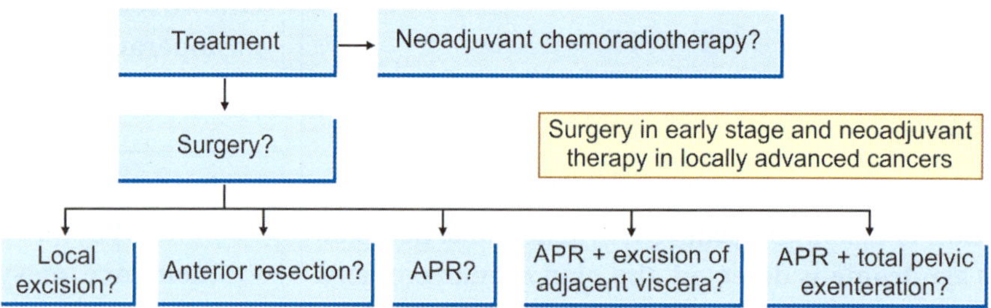

Type of Surgery based on Location of the Tumor

Within 8 cm of anal verge and fulfilling other criteria of local excision: Local excision.

Upper third of rectum: Low anterior resection (LAR) with Total mesorectal excision (TME).

Middle and lower third of rectum: Ultralow anterior resection or abdominoperineal resection (APR) with TME.

Very distal rectum: APR with TME (in most patients) or Ultralow anterior resection with TME (in selected group of patients).

Local excision is appropriate for: Tumor size <3 cm, well to moderately differentiated tumors within 8 cm of the anal verge, limited to <30% of the rectal circumference, endoscopically removed polyp with cancer or indeterminate pathology, no evidence of nodal involvement.

Approaches of local excision: (i) Transanal excision (TAE); (ii) Transanal endoscopic microsurgery (TEM); and (iii) Transanal minimally invasive surgery (TAMIS). Local excision involves excision of ≥10 mm grossly normal circumferential margin, depth down to perirectal fat, minimum 2 mm deep margin.

Principles of Total Mesorectal Excision (TME)

- Sharp dissection in the **"holy plane"** by scissors or monopolar diathermy under direct vision.
- Three-directional traction and counter-traction to make the areolar tissue of "holy plane" on "stretch."
- Recognition of autonomic plexuses and nerves during surgery and their preservation.
- Assessment of the specimen for an intact mesorectum (smooth, shiny, lobed surface) and absence of coning (towards the distal margin of the resection specimen).

Advantages of TME:

- Reduce the chance of local recurrence.
- Preservation of autonomic nerves.
- Decreased risk of genitourinary dysfunction (e.g., difficulty in micturition, erectile dysfunction, retrograde ejaculation, impaired vaginal lubrication).
- Reduce intraoperative bleeding.

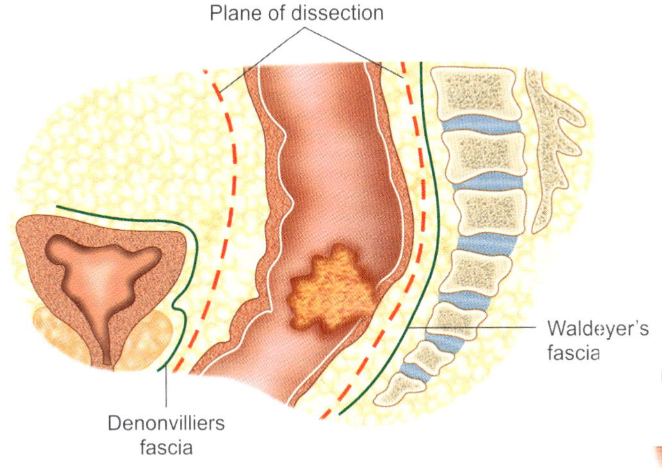

Holy Plane

The avascular plane in between the visceral layer of endopelvic fascia (fascia propria of rectum) and parietal layer of endopelvic fascia overlying the pelvic wall structures is called the **'Holy Plane'**.

TME facilitates en bloc removal of primary tumor along with most of the involved lymph nodes, lymphatics, mesentery, and tumor deposits.

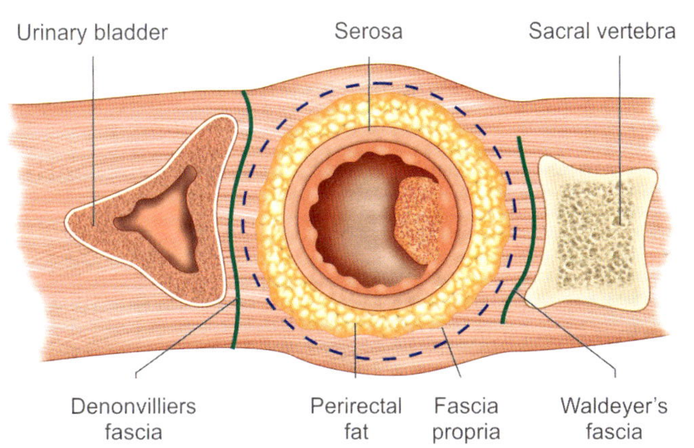

Distal Resection Margin Based on Location of the Tumor

- Upper third of rectum: 5 cm
- Middle and lower third of rectum: 2 cm
- Very distal rectum: 1 cm.
- Propensity of distal mesorectal spread is more than distal intramural spread in rectal cancer.

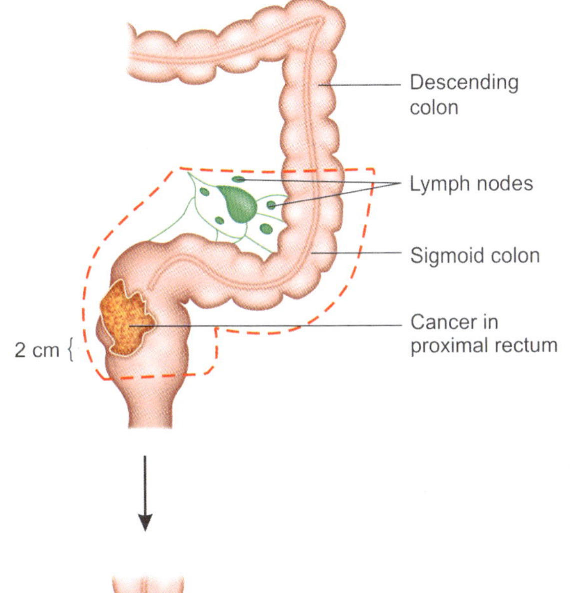

Low Anterior Resection (LAR) with TME

- This surgical technique is particularly indicated in **carcinoma of upper third of rectum**.
- **'Anterior'** term is used to differentiate abdominal (anterior) approach from posterior approach.
- **Anterior resection should not be attempted** if anal sphincter is destroyed or involved by disease.
- **This surgical method includes:** Wide resection of sigmoid colon and proximal rectum with distal clearance margin of at least 2 cm, regional lymphadenectomy and followed by end-to-end colorectal anastomosis.

Low Tie Technique and High Tie Technique

For resection of rectal cancer, **low tie technique** (ligation of the inferior mesenteric artery just distal to the takeoff of the left colic artery at the origin of the superior rectal artery) is appropriate. **High tie technique** (ligation of the inferior mesenteric artery at its takeoff from the aorta) is indicated only if clinically suspicious lymph nodes are present at the level of IMA.

Low tie technique is associated with better genitourinary function but no difference in survival, postoperative complications compared to high tie technique.

Reconstruction Techniques after Low Anterior Resection (LAR)

- End-to-end colorectal anastomosis (handsewn/stapled)
- Colonic J-pouch
- Transverse coloplasty
- Side-to-end (Baker) anastomosis.

Complications of LAR

Anastomotic leakage [A diverting ostomy (loop ileostomy is preferred over loop colostomy) should be considered after LAR to reduce the rate of clinical anastomotic leak].

Bladder dysfunction

Sexual dysfunction

Low anterior resection syndrome

Recurrence.

Low Anterior Resection Syndrome

A constellation of symptoms that includes incontinence, frequency, urgency, or feeling of incomplete emptying, develops most likely due to loss of reservoir function of rectum.

Techniques to augment residual reservoir function: (i) Colonic J-pouch; (ii) Transverse coloplasty; and (iii) Side-to-end anastomosis.

Abdominoperineal Resection (APR) or Abdominoperineal Excision (APE)

Indications:

- **Adenocarcinoma of the lower rectum** (where sphincter preservation is not possible due to direct involvement of anal sphincter or levator muscle or loss of integrity of the intersphincteric plane)
- Squamous cell carcinoma of anal canal, persisting after chemoradiation therapy
- Anal melanoma, sarcoma or GIST.

Complications:

Related to dissection: (i) Ureter injury; (ii) Injury to presacral venous plexus; (iii) Injury to autonomic nerves resulting in genitourinary dysfunction (e.g., bladder dystonia, erectile dysfunction, retrograde ejaculation); and (iv) Recurrence (risk is high if incomplete TME, intraoperative tumor perforation, CRM positivity).

Related to stoma: (i) Stoma retraction and (ii) Parastomal hernia.

Related to perineal wound: (i) Wound infection; (ii) Wound dehiscence; and (iii) Perineal hernia.

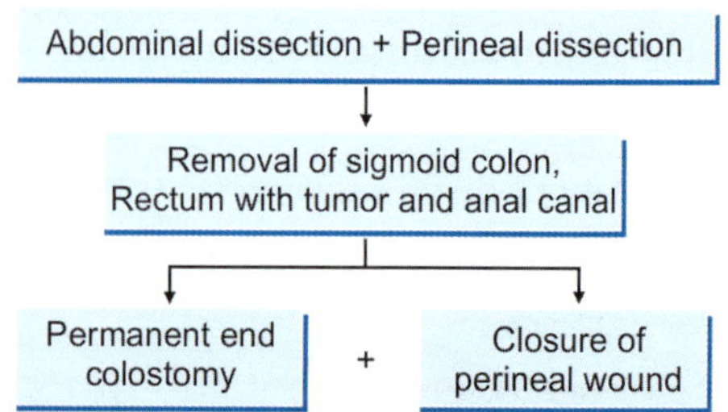

Perineal Positions in Abdominoperineal Resection

- Lithotomy position
- Prone jack-knife position
- Llyod-Davies position
- Left lateral (Sims) position.

Types of Abdominoperineal Excision (APE)

- **Conventional APE**
- **Extralevator APE (ELAPE)**
- Intersphincteric APE
- Ischioanal APE.

Indications of Perineal Reconstruction

- After ELAPE
- Patient with previous radiation therapy
- Patient with risk factors that increase the chance of perineal wound infection or dehiscence.

Reconstruction Options for Perineal Wound

- Vertical rectus abdominis muscle flap (VRAM) Gracilis muscle flap
- Bilateral V-Y advancement gluteal flap.

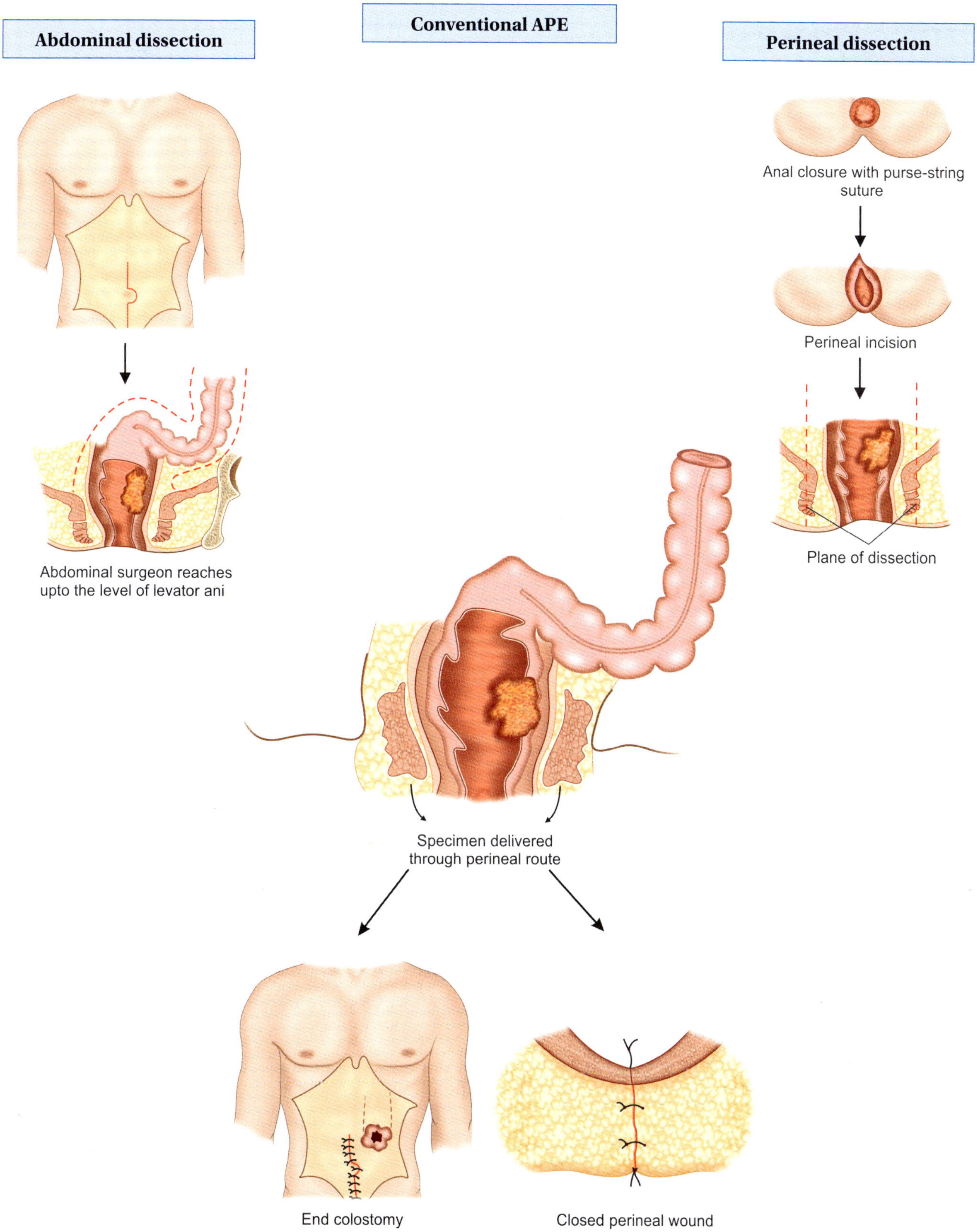

Abdominal dissection

Conventional APE

Perineal dissection

Anal closure with purse-string suture

Perineal incision

Plane of dissection

Abdominal surgeon reaches upto the level of levator ani

Specimen delivered through perineal route

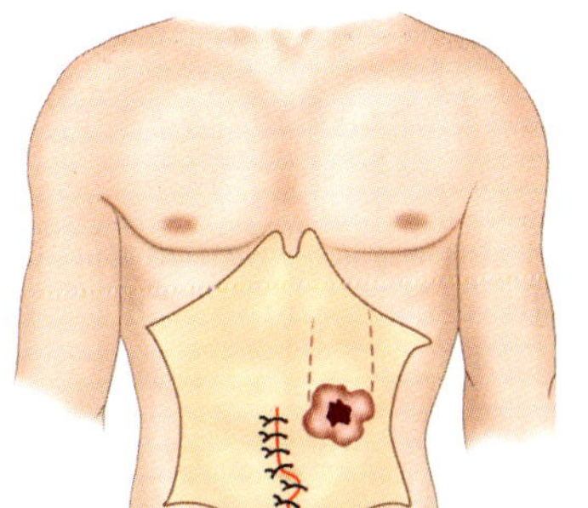

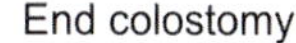

End colostomy

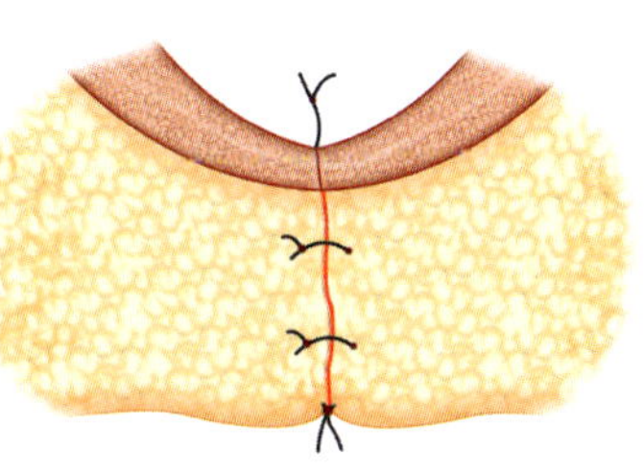

Closed perineal wound

Conventional APE	Extralevator APE (ELAPE)
Indicated in small tumors in middle and lower third of rectum	Indicated in bulky tumor involving levator muscles or high risk of intraoperative perforation
Levator muscles are not excised as part of resection	Levator muscles are excised from their origins on pelvic side walls and removed en bloc with the tumor
Chance of CRM positivity is more	Less chance of CRM positivity
Risk of intraoperative tumor perforation is more	Risk of intraoperative tumor perforation is less
For perineal stage of this operation, patient is placed in lithotomy position	For perineal stage of this operation, patient is placed in prone jack-knife position
A surgical waist exists on the specimen at the level of the tumor	A cylindrical shaped specimen is created
Perineal wound defects can be closed primarily	Perineal wound reconstruction is often indicated.

Grading of TME Specimen

Complete	Nearly complete	Incomplete
Intact bulky mesorectum with a smooth surface	Moderate bulk to the mesorectum	Little bulk to the mesorectum
Only minor irregularities of the mesorectal surface	Irregularity of the mesorectal surface with defects >5 mm, but none extending to the lamina propria	Defects in the mesorectum down to the muscularis propria
No surface defects >5 mm in depth	No areas of visibility of the muscularis propria except at the insertion site of the levator ani muscles	After transverse sectioning, the circumferential margin appears very irregular
No coning toward the distal margin of the specimen	Intermediate coning	Severe coning
After transverse sectioning the circumferential resection margin appears smooth	Intermediate irregularity of circumferential resection margin	Severe irregularity of circumferential resection margin

Transanal Total Mesorectal Excision (TaTME)

It is a technique that combines abdominal and endoscopic transanal approach (using surgical platform used for TAMIS) to overcome the limitations of standard laparoscopic TME.

Indications of TaTME: (i) Mid- or low-rectal cancer (within 8 cm from anal verge); (ii) Obese male patient; and (iii) Bulky tumors.

Principles: (i) Surgical platform used for TAMIS is used; (ii) Sharp dissection in the mesorectal fascial plane in a “down-to-up” approach; (iii) Specimen is delivered transanally or transabdominally; and (iv) Coloanal anastomosis with or without defunctioning loop ileostomy.

Intraoperative adverse events: (i) Difficulty in maintaining pneumopelvis; (ii) Dissection in incorrect tissue plane (during perineal phase) resulting in injuries to urethra, bladder, vagina; and (iii) CO_2 embolism.

Management of Colorectal Cancer (CRC) with Synchronous Resectable (or Potentially Resectable) Liver Metastases

Synchronous metastases are those metastases detected before, at, or within 3 to 6 months after the diagnosis of a primary cancer.

Classic approach

- A staged approach where rectal cancer is treated before the metastatic sites.
- Indicated for symptomatic rectal cancer associated with large extent of metastatic disease
- Not commonly practiced nowadays.

Combined approach

- Indicated in symptomatic rectal cancer with low-volume metastases (four or fewer, less than three segments involved, or all in the same lobe) in a low-risk surgical patient. This is the most preferred approach.
- Increased risk of perioperative morbidity should be considered.

Reversed approach

- A staged approach where metastatic disease is treated before the primary tumor.
- Indicated in patients with asymptomatic rectal cancer with high-volume metastatic disease.

Management of Obstructing Rectal Cancer

Stoma is the most preferable approach for obstructing rectal cancer.

Loop ileostomy may be an option if obstruction is incomplete or ileocecal valve is not patent. If obstruction is complete and ileocecal valve is competent, colostomy is mandatory.

Right-sided loop transverse colostomy is preferred over sigmoid loop colostomy by most surgeons because: (i) Marginal arcade is not disturbed (during definitive resection, oncologic principles can be maintained); (ii) Can be left in place for protection of anastomosis after definitive resection; and (iii) Permanent end colostomy creation is easier if it is indicated after definitive resection.

Loop sigmoid colostomy is particularly indicated in patients at high risk of GA, because this stoma can be created via left side skin incision under LA with IV sedation (Trephine stoma).

Sigmoid end colostomy may be an option if emergency surgeon can predict that abdomino-perineal resection (APR) will be the only option as curative resection.

SEMS is not preferred in low rectal cancer because of chronic pain, tenesmus and increased risk of stent migration and stent-related perforation.

SEMS is not recommended in patients who are being treated with or are expected to be commenced on antiangiogenic drug, Bevacizumab (due to increased risk of stent-related perforation).

Anal Carcinoma

Cancer of the anus (anal canal and perianal skin) is a uncommon cancer of the GI tract.

Anal canal cancer is the tumor that develops from the mucosa that cannot be entirely seen when the buttocks is gently pressed.

Perianal (anal margin) cancer is any tumor within the 5 cm of the anal orifice and can be visualized completely when the buttocks is gently pressed.

Tumors of anus are classified as: (i) Intraepithelial tumors also termed as Anal intraepithelial neoplasia (AIN); and (ii) Invasive tumors.

AIN (AIN-1, AIN-2, AIN-3) are precursors of invasive squamous cell carcinoma.

Invasive carcinomas of the anal canal are—squamous cell carcinoma, adenocarcinoma, small cell carcinoma, undifferentiated cancer, melanoma.

Perianal tumors are—squamous cell carcinoma, verrucous carcinoma (a rare variant of squamous cell carcinoma, also known as Buschke-Lowenstein tumor), basal cell carcinoma, Bowen disease (precursor of squamous cell CA), Paget disease.

Squamous cell carcinoma is the most common histologic type.

Anatomical anal canal—from the dentate line to the anal verge.

Surgical anal canal—from the anorectal ring to the anal verge and length is approximately 3 to 5 cm.

Anorectal ring is composed of external sphincter and puborectalis muscle. This structure can be detected by digital rectal examination (palpable as tight ring-like structure when patient is asked to squeeze the anal sphincter), TRUS or MRI.

Anoderm: The area between the dentate line and the anal verge. Anoderm is lined by nonkeratinized squamous epithelium.

Anal transitional zone (ATZ): This zone is located about 10 mm proximal to the dentate line and extending for 0.5 to 1.5 cm in length. This is the area of transition from the columnar epithelium of distal rectum and the squamous epithelium of the anal canal.

Risk Factors

- HPV infection (HPV-16 and 18)
- History of receptive anal intercourse
- History of cervical, vulvar or vaginal cancer
- History of previous sexually transmitted diseases of any kind
- HIV infection
- Immunosuppression after solid organ transplantation
- Autoimmune disorders (e.g., lupus, sarcoidosis)
- Cigarette smoking.

Role of Human Papilloma Virus (HPV)

- HPV-16 and 18 are strongly associated with high risk of anal cancer.
- HPV infection causes AIN, which progresses from low-grade dysplasia to high-grade dysplasia and then to invasive cancer.

Clinical Presentation

Bleeding per rectum is the most common presentation. Pain, tenesmus and pruritus may be present. Patient can feel a mass in the anus.

Patients may present with mass in the inguinal region due to metastatic inguinal lymph nodes.

Assessment of Tumor

Digital rectal examination (DRE)—Size and location of the tumor, fixity to the adjacent structures are assessed.

Proctoscopy—is essential to assess the size and location of the tumor within the anal canal.

Examination of **inguinal lymph nodes**

Pelvic examination is indicated to rule out presence of other HPV associated cancers

In male patient, **penile examination** should be done to exclude any premalignant or malignant lesions. In female patient, **cervical pap test** should be performed.

Biopsy from the tumor mass (under direct vision or anoscopy guided).

FNAC from the inguinal lymph nodes.

Assessment of the HIV status(if not known).

Clinical Staging

MRI is the imaging modality of choice for locoregional staging (tumor depth, sphincter involvement, perirectal lymph node status).

Endoanal ultrasound (EAUS) is another useful imaging modality for clinical staging.

For metastatic workup: Contrast enhanced CT abdomen with pelvis, CT chest. CT head is indicated if present with symptoms and signs of CNS involvement.

Management

Concurrent chemoradiotherapy (Nigro regime) is the recommended primary treatment for **nonmetastatic anal canal cancer**.

Mitomycin and 5-FU or mitomycin and capecitabine is administered concurrently with radiation.

Treatment of perianal cancer

T1N0, well differentiated perianal cancers, not involving the sphincter is treated by wide local excision with 1 cm margin. All other perianal cancers are treated by CRT.

Treatment of biopsy proven persistent or recurrent disease

Abdomino-perineal resection (APR) with groin dissection if any clinical evidence of inguinal lymph node metastasis.

Treatment of anal intraepithelial neoplasia (AIN)

Electocautery, topical imiquimod, and topical fluorouracil.

Surgical Staplers

Principles of Mechanical Stapling

- Tissue compression
- Placing of metal staples in a closed "B" shape
- Staggered positioning of the staple lines.

Aim of Surgical Stapling

- Transection and/or anastomosis in a accurate and reproducible manner
- Maintaining adequate tissue vascularization
- Achieving good hemostasis
- Proper tissue apposition
- Minimizing postoperative leakage.
- Modern staplers bend each staple into a 'B'-shape. 'Unacceptable' forms of bend staple can compromise integrity and strength of the staple line resulting in increased risk of bleeding and postoperative leaks. Staples are made of titanium. Staples are made available in various sizes and heights.

Types of Staplers

Linear noncutting staplers [Thoracoabdominal (TA) staplers]

- Deliver a double-staggered row of staples
- A specific vascular cartridge (30 mm-V3; white) used for TA stapler places three staggered rows of staples. This is used for closure of large vessels or resection of highly vascularized tissues.
- TA staplers are commonly used in lung lobectomy, liver lobectomy.

Linear cutting staplers [Gastrointestinal Anastomosis (GIA) staplers]

- GIA stapler is made of two interlocking pieces.
- This stapler first delivers double-staggered or triple-staggered rows of staple lines and then deploying a knife to divide the tissue between the staple lines.
- This type of stapler is used to transect tubular structures, create side-to-side anastomosis (e.g., gastrojejunostomy, jejunojejunostomy).

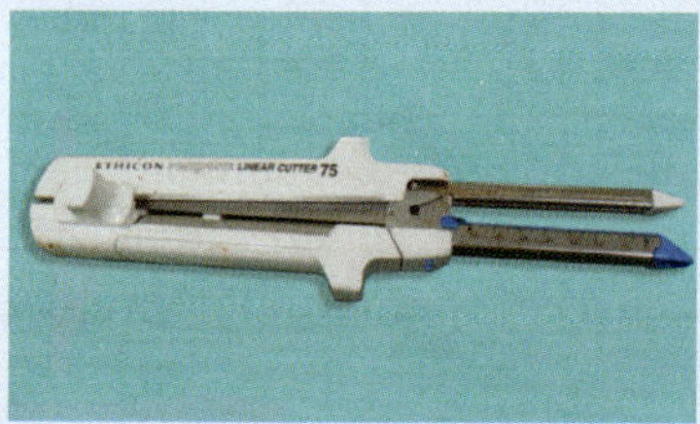

Linear cutter stapler

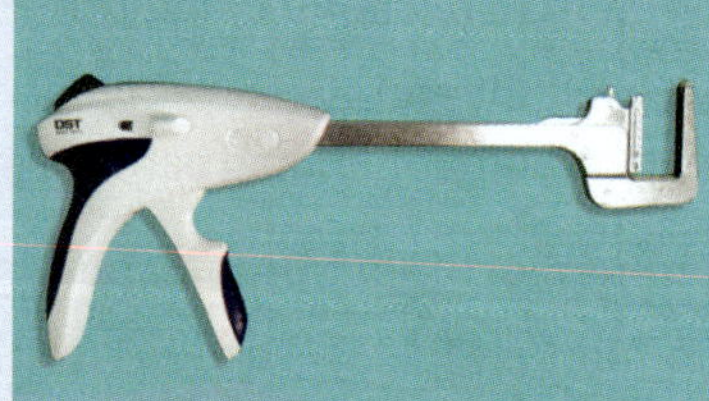

GI linear stapler

Circular staplers

- This stapler fires circular, double-staggered row of staples. Then an integrated circular scalpel resects overlaying tissue as "donuts" of tissue and creates an end-to-end anastomosis.
- These staplers are used primarily for end-to-end anastomosis (e.g., anterior resection, esophagogastrostomy).

Circular stapler

Factors to be Considered for Stapling

- Type of stapler (Linear noncutting/GIA/Circular)
- Type of anastomosis (end-to-end, side-to-side, end-to-side)
- Staple height
- Lumen diameter in circular stapler
- Tissue property (e.g., tissue thickness, compressibility)
- Compression time.

Possible Technical Error

(i) Surgeon misfiring and (ii) Incomplete anastomosis (inadequate donuts, staple line defects).

Complications

(i) Bleeding; (ii) Anastomotic leak; and (iii) Stricture.

Staple Line Reinforcement (SLR): may be done by

- Synthetic bioabsorbable copolymer of glycolic acid and trimethylene carbonate
- ePTFE
- Dry-collagen matrix
- Absorbable synthetic polyester

Color of cartridge	Tissue type	Open staple height	Closed staple height
Grey	Mesentery	2.0 mm	0.75 mm
White	Vascular	2.5 mm	1.0 mm
Blue	Standard	3.5 mm	1.5 mm
Gold	Standard/thick	3.8 mm	1.8 mm
Green	Thick	4.1 mm	2.0 mm

Case 1

History and Physical Examination

A 49-year-old female patient presented in the surgical OPD with complain of painless bleeding after defecation and something coming out per rectum (requiring manual reduction) for last 2 months. Patient suffered from similar complaint about 3 years back which relieved after conservative management. Patient was suffering from chronic constipation. Patient was diabetic and hypertensive. Menstrual and obstetric history were normal.

Physical Examination

Pallor: present; Pulse: 88/min; BP: 150/98 mm Hg

Examination of the rectum and anus—After straining, hemorrhoids were detected at 3 o'clock and 9 o'clock position. Digital rectal examination (DRE) and proctoscopy confirmed the diagnosis. Sphincter tone was normal, no palpable growth.

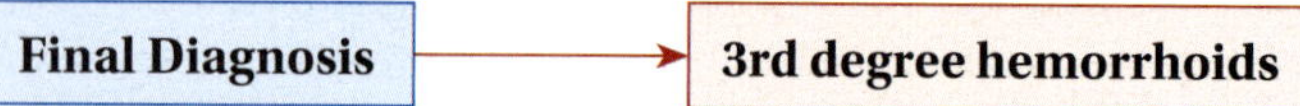

Investigations

Hb: 7.5 gm%; Blood sugar (F): 140 mg/dL; Postprandial blood sugar: 208 mg/dL; Serum urea and creatinine: within normal limit. Echocardiography: normal.

Discussion

History of painless bleeding and something coming out per rectum is highly suggestive of hemorrhoids. DRE and proctoscopic examination confirmed the diagnosis. Investigations were not required for diagnosis. Colonoscopy was also not indicated as criteria for colonoscopy was not fulfilled and patient had a history suggestive of hemorrhoids for last 3 years. Investigations were indicated as preoperative workup. Decision of open hemorrhoidectomy was taken after optimization of the patient.

Management Algorithm

- Correction of anemia (by blood transfusion)
- Control of diabetes and hypertension

→ Open hemorrhoidectomy

Case 2

History and Physical Examination

A 58-year-old male patient presented in the surgical emergency with history of abdominal distension and absolute constipation for last 2 days. Patient had history of alteration of bowel habit and passage of mucus with stool for last 4 months and for these patient was treated by local physician. No history of diabetes or hypertension. Patient was chronic smoker for last 20 years.

Physical Examination

Patient alert, conscious, cooperative

Patient dehydrated, pulse: 114/min; BP: 100/68 mm Hg

Examination of abdomen: Abdomen distended, diffuse tenderness all over the abdomen, hernial orifices normal, no lump palpable, IPS absent.

Digital rectal examination: A proliferative growth involving almost whole of the circumference of the rectum, lower margin was palpable about 4 cm proximal to anal verge, finger could not be negotiated up to the upper limit of the growth.

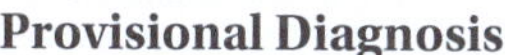

Provisional Diagnosis

→ Acute intestinal obstruction due to annular rectal growth

Investigations

Straight X-ray abdomen revealed dilated large bowel loops.
Hb: 7.8 gm%; Total WBC count: 10,000/cumm; Serum creatinine: 1.5 mg/dL

Discussion

History of alteration of bowel habit and passage of mucus with stool for last 4 months were highly suggestive of colorectal cancer. History of abdominal distension and absolute constipation for last 2 days suggestive of acute intestinal obstruction. Digital rectal examination revealed annular growth in rectum. So, history and clinical findings suggestive of obstructing rectal cancer. Plan of exploratory laparotomy followed by stoma was planned.

Management Algorithm

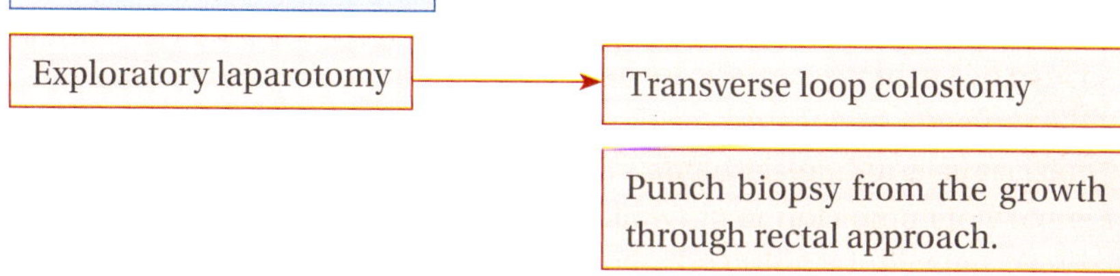

Chapter 13

Breast

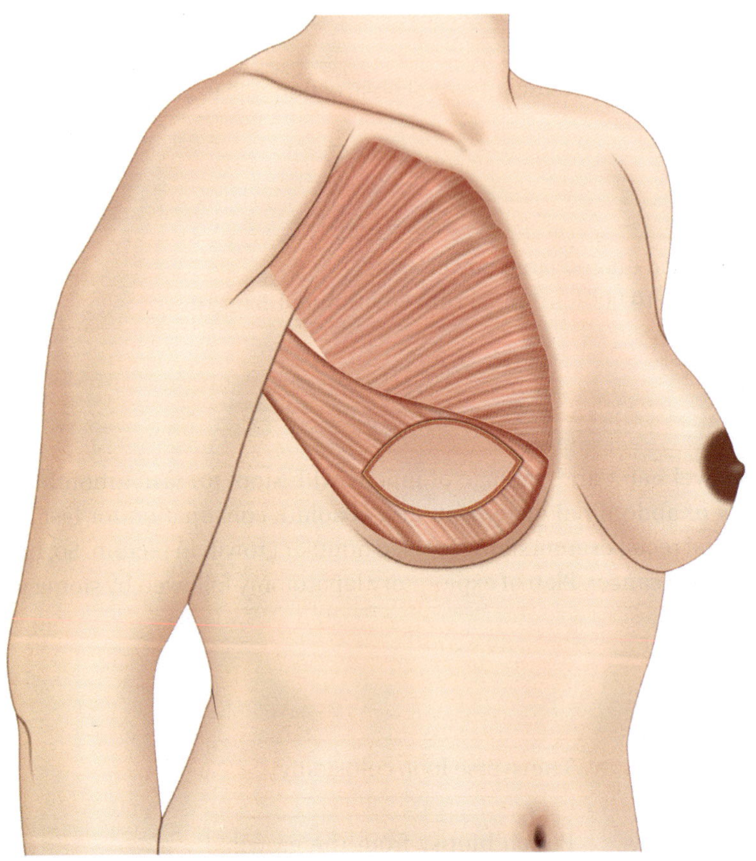

Important Topics

- Developmental Anomalies
- Mastitis and Breast Abscess
- Inflammatory and Benign Breast Lesions
- Gynecomastia
- Nipple Discharge
- Mastalgia
- Breast Carcinoma
- Male Breast Cancer
- Axillary Breast Cancer
- Breast Cancer in Pregnancy
- Inflammatory Breast Cancer
- Paget's Disease of the Nipple

> *'Surgical knowledge depends on long practice, not from speculations.'*
>
> **M Malpighi**
> **Italian Physician, Physiologist and Microscopist**

Diseases of the Breast

Developmental Anomalies

Amastia

It is a rare condition characterized by absence of the breast and nipple due to failure of the milk line to develop. Unilateral amastia is more common than bilateral amastia. Associated ectodermal defects such as cleft palate, isolated pectoral muscle, upper limb deformities are often present. It can also be associated with Poland syndrome.

Amazia

This condition is characterized by presence of nipple without breast tissue. Amazia may be congenital or acquired. Acquired amazia may be due to inadvertent biopsy of breast bud during childhood, chest wall radiation or surgery.

Athelia

It is a rare congenital anomaly characterized by absence of nipple. It may be presented as isolated anomaly or may be presented as a component of syndromes such as scalp-ear-nipple (SEN) syndrome, ectodermal dysplasia complex.

Polymastia

This condition is characterized by presence of accessory breast tissue, commonly in the axillary, abdominal or groin region (along the milk lines). Axilla is the most common site of accessory breast tissue. Accessory breast tissue can respond to hormonal changes during puberty, pregnancy and lactation similar to a normal breast. This accessory breast tissue may undergo benign or malignant changes like normal breast tissue.

Polythelia

This condition is characterized by presence of supernumerary nipples along the milk lines. Most common site is just inferior to normal breast. Renal anomalies may be associated with this congenital anomaly.

Poland Syndrome

This is the best known inherited disorder of breast development. **The main feature** is hypoplasia or absence of the pectoral muscles (particularly sternocostal head of pectoralis major). Serratus anterior or latissimus dorsi muscles may also be affected. Other manifestations are amastia, athelia, and cartilage agenesis of the second to fifth ribs on ipsilateral side, syndactyly, scoliosis. It is common in males and in the right side.

Syndromes Associated with Developmental Anomalies of Breast

- Poland syndrome and ulnar-mammary syndrome (associated with amastia)
- Turner's syndrome and Fleischer's syndrome (associated with polymastia)
- Scalp-ear-nipple (SEN) syndrome (associated with athelia)

Lactational Mastitis and Lactational Breast Abscess

Lactational mastitis develops during breastfeeding, either during the commencement of breastfeeding (during the 2nd and 3rd weeks postpartum) or during weaning. **Milk stasis and infection** are primarily responsible for mastitis. Ineffective suckling, sore nipple, inadequate duration and frequency of breastfeeding are responsible for milk stasis. **Cracked nipple** is the most likely port of entry of infection. Most of the lactational mastitis is caused by **coagulase negative *S. aureus***, but also may be caused by *S. epidermidis* and *Streptocococcus* species. Breast abscess develops as a complication of mastitis.

Clinical Presentation

Patients present with discomfort in the breast, pain, erythema, swelling, tenderness, systemic signs of infection. If abscess develops, a fluctuant swelling with overlying erythematous, shiny skin may be present.

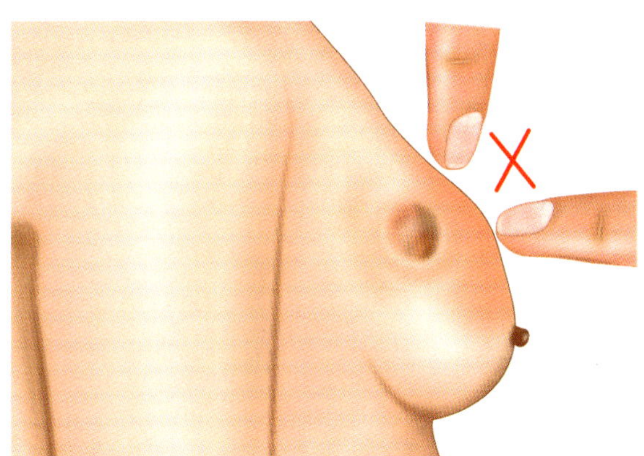

Don't depend on **fluctuation** to differentiate between mastitis and abscess

Fluctuation is a late sign

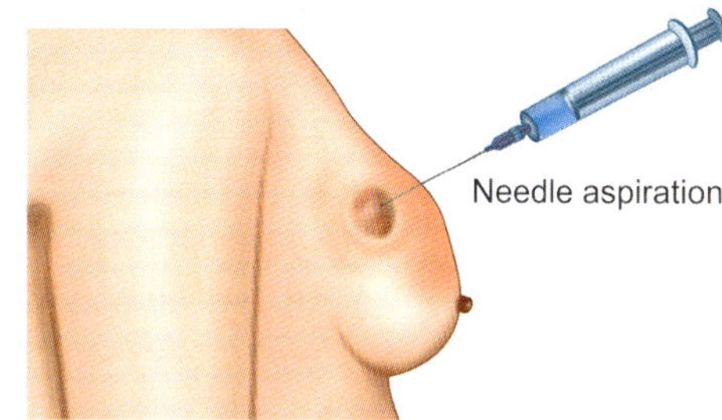

Management

In many patients, abscesses can be difficult to differentiate from mastitis, particularly for deep-seated abscesses. Needle aspiration or USG is often helpful to detect abscess. Sometimes, inflammatory carcinoma can be difficult to differentiate from abscesses. If any suspicion of **inflammatory carcinoma**, full thickness skin biopsy and cytology of aspirated material should be performed.

Treatment of mastitis includes antibiotics (coverage against penicillinase producing *S. aureus*, continuing breastfeeding on the opposite breast, emptying of milk from diseased breast either manually or by breast pump, care of the cracked nipple.

Treatment of breast abscess is either repeated pus aspiration under antibiotic coverage or incision and drainage. Repeated aspiration under oral antibiotic coverage is the treatment of choice for most of the lactational breast abscesses. Aspiration should be repeated every 2–3 days until no pus on aspiration.

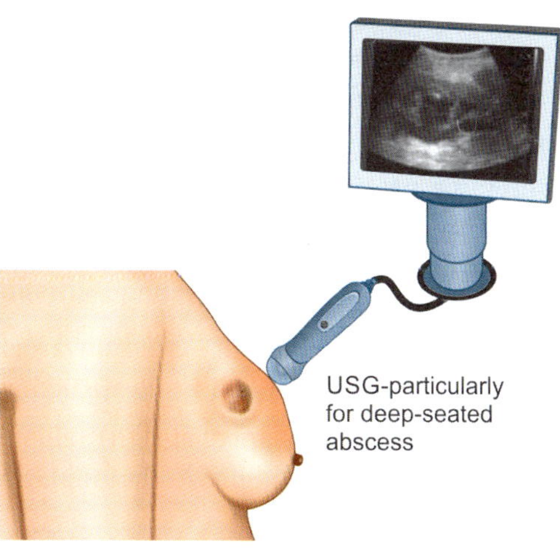

Incision and Drainage of Breast Abscess

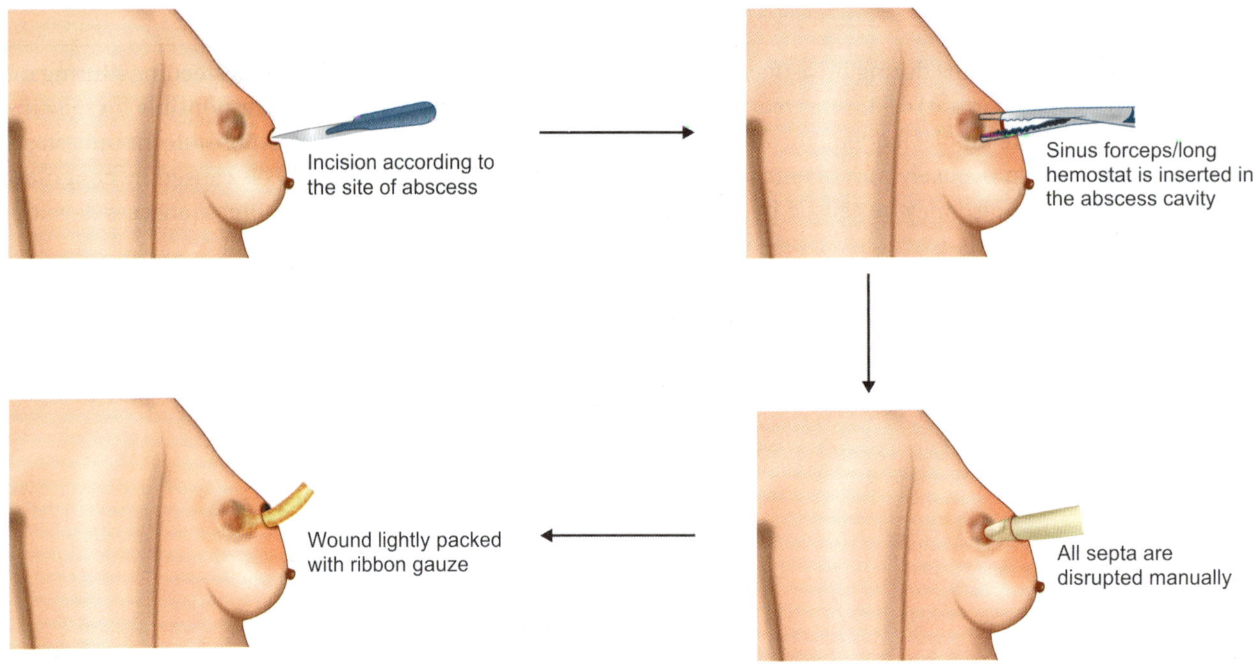

Nonlactational Breast Abscess

Nonlactational breast abscesses are either central (peri-areolar) or peripheral. **Central abscesses** are the most common form of nonlactational abscess. These abscesses are most commonly seen in young women who smoke and arise as a complication of periductal mastitis. These abscesses have high recurrence rate and often associated with cutaneous fistula. Treatment is repeated aspiration and oral antibiotics or incision and drainage.

Mammography is indicated after resolution of infective process. In refractory cases, total duct excision is indicated. **Peripheral abscesses** commonly seen in older women and often associated with diabetes mellitus, rheumatoid arthritis, steroid therapy. *S. aureus* is the most commonly isolated organism. Recurrent aspiration with oral antibiotics or incision and drainage is the treatment. Mammography is indicated after resolution of infective process.

Central (peri-areolar) Abscess

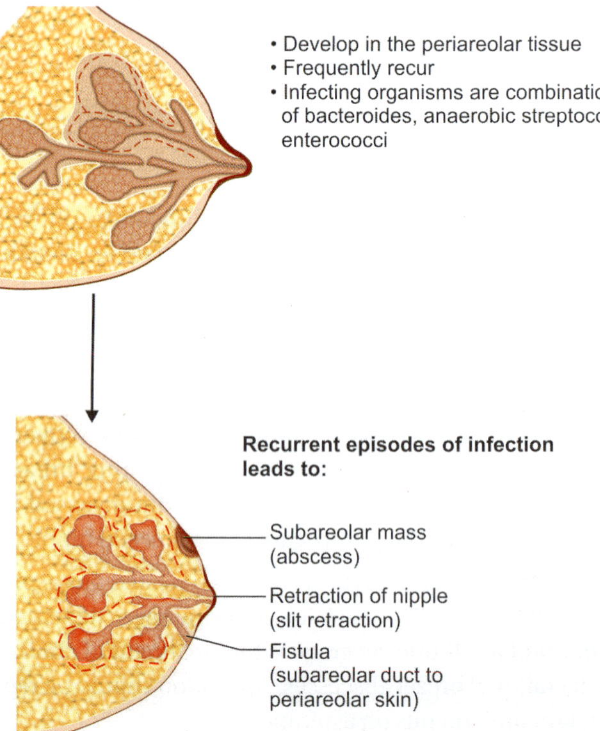

Duct Ectasia and Periductal Mastitis

Duct ectasia is an involutional and age-related condition characterized by dilation of larger periareolar ducts, followed by inflammation and fibrosis.

Clinical presentation of duct ectasia includes (i) unilateral or bilateral off-white, creamy or cheesy, viscous, tooth-paste like nipple discharge. Sometime, greenish nipple discharge may present and (ii) Slit retraction of nipple.

Periductal mastitis is an pathological, inflammatory condition characterized by periareolar inflammation with or without subareolar mass or abscess, nipple retraction or mammary duct fistula. Duct ectasia commonly coexists with periductal mastitis. Smoking is a risk factor for development of periductal mastitis. Clinical presentation of periductal mastitis includes: (i) Episodes of periareolar inflammation; (ii) Periareolar mass or abscess; (iii) Purulent nipple discharge; (iv) Nipple retraction; and (v) Mammary duct fistula.

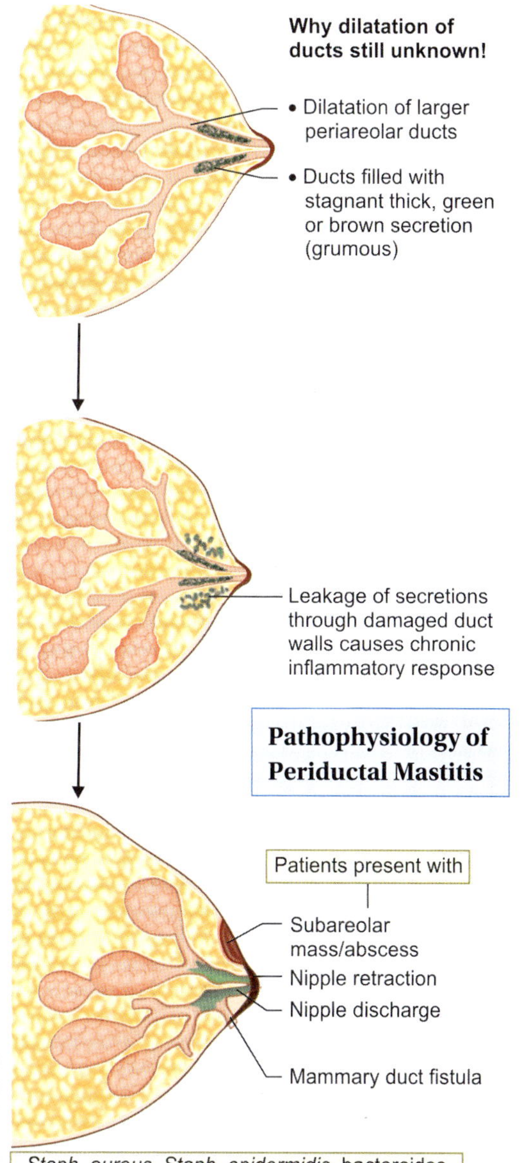

Pathophysiology of Periductal Mastitis

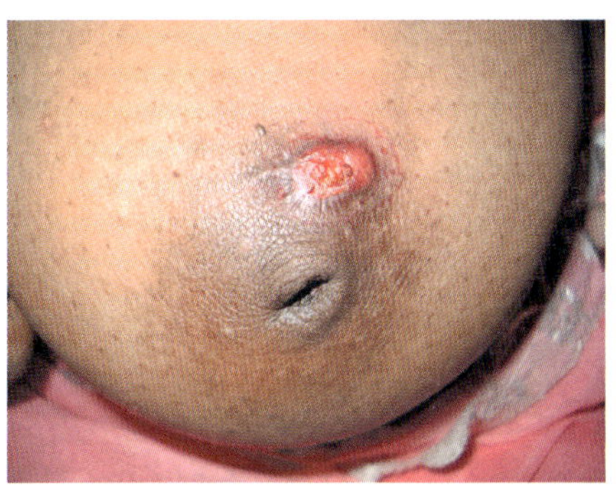

Periductal mastitis with fistula and nipple retraction.

Causes of Nipple Retraction

- Breast carcinoma
- Duct ectasia
- Periductal mastitis
- Tuberculosis

Investigations

- **USG of breast** can detect dilated ducts and architectural changes within parenchyma.
- **Mammography** can detect coarse, large calcifications along prominent ducts.
- **Galactography (Ductography)** is only indicated in patients with single duct discharge.
- **Biopsy (FNAC or core-cut biopsy)** is indicated if patients present with a mass.

Zuska Disease (Recurrent Periductal Mastitis or Recurrent Subareolar Abscess)

Characterized by: (i) Recurrent retroareolar infections and abscesses due to blockage of lactiferous duct by keratin plug; (ii) Presence of slit-type nipple retraction; (iii) Single fistula tract opening at the edge of the areola beneath the smooth muscle of the nipple; and (iv) Strongly associated with smoking. **Treatment:** (i) Smoking cessation; (ii) Incision and drainage of abscess; and (iii) Excision of terminal duct (for long-term control).

USG of Breast

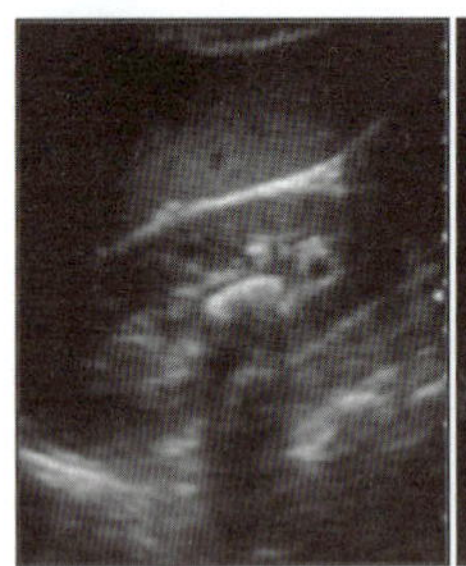

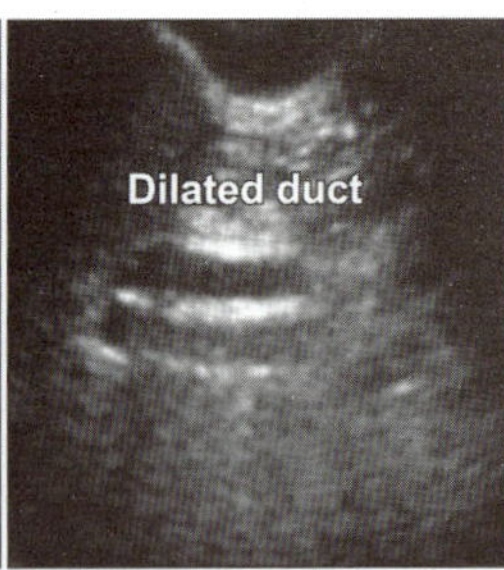

- Can identify dilated ducts leading to the nipple
- Can detect calcification
- Usually detect any abcess, if present

Mammography

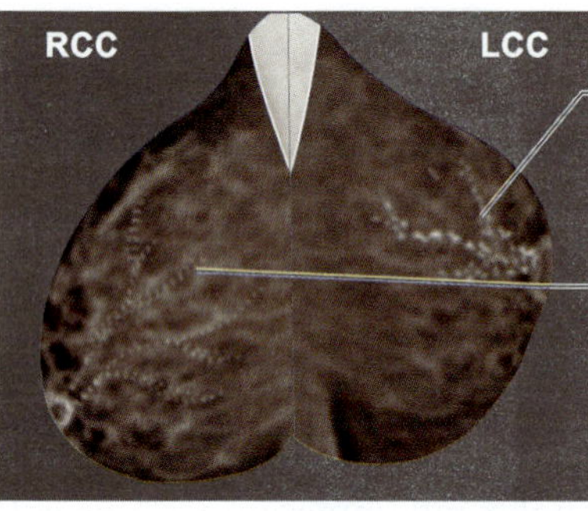

Treatment For duct ectasia, no specific treatment is indicated. Only symptomatic treatment is required. If duct ectasia is associated with periductal mastitis, oral antibiotic therapy coverage against *S. aureus*, *S. epidermidis*, anaerobic *Streptococcus*, *Bacteroides* is indicated. If patient presents with periareolar abscess, repeated aspiration with oral antibiotics or incision and drainage is indicated. If patient presents with recurrent symptoms with single duct discharge, **microdochectomy** (excision of the involved duct and surrounding involved breast parenchyma) may be considered. **Radical duct excision (Modified Hadfield's operation)** may be considered in patients with recurrent periductal mastitis and multiple duct discharge. **All patients are advised to stop smoking.**

Ductography

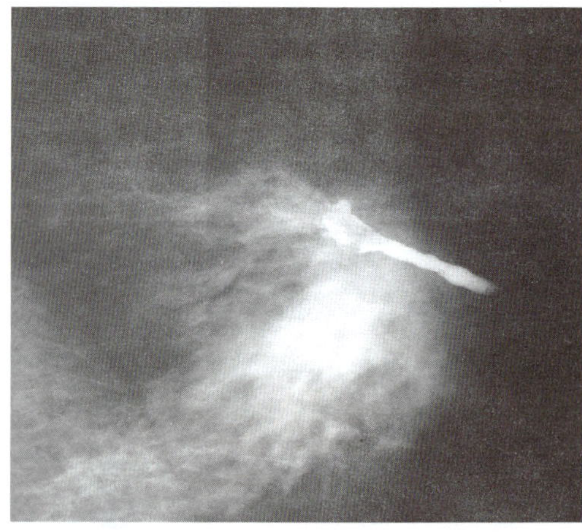

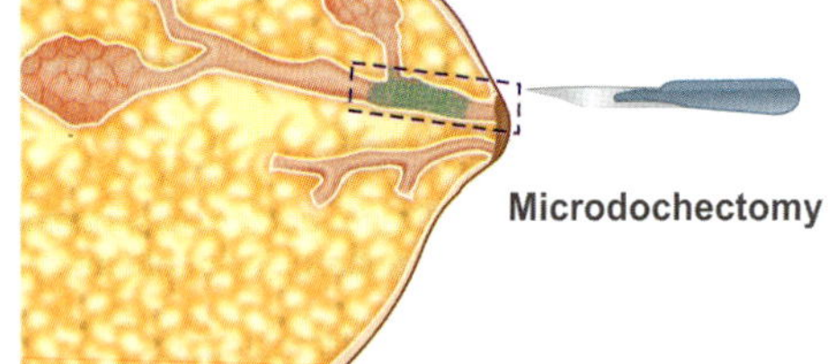

Radical duct excision (modified Hadfield's operation)

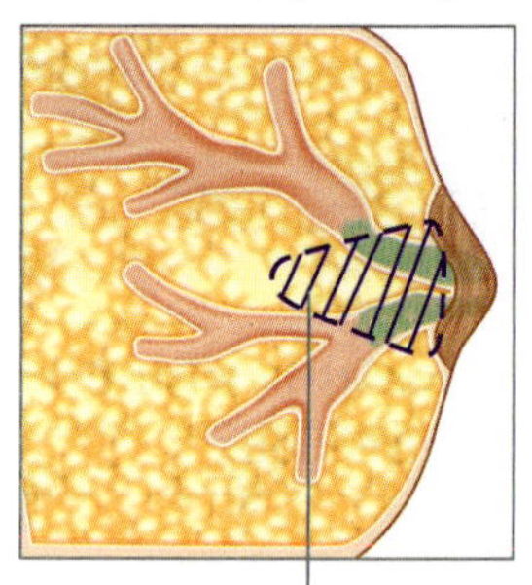

Tuberculosis of the Breast

Tuberculosis of the breast is a rare disease. It most commonly affects lactating women. Most commonly, patient presents with a lump. Patient may present with skin tethering, sinus formation or abscess. Workup is focused on to exclude breast carcinoma and to reach definitive diagnosis of tuberculosis. Mammography and USG are helpful imaging modalities to exclude carcinoma. FNAC, core cut biopsy or open biopsy are useful diagnostic modalities for definitive diagnosis by detecting epithelioid cell granulomas, caseation necrosis, Langhans-type giant cells. Treatment is antitubercular therapy. Surgical intervention is indicated for drainage of abscess, residual sinus tracts after ATD therapy. Simple mastectomy may be considered for painful ulcerated mass involving the whole breast.

Hidradenitis Suppurativa

Hidradenitis suppurativa is a chronic debilitating skin disorder involving mainly the apocrine-gland bearing regions. This condition most commonly affects axilla, but may involve inframammary fold. Conservative management rather than excision is the preferred treatment option.

Pilonidal Abscess

Pilonidal sinus may develop in the periareolar region in roustabouts (Sheepshearers' assistants, who carry shorn wool close to their breast), in hairdressers and canine beauticians.

Mondor's Disease

Mondor's disease is the superficial thrombophlebitis involving the superficial veins of anterior chest wall. Veins involved are lateral thoracic vein, thoracoepigastric vein, and superficial epigastric vein. Patients present with pain in anterior chest wall and lateral part of the breast. On examination, tender cord-like structure is palpable along the course of the superficial vein. Avoidance of strenuous work on diseased side, warm compress, anti-inflammatory agents are sufficient for the management. In Penile Mondor's disease (PMD), superficial dorsal vein of penis is involved.

Histologic Classification of Benign Breast Lesions

Nonproliferative lesions (No relative risk)	Proliferative lesions without atypia (Relative risk 1.5–2.0 fold)	Proliferative lesions with atypia (Relative risk 4-fold)
Cyst	Sclerosing adenosis	Atypical ductal hyperplasia
Mild hyperplasia of the usual type	Moderate or florid ductal hyperplasia of the usual type	Atypical lobular hyperplasia
Papillary apocrine change	Radial scar	Lobular carcinoma in situ
Duct ectasia	Intraductal papilloma	
Fibroadenoma	Flat epithelial atypia	

Fibroadenoma

Fibroadenoma is the most common breast neoplasm in adolescent girls and young women. It may also be considered as an aberration of normal lobular development rather than a true neoplasm. This tumor most commonly develops between second and third decades of life, but not uncommon during postmenopausal period.

Classic clinical presentation is solitary, discrete, non-tender, smooth, mobile lump of 1–3 cm in diameter.

Diagnosis: In most of the patients, diagnosis can be made by characteristic clinical findings. A 'triple assessment approach' [clinical examination, imaging (USG) and tissue diagnosis (Fine-needle aspiration or core-needle biopsy)] is highly accurate for diagnosis.

Management: In women under 35 years of age, reassurance (no cancer, chance of malignant transformation is rare) and close clinical and imaging follow-up is the recommended treatment unless patient wants excision. Surgical excision is indicated if the tumor size is increasing during follow-up or not completely regressed after 35 years. In patients of older age group, surgical excision is indicated. **Newer treatment approach includes:** (i) Percutaneous treatment (USG-guided cryoablation and USG-guided percutaneous excision) and (ii) Transcutaneous ablative therapy (Focused ultrasound ablation and focused microwave thermotherapy).

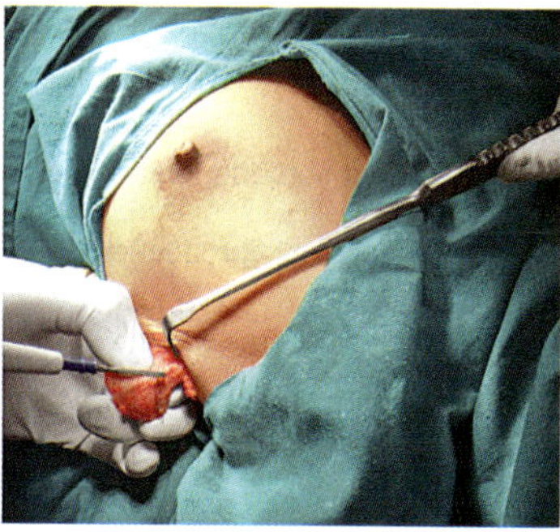

Excision of fibroadenoma.

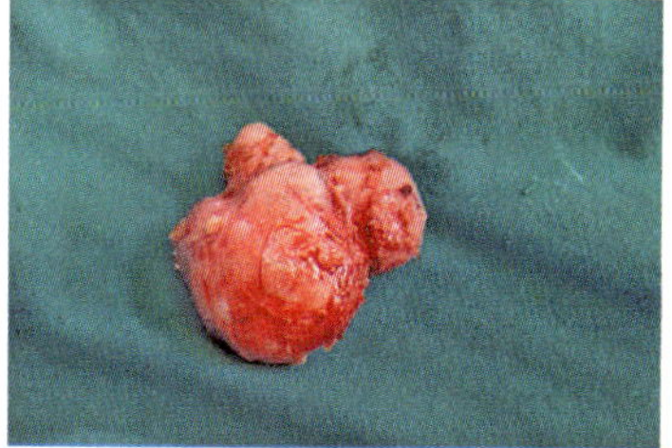

Operated specimen of fibroadenoma.

Criteria to be Fulfilled for Cryoablation or Percutaneous Excision of Fibroadenoma

- Lesion must be visualized on USG.
- Diagnosis must be confirmed histologically on core biopsy.
- Diagnosis must be concordant with the imaging findings, history and physical examination.
- Lesion must be less than 4 cm in largest diameter.

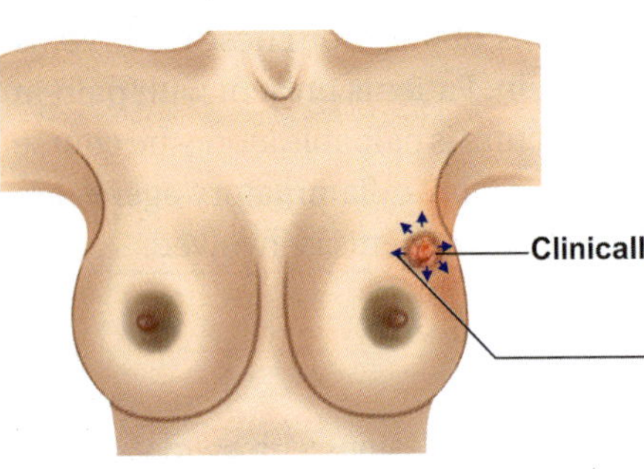

- Basically an aberration of normal lobular development
- That is why, it is more common in breast of young women

Clinically:
- Smooth or slightly lobulated well-encapsulated firm lump
- Extremely mobile—So termed as 'breast mouse'

- Etiology is unknown

- ***Microscopically***

Intracanalicular

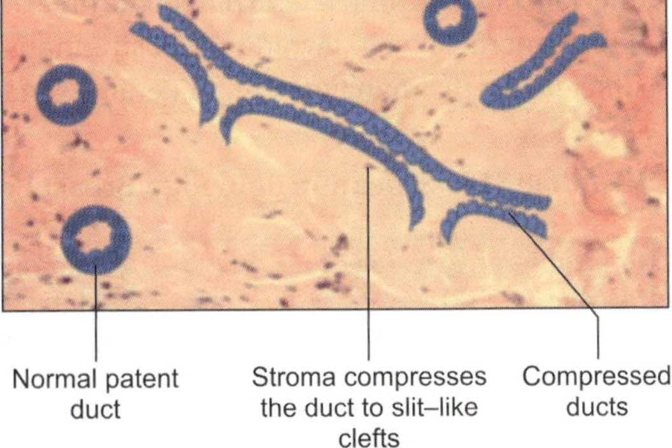

- **Macroscopically**

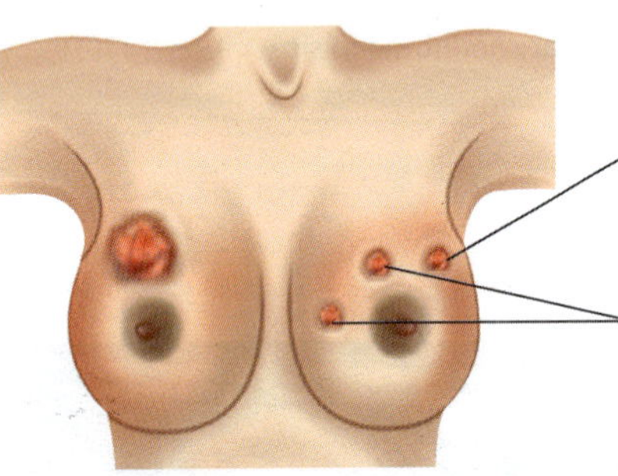

- Simple fibroadenoma (**<5 cm**)
- Multiple fibroadenoma (**>5 in a single breast**)
- Juvenile fibroadenoma — Uncommon variant of fibroadenoma which is large and more cellular than usual fibroadenoma

- Giant fibroadenoma (**>5 cm**)
- Recurrent fibroadenoma

Pericanalicular

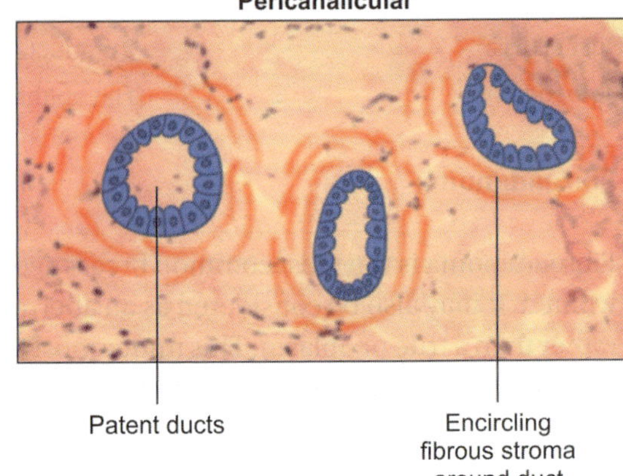

Giant Fibroadenoma

A fibroadenoma is considered as giant fibroadenoma when it is more than 5 cm in diameter or weighing more than 500 g. Giant fibroadenomas are more common in adolescent girls but may develop in mature women. This tumor has propensity to rapid growth and causes asymmetry of breast. It is histologically different from phyllodes tumor (phyllodes tumor exhibit more cellularity, pleomorphism, and mitotic activity). Treatment is enucleation through an appropriately placed cosmetic incision.

Differential Diagnosis

- Phyllodes tumor
- Juvenile breast hypertrophy

Phyllodes Tumor

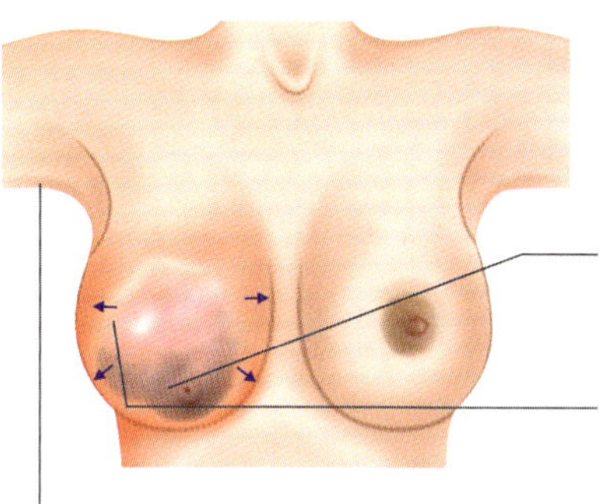

- Arises from periductal stroma
- Histologically, both epithelial and fibrous stromal elements are present. Stroma showing more hypercellularity, much atypia numerous mitoses
- Large, 10–15 cm in diameter, well-circumscribed, bosselated, irregular surface projections (leaf-like appearance)
- A degree of mobility is present even in large phyllodes (compare carcinoma)—in carcinoma, often the lump is fixed
- Axillary lymphadenopathy is uncommon, if present, it indicates extremely aggressive form of the disease
- Based on mitotic index and degree of polymorphism, this tumor is classified into:

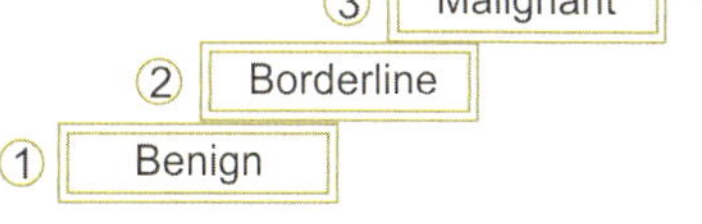

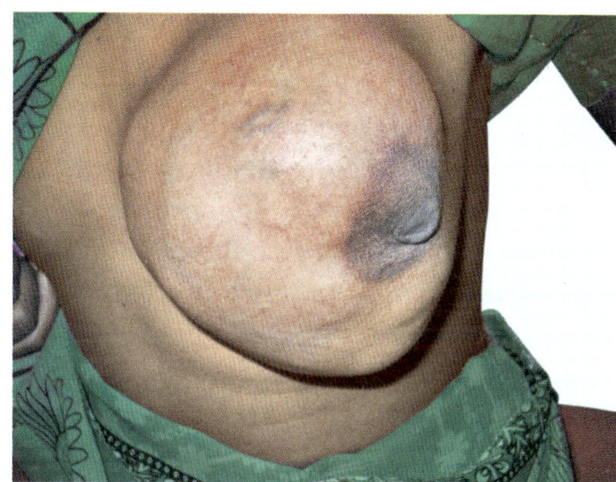

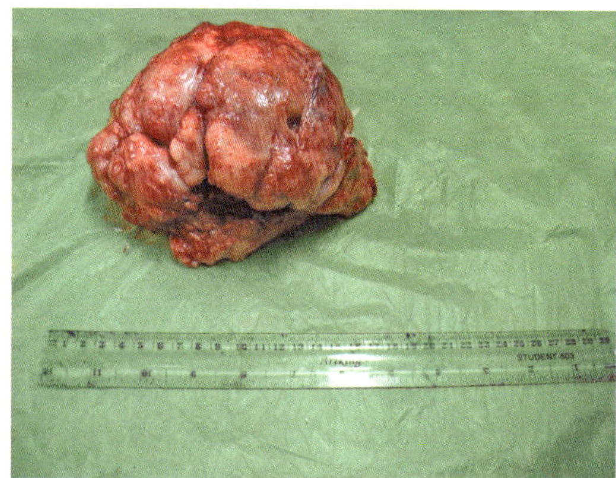

WHO Criteria for Classifying Phyllodes Tumor

Criteria	Benign	Borderline	Malignant
Stromal cellularity and atypia	Minimal	Moderate	Marked
Stromal overgrowth	Minimal	Moderate	Marked
Mitoses/10 HPF	0–4	5–9	≥10
Tumor margins	Well circumscribed with pushing tumor margins	Zone of microscopic invasion around tumor margins	Infiltrative tumor margins

FNA or core biopsy cannot differentiate fibroadenoma from phyllodes tumor. Excisional biopsy should be considered to exclude phyllodes tumor.

Surgical excision (lumpectomy or partial mastectomy) with tumor-free margin of 1 cm or more is recommended for benign, borderline and malignant phyllodes.

Total mastectomy is only indicated if negative margins cannot be obtained by lumpectomy or partial mastectomy. Axillary lymph node sampling or axillary dissection is not routinely indicated.

For locally recurrent phyllodes, re-excision with wide margins is recommended.

Patients with **Li-Fraumeni syndrome** are at increased risk of phyllodes tumor.

Most common site of recurrence is local recurrence.

Most common site of distant metastasis is lungs.

No role of **endocrine therapy** and **chemotherapy**. Role of postoperative radiation following resection of chest wall recurrence is controversial.

Breast Cyst

Breast cyst is one of the common causes of breast lump. Breast cysts most commonly develop in the last decade of reproductive life. Breast cysts are of two types: (i) Simple cyst and (ii) Apocrine cyst. **Based on USG, breast cysts are of three types:** (i) Simple cyst; (ii) Complicated cyst; and (iii) Complex cyst.

Simple cyst: Anechoic, well-circumscribed lesion. Not associated with any risk of malignancy. No need of active management, routine follow-up only.

Complicated cyst: Low-level echoes, intracystic debris. Low risk of malignancy (<2%). Management includes aspiration or follow-up; biopsy if cyst increase in size.

Complex cyst: Diagnosis is confirmed by aspiration and/or USG. Both cystic and solid components are present. High risk of malignancy. Management includes tissue biopsy (core needle biopsy). If the palpable mass is completely disappearing after USG-guided aspiration and aspirated fluid is not gross bloody, no need of cytological analysis and further treatment. Simple cysts usually disappear after aspiration. If aspirated fluid is blood stained, fluid should be sent for cytological analysis to exclude intraduct papilloma or intracystic carcinoma. If USG shows solid components or cyst recurs, then core needle biopsy should be done.

Management of cyst: Surgical excision should be considered if cyst continues to recur or core needle biopsy findings are inconclusive. If histopathology report is benign, follow-up imaging should be done every 6–12 months for 2 years.

Pathophysiology

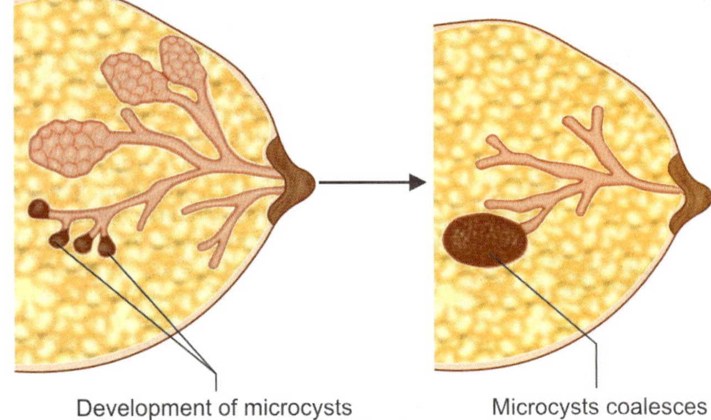

Apocrine cyst

- Classically seen in perimenopausal women.
- New cyst formation in postmenopausal women is often associated with HRT

- Often multiple
- Often painful on palpation, smooth tense lumps with limited mobility

Diagnosis is confirmed by aspiration and/or USG

Fluid in cyst contains unusual amounts of biologically active substances, including hormones and metabolites

Galactocele

Galactocele is the most common benign breast lesion during lactation characterized by encysted collection of milk. It commonly develops in women who recently stopped breastfeeding.

Pathophysiology: Galactocele most likely develops following lactiferous duct occlusion by the protein plug, resulting in extravasation of milk into the surrounding stroma.

Clinical presentation: Patients present with round, well-circumscribed, smooth, mobile, nontender lump, commonly located in the subareolar region.

Diagnosis: USG features are suggestive of simple or complex cyst. Aspiration is both diagnostic and therapeutic.

Treatment: Spontaneous resolution occurs in most of the patients. Therapeutic aspiration is indicated if patient presents with significant symptoms.

Differential Diagnosis

- Breast abscess
- Lactating adenoma
- Fibroadenoma
- Breast carcinoma

Fat Necrosis

Fat necrosis is an inflammatory process mostly secondary to trauma. Diagnosis of fat necrosis is important because it closely mimic carcinoma both clinically and on mammography.

Etiology: Fat necrosis develops due to lipase-induced aseptic saponification of adipose tissue. Fat necrosis is particularly associated with surgery or trauma, but may be idiopathic. Surgeries related to fat necrosis includes lumpectomy, reduction mammoplasty, implant removal.

Clinical presentation: Patient commonly presents with painless irregular lump, often periareolar in location. Sometimes, skin tethering and nipple retraction are present.

Diagnosis: If radiologic findings strongly suggestive of fat necrosis, tissue diagnosis may not be necessary. If any suspicion of malignancy, FNA or core needle biopsy is indicated.

Treatment: Excision of the lump is indicated if patient complaining of any pain or distortion of shape, otherwise close follow-up is sufficient.

Characteristic Microscopic Findings

- Lipid-laden macrophages
- Foreign-body giant cells

Mammographic Features of Fat Necrosis

- Multiple clustered pleomorphic micro-calcifications
- Radiolucent oil cysts (Pathognomonic finding)
- Ill-defined spiculated mass

Gynecomastia

Gynecomastia is generalized enlargement of male breast tissue. Types of gynecomastia are: (i) Physiological; (ii) Pathological.

Pathophysiology of Physiological Gynecomastia

Neonatal gynecomastia: During pregnancy, dehydroepiandrosterone (DHEA) and dehydroepiandosterone-sulfate (DHEA-SO_4) are converted to estrone and estradiol in placenta, respectively. Then these estrone and estradiol enter fetal circulation and stimulate neonatal breast tissue. This type of gynecomastia commonly regresses within 2–3 weeks of delivery.

Puberty gynecomastia: In early puberty, estradiol increases more rapidly than testosterone, resulting in elevated estrogen/androgen ratio. This type of gynecomastia commonly regresses within two years of onset.

Senile gynecomastia: With aging, adiposity increased. In adipose tissue, androgens are converted to estrogens. Decreased testosterone synthesis is also responsible.

Pathophysiology of Pathological Gynecomastia

Due to estrogen excess: (i) True hermaphroditism; (ii) Germ cell tumors of testis; (iii) Stromal tumors of testis (e.g., Leydig cell tumor, Sertoli cell tumor); (iii) Adrenal cortical tumors; (iv) Carcinoma of liver; (v) Nonalcoholic and alcoholic cirrhosis; and (vi) Malnutrition.

Due to androgen deficiency (i) Primary testicular failure (e.g., Klinefelter's syndrome, Kallmann syndrome, ACTH deficiency) and (ii) Secondary testicular failure (e.g., Trauma, irradiation, orchitis).

Medications: (i) Due to estrogenic activity (Digoxin, estrogen, anabolic steroids); (ii) Due to inhibition of testosterone synthesis (Phenytoin, ketoconazole, spironolactone); and (iii) Unknown mechanism (Phenothiazines, Theophylline, verapamil, and furosemide).

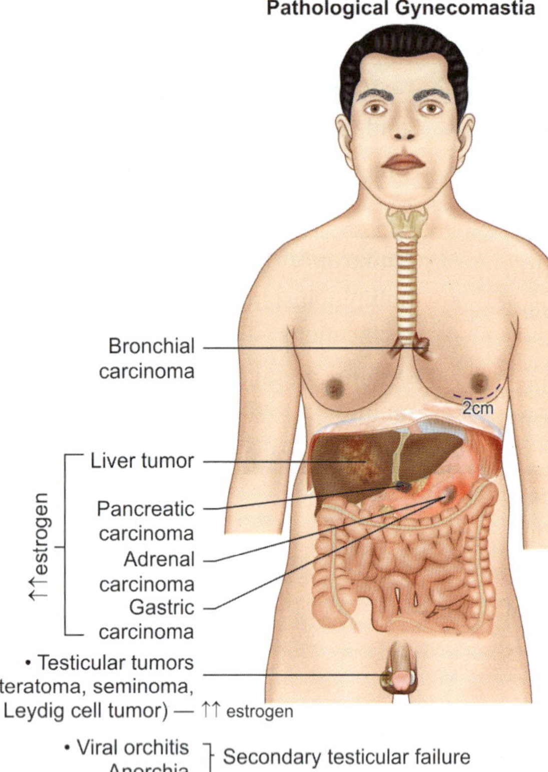

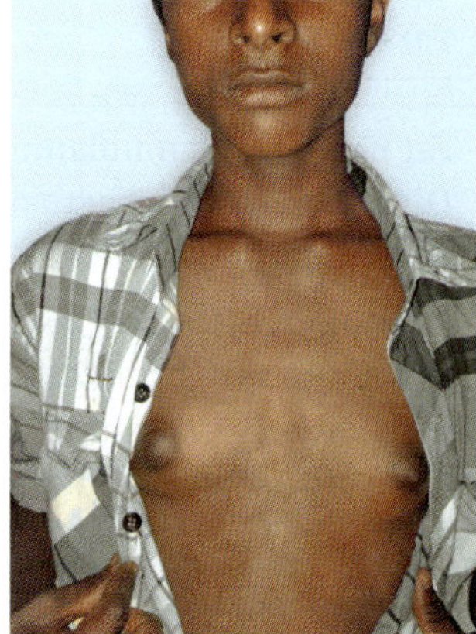

- Among calcium-channel blockers, **diltiazem** has least correlation with gynecomastia.
- Among H_2 blockers, **cimetidine** has the highest and **ranitidine** has the lowest correlation with gynecomastia.

Clinically, gynecomastia is diagnosed by subareolar breast tissue of 2 cm or more.

Grading of Gynecomastia

(based on degree of breast enlargement and skin redundancy) by Simon et al:

- **Grade I:** Mild breast enlargement without skin redundancy
- **Grade IIa:** Moderate breast enlargement without skin redundancy
- **Grade IIb:** Moderate breast enlargement with skin redundancy
- **Grade III:** Marked breast enlargement with skin redundancy and ptosis

Differential Diagnosis of Gynecomastia

- Pseudogynecomastia
- Breast carcinoma
- Lipoma
- Sebaceous cyst
- Fat necrosis

Refeeding Gynecomastia

Development of gynecomastia after recovering from malnourished state.

Gynecomastia	Pseudogynecomastia
Composed of glandular tissues of breast	Composed of fatty tissue
Firm in consistency	Soft in consistency
On palpation, breast tissue may be tender	On palpation, breast tissue nontender
Breast size, not fluctuate with weight gain or loss	Breast size significantly fluctuates with weight gain or loss

Work-up

Work-up is indicated in pathological gynecomastia. Work-up includes: (i) Liver function test; (ii) Testicular USG; (iii) Chest X-ray; and (iv) Hormonal profile (estrogen, testosterone, LH, hCG). If clinical findings are suggestive of malignancy (e.g., Eccentric breast mass, bloody nipple discharge, nipple retraction, axillary lymphadenopathy), biopsy is indicated.

Treatment

- **Observation:** If after work-up, no underlying pathology is detected.
- **Androgen therapy:** In hypogonadism
- **Danazol therapy:** In adult idiopathic gynecomastia
- **Tamoxifen therapy:** In acute painful gynecomastia
- **Surgery** is indicated for cosmetic reasons, suspected malignancy. Subcutaneous mastectomy is the most common surgical approach.

Nipple Discharge

Nipple discharge is one of the most common breast symptoms like mastalgia and breast lump. Nipple discharge is either physiologic or pathologic.

Nipple discharge is pathologic if it is spontaneous, unilateral, from a single duct, serous or blood-stained, persistent (more than twice per week) and a dominant symptom.

Nipple discharge is physiologic if it is nonspontaneous, bilateral, from multiple duct orifices, and white, green or yellowish in color.

Assessment of nipple discharge:

- Spontaneous or induced
- Arises from single duct or multiple ducts
- Unilateral or bilateral
- *Characteristic of discharge:* Serous, serosanguineous, bloody, milky, greenish

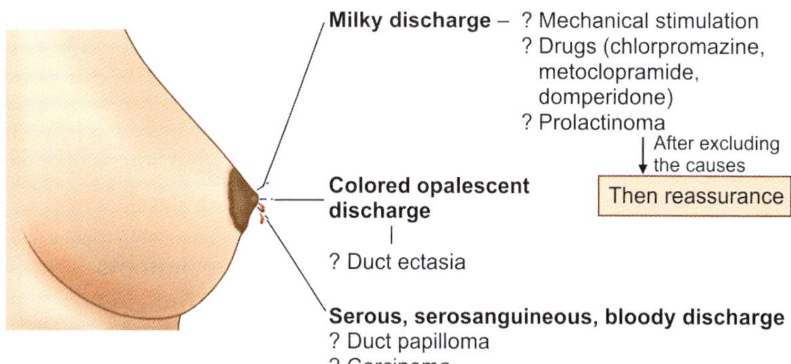

Causes of Nipple Discharge

- Intraductal papilloma (Bloody discharge)
- Duct ectasia (Greenish discharge)
- Breast carcinoma
- Galactorrhea (bilateral milky discharge not associated with pregnancy or lactation)
- Fibrocystic breast disease

Intraductal papilloma is the most common cause of pathologic nipple discharge.

Work-up

Work-up of pathologic nipple discharge includes clinical examination and imaging.

Diagnostic mammography is preferred initial imaging modality for nipple discharge, particularly if no mass is palpable.

Ultrasonography is also a useful imaging modality if mammography is negative.

Ductography (Galactography) is indicated if mammography and sonography both are negative.

MRI may be considered if mammography, sonography, and ductography are negative.

Ductoscopy is a useful modality for evaluation of pathologic nipple discharge, but it is not widely accepted due to lack of availability and expertise.

Image-guided FNA or core-needle biopsy is indicated if any mass lesion is detected on imaging.

Cytologic examination of nipple discharge has no proven value in evaluation of pathologic nipple discharge.

Management

Major duct excision should be considered in patients with pathological nipple discharge and negative imaging evaluations. Nonoperative management may be considered if nipple discharge is non-bloody, normal imaging, and no history of ipsilateral breast cancer, BRCA mutation.

Nipple Discharge of the Male Breast

- Nipple discharge in male breast is rare, but it warrants further work-up because it is strongly associated with underlying breast malignancy.
- Work-up includes clinical examination, mammography, and/USG.

Causes of Galactorrhea

- Prolactinoma
- Drugs (chlorpromazine, metoclopramide, ranitidine)

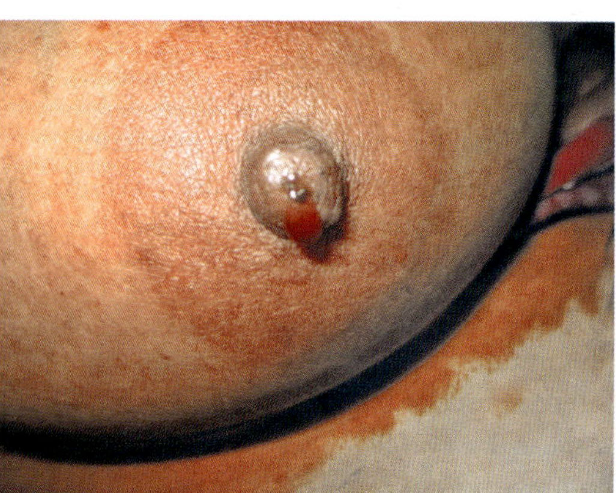

Blood-stained nipple discharge

Ductography: A mammographic imaging technique (standard two-view) after cannulation (with 30-gauge sialogram needle) and filling of the lactiferous duct with contrast medium (1–2 mL). The primary role of ductography is to precisely detect the site of intraductal lesion.

Contraindications of ductography: (i) Lactating women; (ii) Active mastitis; and (iii) Known hypersensitivity to iodinated contrast agents.

Mammary ductoscopy: A method of direct visualization of ductal epithelium of the lactiferous ducts using microendoscope inserted through the ductal opening onto the nipple surface. This modality also allows ductal lavage for cytological analysis.

Advantages of ductoscopy: (i) Accurate identification of intraductal pathologies and (ii) Limiting the extent of resection by precise localization of the lesion.

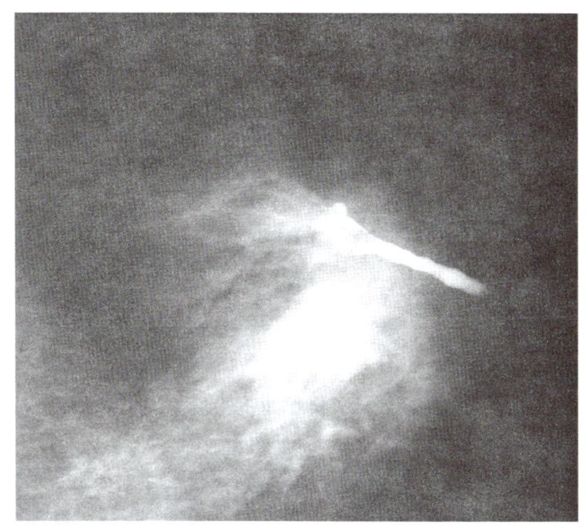

Ductogram

Breast Pain

Breast pain (Mastalgia) is the most common breast symptom. It is more common in pre-menopausal women and rarely associated with cancer. Most of the women consult a health practitioner related to anxiety about cancer.

Mastalgia can be classified into three categories:

Cyclical Mastalgia

Cyclical mastalgia is related to menstrual cycle. It is usually **bilateral aching pain or heaviness** commonly in upper outer quadrants of breast, pain starts during the luteal phase and increases in intensity until menstruation begins and decreasing after onset of mestruation. The pain may radiate to the upper arm and axilla.

The exact etiology is unknown.

Non-cyclical Mastalgia

Non-cyclical mastalgia is not related to menstrual cycle. It is usually unilateral sharp burning pain localized in one quadrant of the breast. Causes of non-cyclical mastalgia are usually localized breast pathology, i.e., periductal mastitis, breast cyst, breast abscess. It is more common in older age group and postmenopausal women.

Extramammary Pain

Causes of extramammary pathologies presenting as mastalgia are:

- Tietze syndrome (costochondritis)
- Pleuritic chest pain
- Mondor disease
- Fibromyalgia
- Herpes zoster
- Biliary pain

Workup

Investigations, particularly imaging (mammography or ultrasonography) are indicated to rule out breast cancer. **However, imaging is not indicated in young female with cyclical, non-focal mastalgia with no risk factors of breast carcinoma and a normal breast examination.**

Ultrasound of breast may considered for evaluation of focal and noncyclical mastalgia in female patients of less than 30 years. Mammography is less accurate than US in these age group due to greater breast density.

Mammography including digital breast tomosynthesis (DBT) and US may be used to rule out malignancy in female patients of 30–39 years. In female patients of 40 years or older with focal and noncyclical mastalgia, **mammography and DBT** are preferred options.

Management

Reassurance: After clinical examination and proper work-up, reassurance is the mainstay of management. Most of the patients are relieved from anxiety once she is informed that it is not a serious pathology and not associated with underlying breast cancer or increased risk of cancer. It is also important to inform the patient that it is often self-limiting and role of medications are limited. Reassurance is helpful in most of the patients. A few percentage of patients need treatment because of negative impact of pain on her daily activities, sleep and sexual life.

Maintenance of breast pain chart: Maintenance of Cardiff breast pain chart for 2 months allows patients to document the nature of their symptoms and the impact on their daily lives. Mastalgia can be defined as cyclical or non-cyclical based on the chart.

Lifestyle modification: Reduction of caffeine intake, consumption of low-fat diet, inculcation of exercise regime are helpful in few groups of patients.

Well-fitting brassiere: Well-fitting sports brassiere is helpful to relief pain by reducing the tension on overstretched Cooper's ligaments, particularly patients with pendulous, heavy breasts.

Topical application of NSAIDs: Topical application of diclofenac gel provides symptomatic relief in most of the patients.

Evening primrose oil (72% Linoleic acid, 7% Linolenic acid): This therapy is the first-line treatment for patients with cyclical mastalgia. If no significant improvement of symptoms after 4–6 months, this therapy should be discontinued.

Tamoxifen: Low-dose tamoxifen (10 mg daily on 15–25 days of menstrual cycle) for 3 months is highly effective for severe refractory mastalgia. The therapy should be stopped if no significant improvements after 3 months. Side effects include headache, nausea, vaginal dryness, and hot flashes.

Danazol: Danazol is a synthetic androgen derived from ethinyl testosterone. It is effective for treatment of cyclical mastalgia (dose is 100–400 mg in two divided doses for 3–6 months), but not well tolerated by the patients due to significant side-effects (e.g., acne, amenorrhea, weight gain, hirsutism, depression). It is also teratogenic and interfere the efficacy of OCP. It is reserved as a second line agent.

Bromocriptine: Bromocriptine blocks the release of prolactin from pituitary by dopaminergic receptor stimulation. This agent is also not well tolerated by the patients due to significant side-effects (e.g., headache, dizziness, and postural hypotension).

Centchroman (Ormeloxifene): Centchroman is a non-steroidal, selective estrogen receptor modulator. It is effective in mastagia (dose is 30 mg alternate day for 3 months) with minimal side-effects. Contraindications are polycystic ovarian disease, cervical dysplasia, pregnancy, and lactation.

ANDI (Aberrations of Normal Development and Involution)

A concept first suggested at Cardiff breast clinic to allow all benign breast problems within an overall framework of pathogenesis. By this comprehensive classification, most of the benign problems can be explained as **mild abnormality (disorder) to severe abnormality (disease) of development, cyclical change, or involution.**

In the ANDI classification, **the vertical component** indicates the period when the breast problem develops, and **the horizontal component** indicates the spectrum—normal to disorder to disease.

	Normal	Disorder	Disease
Early reproductive years (15–25 years)	• Lobular development • Stromal development • Nipple eversion	• Fibroadenoma • Adolescent hypertrophy	• Giant fibroadenoma • Gigantomastia • Subareolar abscess • Mammary duct fistula
Later reproductive years (25–40 years)	• Cyclical changes of menstruation • Epithelial hyperplasia of pregnancy	• Cyclical mastalgia • Nodularity • Bloody nipple discharge	Incapacitating mastalgia
Involution (35–55 years)	• Lobular involution • *Duct involution:* – Dilatation – Sclerosis • Epithelial turnover	• Macrocysts • Sclerosing lesions • Duct ectasia • Nipple retraction • Epithelial hyperplasia	• Periductal mastitis • Epithelial hyperplasia with atypia

Breast Carcinoma

Risk Factors

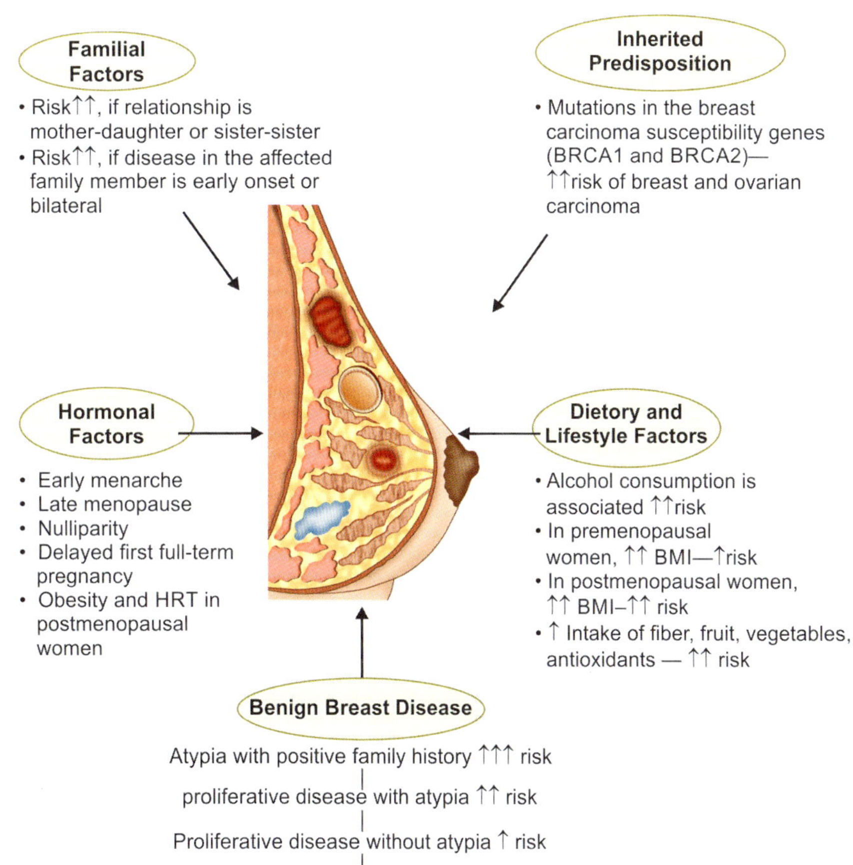

BRCA1	*BRCA2*
Tumor-suppressor gene	Tumor-suppressor gene
Located on chromosome arm 17q	Located on chromosome arm 13q
Female mutation carriers have lifetime risk for: Breast CA 85%, Ovarian CA 40%	Mutation carriers have lifetime risk for: Breast CA 85%, Ovarian CA 20%
No increased risk of breast cancer in male mutation carriers	Male mutation carriers have life-time risk for breast cancer is 6%
Associated breast cancers are invasive ductal carcinoma, poorly differentiated	Associated breast cancers are invasive ductal carcinoma, well differentiated
Most of the tumors are hormone receptor negative or triple negative	Most of the tumors are hormone receptor positive
Presence of associated cancers, commonly ovarian cancer and other cancers (e.g., colon, prostate) in some mutation carriers	Presence of associated cancers, ovarian, colon, prostate, pancreas, gallbladder, stomach, and melanoma in some mutation carriers
Early age of onset (compared to sporadic cancer)	Early age of onset (compared to sporadic cancer)
Bilateral involvement is common	Bilateral involvement is common

Other Cancers Associated with BRCA1 and BRCA2 Mutations

- **In women:** Ovarian cancer, fallopian tube cancer, primary peritoneal cancer.
- **In men:** Breast cancer and prostate cancer.
- **In both men and women:** Pancreatic cancer.

Genetic Predisposing Conditions Associated with High Risk for Breast Carcinoma

- Hereditary breast and ovarian cancer (BRCA1/2)
- Hereditary diffuse gastric cancer (CDH1)
- Li-Fraumeni syndrome (TP53)
- Peutz-Jeghers syndrome (STK11)
- Cowden syndrome (PTEN)

Other Genes Related to Breast Cancer

- PALB2 ("Partner and Localizer of BRCA2")
- CHEK2 ("Checkpoint kinase 2")
- CDH1 ("CaDHerin 1")
- PTEN ("Phosphatase and TENsin homolog")
- STK11 ("Serine/Threonine kinase 11")
- TP53 ("Tumor Protein 53")

High risk for BRCA mutations if one has a family history of:

- Breast cancer diagnosed before age 50
- Male breast cancer at any age
- Multiple relatives on the same side of the family with breast cancer
- Multiple breast cancers in the same woman
- Both breast and ovarian cancers in the same woman
- Ashkenazi Jewish heritage

Risk Assessment Models

Gail model 1	• This risk-assessment model focuses on nongenetic risk factors. • The risk factors include age at menarche, age at first live birth, number of previous breast biopsies, number of first-degree relatives with breast cancer. • The limitations of this model: (i) includes only first-degree relatives; (ii) does not consider age at diagnosis of breast cancer; and (iii) does not consider history of ovarian cancer. • This model estimates the probability of invasive ductal carcinoma, ductal carcinoma in situ, and lobular carcinoma in situ. • Gail risk score ≥1.66 have higher risk for developing breast cancer.
Gail model 2	• This model estimates the absolute risk of developing only invasive breast cancer. • Gail model 1 is modified by involving atypical hyperplasia in breast biopsy, race, and ethnicity.
Claus model	• This model estimates the lifetime risk of breast cancer (both invasive and DCIS). • The risk factors include—age of the person, age at menarche, age at first live birth, history of breast cancer in first-degree and second-degree relatives. • **Limitations:** Discrepancy in results between published tables and computer model.
Claus extended	• It is an extension of the Claus model. • This model adds risk factors—presence of ovarian cancer, bilateral breast cancer, more than two affected relatives with breast cancer.
BRCAPRO model	• This risk assessment tool assesses the probability of an individual carries a germline deleterious mutation of the *BRCA1* and *BRCA2* genes. • This model is based on family history (1st degree, 2nd degree relatives) of breast and ovarian cancer, male breast cancer, bilateral breast cancer, age of diagnosis of breast and/or ovarian cancer, ages of unaffected family members. • **Limitation:** (i) Underestimate the importance of ovarian cancer and (ii) Other genetic element is not incorporated in this model.
Tyrer-Cuzick model	• It is the most sensitive model for detecting risk for breast cancer. • This model incorporates personal risk factors for breast cancer (advancing age, older age at first live birth >30 years, younger age at menarche <12 years, older age at menopause >55 years, hormone replacement therapy), benign breast disease, family history of 1st and 2nd degree relatives (age at onset of breast cancer, bilateral breast cancer, ovarian cancer), *BRCA* gene mutation. • **Limitations:** This model accounts only for hereditary breast and ovarian cancer. • If a woman's life-time risk ≥20%, annual screening breast MRI should be considered.
BOADICEA [Breast and Ovarian Analysis of Disease Incidence and Carrier Estimation Algorithm] **model**	• It is the first polygenic breast cancer risk model. • It is used to: (i) to calculate the risks of breast and ovarian cancer in women based on their family history; and (ii) to calculate the probability that they are carriers of mutation of *BRCA1* and *BRCA2* genes. • Different versions are available; BWA v3, BWA v4Beta, BOADICEA v5. • It is used only for research purposes.

Genetic Risk Model: To Calculate Probability of BRCA Mutation Carrier

- BOADICEA
- BRCAPRO
- IBIS
- Extended Claus model (eCLAUS)

Risk Assessment Model Mostly Based on Family History

- Claus model
- BRCAPRO
- BOADICEA
- Tyrer-Cuzick model

Pathology

• Breast carcinoma may arise from the epithelium of the duct system from the nipple end of the major lactiferous duct to the terminal duct-lobular unit

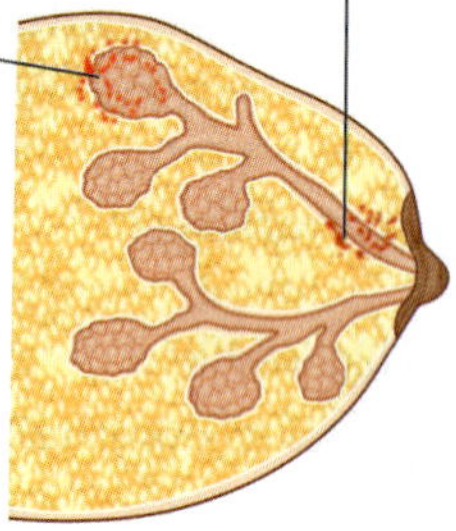

Malignant cells have breached the basement membrane or not?

Noninvasive cancer (Carcinoma in situ)

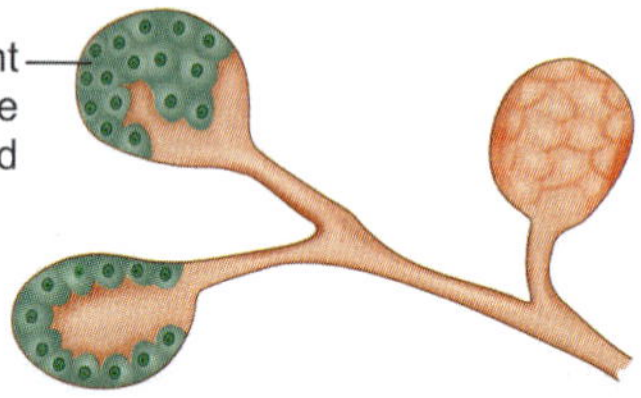

Invasive cancer

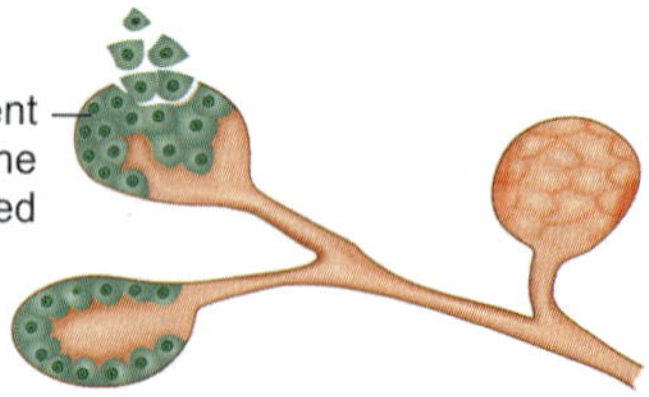

Basement membrane not breached

Basement membrane is breached

Carcinoma in situ

Lobular carcinoma in situ (LCIS)
- It is a increased risk factor
- Not a anatomic precursor

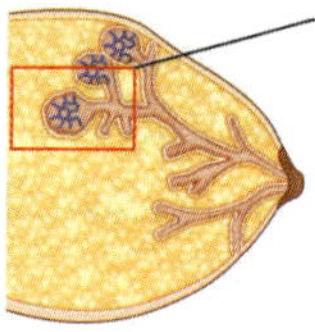

Ductal carcinoma in situ (DCIS)
- Anatomic precursor of invasive ductal carcinoma
- Predominantly seen in female breast, but seen in about 5% of male breast.

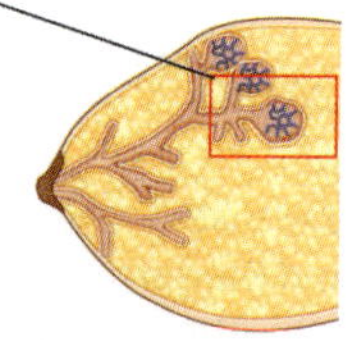

• Originates from terminal duct lobular unit

• Multifocal, multicentric and also bilateral in more than 50% of patients

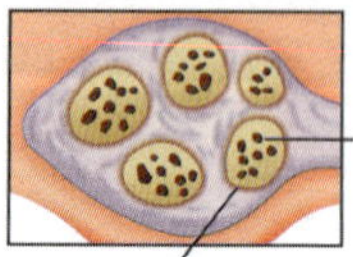

• Neoplastic cells fill up the acini but preserving the cross-sectional architecture of the lobular unit

• Basement membrane intact

Only develops in female breast

It must be remembered that most tumors arise from terminal duct-lobular unit

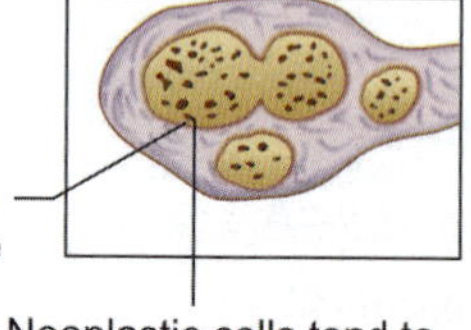

• Basement membrane intact

• Neoplastic cells tend to fill, distort, and unfold involved lobules—thus appears to involve duct-like spaces

Multicentricity: Presence of a second breast cancer in other quadrant of the same breast or atleast 4 cm away.

Multifocality: Presence of a second breast cancer in the same quadrant or within 4 cm of the primary tumor.

Lobular carcinoma *in situ* is not included as a type of ***in situ*** carcinoma in recent NCCN guideline.

Invasive Cancer

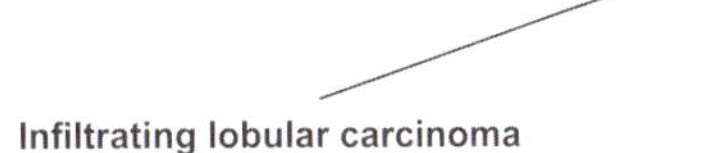

Infiltrating lobular carcinoma

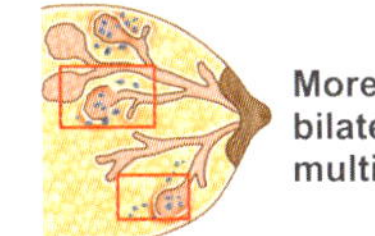

More frequently bilateral and multicentric

- Most of the lobular carcinomas express hormone receptors (ER, PR), but HER 2-neu overexpression is rare

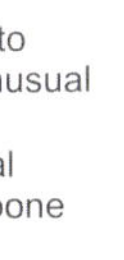

- Invasive lobular carcinomas tend to metastasize to unusual sites (e.g., CSF, meninges, serosal surfaces, ovary, bone marrow)

Stromal invasion by tumor cells (Indian file arrangements)

Less coherent tumor cells make tumor clinically occult and less detectable on mammography

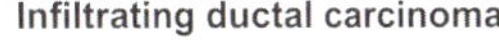

Infiltrating ductal carcinoma

Different types

1) Infiltrating ductal carcinoma—Not Otherwise Specified (NOS)
2) Medullary carcinoma
3) Tubular carcinoma
4) Papillary carcinoma
5) Mucinous carcinoma
6) Invasive cribriform carcinoma

Infiltrating Ductal CA-NOS

Most common histologic pattern (about 70–80%)

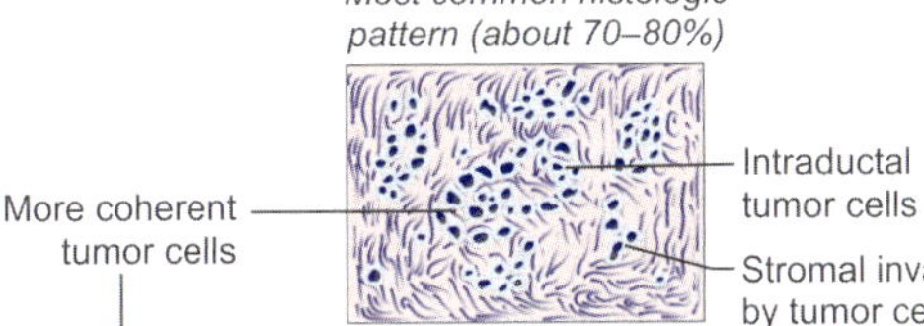

- Usually assoicated with DCIS
- Significant desmoplastic response is present, so this histologic type usually presents as hard mass and gritty when transected
- Most of these type of tumors express ER/PR or both, few of these tumors (about 25%) overexpress HER2-neu

Invasive ductal carcinoma of no special type (NST) is the most common type of invasive breast cancer. This type has worse prognosis than other special-type of invasive cancers (e.g., medullary carcinoma, mucinous carcinoma, papillary carcinoma, etc.).

Histologic Grading

Histologic grading is determined for all invasive breast carcinomas by totaling the values of all three morphologic features **(tubule formation, nuclear polymorphism and calibrated mitotic count)**. This is the Nottingham modification of the SBR (Scarff-Bloom-Richardson) grading system.

Value of each morphologic feature ranges from **1 (favorable), 2 (moderately favorable) and 3 (unfavorable)**.

For ductal carcinoma in situ, only nuclear grading is determined.

Nottingham Modification (Elston-Ellis modification) of the SBR (Scarff-Bloom-Richardson) Grading System

- **GX:** Grade cannot be assessed
- **G1:** Low combined histologic grade (favorable); SBR score of 3–5 points
- **G2:** Intermediate combined histologic grade (moderately favorable); SBR score of 6–7 points
- **G3:** High combined histologic grade (unfavorable); SBR score of 8–9 points

Nuclear Grading of Ductal Carcinoma in Situ

- **GX:** Grading cannot be assessed
- **G1:** Low nuclear grade
- **G2:** Intermediated nuclear grade
- **G3:** High nuclear grade

Spread of Breast Carcinoma

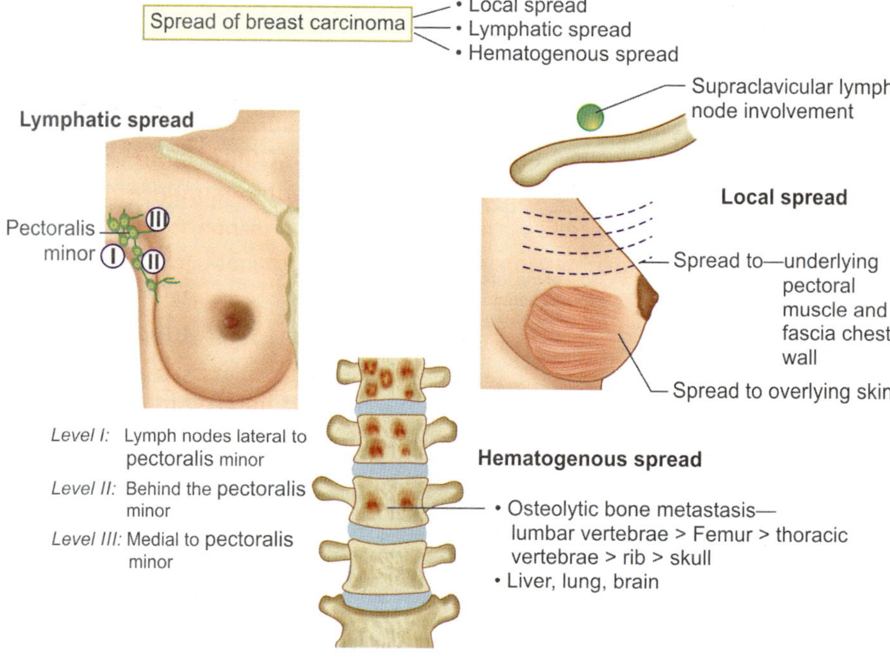

Clinical Presentation

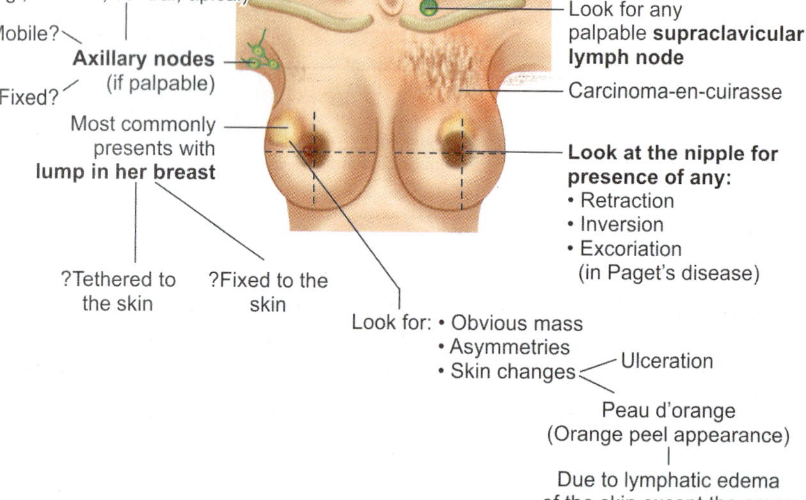

History: Age at menarche and menopause, history of breastfeeding, drug history (OCP, HRT), family history of carcinoma breast (age at diagnosis and whether bilateral or not) and ovary, diagnosis of atypical hyperplasia or lobular carcinoma in situ are important.

Clinical Presentations due to Distant Metastasis

- Cough, respiratory distress—**in lung metastasis**
- Localized bone pain and tenderness, pathological fracture—**in bone metastasis**
- Drowsiness, convulsion—**in brain metastasis**

Unilateral circumferential nipple retraction within a short period—**suggestive of breast carcinoma.**

Bilateral slit retraction for a long period—**suggestive of periductal mastitis.**

Peau d'orange (French for 'orange peel) appearance is due to subcutaneous edema with associated tethering and retraction of the hair follicles and sweat glands.

Tethering: Dimpling of the skin of overlying skin during movement of the lump from side to side. Tethering is due to infiltration of the Cooper's (Astley) ligaments by the tumor make them short and inelastic.

Diagnostic Work-up

Diagnostic workup includes: (i) Clinical examination; (ii) Imaging; and (iii) Biopsy. Imaging should always be performed before biopsy because biopsy-related tissue changes may alter the image interpretation. Imaging evaluation is indicated to characterize the palpable lesion and to establish the concordance between the imaging findings and the clinical findings. Any suspicious mass detected by clinical examination or by imaging or both should undergo biopsy.

Diagnostic mammography is recommended for **women of 40 years or more with palpable breast lesion**. Digital breast tomosynthesis (DBT) is also a useful imaging modality in these group of patients. Ultrasound is indicated if mammography is negative or equivocal.

US or diagnostic mammography or DBT may be used as imaging modality for **women of 30–39 years with palpable breast lesion**.

Ultrasound is recommended for **women of less than 30 years with palpable breast lesion**. Diagnostic mammography or DBT is warranted if any suspicious findings in US.

Biopsy techniques includes: (i) Fine-needle aspiration biopsy (FNAB); (ii) Core-needle biopsy; and (iii) Excision biopsy. In palpable lesion, biopsy can be performed by palpation or image-guided. Advantages of image-guided biopsy are better accuracy and ability to place biopsy marker clip.

	FNA	Core-cut biopsy	Excision biopsy
Nature of procedure	Few cells are retrieved from the lesion—only cytology	Multiple cores of tissues obtained from the lesion—histological assessment	Excision of entire lesion—histological assessment
Instruments used	22G needle with syringe	Core-cut biopsy gun	Operative setup
Performed by	Pathologist	Pathologist or Surgeon	Surgeon
Invasiveness	Minimal	More invasive than FNA	More invasive than FNA and core-cut biopsy
Interpretation	Needs an experienced cytopathologist	Can be done by any pathologist	By any Pathologist
ER, PR, HER2 neu study	Not possible	Can be done	Can be done
Differentiating invasive from carcinoma in situ	Cannot be done	Differentiation can be done	Differentiation can be done

Fine Needle Aspiration Cytology (FNAC)

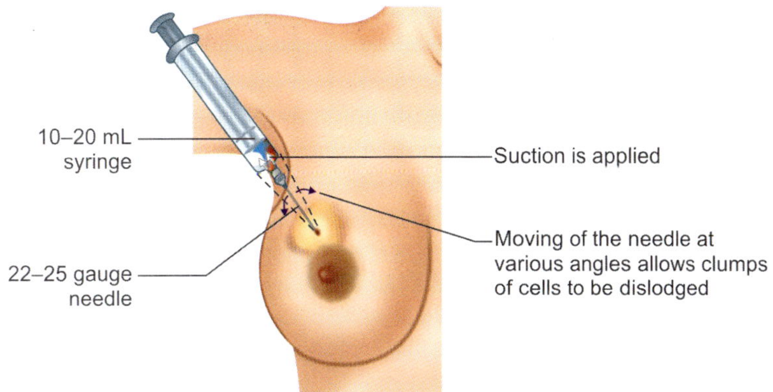

Core-needle Biopsy

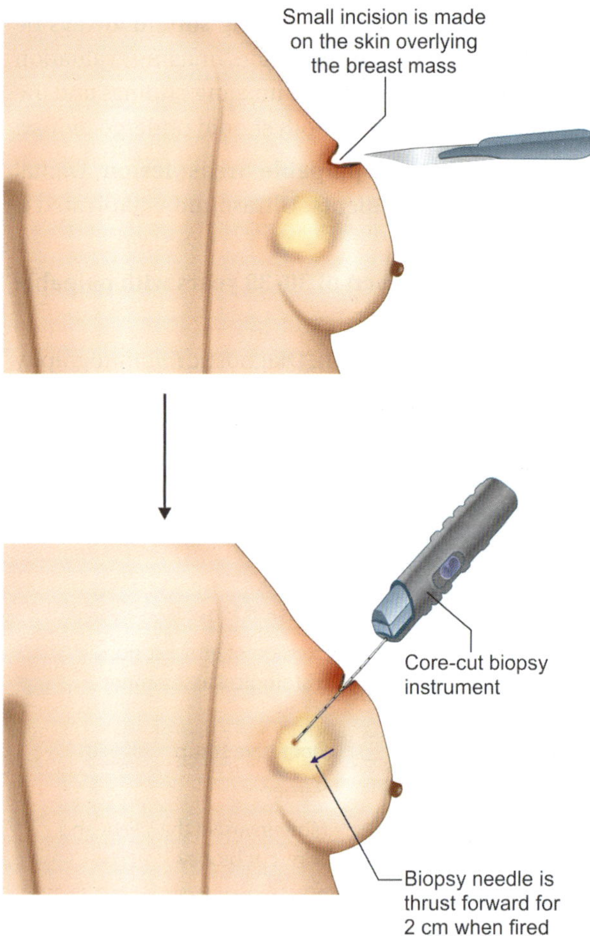

Excision Biopsy

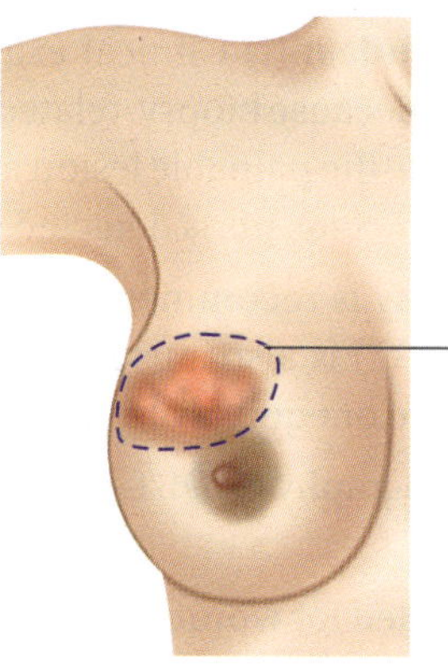

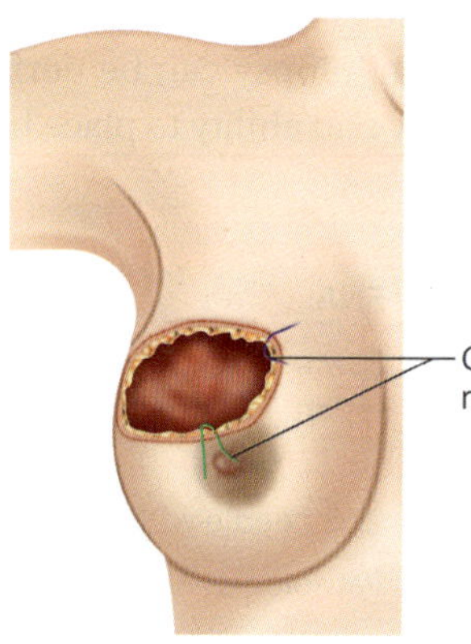

Indications for Excisional Breast Biopsy [as per ASBrS guidelines]

- Atypical ductal or lobular hyperplasia, LCIS on core biopsy
- Papillary and/or sclerosing lesion on core biopsy
- "Fibroepithelial lesion" on core biopsy
- Imaging findings and core biopsy histology are not corroborating.
- Insufficient tissue material from core biopsy.

Image-guided Localization for Nonpalpable Breast Lesions

- **Wire-guided localization (WGL):** Most widely adopted approach for localizing non-palpable breast lesions for surgical excision. A 3–5 cm wire, usually with a terminal hook or pigtail, is inserted to localize the lesion to be excised, under stereotactic or USG guidance or MRI guidance. *Complications:* (i) Wire transection; (ii) Wire migration; (iii) Pneumothorax; and (iv) Injury associated with barbs.
- **Radio-guided occult lesion localization (ROLL):** This technique utilizes a non-specific radioisotope technetium-99m (^{99m}Tc) labeled human serum albumin injected intratumorally under stereotactic or US guidance preoperatively. Intraoperatively, the lesion is detected by handheld gamma probe.
- **Sentinel node and occult lesion localization (SNOLL):** This is a technique of radio-guided occult lesion localization along with localization of sentinel node. The technique of occult lesion localization is similar to ROLL technique. For localization of sentinel node, another radiotracer is injected near to the tumor, and sentinel node is identified by gamma probe and biopsied in same surgical session.

- **Radioactive seed localization (RSL):** In this technique, radioactive seeds (^{125}I) are placed inside the tumor under USG, mammography/tomosynthesis, or MRI guidance. On the day of surgery, the seeds are localized by gamma probe and excised along with breast tissue. The seeds can be implanted upto 5 days before surgery.
- **Magnetic seed localization:** This localization method uses paramagnetic steel and iron oxide seeds placement inside the lesion under mammography/tomosynthesis or USG. During surgery, surgeon localize the seed using dedicated magnetic probe.
- **Other localization methods:** (i) ROLL technique in combination with methylene dye (RCML); (ii) Intraoperative ultrasound-guided lumpectomy (IOUS); and (iii) Cryoprobe-assisted localization (CAL).

Wire-guided Localization

1. In Radiology Suite

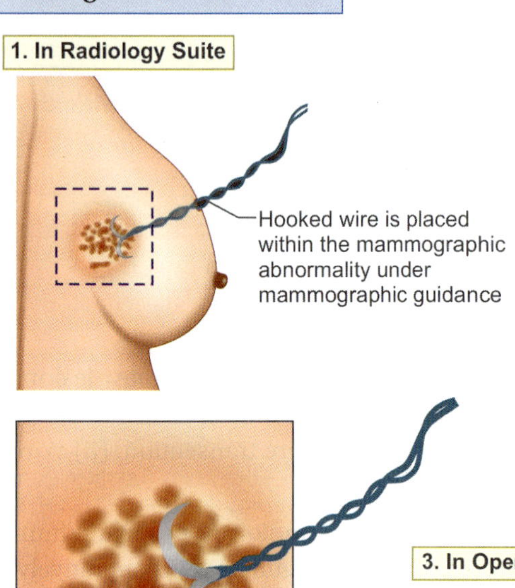

2. Transportation

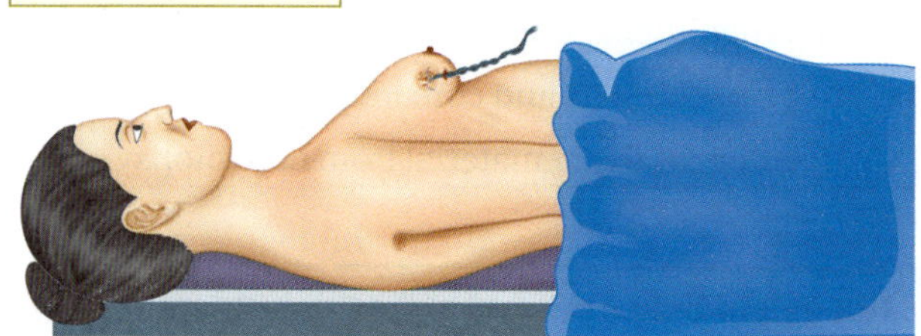

Careful transportation to the operating room-wire must be secured on the surface of the breast

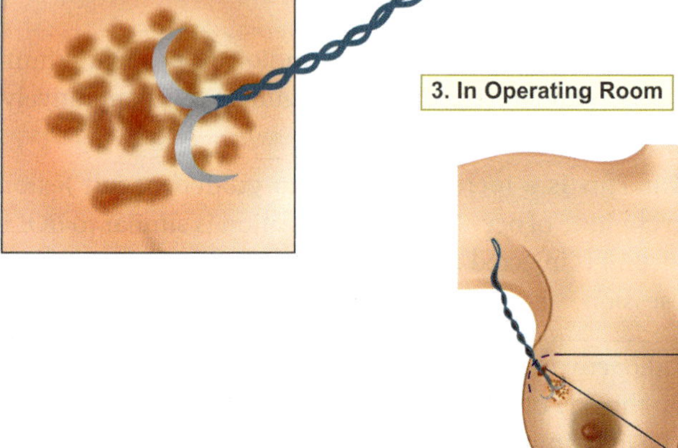

3. In Operating Room

Wire and tissue around microcalcifications are removed en bloc by sharp dissection. During dissection, electrocautery should be avoided

4. In radiology suite

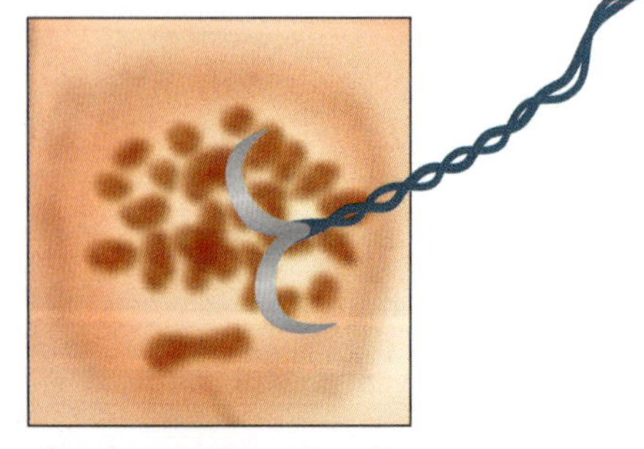

Specimen radiography with wire intact is done to confirm full excision of the mammographic abnormality

Biopsy Techniques for Nonpalpable Breast Lesions

- **US-guided biopsy:** This biopsy technique is particularly useful for US-detected lesions. If the lesion is detected in both US and mammography, US-guided biopsy is preferred because it is: (i) technically easier; (ii) absence of ionizing radiation; and (iii) real-time visualization of the biopsy needle within the lesion.
- **Stereotactic biopsy:** This biopsy technique is indicated for mammographically detected lesions.
- **Vacuum-assisted biopsy:** This technique uses vacuum-assisted instrument (e.g., Mammotome) for tissue retrieval under US or stereotactic guidance.

Stereotactic Breast Biopsy

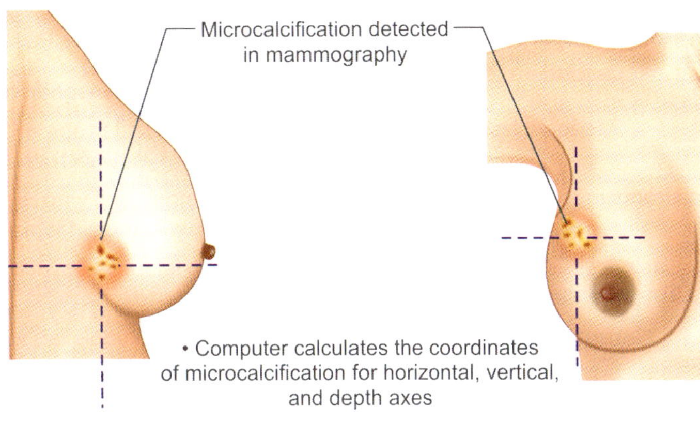

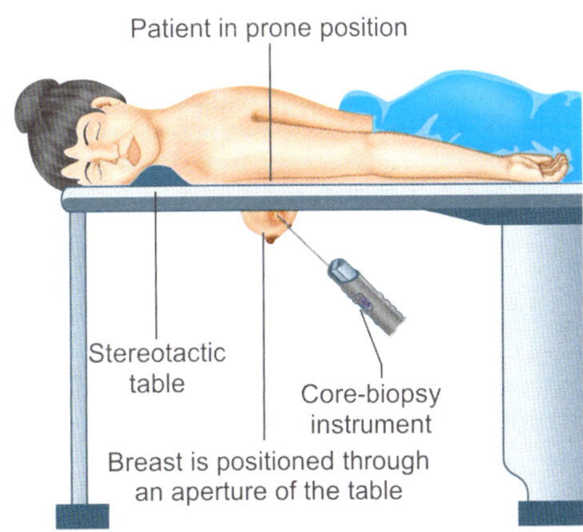

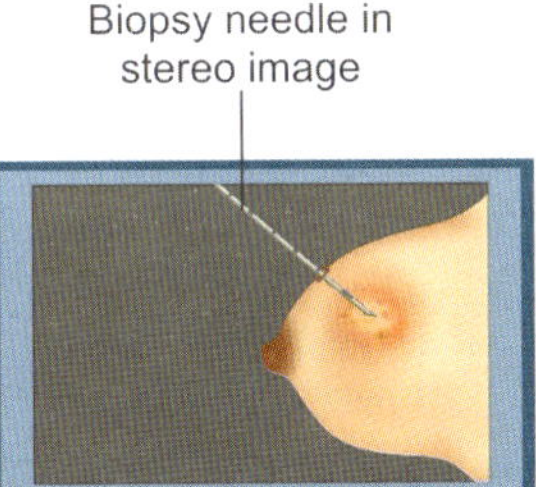

Stereo images are seen to ensure correct position of the needle tip

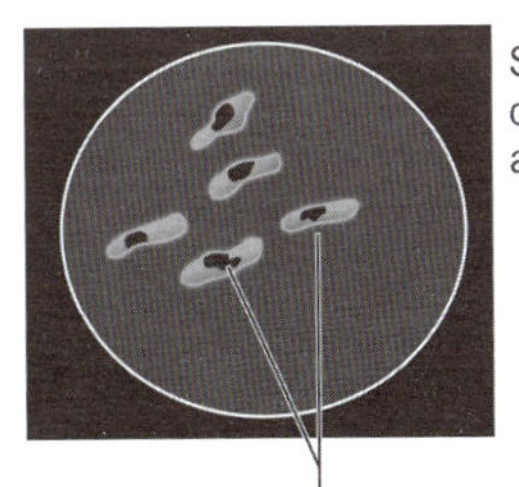

Specimen radiography of multiple tissue samples are performed

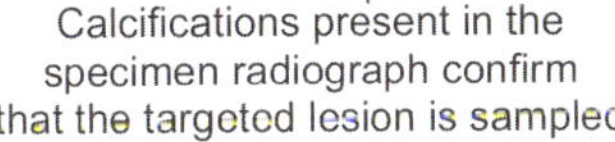

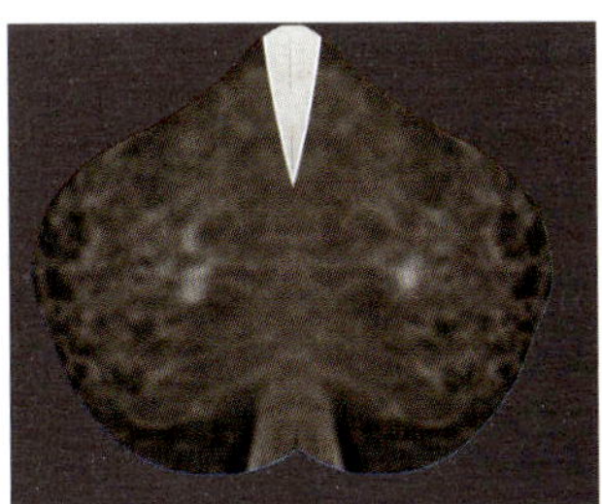

Postbiopsy mammogram is done to confirm that a defect is created within the target lesion and marking clip is in position

Mammography

Mammography is used for both **screening** and **diagnostic** purposes. Mammography remains the most important imaging modality for detecting breast cancer. Mammogram allows assessment of contralateral breast and multifocal lesion. Mammography delivers a radiation dose of 0.1 centigray (cGy).

Components of Breast Cancer Screening

- Complete medical history
- Breast awareness
- Clinical breast examination
- Breast cancer risk assessment
- *Imaging:* Mammography; US and MRI (in specific indications)

Screening Mammography

Screening mammography is performed in asymptomatic women with the goal of detecting breast cancer which is not yet clinically evident. Clinically not detected but mammographically detected cancers have a better prognosis and require less aggressive treatment.

Screening Protocol (as per NCCN Guideline)

Women with average risk: Annual screening mammography beginning at age 40. No upper age limit for screening.

Women at increased risk:

- **Women with prior history of breast cancer:** Mammography every 12 months to begin 6–12 months after completion of radiation therapy. Routine imaging of reconstructed breast is not indicated.
- **Women of ≥35 years of age with 5-year risk of invasive breast cancer ≥1.7% (as per Gail model):** Mammography every 12 months to begin at the age identified as being at increased risk.
- **Lifetime risk >20% based on history of LCIS/ADH/ALH:** Mammography every 12 months beginning at age of diagnosis but not less than 30 years of age and annual MRI beginning at age of diagnosis but not less than 25 years of age.
- **Life-time risk >20% as defined by models that are mostly dependent on family history:** Annual mammography and annual MRI starting 10 years prior to the youngest family member diagnosed.
- **Women between ages 10 and 30 with prior thoracic irradiation:** Annual mammogram and annual MRI to begin 8–10 years after radiation exposure in women aged 25 years and older.
- **Advantages:** (i) Early detection of cancer; (ii) Reduction in breast cancer mortality; and (iii) Required less aggressive treatment.
- **Disadvantages:** (i) Cost and (ii) Overdiagnosis.
- **Views of screening mammography:** (i) Craniocaudal (CC) view and (ii) Mediolateral oblique (MLO) view.
- **Types of mammography:** (i) Film-screen mammography and (ii) Digital mammography. Advantages of digital mammography: (i) Images can be stored digitally and (ii) Images can be enhanced, that facilitates better interpretation.

Increased Risk Category Patients (for the Purpose of Breast Cancer Screening)[adapted from NCCN guideline]

- Women with prior history of breast carcinoma
- Women of ≥35 years of age with 5-year risk of invasive breast cancer ≥1.7% (as per Gail model)
- Lifetime risk >20% based on history of LCIS/ADH/ALH
- Lifetime risk >20% as defined by models that are mostly dependent on family history.
- Women between ages 10 and 30 with prior thoracic irradiation
- Women with a pedigree suggestive of or known genetic predisposition.

Indications of Annual MRI Screening of Breast (as an Adjunct to Mammography)

- First-degree relative of breast cancer genetic mutation carrier, but untested.
- Lifetime risk 20% or greater primarily based on mathematical models that are mostly based on family history (e.g., Claus model, BRCAPRO, BOADICEA, Tyrer-Cuzick model)
- History of chest irradiation between the ages of 10–30
- Women with other germline mutations known to predispose to a high risk of breast cancer: Li-Fraumeni syndrome, Cowden's disease; ATM; CDH1; PALB2; CHEK2; STK11; NF1.
- Women with LCIS or ALH/ADH with a lifetime risk of ≥20%.

Position of the Breast in CC View

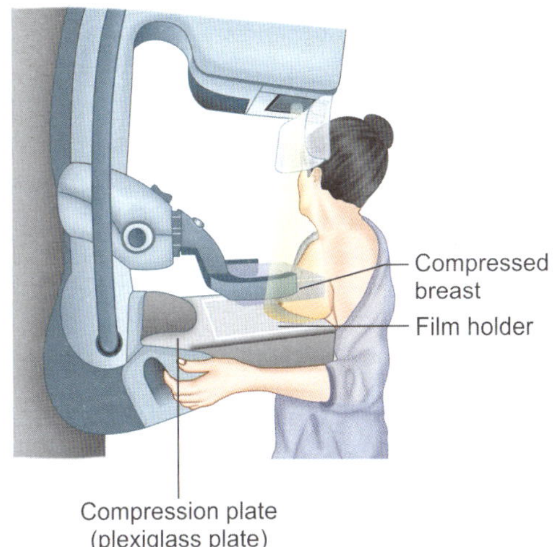

Compression device – Minimizes motion artifact
– Improves definition
– Separates overlying tissues
– Decreases radiation dose
– Reduces geometric unsharpness

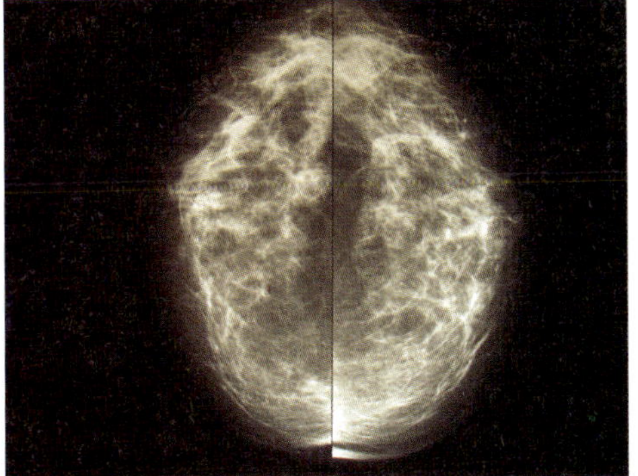

Position of the Breast in MLO

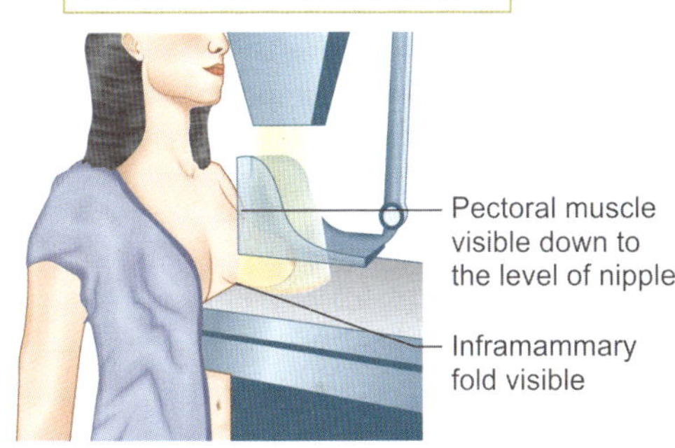

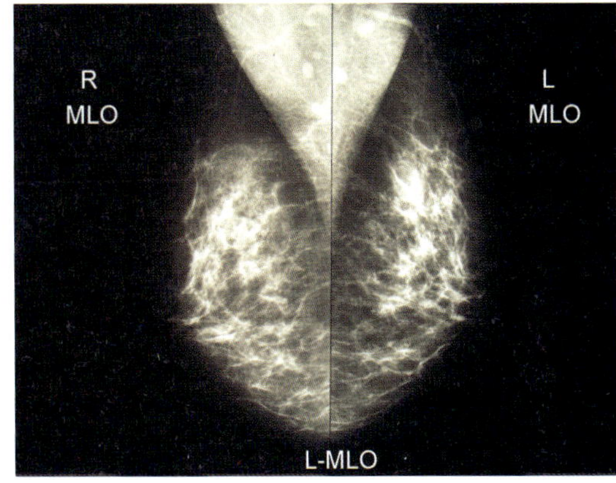

- **In craniocaudal view,** medial aspect of the breast is better visualized.
- **In mediolateral oblique view,** upper outer quadrant and axillary tail of Spence is visualized.

Indications of Diagnostic Mammography

(i) For evaluation in patients with breast mass or nipple discharge in women of 40 years or more; (ii) Diagnostic imaging after screening mammography recall; and (iii) In diagnosed breast carcinoma patient, for assessment of nonpalpable lesion in ipsilateral and contralateral breast.

Standard mammographic views: (i) Craniocaudal and (ii) Mediolateral oblique.

Additional mammographic views: (i) Spot compression view; (ii) 90° lateral view; (iii) Craniocaudal exaggerated; (iv) Cleavage view; and (v) Step-oblique view.

Indications of Diagnostic MRI of Breast

- In Paget's disease of the nipple, to search for occult breast cancer when conventional imaging findings are inconclusive.
- In patients with axillary node metastasis, to search for occult breast cancer when conventional imaging (e.g., mammography or USG) fail to detect primary lesion.
- To assess response to neoadjuvant endocrine therapy or chemotherapy.
- For evaluation of suspected implant rupture, particularly silicone implants.

Concordance between BI-RADS Assessment Categories and Management Recommendations

Assessment	Management	Likelihood of cancer
Category 0: Incomplete-need additional imaging evaluation and/or prior mammograms for comparison	Recall for additional imaging and/or comparison with prior examination(s)	N/A
Category 1: Negative	Routine mammography screening	Essentially 0% likelihood of malignancy
Category 2: Benign	Routine mammography screening	Essentially 0% likelihood of malignancy
Category 3: Probably benign	Short interval (6-month) follow-up or continued surveillance mammography	>0% but ≤2% likelihood of malignancy
Category 4: Suspicious *Category 4A:* Low suspicion for malignancy *Category 4B:* Moderate suspicion for malignancy *Category 4C:* High suspicion for malignancy	Tissue diagnosis	>2% but <95% likelihood of malignancy >2% to ≤10% likelihood of malignancy >10% to ≤50% likelihood of malignancy >50% to <95% likelihood of malignancy
Category 5: Highly suggestive of malignancy	Tissue diagnosis	≥95% likelihood of malignancy
Category 6: Known biopsy-proven malignancy	Surgical excision when clinically appropriate	N/A

The ACR BI-RADS (Breast Imaging-Reporting and Data System)

These assessment categories are developed by American College of Radiology (ACR) to standardize the reporting of mammography, US and MRI findings and the recommendations for further management.

BI-RADS Breast Density Category

a. The breasts are almost entirely fatty.
b. There are scattered areas of fibroglandular density.
c. The breasts are heterogeneously dense, which may obscure small masses
d. The breasts are extremely dense, which lowers the sensitivity of mammography.

Determination of ER, PR and HER2 Status

- Determination of ER, PR and HER2 status is recommended for all newly diagnosed invasive breast cancers.
- Determination of ER status is recommended for all ductal carcinoma in situ (DCIS).

Additional Work-up Prior to Neoadjuvant Systemic Therapy

- Core biopsy of the tumor with placement of image-detectable markers
- USG of axilla and biopsy of clinically detected or image-detected axillary lymph nodes
- Pregnancy test in all patients with child-bearing potential
- Counseling for fertility-related complications due to systemic therapy

Metastatic Work-up

Early Breast Cancer

- Routine metastatic work-up is not indicated in early breast cancer without symptoms.
- Chest CT with contrast is indicated if pulmonary symptoms (e.g., cough, hemoptysis) are present.
- *Abdominal and pelvic CT with contrast or MRI with contrast:* If abdominal symptoms, clinical findings in abdomen or pelvis suggestive of metastasis, abnormal liver function tests, elevated alkaline phosphatase.
- *Bone scan:* If localized bone pain or elevated alkaline phosphatase.

Locally Advanced Breast Cancer

- Chest CT with contrast
- Abdominal and pelvic CT with contrast or MRI with contrast
- FDG PET/CT
- Bone scan is not indicated if FDG-PET/CT shows bone metastasis.

Molecular Subtypes of Breast Cancer

Luminal A

- ER positive, PR positive, HER2neu negative, low Ki-67 level
- Low grade
- Most common subtype
- Best prognosis
- Less sensitive to cytotoxic chemotherapy

Luminal B

- ER positive, PR positive, HER2neu negative, high Ki-67 level
- Less expression of ER, PR than luminal A type, about 30% are HER2neu positive
- Intermediate-to-high grade
- Prognosis poorer than luminal A
- Less sensitive to cytotoxic chemotherapy.

Ki-67 is a proliferation index; Ki-67>15–20% indicates high proliferation rates, is associated with more aggressive behavior.

HER2-enriched

- ER negative, PR negative, HER2neu positive
- 30–40% tumors express ER, PR
- Mid-to-high grade
- Responsive to trastuzumab therapy

Claudin-low

- ER-negative, PR-negative, HER2-neu negative
- Low expression of Claudin 3, 4, 7, E-cadherin (cell-cell adhesion genes)
- Overexpression of genes associated with epithelial to mesenchymal transition (EMT).

Basal-like

- ER negative, PR negative, HER2neu negative (triple negative)
- Overexpression of oncogenes (e.g., c-kit, c-myc, EGFR)
- Associated with high incidence of p53 mutation
- More common in BRCA1 mutation carriers
- Worst prognosis

Staging

TNM Staging System for Breast Cancer (AJCC, 8th edition)

T category is based on the largest dimension of the invasive component of the tumor. The size of the tumor is measured based on the physical examination and imaging (mammography, US and MRI).

Tis only includes DCIS (Ductal carcinoma *in situ*). LCIS (Lobular carcinoma *in situ*) is removed from TNM staging and categorized as a benign pathology.

Clinical N category (cN) is based on metastases of regional lymph nodes (ipsilateral axillary, internal mammary, infraclavicular, and supraclavicular lymph nodes), involvement of level of axillary lymph nodes (level I, II or III) and whether they are fixed/matted or movable.

Pathologic N category (pN) is based on number of axillary lymph nodes involved by metastases and the size of metastases.

M category is based on clinical or radiological evidence of distant metastases. Any M0 is clinical, pM0 is invalid terminology.

"yc" prefix is used for clinical staging and **"yp" prefix** is for pathologic staging after neoadjuvant therapy for T and N classification.

The anatomic stage group table includes T, N, and M categories and categorizes into following stages: 0, IA, IB, IIA, IIB, IIIA, IIIB, IIIC, IV.

Clinical prognostic stage is applicable to all patients with breast cancer and includes Clinical tumor (T), Node (N), Metastases (M), Histologic grade and biomarkers (ER, PR, HER2) information.

Pathological prognostic stage is applicable only to the patients treated with surgery as the initial treatment. This stage includes T, N, M, histological grade, biomarkers, findings from surgery and pathological findings from resected tissue.

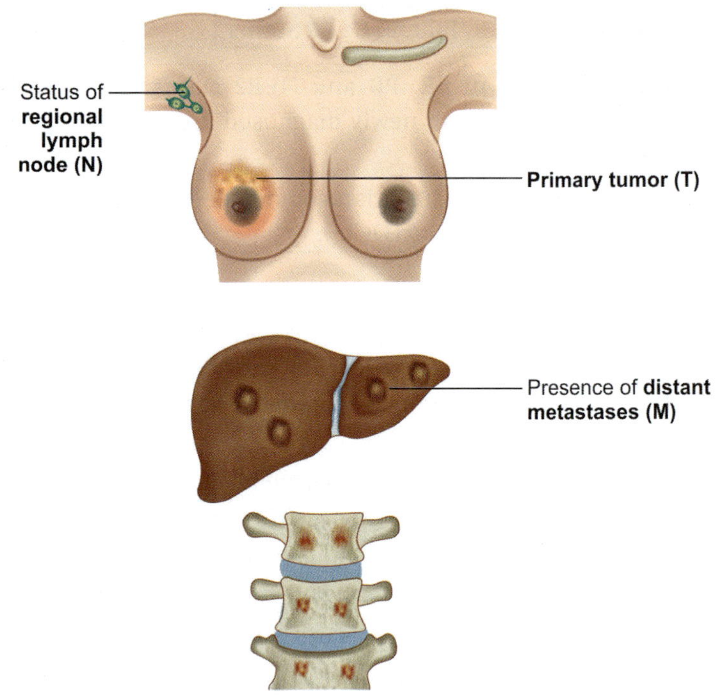

Anatomic Stage Group Table			
Stage 0	Tis	N0	M0
Stage IA	T1	N0	M0
Stage IB	T0	N1mi	M0
	T1	N1mi	M0
Stage IIA	T0	N1	M0
	T1	N1	M0
	T2	N0	M0
Stage IIB	T2	N1	M0
	T3	N0	M0
Stage IIIA	T0	N2	M0
	T1	N2	M0
	T2	N2	M0
	T3	N1	M0
	T3	N2	M0
Stage IIIB	T4	N0	M0
	T4	N1	M0
	T4	N2	M0
Stage IIIC	Any T	N3	M0
Stage IV	Any T	Any N	M0

Classic prognostic factors of breast carcinoma:

(i) Age of the patient; (ii) TNM stage; (iii) Number of positive axillary lymph nodes; (iv) Tumor grade; (v) Mitotic rate; and (vi) ER/PR status.

Treatment of Ductal Carcinoma in Situ (Tis, N0, M0)

Primary Treatment of DCIS

Options are:

1. Lumpectomy (with atleast 2 mm margin) plus whole breast radiation therapy with or without RT boost
2. Total mastectomy with or without sentinel lymph node biopsy
3. Lumpectomy only (least preferred option).

Atleast 2 mm margin, whole breast radiation therapy (WBRT) and RT boost decrease the risk of *in-breast tumor recurrence (IBTR)*.

To confirm complete resection, analysis of specimen margins, specimen radiography and post-excision mammography should be performed.

Management of DCIS after Primary Treatment (To Reduce the Risk of Ipsilateral Breast Cancer Recurrence)

Premenopausal and postmenopausal women with ER-positive DCIS treated with lumpectomy followed by WBRT—**Endocrine therapy with tamoxifen for 5 years**.

Postmenopausal women: Aromatase inhibitor therapy may be considered.

Follow-up: Physical examination every 6–12 months for 5 years and then annually and yearly diagnostic mammography.

In-breast Tumor Recurrence (IBTR)

IBTR may occur following BCT. It may develop either as true recurrence or as a second primary.

Risk factors: (i) Young age; (ii) Tumor with higher grade; (iii) Lymphovascular invasion; and (iv) Neo-adjuvant radiotherapy.

Treatment is re-excision or mastectomy.

Treatment of Invasive Breast Cancer

Treatment of Early-stage Breast Cancer [stage I, II and operable stage III (T3N1)]

Surgery (lumpectomy or mastectomy) with or without radiation therapy followed by adjuvant systemic therapy (chemotherapy, endocrine therapy, HER2-targeted therapy) based on tumor size, grade, lymph node involvement, ER/PR and HER2 status. Lumpectomy is alternatively called breast conserving therapy (BCT), partial mastectomy, wide local excision, tylectomy. Lumpectomy is excision of the tumor along with an envelope of normal-appearing breast tissue to achieve a cancer-free margin ("no ink on a tumor").

In patients with clinically palpable axillary nodes, NCCN panel recommends pathologic confirmation of malignancy using USG-guided FNAC or core biopsy of suspicious nodes. **For biopsy proven axillary metastases, axillary dissection of level I & II** is indicated. **Level I & II axillary dissection requires atleast 10 lymph nodes** be provided for accurate staging of axilla. Axillary dissection should be extended to level III if level I & II are grossly involved.

In patients with clinically negative nodes or if FNA/core biopsy result is negative, NCCN panel recommends **sentinel lymph node biopsy**.

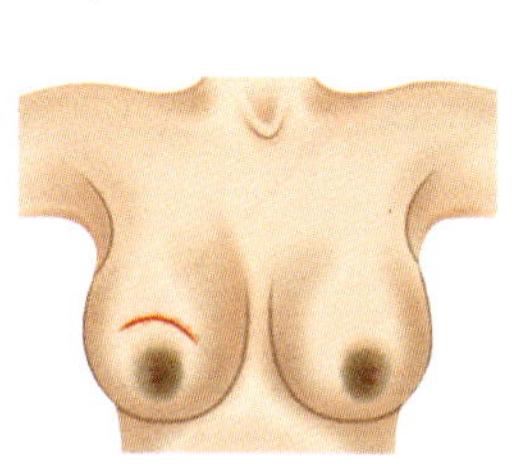

After BCT

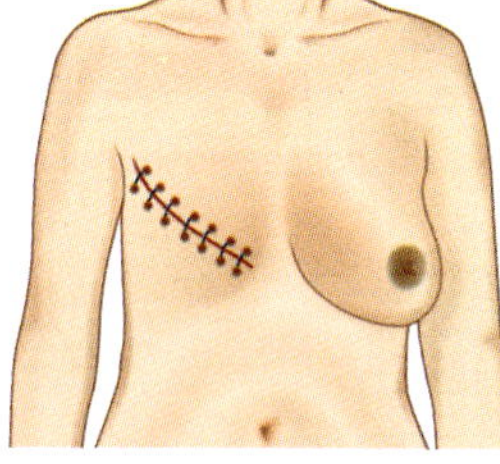

After mastectomy

Advantages of Breast Conserving Therapy (lumpectomy)

- Preservation of cosmesis
- Less anxiety and depression
- Improved body image, sexuality, self-esteem than mastectomy.
- Survival and recurrence almost similar to mastectomy.

Complications of BCS

- Hematoma
- Incomplete excision
- Infection
- Poor cosmetic outcome
- In-breast tumor recurrence

Absolute contraindications for BCS	Relative contraindications for BCS
Early pregnancy	Collagen-vascular disease
Multicentric tumor involving two or more quadrants of the breast	Large tumor size relative to breast volume
Diffuse suspicious or malignant-appearing microcalcifications	Prior radiation to the chest wall or breast
Diffusely positive pathologic margins	Known or suspected genetic predisposition to breast cancer
Inflammatory breast cancer	

Indications for Mastectomy

- Inflammatory breast cancer
- Multicentric tumor
- Extensive malignant/indeterminate microcalcifications
- Inadequate response to neoadjuvant chemotherapy or endocrine therapy
- Local recurrence following BCS
- Proven or suspected genetic susceptibility
- Early pregnancy
- Large tumor size relative to breast volume
- Collagen-vascular disease
- Patient's choice.

Types of Mastectomy

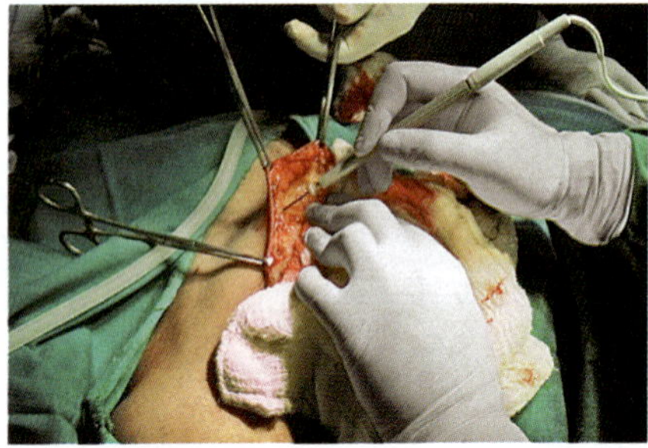
Creation of superior skin flap.

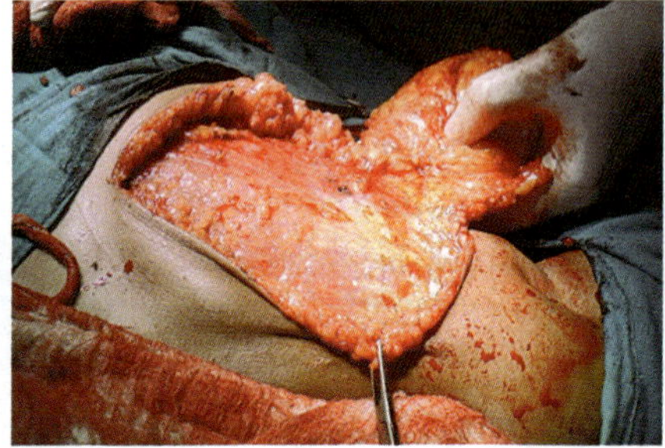
Whole breast tissue is dissected from the pectoralis muscle.

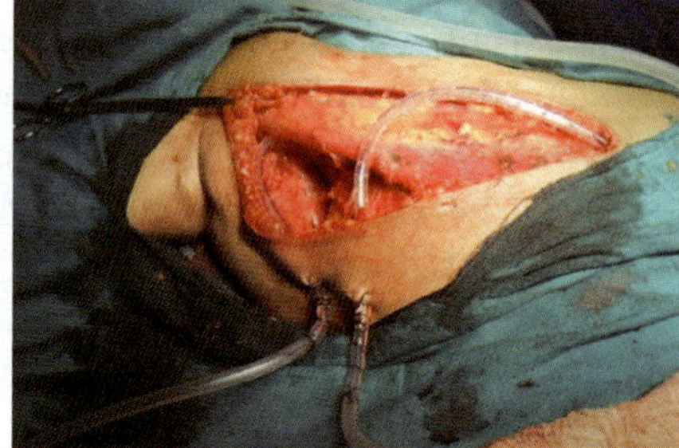
One drain is placed over the pectoralis muscle; another drain is placed in the axilla.

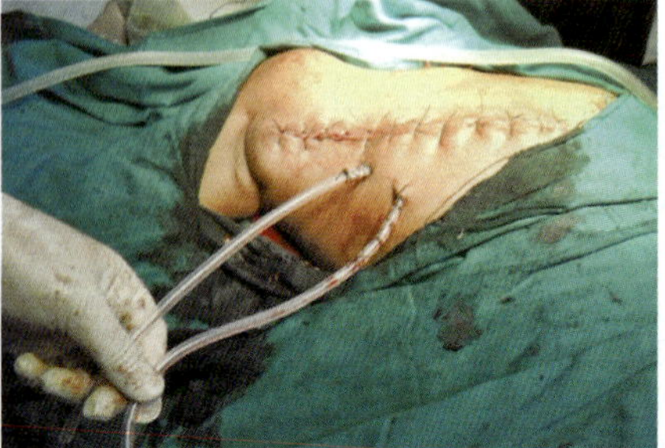
Skin is closed with nonabsorbable monofilament suture.

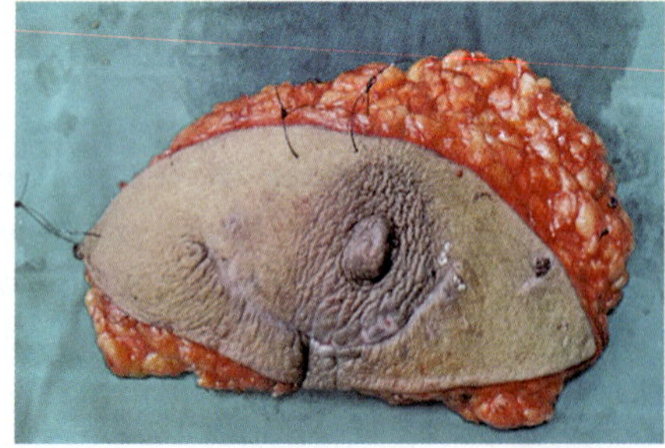
Operated specimen of simple mastectomy (note the previous operative scar mark). Sides are marked by sutures.

Radical mastectomy Based on the idea that breast cancer spread first by locally or "centrifugally".	• Involves removal of all breast tissue, overlying skin, both pectoralis major and minor, with complete en bloc removal of axillary lymph nodes. • **Complications:** (i) Large wound; (ii) Severely restricted movement; (iii) Chronic pain; and (iv) Lymphedema
Patey-Dyson mastectomy Patey believed that without removing pectoralis minor, complete clearance of axillary lymph nodes not feasible.	• Involves removal of all breast tissue, overlying skin, pectoralis minor, enbloc removal of axillary lymph nodes. • No difference in survival or local recurrence between standard radical mastectomy and this technique.
Madden-Auchincloss mastectomy	• Involves removal of all breast tissue, overlying skin, removal of axillary lymph nodes (Level I & II) • Apical nodes (Level III) should be removed when evidently invaded.
Simple mastectomy	Involves removal of all breast tissue along with pectoral fascia, overlying skin
Skin-sparing mastectomy	Includes removal of all breast tissue, nipple-areola complex, biopsy scar, overlying skin (if tumor is superficial) with preservation of remaining skin and inframammary fold **Advantages:** (i) Less mastectomy scar; (ii) More natural breast shape (particularly after autologous tissue reconstruction); and (iii) Immediate reconstruction is feasible **Contraindications:** (i) Skin involvement; (ii) Previous irradiation; (iii) Adjuvant radiotherapy; and (iv) Smoking **Complications:** (i) Infection; (ii) Hematoma; and (iii) Skin necrosis
NAC-sparing mastectomy	Includes removal of all breast tissue, biopsy scar with preservation of skin and nipple-areolar complex **Indications:** (i) Risk-reduction procedures; (ii) Ductal carcinoma in situ; and (iii) Early breast carcinoma **Advantages:** (i) Excellent cosmetic outcome and (ii) Preservation of nipple-areolar complex sensitivity **Contraindications:** (i) Preoperative clinical evidence of nipple involvement; (ii) Paget's disease of the nipple; (iii) Palpable tumor less than 1 cm from the nipple; (iv) Nipple discharge associated with malignancy; (v) Imaging features suggestive of malignant involvement of nipple or subareolar tissue; and (vi) Inflammatory breast cancer. **Ideal candidate:** Patient with small-to-moderate breast volume with good nipple position. **Complications:** Necrosis of nipple-areolar complex.

Simple mastectomy with or without reconstruction is the surgical approach for the patients who has contraindications to BCT or who prefer treatment with mastectomy.

Breast Reconstruction

Types of Breast Reconstruction

- Implant-based reconstruction
- Autologous (tissue-based) reconstruction
- Composite reconstruction (using implant in combination with autogenous reconstruction)

Implant-based Reconstruction

- Silicone/saline implants
- Round/anatomic implants
- Textured/smooth implants
- Integrated part/distant part tissue expanders

Free Flap

- Deep inferior epigastric artery perforator (DIEP) flap—**most preferred autologous reconstruction method**
- Free TRAM flap
- Superior gluteal artery perforator (sGAP) flap
- Inferior gluteal artery perforator (iGAP) flap
- Fasciocutaneous infragluteal (FCI) flap
- Profunda femoral artery perforator (PAP) flap
- Transverse myocutaneous gracilis (TMG) flap

Autologous (Tissue-based Reconstruction)

- **Pedicled myocutaneous flap:** (i) Latissimus dorsi myocutaneous flap (supplied by thoracodorsal artery) and (ii) Transverse rectus abdominis myocutaneous (TRAM) flap (supplied by deep inferior epigastric artery)
- Free flap (using microvascular techniques)
- Hybrid flap
- Fat grafting

Hybrid Flap

- Stacked DIEP flap
- Stacked/"Hybrid" GAP flap
- Body lift perforator flap

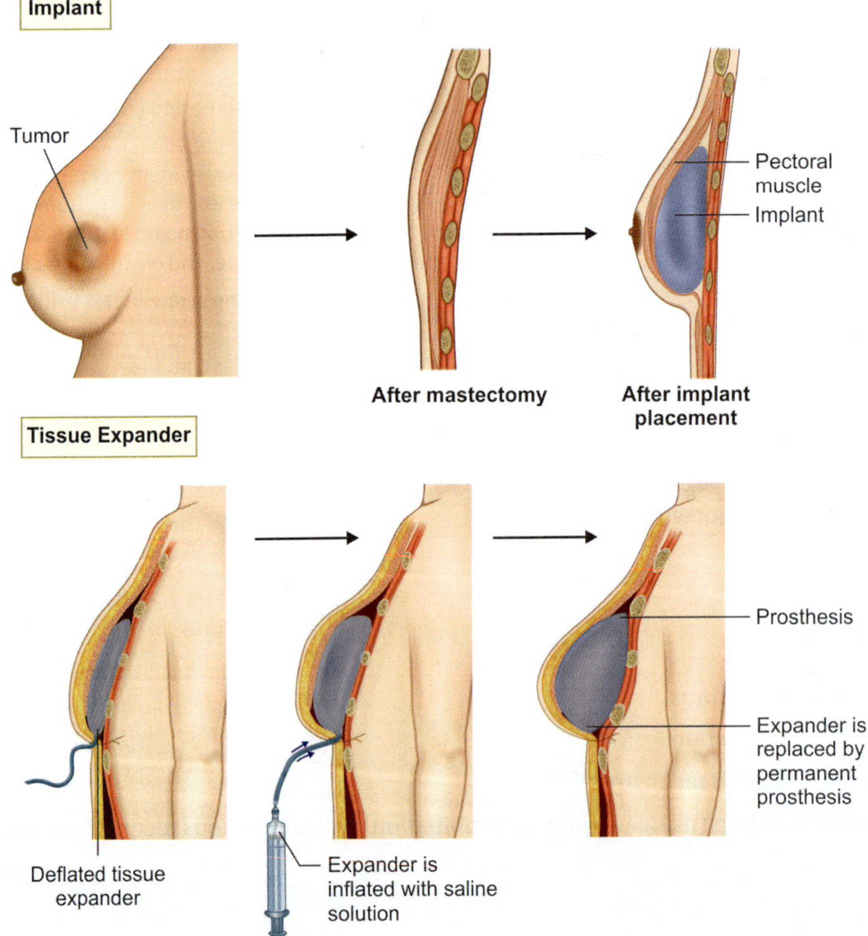

Latissimus Dorsi Flap

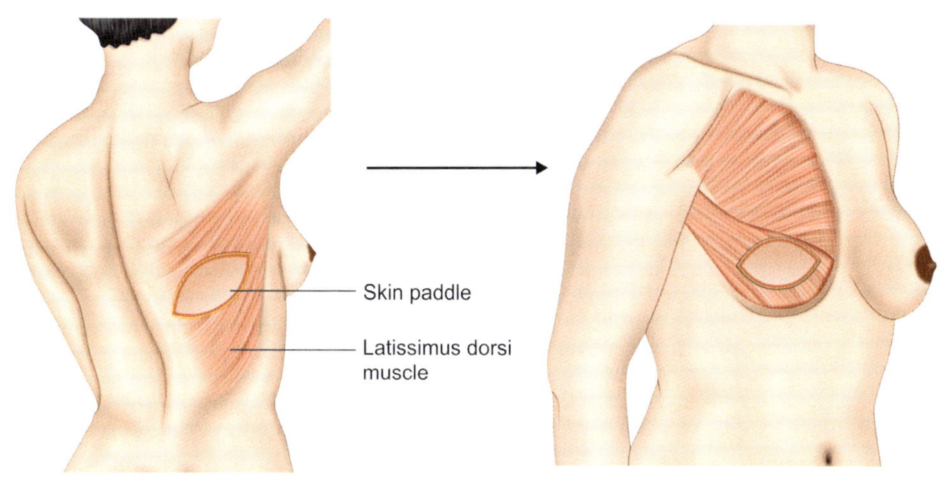

Transverse Rectus Abdominis Myocutaneous Flap

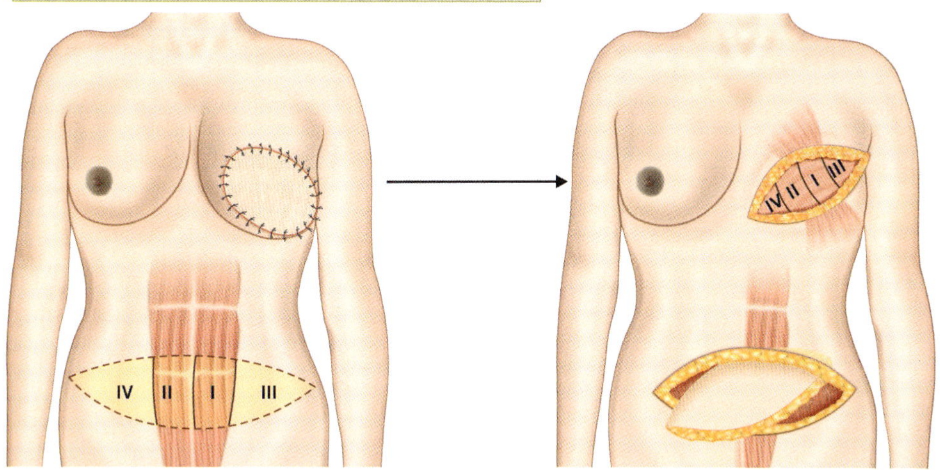

Deep Inferior Epigastric Perforator (DIEP) Flap

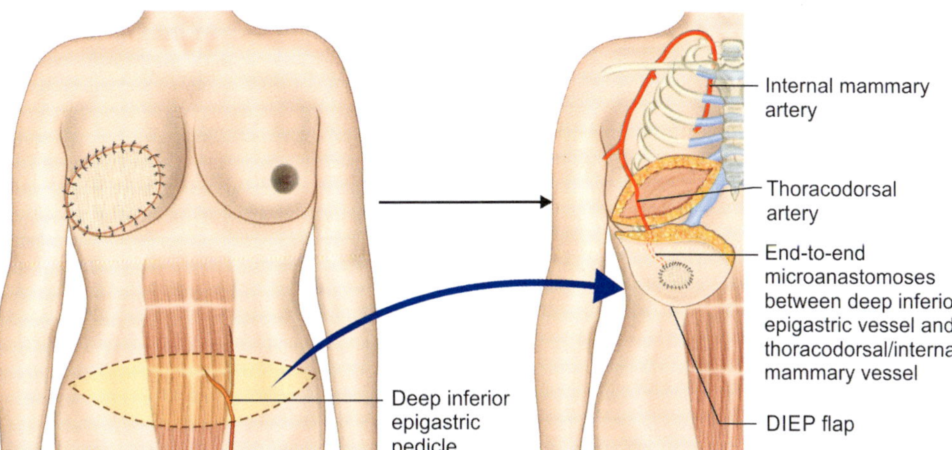

Complications of Reconstruction

Implant-based reconstruction	Tissue-based reconstruction
Capsular contracture	Partial or complete flap failure
Rupture of implant	Flap necrosis
Malposition	Donor-site morbidity (wound dehiscence, weakness, hernia)
Implant rippling or visibility	
Deflation	
Breast implant-associated anaplastic large cell lymphoma (BIA-ALCL)—associated with textured breast implants	
Breast implant illness (BII)	

Advantages of Pedicled Flap

- Lower risk of flap failure
- Technically easier
- Shorter operative time

Disadvantages of Pedicled Flap

- Donor-site morbidity
- Weakness of muscles

Advantages of Free Flap

- No loss of function of muscles
- Larger amount of tissue can be harvested

Disadvantages of Free Flap

- Technically demanding
- Need microvascular surgery facility
- Longer operative time

Important Facts Related to Reconstruction

- Immediate reconstruction is contraindicated after mastectomy for inflammatory breast cancer.
- Patients with chronic smokers are at increased risk of complications (e.g., delayed wound healing, flap necrosis) following autologous tissue reconstruction (due to underlying microvascular disease).
- Patients who received radiation therapy are at increased risk of implant-related complications.
- Autologous tissue reconstruction is the preferred breast reconstruction method for patients received radiation therapy.
- Smoking and obesity are relative contraindication to breast reconstruction.
- Obese patients (WHO class 2 and 3) are at increased risk of total flap failure.
- Revision surgery (e.g., fat grafting, mastopexy, excision/suction-assisted lipectomy, etc.) may be indicated after breast reconstruction.
- Patient with thrombophilia is at increased risk of failure of microsurgical reconstruction.

Management of Axilla

- In patients with clinically palpable axillary nodes, NCCN panel recommends pathologic confirmation of malignancy using USG-guided FNAC or core biopsy of suspicious nodes. **For biopsy proven axillary metastases, axillary dissection of level I&II is indicated**.
- **Level I & II axillary dissection requires atleast 10 lymph nodes** be provided for accurate staging of axilla. Axillary dissection should be extended to level III if level I & II are grossly involved.
- In patients with clinically negative nodes or if FNA/core biopsy result is negative, NCCN panel recommends **sentinel lymph node biopsy**.

Level of Axillary Lymph Nodes (Berg's level)

Level I: Lymph nodes lateral and inferior to the pectoralis minor (anterior, posterior and lateral group)

Level II: Lymph nodes behind the pectoralis minor (Central group)

Level III: Lymph nodes medial and superior to the pectoralis minor (apical and infraclavicular group)

Indications of axillary lymph node dissection (ALND) [as per ASBrS guidelines]:

- Clinically node-positive axilla, confirmed by FNA or core biopsy, in a patient for whom neoadjuvant chemotherapy is not planned
- Occult breast cancer presenting as axillary node mestastasis
- Axillary recurrence following previous breast cancer treatment
- Sentinel or axillary nodes which remain positive after neoadjuvant chemotherapy
- Inadequate prior ALND with residual clinically suspicious nodes
- Sentinel lymph node positive patients who fall outside the ACOSOG Z0011 trial and IBCSG 23-01 trial selection criteria
- Failed SLN mapping
- Inflammatory, clinical stage T4, or high-risk T3 breast cancer.

Complications of axillary dissection:

- Seroma
- Lymphedema
- Paresthesia of the upper, inner arm (due to injury of the intercostobrachial nerve)
- Atrophy of latissimus dorsi muscle (due to injury of the thoracodorsal nerve)
- Winged scapula (due to injury of long thoracic nerve)

Indications for Sentinel Lymph Node (SLN) Biopsy [as per ASBrS guidelines]

- T1-2 invasive breast cancer with clinically negative axilla
- Clinically negative axilla following neoadjuvant chemotherapy
- DCIS sufficient to require mastectomy, or DCIS with suspected/proved microinvasion.

Tracers (Mapping agents) for Sentinel Node Biopsy in Breast Cancer

Blue dye:

- Isosulfan blue
- Methylene blue
- Patent blue V

Radioisotope:

- Technetium 99m
- 99mTc-sulfur colloid
- 99mTc-nanocolloid human serum albumin

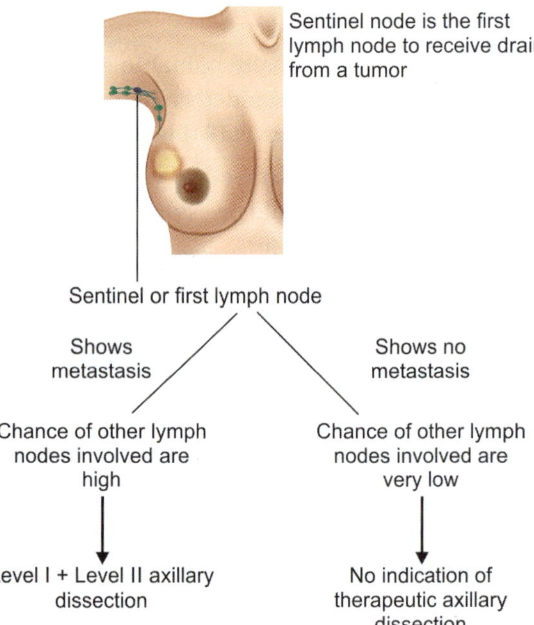

Axillary reverse mapping (ARM): A minimally invasive technique to differentiate upper extremity lymph nodes from lymphatic drainage of breast, thereby reducing upper extremity lymphedema following axillary lymph node dissection (ALND) or sentinel lymph node biopsy (SLNB).

Technique of Sentinel Lymph Node Biopsy (SLNB)

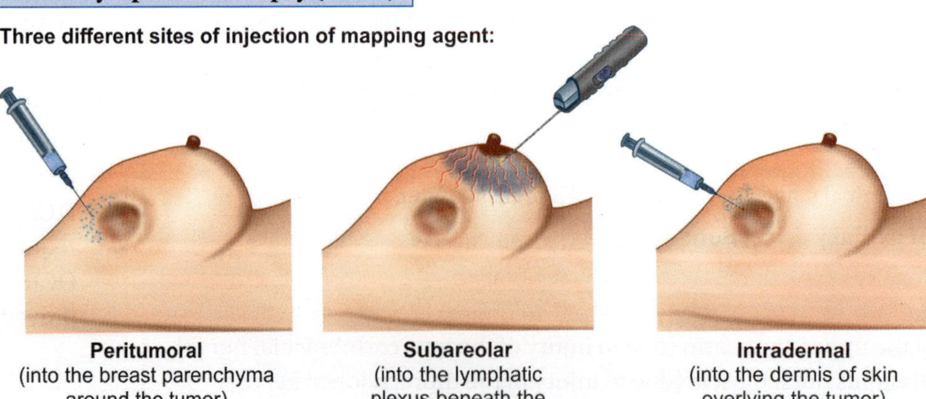

- **Blue dye, radioisotope or both blue dye and radioisotope** can be used as mapping agent in sentinel lymph node biopsy.
- The success rate of radioisotope plus blue dye mapping is superior to any of the methods.
- Blue dye must be injected at the start of surgery. Radioisotope may be injected the day before or the morning of surgery.

The incision for sentinel lymph node biopsy is separate from that of mastectomy or lumpectomy.

In blue dye mapping, all blue nodes, and nodes contiguous with blue-stained lymphatics are removed.

In isotope mapping, "hottest" node, and all nodes whose counts are 10% or more of the hottest node, are removed.

Neither blue nor hot, but palpably suspicious nodes must be removed.

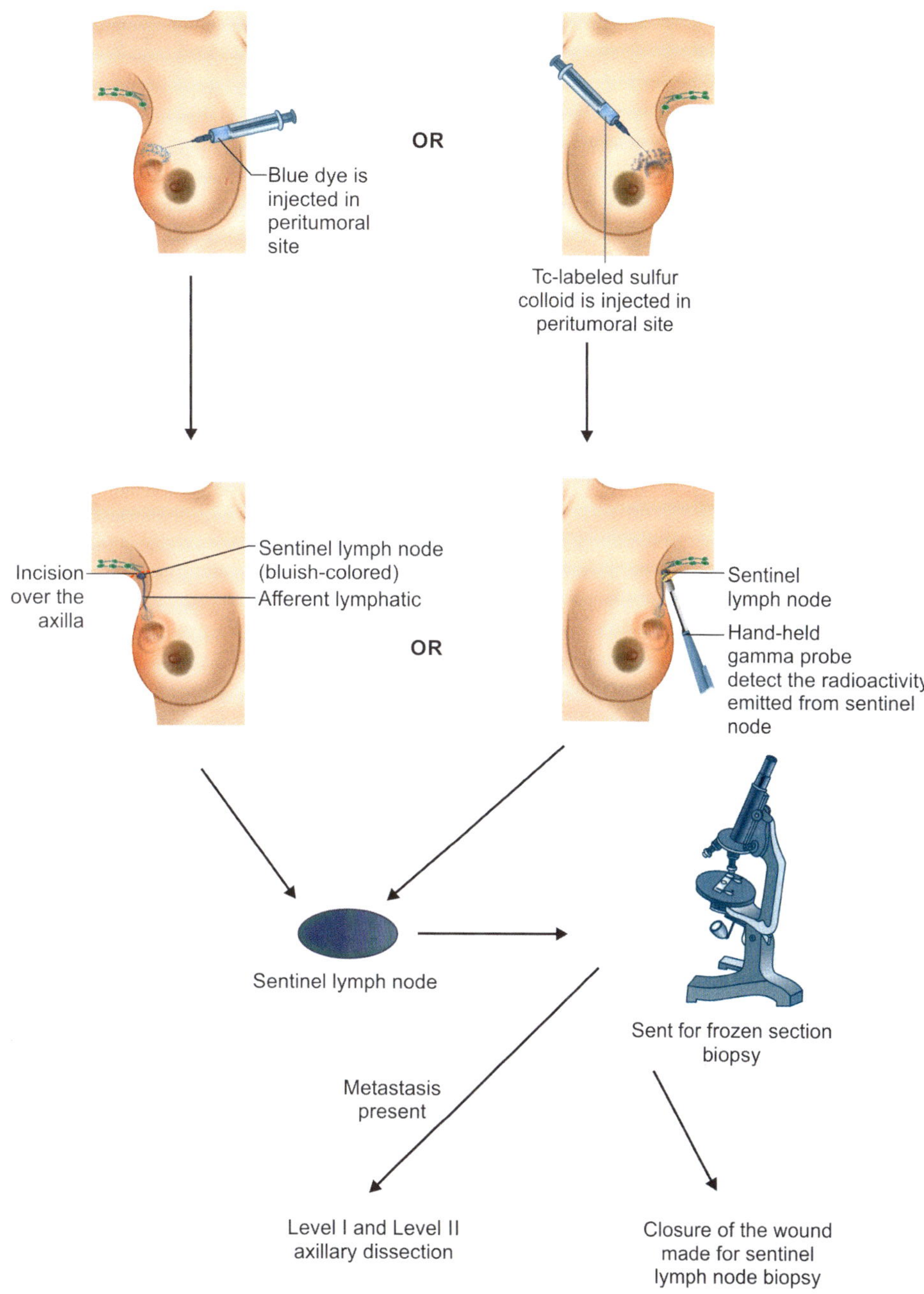

Adjuvant systemic therapy should be considered in early stage breast cancer to reduce the risk of recurrence. The decision to use adjuvant systemic therapy depends on patient's age, tumor size, tumor grade, number of involved axillary lymph nodes, hormone receptor status, HER2 expression.

'Adjuvant! Online' is a validated, computer-based model that is useful to estimate benefits of systemic adjuvant endocrine therapy and chemotherapy.

Multigene assays are useful to predict the advantage of adding adjuvant chemotherapy to further reduce the risk of recurrence.

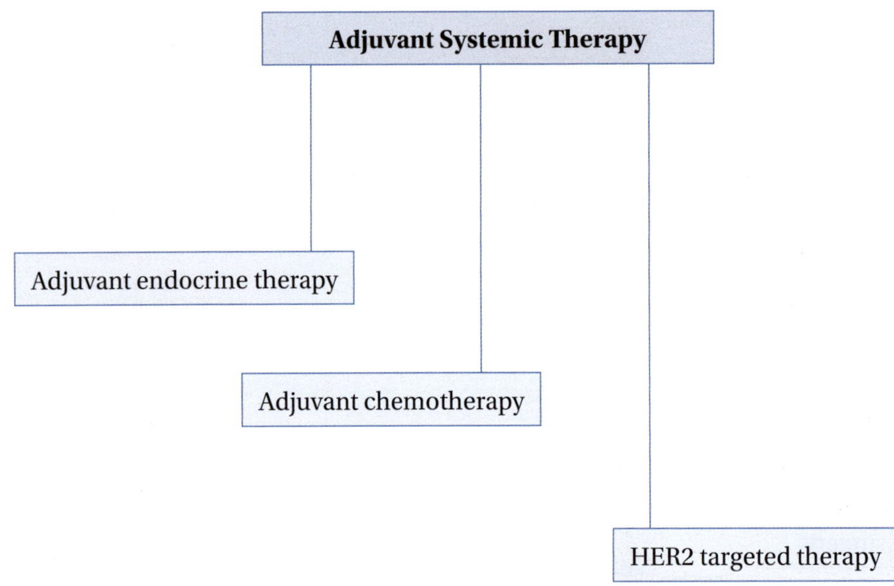

Adjuvant Endocrine Therapy

Selective Estrogen Receptor Modulators (SERMS) • **Tamoxifen** is chemically similar to estradiol, a competitive inhibitor of estradiol. It exerts antiestrogenic effect on breast tissue and estrogenic effect on skeletal system. • **Raloxifene** acts as an estrogen antagonist on breast tissue and agonistic effect on skeletal system. It increases bone mineral density in postmenopausal patients.	• **Indications:** (i) As an adjuvant therapy in hormone receptor-positive breast cancer in both pre- and postmenopausal women and (ii) In hormone-receptor positive breast cancer in men. • **Dose:** Tamoxifen 20 mg/day for 5 years; Raloxifen 60 mg/day for 5 years. • **Contraindications:** (i) Pregnancy; (ii) Breastfeeding; (iii) History of thrombotic events (e.g., DVT, TIA, CVA, pulmonary embolism); and (iv) History of clotting disorder • **Adverse effects:** (i) Hot flash; (ii) Venous thromboembolism—in both tamoxifen and raloxifene; and (iii) Increased risk of endometrial cancer and cataract—in tamoxifen.
Aromatase Inhibitors (AIs) • **Nonsteroidal AIs:** Anastrozole and Letrozole. Both bind aromatase enzyme reversibly. • **Steroidal AIs:** Exemestane. It binds aromatase enzyme irreversibly. • Aromatase enzyme is responsible for conversion of androgens into estrogen.	• **Indication:** As an adjuvant therapy in hormone receptor-positive breast cancer in postmenopausal patients. • **Dose:** Anastrozole: 1 mg/day; Letrozole: 2.5 mg/day; Exemestane: 25 mg/day. AIs should be continued for 5 years. • **Adverse effects:** (i) Hot flashes; (ii) Arthralgia and myalgia; (iii) Osteoporosis; and (iv) Loss of libido.
Selective Estrogen Down Regulators (SERDs) Fulvestrant, an estrogen receptor antagonist that downregulates ER. It competitively inhibits binding of estradiol to the estrogen receptor.	• **Indication:** As a second-line treatment option for postmenopausal women with hormone-receptor positive advanced breast cancer who have progressed on prior tamoxifen or AI therapy. • **Dose:** 500 mg monthly—intramuscular injection • **Adverse effects:** (i) Hot flashes; (ii) Nausea; (iii) Vomiting; (iv) Headache; and (v) Injection site pain

Selection of Adjuvant Endocrine Therapy

Adjuvant endocrine therapy should be considered in all patients with invasive breast cancer that are hormone receptor positive regardless of age and lymph node status.

Premenopausal, low-risk group: Tamoxifen for 5 years

Premenopausal, high-risk group: Tamoxifen for 5 years followed by aromatase inhibitors for 5 years (if patient become postmenopausal) or Tamoxifen with ovarian suppression.

Postmenopausal, low-risk group: Aromatase inhibitor therapy for 5 years or Tamoxifen for 2 years followed by aromatase inhibitor therapy for 3 years (in patients with significant osteoporosis).

Postmenopausal, high-risk group: Aromatase inhibitor therapy for 5–10 years.

Adjuvant bisphosphonate therapy is indicated in postmenopausal patients receiving adjuvant endocrine therapy to delay the development of osteoporosis associated with aromatase inhibitor therapy.

Adjuvant!online

Adjuvant!online *(https://www.adjuvantonline.com)* is the most widely used Internet tool for estimating the benefits of adjuvant endocrine therapy and chemotherapy.

This tool assesses 10-year disease-free survival and overall survival, by using information of age and selected tumor characteristics (tumor size and grade, number of positive axillary nodes, hormone receptor status).

This tool provides information on death from both breast cancer and non-breast cancer causes.

Limitations: (i) Relapse estimates both loco-regional recurrence and distant metastases and (ii) Benefits of adjuvant trastuzumab cannot be estimated.

Adjuvant Chemotherapy

- If patient is a potential candidate for adjuvant chemotherapy based on clinical characteristics, tumor stage, pathology, comorbid conditions, **systemic adjuvant chemotherapy** is recommended if **multigene assay (preferably Oncotype DX)** is not available. If it is available, it should be considered for predicting the benefit of adding adjuvant chemotherapy.
- **Chemotherapy regimens:** (i) Dose-dense doxorubicin and cyclophosphamide (AC) with dose-dense sequential paclitaxel; (ii) Dose-dense AC followed by sequential weekly paclitaxel; (iii) CMF (Cyclophosphamide, Methotrexate, Fluorouracil); (iv) FEC (Fluorouracil, Epirubicin, Cyclophosphamide); and (v) TAC (Docetaxel, Doxorubicin, Cyclophosphamide).

Multigene Assays (for Assessment of Prognosis and for Prediction of Response to Adjuvant Systemic Chemotherapy)

Oncotype DX:

- It is a 21-gene qRT-PCR based assay and the only one clinically validated gene-based assay for breast cancer. It is used for newly diagnosed, early stage node-negative, ER-positive, HER2-negative breast cancer. This recurrence score also can be used in postmenopausal patients with ER-positive tumors and 1-3 involved axillary lymph nodes. Recurrence score ranges from 0–100.
- Postmenopausal patient, pT1-3, HR-positive, HER2-negative, risk score (RS) <26—no benefit from addition of chemotherapy to endocrine therapy. Postmenopausal pt, pT1-3, HR-positive, HER2-negative, pN0 and pN1 (1–3 positive nodes) and RS ≥26—addition of chemotherapy is recommended.
- Premenopausal patient, pT1-3 and pN1 (1–3 positive nodes) and RS <26—additional of chemotherapy may be considered. Premenopausal patient, pT1-3, pN0, HR-positive, HER2-negative and RS ≥26—addition of chemotherapy is recommended.
- Patients with intermediate recurrence score (16–25) may benefited from chemotherapy depending on other clinicopathologic variables.
- Patients with high recurrence score (>25) greatly benefit from chemotherapy.

Mammaprint:

70-gene, DNA microarray test. For stage I and II, node-negative, ER-positive, ER-negative breast cancers to identify patients with high- or low-risk of recurrence

Prosigna PAM50 ROR:

50-gene, qRT-PCR and DNA microarray based test. For guiding adjuvant chemotherapy decisions in early-stage ER-positive, HER2-negative tumors

Endo-Predict:

12-gene (8 target + 4 reference), qRT-PCR based assay

Adjuvant HER2-targeted Therapy

Trastuzumab (for 12 months) is recommended in patients with HER2-positive tumors of 1 cm or more, along with chemotherapy.

Trastuzumab is a humanized monoclonal antibody binds to the extracellular domain of HER2 (Human epidermal growth factor receptor). It is the first monoclonal antibody approved for breast cancer treatment. Most significant side effect is carditoxicity.

Pertuzumab is a humanized recombinant monoclonal antibody binds to the HER2 at a different extracellular domain.

Lapatinib is a dual tyrosine kinase inhibitor of HER2 and EGFR.

Adjuvant Radiation Therapy

After breast conserving therapy in node-positive patients: Whole breast irradiation with or without boost dose of radiation after BCT is recommended. Regional nodal irradiation (infraclavicular, supraclavicular, internal mammary, suspicious area of the axillary bed) is indicated for 4 or more positive ALNs.

After BCT in node-negative patients: Whole breast irradiation may be considered without any regional nodal irradiation.

After mastectomy in node-positive patients: Chest wall radiation is recommended in node-positive disease. Regional nodal irradiation (infraclavicular, supraclavicular, internal mammary, suspicious area of the axillary bed) is indicated for 4 or more positive ALNs.

After mastectomy in node-negative patients: Chest wall irradiation is not indicated if tumor is less than 5 cm and negative margin of 1 mm or more. Chest wall irradiation may be considered in high-risk patients.

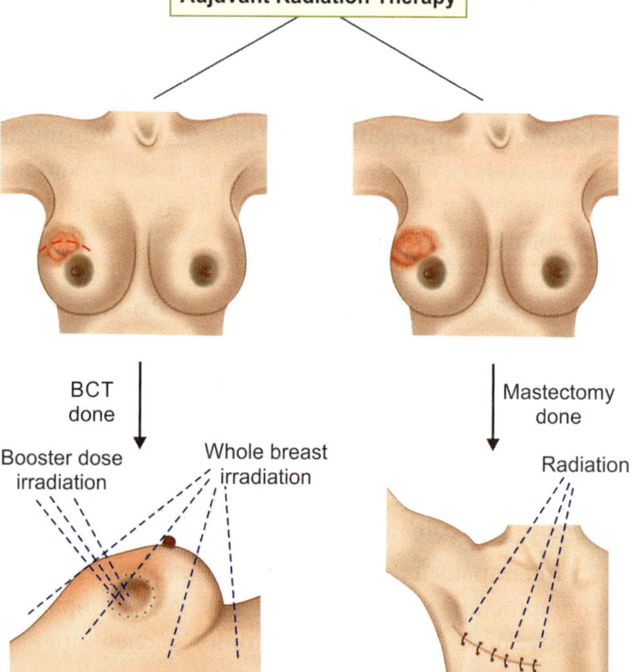

Whole breast irradiation decreases the risk of local recurrence and **boost dose of radiation** decreases the risk of in-breast recurrence.

Management of Inoperable Locally Advanced Breast Carcinoma

Management of locally advanced breast carcinoma is **neoadjuvant systemic therapy followed by surgery followed by adjuvant therapy**.

Neoadjuvant systemic therapy comprises chemotherapy, endocrine therapy and HER2 targeted therapy.

The primary goal of neoadjuvant systemic therapy is to **tumor or nodal downstaging**.

The optimal tumor response to neoadjuvant systemic therapy is clinical complete response (cCR) and pathological complete response (pCR) as per **RECIST criteria**.

Neoadjuvant chemotherapy:

Anthracycline-based regimen with or without taxane is the standard neoadjuvant chemotherapy. If surgery is performed before completion of planned chemotherapy regimen, it should be completed as adjuvant therapy.

Neoadjuvant HER2 targeted therapy:

In patients with HER2-positive tumor, dual HER2 targeted therapy (pertuzumab and trastuzumab) is indicated along with chemotherapy. Trastuzumab-based therapy should be continued as adjuvant therapy and total 12 months therapy should be completed.

Neoadjuvant endocrine therapy:

Neoadjuvant endocrine therapy (tamoxifen for premenopausal and aromatase inhibitors for postmenopausal patients) may be considered for hormone receptor-positive patients. Adjuvant endocrine therapy should be same as early stage invasive cancer.

During neoadjuvant systemic therapy, tumor response should be monitored regularly by clinical examination. If disease progression is evident during neoadjuvant therapy, palliative irradiation should be considered.

Indications of neoadjuvant systemic therapy:

- Locally advanced or inoperable breast cancer
- Inflammatory breast cancer
- N2 and N3 nodal disease
- T4 tumors
- Operable breast CA but patient desires BCS (not feasible due to size of the tumor relative to size of the breast)

Advantages of neoadjuvant systemic therapy:

- Make inoperable tumor to operable
- Provides prognostic information particularly in patients with triple-negative and HER2-positive breast cancer
- Breast conservation become feasible
- Decrease the extent and morbidity related to axillary dissection
- Allows time for genetic testing

Neoadjuvant systemic therapy is not appropriate in:

- Extensive in situ disease when extent of disease is not well defined
- Tumors are not palpable or clinically assessable

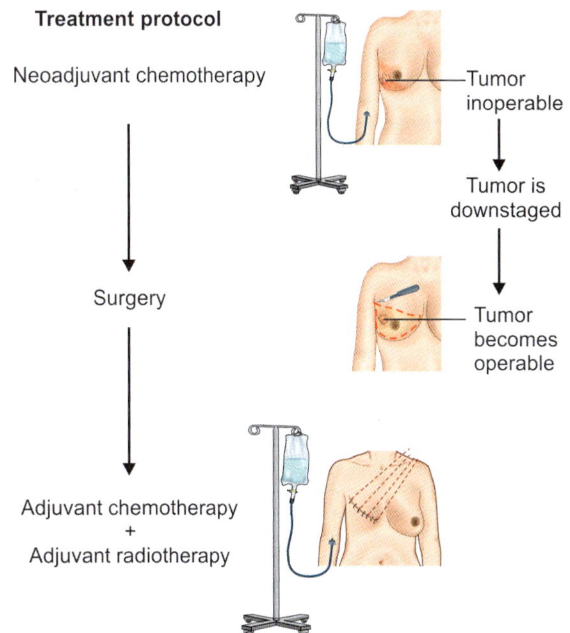

Management of Stage IV Breast Carcinoma

Primary management of metastatic breast carcinoma is systemic therapy. Systemic therapy prolongs the survival of the patient and improves the quality of life. Surgery (Palliative mastectomy) is indicated after systemic therapy if patients present with skin ulceration, tumor bleeding or fungation.

In hormone receptor-positive and HER2-negative postmenopausal and premenopausal patients with ovarian ablation or suppression (by LHRH agonist), aromatase inhibitor in combination with CDK 4/6 inhibitors (palmocicib, ribicicib) is the first-line therapy.

In hormone receptor-negative and HER2-positive patients, preferred treatment option is pertuzumab plus trastuzumab in combination with systemic chemotherapy (Docetaxel or Paclitaxel).

In hormone receptor-positive and HER2-positive patients, either HER2-targeted therapy in combination with endocrine therapy or HER-targeted therapy in combination with chemotherapy is the treatment option.

Male Breast Cancer

- **Risk factors:** (i) Family history of breast cancer in a first-degree male or female relative; (ii) BRCA2 mutation; (iii) Advanced age; (iv) Klinefelter syndrome; (v) History of chest irradiation; and (vi) Exogenous estrogen treatment (for feminization purpose).
- **Characteristic features:** (i) Typically diagnosed about 5–10 years after the age of presentation in female and (ii) Present at a more advanced stage.
- **Histology:** Infiltrating ductal carcinoma not otherwise specified is the most common histologic subtype. Ductal carcinoma in situ (DCIS) is the second most common subtype.
- **Clinical presentation:** Painless palpable mass with palpable axillary lymph nodes in most of the cases. Nipple retraction, nipple ulceration or skin changes may be present.

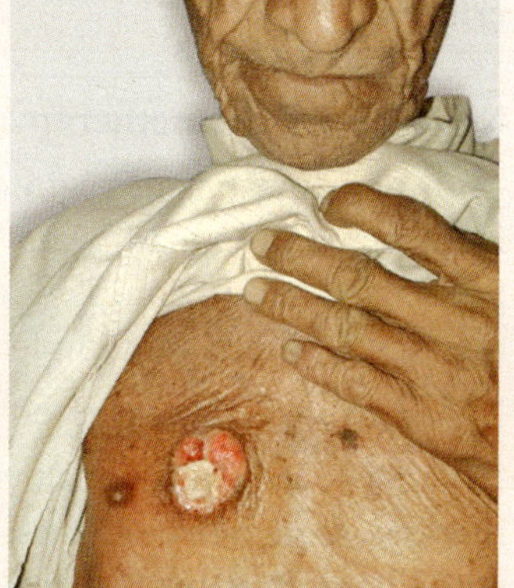

Male breast cancer.

- **Diagnosis:** Mammography is the imaging modality of choice. For tissue diagnosis, USG-guided biopsy is indicated. Estrogen and progesterone receptors are expressed in majority of patients.
- **Treatment:** Treatment depends on the stage of the disease and hormone receptor status. Management is similar to management of breast cancer in postmenopausal women. Aromatase inhibitor therapy should be considered only if concomitant testicular steroidogenesis is planned.

Axillary Breast Cancer

- MRI of the breast is helpful for detection of occult breast cancer. MRI-positive disease should be evaluated with MRI-guided biopsy. Chest and abdominal CT is recommended to evaluate presence of distant metastases. ER/PR and HER2neu status should be evaluated.
- MRI-positive disease is evaluated with MRI-guided biopsy and further treatment is based on clinical staging. Treatment of MRI-negative disease is based on nodal status.
- Treatment of T0N1M0 disease is mastectomy along with axillary nodal dissection or axillary nodal dissection along with whole breast irradiation with or without nodal irradiation. Chemotherapy, endocrine therapy or trastuzumab therapy as per recommendations.
- Treatment of T0N2-3M0 disease is neoadjuvant chemotherapy or endocrine therapy followed by axillary nodal dissection and mastectomy.

Breast Cancer during Pregnancy

- Breast cancer during pregnancy is characterized by: (i) Larger size of the tumor; (ii) Axillary lymph nodes commonly involved; (iii) Poorly differentiated tumor; and (iv) Often ER/PR negative.
- USG of the breast and axillary lymph nodes is helpful to evaluate the extent of disease and to guide biopsy. Mammogram can be done if proper shielding can be ensured.
- Surgical procedure of choice is modified radical mastectomy. BCS may be considered if only adjuvant radiation therapy can be delayed upto postpartum period. Sentinel lymph node biopsy should be avoided before 30 weeks. Use of isosulfan blue and methylene blue dye is contraindicated during pregnancy.
- Endocrine therapy, Radiation therapy and Trastuzumab therapy are contraindicated during pregnancy. Chemotherapy should not be given during the first trimester, after 35 weeks or within 3 weeks of planned delivery.
- FAC chemotherapy may be considered in 2nd and 3rd trimesters of pregnancy.

Inflammatory Breast Cancer

- Inflammatory breast cancer is a aggressive form of breast cancer, characterized by erythema and dermal edema of the skin of the breast. These characteristic features are due to blockage of dermal lymphatics by tumor emboli.
- Inflammatory breast cancer is a clinical diagnosis, biopsy is not essential.
- These cancers are commonly ER/PR-negative and HER2-positive. Basal and HER2 overexpressed molecular subtypes are more common.
- Workup includes diagnostic mammogram and hormone receptor and HER2neu status.
- Modified radical mastectomy is the recommended surgical management in patients who respond to neoadjuvant chemotherapy (anthracycline-based regimen with or without taxanes). Sentinel lymph node biopsy is not recommended. If breast reconstruction is to be considered, it must be delayed reconstruction. Surgery should not be considered who do not respond to neoadjuvant chemotherapy. Additional systemic chemotherapy and/or radiation therapy should be considered.

Paget's Disease of the Nipple

- Paget's disease of the nipple is characterized by neoplastic cells in the epidermis of the Nipple-areolar complex. Associated cancer (DCIS or invasive cancer) may present in about 80–90% of patients and they are categorized based on the size and characteristics of the parenchymal disease. Most of the patients present with eczema of areola, bleeding, ulceration and itching of the nipple.
- Biopsy (including full thickness of epidermis) of the skin of NAC is indicated. If biopsy is suggestive of Paget's disease, breast MRI is recommended to evaluate the extent of disease and to detect any associated cancer.
- Treatment is total mastectomy or BCS (if no evidence of invasive cancer). BCS includes removal of the entire NAC with a negative margin of underlying breast tissue. Axillary lymph node staging is indicated in presence of underlying invasive breast cancer.

Case 1

History and Physical Examination

A 25-year-old female patient presented in the surgical OPD with complain of swelling in the right breast for last 4 months not associated with pain. Patient consulted with local physician and as per his advice she attended surgical OPD for opinion. No history of alteration of size or appearance of pain related to menstrual cycle. No history of nipple discharge. No history of breast cancer in first-degree relatives.

Physical Examination

- No pallor, cervical lymph nodes not palpable
- *Examination of the breast and axilla:* A 2 cm × 2 cm, solitary, discrete, non-tender, mobile lump palpable in the upper inner quadrant of the right breast. No lump palpable in the other quadrant of the same breast or contralateral breast. No lymph nodes were palpable in both axilla.

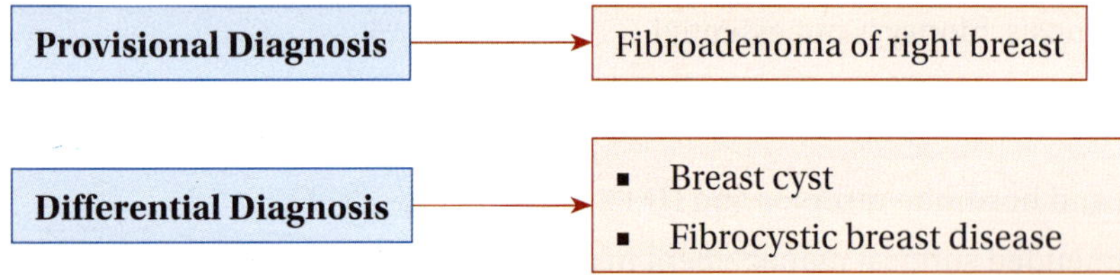

Investigations

- *USG breast:* Well-circumscribed, round mass with uniform hypoechogenicity, dimension of 2 cm × 2.5 cm × 2 cm, in the right breast
- FNAC of right breast lump revealed fibroadenoma without any atypia.

Discussion

Young female patient presented with solitary, discrete, non-tender mobile lump in her breast was suggestive of fibroadenoma. USG findings and FNA confirmed the diagnosis. No need of mammography or other investigations for confirmation of diagnosis. As the patient was young and the fibroadenoma was small (maximum dimension 2.5 cm), we planned for reassurance and follow-up, but patient was anxious and wanted surgery.

Management Algorithm

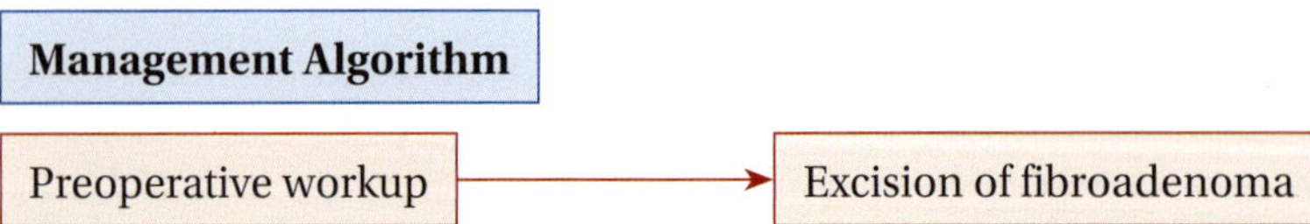

Case 2

History and Physical Examination

A 48-year-old female patient attended surgical OPD with a lump in the right breast and right axillary swelling for last 6 months. Patient had taken some medicines for this swelling without any diagnostic workup. Now she concerned about the swelling as it was increasing in size and causing pain and discomfort. No history of nipple discharge but patient noticed some changes in nipple and skin overlying the swelling. Her mother died about 10 years back from breast cancer. Patient attained menopause 1 year back. Patient had taken OCP for about 20 years. No significant menstrual or obstetric history.

Physical Examination

Patient alert, conscious, cooperative

Pallor present, cervical lymph nodes—not palpable

Examination of breast and axilla: A 6 cm × 5.5 cm lump in the upper and outer quadrant of right breast also involving the upper inner quadrant, firm in consistency, margin well-defined, overlying skin fixed with Peau d'orange appearance, lump not fixed to the underlying pectoral muscle, nipple retracted. One fixed medial group of lymph node palpable in right axilla. No abnormal clinical findings in left breast and axilla.

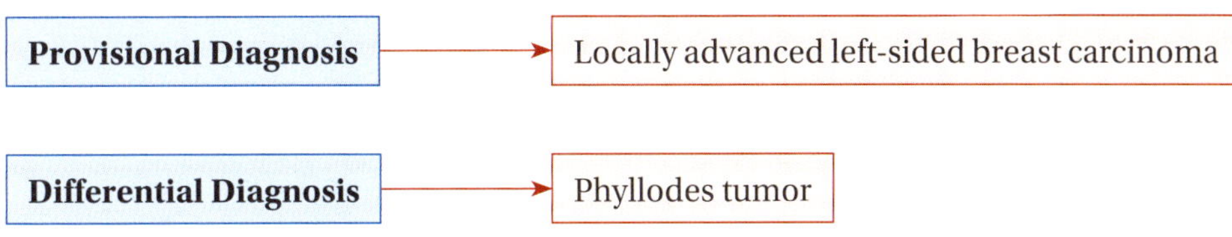

Investigations

- Mammographic features consistent with carcinoma without any microcalcification in other quadrant of the same breast or contralateral breast.
- Tru-cut biopsy from the breast lump revealed invasive ductal carcinoma. FNA of axillary lymph nodes revealed metastatic deposit. ER, PR positive, Her2neu negative.
- CT abdomen and pelvis, CT chest revealed no distant metastasis. PET/CT also revealed no distant metastasis.

Discussion

A postmenopausal patient presented with breast lump along with axillary lymphadenopathy for last 6 months. Triple assessment revealed it as a invasive ductal carcinoma with axillary lymph node positive. Hormonal receptor study report was ER, PR positive and Her2neu negative. No distant metastasis was detected in metastatic work-up. Clinical staging was cT3N2M0. Neoadjuvant chemotherapy was planned for downstaging.

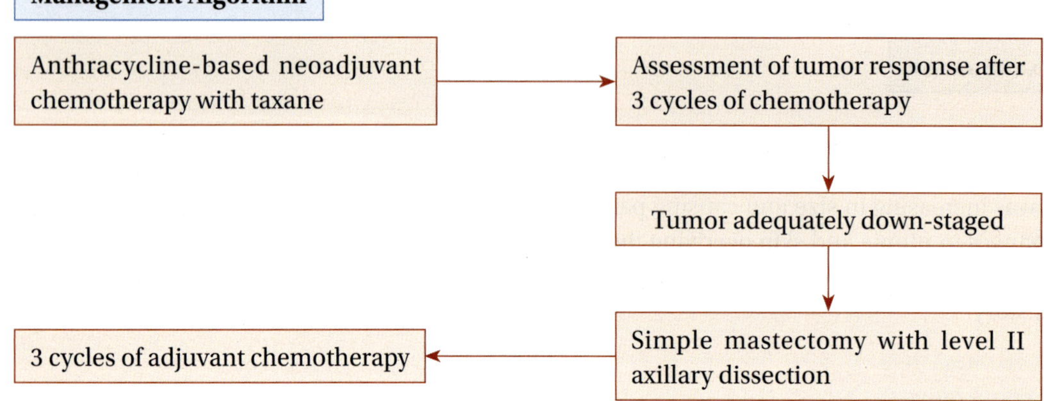
Management Algorithm
Anthracycline-based neoadjuvant chemotherapy with taxane
Assessment of tumor response after 3 cycles of chemotherapy
Tumor adequately down-staged
Simple mastectomy with level II axillary dissection
3 cycles of adjuvant chemotherapy

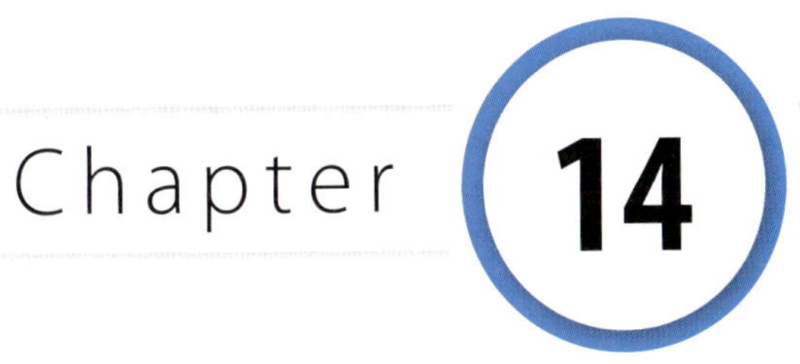

Disorders of Thyroid

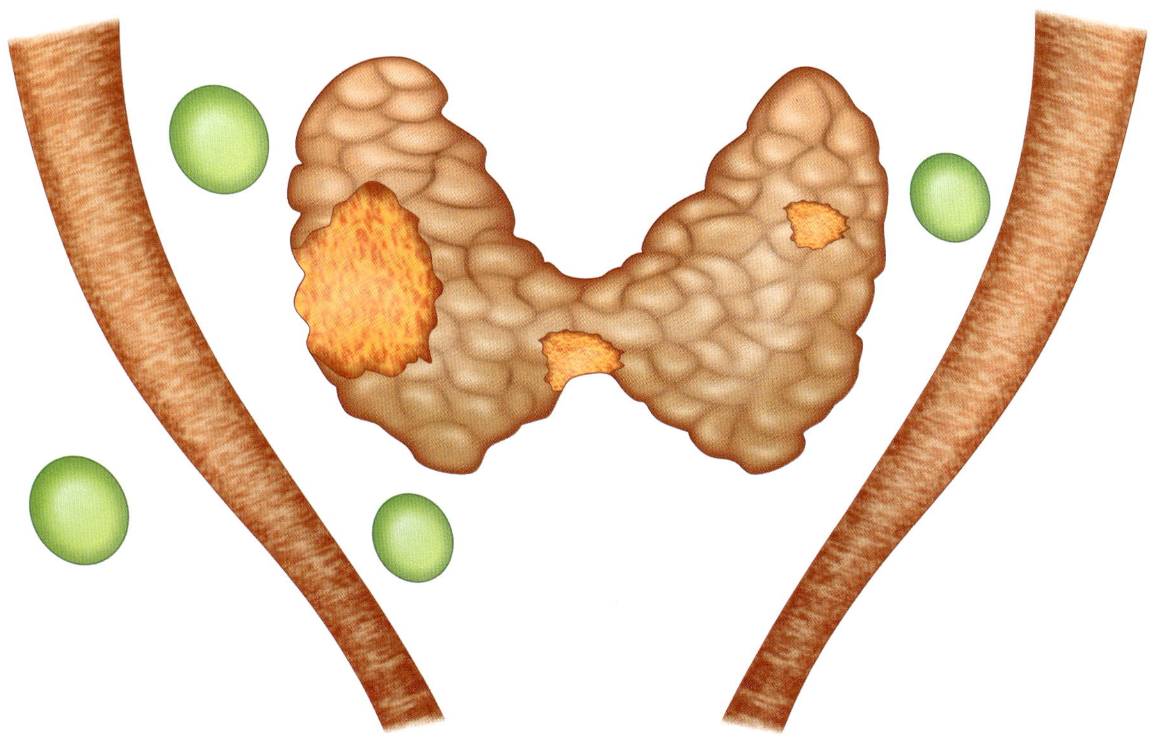

Important Topics

- Hypothyroidism
- Thyrotoxicosis
- Thyroid Nodule
- Thyroiditis
- Thyroid Neoplasm
- Surgical Approaches to Thyroid
- Remote Access Thyroid Surgery

'Scientific reasoning is a kind of dialogue between the possible and the actual, between what might be and what is in fact the case.'

Peter Brian Medawar (1915–1987)
Brazilian-born British Immunologist

Disorders of Thyroid

Disorders of thyroid

- Disorders of thyroid metabolism
  - Hypothyroidism
  - Hyperthyroidism
- Thyroiditis
  - Hashimoto's thyroiditis
  - Riedel's thyroiditis
  - de Quervain's thyroiditis
- Neoplasm
  - Benign
    - Follicular adenoma
  - Malignant
    - Papillary carcinoma
    - Follicular carcinoma
    - Anaplastic carcinoma
    - Medullary carcinoma

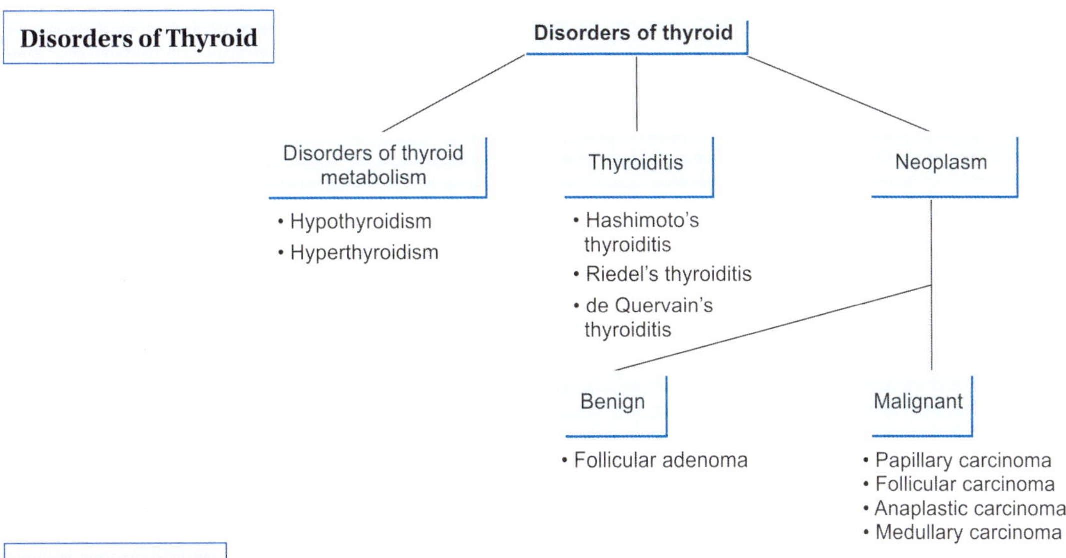

Hypothyroidism

Hypothyroidism is deficiency of circulating level of thyroid hormones (T3, T4). **Iodine deficiency** is the most common cause of hypothyroidism worldwide. **Hashimoto's thyroiditis** is the most common cause of hypothyroidism in the areas of iodine sufficiency.

Causes of Hypothyroidism

Causes of hypothyroidism
Primary
[intrinsic abnormality of thyroid]
Secondary
[Hypothalamic or pituitary abnormality]
Hypothalamus
↑↑TRH
Pituitary
↑↑TSH
↓↓T3
↓↓T4
↓↓T3
↓↓T4
↓↓TRH
Hypothalamic disease (tumor and trauma)
↓↓TSH
Hypopitutarism (tumor, trauma, surgery, and irradiation)
↓↓T3
↓↓T4
• Iodine deficiency
• Hashimoto's thyroiditis
• Postablative – Surgery
– Radioiodine therapy
– External radiation
• Drugs – Lithium
– Amiodarone
– Antithyroid drugs
• Congenital – Absent/ectopic thyroid gland
– Dyshormonogenesis
• Infiltrative disorders – Amyloidosis
– Sarcoidosis
– Riedel's thyroiditis

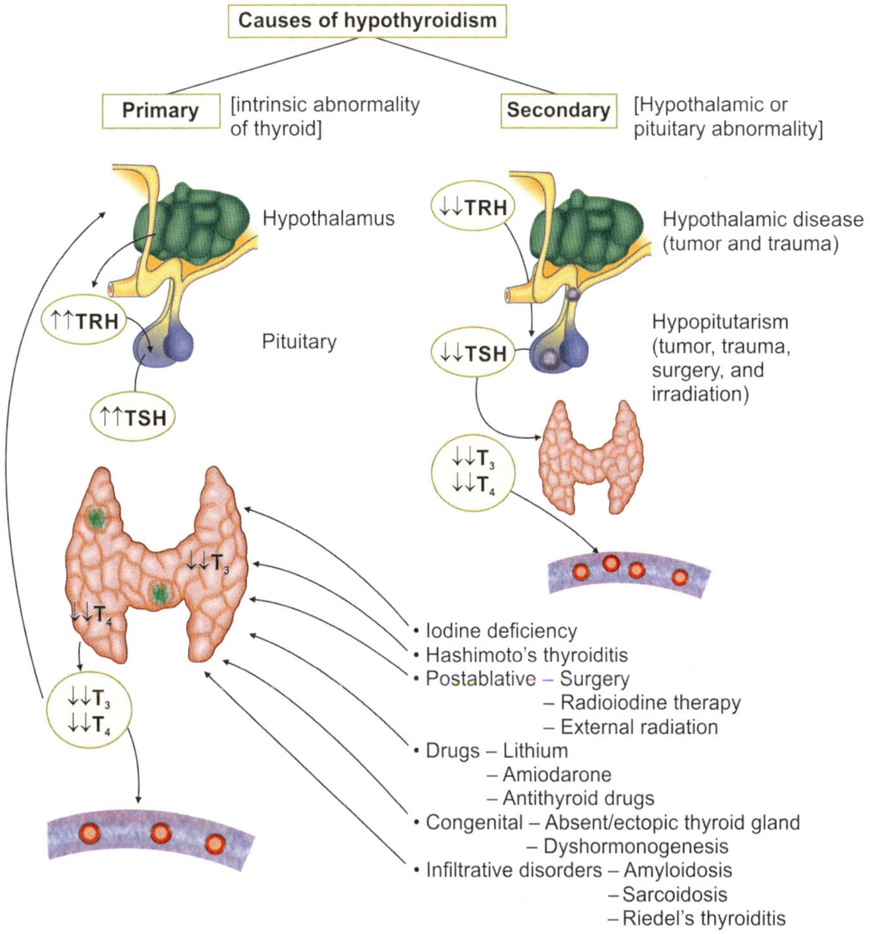

Drugs Causing Hypothyroidism

- Radioactive iodine therapy
- Antithyroid drugs
- Lithium
- Amiodarone
- Tyrosine kinase inhibitors (Sunitinib, vandetanib).

Congenital Hypothyroidism (Cretinism)

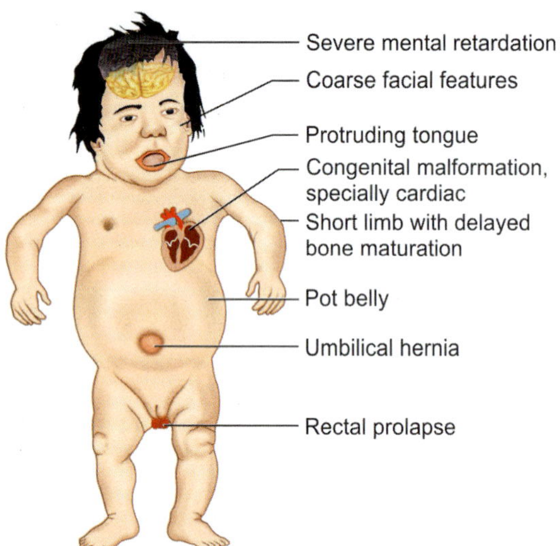

Cretinism is hypothyroidism in infancy or early childhood.

Classification

- Primary (due to dysgenesis of thyroid gland or dyshormonogenesis)
- Secondary (isolated TSH deficiency due to mutations in the TSH β-subunit gene or as a part of congenital hypopituitarism).
- Neurological cretinism
- Myxoedematous cretinism
- Transient hypothyroidism
- Permanent

Causes

- Thyroid gland dysgenesis **(most common cause)**
- Inborn errors of thyroid hormone synthesis
- Maternal iodine deficiency
- Antithyroid medication during pregnancy **(Transient hypothyroidism)**
- Mother with TSH-R blocking antibody **(Transient hypothyroidism)**

Clinical Presentation

Neurological cretinism is manifested as severe mental retardation, deaf mutism, squint, disorders of stance and gait.

Myxoedematous cretinism is manifested as less severe form of mental retardation, dwarfism, coarse and dry skin, delayed sexual maturation.

Associated cardiac malformations (most common congenital malformation in cretinism)

- Pulmonary stenosis
- Atrial septal defect
- Ventricular septal defect.

Treatment

Treatment with **levothyroxine (LT_4)** should be started at a dose of **10–15 μg/kg/day** as early as possible after diagnosis. Initially, higher recommended dose is indicated for rapid normalization of serum T4, which is essential for optimal neurodevelopmental outcome.

Diagnosis

Most of the newborn infants with congenital hypothyroidism remain undiagnosed at birth. Delay in diagnosis may lead to mental retardation, the most severe outcome of congenital hypothyroidism.

Screening

Screening is the most effective method to detect congenital hypothyroidism earliest. Neonatal screening is done by **estimation of TSH/T4 in heel-prick blood specimen between 2 and 5 days of age**.

If screening T4 value is below the 10th percentile of cutoff and/or the TSH is greater than 30 mU/L, **serum TSH and T4 estimation is indicated for confirmation.**

Important Facts about Thyroid Hormone

- Daily production of **T_4 is about 84 μg**, secreted by the thyroid gland. Daily production of **T_3 is about 33 μg**, of which **approximately 80% (about 26 μg) is derived from peripheral conversion of T_4**, about 20% derived from secretion from thyroid.
- Pro-hormone T_4 is converted into active metabolite, T_3 by D1 and D2 deiodinases. **Most of the T_4 to T_3 conversion occurs by D2 deiodinase**.
- **T_4 is the major secretory product** of thyroid gland, whereas effects of thyroid hormone on peripheral tissues depend on **binding of T_3 to its nuclear receptor**.
- The half-life of LT_4 is **approximately 7 days**. Serum T_4 and TSH levels achieve steady-state level after about **six weeks of therapy**.

Adult Hypothyroidism

Clinical Presentation

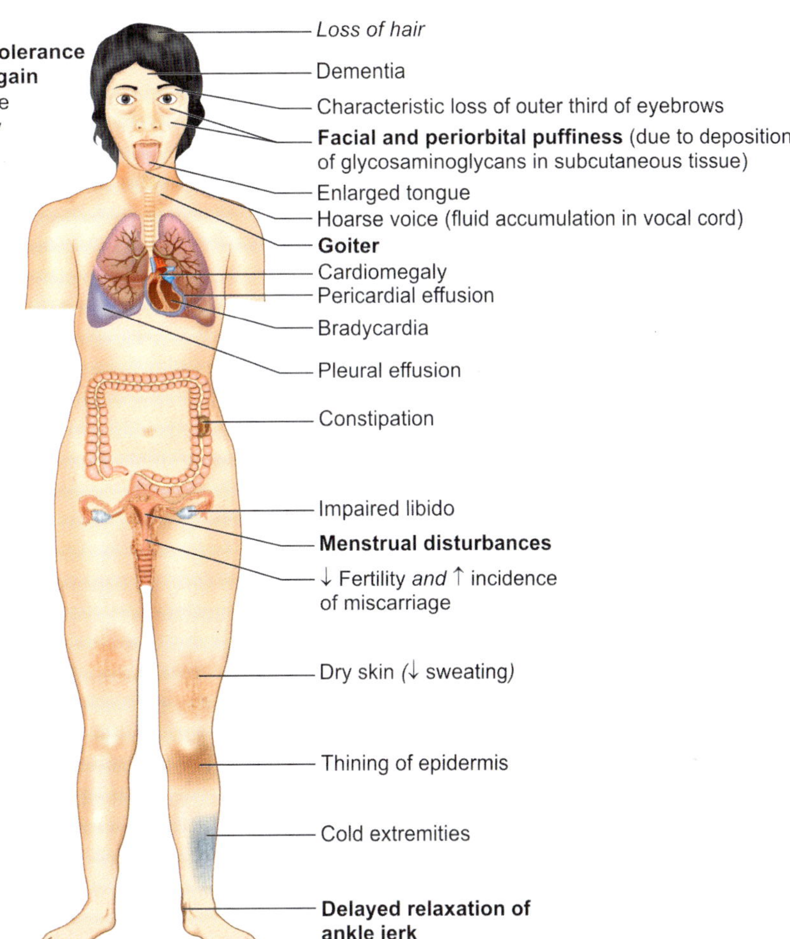

Achilles reflex time has a high sensitivity and specificity to confirm or exclude hypothyroidism.

Diagnosis

- Decreased T3 and T4 and increased TSH level is suggestive of **primary thyroid failure**. Decreased level of T3, T4, and TSH is suggestive of **secondary hypothyroidism**.
- Once clinical or subclinical hypothyroidism is confirmed, **anti-TPO antibody** should be assessed to rule out autoimmune hypothyroidism (TPO antibodies are present in more than 90% patients with autoimmune hypothyroidism).
- **FNA** is also indicated to confirm the diagnosis of Hashimoto's thyroiditis.

Treatment

- **In clinical hypothyroidism**, the replacement dose of levothyroxine is 100–150 μg daily 30 minutes before breakfast.
- The dose should be adjusted based on TSH level. The goal of treatment being a normal TSH (Lower half of the reference range). TSH should be assessed about 2 months after initiating treatment.
- **In subclinical hypothyroidism**, levothyroxine therapy is indicated in: (i) Pregnant patient; (ii) Patient wants to conceive; and (iii) Serum TSH >10 mIU/L.

In hypothyroid patient, elective surgery should be deferred until patient becomes euthyroid.

Thyrotoxicosis

Thyrotoxicosis: A clinical state that results from inappropriately high thyroid hormone action in tissues generally due to inappropriately high tissue thyroid hormone levels [ATA guideline].

Hyperthyroidism: A form of thyrotoxicosis due to inappropriately high synthesis and secretion of thyroid hormone(s) by the thyroid [ATA guideline].

Pathophysiology

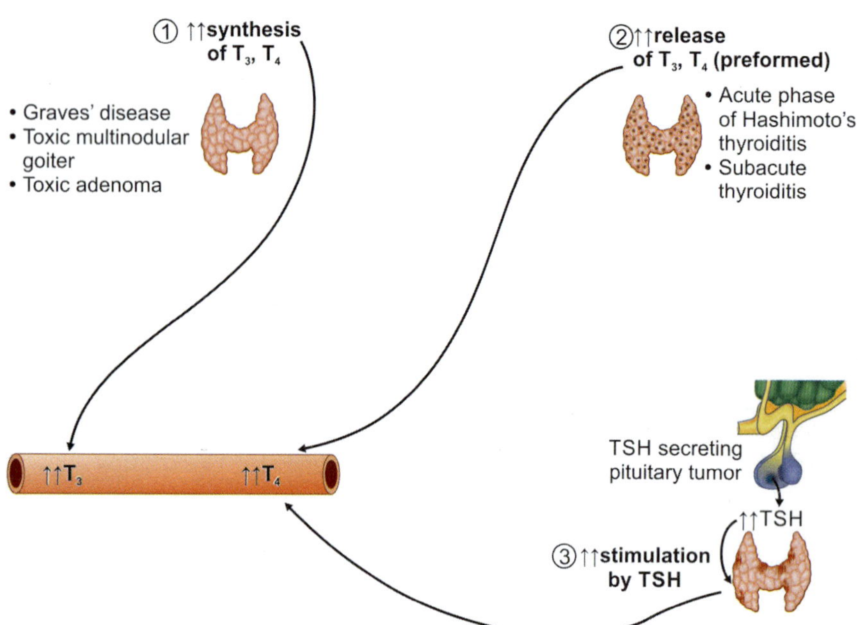

Common Causes of Thyrotoxicosis

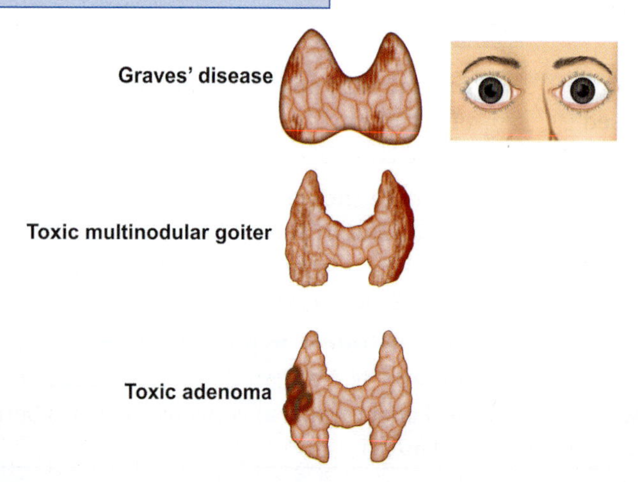

Thyrotoxicosis with Hyperthyroidism

- Graves' disease
- Toxic multinodular goiter
- Toxic adenoma

Thyrotoxicosis without Hyperthyroidism

- Subacute (granulomatous, de Quervain's) thyroiditis
- Painless (silent) thyroiditis
- Amiodarone-induced thyroiditis
- Factitious ingestion of thyroid hormone.

Graves' Disease

- An autoimmune disease of unknown cause with a strong familial predisposition.
- Most common cause of thyrotoxicosis
- Female preponderance
- Peak incidence between 20 and 40 years of age.

Pathophysiology

Genetic Factors Associated with Graves' Disease

- HLA-B8, HLA-DR3
- Polymorphisms of *CTLA-4* gene

Other Autoimmune Diseases that may be Associated with Graves' Disease

- Hashimoto thyroiditis
- Rheumatoid arthritis
- Addison disease
- Pernicious anemia.

The presence of **TSI (Thyroid-stimulating immunoglobulin)** is diagnostic of Graves' disease.

TPO antibodies are present in about 80% of patients with Graves' disease.

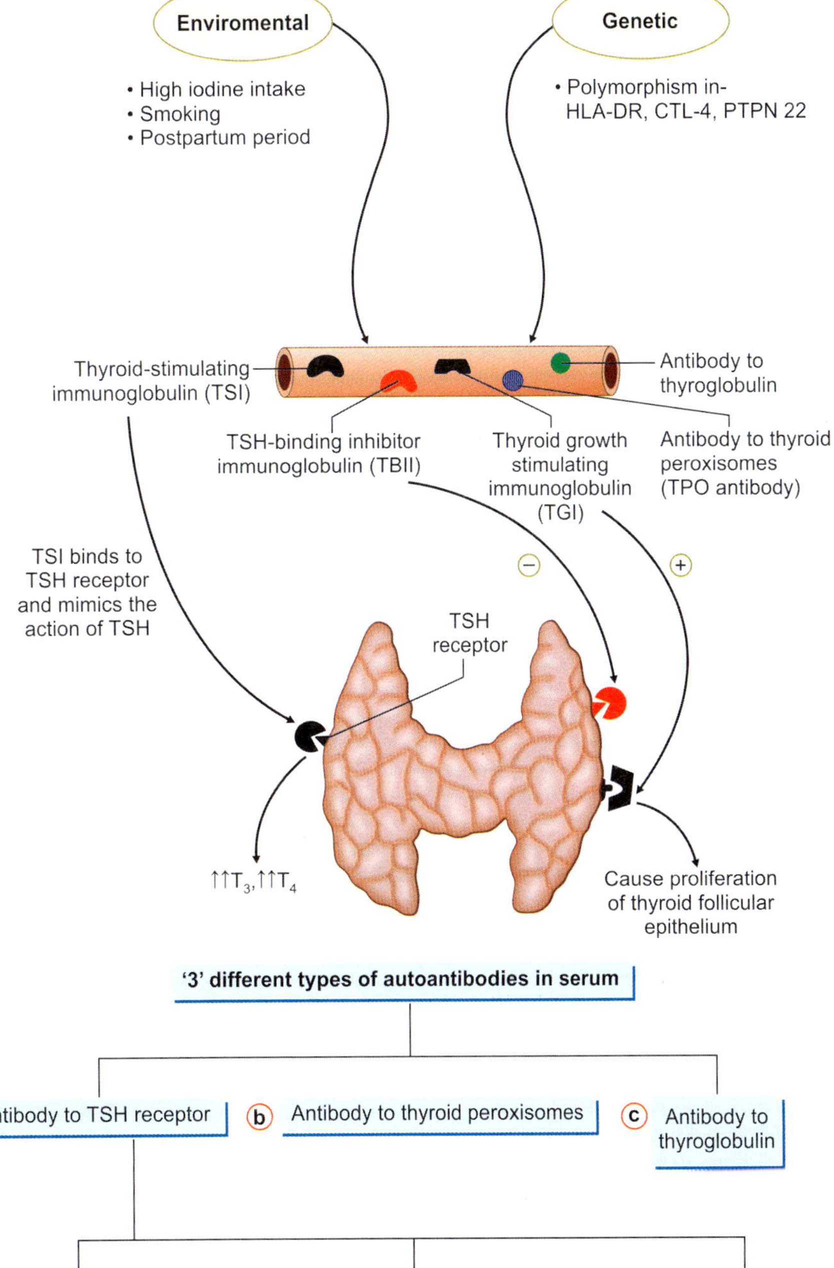

Microscopic Appearance

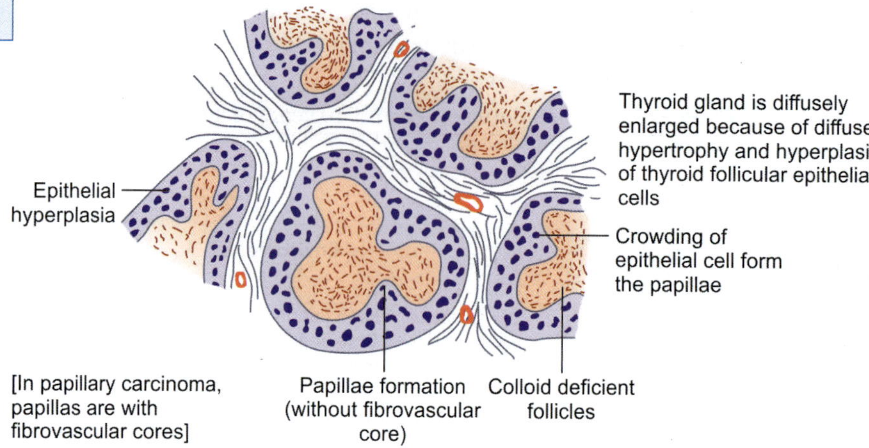

Clinical Manifestations

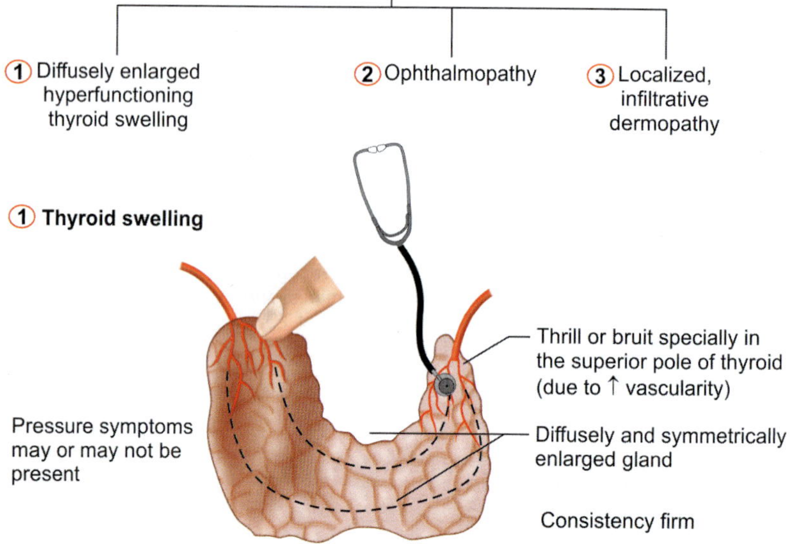

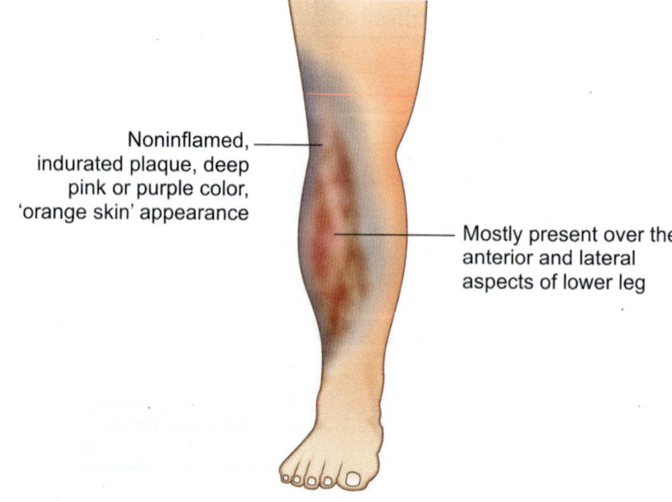

- **This dermopathy is due** to deposition of glycosaminoglycans and lymphocyte infiltration in the dermis leads to thickening of dermis.
- This dermopathy most commonly develop over the **anterior and lateral aspects of lower leg ('Pretibial myxedema')**.

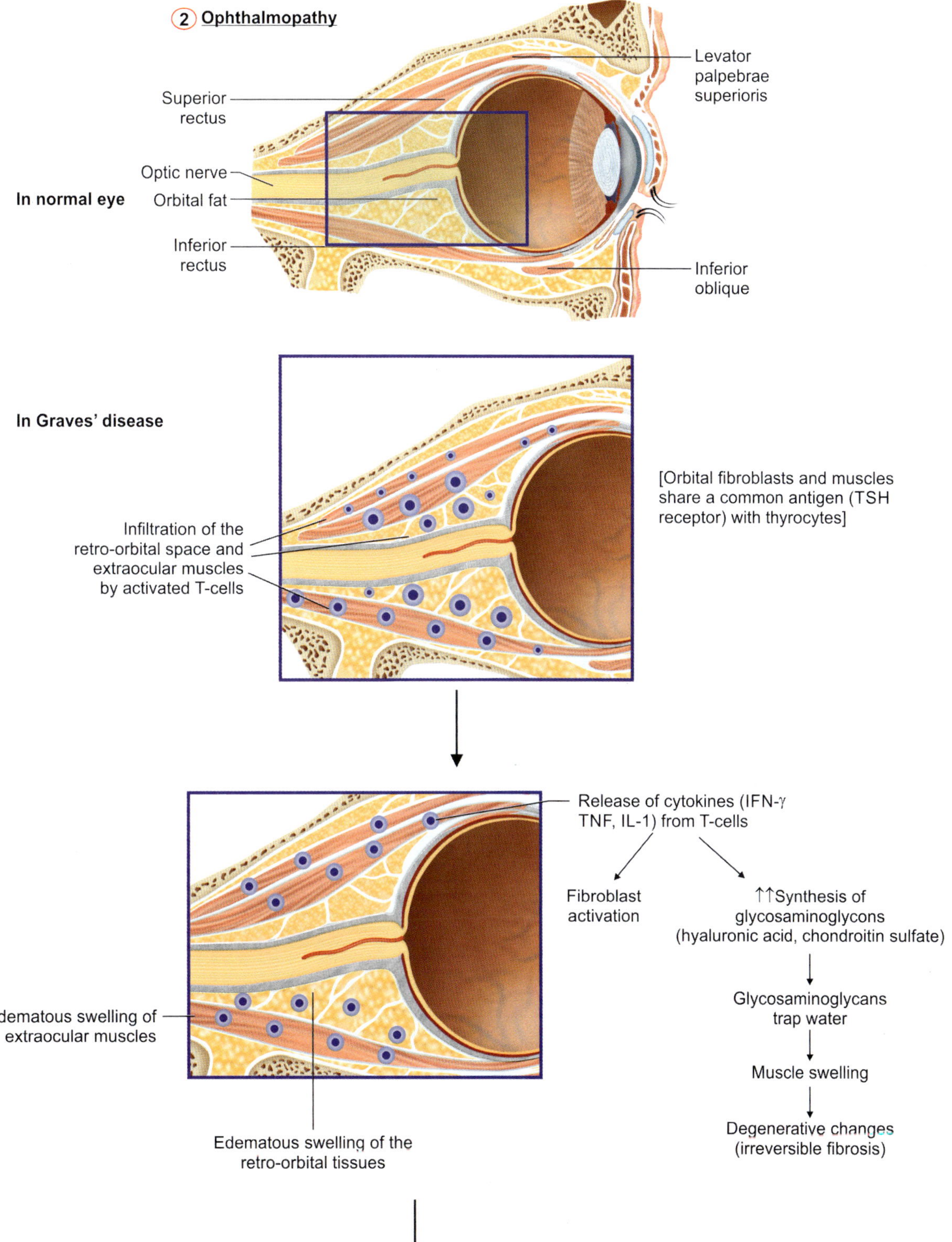
2 Ophthalmopathy
In normal eye
Superior rectus
Optic nerve
Orbital fat
Inferior rectus
Levator palpebrae superioris
Inferior oblique
In Graves' disease
Infiltration of the retro-orbital space and extraocular muscles by activated T-cells
[Orbital fibroblasts and muscles share a common antigen (TSH receptor) with thyrocytes]
Release of cytokines (IFN-γ TNF, IL-1) from T-cells
Fibroblast activation
↑↑Synthesis of glycosaminoglycons (hyaluronic acid, chondroitin sulfate)
Glycosaminoglycans trap water
Muscle swelling
Degenerative changes (irreversible fibrosis)
Edematous swelling of extraocular muscles
Edematous swelling of the retro-orbital tissues

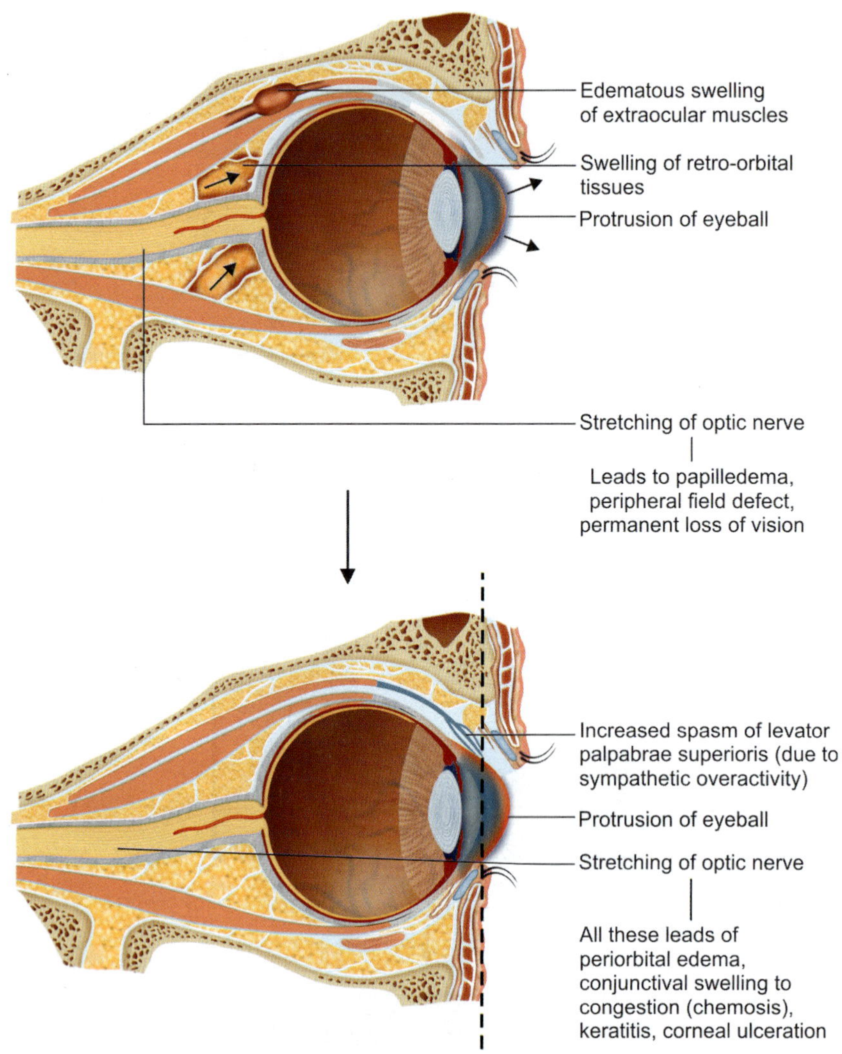

Other Clinical Manifestations

Symptoms

- Heat intolerance
- Increased sweating and thirst
- Increased appetite but weight loss
- Hyperactivity
- Palpitations
- Nervousness
- Diarrhea
- Oligomenorrhea or amenorrhea
- Swelling of the digits with clubbing (Thyroid acropachy)

Signs

Neurologic manifestations

- Fine tremor
- Muscle wasting
- Hyperreflexia
- Proximal myopathy without fasciculation

Cardiovascular manifestations

- Sinus tachycardia
- Atrial fibrillation
- Congestive cardiac failure.

Graves' Ophthalmopathy (Graves' Orbitopathy, Thyroid-associated Orbitopathy)

About half of the patients with Graves' disease have symptoms and/or signs of Graves' ophthalmopathy.

Two types of Graves' orbitopathy: (i) Type I (lipogenic) and (ii) Type II (myogenic). **Type I orbitopathy** is characterized by increase in orbital fat and soft tissue edema and more common in young women. **Type II orbitopathy** is characterized by extraocular muscle enlargement resulting in restrictive myopathy and compressive neuropathy and more common in males.

GO follows a biphasic course. Active phase persists for 18–36 months, followed by a stable or inactive phase.

The active phase is best described by **the Clinical Activity Score (CAS)**. One point is given for the presence of each of the parameters assessed. The sum of all patients defines clinical activity: active ophthalmopathy if the score is above 3/7 at the first examination or above 4/10 in successive examination.

For initial CAS, only score item 1–7

1. Spontaneous orbital pain
2. Gaze evoked orbital pain
3. Eyelid swelling that is considered to be due to active GO
4. Eyelid erythema
5. Conjunctival redness that is considered to be due to active GO
6. Chemosis
7. Inflammation of caruncle or plica

Patients assessed after follow-up (1–3 months) can be scored out of 10 by including items 8–10

8. Increase of >2 mm in proptosis
9. Decrease in unilocular ocular excursion in any one direction of >8 degree
10. Decrease of acuity equivalent to 1 Snellen line.

EUGOGO (European Group of Graves' Orbitopathy) classification of the severity of the ophthalmopathy

GO is classified as mild, moderate to severe and sight-threatening depending on the severity of ophthalmopathy.

(1) Mild: Characteristics of have a minimum impact on the patient's life, generally insufficient to justify immunosuppressive or surgical treatment. They usually present one or more of the following signs: (i) Minor lid retraction (<2 mm); (ii) Mild soft tissue involvement; (iii) Exophthalmos <3 mm (above the normal range for the race and gender); (iv) Transient or no diplopia; and (v) Corneal exposure responsive to lubricants.

(2) Moderate to severe: Patients without sight-threatening GO whose eye disease has sufficient impact on daily life to justify the risks of immunosuppression (if active) or surgical intervention (if inactive). Patients usually present one or more of the following signs: (i) Lid retraction (>2 mm); (ii) Moderate or severe soft tissue involvement; (iii) Exophthalmos ≥3 mm (above the normal range for the race and gender); and (iv) Inconstant, or constant diplopia.

(3) Sight-threatening GO: Patients with dysthyroid optic neuropathy or corneal breakdown due to severe exposure. This category warrants immediate intervention.

Exophthalmos is protrusion of eyes secondary to thyrotoxicosis.

Eye Signs

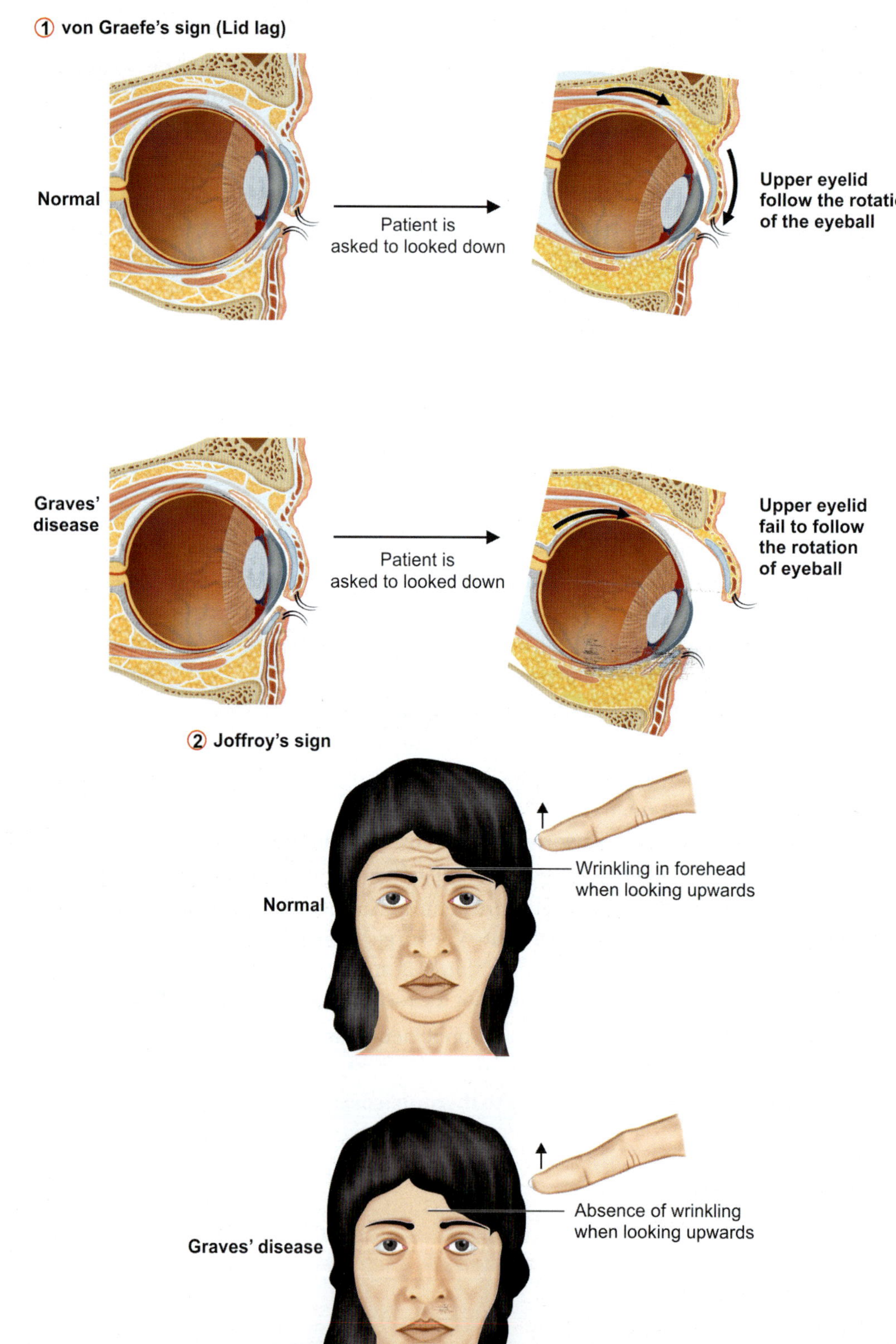

① von Graefe's sign (Lid lag)
Normal
Patient is
asked to looked down
Upper eyelid
follow the rotation
of the eyeball
Graves'
disease
Patient is
asked to looked down
Upper eyelid
fail to follow
the rotation
of eyeball
② Joffroy's sign
Normal
Wrinkling in forehead
when looking upwards
Graves' disease
Absence of wrinkling
when looking upwards

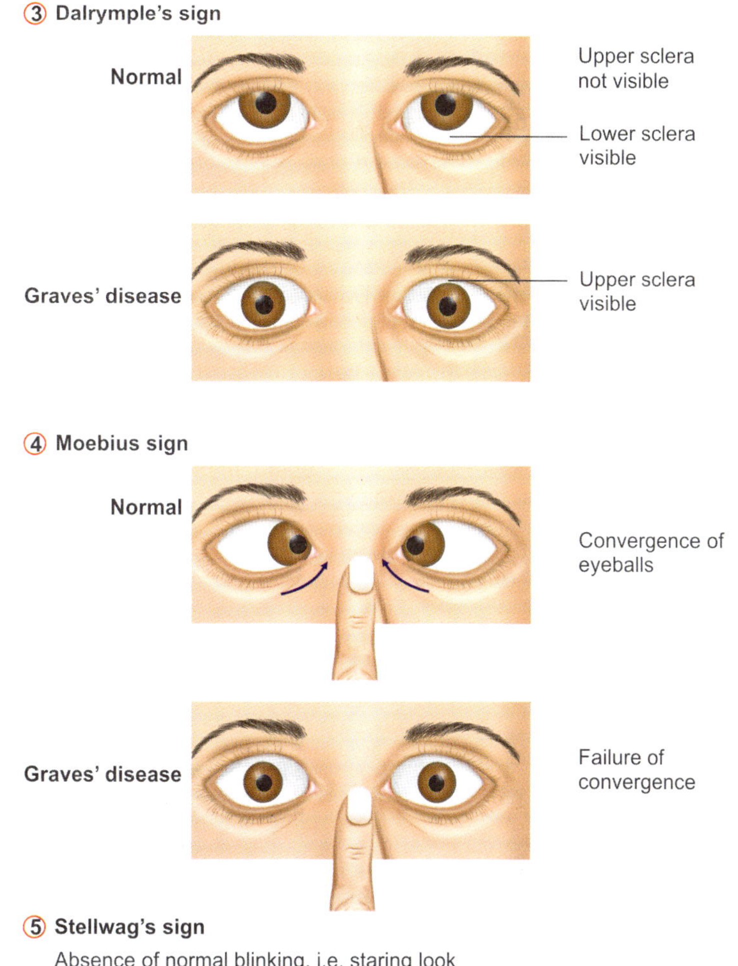

⑤ **Stellwag's sign**

Absence of normal blinking, i.e. staring look

> **Naffziger test:** A clinical method to evaluate proptosis or exophthalmos.
>
> **Exophthalmometer:** An instrument to measure proptosis.

Investigations

- Presence of **signs and symptoms of thyrotoxicosis, diffusely enlarged thyroid gland along** with **ophthalmopathy** and **biochemically confirmed thyrotoxicosis** (suppressed TSH with or without an elevated free T_4 or T_3) are diagnostic of Graves' disease.
- In the absence of ophthalmopathy, **a radionuclide scan** (^{99m}Tc, ^{123}I, ^{131}I) is indicated to confirm the diagnosis and to exclude other causes of hyperthyroidism. A diffuse, high uptake is diagnostic of Graves' disease.
- **Elevated thyroid-stimulating antibodies (TSAb)** is diagnostic of Graves' disease.
- If ophthalmopathy is present, **CT or MRI of the orbit** is indicated for evaluation.

Overt hyperthyroidism: Serum free T4 and T3 elevated, Serum TSH undetectable.

T3-toxicosis: Serum T4, free T4 normal; Serum T3 elevated; Serum TSH <0.01 mU/L (or undetectable).

Subclinical hyperthyroidism: Serum free T4, total T3 or free T3 normal; Serum TSH subnormal.

Euthyroid hyperthyroxinemia: Elevated serum total T4 and T3 but normal serum TSH, no clinical features of hyperthyroidism. This condition is due to elevated T4 binding globulin (TBG) or transthyretin (TTR).

Treatment

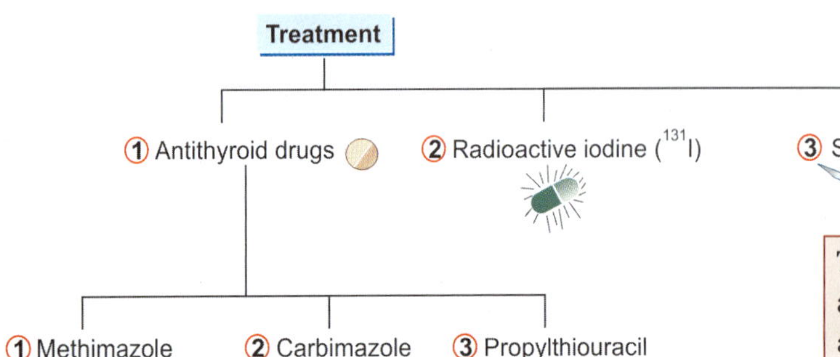

The three treatment options for Graves' disease are antithyroid drugs, Radioactive iodine (RAI) ablation and surgery.

Antithyroid Drugs

- The antithyroid drugs are **propylthiouracil, carbimazole,** and **methimazole** (active metabolite of carbimazole). All antithyroid drugs inhibit TPO, thereby oxidation and organification of iodide are reduced.
- **Propylthiouracil** also inhibits peripheral conversion of T_4 to T_3. This drug has a lower risk of transplacental transfer but increased risk of hepatotoxicity. Due to its hepatotoxicity, use of propylthiouracil as antithyroid drug is restricted except in certain situations, e.g., first trimester of pregnancy, thyroid storm management.
- **Dosage of carbimazole or methimazole** is 10–30 mg three times daily, once-daily after euthyroid state is achieved. **Dosage of propylthiouracil** is 100–200 mg three times daily. The dose should be titrated according to TSH and T_4 level. Euthyroid state is achieved after about 6–8 weeks of initiation of treatment.

Antithyroid drugs are favored in:

- Female patient with mild disease, small goiter, and negative or low-titer TRAb
- Patient with poor surgical risk or with limited life expectancy
- Moderate-to-severe active Graves' ophthalmopathy
- Previously operated or irradiated neck.

Antithyroid drugs are contraindicated in:

Past history of known major adverse reaction to antithyroid drugs.

Side effects of antithyroid drugs:

(i) Pruritic rash; (ii) Arthralgia; (iii) Fatigue; (iv) Fever; (v) Pharyngitis; (vi) Agranulocytosis; (vii) Hepatotoxicity; and (viii) Fulminant hepatic necrosis (in propylthiouracil).

Antithyroid drug should be stopped if major side effects, e.g., hepatitis, agranulocytosis, cholestasis, develops.

Management of agranulocytosis:

Urgent complete blood count should be advised if patient develops fever, sore throat, mouth ulcer. Patient needs immediate hospital admission, discontinuation of antithyroid drug, and broad-spectrum antibiotics.

Radioactive Iodine (RAI) Ablation Therapy

- Radioactive iodine ablation therapy includes administration of ^{131}**I isotope** as oral pill. This radioactive iodine is selectively taken up by thyroid tissue, resulting in progressive destruction of thyroid tissue.
- Antithyroid drug should be started at least 1 month before RAI to minimize the risk of thyrotoxic crisis after ablation therapy.
- Antithyroid drug should be stopped 3–5 days before starting ablation therapy to achieve optimum iodine uptake.
- Patients should avoid close and prolonged contact with children and pregnant women for 5–7 days to avoid transmission of radiation.

Side effects in babies born to mother taking methimazole:

- Aplasia cutis of the scalp
- Syndrome of Methimazole embryopathy (choanal atresia, esophageal atresia).

RAI ablation therapy is favored in:

- Poor surgical candidates
- Contraindications to use of antithyroid drugs
- Previously operated or externally irradiated neck.

RAI ablation therapy is contraindicated in:

- Pregnancy
- Lactation
- Planning pregnancy within 4–6 months
- Coexisting thyroid cancer, or suspicion of thyroid cancer.

Surgery

Surgery causes complete and permanent control of the disease with minimal morbidity. The recommended surgery for Graves' disease is total, near-total thyroidectomy or subtotal thyroidectomy.

Surgery is favored in:

- Presence of compressive symptoms
- Relative low uptake of radioactive iodine
- Suspected or diagnosed thyroid malignancy
- Planning pregnancy in <4–6 months
- Moderate to severe active Graves' ophthalmopathy
- Coexisting hyperparathyroidism requiring surgery.

Surgery is contraindicated in:

- Poor surgical candidates
- Pregnancy.

Total thyroidectomy is indicated in:

- Patient with coexistent thyroid cancer
- Patient with severe ophthalmopathy
- Patients who have life-threatening complications to antithyroid drugs.

Total thyroidectomy

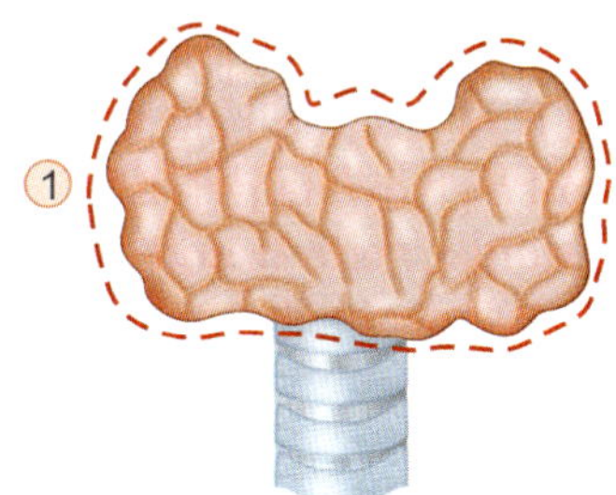

Subtotal thyroidectomy

Subtotal thyroidectomy (Hartley-Dunhill procedure)

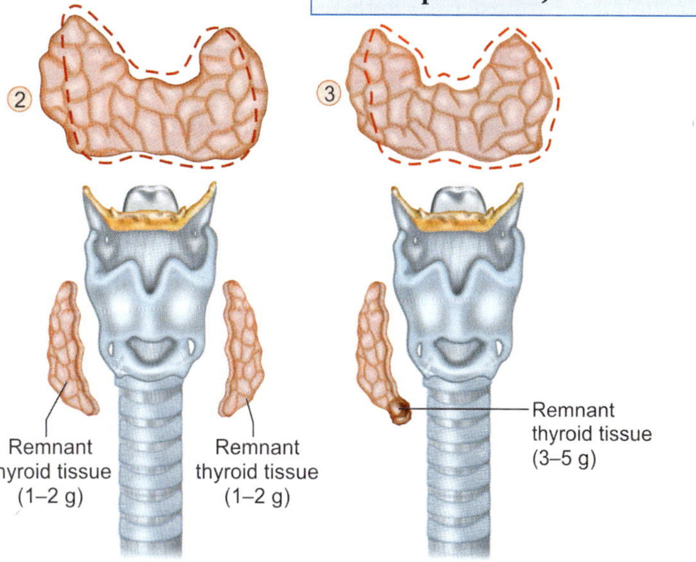

Preoperative Preparation of Patients with Graves' Disease for Thyroidectomy

- Thyrotoxic patients should be rendered euthyroid by antithyroid drugs before thyroidectomy (thyroid storm may be precipitated by surgery, anesthesia, thyroid manipulation).
- If surgery is urgent or antithyroid drugs are contraindicated, patient should be prepared with beta blockers and potassium iodide.
- Preoperative use of potassium iodide, saturated solution of potassium iodide (SSKI) or inorganic iodine decreases vascularity of thyroid gland and therefore decrease intraoperative blood loss. Potassium iodide is given as Lugol's solution (8 mg iodide/drop) 5–7 drops or SSKI (50 mg iodide/drop) 1–2 drops three times daily (mixed in water or juice) for 10 days before surgery.

Management of Graves' Ophthalmopathy

Patients with uncontrolled thyroid dysfunctions (both hypo and hyperthyroid state) are more likely to experience severe GO. Therefore, patient must be in euthyroid state.

Cessation of smoking: Smoking is associated with progression to more severe GO, impaired response to IV corticosteroids and immunosuppressant therapies.

General measures include use of artificial tears, sunglasses, sleeping with the head of the bed slightly elevated.

In mild ophthalmopathy, ^{131}I therapy with or without concurrent glucocorticoids.

In moderate to severe ophthalmopathy, immunosuppressive therapy (systemic corticosteroids or orbital radiation) for active disease and surgical intervention for inactive disease is indicated. Rehabilitative surgical procedures for inactive disease are orbital decompression (for disfiguring proptosis), strabismus surgery (for symptomatic ocular motility restriction), eyelid recession (for eyelid retraction), blepharoplasty (for excessive soft tissue prominence of the eyelids).

In sight-threatening ophthalmopathy due to dysthyroid optic neuropathy: Is treated with high-dose IV glucocorticoids, if no response, then orbital decompression. Corneal exposure keratopathy is treated by topical lubrication, botulinum toxin, levator recession surgery, tarsorrhaphy, or even orbital decompression.

Thyroid Storm

A life-threatening thyrotoxicosis characterized by multisystem involvement.

Precipitating factors: (i) Abrupt stoppage of antithyroid drugs; (ii) Thyroid or nonthyroid surgery in a undiagnosed or inadequately treated thyrotoxicosis patient; and (iii) Following radioactive iodine therapy.

Diagnosis: Precise criteria includes tachycardia, arrhythmia, congestive heart failure, hypotension, hyperpyrexia, agitation, delirium, psychosis, stupor, coma, nausea, vomiting, diarrhea, hepatic failure. In Point scale (Burch and Wartofsky, 1993), Score >45 indicates thyroid storm, score 25–44 is impending storm and score <25 indicates that storm is unlikely.

Treatment: (i) Early diagnosis and prompt intervention; (ii) Treatment should be in intensive care unit; (iii) Fluid resuscitation; and (iv) Aggressive cooling with cooling blankets and acetaminophen.

Treatment is based on– (i) Immediate blockade of thyroid hormone synthesis (by high doses of antithyroid drugs); (ii) Blockade of release of hormones (by inorganic iodide); (iii) Blockade of T4 into T3 conversion (by high-dose propylthiouracil, propranolol, corticosteroids); and (iv) Inhibition of peripheral effects of excess thyroid hormone (by propranolol, esmolol, metoprolol).

Toxic Multinodular Goiter

Toxic multinodular goiter is also known as **plummer disease**. It is the second most common cause of thyrotoxicosis. This disease commonly occur in older individuals and has a female preponderance.

Pathophysiology

One or more nodules become autonomous resulting in secretion of thyroid hormones, but how they become autonomous still unknown. Recent exposure to iodinated contrast media or amiodarone may precipitate thyrotoxicosis.

Clinical Manifestations

Patients commonly present with subclinical hyperthyroidism, but may present with palpitation, tremor, tachycardia, atrial fibrillation, congestive heart failure.

Investigations

Thyroid function test shows suppressed TSH level with elevated T_4 or T_3. Thyroid antibodies including TRAb is indicated to exclude Graves' disease and to detect coexisting autoimmune thyroiditis.

Radioiodine scan is indicated to identify the nodules with increased and decreased uptake.

Ultrasound is indicated to characterize any discrete nodule with decreased uptake ("cold nodule") and FNA may be required based on sonographic findings.

Treatment

Treatment options are RAI, surgery and antithyroid drugs. Antithyroid drugs are not preferred except in elderly and otherwise ill patients with limited life expectancy.

RAI is the treatment of choice but dose of radiation is higher than Graves' disease because of decreased uptake.

Total or near-total thyroidectomy is the recommended surgical option for toxic multinodular goiter. Preoperative treatment with antithyroid drugs with or without beta blockers is indicated before surgery. SSKI and Lugol's solution are not indicated because they induce hyperthyroidism from Jod-Basedow phenomenon.

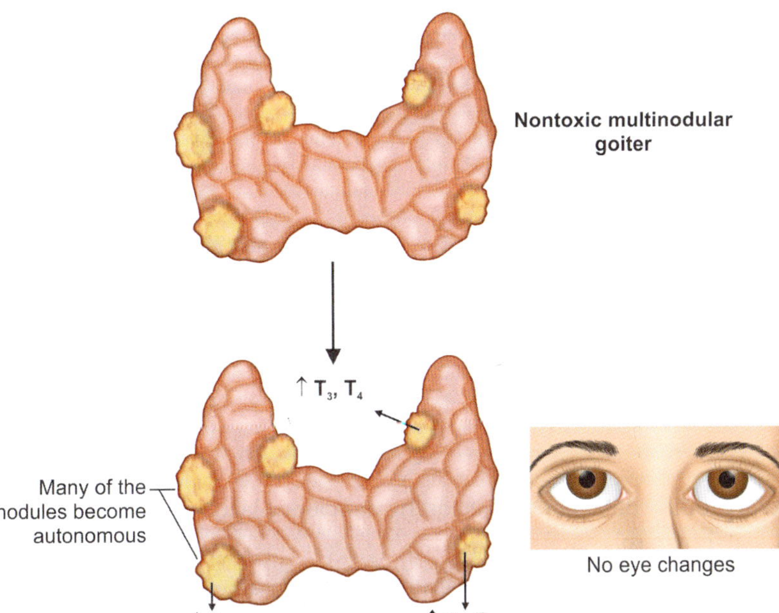

Jod-Basedow Phenomenon

Also known as iodine-induced hyperthyroidism, is a rare cause of thyrotoxicosis. It usually develops after exogenous administration of iodine.

Wolff-Chaikoff Effect

Excess amount of ingested iodine inhibits thyroid hormone synthesis by inhibiting the organification of iodine.

Toxic Adenoma

Toxic adenoma is autonomously functioning solitary thyroid nodule.

Pathophysiology

Somatic mutation in TSH receptor (TSH-R) gene resulting in stimulation of TSH-R signaling pathway. These result in enhanced follicular cell proliferation and function.

Clinical manifestations

Clinical features include solitary thyroid nodule with mild thyrotoxicosis.

Investigations

Thyroid function test shows suppressed TSH level with elevated T_4 or T_3. Thyroid scan reveals "hot nodule" with decreased uptake in the remaining gland.

Treatment

The treatment options are RAI or thyroidectomy. Radioiodine ablation is preferred because radioactive iodine is mostly concentrated in the hyperfunctioning nodule with minimal uptake by surrounding tissue. Lobectomy with isthmusectomy is the surgery of choice and preferred in young patients. Percutaneous ethanol injection and radiofrequency ablation are other treatment options.

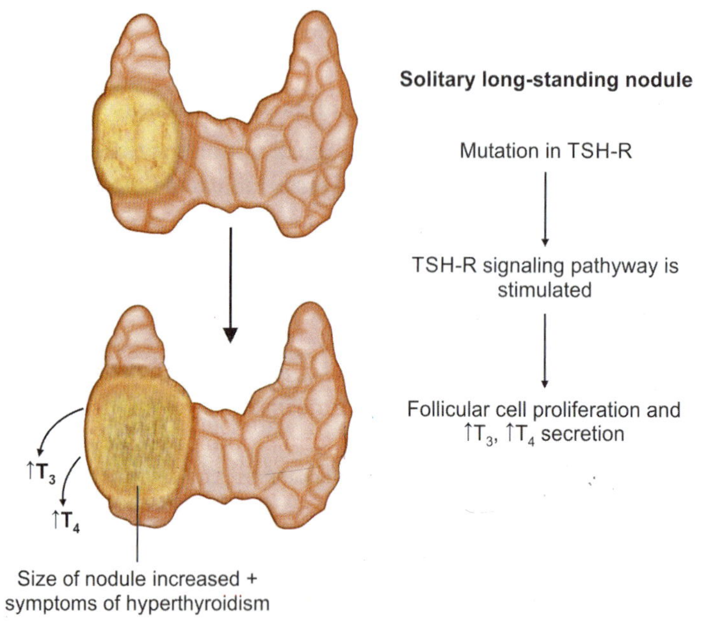

Diffuse Nontoxic Goiter

Diffuse nontoxic goiter is also called **colloid goiter** due to presence of colloid-distended follicles. It is more common in women.

Etiopathology

Colloid goiter is most commonly caused by dietary iodine deficiency. This iodine deficiency leads to persistent TSH stimulation of the gland, resulting in diffuse follicular hyperplasia.

Colloid goiter is also caused by environmental goitrogens, e.g., cassava root, cruciferous vegetables (Brussels sprouts, cauliflower, cabbage).

Clinical Manifestations

Most of the patients with diffuse goiter are asymptomatic except a symmetrically enlarged, nontender, soft thyroid swelling. A large goiter or substernal goiter may cause symptoms.

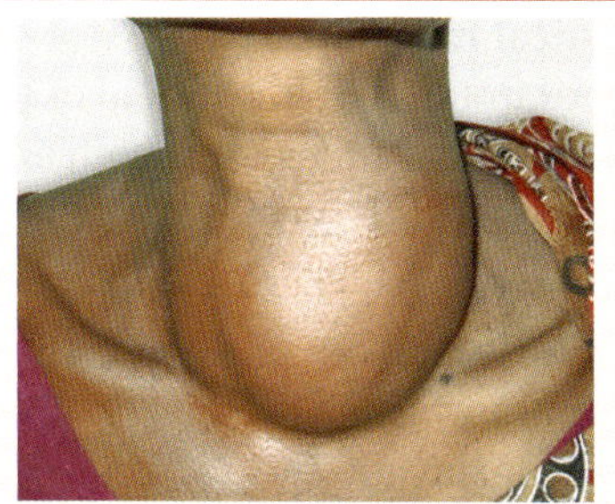

Thyroid swelling.

Investigations

Thyroid function test commonly reveals low total T_4 with normal T_3 and TSH. USG of thyroid is indicated to rule out presence of any nodule. CT or MRI of neck is indicated in substernal goiter or in any patient presenting with compressive symptoms.

Treatment

Treatment options include TSH-suppressive therapy, RAI ablation and thyroidectomy. TSH-suppressive therapy with thyroxine is particularly indicated in small goiters. RAI ablation is a preferred treatment option where surgical resources are limited. Surgery (Subtotal or near-total or total thyroidectomy) is indicated if; (i) Substernal goiter; (ii) Presence of compressive symptoms; (iii) Presence of nodules; and (iv) Patient wants surgery.

Nontoxic Multinodular Goiter

Nontoxic multinodular goiter occurs in both iodine-deficient and in regions with iodine sufficiency. This goiter is more common in women.

Pathophysiology

The etiology of most of the multinodular goiters are not known.

Clinical Presentations

Most of the patients are asymptomatic. Large goiter may cause difficulty in swallowing, difficulty in respiration (due to tracheal compression).

Investigations

Thyroid function test commonly reveals normal total T_4 with normal T_3 and TSH. USG is indicated to characterize the nodules and to decide which nodule should be biopsied by FNA. CT or MRI is indicated for large goiter to exclude substernal extension and to evaluate the extent of tracheal compression.

Treatment

Radioiodine ablation therapy is very much effective by selectively ablating the autonomous nodules. Surgery is another treatment option if patient not responding to radioiodine ablation therapy.

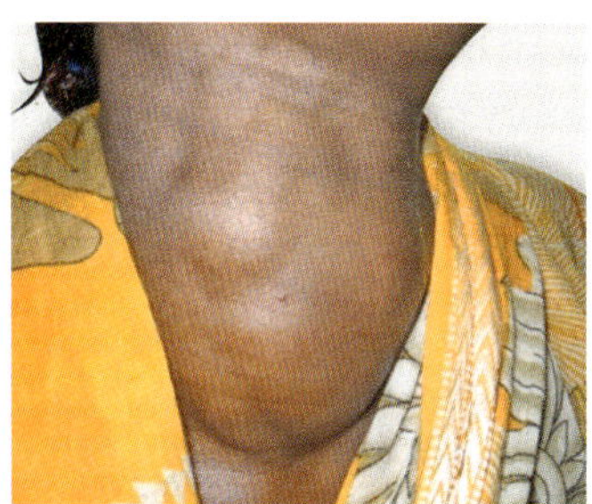

Multinodular goiter.

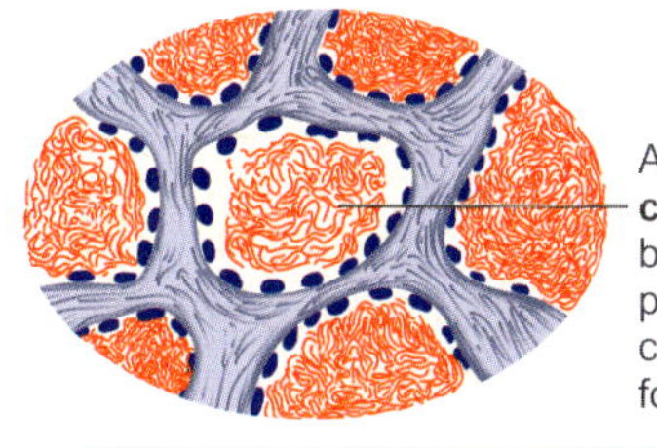

Histology of diffuse goiter.

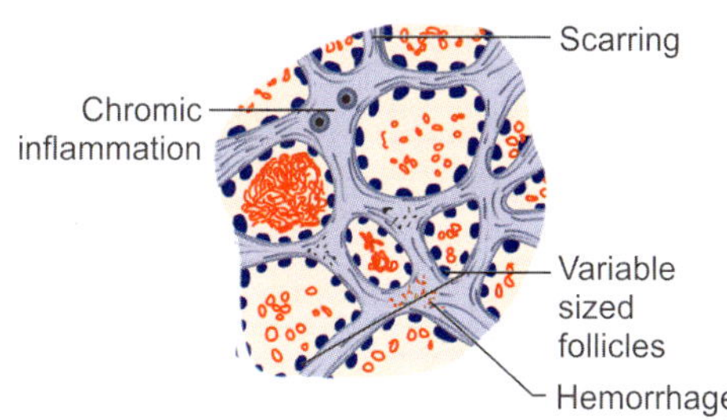

Histology of multinodular goiter.

Substernal Goiter

Substernal or retrosternal goiter is defined as goiter with a significant proportion of its mass lies inferior to the thoracic inlet.

Subtypes: (i) Goiter extends into the anterior mediastinum (most common); (ii) Goiter extends posteriorly to the trachea, recurrent laryngeal nerve, great vessels; and (iii) Isolated mediastinal goiter (least common). Most of the substernal goiter found in fifth decades of life with female predominance.

Clinical manifestations: Most of the patients present with cervical mass, dyspnea, stridor, dysphagia, hoarseness. On examination, lower pole of thyroid cannot be palpated and pemberton sign (appearance of facial flushing and dilated veins after raising both arms) may be present.

Investigations: Workup for substernal goiter is same as cervical goiter. Chest CT is particularly indicated to assess the extension of substernal goiter and its compression effect on adjacent structures.

Treatment: Most of the substernal goiters can be resected via standard cervical approach. Partial or total median sternotomy is required if goiter extends into the posterior mediastinum or extends inferiorly to the aortic arch, goiter crossing the midline.

Thyroid Nodule

A thyroid nodule is a discrete lesion within the thyroid gland that is radiologically distinct from the surrounding thyroid parenchyma (ATA guideline).

History includes: (i) Head and neck radiation therapy in childhood; (ii) Total body radiation for bone marrow transplantation; (iii) History of familial thyroid carcinoma; (iv) Any rapid growth of nodule; and (v) Hoarseness of voice.

Physical examination includes: (i) Examination of neck to search for cervical lymphadenopathy and (ii) Examination of the nodule.

Diagnostic workup and management:

- Initially, **serum TSH evaluation** should be done in any patients with **solitary thyroid nodule more than 1 cm** in any diameter.
- **Radionuclide thyroid scan** is indicated if serum TSH level is subnormal. Based on thyroid scan, thyroid nodules are classified into **hot, warm, and cold nodule**. No cytological evaluation is required for hot nodule. If serum TSH is normal or elevated, USG of thyroid is indicated.
- Based on sonographic pattern and size of the nodule, **decision of FNA** is taken.
- If sonographic pattern is 'high suspicion' or 'Intermediate suspicion', then FNA is indicated for nodule size 1 cm or more. If sonographic pattern is 'Low suspicion', then FNA is indicated for nodule size 1.5 cm or more. For 'Very low suspicion' pattern, size cutoff is 2 cm or more. FNA is not required for 'Benign' sonographic pattern.
- Based on thyroid cytopathology (The Bethesda system), decisions of further interventions (e.g., repeat FNA, molecular profiling tests, surgery) are taken.
- For **cytologically nondiagnostic nodule**, repeat FNA with USG-guidance is indicated. Surgery may be considered for this category if 'high suspicion' sonographic pattern is present during US surveillance or clinical risk factors for malignancy are present.
- For nodules of '**Benign' category**, no further diagnostic workup or treatment is indicated.
- For **'Malignant' category**, surgery is recommended.

Types of Thyroid Nodule Based on Radionuclide Thyroid Scan

Hot nodule: Tracer uptake is greater than surrounding normal thyroid tissue.

Warm nodule: Tracer uptake is same as surrounding thyroid tissue.

Cold nodule: Tracer uptake less than the surrounding thyroid tissue.

Sonographic Pattern of Thyroid Nodule (Adapted from ATA Classification)

High suspicion: Solid hypoechoic nodule or solid hypoechoic component of a partially cystic nodule with one or more of the following features: irregular margins (infiltrative, microlobulated), microcalcifications, taller than wide shape, rim calcifications with small extrusive soft tissue component, evidence of extrathyroidal extension.

Intermediate suspicion: Hypoechoic solid nodule with smooth margins without microcalcifications, extrathyroidal extension, or taller than wide shape.

Low suspicion: Isoechoic or hyperechoic solid nodule, or partially cystic nodule with eccentric solid areas, without microcalcification, irregular margin or extrathyroidal extension, or taller than wide shape.

Very low suspicion: Spongiform or partially cystic nodules without any of the sonographic features described in low, intermediate, or high suspicion patterns.

Benign: Purely cystic nodules (no solid component).

Management of Nodule with Indeterminate Cytology

- For nodules with indeterminate cytology [Atypia of undetermined significance (AUS) or follicular lesion of undetermined significance (FLUS), follicular neoplasm (FN), or suspicious for a follicular neoplasm (SFN), suspicious for malignancy (SUSP)], molecular profiling tests are recommended.
- Recommended molecular profiling tests are:
  - 7-Gene MT panel [a panel of mutations (BRAF, N-/H-/K-RAS) and for translocations of the RET/PTC and PAX8/PPAR/genes]
  - A gene expression classifier (167 GEC; mRNA expression of 167 genes).
- No single optimal molecular test can definitively rule in or rule out malignancy in all cases of indeterminate cytology.
- Role of surgery in cytologically indeterminate thyroid nodule: (i) To establish a histological diagnosis and (ii) Definitive removal of nodule.
- Surgical options: (i) Lobectomy (hemithyroidectomy) with or without isthmusectomy; (ii) Near-total thyroidectomy; and (iii) Total thyroidectomy.

The Bethesda System for Reporting Thyroid Cytopathology

Diagnostic category	Estimated/predicted risk of malignancy by the Bethesda system (%)
Nondiagnostic or unsatisfactory	1–4
Benign	0–3
Atypia of undetermined significance (AUS) or follicular lesion of undetermined significance (FLUS)	5–15
Follicular neoplasm or suspicious for a follicular neoplasm	15–30
Suspicious for malignancy	60–75
Malignant	97–99

ACR-TIRADS (American College of Radiology Thyroid Imaging Reporting and Data System) is a scoring system of USG reporting of thyroid nodules with recommendations for when to use FNA or followup. **The scoring system is based on certain sonographic features:** (i) Composition; (ii) Echogenicity; (iii) Shape; (iv) Margin; and (v) Echogenic foci.

Composition
(Choose 1)
Cystic or almost completely cystic
0 point
Spongiform
0 point
Mixed cystic and solid
1 point
Solid or almost completely solid
2 points

Echogenicity
(Choose 1)
Anechoic
0 point
Hyperechoic or isoechoic
1 point
Hypoechoic
2 points
Very hypoechoic
3 points

Shape
(Choose 1)
Wider than tall
0 point
Taller than wide
3 points

Margin
(Choose 1)
Smooth
0 point
Ill-defined
0 point
Lobulated or irregular
2 points
Extrathyroidal extension
3 points

Echogenic foci
(Choose all that apply)
None or large comet-tail artifacts
0 point
Microcalcification
1 point
Peripheral (rim) calcifications
2 points
Punctate echogenic foci
3 points

Points from all categories are added to determine TI-RADS level.

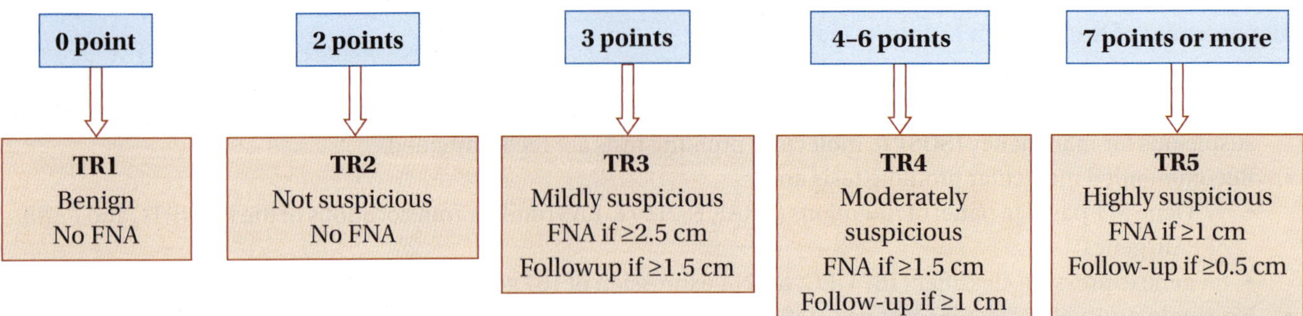

Thyroiditis

Acute (Suppurative) Thyroiditis

- A rare type of thyroiditis but potentially life-threatening condition. Most commonly caused by gram-positive aerobic bacterial infection.
- More common in children, mostly due to presence of a pyriform sinus (a remnant of the fourth branchial pouch that connects the oropharynx with the thyroid).
- Patients present with severe neck pain radiating to the jaws or ear, fever, odynophagia, and dysphonia.
- White cell count and ESR are raised, but thyroid profile is normal.
- FNA shows neutrophilic infiltration.
- CT scan is helpful to delineate the extent of infection.
- Treatment is parenteral antibiotics and drainage of abscess.

If pyriform sinus fistula is detected, the fistula tract must be resected including the area of thyroid attachment.

Thyroid gland is resistant to infection because:

- Extensive blood and lymphatic supply
- High iodine content
- Fibrous capsule around the gland that protects the gland from infection of other adjacent neck structures.

Pyriform sinus fistula begins at the apex of pyriform sinus, coursed anteroinferiorly through the thyroid gland into the perithyroidal space. This fistula is almost always in the left side.

Subacute Thyroiditis

Subacute Lymphocytic Thyroiditis (Silent Thyroiditis)

Subacute Granulomatous (de Quervain's thyroiditis) Thyroiditis

Pathophysiology: It is most likely caused by viral infection (mumps, coxsackie, influenza, adenovirus, and echovirus) or postviral inflammatory process.

Clinical manifestation: Sudden onset or chronic onset neck pain radiating towards mandible or ear is the cardinal symptom of subacute thyroiditis. History of a preceding upper respiratory tract infection is often present.

The thyroid gland is tender and become enlarged.

The disease progresses through 3 stages: (i) Thyrotoxic phase; (ii) Hypothyroid stage; and (iii) Recovery phase.

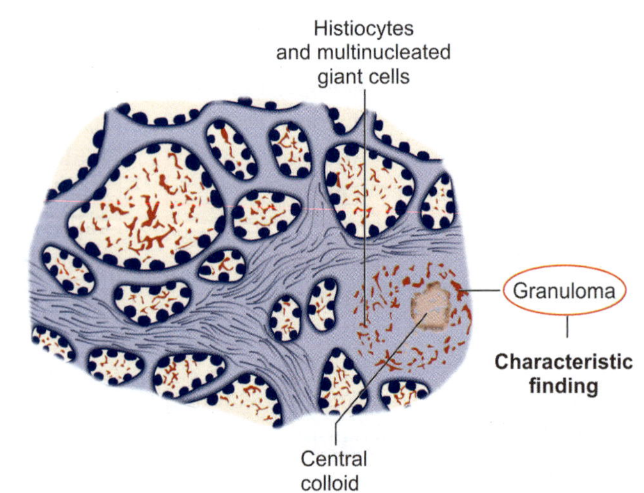

This disorder progresses through three stages:

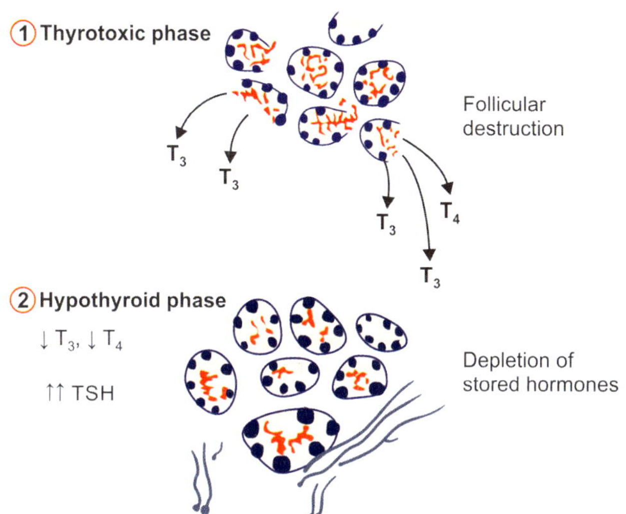

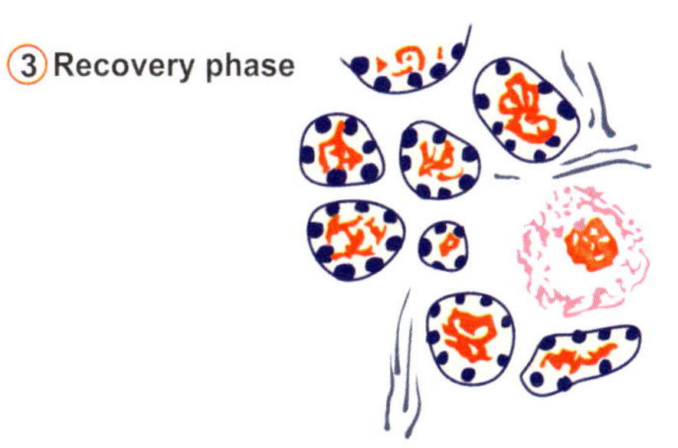

Treatment

- The disease is self-limited, so symptomatic treatment is all that needed.
- Aspirin or NSAIDs are usually indicated to control pain.
- If patient has marked local or systemic symptoms, steroid is indicated.
- Levothyroxine replacement (in low dose) may be necessary if hypothyroid phase is prolonged.

Antithyroid drugs have no role in treatment of thyrotoxic phase.

Subacute Lymphocytic Thyroiditis

- This disease is most likely autoimmune in etiology.
- It may occur sporadically or in the postpartum period (3-6 months after pregnancy)-**postpartum thyroiditis**.
- It also progresses through three stages: (i) Thyrotoxic phase; (ii) Hypothyroid phase; and (iii) Resolution phase.
- Clinical examination reveals a normal or minimally enlarged nontender thyroid gland.
- Thyroxine replacement is indicated in hypothyroid phase and propranolol, if severe thyrotoxic symptoms are present.

Silent thyroiditis can be distinguished from de Quervain's thyroiditis by:

- Painless goiter
- Normal ESR
- Presence of TPO antibodies.

Chronic Lymphocytic (Hashimoto) Thyroiditis

Hashimoto thyroiditis is the most common cause of hypothyroidism in world where iodine levels are sufficient.

It is a autoimmune thyroiditis characterized by **'3' cardinal features**:

1. Diffuse enlargement of thyroid
2. Lymphocytic infiltration of thyroid
3. Presence of thyroid autoantibodies

Pathophysiology

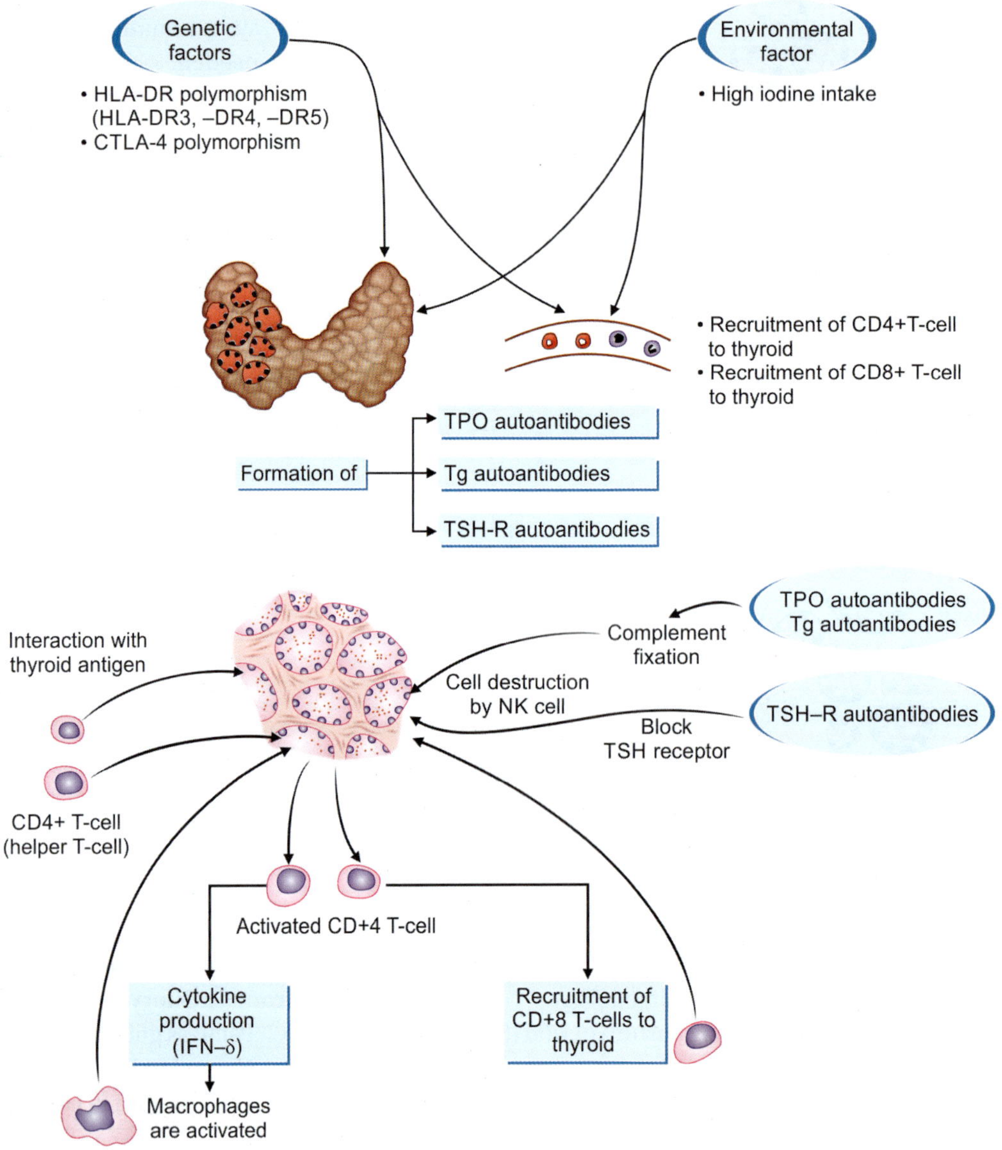

Genetic factors
• HLA-DR polymorphism (HLA-DR3, –DR4, –DR5)
• CTLA-4 polymorphism
Environmental factor
• High iodine intake
• Recruitment of CD4+T-cell to thyroid
• Recruitment of CD8+ T-cell to thyroid
Formation of
TPO autoantibodies
Tg autoantibodies
TSH-R autoantibodies
TPO autoantibodies Tg autoantibodies
Complement fixation
Cell destruction by NK cell
TSH–R autoantibodies
Block TSH receptor
Interaction with thyroid antigen
CD4+ T-cell (helper T-cell)
Activated CD+4 T-cell
Cytokine production (IFN–δ)
Recruitment of CD+8 T-cells to thyroid
Macrophages are activated

Microscopic Appearance

Lymphoid cell infiltration
Lymphoid follicle with germinal center
Hurthle cell
(Follicular epithelial cells are transformed to cells that contain large number of mitochondria and large bizarre nuclei)
Colloid deficient follicles
Also called
'Oxyphil cell or Askanazy cell'

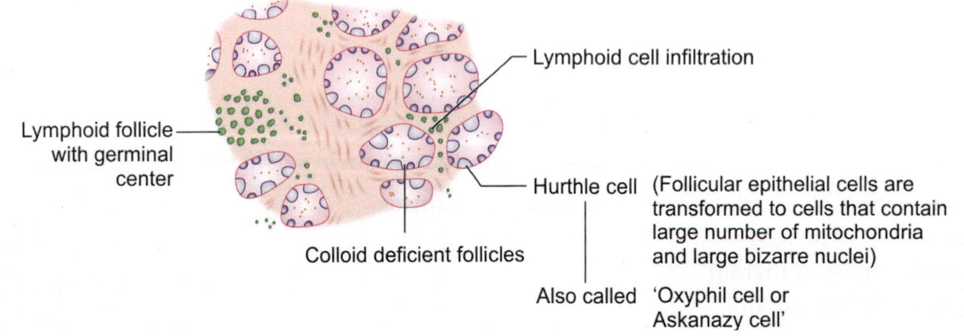

Clinical Presentation

- More common in women (10:1) between 30 and 50 years of age.
- Most commonly presented as painless diffuse enlargement of thyroid, usually associated with hypothyroidism.
- In some patients, it may be preceded by transient thyrotoxicosis due to disruption of thyroid follicles (Hashitoxicosis).

Investigations

- Elevated TSH with low T_3 and T_4, presence of thyroid autoantibodies confirm the diagnosis.
- FNA is indicated in patient presents with solitary suspicious nodule or rapidly enlarging goiter.

Autoimmune diseases that may be associated with Hashimoto thyroiditis:

- Type I diabetes mellitus
- Addison's disease
- Pernicious anemia
- Vitiligo.

Treatment

- Thyroxine replacement therapy should be initiated in patients with overt hypothyroidism (elevated TSH and low free T_4).
- Replacement therapy is particularly indicated when TSH >10 mu/L or in euthyroid patients with large goiter.
- Surgery is indicated for suspicion of malignancy, for pressure symptoms and cosmetic reason.

Riedel's Thyroiditis (Invasive Fibrous Thyroiditis)

- A rare type of thyroiditis.
- Etiology is unknown, but most likely this disease is a part of multifocal idiopathic fibrosclerosis.
- Patients present with hard, nontender, asymmetric goiter with pressure symptoms (dysphagia, dyspnea, dysphonia).
- Usually FNA biopsy is inadequate, the diagnosis is confirmed by open biopsy.
- Surgery is the treatment. The goal of surgical intervention is to decompress the trachea by excision of isthmus. More extensive resections are not attempted because extensive fibrosis obscures anatomical landmarks and structures.

Components of Multifocal Idiopathic Fibrosclerosis

- Retro-orbital fibrosis
- Riedel's thyroiditis
- Mediastinal fibrosis
- Sclerosing cholangitis
- Idiopathic retroperitoneal fibrosis.

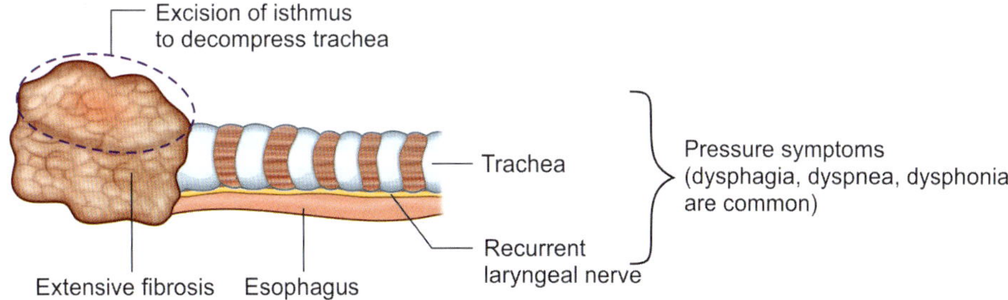

Thyroid Neoplasms

Follicular Adenoma

- **Most common benign thyroid neoplasm.**
- This neoplasm is derived from follicular epithelium.
- The TSH receptor signaling pathway plays an important role in the pathogenesis of adenoma.
- A typical thyroid adenoma is a solitary, spherical lesion that compresses adjacent normal tissue.
- Clinically, most adenomas present as painless nodules.
- **FNA cannot differentiate between follicular adenoma and follicular carcinoma**. Follicular adenoma is diagnosed after lobectomy for follicular neoplasia detected by FNA.
- Lobectomy with isthmusectomy is the treatment of follicular adenoma. No follow up is necessary.

Histological types of follicular adenoma:

- Microfollicular adenoma
- Macrofollicular adenoma
- Normofollicular adenoma
- Trabecular adenoma
- Hürthle cell adenoma
- Atypical adenoma.

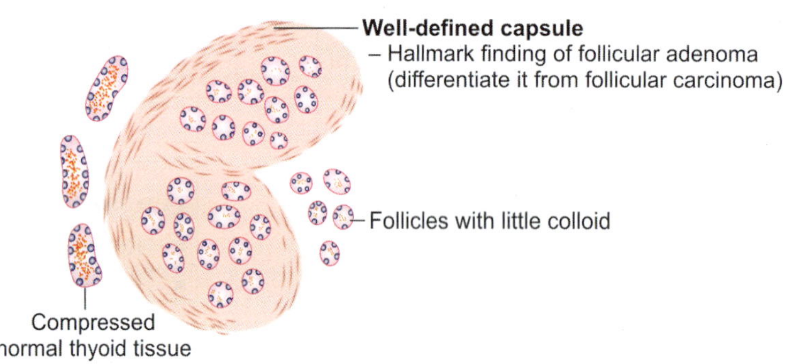

Malignant Neoplasms of Thyroid

Malignant tumors of thyroid is classified into **primary thyroid malignancy** and **secondary thyroid malignancy**. About 95% of all primary thyroid malignancies are **carcinomas**. Primary lymphoma constitutes <5% of malignancies. Most of them evolve from autoimmune thyroiditis. Sarcoma is extremely rare. Secondary thyroid malignancies (most commonly from renal cell carcinoma) are also rare.

Follicular cells: (i) Form the lining of colloid follicles; (ii) Produce thyroid hormones; and (iii) Concentrate iodine.

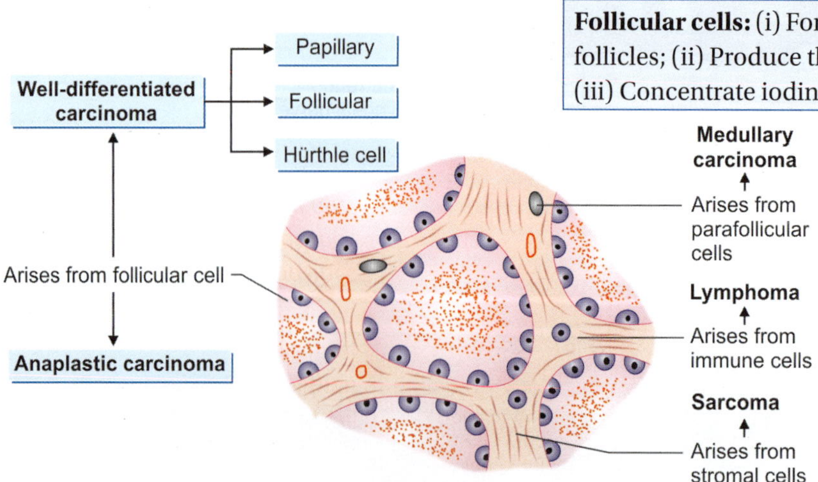

Pathogenesis of Primary Thyroid Malignancy

Radiation: Differentiated thyroid carcinoma, particularly papillary carcinoma follows radiation exposure of neck in childhood. Radiation derived from ^{131}I therapy may contribute minimal increased risk of carcinoma.

TSH and growth factor: Many differentiated thyroid cancers express TSH receptors. The incidence of follicular carcinoma is high in endemic goitrous areas, particularly due to TSH stimulation. Anaplastic carcinoma is also associated with iodine deficiency.

Oncogenes and tumor-suppressor gene: Distinct mutations are seen in different histologic types.

- *Papillary carcinoma:* Mutation in RET protooncogene (located on chromosome 10)
- Gene rearrangement in *NTRK1* gene.
- *Follicular carcinoma:* Mutation in RAS oncogenes (HRAS, NRAS, and KRAS).
- *Medullary carcinoma:* Point mutation in RET-protooncogene.
- *Anaplastic carcinoma:* Inactivation of point mutation in p53 tumor suppressor gene
- Mutation in gene coding for β-catenin pathway.

Radiation-induced thyroid carcinoma:

- Papillary carcinoma is most commonly associated with radiation-induced thyroid carcinoma.
- Children, certain Jewish population and patients with family history of thyroid carcinoma are at increased risk.
- Radiation-induced papillary carcinoma is more aggressive and associated with high recurrence rate.

Differentiated thyroid carcinomas can concentrate iodine, express TSH receptor, and produce thyroglobulin, whereas **poorly differentiated or undifferentiated carcinomas** do not.

Prognostic Systems in Differentiated Thyroid Cancer

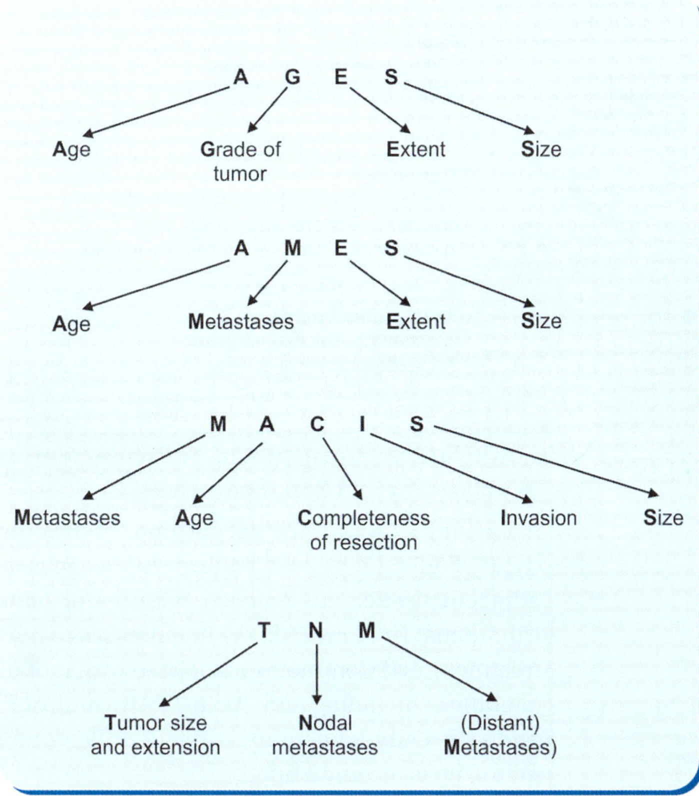

Risk Stratification

Low Risk

- <55 years
- Tumor size <2 cm
- Female
- No local extension, intrathyroidal, no capsular invasion
- No metastasis
- Well-differentiated.

High Risk

- >55 years
- Tumor size >4 cm
- Male
- Extrathyroidal extension, capsular invasion
- Regional/distant metastases
- Poorly differentiated.

Papillary Thyroid Carcinoma

- Most common type of thyroid cancer, constitutes about 70–90% of well-differentiated thyroid malignancies.
- Predominant thyroid cancer in individuals exposed to external radiation in neck during childhood.
- More common in females (2:1), mean age at presentation is 30–40 years.
- Slow growing malignant tumor, tends to be multifocal.
- Propensity to spread by lymphatics, leads to involvement of regional lymph nodes.
- Most of the patients are euthyroid.
- Hematogenous spread is not so common, metastases is most common in lungs followed by bone, liver, and brain.

Differentiated thyroid carcinomas can concentrate iodine, express TSH receptor, and **produce thyroglobulin, whereas poorly differentiated or undifferentiated carcinomas** do not.

'Microcarcinoma'

- Papillary thyroid carcinomas smaller than 1 cm are termed as **'microcarcinomas' or 'incidentalomas'**.
- These type of PTCs are typically diagnosed after surgery for benign thyroid pathologies.
- These PTCs are less commonly associated with recurrence and distant metastases.

Slow growing malignant tumor, tends to be multifocal

Propensity to spread by lymphatics, leads to involvement of regional lymph nodes

Microscopic Appearance

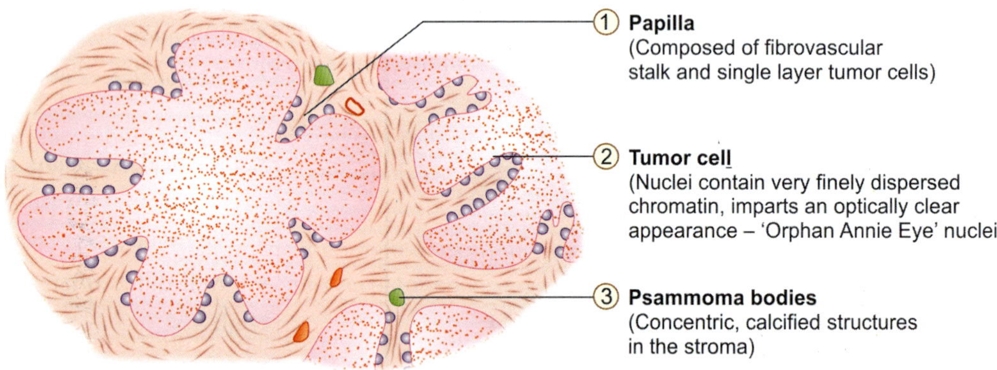

Papillary Carcinoma with High-risk Histopathology

- Tall cell
- Insula
- Hobnail
- Columnar
- Diffuse sclerosing
- Trabecular
- Solid
- Poorly differentiated.

Noninvasive Encapsulated Follicular Variant of Papillary Thyroid Carcinoma (NIFTP)

A variant of papillary carcinoma, characterized by: (i) Follicular growth pattern; (ii) No invasion of adjacent tissue; (iii) Nuclear features of papillary carcinoma; (iv) Low risk; (v) Requires less aggressive treatment; (vi) Commonly associated with mutations/alterations including RAS, PAX8/PPARγ, and/or BRAF; and (vii) Only lobectomy is needed. Postoperative follow-up is recommended.

Clinical Presentation

Most of the patients present with a painless mass in the neck, either in the thyroid or as metastasis in cervical lymph node (in about 20–50% patients). Locally invasive tumors may present with progressive dysphagia, dyspnea, voice change.

Investigations

- USG of the neck, including the thyroid and the central and lateral compartment of the neck is recommended imaging modality. USG is helpful to assess the size of the tumor, can assess the status of cervical lymph nodes (both palpable and nonpalpable). USG-guided FNA should be considered for sonographically suspicious lymph nodes ≥8–10 mm. Tg washout assay may be considered as an adjunct to FNA biopsy if cytology is negative.
- **FNA biopsy** can confirm the diagnosis of papillary carcinoma as well as metastasis in cervical lymph node.
- **Contrast-enhanced CT or MRI of neck is indicated if**: (i) Swelling is fixed, bulky; (ii) USG shows extrathyroidal extension especially with posterior capsular extension and extension into mediastinum; and (iii) Bulky neck nodes.
- **Assessment of vocal cord** by indirect laryngoscopy, fiberoptic laryngoscopy should be considered in patients with voice change, invasive disease, bulky disease of the central compartment.
- Routine preoperative assessment of **serum thyroglobulin** is not recommended.

Treatment

- Primary treatment is surgery.
- **Lobectomy plus isthmusectomy** should be the surgical procedure for tumor <1 cm without extrathyroidal extension and without cervical lymph node metastases.

Lobectomy plus isthmusectomy may be considered if tumor size is more than 1 cm and less than 4 cm, extrathyroidal extension is absent and without clinical evidence of cervical lymph node metastases. In patients who undergo lobectomy plus isthmusectomy for papillary carcinoma, **completion thyroidectomy** is recommended for any one of the following factors: (i) Tumor >4 cm; (ii) Positive resection margin; (iii) Gross extrathyroidal extension; and (iv) Vascular invasion. **Total thyroidectomy is recommended with any one of the following factors:** (i) Tumor >4 cm in diameter; (ii) Poorly differentiated histology; (iii) Extrathyroidal extension; (iv) Cervical lymph node metastases; and (v) Known distant metastases. **Total thyroidectomy may be considered in:** (i) Bilateral nodularity and (ii) In patients with prior exposure to radiation.

FNAB can confirm the diagnosis of most primary thyroid cancers—Papillary, medullary, anaplastic, lymphoma.

FNAB cannot confirm the diagnosis of follicular carcinoma and Hurthle cell carcinoma.

USG Features Suggestive of Metastatic Lymph Nodes

- Loss of fatty hilum
- Rounded rather than oval shape
- Hyperechogenicity
- Cystic change
- Microcalcification
- Peripheral vascularity.

Disadvantages of Lobectomy plus Isthmusectomy

- Tumor may be multifocal
- Adjuvant radioiodine therapy not feasible
- Follow up with serum thyroglobulin is not possible.

Follow-up after Lobectomy

- Physical examination
- TSH assessment
- Periodic neck USG

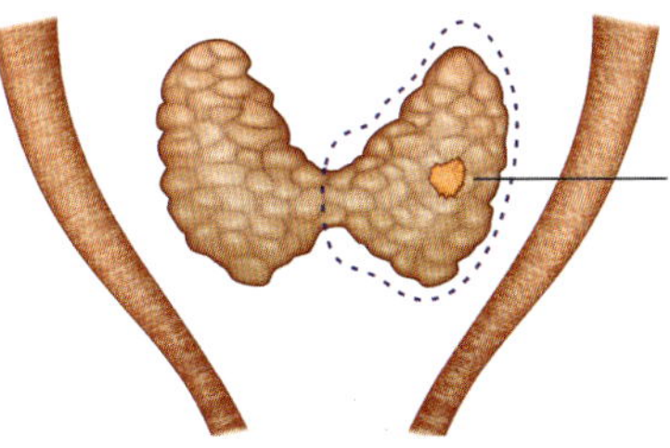

Lobectomy Plus Isthmusectomy

Advantages of Total Thyroidectomy

- Any occult tumor, if present in contralateral lobe can be resected.
- Adjuvant radioiodine therapy can be done.
- Follow up with thyroglobulin estimation is feasible.

Modified radical neck dissection (level II, III, IV, and Vb) should be considered for clinically positive and/or biopsy-proven nodal metastases in lateral neck compartment. Level I and Va lymph node dissection may be considered if these lymph nodes are clinically involved. **Therapeutic central neck dissection (level VI)** is indicated for clinically involved central nodes.

'Cherry picking' (selective dissection of metastatic nodes) is not recommended for patients with clinically or biopsy-proven nodal metastatic disease.

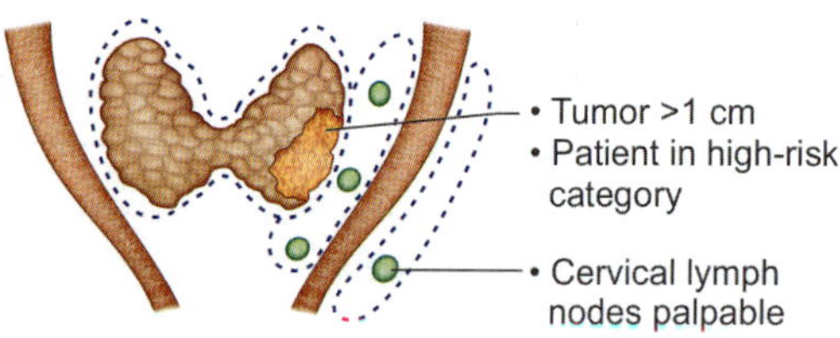

Total Thyroidectomy with Modified Radical Neck Dissection

Detectable Tg level after total thyroidectomy suggests residual disease or recurrence of tumor.

Postoperative thyroglobulin (Tg) estimation: Tg and anti-Tg antibodies should be measured 6–12 weeks after total thyroidectomy to obtain a postoperative baseline. After total thyroidectomy, Tg level should be undetectable (<2 ng/mL).

Postoperative thyroid hormone replacement (T_4 or T_3) withdrawal should be planned before diagnostic imaging or RAI therapy. T_4 should be withdrawn for 3–4 weeks, whereas T3 should be withdrawn for at least 2 weeks. The goal is to achieve TSH >30 mIU/L for optimal RAI uptake. **Recombinant human TSH (rhTSH) is an alternative approach to thyroid hormone withdrawal**, particularly indicated in patients with significant comorbidities to avoid the hypothyroidism-related side effects (e.g., aggravation of CHF, respiratory compromise, psychiatric illness).

Diagnostic whole body ^{123}I or ^{131}I imaging may be considered to assess the residual disease and to assess distant metastatic disease before the RAI therapy.

Radioactive iodine therapy is recommended (if any present): (i) Gross extrathyroidal extension; (ii) Primary tumor >4 cm; (iii) Postoperative unstimulated Tg >5–10 ng/mL; and (iv) Bulky or >5 positive lymph nodes.

Postablation whole body iodine scan should be considered to detect residual disease after ablation. Periodical serum Tg measurement should be done.

TSH-suppression is recommended and the optimal serum level of TSH is tailored based on risk of recurrence.

Thyroid hormone withdrawal for preparation of RAI ablation therapy is preferred over rhTSH by most of the oncologists due to increased chance of augmentation of the delivered radiation dose.

Radioactive iodine therapy is not recommended (if all present):

- Classic papillary carcinoma
- Largest primary tumor <2 cm
- Intrathyroidal tumor
- Unifocal or multifocal (all foci ≤1 cm)
- No detectable Anti-Tg antibodies
- Postoperative unstimulated Tg <1 ng/mL
- Negative postoperative USG, if done.

Recommended TSH level after TSH-suppressive doses of levothyroxine

- High-risk for recurrence—TSH <0.1 mU/L
- Intermediate-risk—TSH 0.1–0.5 mU/L Low-risk- TSH 0.5-2.0 mU/L.

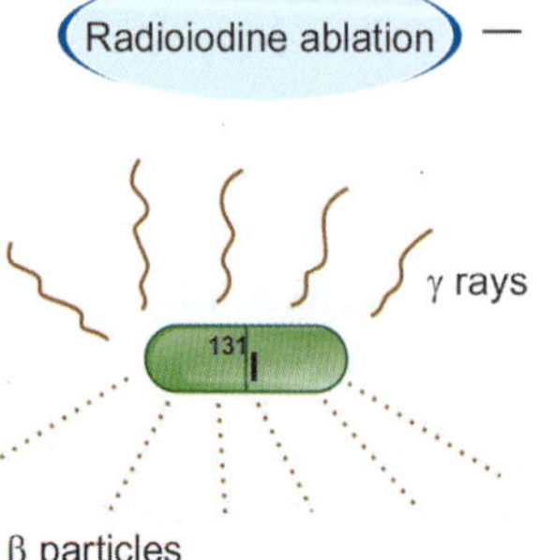

- This ablation therapy destroys any residual thyroid tissue after surgery, thereby almost prevents locoregional recurrence
- Radioiodine ablation is performed about 6 weeks after total thyroidectomy
- Postoperative thyroid hormone placement with T_3 is preferred as it has shorter half life than T_4
- T_3 replacement should be discontinued 2 weeks before ablation so that TSH level is elevated (>50 mu/L). T_4 replacement should be discontinued 6 weeks prior to ablation
- A low iodine diet is recommended 1–2 weeks before ablation

RAI ablation therapy should not be considered for at least 2 months after an **imaging with iodine contrast agent**.

A low iodine diet is recommended for 1–2 weeks before ablation.

Time interval between diagnostic I-131 and therapeutic I-131 should be less than 48–72 hours to avoid the "stunning" effect.

Medications or Contrast Agents Blocking RAI Uptake (adapted from Society of Nuclear Medicine)

Medications	Time of withdrawal
Antithyroid drugs	3 days
Thyroid hormone supplements	10–14 days (for triiodothyronine) 3–4 weeks (for thyroxine)
Lugol solution, saturated solution of potassium iodide	4 weeks
Topical iodine (as used for surgical skin preparation)	2–3 weeks
IV contrast agents • Water soluble • Lipophilic	 6–8 weeks 1–6 months

Therapeutic Indications of ^{131}I Therapy

Benign	Malignant
Graves' disease	Differentiated papillary and follicular thyroid cancer (after total thyroidectomy)
Toxic nodular goiter	Recurrent thyroid cancer
Nontoxic nodular goiter	Metastatic disease after near-total thyroidectomy

Complications of ^{131}I Therapy

Early	Late
Oral mucositis	Diminished spermatogenesis (transient)
Sialadenitis	Xerostomia
Loss of taste	Sialolithiasis
Nausea	Dental caries
Painful thyroiditis (if sizeable postsurgical remnant present)	Dysgeusia
Recurrent laryngeal nerve paralysis	Xerophthalmia or epiphora (rare)
	Secondary malignancies (stomach, bladder, colon, salivary glands, melanoma)

Thyroid Scintigraphy

Indications:

- Evaluation of solitary toxic nodule
- Evaluation of congenital thyroid abnormalities
- To locate the ectopic thyroid tissue (e.g., lingual thyroid)

Assessment of function of thyroid nodule:

- Differentiating hyperthyroidism from other forms of thyrotoxicosis (e.g., thyroiditis, thyrotoxicosis factitia)
- Calculating iodine-131 administered activity for patients to be treated for ablative therapy
- Whole-body imaging for determining the presence and location of metastases.

Contraindications: (i) Pregnancy and (ii) Lactation

Radiopharmaceuticals used for thyroid scintigraphy: (i) ^{123}I; (ii) Tc-99m Pertechnetate; and (iii) ^{131}I

^{123}I	Tc-99m Pertechnetate
Trapped and organified	Trapped but not organified
Yields better images when uptake is low	Poor image quality when uptake is low
Imaging time longer	Imaging time shorter
Higher cost and less readily available	Readily available

Follicular Carcinoma

- Follicular carcinoma account for about 10% of thyroid cancers and more commonly in iodine-deficient areas.
- Older population (50 years or more) are commonly affected.
- More common in females (3:1).

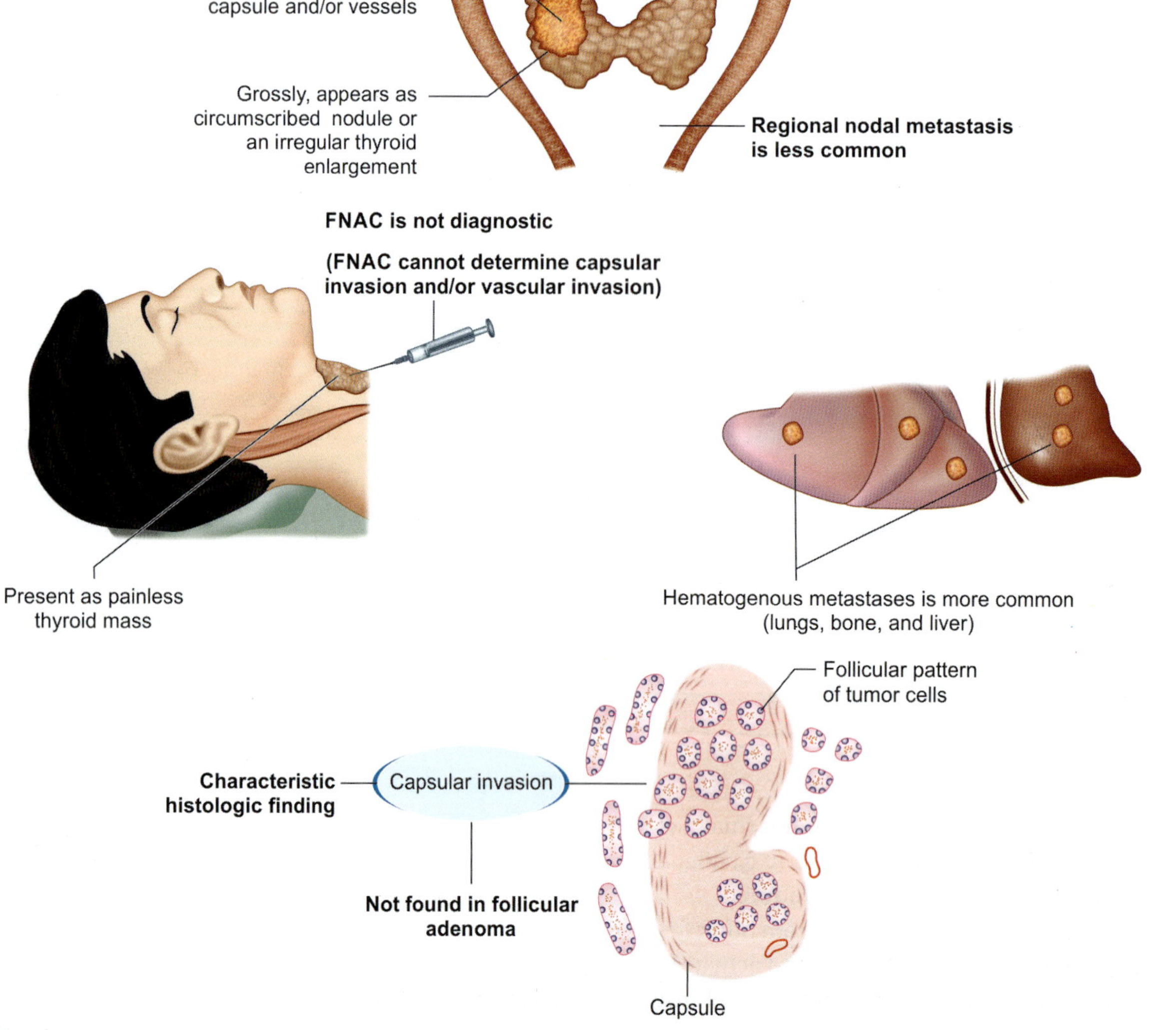

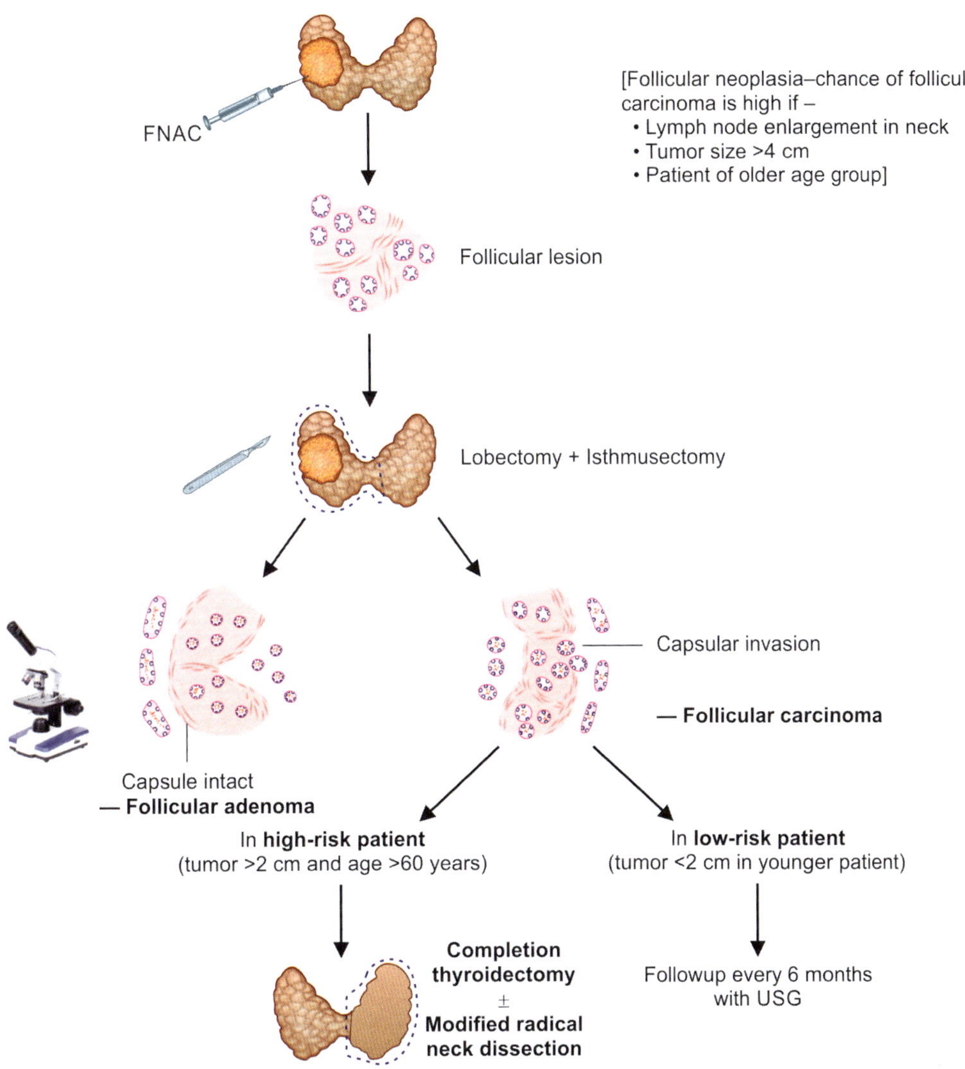

Total thyroidectomy is recommended for follicular neoplasm only if: (i) Extrathyroidal invasion or metastatic disease is apparent at the time of surgery; (ii) Imaging findings suggestive of extrathyroidal invasion; and (iii) Patient wants total thyroidectomy to avoid a second procedure.

Completion thyroidectomy is recommended if after lobectomy plus isthmusectomy, histology reveals invasive follicular thyroid carcinoma. If histology reveals minimally invasive follicular thyroid carcinoma, completion thyroidectomy or follow-up may be considered.

Radioactive iodine therapy is recommended in follicular carcinoma (if any present): (i) Gross extrathyroidal extension; (ii) Primary tumor >4 cm; (iii) Extensive vascular invasion; (iv) Postoperative unstimulated Tg >5–10 ng/mL; and (v) Bulky or >5 positive lymph nodes.

Radioactive iodine therapy is not recommended in follicular carcinoma (if all present): (i) Largest primary tumor<2 cm; (ii) Intrathyroidal; (iii) No vascular invasion; (iv) Clinically N0; (v) No detectable anti-Tg antibodies; (vi) Postoperative unstimulated Tg <1 ng/mL; and (vii) Negative postoperative USG, if done.

Hurthle Cell Carcinoma

- Hurthle cell carcinoma (also known as **oxyphilic cell carcinoma**) is a type of differentiated thyroid carcinoma. Previously, it was considered as a variant of follicular carcinoma. This tumor contains abundance of oxyphilic cells or oncocytes and characterized by vascular or capsular invasion.
- More often **multifocal, bilateral and more likely metastasize to regional nodes and distant sites.**
- Work-up and management are similar to follicular carcinoma. **FNAB cannot differentiate between benign Hurthle cell tumor and Hurthle cell carcinoma.**
- Therapeutic neck dissection may be considered for clinically-apparent biopsy-proven nodal metastases. **Prognosis is worse in comparison to follicular carcinoma.**
- Most of the Hurthle cell carcinomas are **noniodine avid, hence response to RAI therapy is lower in comparison to papillary or follicular carcinomas**. In patients with high-risk features, FDG-PET scan is indicated instead of RAI scan to rule out distant metastases.

Medullary Thyroid Carcinoma

Medullary thyroid carcinoma (MTC) arises from **neural crest-derived parafollicular C-cells** of the thyroid. Most of the sporadic MTC presents as nodule in the upper part of thyroid lobe. About half of the patients present with neck node metastases. Patients with advanced disease may present with diarrhea, facial flushing, cushing syndrome.

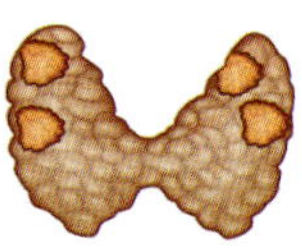

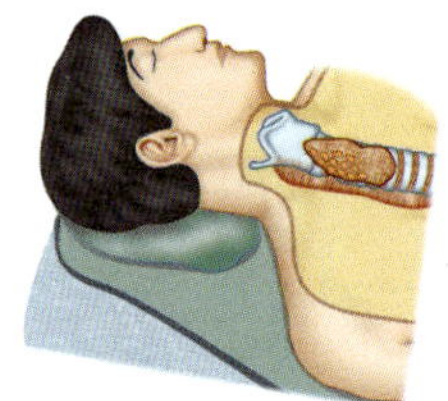

- MTC usually found in **upper and middle thirds of thyroid lobe** (Because, parafollicular or C cells are concentrated in these regions)

Also found particularly in the posterior part of lobe

Derived from neural crest

Distinctive Features of MTC

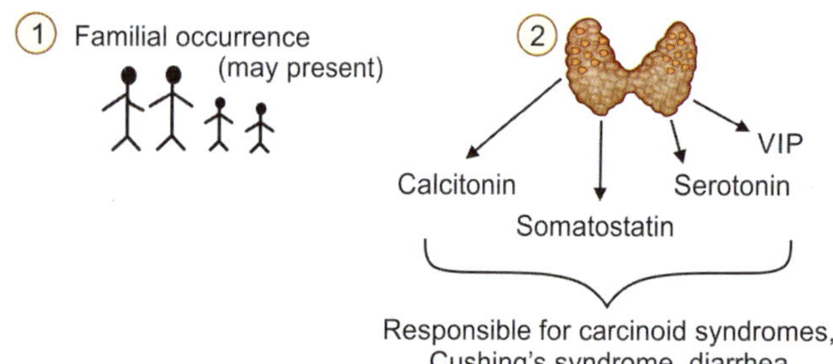

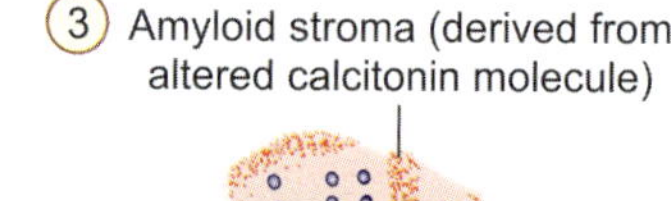

Tumor cells

Types of MTC

Sporadic medullary thyroid carcinoma accounts for about 80% of all medullary carcinoma, remainder consists of- **MEN type 2A (MEN2A), MEN2B**. Familial MTC is now classified as a variant of MEN2A. Sporadic MTC typically occurs between the fourth and sixth decades of life, whereas inherited form of MTC presents as earlier age (between the second and third decade).

Inherited forms of MTC are more aggressive than sporadic MTC.

Genetic event in MTC is mutation in RET protooncogene. Almost all MTC patients related to MEN2A, MEN2B, familial MTC have RET germline mutations. About 50% of sporadic MTCs have somatic RET mutations.

RET is a protooncogene (located in chromosome 10q11.2), expressed in cells derived from neural crest, the branchial arches, and the urogenital system.

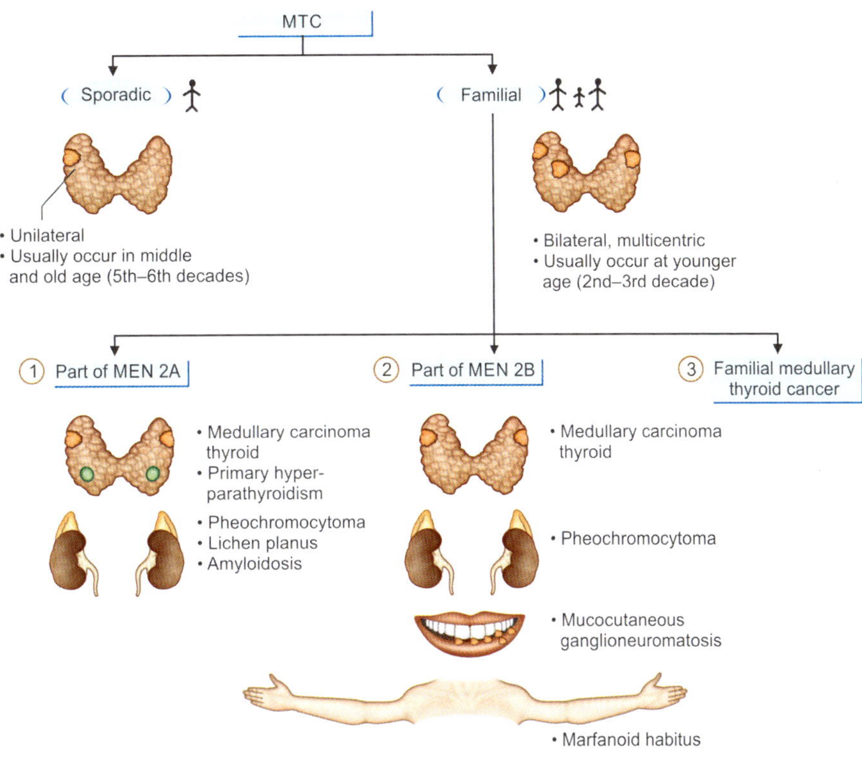

Diagnostic Workup

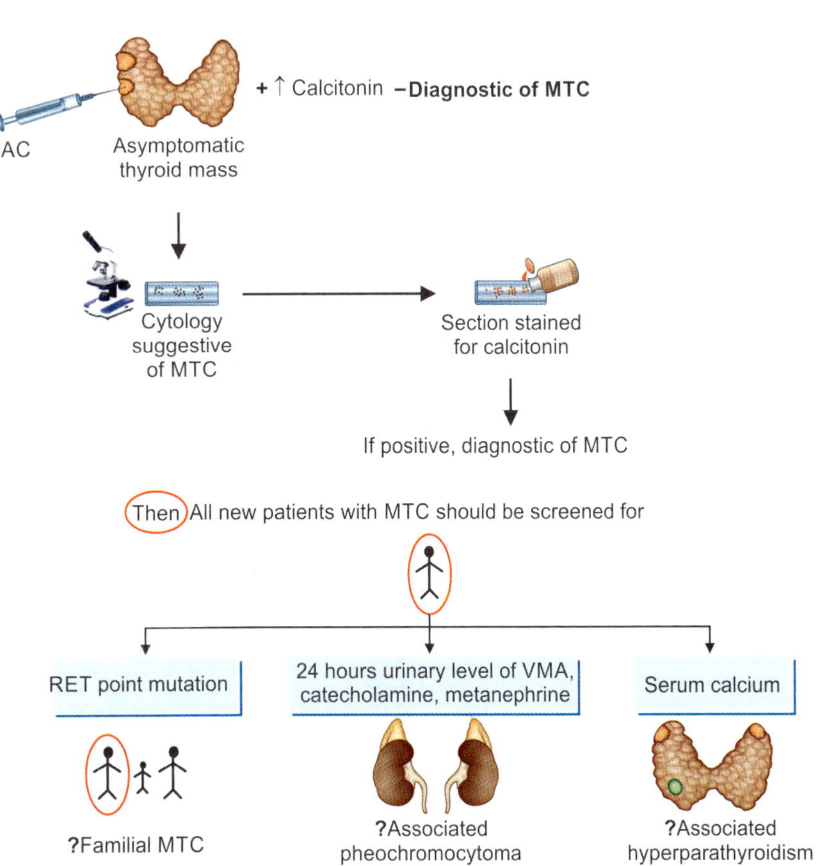

Most of the sporadic MTC are diagnosed after FNA of solitary nodule.

MTC associated with inherited syndromes are detected by family screening for mutant RET protooncogene.

Diagnostic work-up for MTC:
- Basal serum calcitonin level
- CEA
- Pheochromocytoma screening
- Serum calcium
- Screening for germline RET proto-oncogene mutations (exon 10,11,13-16).

Treatment

Primary treatment of MTC is **total thyroidectomy with prophylactic bilateral central neck dissection (level VI)**. Therapeutic ipsilateral or bilateral modified neck dissection is also indicated for clinically or radiologically identifiable disease (level II–V).

Work-up to rule out pheochromocytoma and hyperparathyroidism should be done before surgery for MTC. Adrenalectomy should be done before thyroid surgery to avoid hypertensive crisis during surgery.

RAI treatment is not effective in MTC. TSH suppression is not appropriate because C cells lack TSH receptors. Dose of levothyroxine therapy is adjusted to keep the TSH level in normal range.

Prophylactic total thyroidectomy is indicated in RET mutation carriers. In MEN 2A, prophylactic thyroidectomy (along with therapeutic unilateral or bilateral central node dissection if increased calcitonin or CEA) recommended by age 5 and in MEN 2B (total thyroidectomy along with prophylactic bilateral central neck dissection) during the first year of life or at diagnosis.

Surgery for Sporadic MTC

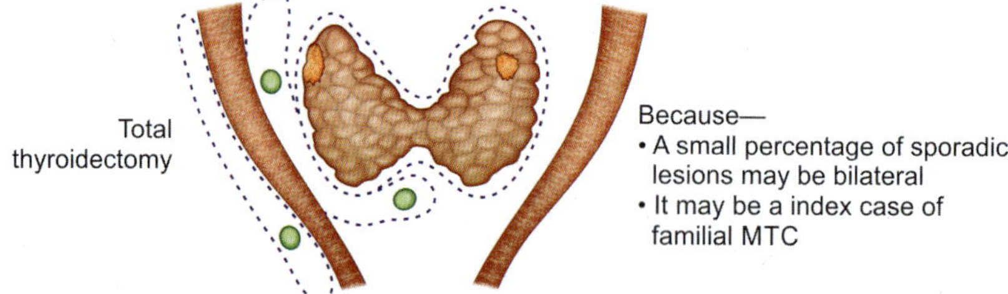

Total thyroidectomy with prophylactic bilateral central neck dissection (level VI).

Surgery for MTC along with Pheochromocytoma

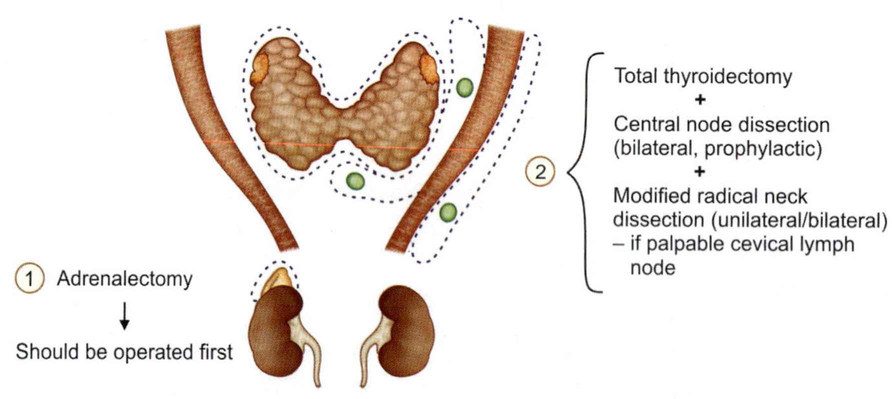

Anaplastic Thyroid Carcinoma

- Anaplastic thyroid carcinoma (ATC) is an **aggressive undifferentiated, highly lethal type** of **rare** thyroid cancer.
- This tumor predominantly found in 7th–8th decades.
- It is commonly related to a **prior or concurrent diagnosis of well-differentiated thyroid cancer** or **benign nodular thyroid disease**. Iodine deficiency is also associated with ATC.

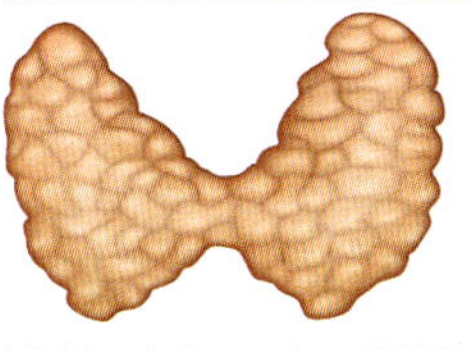

Multinodular goiter (50%)

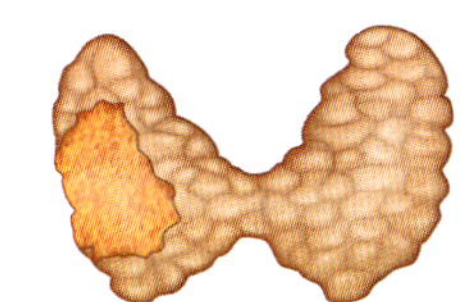

Differentiated carcinoma (20%)

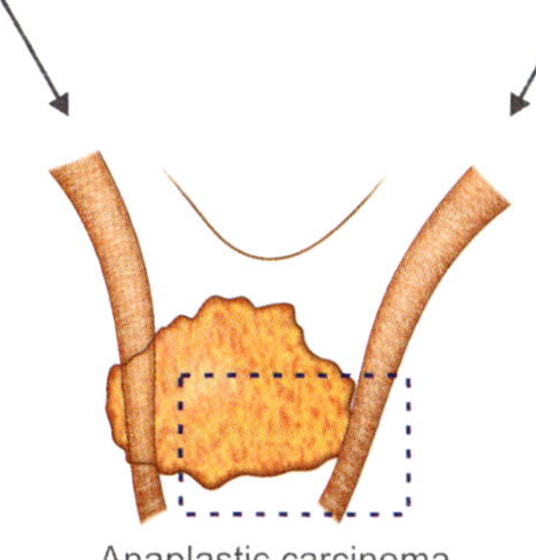

Anaplastic carcinoma

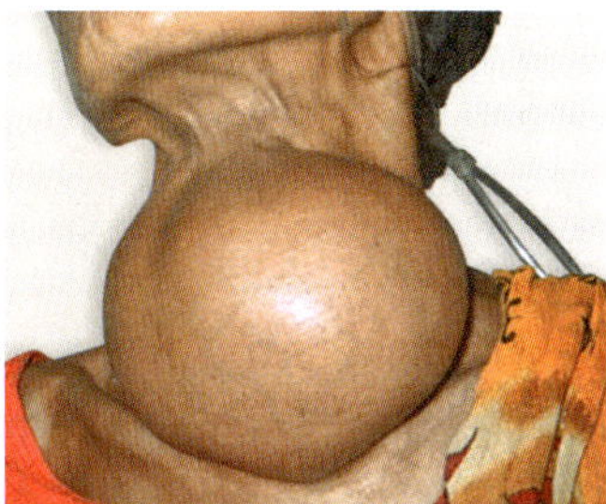

Large thyroid swelling causing dyspnea.

- **Patients may present** with rapidly enlarging thyroid swelling, dyspnea, dysphagia, and hoarseness of voice due to extensive local invasion. A few percentage of patients present with distant metastases.
- **Diagnosis** is confirmed by FNA biopsy revealing characteristic giant cell and multinucleated cells. If FNA is suspicious or nondiagnostic, core biopsy or open biopsy should be considered to establish the diagnosis.

High resolution USG of the neck is indicated to assess the primary tumor, involvement of neck nodes and airway patency.

Contrast-enhanced-CT scan or MRI (with gadolinium contrast) of neck and chest is essential to determine the extent of tumor and to assess the involvement of great vessels and aerodigestive tract. **CT or PET/CT** is helpful to rule out distant metastases.

Surgery should be considered if tumor is resectable (no local invasion of internal jugular vein, carotid artery, recurrent laryngeal nerve, vagus, spinal accessory and phrenic nerve, trachea, esophagus) and distant metastases is not present.

Total or near-total thyroidectomy with therapeutic lymph node dissection of central and lateral neck node compartments should be considered for resectable disease.

Tracheostomy may be considered for impending airway obstruction.

- All patients of ATC are **classified as stage IV (A, B, or C)** by AJCC TNM system.
- About half of the anaplastic thyroid carcinomas develop **following dedifferentiation of differentiated thyroid carcinomas**.
- Most common coexistent differentiated carcinoma is well-differentiated papillary carcinoma (often the tall cell type), followed by follicular carcinoma and Hurthle cell carcinoma.

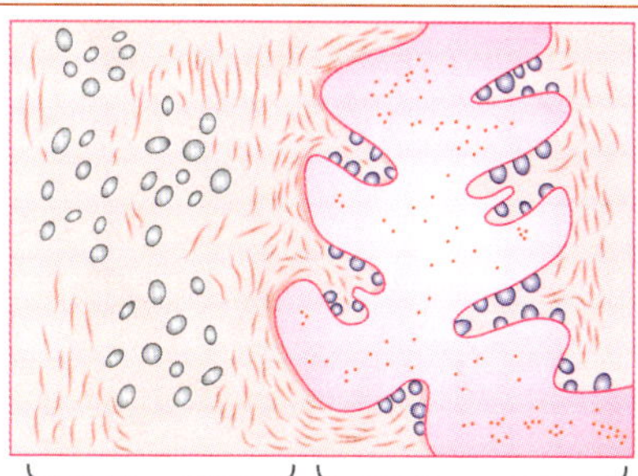

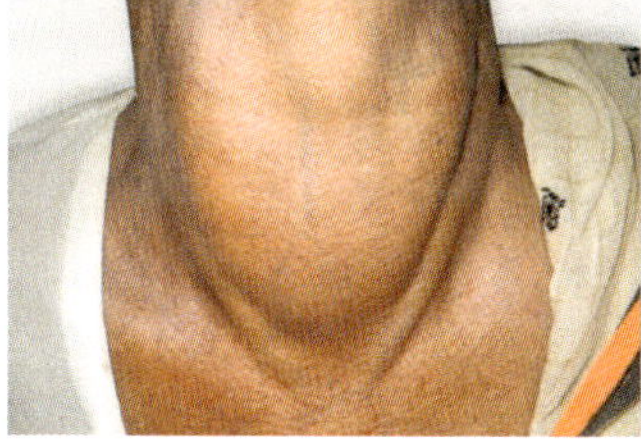

Diffuse thyroid swelling.

- Anaplastic thyroid carcinoma should be suspected if an elderly patient with longstanding thyroid swelling which rapidly enlarged and becomes painful.
- Most common site of metastases are lungs and pleura. Other sites of metastases are bone and brain.
- **Anaplastic carcinomas cannot concentrate iodine.**

Genetic mutations in different type of thyroid cancer:

- Well-differentiated thyroid carcinoma—BRAF, RAS, PAX8/PPARγ
- Medullary carcinoma—RET
- Anaplastic carcinoma—TP53, β-catenin, BRAF, RAS.

Radiation therapy with or without systemic therapy should be considered for patients with locoregionally confined but unresectable disease.

Systemic therapy includes targeted therapy (Dabrafenib/trametinib, larotrectinib, pralsetinib) and cytotoxic chemotherapy (Paclitaxel, doxorubicin). **^{131}I therapy has no role in treatment of anaplastic carcinoma.**

Surgical Approaches to Thyroid

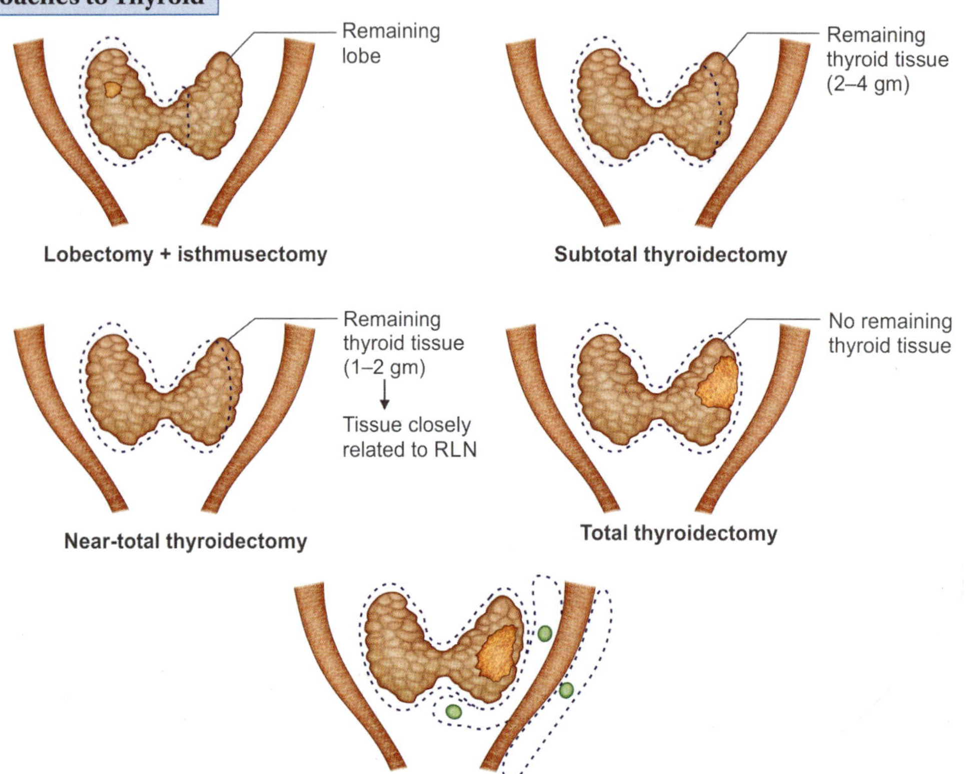

Preoperative Preparation

Patient should undergo vocal cord assessment by indirect laryngoscopy if:

- History of recent change in voice
- Malignancy is suspected
- History of previous thyroid surgery

Thyrotoxic patients need to be euthyroid before surgery.

Preoperative Investigations

- Hb, TC, DC, ESR
- Blood sugar, urea, creatinine
- Serum T_3, T_4, TSH.
- Chest X-ray, ECG
- X-ray of neck
- High resolution USG of neck
- CT scan of neck (if only suspicion of invasion of adjacent structures by thyroid mass)

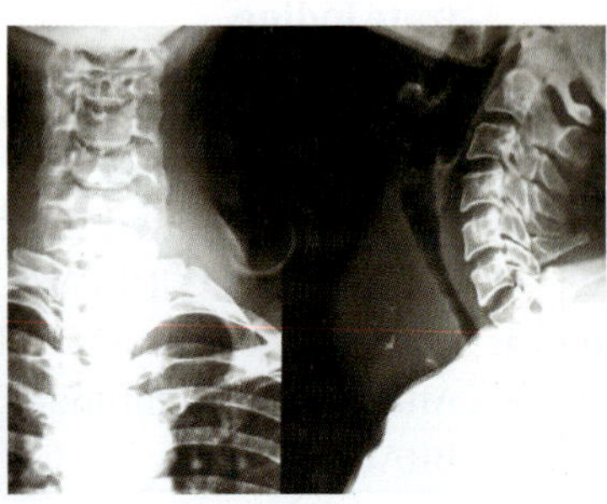

X-ray of Neck

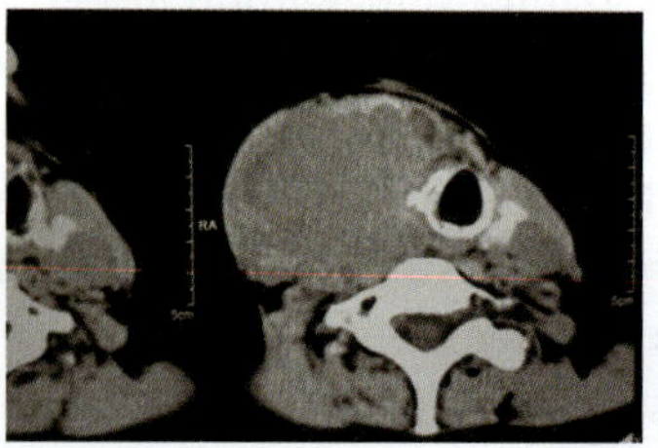

CT scan of Neck

Basic Steps of Thyroidectomy

Positioning of the Patient

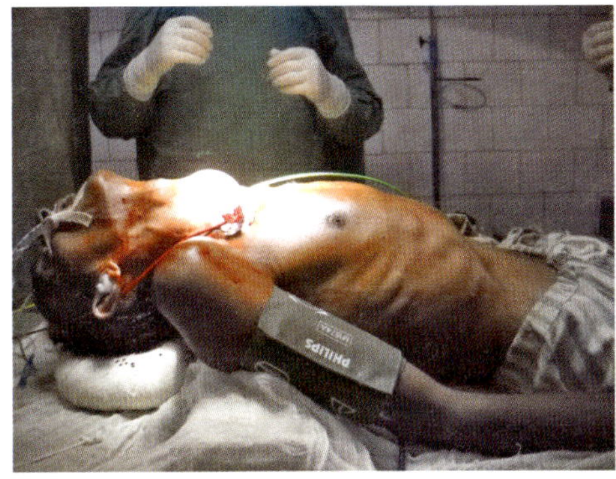

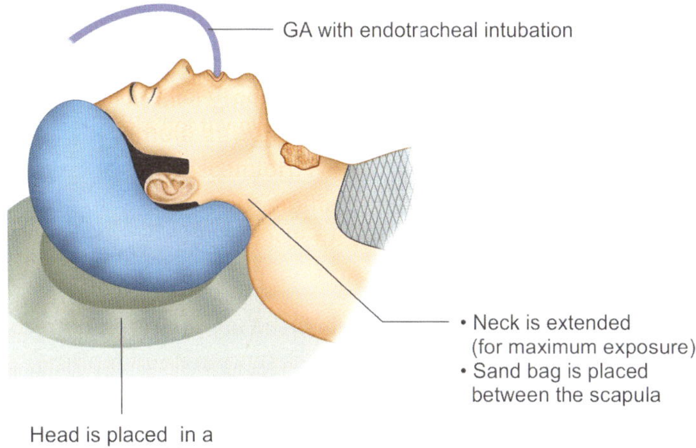

Incision

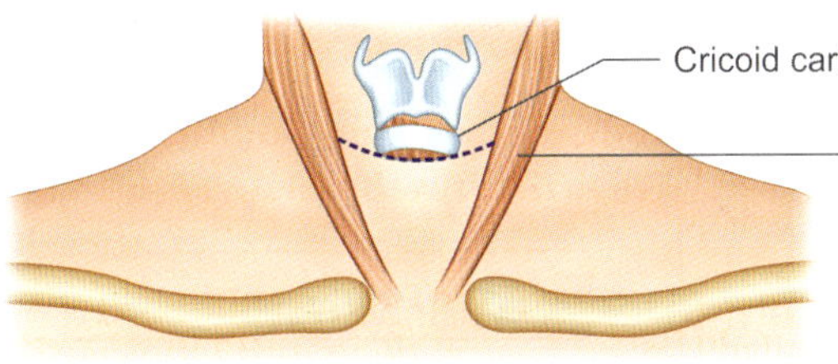

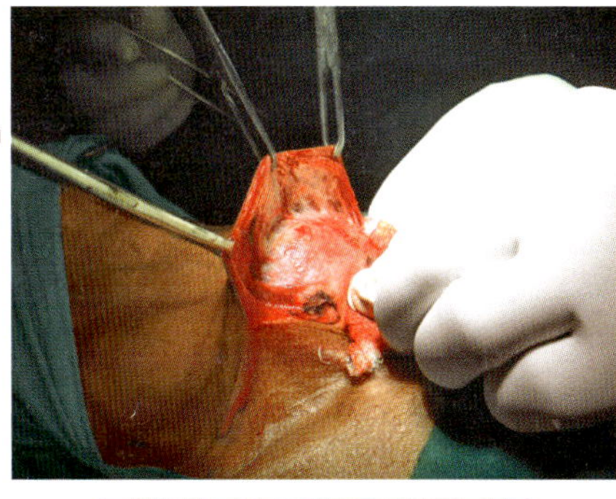

Superior flap is raised.

Raising the Flaps

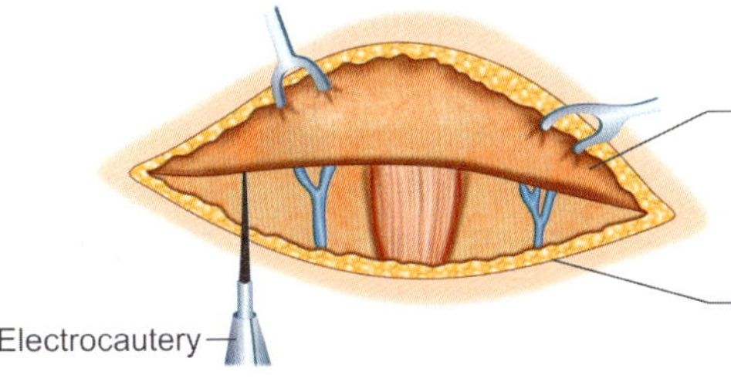

Identification and Ligation of Middle Thyroid Vein

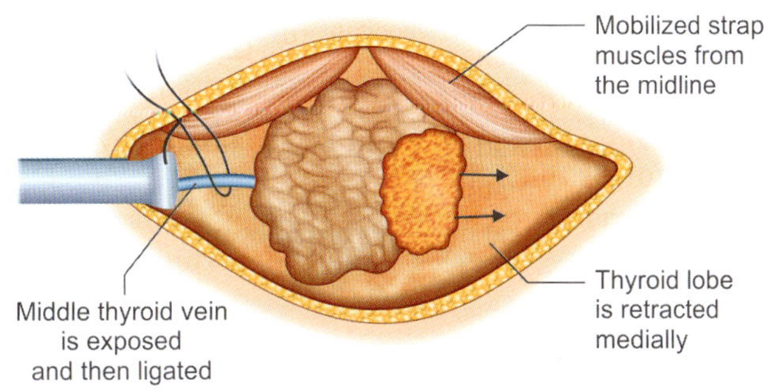

Dissection and Ligation of Superior Thyroid Vessels

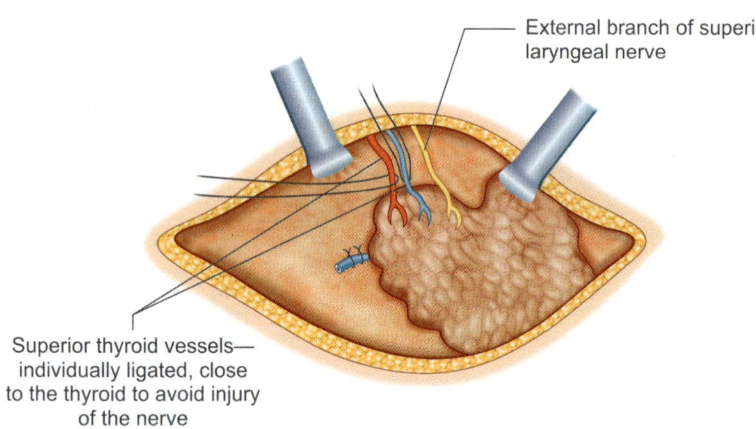

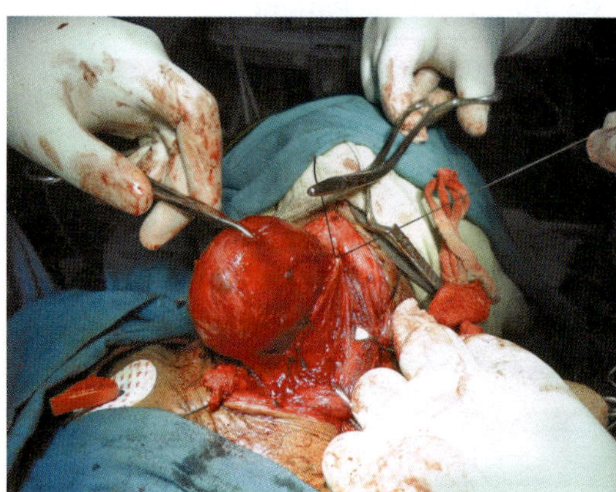

Dissection and Ligation of Inferior Thyroid Vessels

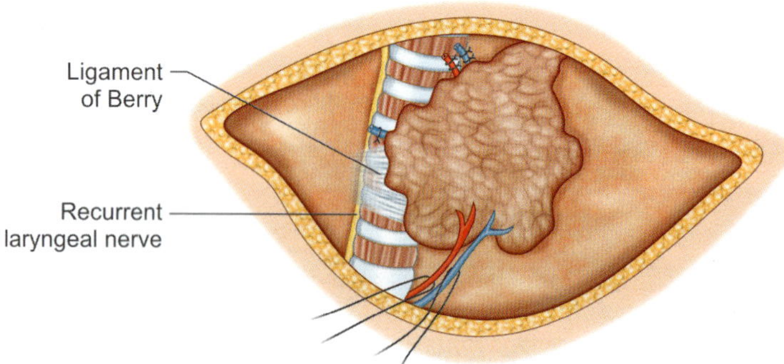

Skin Closure with Drain Placement

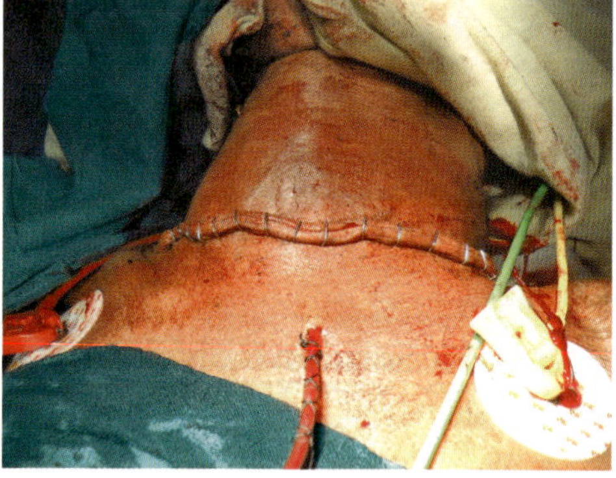

Complications of Thyroid Surgery

- Hemorrhage (from middle thyroid vein, superior or inferior thyroid vessels)
- Airway obstruction (due to hematoma)
- Nerve injury (Recurrent laryngeal nerve, External branch of superior laryngeal nerve)
- Hypocalcemia
- Hypothyroidism
- Hypertrophic scar or keloid

Measures to decrease the chance of external branch of superior laryngeal nerve (EBSLN) injury:

- Visualization during surgery
- If EBSLN is not visualized during surgery, dissection to be done close to thyroid capsule at the superior pole and skeletonizing the superior vascular pedicle.
- Intraoperative nerve monitoring.

Cernea classification (Classification of EBSLN based on its relationship with superior thyroid vessels):

Type 1: Nerve crossing the superior thyroid pedicle more than 1 cm above the superior thyroid pole

Type 2a: Nerve crosses the superior thyroid pedicle less than 1 cm above the superior thyroid pole

Type 2b: ("high risk") Nerve crossing the vessels below the upper border of the superior thyroid pole.

Causes of Voice Changes related to Thyroid Surgery (adapted from AAOL Guideline)

- Recurrent laryngeal nerve injury (complete/partial, transient/permanent)—Hoarseness, vocal fatigue
- External branch of superior laryngeal nerve (complete/partial, transient/permanent)—Decreased ability to raise pitch, inability to project voice, decreased pitch flexibility and range.
- Intubation related injuries—Hoarseness, odynophagia
- Cricothyroid muscle injury—similar to EBSLN injury.

Recurrent Laryngeal Nerve Injury

Risk factors for recurrent laryngeal nerve injury during thyroidectomy:

- Revision procedure
- Thyroidectomy for malignancy
- Thyroidectomy for Graves' disease, recurrent goiter, substernal goiter.

Symptoms of recurrent laryngeal nerve injury:

- Dyspnea
- Dysphonia (hoarseness, vocal fatigue, breathy voice)
- Dysphagia with potential aspiration
- If bilateral injury—Stridor, respiratory distress, and airway compromise.

Surgical approaches to identify RLN during thyroid surgery:

- Lateral approach (most common)
- Inferior approach—preferred approach in revision surgery
- Superior approach—preferred approach in large goiter with significant substernal component
- Medial approach—useful for large goiters.

Anatomical landmarks related to identification of recurrent laryngeal nerve:

- Suspensory ligament of Berry
- Inferior thyroid artery
- Inferior horn of the thyroid cartilage
- Tubercle of Zuckercandl.

Measures to avoid RLN injury:

- Visual identification of RLN
- Intraoperative neuromonitoring (IONM)—Intermittent IONM (I-IONM) and Continuous-IONM (C-IONM).

Mechanisms of RLN injury during thyroidectomy:
- Traction injury (at the point of fixation)
- Compression (by surgical instrument, ligature, clip)
- Transection (by sharp instrument)
- Thermal injury.

Management:
- Voice therapy
- Vocal cord injection technique (injection of autologous fat, minced autologous fascia lata)
- Open vocal cord medialization (Medialization thyroplasty)
- Tension-free primary anastomosis of the nerve
- Nerve transfer (ansa cervicalis-to-RLN anastomosis) with epineural microsuturing
- Arytenoid cartilage resection.

Remote Access Thyroid Surgery

Criteria ideal for remote-access techniques (adapted from ATA statement 2016)
- Well-circumscribed thyroid nodule ≤3 cm
- Thyroid lobe <5–6 cm in largest dimension
- No associated thyroiditis on ultrasound
- Thin body habitus (except for facelift approach)
- Absence of excessive body fat along the flap trajectory (except for the facelift approach)
- Distance between the axilla and the sternal notch should be <15–17 cm (for an axillary approach)

Absolute contraindications: (i) Thyroid malignancy with extrathyroidal extension or lymph node involvement; (ii) Graves' disease; (iii) Substernal extension of thyroid swelling; and (iv) Previous neck surgery.

Different approaches:

Endoscopic breast approach:
- First remote-access technique.
- Involves two circumareolar incisions (12–15 mm) for 8–12 mm port and another 5 mm port 3 cm below the clavicle on the side of the pathology.
- CO_2 insufflation (5–6 mm Hg) is necessary.

Axillo-bilateral breast approach (ABBA):
- Involves two circumareolar ports and one axillary port (8–12 mm).
- Gland is removed through the axillary port.
- CO_2 insufflation (5–6 mm Hg) is necessary.

Bilateral axillo breast approach (BABA):
- Modification of the axillo bilateral breast approach (ABBA)
- Involves 8–12 mm ports placed around both areola and axilla.
- CO_2 insufflation (5–6 mm Hg) is necessary.

Da Vinci Robotic system is now adapted to this approach. This approach closely resembles conventional thyroid surgery (as it provides a midline access to the gland) and better visualization of critical structures (e.g., RLN, parathyroid glands, superior and inferior thyroid vessels).

Endoscopic and Robotic facelift approach:
- Involves a facelift incision that is marked out in or adjacent to the postauricular crease.
- Flap distance is the shortest of all the remote-access techniques.
- CO_2 insufflation not necessary.
- Access to the contralateral lobe is limited, therefore only lobectomy is feasible.

Transoral endoscopic approach:

- Includes completely vestibular access (safer) and floor-of-the mouth access.
- CO_2 insufflation (5–6 mm Hg) is necessary.
- This approach is contraindicated in; (i) Intraoral infection; (ii) Previous neck surgery or neck irradiation; and (iii) Recurrent disease.

Complications:

- Seroma
- Transient hypocalcemia
- Transient RLN injury
- Specific for transoral endoscopic approach—mental nerve injury, chin paresthesia, flap perforation, mediastinal emphysema.

Case 1

History and Physical Examination

A 36-year-old female patient presented with a painless swelling in the neck just lateral to the midline for last 8 months. Patient had no symptoms of hypo- or hyperthyroidism. No history of dysphagia, dyspnea or alteration of voice. Menstrual and obstetric history were normal.

Physical Examination

Patient alert, conscious, cooperative

Pulse: 88/min, BP: 114/86 mm Hg

Examination of neck: A 3.5 cm × 3 cm non-tender, solitary, firm nodule was palpable slightly right to the midline, that moves with deglutition, but not moves with protrusion of tongue. Cervical lymph nodes were not palpable.

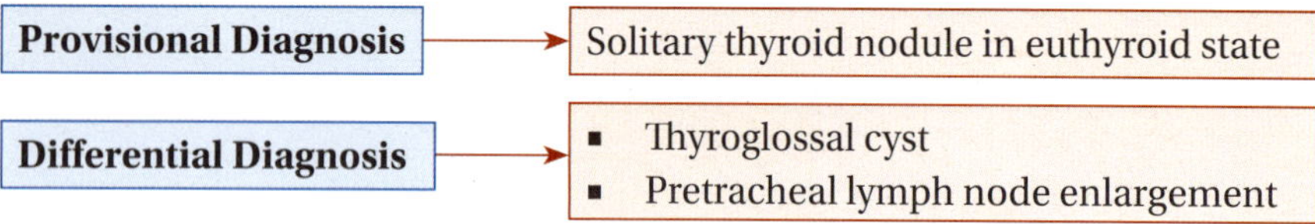

Investigations

- Serum TSH: 4.0 mIU/L
- USG of thyroid and neck: 3.5 cm × 3.2 cm solitary nodule in right lobe, TIRADS 3
- FNA of thyroid nodule revealed follicular neoplasia.

Discussion

A middle aged female patient presented with discrete thyroid swelling without any features of hypo- or hyperthyroidism. Serum TSH was within normal limit, USG revealed a solitary thyroid nodule of 3.5 cm with TIRADS 3 grading. FNA revealed follicular neoplasia. Lobectomy along with isthmusectomy was planned as no extrathyroidal invasion detected on imaging.

Management Algorithm

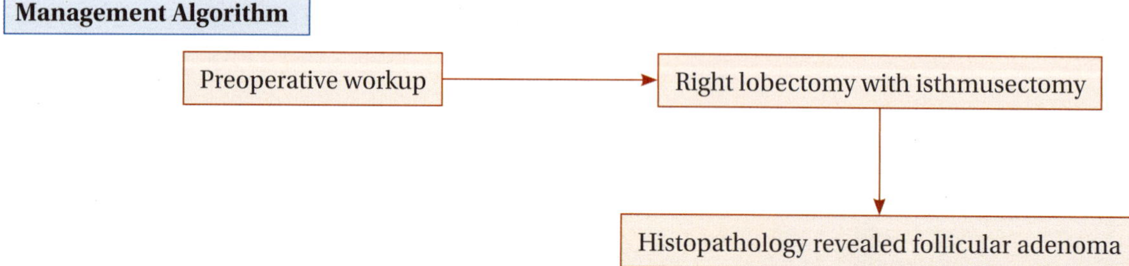

Case 2

History and Physical Examination

A 40-year-old female patient presented with a painless swelling in the thyroid region for last 3 months. Patient had no history suggestive of hypothyroidism or hyperthyroidism. No history suggestive of pressure symptoms. Menstrual and obstetric history were normal.

Physical Examination

Patient alert, conscious, cooperative

Pulse: 84/min, BP: 112/80 mm Hg

Examination of neck: A 4.0 cm × 3.2 cm non-tender, solitary, firm nodule was palpable slightly right to the midline, that moves with deglutition, but not moves with protrusion of tongue. Multiple cervical lymph nodes were palpable at level II and III.

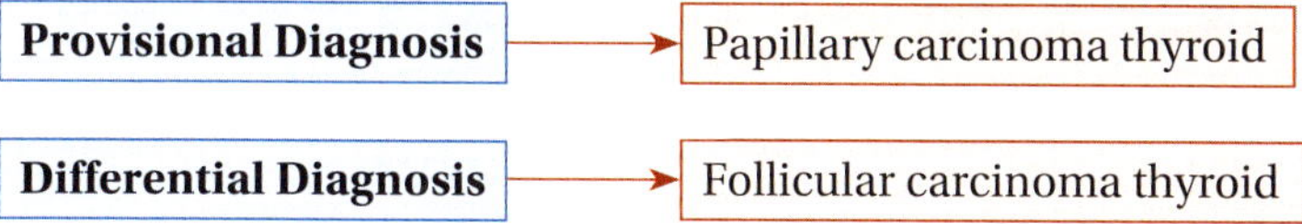

Investigations

- Serum TSH, T3 and T4 level were normal.
- USG revealed 4.2 cm × 3.5 cm, hypoechoic nodule within the thyroid parenchyma—TIRADS 4. Multiple lymph nodes were found in level II, III, and IV.
- FNA of thyroid nodule revealed papillary carcinoma. USG-guided FNA of cervical lymph nodes revealed metastatic lymph nodes.
- CT scan of neck revealed no extrathyroidal invasion.

Discussion

A middle-aged female patient presented with painless thyroid swelling with cervical lymphadenopathy highly suggestive of papillary carcinoma thyroid. USG findings of hypoechoic nodule with TIRADS grading of 4 and multiple cervical lymph node enlargement also suggestive of papillary carcinoma. FNA of thyroid nodule confirmed the diagnosis and USG-guided FNA confirmed the lymph node metastases. Total thyroidectomy with modified radical neck dissection (level II, III, IV, and Vb) should be planned.

Management Algorithm

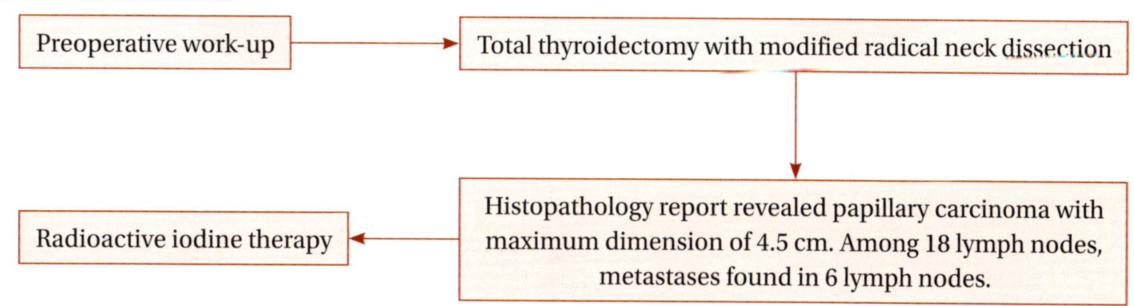

Chapter 15

Parathyroid, Adrenal, Endocrine Pancreas, and MEN

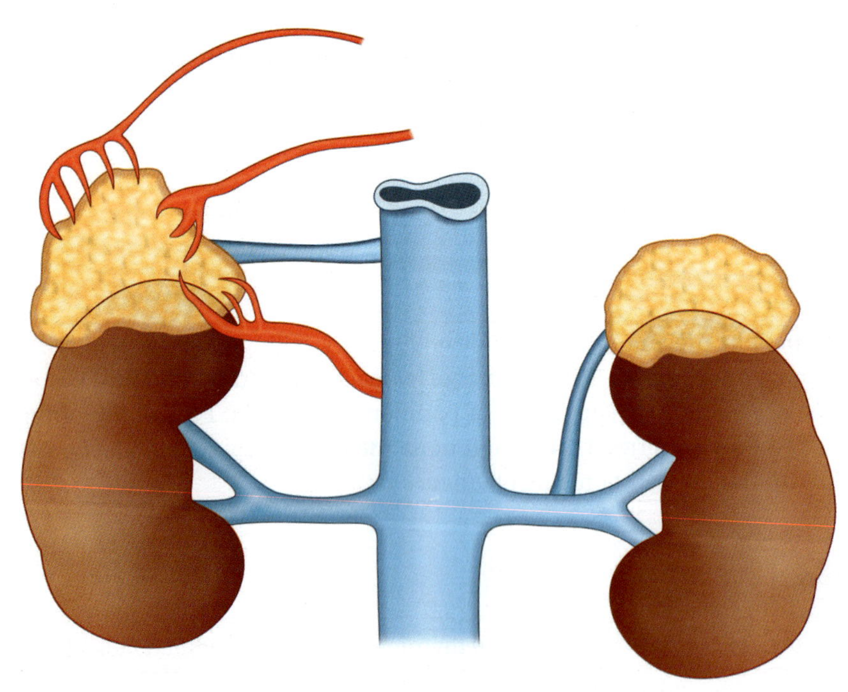

Important Topics

- Surgical Anatomy of Parathyroid Gland
- Microscopic Features
- Calcium Homeostasis
- Primary Hyperparathyroidism
- Secondary Hyperparathyroidism
- Tertiary Hyperparathyroidism
- Hypoparathyroidism
- Surgical Anatomy of Adrenal Gland
- Microscopic Features
- Conn's Syndrome
- Cushing Syndrome
- Adrenogenital Syndrome
- Adrenal Insufficiency
- Pheochromocytoma
- Incidentaloma
- Principles of Adrenal Surgery
- Neuroendocrine Tumors of Pancreas
- Multiple Endocrine Neoplasia Syndromes

'Let people who have to observe sickness and death look back and try to register in their observation the appearances which have preceded relapse, attack or death, and not assert that there were none, or that there were not the right ones. A want of the habit of observing conditions and an inveterate habit of taking averages are each of them often equally misleading.'

Florence Nightingale (1820–1910)
British Nurse and Reformer

Relevant Surgical Anatomy of Parathyroid

- Four parathyroid glands on the posterior surface of thyroid

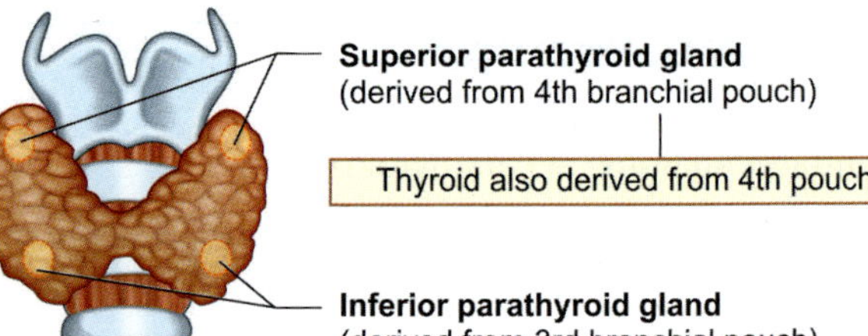

Site of the glands are very variable

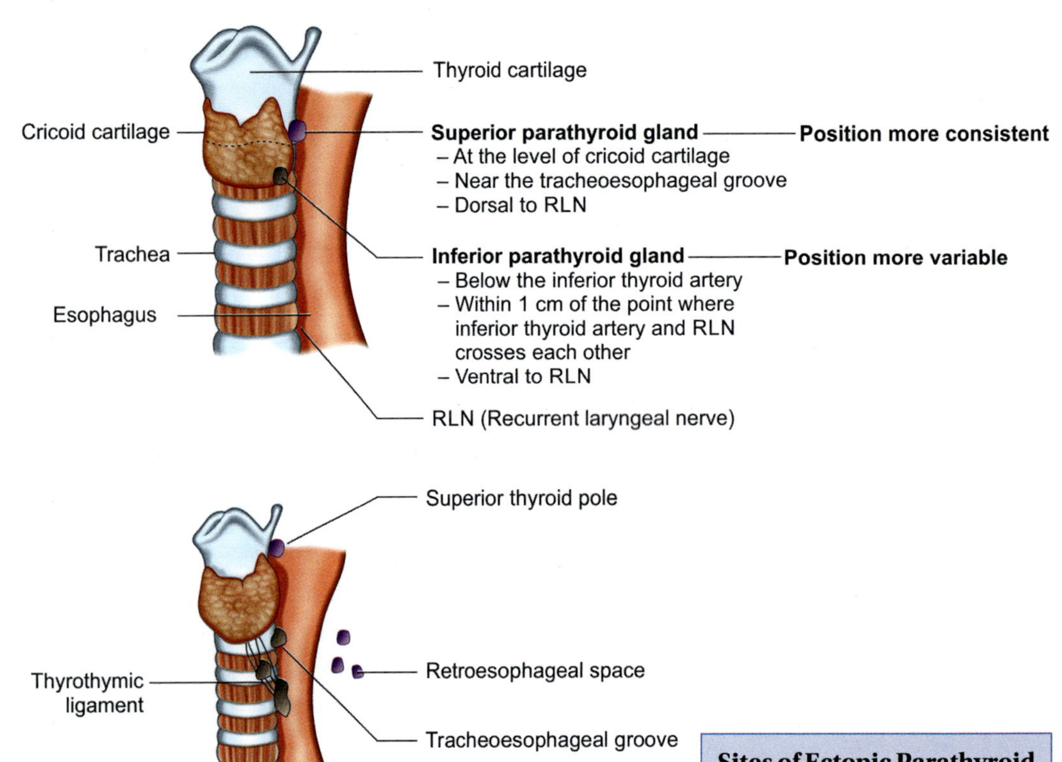

Sites of Ectopic Parathyroid

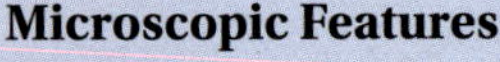

Microscopic Features

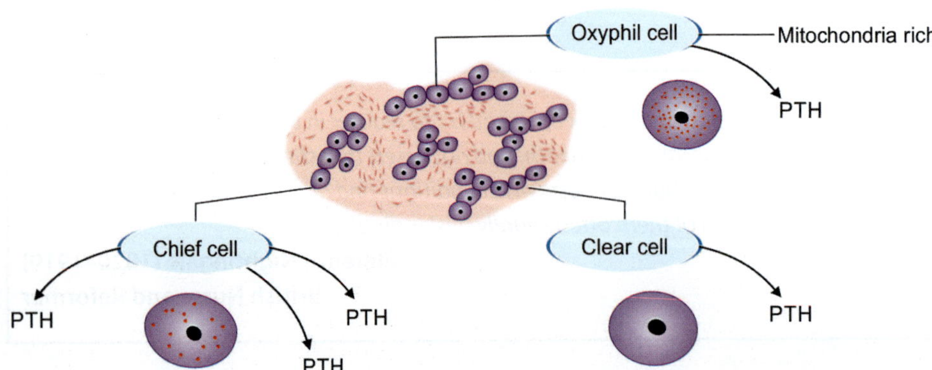

- Most numerous is **chief cell**
- Chief cells are rich in mitochondria
- **Oxyphil and clear cells** are derived from chief cell
- Chief cell is the major source of PTH
- Chief cell is most sensitive to changes in ionized calcium

Key components of calcium homeostasis:
- Serum calcium
- Serum phosphate
- 1,25-dihydroxyvitamin D-3
- Parathyroid hormone (PTH)

Hormones Involved in Calcium Homeostasis
- *Parathyroid hormone:* Responsible for rise in serum calcium
- 1, 25-dihydroxyvitamin-D3
- *Calcitonin:* Responsible for decrease in serum calcium

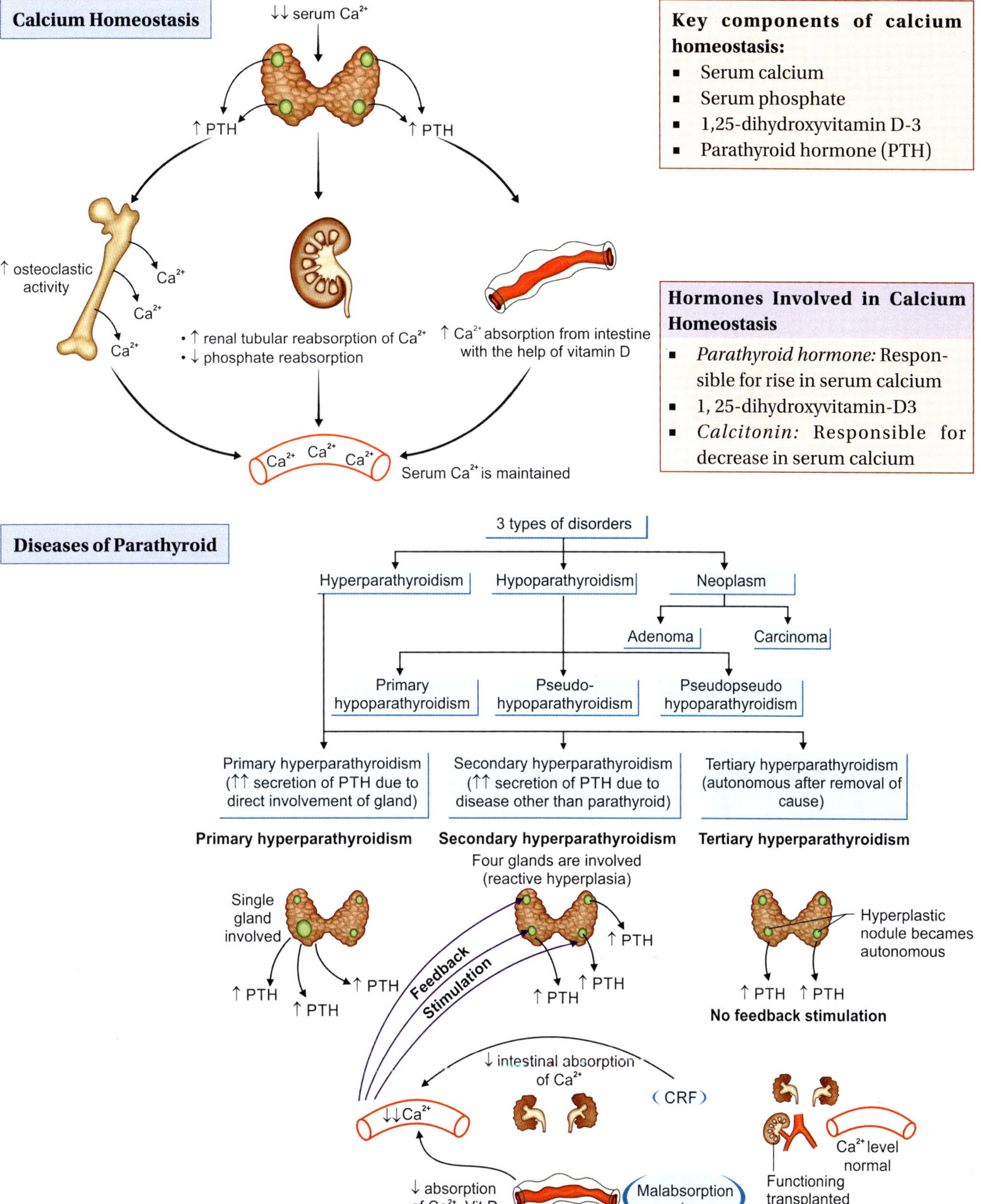

Primary Hyperparathyroidism

- Primary hyperparathyroidism (PHPT) is the 3rd most common endocrine disorder after diabetes mellitus and thyroid disease.
- A generalized disorder of calcium, phosphate and bone metabolism.
- Most cases of primary hyperparathyroidism are sporadic.
- *PHPT may present as inherited disorder:* (i) As part of MEN1, MEN 2A; (ii) Isolated familial HPT; and (iii) Familial HPT with jaw-tumor syndrome. The last two disorders are inherited as autosomal dominant disorder.

Causes

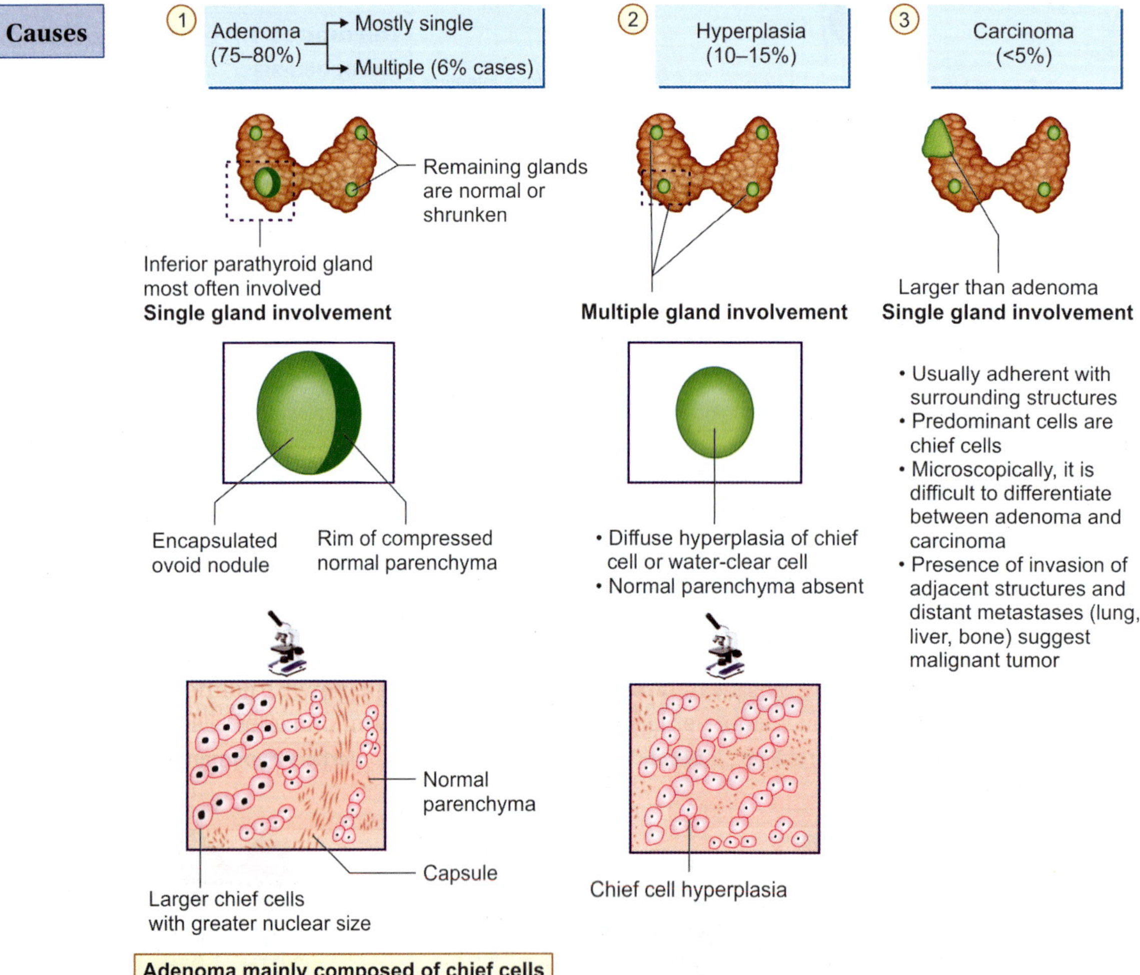

Clinical Presentation

- About half of the patients are asymptomatic. Classic pentad of symptoms ("Kidney stones, painful bones, abdominal groans, psychic moans, fatigue overtones") are rare nowadays due to early diagnosis.
- Diagnosis of clinically silent hyperparathyroidism is common nowadays due to routine assessment of serum calcium for work-up of many diseases.

Renal Disease
- Nephrolithiasis
- Nephrocalcinosis

Hyperparathyroidism must be considered in every patient presenting with renal stone or nephrocalcinosis.

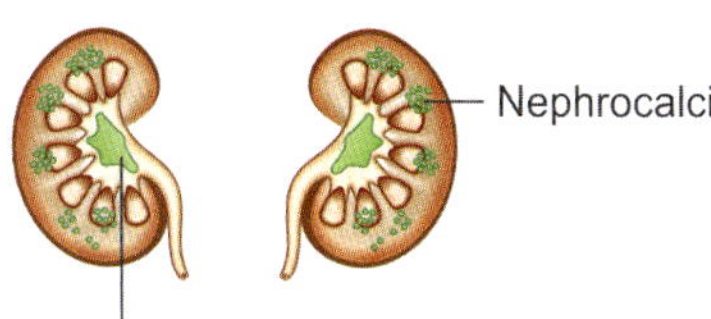

Bone Disease
- Osteopenia
- Osteoporosis
- Bone cysts
- *Osteitis fibrosa cystica:* It is due to osteoclastic resorption of bone and its replacement by connective tissue.
- Skull bone may also affected, X-ray shows mottled (salt and pepper) appearance with loss of definition of the inner and outer cortex.

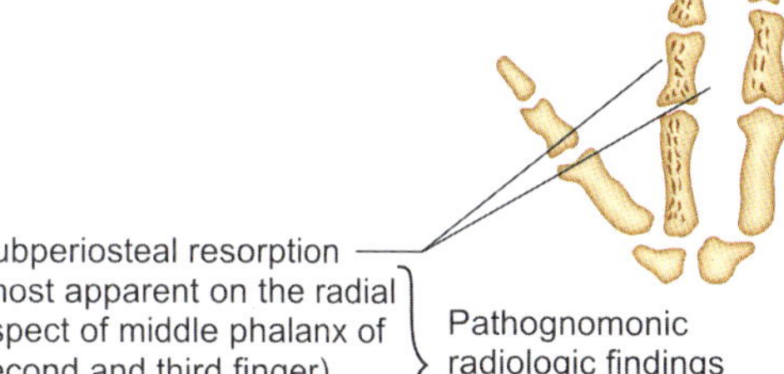

Gastrointestinal Manifestations

Increased incidence of cholelithiasis, pancreatitis, and peptic ulcer disease.

Neuromuscular Manifestations
- Proximal muscle weakness
- Easy fatigability
- Atrophy of muscles

Neuropsychiatric Manifestations

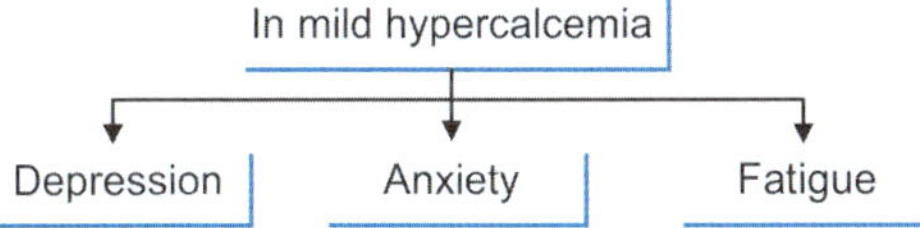

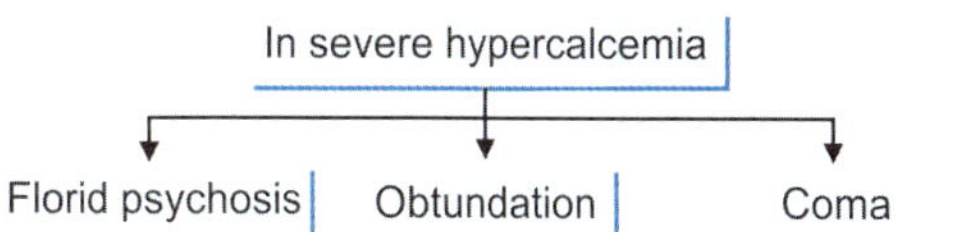

Metastatic Calcification in Different Organs
- Corneal calcification
- Conjunctival calcification
- Chondrocalcinosis
- Calcification in blood vessels and cardiac valves

Workup for Suspected Primary Hyperparathyroidism
- Serum total calcium
- Serum PTH
- Serum creatinine
- 25-hydroxyvitamin D
- 24-hour urine measurement of calcium and creatinine
- Bone mineral density of lumbar spine, hip and distal radius.
- **High serum calcium and PTH level is diagnostic of primary hyperparathyroidism.** 24-hour urinary calcium is also increased in PHPT.
- **Normocalcemic primary hyperparathyroidism** is a recently recognized variant, presents with high PTH level and normal total and ionized serum calcium levels.

Hypercalcemic Crisis

Rapid-onset, albumin-corrected serum calcium level greater than 14 mg/dl and signs or symptoms of multiorgan dysfunction.

Genetic counseling is indicated in:
- Patients younger than 40 years with primary hyperparathyroidism
- Multigland disease (MGD)
- Patient with family history of PHPT or syndromic manifestations

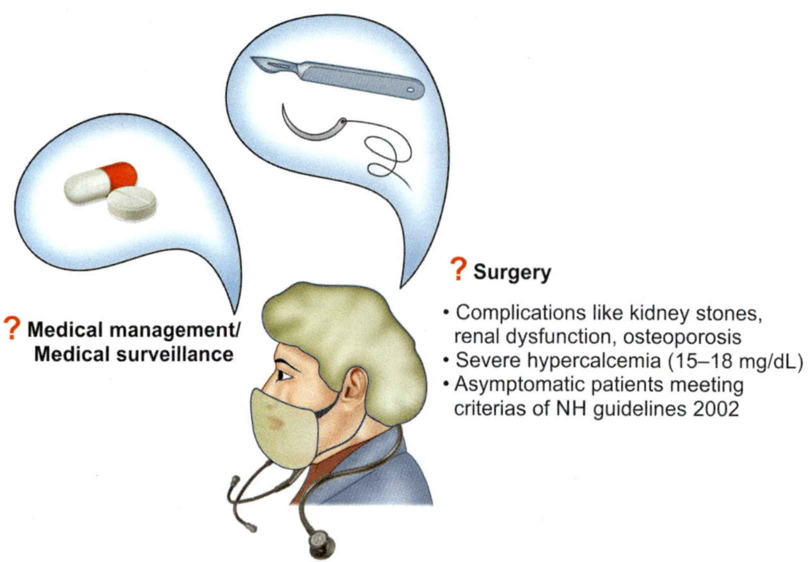

Treatment

Indications of Parathyroidectomy in Primary Hyperparathyroidism

- Serum calcium >1 mg/dL above normal, regardless of whether objective symptoms are present or absent.
- Objective evidence of renal involvement, including silent nephrolithiasis on renal imaging, nephrocalcinosis, hypercalciuria (24-hr urine calcium level >400 mg/dL) with increased stone risk, or impaired renal function (GFR <60 mL/min).
- Patient with osteoporosis, fragility fracture, or evidence of vertebral compression fracture on spine imaging.
- PHPT is diagnosed at 50 years or younger regardless of whether objective or subjective features are present or absent.
- Patients with neurocognitive and/or neuropsychiatric symptoms that are attributable to PHPT.
- Clinical or biochemical evidence consistent with parathyroid carcinoma.

Asymptomatic patients not meeting these criterias may be monitored regularly and surgical intervention must always be undertaken when indicated. The goals of strict monitoring are early detection of worsening hypercalcemia deteriorating bone or renal status or development of other complications of hyperparathyroidism.

- **Parathyroid surgery:** Experienced surgeon with thorough knowledge of parathyroid anatomy and meticulous technique is crucial for a desirable surgical outcome.
- **Parathyroidectomy can be performed by:** (i) Bilateral neck exploration and (ii) Unilateral neck exploration.
- **Bilateral neck exploration** is the classic and traditional approach for PHPT.
- **Planned bilateral exploration is the preferred operative strategy if:** (i) Discordant or nonlocalizing preoperative imaging; (ii) High suspicion of multiglandular disease; (iii) Concomitant thyroid disorders; (iv) Intraoperative PTH monitoring facility is not available; and (v) Surgeon's choice.
- **Unilateral neck exploration** can be planned if localization study and intraoperative PTH assay facilities are available.

Patients undergoing parathyroidectomy should have preoperative thyroid evaluation because of high rate of concomitant disease. In patients with concomitant pHPT and thyroid disease that requires resection, thyroid resection should be performed at the time of parathyroidectomy.

Surgical Adjuncts

- Intraoperative PTH monitoring
- Confirmation of resected parathyroid tissue (by frozen section biopsy, ex-vivo parathyroid aspiration)
- Gland visualization (by methylene blue, near infrared fluorescence or infrared spectroscopy)
- Gland localization (by intraoperative USG, bilateral jugular venous sampling)

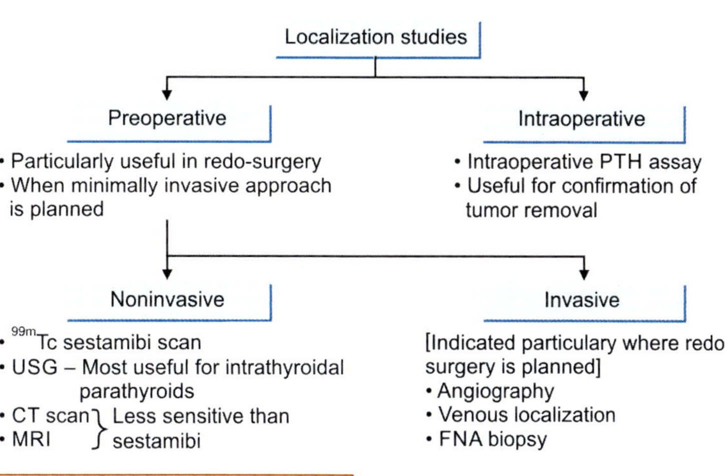

- **^{99m}Tc sestamibi scan** is the most widely used localization study method for detection of parathyroid adenoma (sensitivity >80%).
- It is also known as cardiolite (initially introduced for cardiac imaging)
- It is concentrated in mitochondria rich tissues.

Cervical USG (by an experienced parathyroid sonographer) combined with sestamibi or 4-dimensional computed tomography is the most cost-effective strategy for parathyroid localization.

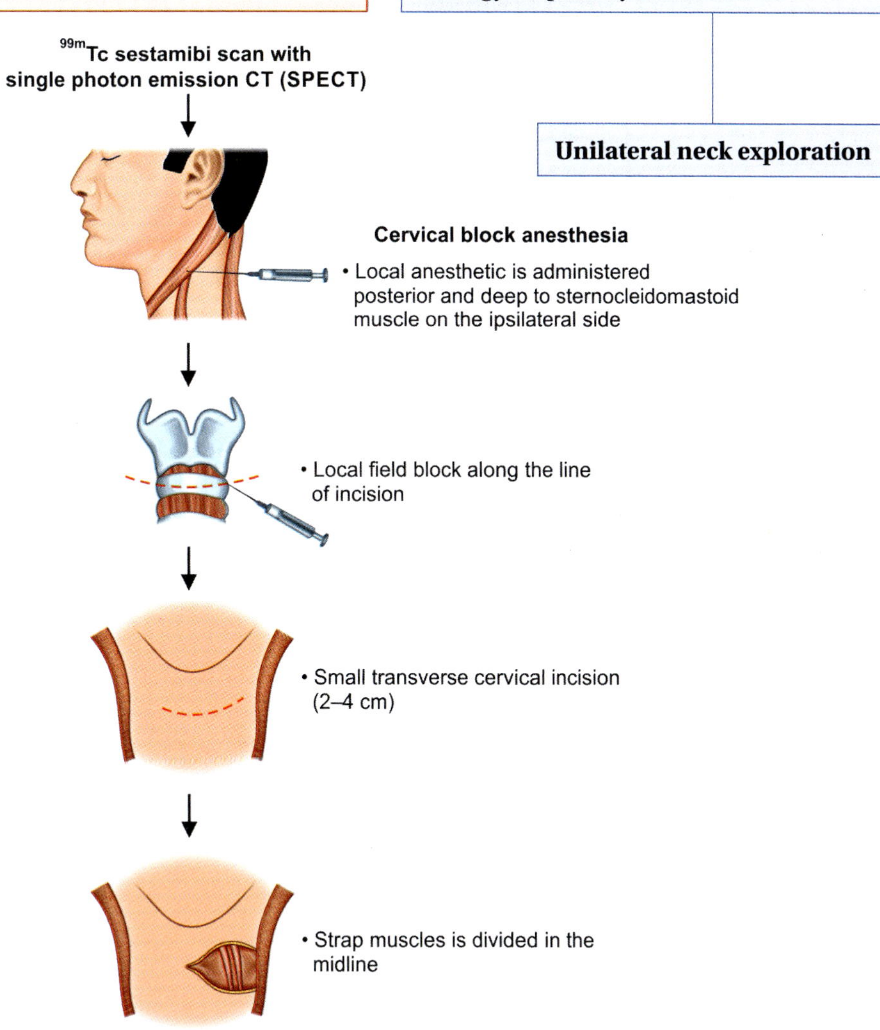

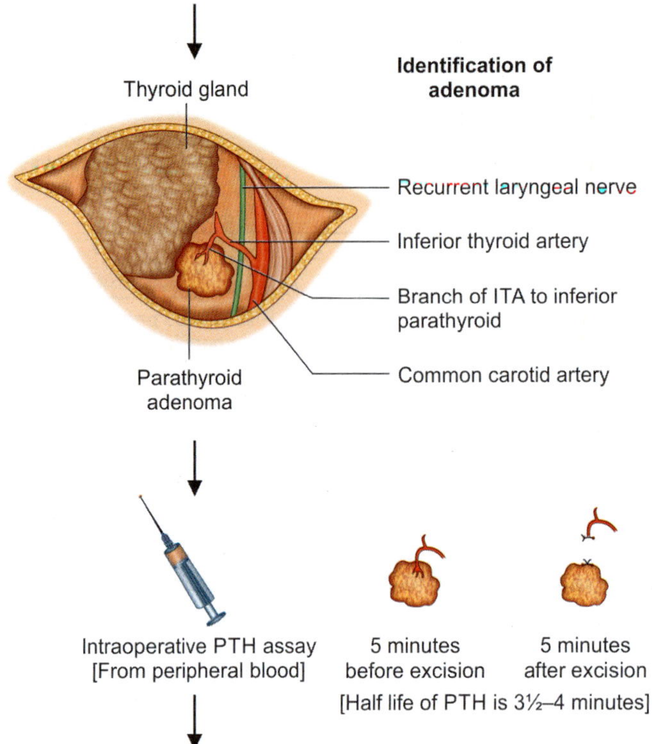

Bilateral Neck Exploration

- Patient's positioning, incision and initial dissection and exposure are similar to thyroidectomy.
- In most cases, parathyroid tumor is found attached to the posterior capsule of the thyroid gland.
- Superior parathyroid glands lie posterior to the RLN, where it enters the cricothyroid muscle. Inferior parathyroid glands lie anterior to the RLN.
- Care must be taken to avoid bleeding and not to traumatize the parathyroid gland, because the color of the gland is useful in distinguishing it from surrounding thyroid, thymus, lymph node and fat.
- Care must be taken to avoid rupture of the gland (rupture results in parathyromatosis and recurrent hyperparathyroidism).

In Patients with Familial HPT and MEN1 and 2A

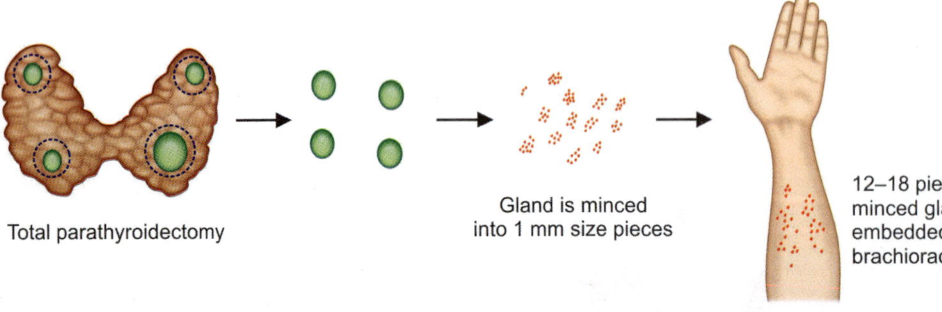

Secondary Hyperparathyroidism

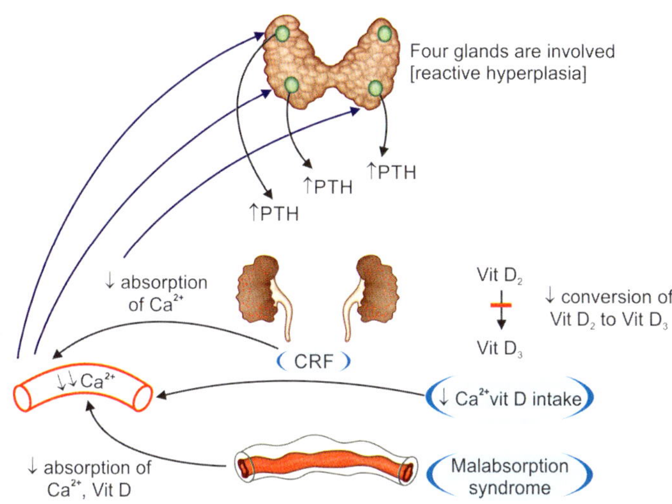

Surgical Approach

- **Preoperative localization is not indicated** because there is compensatory hyperplasia of all parathyroids.
- **Bilateral neck exploration** is required for identification of all glands.
- Either **subtotal parathyroidectomy or total parathyroidectomy with autotransplantation** is performed for secondary hyperparathyroidism.

Causes

- Chronic kidney disease
- Vitamin D deficiency
- Malabsorption syndrome

Treatment

Conservative management:

- Low-phosphate diet
- Phosphate binders
- Calcium and Vit D3 supplementation

Surgery is indicated when:

- Renal osteodystrophy (osteitis fibrosa cystica, osteomalacia, adynamic bone disease).
- Ca^{2+} >11 mg/dL with markedly elevated PTH
- Soft tissue calcification and tumoral calcinosis
- Calciphylaxis (rare, severe complication characterized by calcification of the media of small to medium sized arteries).

Subtotal parathyroidectomy OR **Total parathyroidectomy with autotransplantation**

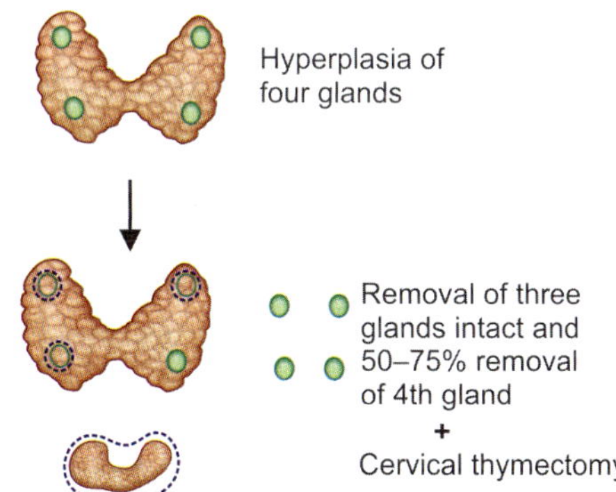

[Supernumerary intrathymic parathyroid gland is a common cause of recurrence]

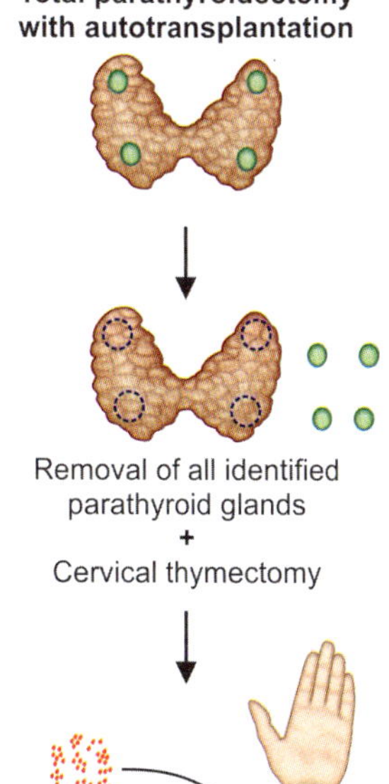

Tertiary Hyperparathyroidism

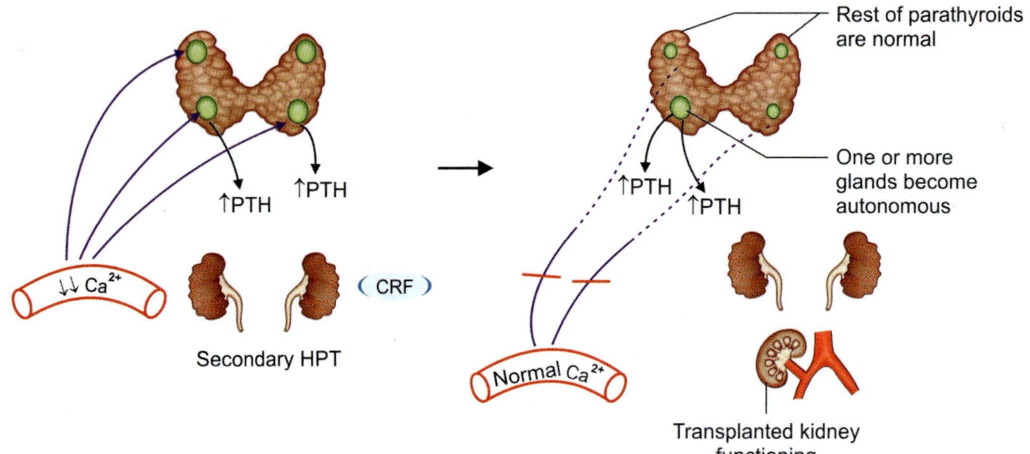

- **Surgical intervention is indicated for symptomatic disease** (renal stones, pathologic fractures, bone pain, mental status changes) or increased PTH secretion persisting for more than 1 year after successful transplant.
- **Subtotal parathyroidectomy** is the preferred surgical approach, if all of the glands become autonomous.

Hypoparathyroidism

Hypoparathyroidism is characterized by **decreased PTH secretion or action.**

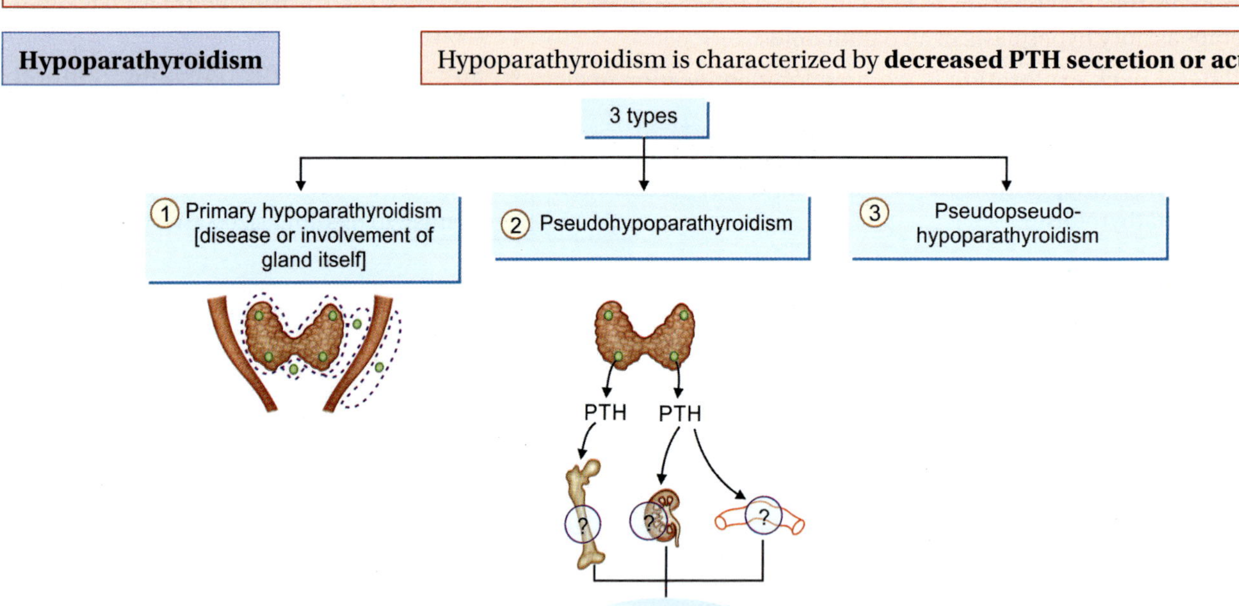

Primary Hypoparathyroidism

- After thyroid surgery, particularly after total thyroidectomy with neck dissection **(Most common cause)**
- After parathyroid exploration
- Hereditary polyglandular deficiency syndrome (beside parathyroid, thyroid, adrenal, pancreas also affected)
- Infiltrative disease (hemochromatosis, Wilson's disease, sarcoidosis, and tuberculosis)
- Congenital absence of parathyroids and thymus—DiGeorge syndrome

Primary hypoparathyroidism is characterized by hypocalcemia, hyperphosphatemia, hypocalciuria.

Pseudohypoparathyroidism

- Pseudohypoparathyroidism is a rare inherited disorder characterized by resistance to parathyroid hormone.
- This disorder is manifested by signs and symptoms of hypoparathyroidism.
- Albright's hereditary Osteodystrophy (Short stature, short metacarpals and metatarsals, flat nose, round face, multiple exostoses) phenotype is commonly observed in pseudohypoparathyroidism type 1A and 1C.

Pseudopseudohypoparathyroidism

- Rare familial disorder with clinical features of pseudohypoparathyroidism
- Tissues normally respond to PTH
- No hypocalcemia or hyperphosphatemia

Clinical Presentation of Hypoparathyroidism

- Signs and symptoms of hypocalcemia are due to neuromuscular excitability from reduced ionized calcium in plasma
- Early symptoms are tingling and numbness in fingertip and circumoral region
- Late symptoms are anxiety, confusion, depression and tetany
- In extreme cases, carpopedal spasms and tetany

Tetany

Clinical presentations of tetany are tonic-clonic seizures, carpopedal spasm, laryngeal stridor.

Latent tetany may be elicited by: **Chvostek's sign** and **Trousseau's sign**.

Chvostek's Sign

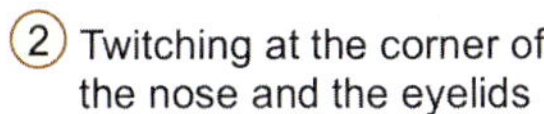

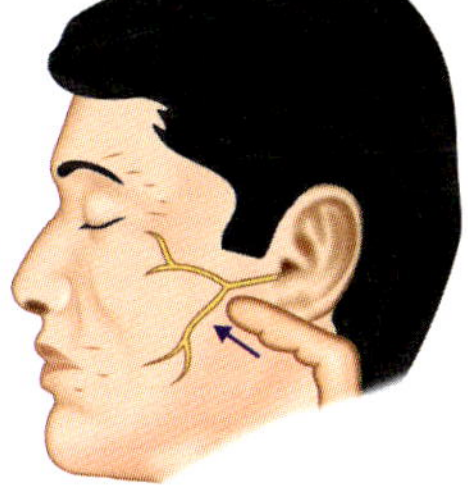

Trousseau's Sign

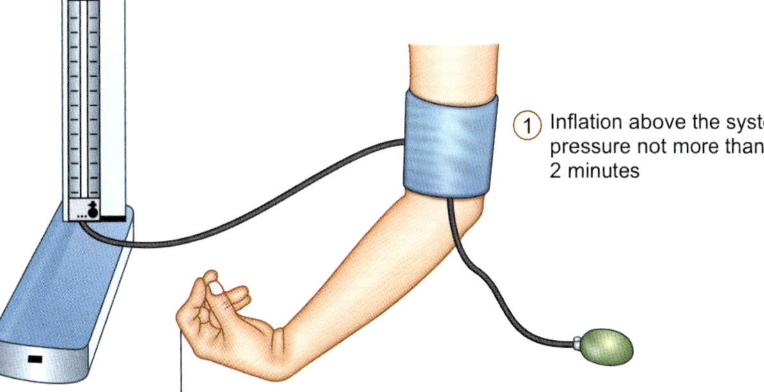

Treatment of Hypoparathyroidism

- In acute cases, slow IV Ca gluconate (10%) 10–20 mL
- For long-term management, 1, 25 $(OH)_2$ D_3 combined with high oral calcium
- Thiazide diuretics help to lower urinary calcium and thereby decreasing the chance of kidney stone formation

Diseases of Adrenal Gland

Anatomy and Anatomical Variations

- Right adrenal gland is pyramidal shaped and left adrenal gland is crescentic in shape.
- Each gland is drained by 'single' vein.
- Right adrenal vein drains into IVC (80% cases), left adrenal vein drains into left renal vein.
- Each gland is supplied by '3' arteries:
  - **Superior adrenal artery:** Branch of inferior phrenic artery.
  - **Middle adrenal artery:** Branch of abdominal aorta.
  - **Inferior adrenal artery:** Branch of renal artery.
- Inferior adrenal artery is the most prominent artery and can be distinctly identified during operation.

Arteries supply to the adrenals branch into numerous arterioles to form an arterial plexus beneath the glandular capsule. Therefore, careful dissection, ligation and division is necessary during adrenalectomy.

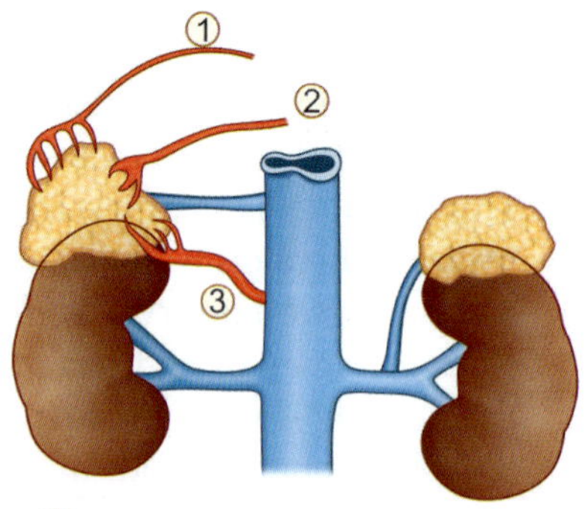

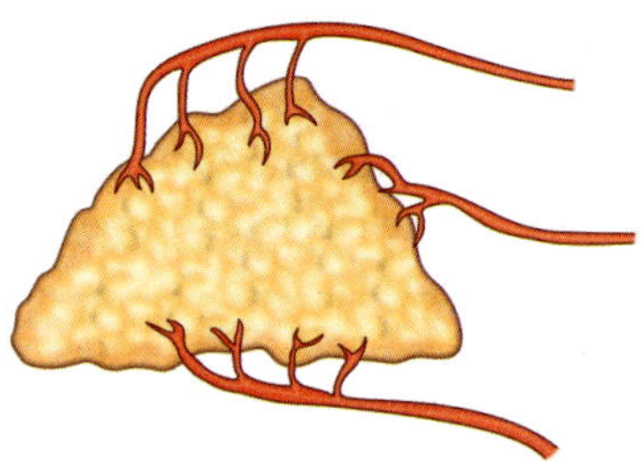

Variant Drainage of Right Adrenal Vein

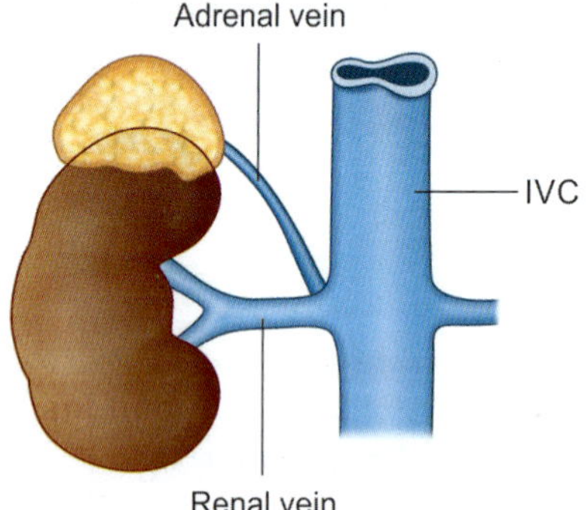

Adrenal Vein Drains into Renal Vein-IVC Confluence

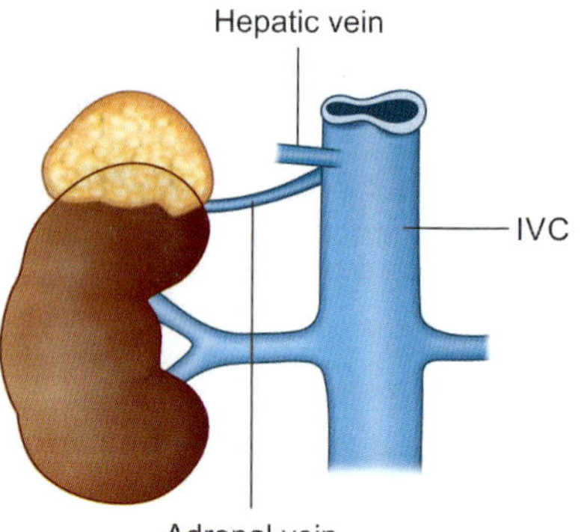

Adrenal Vein Drains into Right Hepatic Vein-IVC Confluence

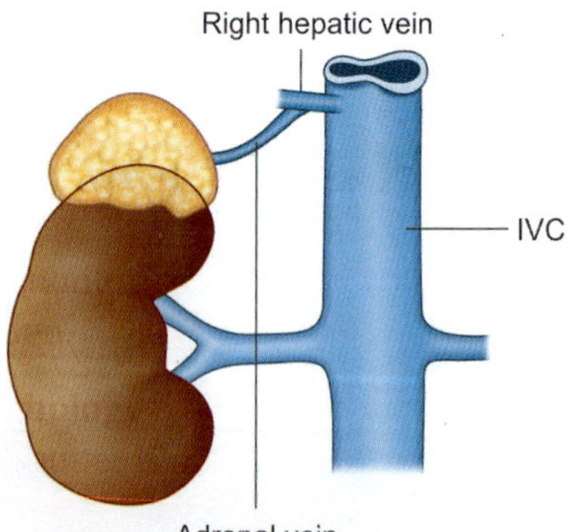

Adrenal Vein Drains into Right Hepatic Vein

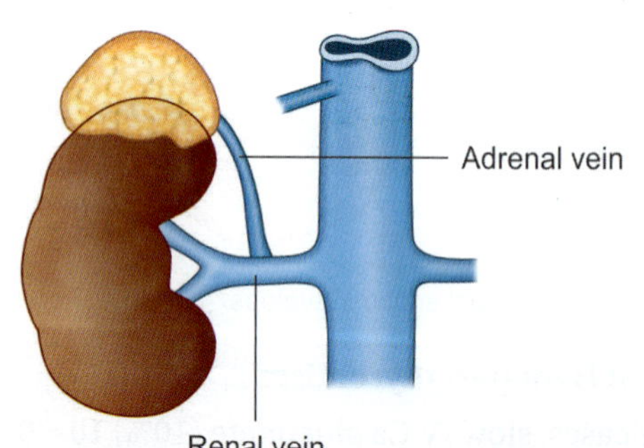

Adrenal Vein Drains into Right Renal Vein

Microscopic Features of Adrenal Gland

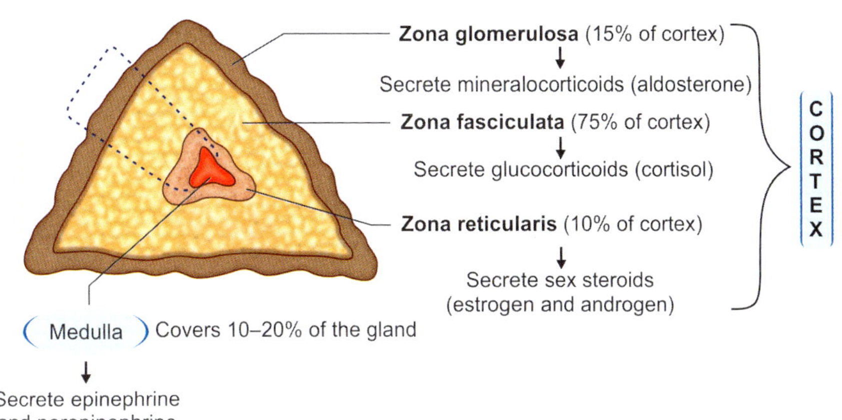

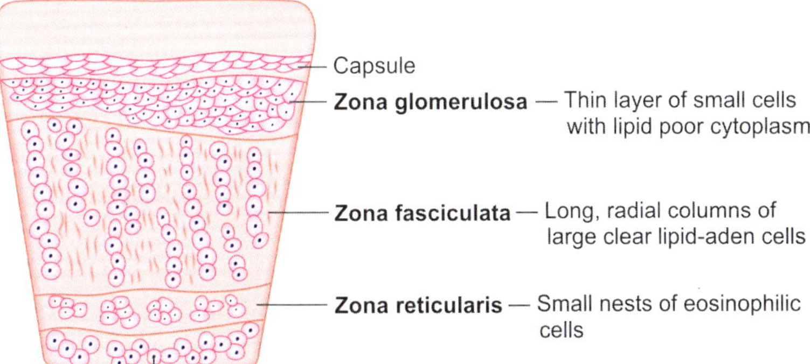

- **Cortex and medulla** differ in their **development, structure, and function.**
- Sympathetic fibers synapse directly with the **chromaffin cells. These cells are called 'chromaffin cells' because** the secretory granules yield a brown colored reaction when treated with chromium salts.

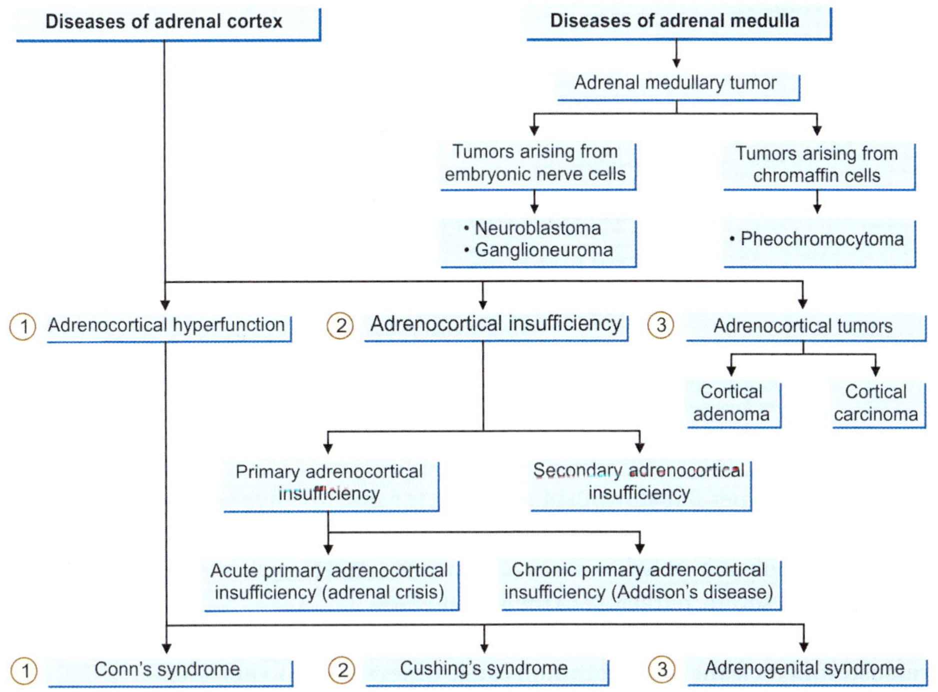

Conn's Syndrome (Hyperaldosteronism)

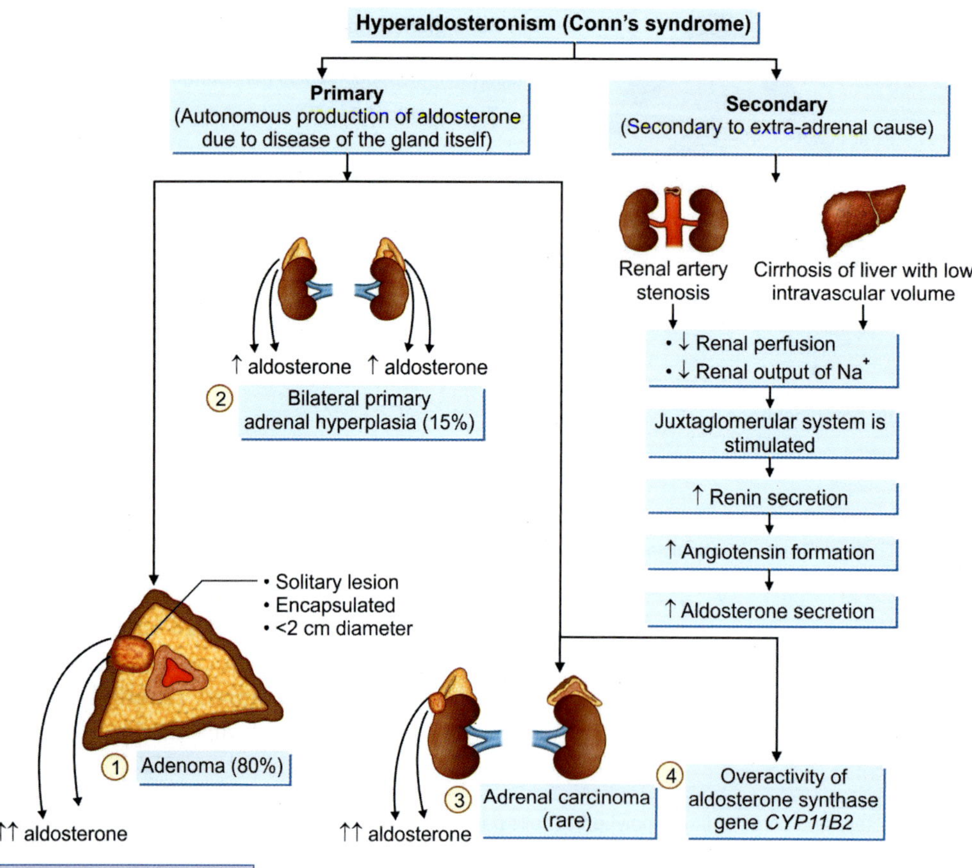

Microscopic Features of Adenoma

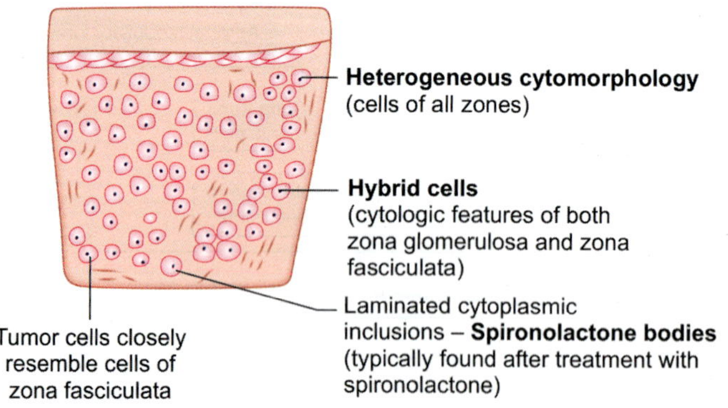

Clinical Presentation

- **Classic findings in primary hyperaldosteronism are hypertension and hypokalemia**
- Disease is most commonly found in mid-adult life, more common in females
- Malaise, muscle weakness, polyuria, polydipsia, muscle cramps, paresthesia's are usual presentations
- Hypertension is moderate to severe, refractory to medical therapy
- Primary hyperaldosteronism is associated with significantly increased risk for stroke, AMI and atrial fibrillation
- **Primary hyperaldosteronism is the most common cause of secondary hypertension**

Pathophysiology of Hypertension and Hypokalemia

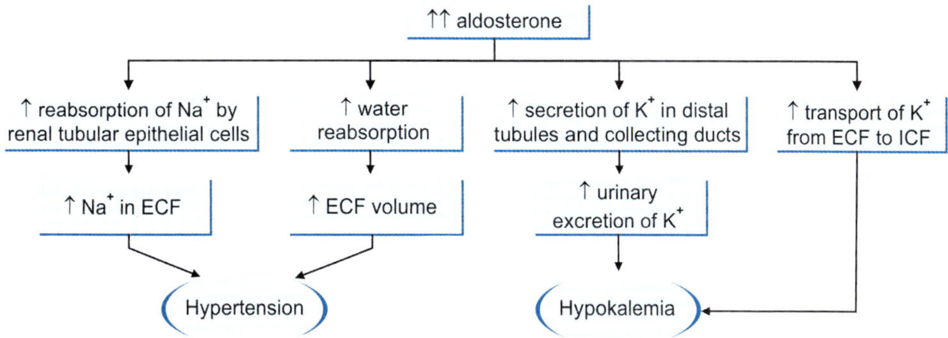

Biochemical screening:

- Biochemical screening is indicated if clinical presentations are suggestive of primary hyperaldosteronism.
- The screening is based on the fact that primary hyperaldosteronism suppresses rennin secretion.
- *Screening tests are:* Plasma aldosterone conc (ng/dl): Plasma renin activity (ng/ml/h) >20
- Setting of absolute plasma aldosterone conc. >15 ng/dl.

Confirmatory test:

- If biochemical screening tests suggest primary hyperaldosteronism, then confirmatory test is indicated.
- Failure to suppress aldosterone secretion with sodium loading (oral salt/IV Nacl infusion) confirm the diagnosis of primary hyperaldosteronism.

Localization of the pathology:

- After confirmation of diagnosis, localization of the pathology is the next step.
- Localization is important because surgical management is indicated for unilateral pathology whereas medical management is preferred for bilateral pathology.
- Thin-cut (3 mm) adrenal CT is the imaging modality of choice for localization.

Finding of a solitary adrenal mass (>1 cm) and a normal contralateral adrenal in CT is sufficient to proceed to adrenalectomy without further testing.

- If, CT scan is equivocal or negative, adrenal vein sampling is indicated. This is the most certain way to localize an aldosteronoma.

Treatment

Medical management:

- Indicated for bilateral pathology, idiopathic hyperaldosteronism, surgically unfit patients
- Goal of therapy is to control hypertension and hypokalemia
- Spironolactone is the preferred agent
- Amiloride, ACE inhibitors, calcium-channel blockers are also used

Surgical management:

- Indicated for aldosteronoma, unilateral adrenal hyperplasia, cortical carcinoma
- Usually aldosteronomas are small and benign, so **laparoscopic adrenalectomy is the surgery of choice**
- In open approach, lateral transabdominal approach is thc preferred approach
- Bilateral adrenalectomy is not indicated

Blood pressure and hypokalemia should be corrected before surgery.

Spironolactone is the drug of choice for treating the manifestations.

Hypercortisolism (Cushing Syndrome)

Cushing syndrome is characterized by raised serum cortisol level, regardless of etiology.

Types: (i) Pituitary Cushing's syndrome; (ii) Adrenal Cushing's syndrome; (iii) Ectopic ACTH syndrome; and (iv) Iatrogenic Cushing's syndrome.

Pituitary Cushing's Syndrome

- **Also known as Cushing disease**
- Females are more affected (5:1)
- ACTH dependent

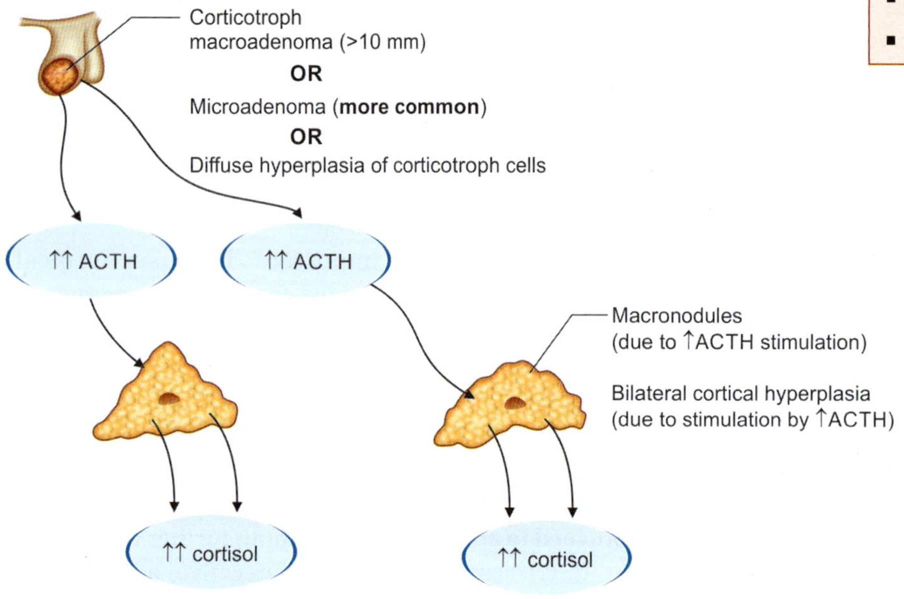

Corticotroph macroadenoma (>10 mm)
OR
Microadenoma (**more common**)
OR
Diffuse hyperplasia of corticotroph cells

↑↑ ACTH

↑↑ ACTH

Macronodules (due to ↑ACTH stimulation)

Bilateral cortical hyperplasia (due to stimulation by ↑ACTH)

↑↑ cortisol

↑↑ cortisol

Adrenal Cushing's Syndrome

ACTH-independent

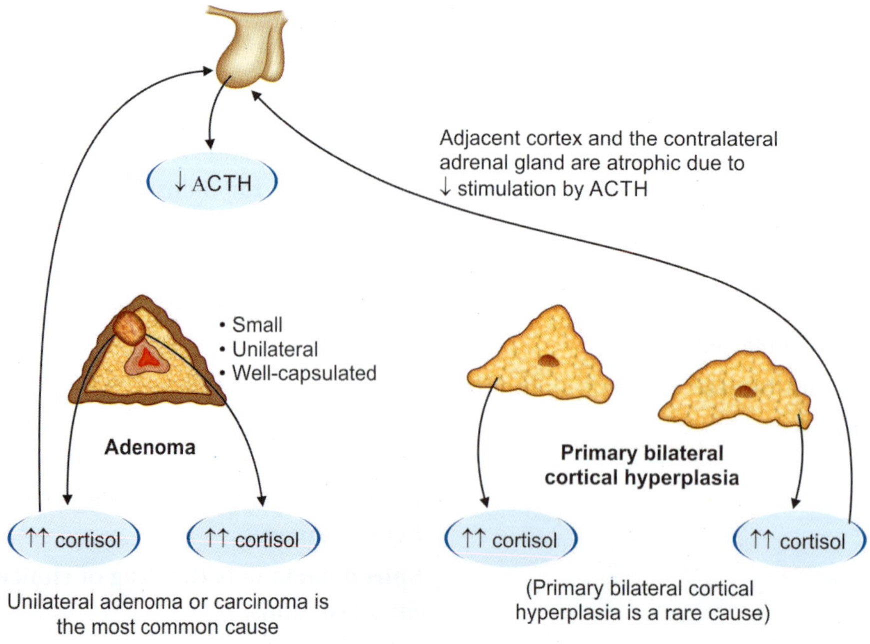

↓ ACTH

Adjacent cortex and the contralateral adrenal gland are atrophic due to ↓ stimulation by ACTH

- Small
- Unilateral
- Well-capsulated

Adenoma

Primary bilateral cortical hyperplasia

↑↑ cortisol

↑↑ cortisol

↑↑ cortisol

↑↑ cortisol

Unilateral adenoma or carcinoma is the most common cause

(Primary bilateral cortical hyperplasia is a rare cause)

Ectopic ACTH Syndrome

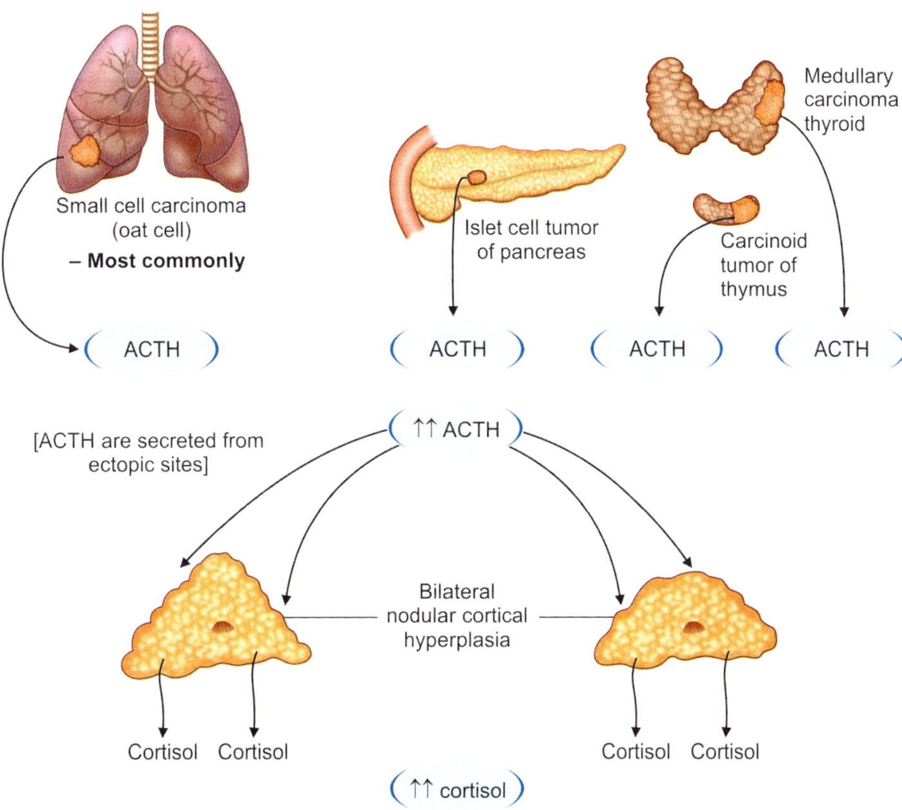

Iatrogenic Cushing Syndrome

Most common cause of Cushing syndrome

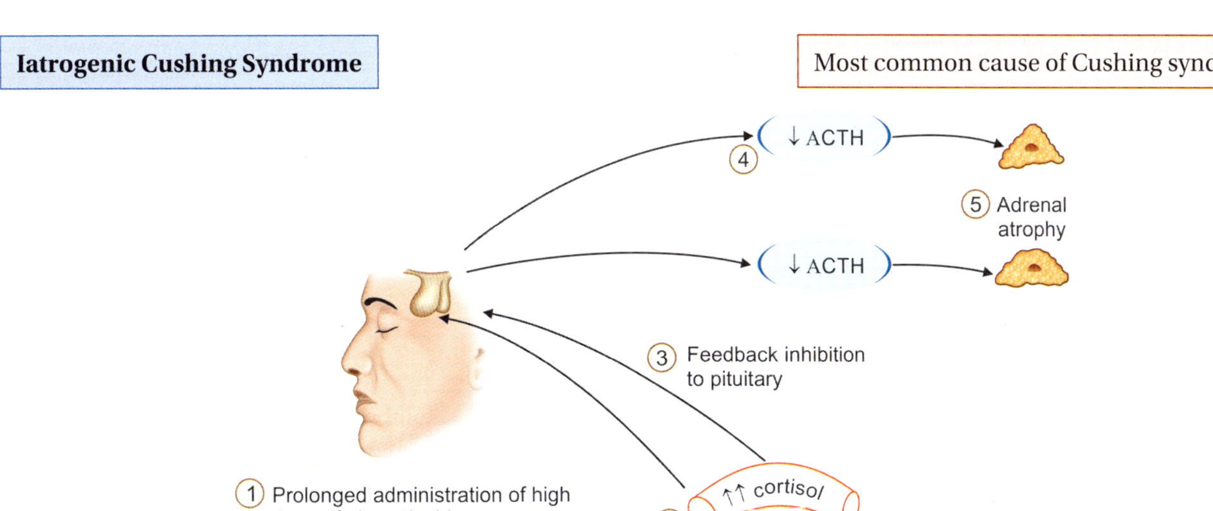

Clinical Presentation

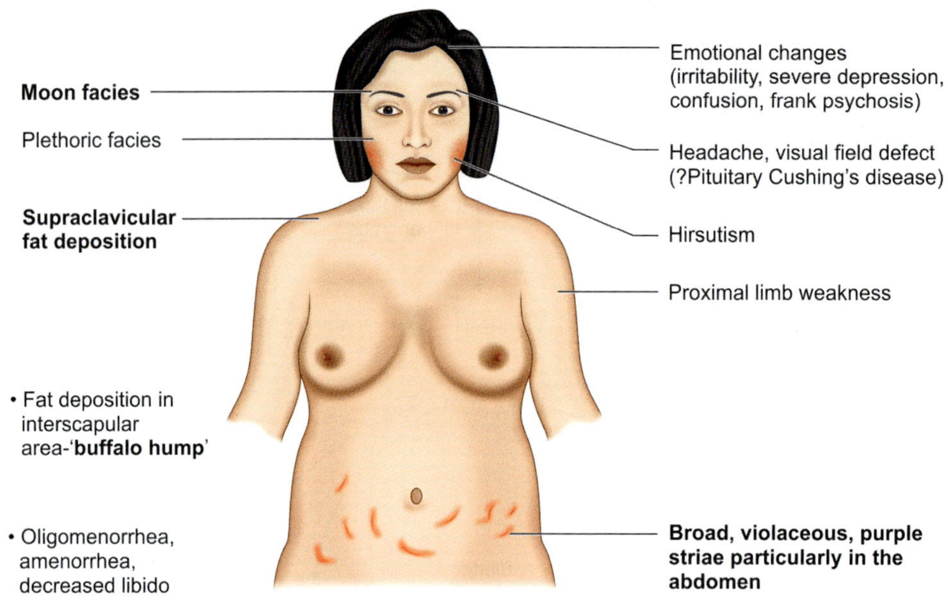

- Progressive truncal obesity is the **most common symptom.**
- Osteoporosis leads to collapse of vertebral bodies and pathologic fractures of bones
- Hypertension
- Hyperglycemia, glucosuria, polydipsia (due to increased hepatic gluconeogenesis and insulin resistance)
- Hyperpigmentation of the skin (due to melanocyte stimulating activity of ACTH precursor molecule)
- Possibility of ectopic ACTH syndrome must be keep in mind.
- **Typical striae, myopathy, easy bruising, virilizing signs are suggestive findings of Cushing's syndrome.**

Diagnosis

- If clinical features are suggestive of Cushing syndrome, **overnight dexamethasone suppression test** is indicated. If the test is positive, the diagnosis is established.
- If the test is negative, classic low dose dexamethasone suppression test is indicated.
- **Positive overnight dexamethasone suppression test** or positive classic low dose dexamethasone suppression test along with **24 hours elevated urinary cortisol—diagnostic of Cushing's syndrome**

Once the diagnosis of Cushing's syndrome is established, **then it should be determined whether Cushing syndrome is ACTH dependant or ACTH independent.**

Dexamethasone Suppression Tests

- **These tests are done based on the fact** that in Cushing syndrome, increased glucocorticoid level is not suppressed by exogenous cortisol administration.
- **In overnight dexamethasone suppression test,** 1 mg dexamethasone is administered orally at 11 pm, then serum cortisol is measured at 8 am.
- In normal adults, serum cortisol will be less than 3 μg/dL. In Cushing syndrome, serum cortisol will be normal.
- Classic low dose dexamethasone suppression test is not preferred nowadays due to low sensitivity and specificity.

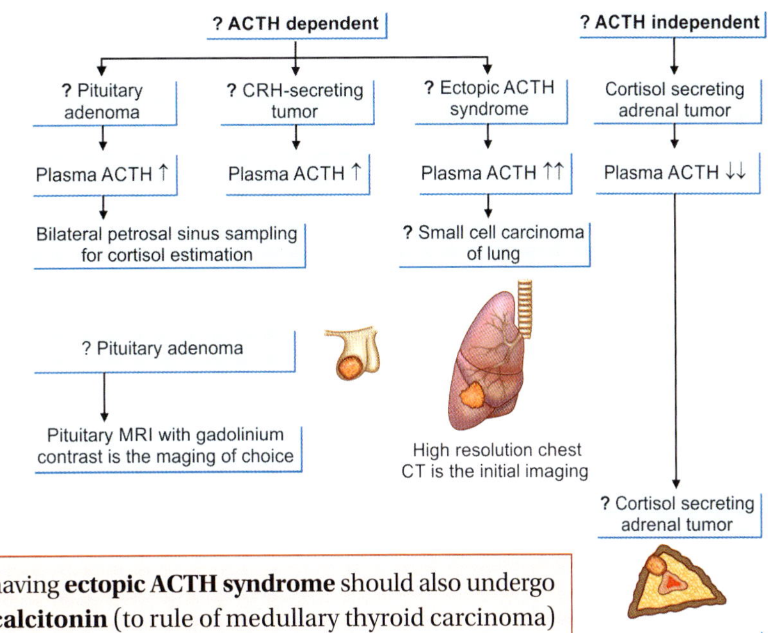

[Patients suspected of having **ectopic ACTH syndrome** should also undergo **estimation of serum calcitonin** (to rule of medullary thyroid carcinoma) and **urinary catecholamines** (to rule out pheochromocytoma)].

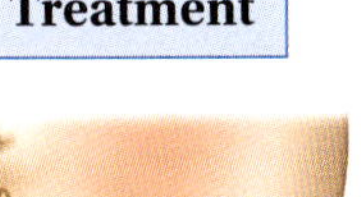

Surgery for Adrenal Cushing Syndrome

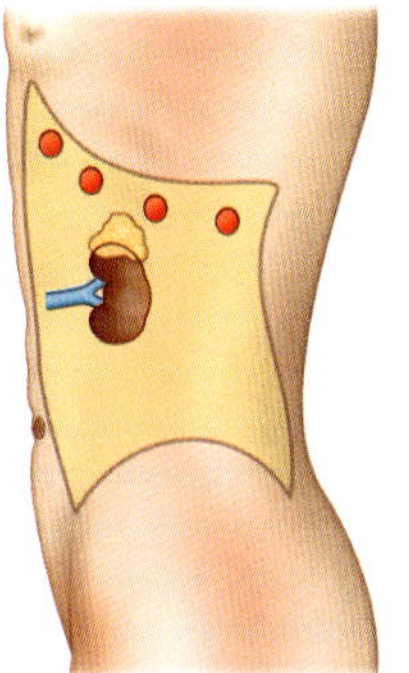

Lap adrenalectomy for small adenoma (<6 cm)

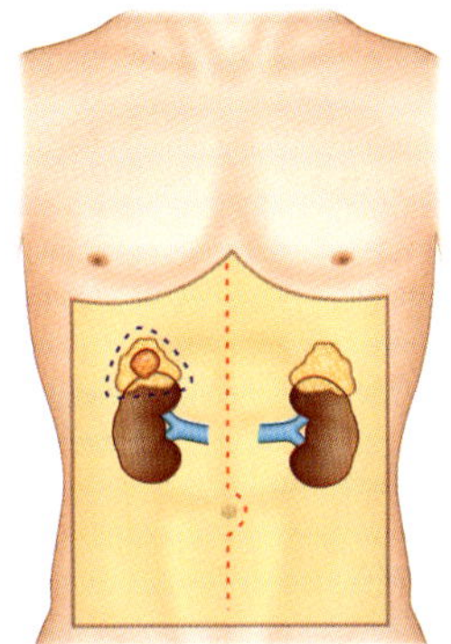

Large adenoma or Carcinoma — Open adrenalectomy

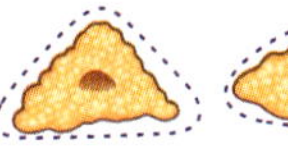

Bilateral adrenalectomy for primary adrenal hyperplasia

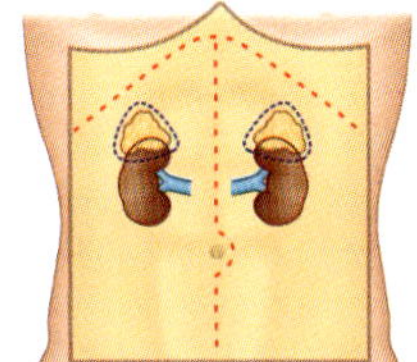

Treatment for Pituitary Cushing Syndrome

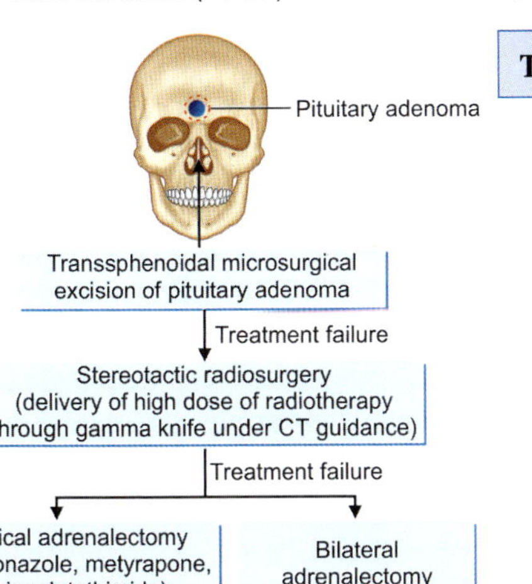

Treatment for Ectopic ACTH Syndrome

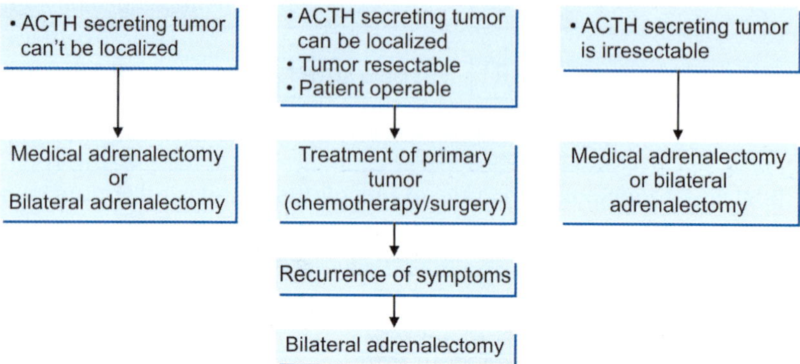

- In patients undergoing adrenalectomy, **perioperative 'stress dose' steroid** (hydrocortisone, 100 mg every 8 hours for 24 hours) is recommended.
- After total adrenalectomy, **lifelong corticosteroid maintenance therapy** is necessary.

Adrenogenital Syndrome

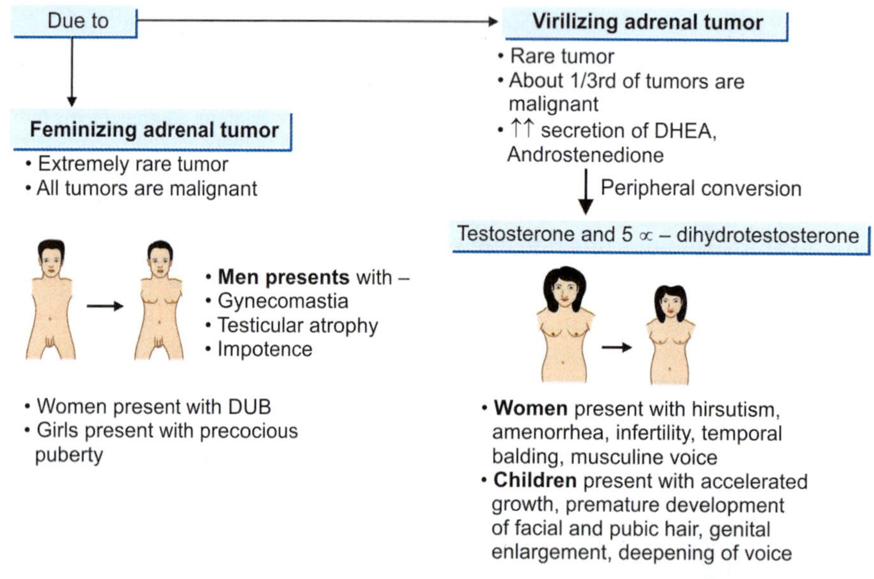

Diagnosis

Diagnosis is established by increased level of plasma or urinary 17-ketosteroids.

Treatment

- Feminizing adrenal tumors are all malignant, so radiographic and intraoperative assessment for evidence of metastasis are necessary.
- **For benign tumor:** Laparoscopic adrenalectomy
- **For malignant tumor:** Open adrenalectomy

Adrenal Insufficiency

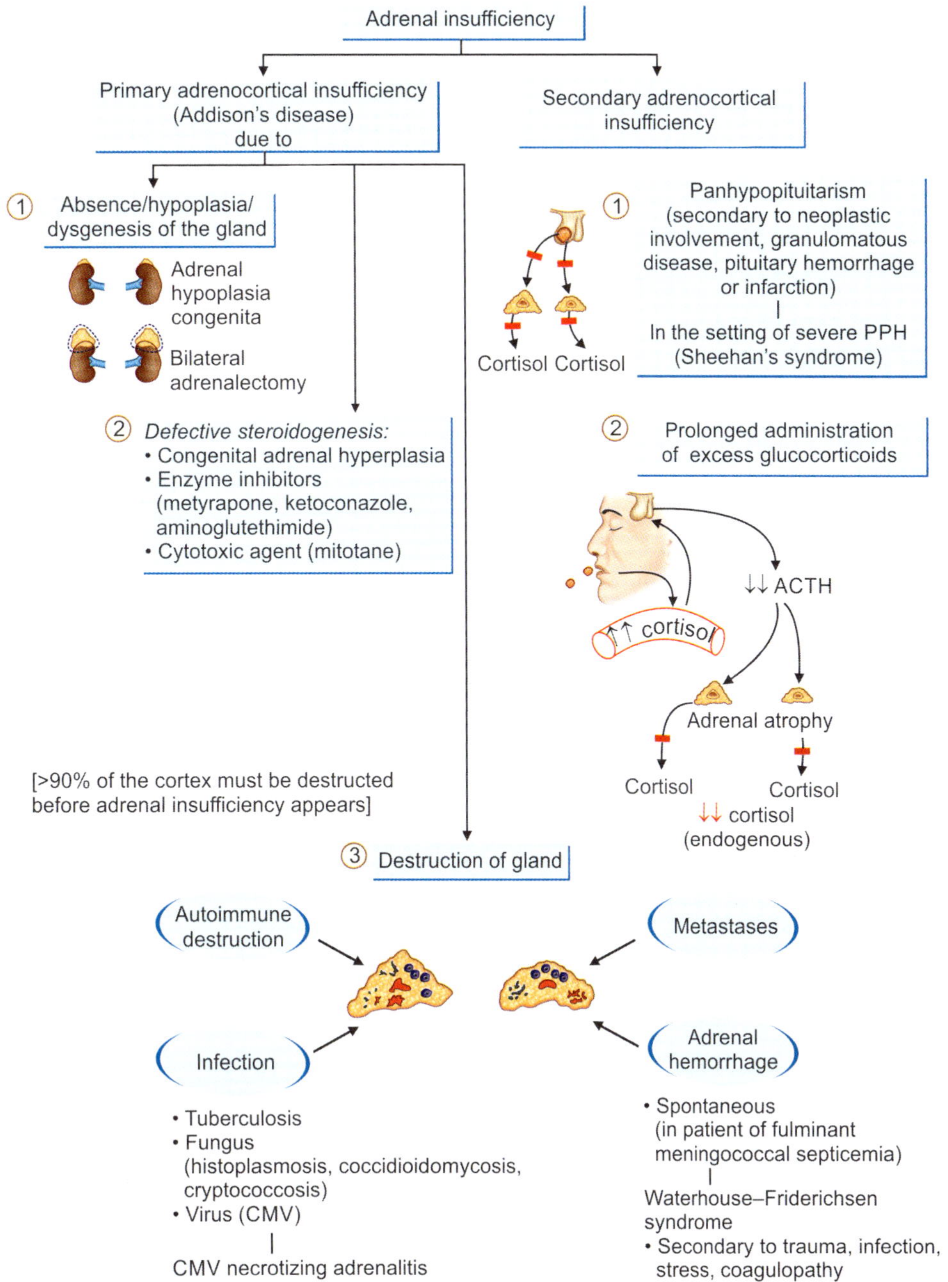

Clinical Presentations

- Both in primary and secondary adrenocortical insufficiency, most of the symptoms and signs are similar except hyperpigmentation, which is absent in secondary adrenocortical insufficiency.
- Insidious onset of fatigability, weakness, anorexia, nausea, vomiting, weight loss, cutaneous and mucosal pigmentation and hypotension.

Diagnosis

- **Characteristic laboratory findings:** (i) Hyponatremia; (ii) Hyperkalemia; (iii) Fasting or reactive hypoglycemia; and (iv) Eosinophilia.
- **ACTH stimulation test** is indicated for diagnosis of adrenal insufficiency.

Treatment

Hormone replacement therapy:

Glucocorticoid replacement:

- Cortisol (hydrocortisone)—(20-30 mg/day)
- 2/3rd of dose in the morning
- 1/3rd of dose in the late afternoon

Mineralocorticoid replacement:

- Fludrocortisone
- Ample intake of sodium (3-4 g/day)

(Mineralocorticoid therapy is not necessary in secondary insufficiency)

- Patients must know about his/her disease
- He/she should carry medical identification and must know the method of parenteral self-administration of steroids

Adrenal Crisis

Acute adrenal insufficiency may cause life-threatening condition.

Risk factors:

- Stress, infection or trauma in patients of Addison's disease
- Waterhouse—Friderichsen syndrome
- Anticoagulant therapy or coagulation disorders causing bilateral adrenal hemorrhage
- Rapid withdrawal of steroids from patient with adrenal atrophy

Clinical presentation:

- Nausea, vomiting and abdominal pain
- Hypovolemic shock

Treatment:

- Replacement of sodium and water deficit (>2l)
- Replacement of Glucocorticoid (hydrocortisone/dexamethasone)
  [Initially mineralocorticoid replacement is not necessary]

Diseases of Adrenal Medulla

Pheochromocytomas and **paragangliomas** are catecholamine-producing neuroendocrine tumors. Pheochromocytomas arise from chromaffin cells of the adrenal medulla, paragangliomas arise from extra-adrenal autonomic paraganglia.

Pheochromocytoma

Pheochromocytoma is a catecholamine-producing tumor arising from chromaffin cells and a surgically correctable cause of hypertension.

- **It is often called '10% tumor'** because—10% bilateral, 10% malignant, 10% in pediatric patients, 10% are extra-adrenal, 10% familial.
- **Etiology** of sporadic pheochromocytoma is unknown, but in familial cases, various germline mutations are detected-RET, VHL, NF1, SDHB, SDHC, SDHD.
- **Grossly**, pheochromocytoma appears as circumscribed lesion. On cut section, areas of hemorrhage and necrosis are seen.
- **Microscopically**, it looks—Tumor cells arranged as well-defined nests (Zell-Ballen pattern). Tumor cells are large, polyhedral, pleomorphic with abundant granular cytoplasm.

Clinical presentation:

- Presentation is so variable, from an incidentaloma to hypertensive crisis with CVS and cardiac complications, termed as 'the **great masquerader**'.

Classic triad: 1. Palpitation; **2.** Headache; and **3.** Profuse sweating.

- Episodic presentation along with hypertension almost confirms the diagnosis.
- Hypertension is the most common clinical sign.
- Hypertension may be presented as paroxysmal with intervening normotension or sustained hypertension with paroxysms or sustained hypertension alone.
- Paroxysms (episodes of hormone release) usually lasts for less than an hour.
- During paroxysms, patients become anxious and pale, suffering from palpitation and profuse sweating. Paroxysms precipitated by positional changes, exercise, pregnancy, surgery, urination and medications (tricyclic antidepressants, opioids, metoclopramide).

Anxiety, tremulousness, flushing, chest pain, shortness of breath, abdominal pain, nausea, vomiting are nonspecific symptoms.

- **Paragangliomas** are non-epithelial neuroendocrine neoplasms derive from paraganglia.
- Paragangliomas arise from either sympathetic paravertebral ganglia of thorax, abdomen, and pelvis or may arise from parasympathetic ganglia along the glossopharyngeal and vagal nerves in the neck and at the base of the skull.
- About 40% of paragangliomas secrete catecholamines. About 5% of head and neck paragangliomas secrete catecholamines, mostly it is dopamine.

Extra-adrenal Sites of Pheochromocytoma

- Organ of Zuckerkandl at the aortic bifurcation (most common extra-adrenal site)
- Urinary bladder
- Renal hilum
- Chest
- Neck

Familial Syndromes Associated with Pheochromocytoma and Paraganglioma

- Multiple endocrine neoplasia type 2A and 2B (RET proto-oncogene mutation)
- Neurofibromatosis type 1 (NF1, a tumor suppressor gene)
- Von Hippel-Lindau disease (VHL, a tumor suppressor gene)
- Familial paraganglioma syndromes (genes encoding SDH complex subunits)
- Renal cell carcinoma with SDHB mutation
- Carney triad
- Osler-Weber-Rendu syndrome

Syndrome associated pheochromocytomas are usually bilateral.

Diagnosis

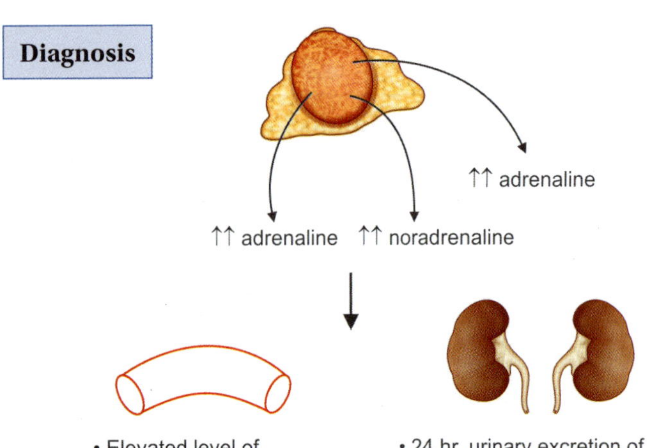

If biochemical studies confirm the presence of catecholamine secreting tumor, then localization study is to be done to know whether the tumor is unilateral or bilateral or extra-adrenal.

Localization study:

- CT scan is the imaging of choice.
- If CT scan showing normal adrenals, then ^{131}I or ^{123}I labelled metaiodobenzylguanidine (MIBG) scanning is valuable, because only ectopic areas of adrenergic tissue show uptake of MIBG.
- T2-weighted MRI with gadolinium contrast is also helpful to detect extra-adrenal pheochromocytomas and paragangliomas.

By documentation of catecholamine excess

Biochemical Tests

- Plasma metanephrines measurement is the most sensitive assay
- Plasma free metanephrines and normetanephrines—3 times above the upper limit of normal is diagnostic

Medications that interfere with plasma metanephrines evaluation:

- Acetaminophen
- Serotonin-reuptake inhibitors
- Monoamine oxidase inhibitors

^{131}I or ^{123}I labelled Metaiodobenzylguanidine (MIBG) Scanning

- This imaging modality can be used for functional assessment and localization of pheochromocytoma. MIBG is the imaging of choice if metastatic extra-adrenal pheochromocytoma is suspected.
- MIBG is a structural and functional analog of norepinephrine and guanethidine. MIBG is also concentrated in neuroblastomas and carcinoid tumors.

Treatment

Complete tumor removal without any hypertensive crisis should be the goal of management.

Preoperative preparation in pheochromocytoma:

α-adrenergic blockers (Phenoxybenzamine, doxazosin, terazosin, prazosin):

- Should be started 1–3 weeks preoperatively
- Most commonly used alpha blocker is phenoxybenzamine
- Therapy is started at a dosage of 10 mg twice daily and the dosage is titrated to 300–400 mg daily in divided doses until patient becomes normotensive, hypertension is well controlled, or intolerable side effects develop (orthostatic hypotension, tachycardia, nasal congestion).

α-methyltyrosine:

- Inhibits tyrosine hydroxylase (rate-limiting enzyme in catecholamine synthesis)
- May be used in combination with phenoxybenzamine when standard alpha-blockade is ineffective in reaching target blood pressure.

β-blockers:

- β-blockers should be given only after adequate alpha-adrenergic blockage (to avoid the effects of unopposed α-stimulation, i.e. hypertensive crisis, congestive heart failure.
- Indicated for persistent tachycardia, extrasystoles, or arrhythmias
- Most commonly used beta blocker is propranolol, dosage of 10–40 mg every 6–8 hours

Calcium-channel Blockers

- Most commonly used calcium channel blocker is Nicardipine
- Calcium channel blockers are not recommended as monotherapy unless the patient cannot tolerate alpha-blockade, liberal fluid and salt intake.

Roizen criteria: To objectively assess the adequate preoperative alpha blockade.

Criteria's are:

- No in-hospital blood pressure >160/90 mm Hg for 24 hour prior to surgery
- No orthostatic hypotension with blood pressure <80/45 mm Hg
- No ST or T wave changes for 1-week prior to surgery
- No more than 5 premature ventricular contractions per minute

Intraoperative Management of Pheochromocytoma

- An arterial line (for continuous monitoring of blood pressure) and central venous line (to monitor intravascular volume status). Pulmonary arterial line may be indicated in patients with cardiac disease.
- **Inhalation agents:** Isoflurane and enflurane are preferred (minimal cardiac depressant effects).
- **Intraoperative hypertension:** Controlled with nitroprusside, nicardipine, nitroglycerine, phentolamine.
- **Tachyarrhythmia:** Treated with β-adrenergic blocker (Esmolol), ventricular arrhythmia is treated with lidocaine.
- Minimal tumor manipulation and avoidance of rupture of tumor capsule.
- After removal of tumor, severe hypotension may develop- treated with large volume of IV fluid and α-adrenergic agonist.
- In immediate postoperative period- patient should be monitored for hypotension and hypoglycemia.

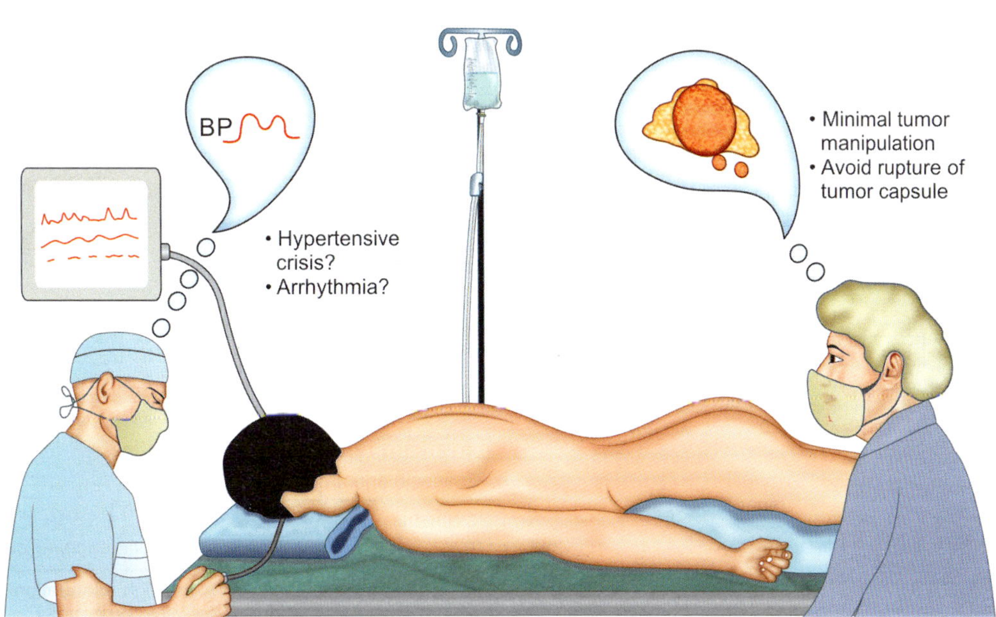

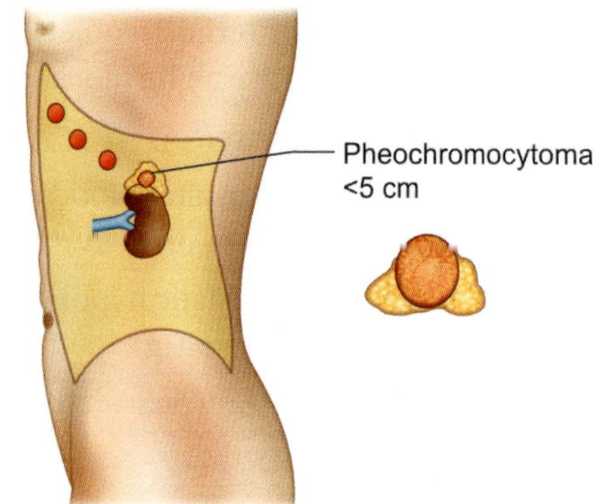

Lap adrenalectomy – for <5 cm

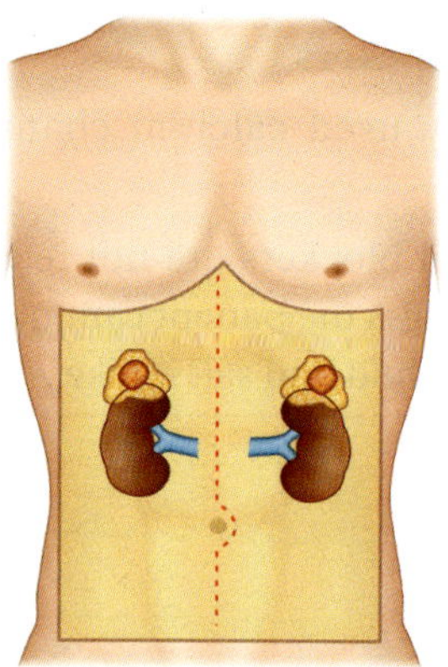

Open anterior approach
For – Bilateral tumors
– Extra-adrenal tumor
– Metastatic lesions

Approaches for Open Adrenalectomy

- Transperitoneal approach (Anterior transabdominal and Thoracoabdominal)
- Retroperitoneal approach (Flank approach and Posterior lumbodorsal approach)

In Patients of MEN2 and Bilateral Pheochromocytoma

Total adrenalectomy on the side of larger tumor and Cortical sparing subtotal adrenalectomy on the side of smaller tumor.

Transperitoneal Approach

- **Advantages:** (i) Excellent exposure and (ii) Better access to hilum and great vessels.
- **Disadvantages:** (i) Chance of postoperative ileus is more; (ii) Risk of intra-abdominal organ injury; and (iii) Longer hospitalization

Retroperitoneal Approach

- **Advantages:** (i) Less chance of postoperative ileus; (ii) Shorter hospitalization; and (iii) Particularly ideal approach for morbidly obese patients
- **Disadvantages:** Exposure is limited

Adrenal Incidentaloma

Nonadrenal related work-up → **Incidentally detected adrenal mass**

Adrenal incidentaloma includes [adapted from AACE/AAES guidelines]; (i) Nonfunctioning adenoma (80%); (ii) Subclinical Cushing syndrome (5%); (iii) Pheochromocytoma (5%); (iv) Aldosteronoma (1%); (v) Adrenocortical carcinoma (<5%); (vi) Metastatic lesion (2.5%); and (vii) Ganglioneuroma, myelolipoma, benign cysts.

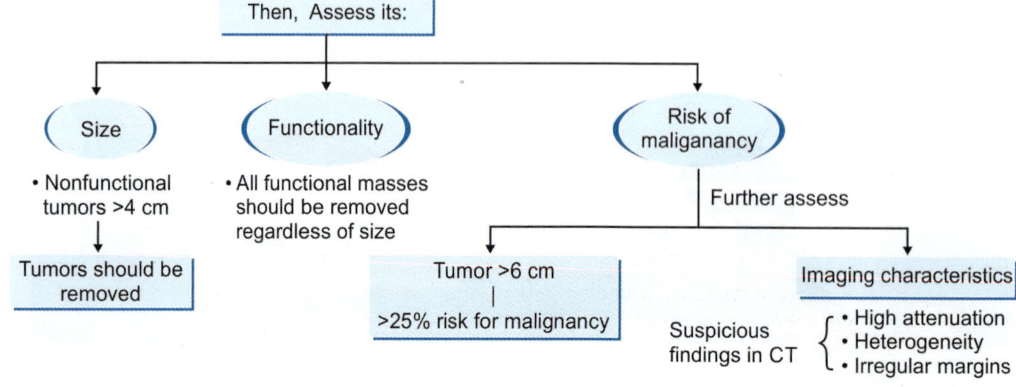

Assessment of Functionality

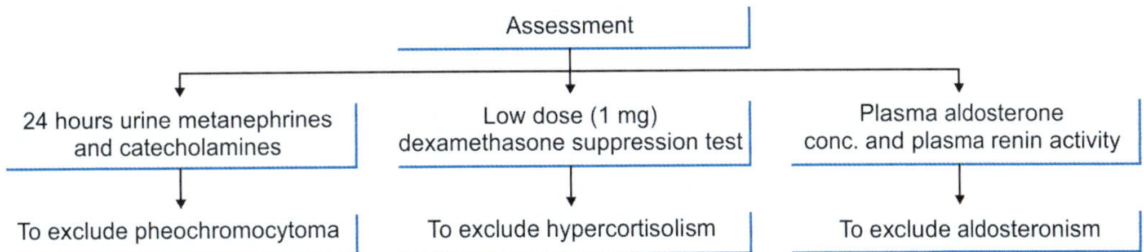

- FNAC should be reserved for patient who are not candidates for surgical resection.
- **Pheochromocytoma must be excluded before attempting FNAC.**

Primary tumors those can metastasize to adrenals:

- Lung cancer
- Breast carcinoma
- Renal cell carcinoma
- Melanoma

Management of Incidentaloma

- All functional adrenal masses should be removed regardless of size
- Nonfunctional lesion, size >6 cm, suspicious features in imaging: Adrenalectomy
- Nonfunctional lesion, size <4 cm, benign features in imaging: Periodic follow-up with 6 monthly interval CT
- Nonfunctional lesion, size 4–6 cm, benign features in imaging: Periodic follow-up or surgery depends on patient's age, surgical risk factors and patient's preference

Approaches of Adrenal Surgery

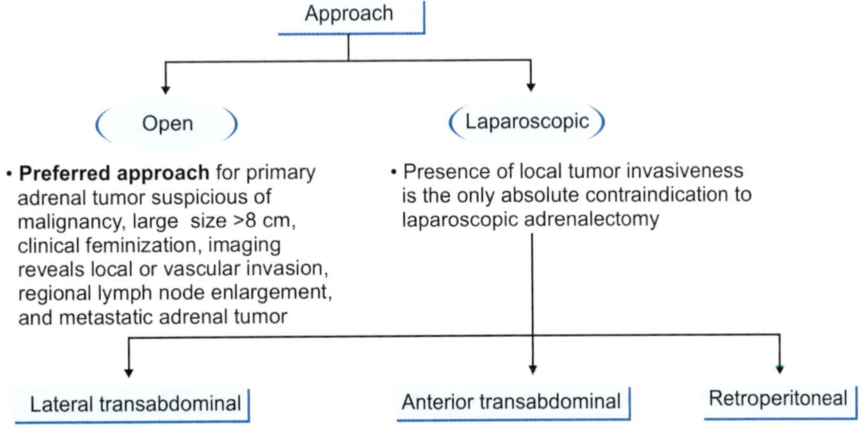

- **Most preferred approach**
  - Good exposure
  - Large working space
  - Access to superior retroperitoneum
  - Anatomical landmarks are clearly identifiable
  - Very large tumors can be handled

Patient Positioning and Port Positioning in Laparoscopic Adrenalectomy

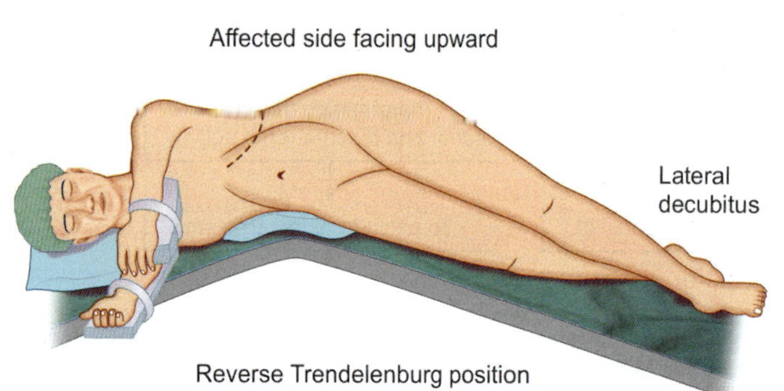

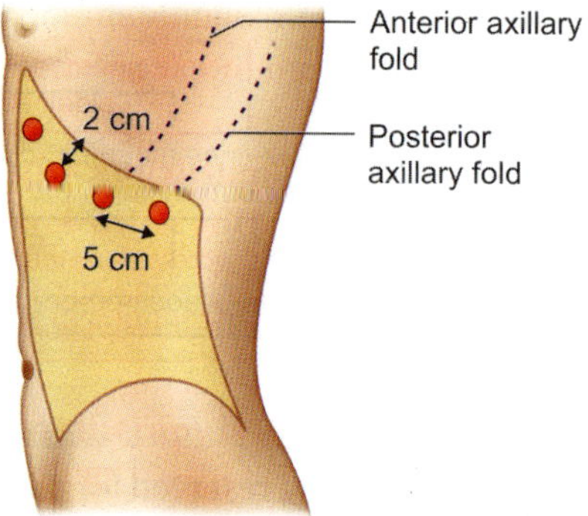

Placement of trocars

Different Approaches of Open Adrenalectomy

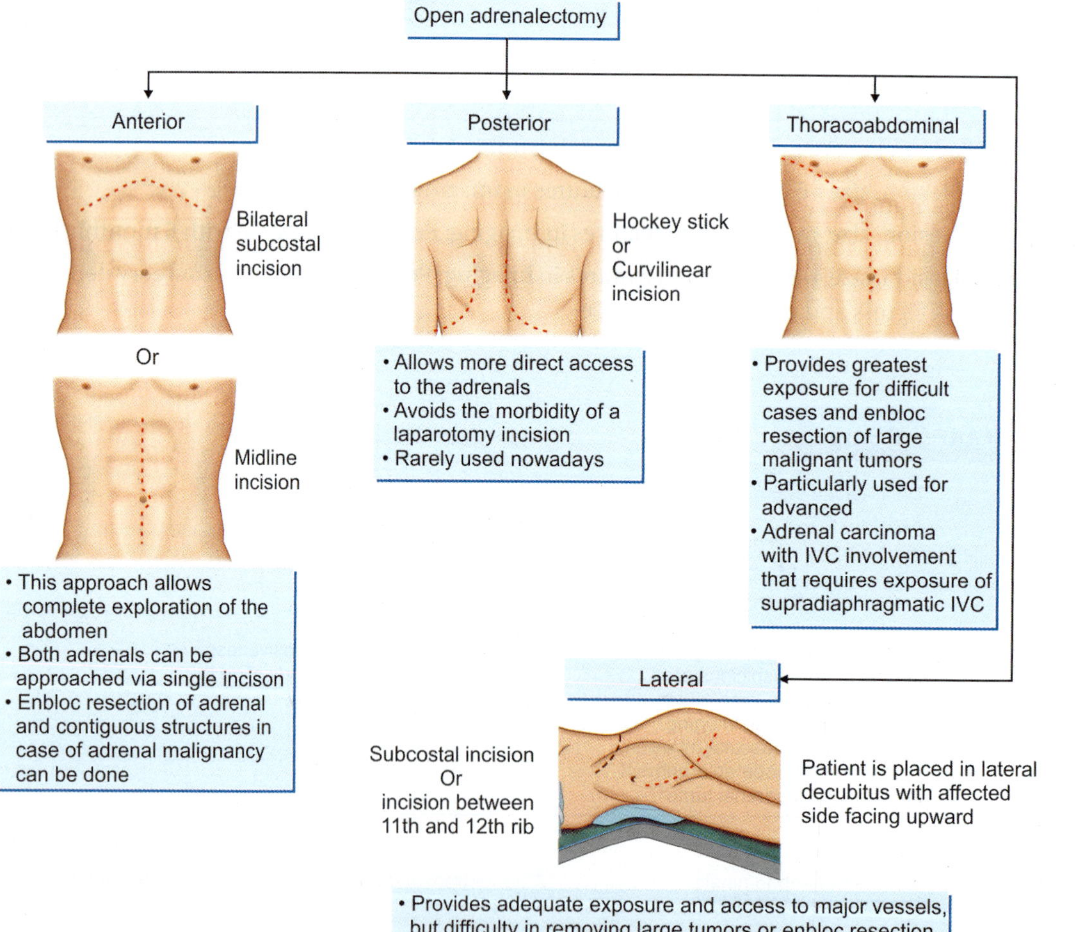

Neuroendocrine Tumors of Pancreas

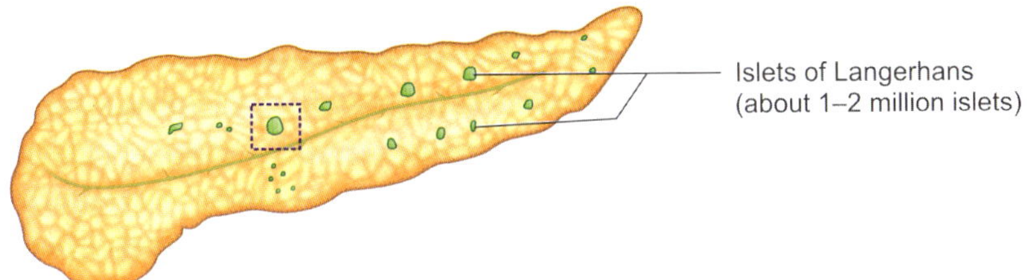

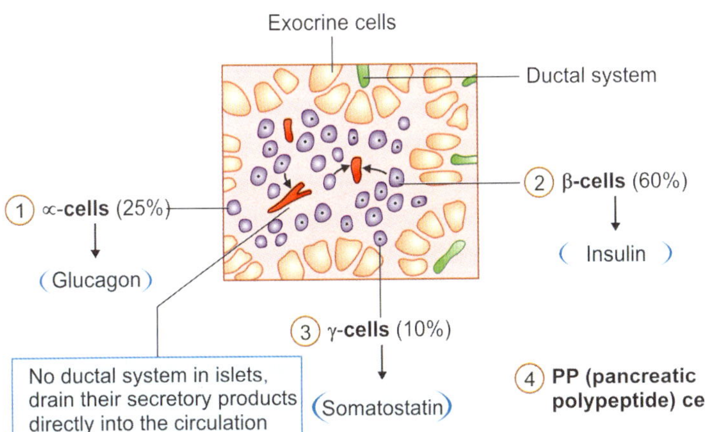

The islets of Langerhans form 1–2% of the pancreatic tissue. The islets are interspersed within the structure of exocrine pancreas.

Pancreatic neuroendocrine tumors (PNETs) are also known as 'islet cell tumor'

These tumors are rare in comparison to exocrine pancreatic tumors.

Feedback mechanism does not exist.

Types according to origin:

- Insulinoma **(most common)**
- Gastrinoma **(most common malignant endocrine tumor)**
- Glucagonoma
- Somatostatinoma
- VIPoma

Types according to functionality: (i) Functional PNETs and (ii) Nonfunctional PNETs.

Familial Syndromes Associated with Pancreatic Neuroendocrine Tumors

- Multiple endocrine neoplasia 1 (MEN1)
- Von Hippel Lindau syndrome (VHL)
- Neurofibromatosis type 1 (NF1)
- Tuberous sclerosis

PNETs with Aggressive Behavior

- Glucagonoma
- Somatostatinoma
- VIPoma
- Most of the nonfunctional PNETs

Grading System for Pancreatic Neuroendocrine Tumors [by ENETS and WHO]

Grade	Mitotic index		Ki-67 index
Low grade (G1)	<2 mitoses/10 HPF	AND	<3%
Intermediated grade (G2)	2–20 mitoses/10 HPF	OR	3–20%
High grade (G3)	>20 mitoses/10 HPF	OR	20%

Insulinoma

Most common pancreatic endocrine neoplasm

- Small <1.5 cm
- Encapsulated, pale to red brown nodules anywhere in the pancreas
- Single (10% multiple)
- Benign (5–10% malignant)
- 90% sporadic and 10% is associated with MEN1
- Almost always in the pancreas

Insulinomas associated with MEN1:

- Tumor size >3 cm
- Multiple
- Increased chance of recurrence.

Whipple Triad

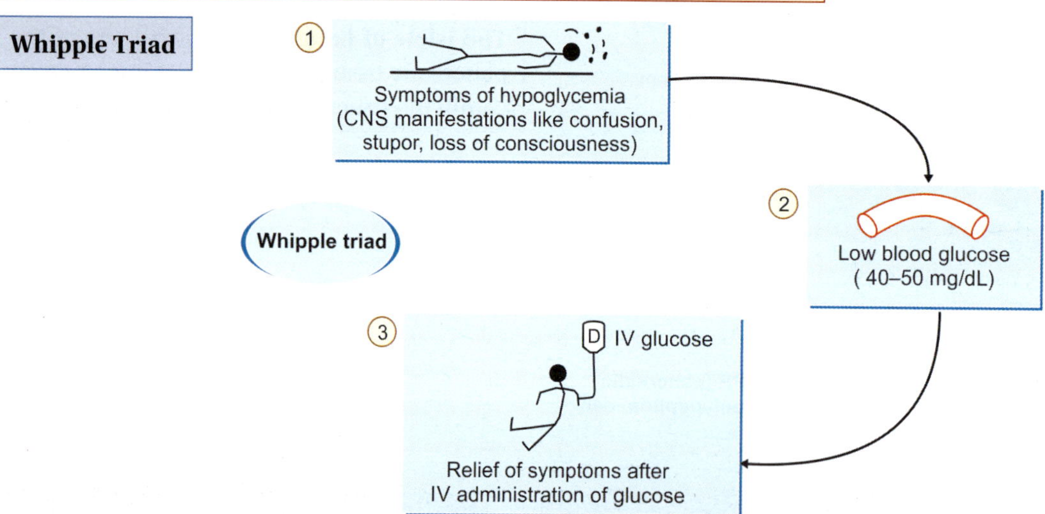

Diagnosis

In a 72-hour fasting period, Insulin level >6 mcIU/mL; C-peptide concentration ≥0.6 ng/mL; Proinsulin level ≥5 pmol/L when, fasting blood glucose <55 mg/dL is suspicious for Insulinoma.

Localization of insulinoma:

- **Thin-cut pancreatic protocol CT with IV contrast:** About 80% of insulinomas can be detected but small tumors (<2 cm) cannot be localized.
- **Magnetic resonance imaging:** Sensitivity is equivalent to CT.
- **Endoscopic ultrasound:** This imaging can localize tumors of 2–3 mm size. Sensitivity is 70%-90%, specificity is almost 100%.
- **Somatostatin Receptor Scintigraphy (Octreoscan):**
  - Uses ^{111}Indium-labeled octreotide which is a somatostatin analogue
  - This radiotracer has a high affinity with the somatostatin receptor 2 (SST2)
  - Can localize primary as well as metastatic neuroendocrine tumors
  - About 90% of NETs can be detected
  - This imaging should be performed if octreotide or lanreotide is being considered as a treatment for metastatic disease.
- **DOTATOC scan:** It is a newer type of somatostatin receptor scintigraphy, often combines with PET/CT.
- **Intraoperative ultrasound**

Imamura-Doppman procedure: Indicated only when other localization tests are equivocal or negative.

This method includes injecting calcium into the gastroduodenal, proximal splenic, superior mesenteric, and proper hepatic arteries and then measuring insulin levels in right (usually) or left hepatic vein.

Management

Prevention of hypoglycemia:
- High-carbohydrate diet
- Medications (that inhibit insulin release or production)- diazoxide, phenytoin, calcium channel blockers.

Insulinoma patients receiving octreotide or lanreotide should be carefully monitored because these medications may increase the risk of hypoglycemia.

Surgical management:
- Enucleation- if solitary with no local invasion
- Pancreatoduodenectomy or distal pancreatectomy- if tumor is invasive or located within the pancreas.

Surgeons operating on insulinomas must be familiar with intraoperative USG.

Gastrinoma

Second most common islet cell tumor.
- Most common symptomatic malignant endocrine tumor of pancreas.
- 60–90% of gastrinomas are found in the **'Gastrinoma triangle'**.
- About 75% of gastrinomas are sporadic, rest are associated with MEN1.

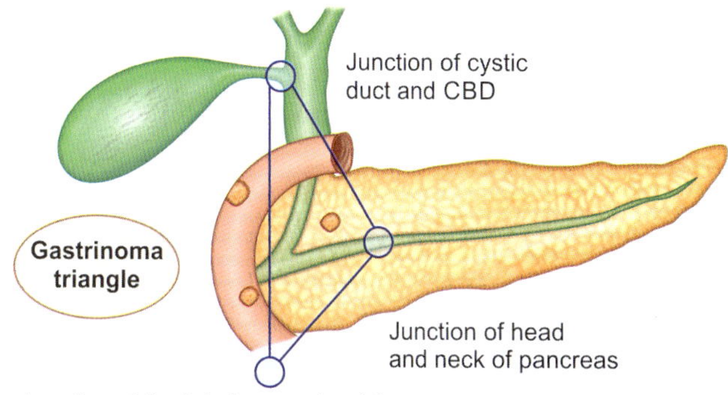

Sporadic gastrinoma:
- Found (50–70%) in the duodenum (1st part >2nd part >3rd part; never in 4th part).
- 20–40% are found in pancreas, rest in other intraabdominal sites.
- Usually single lesion.

Gastrinoma Triangle (Passaro's Triangle)

The triangle is formed by:
- **Superiorly:** Confluence of the cystic and common bile duct.
- **Inferiorly:** Junction of the second and third part of duodenum.
- **Medially:** Junction of the neck and body of pancreas.

Gastrinomas associated with MEN1:
- Gastrinomas are usually in the duodenum (50–90%) or in the pancreas (10–30%).
- Always multiple lesions.

Gastrinoma should be suspected if:

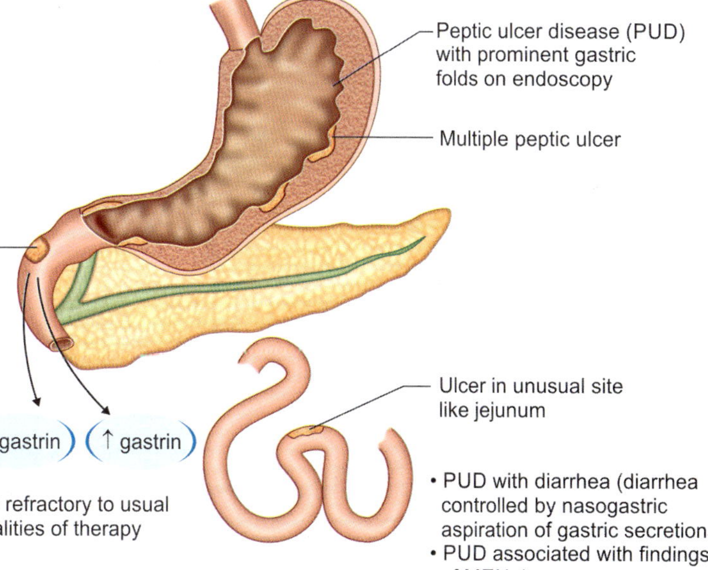

Diagnosis

- Fasting hypergastrinemia (>1000 ng/L) in the setting of gastric pH ≤2, the diagnosis of gastrinoma is established.
- If diagnosis is in doubt, secretin provocation test is indicated.
- If secretin provocation test is equivocal, calcium infusion test is indicated.

Surgical Management

- **Occult gastrinoma** (on imaging, no primary tumor or metastasis)- Observation or exploratory surgery (duodenotomy, intraoperative USG with enucleation, removal of periduodenal nodes). MEN1 syndrome should be ruled out by estimating serum calcium before surgery.
- **Gastrinoma in the duodenum:** Intraoperative USG with local resection or enucleation of tumors and periduodenal node dissection.
- **Gastrinoma in the head of pancreas, not immediately adjacent to pancreatic duct:** Enucleation with periduodenal node dissection. Tumor in pancreatic head with proximity to pancreatic duct- Pancreatoduodenectomy.
- **Gastrinoma in distal pancreas:** Distal pancreatectomy and splenectomy.

Localization of the Tumor

- Accurate localization of the tumor is important for definite therapy and assessment of prognosis.
- **Somatostatin receptor scintigraphy:** Tumor <1 cm can be localized and whole-body imaging can also be done. This imaging modality is sensitive for both primary and metastatic gastrinomas.
- **Endoscopic US** is particularly useful in localizing tumors in pancreatic head or duodenum.

Causes of Hypergastrinemia

Associated with decreased acid production

- PPI therapy
- Atrophic gastritis
- Renal failure
- Vagotomy

Associated with increased or normal acid production

- Zollinger-Ellison syndrome
- Antral G cell hyperplasia
- Retained antrum syndrome
- Gastric outlet obstruction

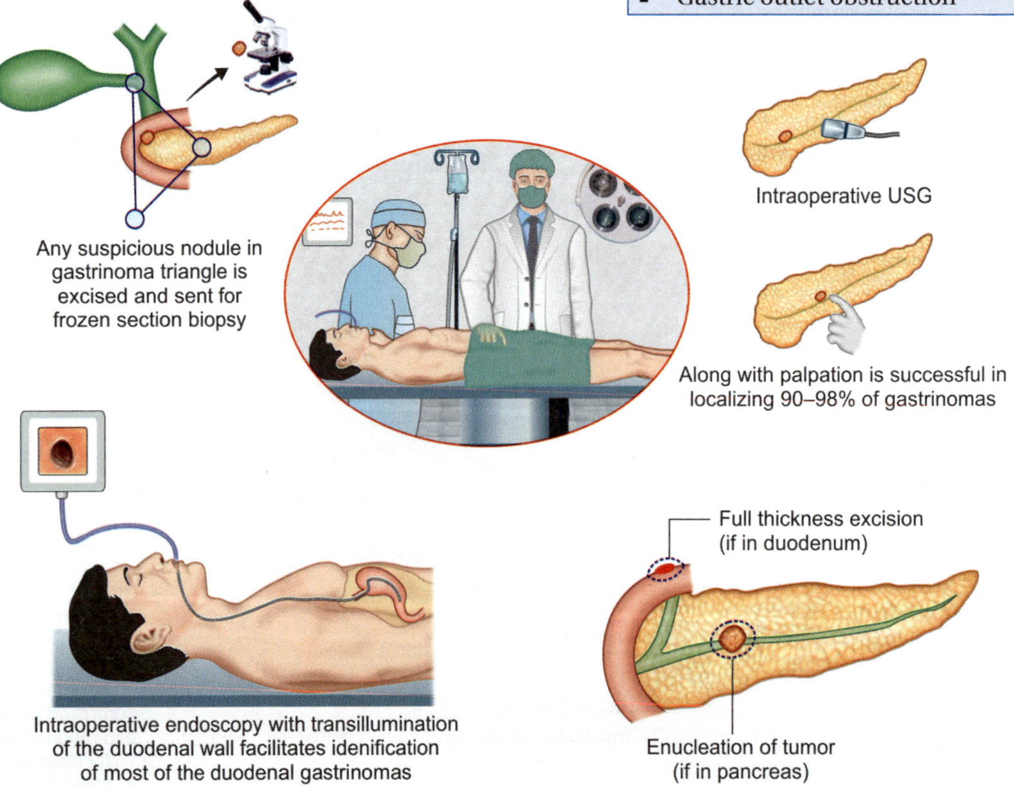

Glucagonoma

This tumor secretes excess amount of glucagon.

- Common symptoms are glucose intolerance, migratory necrolytic erythema and weight loss.
- Other clinical manifestations are glossitis, pulmonary and venous thromboembolism.
- These tumors are almost always found in body and tail of the pancreas.
- About 70% of patients present with liver metastases at the time of diagnosis.
- Plasma glucagon level >1000 pg/mL is diagnostic.

Management: (i) Control of diabetes; (ii) Nutritional support (glucagon is a catabolic hormone); (iii) Peri-operative anticoagulation (to prevent pulmonary and venous thromboembolism); and (iv) Resection of tumor (e.g. distal pancreatectomy with splenectomy) with peripancreatic lymph nodes.

Somatostatinoma

- Somatostatinomas **originate from pancreatic islet D cell or duodenum,** secretes excess amount of somatostatin. [somatostatin inhibits release of other GI hormones]
- **Common presentations are**- Cholelithiasis (due to bile stasis), Diabetes (due to inhibition of insulin secretion), Steatorrhea (due to decreased enzyme secretion and bile secretion). Other clinical features are- weight loss, anemia, diarrhea, hypochlorhydria.
- Most of the somatostatinomas arise in the ampulla and periampullary area.
- These tumors may be associated with MEN1, NF1 or VHL syndrome. Duodenal somatostatinomas commonly associated with Neurofibromatosis type 1.
- Pancreatic somatostatinomas are more malignant than the duodenal somatostatinomas.
- **Diagnosis** is confirmed by elevated serum somatostatin level (10 ng/mL)
- Surgical resection is the treatment of choice.

Other Functional PNETs

- Pancreatic peptide-producing tumor (PPoma)
- Growth hormone-releasing factor-producing tumor (GRFomas)
- Adrenocorticotrophic hormone producing tumors (ACTHomas).

Migratory Necrolytic Erythema

- This clinical presentation is pathognomonic for the glucoganoma.
- The rash is migratory, red, scaly, associated with intense pruritus, tends to start in the perineum and then spreads to the trunk and extremities.
- The rash is due to decreased level of amino acids and is completely reversed after TPN therapy.

Vasoactive Intestinal Peptide-secreting Tumor (VIPoma)

- VIPomas are commonly solitary, intrapancreatic tumors. Most of the tumors are in the body and tail of pancreas.
- About 50% of the VIPomas are benign. The hypersecretion of VIP (intestinal secretagogue) leads to development of **"pancreatic cholera", also known as WDHA syndrome** (watery diarrhea, hypokalemia, achlorhydria) or Verner- Morrison syndrome (first described by Verner and Morrison in 1958).
- **Clinical presentations** include large volume intermittent watery diarrhea (about 4.5 l/day), severe hypokalemia with muscle weakness, achlorhydria, metabolic acidosis, hypercalcemia.
- Measurement of serum VIP level must be done on multiple occasion (VIP secretion from the tumor is episodic).
- **CT scan and EUS** can localize most of the VIPoma's.
- **Treatment includes:** (i) Correction of fluid, dyselectrolytemia and metabolic derangements; (ii) Long-acting somatostatin analogues- for management of diarrhea; and (iii) Surgical resection.

Multiple Endocrine Neoplasia (MEN) Syndromes

A disorder with neoplasms in two or more different hormonal tissues in several members of a family

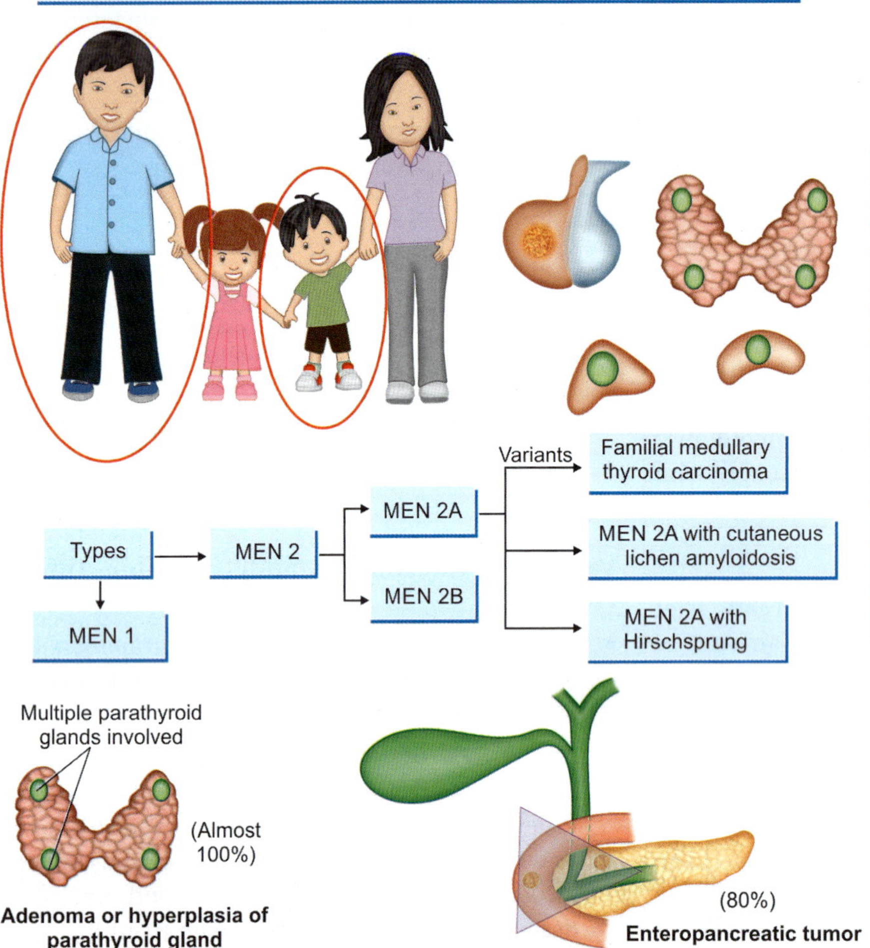

Multiple Endocrine Neoplasia Type 1 (MEN 1)

- MEN 1 is also called **Wermer's syndrome**. It is the **most common type of MEN**.
- Every individual who inherits MEN1 gene develops at least one clinical manifestation during his/her lifetime.
- MEN 1 is Inherited as autosomal dominant trait. MEN 1 gene is a tumor-suppressor gene, located at chromosome 11q13.

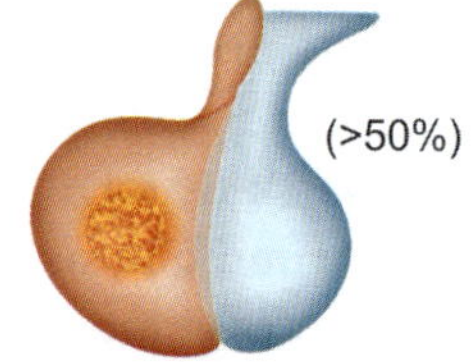

Pituitary tumors

- Primary hyperparathyroidism is the **most common manifestation**.
- It is the earliest manifestation.
- Manifested like sporadic HPT.
- **Management is difficult because:** (i) Early onset; (ii) Significant chance of Recurrence; and (iii) Multiple parathyroid involvement.
- Observation policy for asymptomatic HPT.
- **Parathyroid exploration is indicated if:** (i) Serum Ca^{2+} >12 mg/dL; (ii) Complications of HPT develop; and (iii) Age <50 years.
- **Surgical approaches are:** (i) Total parathyroidectomy and (ii) Subtotal parathyroidectomy.

- Enteropancreatic tumor is the second most common manifestation.
- Gastrinoma is the most common enteropancreatic tumor.
- Insulinoma is the second most common enteropancreatic tumor.
- Tumor producing insulin, glucagon, VIP should be resected.

- Hyperprolactinemia (due to prolactinoma) is the most common manifestation due to pituitary tumor.
- Acromegaly (due to increased GH) and Cushing's disease may present.
- Dopamine agonists are effective for control of prolactin level and for prevention of tumor growth.
- Surgical resection is indicated for mass effects.

Other Tumors in MEN 1
- Bronchial and thymic carcinoids
- Benign thyroid tumor
- Benign and malignant adrenocortical tumors
- Lipoma
- Ependymomas of CNS
- Facial cutaneous angiofibroma.

Multiple Endocrine Neoplasia Type 2

- MEN 2 is inherited as autosomal dominant trait.
- Caused by germline mutations in the RET gene on chromosome 10.
- The **hallmark of these syndrome is MTC, which is bilateral and multifocal.**
- All individuals who carry the disease allele develops MTC.

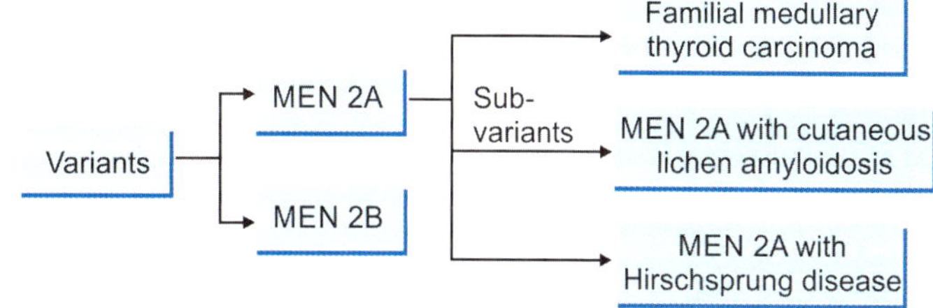

MEN 2A

Multifocal, bilateral involvement of thyroid

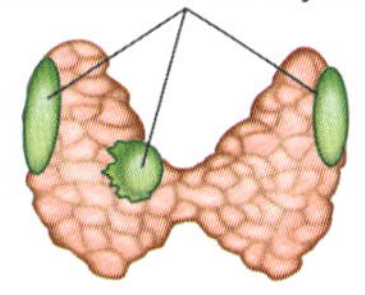

MTC—100%

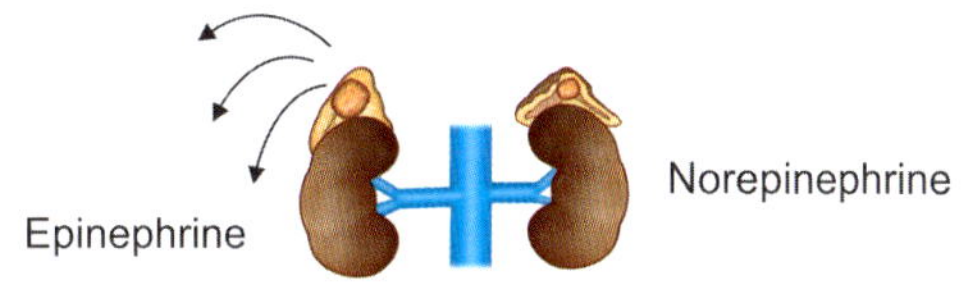

Pheochromocytoma—50%

Multiple parathyroid glands involved

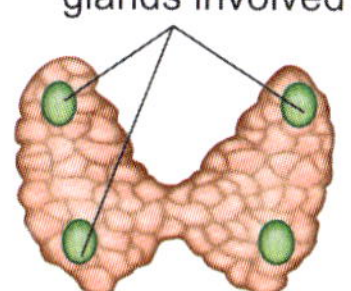

HPT—15–20%

- MTC is the most common manifestation.
- Multifocal, bilateral lesion with C-cell hyperplasia.
- Total thyroidectomy with central lymph node dissection should be performed in children carrying the mutant gene.

- Multifocal, bilateral with adrenal medullary hyperplasia.
- Increased epinephrine secretion in comparison to norepinephrine.
- Rarely malignant.
- Almost never extraadrenal.
- Partial or complete adrenalectomy is the treatment.

- Manifestations are same like primary HPT
- Multiple glands are involved with hyperplasia.
- Total parathyroidectomy with autotransplantation at the time of total thyroidectomy.

MEN 2B

- All MEN2B patients develop MTC. MTC presents at very young age (in infancy); **most aggressive form of MTC.**
- All MEN2B patients develop mucosal neuromas. **Mucosal neuromas** (in tip of tongue, lip, under the eyelid, gingiva, buccal mucosa, nasal mucosa) and **marfanoid habitus** are the most distinctive features and easily identifiable in childhood.
- 40–50% patients develop pheochromocytomas.
- All patients have megacolon, chronic bowel problems (intermittent colic, pseudo-obstruction and diarrhea).

Case 1

History and Physical Examination

A 36 years female patient presented with recurrent upper abdominal pain along with polyuria, polydipsia for last 4 months. Patient also complained of feeling fatigue after normal daily activities for last 3 months. Patient diagnosed as diabetic for last 6 months and on oral antidiabetics.

Physical examination:

- Patient alert, conscious, cooperative
- No obvious clinical findings except mild tenderness in upper abdomen.

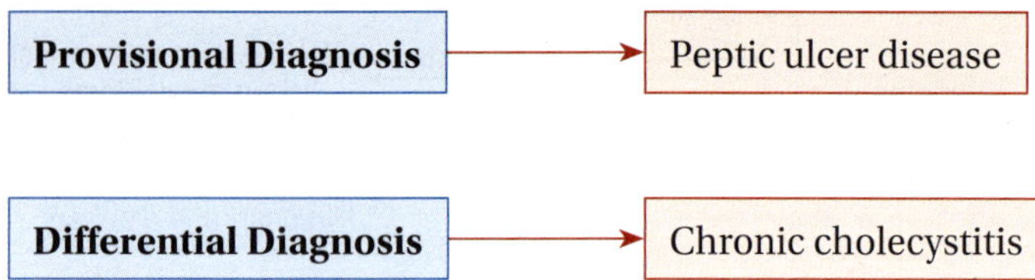

Investigations

- USG abdomen revealed chronic calculous cholecystitis with bilateral nephrocalcinosis.
- Serum calcium 15 mg/dL, Serum PTH 100.6 pg/mL, Serum creatinine 1.2 mg/dL
- ^{99m}Tc sestamibi scan revealed parathyroid adenoma adjoining the lower pole of left thyroid lobe. DEXA scan revealed T score of ≤ 3.0 SD.

Discussion

Patient presented with features of peptic ulcer disease or chronic cholecystitis. Imaging revealed cholelithiasis and bilateral nephrocalcinosis. Bilateral nephrocalcinosis is a characteristic presentation of primary hyperparathyroidism. Biochemical workup revealed primary hyperparathyroidism. Localization imaging study localized the parathyroid adenoma. Excision of left inferior parathyroid adenoma was planned by unilateral neck exploration.

Management Algorithm

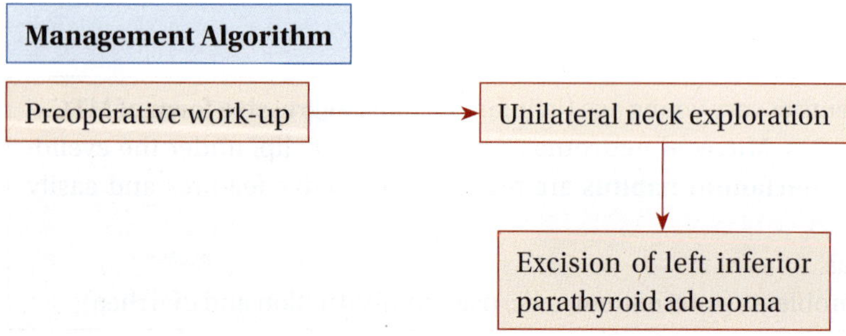

Case 2

History and Physical Examination

A 49 years male patient presented with vague pain in right loin for last 8 months. Patient had no history of acute onset colicky pain in right loin, hematuria or dysuria. Patient had a history of laparoscopic cholecystectomy 2 years back. No history of diabetes and hypertension.

Physical examination:

- Patient conscious, alert, cooperative
- Pulse 82/min, BP 116/86 mm Hg
- Abdominal examination: No specific point of tenderness or lump palpable.

Provisional Diagnosis

Provisional Diagnosis → Right kidney stone

Investigations

- Hb 13.2 gm%, Fasting blood sugar 98 mg/dL, Serum creatinine 0.9 mg/dL
- USG abdomen revealed a space occupying lesion with well-defined borders measuring 5 cm × 4.6 cm in segment V of liver, likely to be a hemangioma.
- CT scan abdomen revealed a right adrenal mass lesion measuring 6.8 cm × 5.5 cm.
- 24-hr urinary cortisol, urinary metanephrines, serum aldosterone, and serum potassium—within normal limit.

Discussion

A middle-aged male patient presented with pain in right loin without any history of hematuria or dysuria. USG revealed a lesion, likely to be a hemangioma. For definitive diagnosis, CT abdomen done, and it revealed a right adrenal mass. Functionality of the incidentaloma was assessed by a series of biochemical tests and diagnosed as a non-functioning adrenal incidentaloma. As per size criteria, decision of adrenalectomy was taken.

Management Algorithm

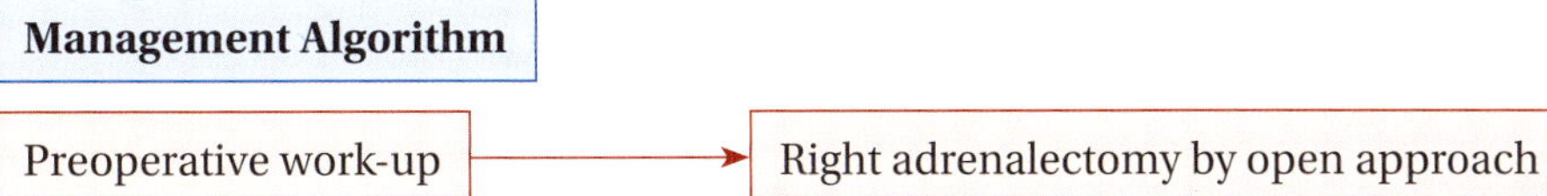

Chapter 16

Trauma

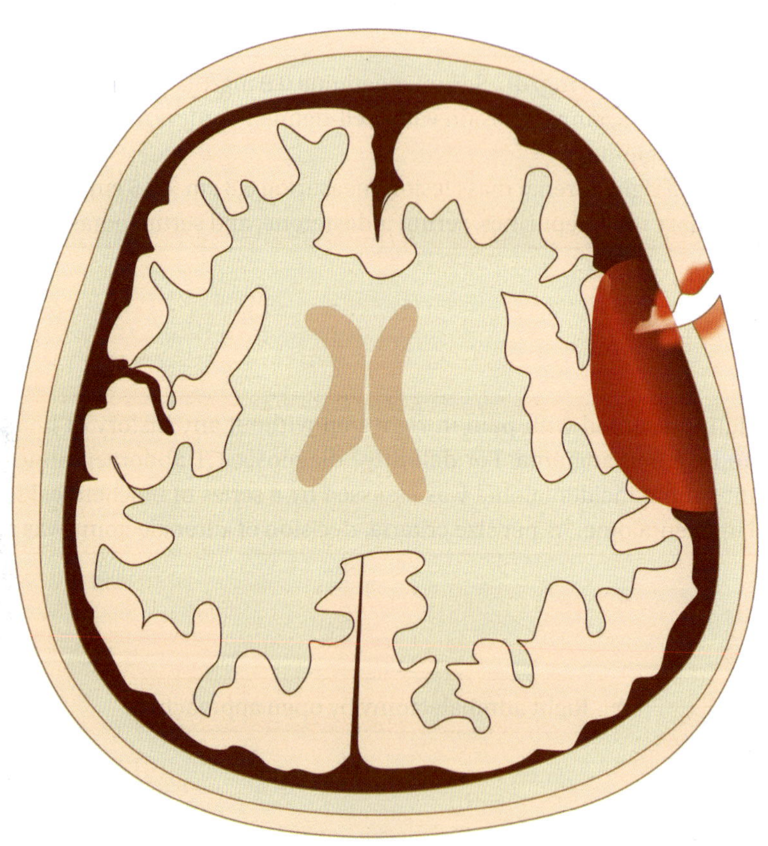

Important Topics

- Types of Injury
- Basic Management of Trauma
- Head Injury
- Maxillofacial Trauma
- Neck Injury
- Spinal Injury
- Thoracic Trauma
- Abdominal Trauma
- Genitourinary Injury
- Damage Control Surgery
- Abdominal Compartment Syndrome
- Open Abdomen

'That man can interrogate as well as observe nature, was a lesson slowly learned in his evolution.'

William Osler (1849–1919)
Canadian Physician

Trauma

- **Trauma is characterized by** a structural alteration and/or physiologic imbalance that results when energy is imported, or vital functions compromised during interaction with physical or chemical agents.
- Trauma is one of the leading causes of death and disability and is the third most common cause of death worldwide.

Types of Injury

- Blunt
- Penetrating
- Blast
- Thermal
- Chemical

Mechanisms of Blunt Trauma

- Motor-vehicle accident
- Fall from height
- Assault by blunt object
- Stampede
- Wild animal injury

Determinants of Impact Force

- Area of application
- Duration of application
- Direction of application

Injury Patterns Depend on Types of Motor-vehicle Accidents

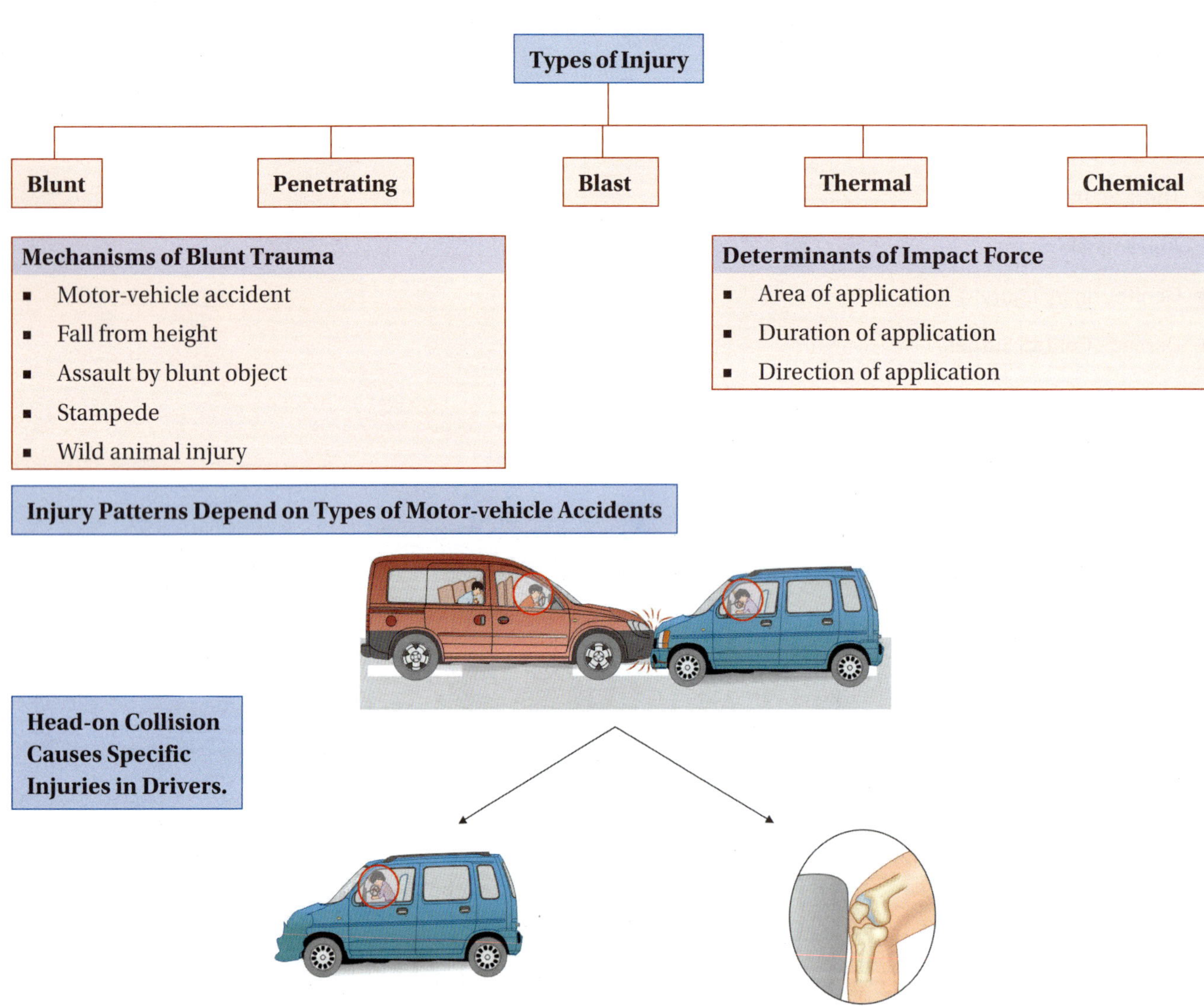

Head-on Collision Causes Specific Injuries in Drivers.

Head strike the windshield causing facial fracture and fracture of cervical spine.

Chest and upper abdomen strike the steering wheel causing the laceration of thoracic aorta, myocardial contusion, injury of liver and spleen.

Seatbelt injury occurs as a result of interaction between the restrained occupant in the front seat and the three-point seatbelt. Injuries commonly develop includes fracture of ribs, clavicle and sternum, abdominal wall disruption and mesenteric tear.

Impact between driver's knee and dashboard causing—patellar fracture, posterior dislocation of knee with popliteal artery injury, fracture of femoral shaft and acetabulum.

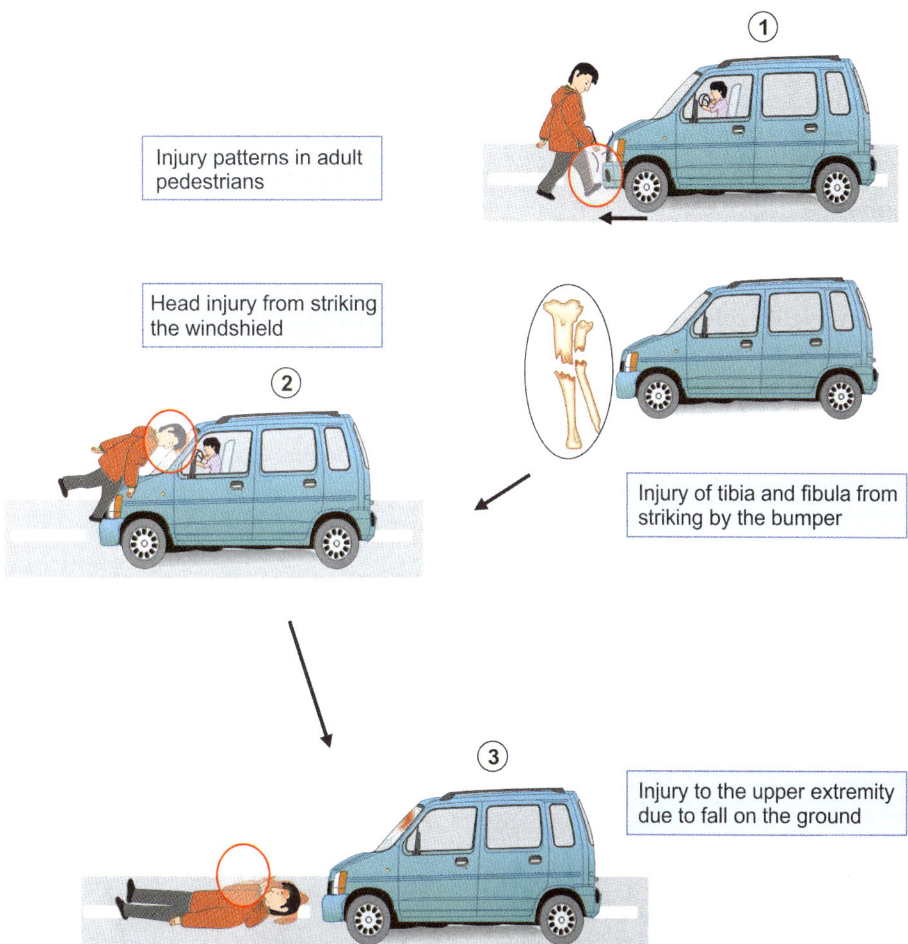

Young Pedestrians have a Distinct Pattern of Injuries (Waddell triad)

- Fracture femur from striking the bumper.
- Abdominal solid organ injury from striking the fender.
- Opposite-side head injury from landing on the pavement.

Trauma deaths have trimodal distribution (according to time interval between injury and death)

Immediate death (50%)—within few minutes

- **Immediate deaths are due** to brain injury, high spinal injury, catastrophic hemorrhage due to major vessel injury.
- **These types of injuries are not treatable, rather preventable.**

Early death (30%)—within few hours

- The first hour after injury is called the **"golden hour".**
- **Early deaths are due to** hemorrhage, airway obstruction, airway injury.
- **Trauma management system is particularly effective for these group of patients.**

Late death (20%)—within days to weeks

Late deaths are due to sepsis, multi-organ failure.

Prehospital Retrieval and Care

Assessment:
- Whether patient needs an emergency treatment at the site of incident or not.
- Distance between the site of incident and a verified trauma center.

Then, choose any one:
- **'Scoop and run'** policy (immediate evacuation)
- **'Stay and play'** policy (scene resuscitation).

If, 'stay and play' policy: Field professionals perform 3 major functions:
1. Assessment of the injury scene
2. Airway maintenance, control of external bleeding and shock, immobilization of the patient
3. Safe and rapid transportation of critically ill patients to the appropriate trauma center.

Providers must obtain information that include time of injury, events related to injury, mechanism of injury, patient's history. These information are helpful for triage at the hospital.
Then, **'Triage'**.

Triage is a dynamic process of sorting casualties to identify the priority of treatment and evacuation of the wounded.

'Triage' came from the French word 'trier', means to shift or to sort.

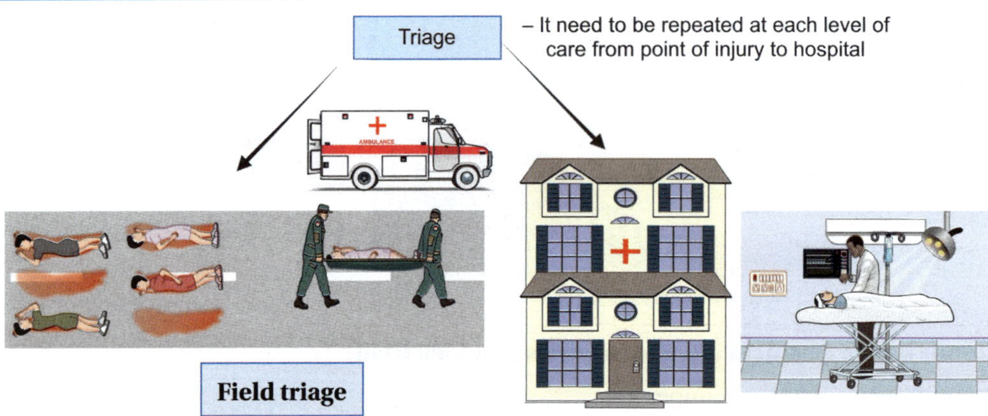

Field triage decision scheme (as per ATLS protocol) consists of step 1, 2 and 3. **Step 1 and 2 attempts are to identify the most seriously injured patients.** These patients should be transported to the highest-level trauma center.

Triage is for access to resuscitation and operating room.

Patients who should be transported to highest-level trauma center.

Step 1:
- Glasgow coma scale ≤13
- Systolic blood pressure <90 mm Hg
- Respiratory rate <10 or >29 breaths/min (<20 in infants <1 year) or need for ventilator support

Step 2:
- All penetrating injuries to head, neck, torso, and extremities proximal to the elbow and knee
- Chest wall instability or deformity (e.g., flail chest)
- Two or more proximal bone fractures
- Crushed, degloved, mangled, or pulseless extremity
- Amputation proximal to wrist or ankle
- Pelvic fractures
- Open or depressed skull fracture
- Paralysis

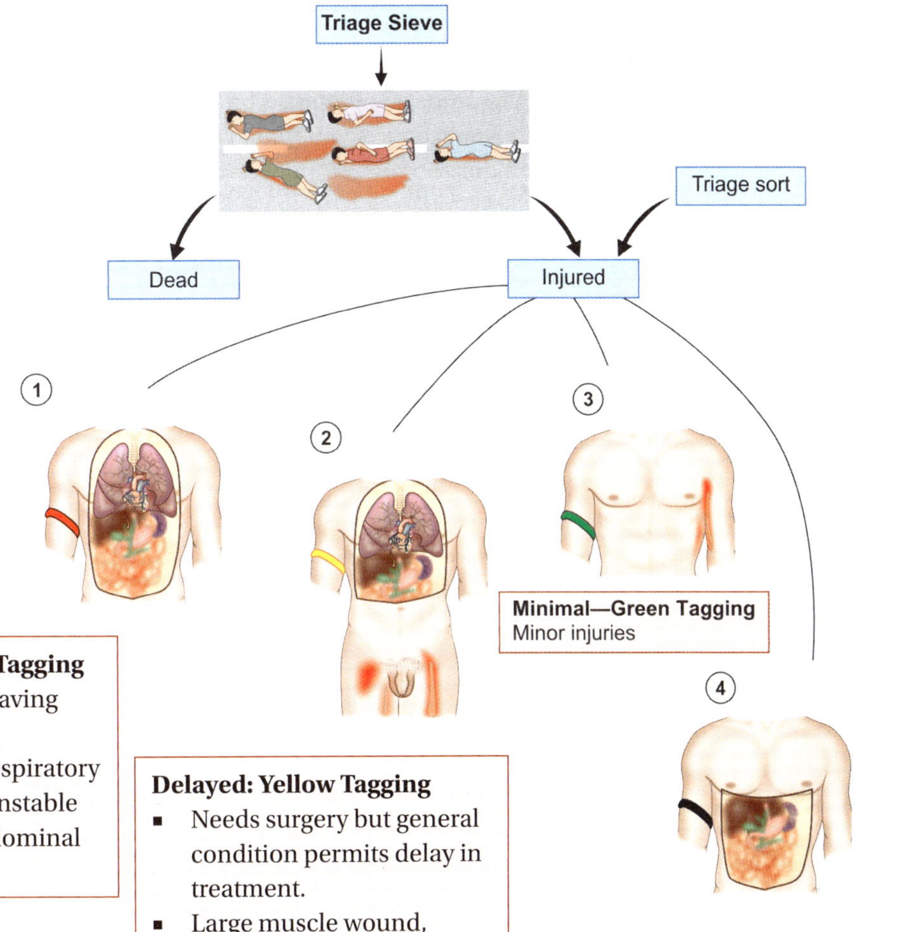

Immediate: Red Tagging

- Requires life-saving surgery
- Patient with respiratory obstruction, unstable chest, and abdominal injuries

Delayed: Yellow Tagging

- Needs surgery but general condition permits delay in treatment.
- Large muscle wound, fracture of long bones, stable abdominal, and thoracic wound.

Expectant: Black Tagging

- Survival unlikely
- Penetrating head injury, high spinal cord injury, mutilating wounds involving multiple organs

Prehospital Management

Prehospital management period should not exceed 30 minutes.

Neck, Spine Immobilization

- All patients with major blunt trauma should be suspected of having spinal injury. Cervical spine is immobilized by Philadelphia collar. Spine immobilization must be ensured to prevent development of or progression of neurologic deficit.
- Soft collars are not recommended for cervical spine immobilization as this type of collar does not effectively immobilize cervical spine.

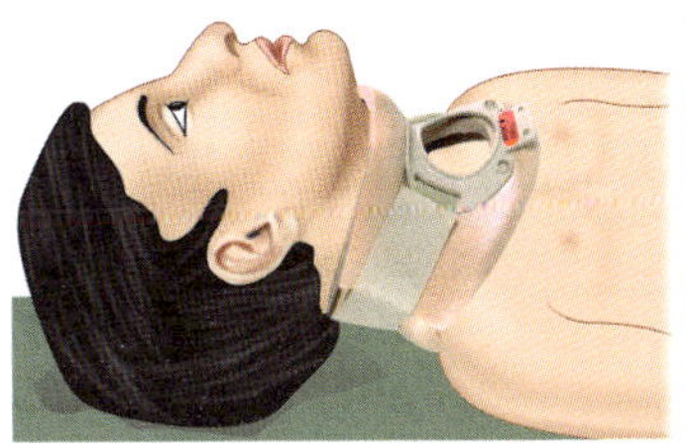

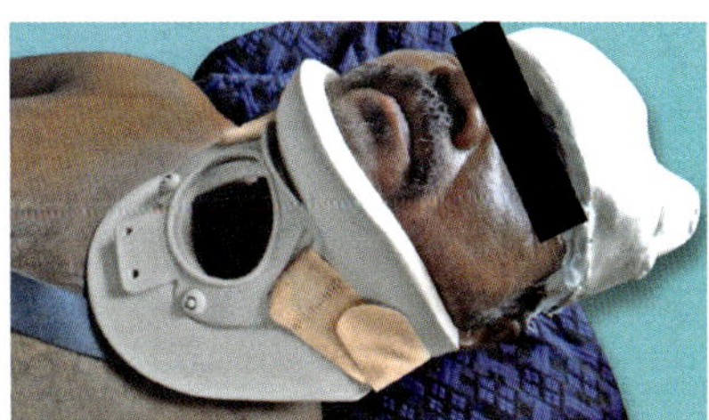

Philadelphia collar for neck immobilization in blunt trauma patient.

Airway Management

- Cleaning of solid debris from mouth and pharynx
- Suctioning of mouth and pharynx to clear blood, mucus, and vomitus
- Insertion of an airway device if field professional has sufficient expertise

Intravenous Access

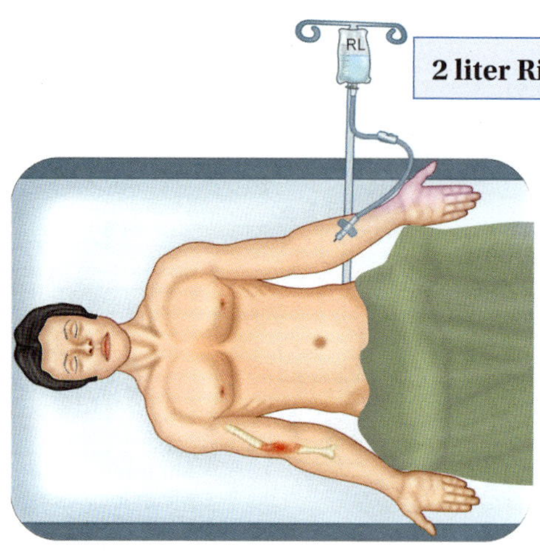

2 liter Ringer lactate

Large bore IV catheter (16/18 gauge)

Fracture Immobilization

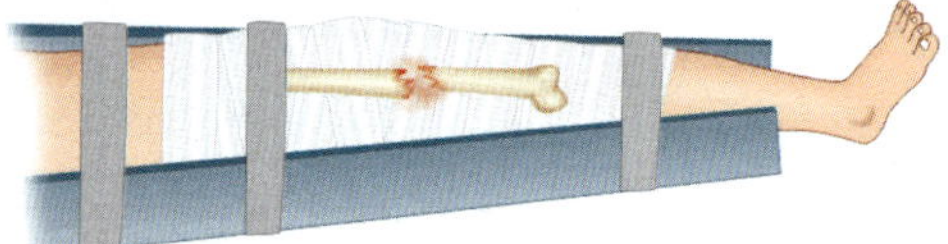

Recognition and splinting of all major fractures before transportation

Cardiac Arrest Management

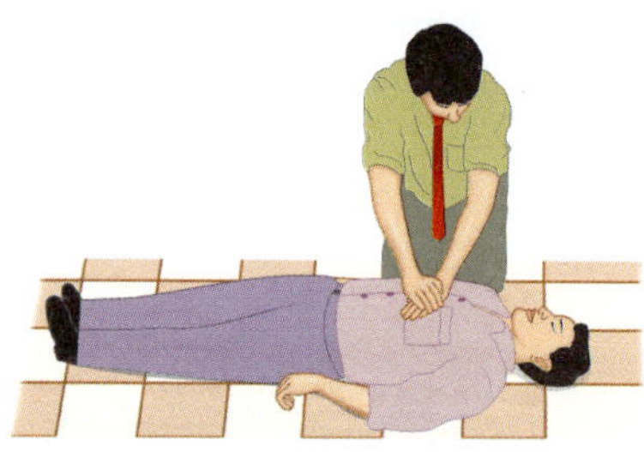

Prehospital Transport

- Ideally by ground or air ambulance.
- Ideally transport time should not exceed 15 minutes.
- Resuscitation should be continued during transportation.
- If no ambulance is available, station wagon or truck is preferable to a passenger car.
- Should be transported in the supine position.

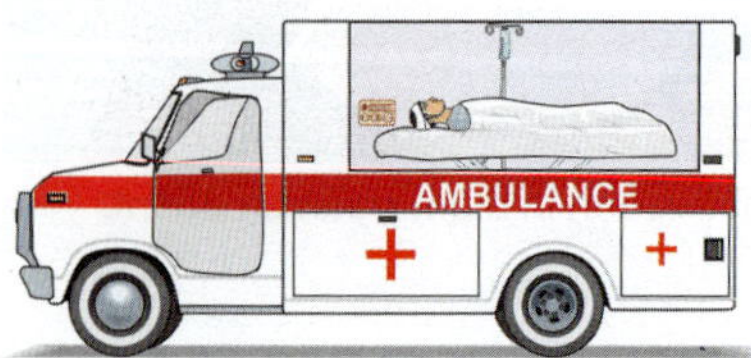

Basic Principles of Resuscitative Measures to Prevent Possible Cardiopulmonary Arrest in Critically Injured Pregnant Patients

- Patient should be in full left lateral position (to relieve aortocaval compression)
- 100% oxygen support
- Intravenous catheter access above the diaphragm
- During CPR, patient should be placed in supine position and manual left lateral and upward displacement of the uterus should be done by a member of trauma team.
- Chest compressions should be done at a slightly higher level.
- Other protocols of CPR are same as non-pregnant patient.

Hospital Care

- Trauma patients require a precise, rapid, and systematic approach.
- The advanced trauma life support (ATLS) system is the best approach to the severely injured patient.
- Management consists of: (i) Primary survey with simultaneous resuscitation; (ii) Secondary survey; and (iii) Definitive care

Primary Survey with Simultaneous Resuscitation

Primary survey is a systematic, rapid evaluation of the injured patient and encompasses the **ABCDE** of trauma management.

- **A** – Airway maintenance with restriction of cervical spine motion
- **B** – Breathing and ventilation
- **C** – Circulation and hemorrhage control
- **D** – Disability (assessment of neurologic status)
- **E** – Exposure and environmental control

Airway Maintenance with Restriction of Cervical Spine Motion

- Establishing a patent airway is the highest priority because irreversible brain damage from hypoxia can occur within minutes.
- A patient who is able to respond verbally has a patent airway, therefore early attention to the airway is not required.
- Rapid assessment should be done to detect any foreign bodies, facial or mandibular fractures, tracheal, or laryngeal injuries that may cause airway obstruction.
- Initially, jaw-thrust or chin-lift maneuver may be effective for relief of airway obstruction.
- Cleaning of solid debris from mouth and pharynx and suctioning of mouth and pharynx to clear blood, mucus, and vomitus should be initiated while restricting cervical spine movement.
- Oxygen is administered via nasal cannula or bag valve facemask at the rate of 10–12 L/minute and oxygen saturation is measured using pulse oximeter.
- Then, orotracheal intubation is done using Rapid-sequence induction. When opening of cervical collar is needed for airway management, neck movement should be restricted by one of the team members.
- When endotracheal intubation is not feasible, cricothyroidotomy is indicated. Open cricothyroidotomy is indicated in adults and needle cricothyroidotomy is indicated below 12 years.

Elective intubation is indicated in these group of patients:

- Penetrating injuries in neck with expanding hematoma
- Complex maxillofacial trauma
- Extensive subcutaneous emphysema in neck
- Chemical or thermal injuries to the mouth and nose.

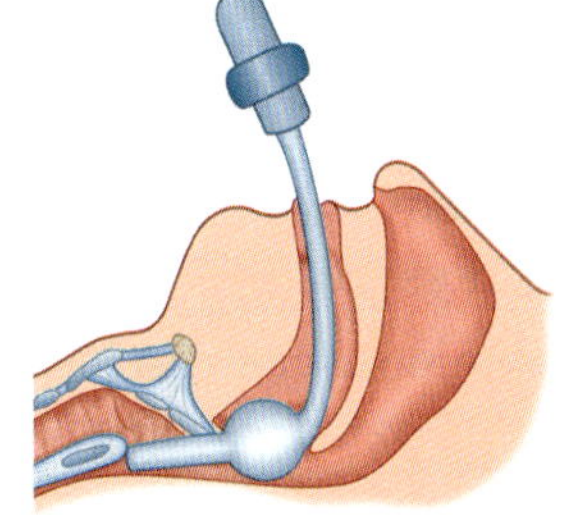

Orotracheal Intubation

Signs of Airway Obstruction

- Agitation
- Cyanosis
- Hoarse voice
- Stridor
- Abnormal breath sounds

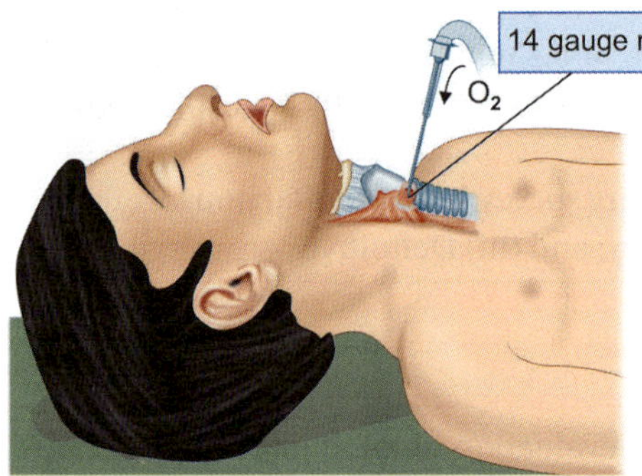

Needle cricothyroidotomy

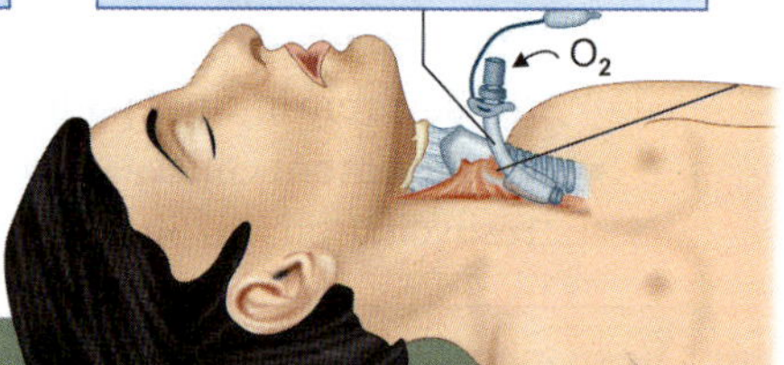

Open cricothyroidotomy

Open cricothyroidotomy is contraindicated below 12 years because of the risk of damage to the cricoid cartilage and subsequent risk of subglottic stenosis.

Patent Airway

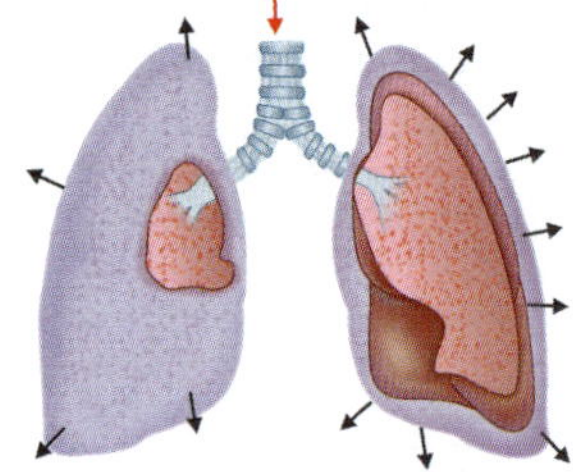

Ventilation impaired | **Ventilation adequate**

Breathing and Ventilation

- Breathing and ventilation function should be maintained in trauma patients for optimal oxygenation and carbon dioxide elimination.
- For evaluation of ventilation, examination of the functions of lungs, chest wall and diaphragm (by clinical examination and chest X-ray) is important.
- **Conditions that significantly impair ventilation:** (i) Tension pneumothorax; (ii) Massive hemothorax; (iii) Open pneumothorax; (iv) Flail chest with pulmonary contusion; and (v) Tracheobronchial disruption. These conditions should be detected during the primary survey and need immediate intervention.

Before initiating positive pressure ventilation, pneumothorax must be excluded because simple pneumothorax can be converted to a tension pneumothorax.

Circulation with Hemorrhage Control

- **Primary goals** are to identify the source of hemorrhage, control of bleeding and initiating resuscitation.
- Hypotension in trauma patients is most likely due to hemorrhage if tension pneumothorax is already excluded.
- Rapid, thready pulse, gray facial skin and pale extremities, altered level of consciousness are indicators of **hypovolemia**.
- **External hemorrhage can be controlled by:** (i) Direct pressure on the wound; (ii) Elevation of the bleeding point and splint application; and (iii) Tourniquet. Tourniquet is only indicated for exsanguinating hemorrhage from the extremities.
- **Sources of internal bleeding** (chest cavity, peritoneal cavity, retroperitoneum, pelvis, long bones) can be detected by imaging or diagnostic peritoneal lavage and need appropriate surgical intervention depending on the injuries.
- **Vascular access** is to be established by two large-bore peripheral venous catheter. If peripheral access cannot be established, venous cutdown or central venous access or intraosseous infusion should be considered.
- Resuscitation should be started with **1 L bolus of crystalloids (Ringer lactate or normal saline)**. Blood transfusion must be started, whenever available.

Blind clamping should not be done to avoid risk of injury to nerve and veins. **Tourniquet** use is associated with risk of irreparable vascular and neurological damage.

- **Permissive hypotension, massive transfusion protocol, preemptive use of tranexamic acid** are the recent changes in concepts regarding the management of traumatic hemorrhage.
- **Aggressive fluid resuscitation is now discouraged.**

Disability (Assessment of Neurologic Status)

The goal of this phase is to identify and treat life-threatening neurologic injuries. In this phase, rapid neurologic evaluation is done to assess **the level of consciousness, pupillary size, reaction and symmetry, presence of any lateralizing signs, spinal cord injury level** (if present).

Level of consciousness is quickly assessed by: 'AVPU'

- **A**—Patient **A**wake
- **V**—Open eyes to **V**oice
- **P**—Open eyes to **P**ainful stimulus
- **U**—**U**narousable

Exposure and Environmental Control

- The purpose of this phase is complete visual inspection of the injured patient along with measures taken to avoid excessive heat loss.
- **For thorough assessment of the patient:** (i) Complete disrobing; (ii) Logrolling to examine the back; (iii) Splaying of the legs to examine the perineum; and (iv) Elevation of the arms to inspect the axilla.
- **Measures to prevent hypothermia:** (i) Covering the patient with warm blanket or external warming device; (ii) Warm IV fluid; and (iii) Warm resuscitation area.

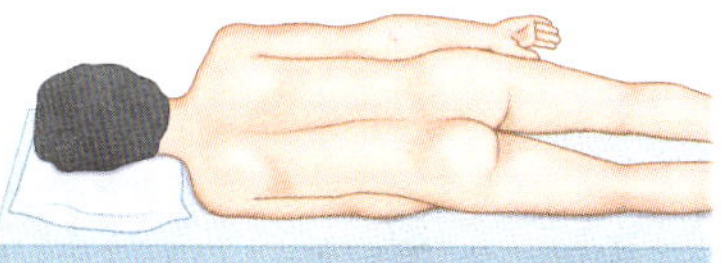

Logrolling to examine the back.

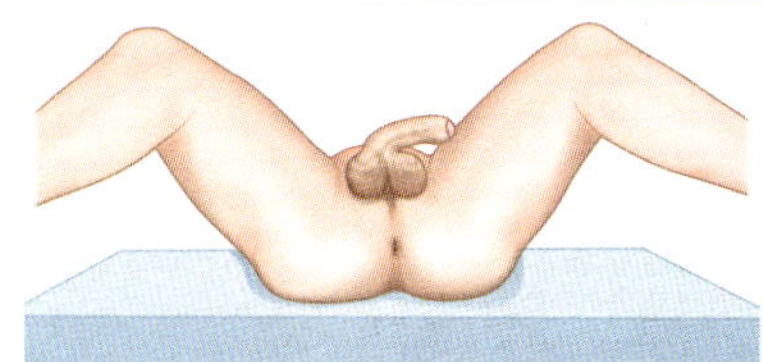

Splaying of the legs to examine perineum.

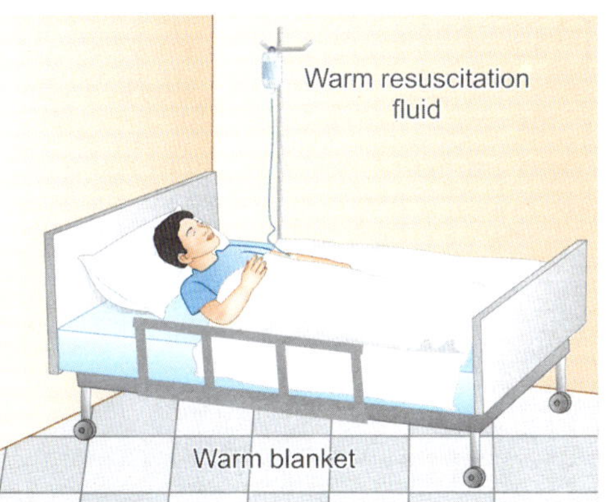

Warm resuscitation room

Adjuncts to the Primary Survey

- ECG monitoring
- Pulse oximetry
- Capnography
- Arterial blood gas (ABG) measurement
- Urinary catheter
- X-ray of chest and pelvis
- FAST and eFAST

- **Pediatric patients** usually have few signs of hypovolemia following severe volume depletion due to abundant physiologic reserve, but the clinical condition may deteriorate very rapidly.
- **Older adult trauma patients** need special consideration due to decreased physiologic reserve, associated comorbidities, long-term use of medications. These factors may alter the physiologic responses to injury.
- **Obese patients** also need special consideration due to associated comorbidities, technical difficulties related to endotracheal intubation, vascular access, FAST, and DPL.

Secondary Survey

- The secondary survey is complete **systematic head-to-toe evaluation** along with **complete history. The head-to-toe evaluation follows the sequence of** head, maxillofacial structures, cervical spine and neck, chest, abdomen and pelvis, perineum/rectum/vagina, musculoskeletal system, neurological system.
- **History includes:** (i) **A**llergies; (ii) **M**edications currently used; (iii) **P**ast illnesses/**p**regnancy; (iv) **L**ast meal; and (v) **E**vents/**e**nvironment related to the injury **(pneumonic 'AMPLE')**
- **Aims of secondary survey are to detect:** (i) Changes in clinical findings; (ii) Missed injuries; and (iii) Response to resuscitation.

Secondary Survey of 'Head'

- Patient's conscious level is evaluated by GCS (Glasgow Coma Scale). It measures: (i) Eye opening; (ii) Best verbal response; and (iii) Best motor response.
- Deep lacerations in scalp should be explored with a gloved finger to rule out depressed fracture.
- Signs of basal skull fracture should be searched.

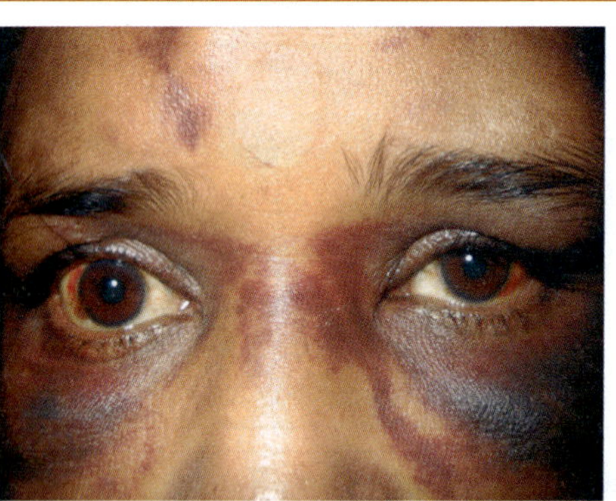

Bilateral periorbital ecchymosis

Patient with GCS <8 should be considered to have severe neurologic deficit.

Signs of anterior cranial fossa fracture:
- CSF rhinorrhea
- Periorbital ecchymosis ('Raccoon eyes')

Signs of middle cranial fossa fracture:
- CSF otorrhea
- Mastoid ecchymosis (Battle sign)

"Halo" sign:
- CSF mixed with blood produces double-ring pattern when dripped on pillow or hospital linen.
- A darker center spot (containing blood components) surrounded by light halo (containing CSF) form this pattern.

Secondary Survey of 'Maxillofacial Structures'

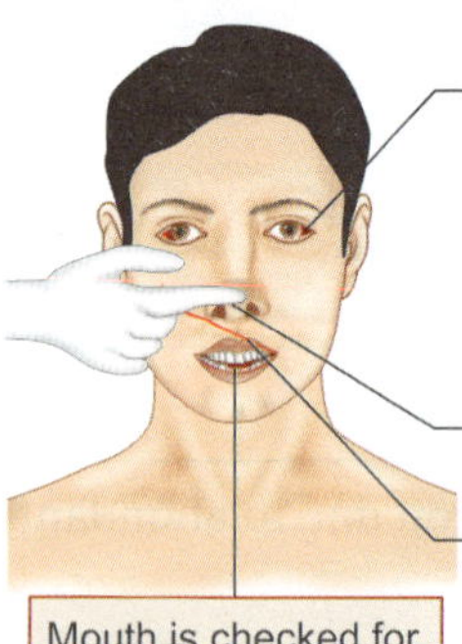

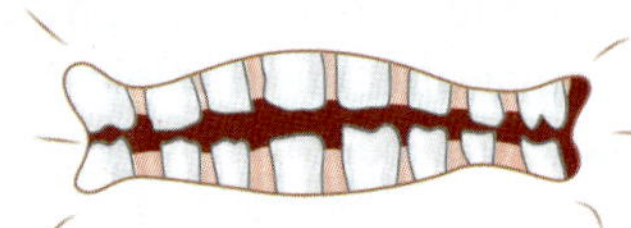

Abnormal dental occlusion if present, is highly suggestive of mandibular or maxillary fracture.

Fracture of the midface may be associated with fracture of the cribriform plate. In these patients, **gastric intubation should be done via oral route.**

Secondary Survey of "Cervical Spine and Neck'

- Neck is inspected, palpated, and auscultated to exclude: Cervical spine injury, aerodigestive tract injury (larynx, trachea, esophagus), vascular injury (carotid arteries, subclavian artery, jugular vein, and subclavian vein).
- In unconscious or intoxicated patient, **cervical spine should be considered unstable** unless excluded by CT or MRI of spine.
- **Spinal cord injury** should be suspected if midline cervical spine tenderness, vertebral step-off are present.
- **Aerodigestive tract injury** must be suspected if subcutaneous emphysema in neck is present.

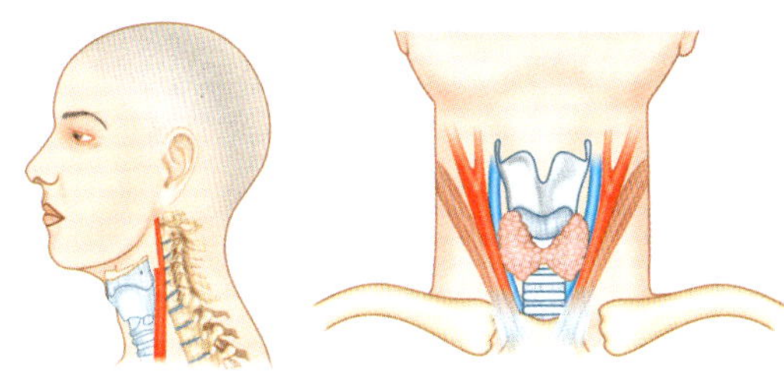

Radiographic evaluation of the cervical spine can be avoided in patients who meet the NEXUS Low-Risk Criteria or Canadian C-spine rule. [ATLS guideline 10th Ed.]

Secondary Survey of "Chest'

Evaluation of the chest includes clinical examination (inspection, palpation, auscultation, and percussion) and chest X-ray. **Inspection** can detect open pneumothorax, large flail segment, tension pneumothorax (distended neck vein). **Palpation** can reveal subcutaneous emphysema, tracheal deviation. **Auscultation** is done for detection of pneumothorax and hemothorax. **Percussion** demonstrates hyperresonance in presence of pneumothorax and dull note in presence of hemothorax.

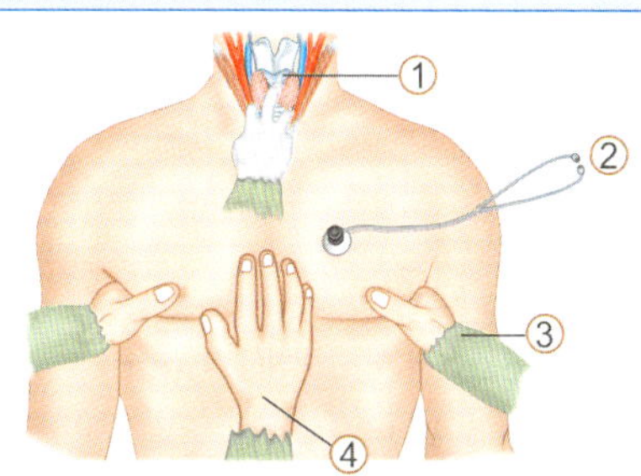

(1) Position of the trachea; (2) Quality and symmetry of breath sound; (3) Excursion of chest; and (4) Palpation for subcutaneous emphysema.

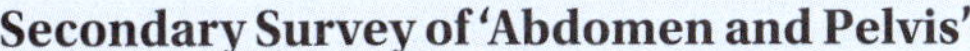

Secondary Survey of 'Abdomen and Pelvis'

- Repeated evaluation of the abdomen preferably by the same observer is important to rule out any significant Intra-abdominal injuries because clinical findings often change with time.
- During secondary survey of the abdomen, decision has to be taken whether surgical intervention is required or not. DPL, FAST, CT abdomen must be considered if any suspicion of Intra-abdominal injuries. Imaging of the pelvis is indicated if clinical findings are suggestive of pelvic fracture.

Clinical Findings Suggestive of Pelvic Fracture

- Ecchymosis over the iliac wings, pubis, labia, scrotum
- Pain on palpation of pelvic ring

Eviscerated bowel should be covered in warm wet packs and must not be returned to the peritoneum.

Secondary Survey of 'Perineum, Rectum, and Vagina'

- Perineum should be inspected for contusions, hematomas, and lacerations.
- Rectal examination is done to assess any injury of rectum, presence of blood in lumen.
- Vaginal examination is indicated if any suspicion of vaginal injury.

Secondary Survey of 'Musculoskeletal System'

Secondary survey is to be done to exclude: (i) Soft tissue injury; (ii) Bony injury; (iii) Vascular injury; and (iv) Neurologic injury. Patient's back should be examined otherwise significant injuries may be missed.

Secondary Survey of "Neurological System'

Secondary survey includes evaluation of sensory and motor functions of the extremities; reevaluation of GCS; pupillary size; symmetry; and response.

Head Injury

Types of Head Injury

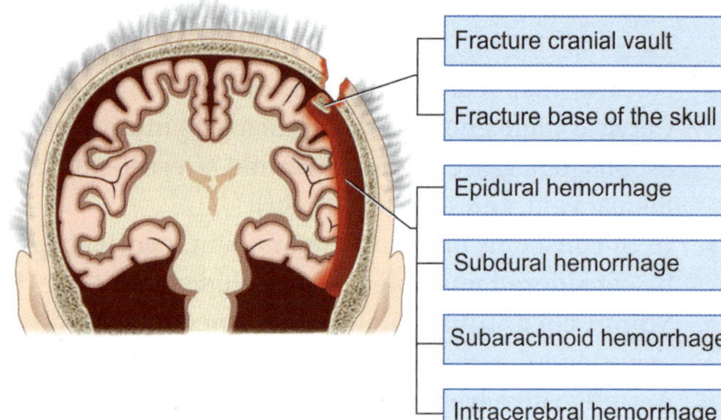

Traumatic brain injury (TBI) is classified into

Primary injury (occurs at the time of impact due to mechanical injury)
- Cerebral concussion
- Cerebral contusion and laceration
- Intracranial hematoma
- Diffuse axonal injury (DAI)
- Skull bone fracture

The primary goal of treatment in patients with TBI is to prevent secondary brain injury.

Secondary injury (occurs as a result of physiologic responses after the initial injury)
- Cerebral ischemia
- Cerebral edema
- Raised intracranial pressure
- Infection
- Epilepsy

Mechanisms of Injury
- **Acceleration/deceleration injury**
- **Impact injury**
- **Penetrating injury**

Acceleration/Deceleration Injury

- Classically seen in high-speed motor vehicle accidents.
- **Types of injuries associated with this mechanism of injury:** (i) Coup-contrecoup injury—due to abrupt deceleration of moving head; (ii) Brain impacts against bony irregularities; and (iii) Shear injuries to neurons and blood vessels.

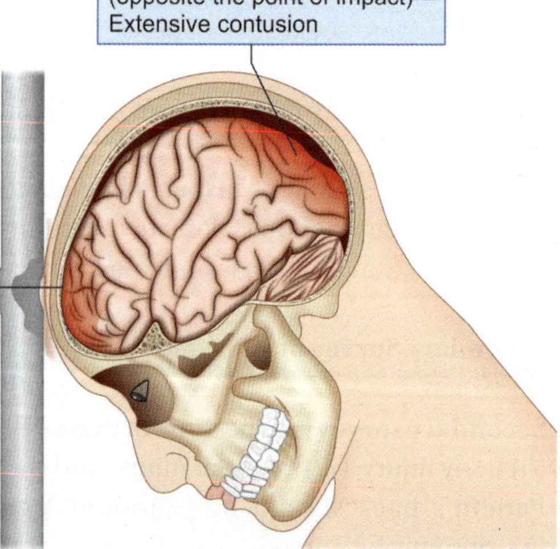

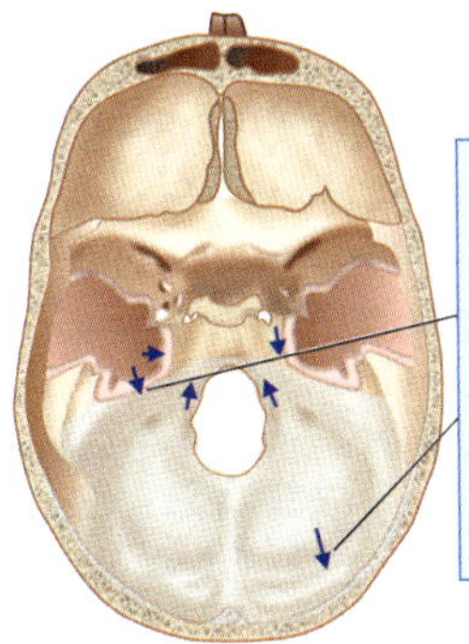

As the skull and brain accelerate and decelerate differentially, **brain moves within the skull and this brain impacts against intracranial bony irregularities** (floor of frontal sinus, sphenoid wing, petrous ridge) leads to contusion and hematoma.

- Differential acceleration and deceleration of skull and brain causes stretching of bridging veins and dural sinuses leads to rupture.
- Kinetic force causes shear injury to neurons and blood vessels lead to DAI and hematoma.

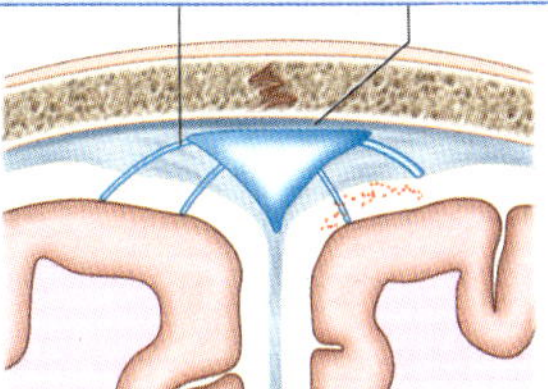

Impact Injury

- Classically seen following injury by blunt objects (e.g., bat, wooden or iron rod).
- Severity of brain injury is less.

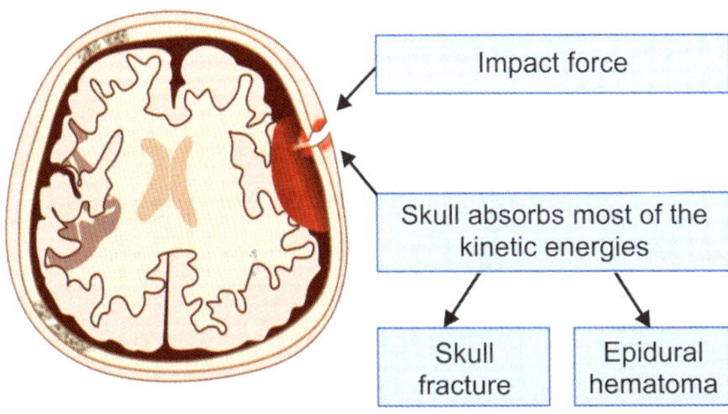

Penetrating Injury

Low Velocity Injuries

- Most low velocity injuries (by pen, pencil, branches, dart) occur through relatively thin skull bone-particularly orbitocranial window.
- Structures along the path are only injured.

High Velocity Injuries

In high velocity injuries, structures along the path are injured along with diffuse injury of the brain due to missile's kinetic energies is absorbed by the skull and brain.

Scalp Injury

Scalp has a rich blood supply, so significant blood loss may occur after injury.

- Treatment of simple laceration of scalp includes copious irrigation of the wound with normal saline followed by primary closure with mattress suture. Separate galeal apposition is recommended for long wounds.
- Scalp injury with tissue loss is treated by debridement followed by advancement flap. **Skull fracture must be excluded in deep lacerations by a gloved finger.**

Skull Fracture

- Fracture of the cranial vault
- Fracture of base of the skull

- Open fracture
- Closed fracture

- Depressed fracture
- Nondepressed fracture

- Linear fracture
- Stellate fracture

Fracture of Base of the Skull

- **Fracture of anterior cranial fossa may present with:** (i) Anosmia (due to damage of olfactory nerve); (ii) Bilateral periorbital ecchymoses ('Raccoon eyes'); and (iii) CSF rhinorrhea.
- **Fracture of middle cranial fossa may present with:** (i) Vertigo, ipsilateral deafness, facial paralysis (due to damage of vestibulocochlear nerve or facial nerve); (ii) CSF otorrhea; and (iii) Ecchymoses behind the ear ('Battle sign').

Management

- Most of the CSF leaks will heal with elevation of head of the bed for several days.
- No proven role of prophylactic antibiotics to prevent meningitis.
- Dura is repaired with autologous, vascularized graft.
- Facial nerve palsy may benefit with steroid. If not responding within 72 hours, surgical decompression of the petrous part of the nerve is indicated.

Fracture of the Cranial Vault

- **Closed, nondepressed fractures** usually do not require any active management. Patients should be admitted for observation.
- **Open, nondepressed fractures** require scalp repair and broad-spectrum antibiotic therapy.
- **In minor depressed fractures**, the risk of dural tear or underlying brain injury is minimal. Elevation of the depressed fragment is indicated for cosmetic reasons, particularly when in the frontal region.
- **In severe depressed fractures**, there is high risk of dural laceration, brain parenchyma and vessels. Surgical intervention is indicated for this type of fracture.
- **Depression of the outer table of the depressed fragment below the level of inner table of surrounding skull is an indication for operative elevation.**
- **Treatment of depressed fracture includes:** (i) Elevation of the depressed fragment; (ii) Duraplasty (if any dural tear).

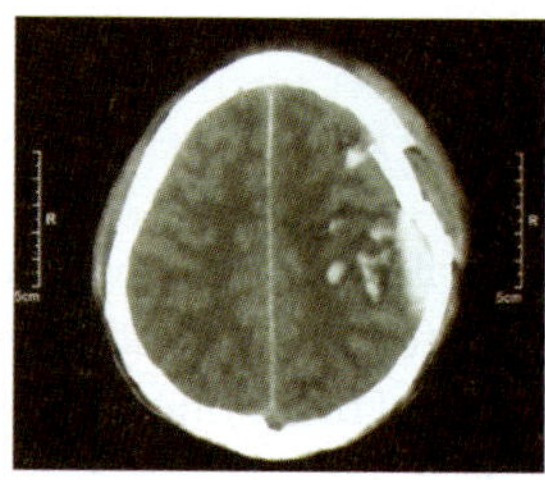

CT brain showing depressed skull bone fracture with underlying brain contusion.

If venous sinus involved in the depressed fracture, surgery is better avoided for risk of excessive bleeding. Only antibiotic therapy is preferred.

Ping Pong Fracture ('Pond Fracture')

- A type of **depressed skull fracture is seen in infants**. This fracture is characterized by smooth depression of cranial vault without any fracture of inner table or dural tear. The risk of underlying brain injury is minimal.
- **Surgery is indicated** to prevent formation of leptomeningeal cyst. Through a burr hole adjacent to depressed fracture, the bone is 'popped' back into normal shape by Adson's periosteal elevator or surgeon's finger.

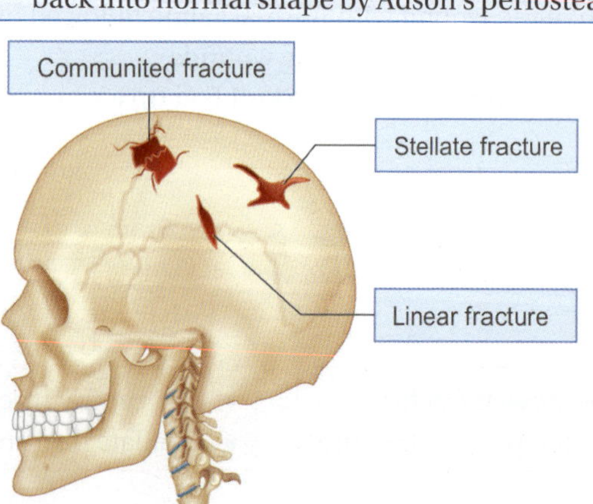

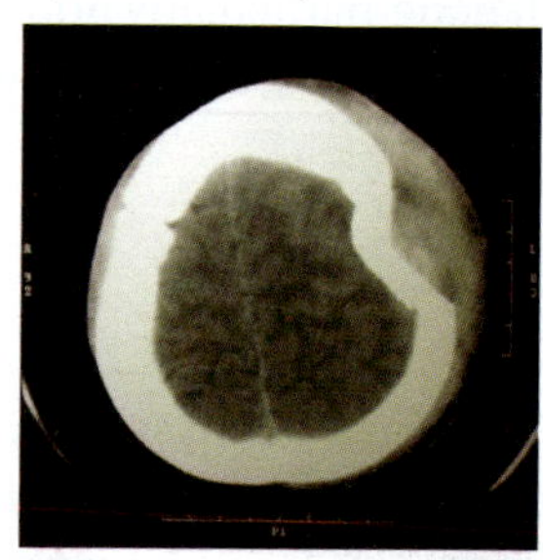

CT brain showing 'Pond fracture'.

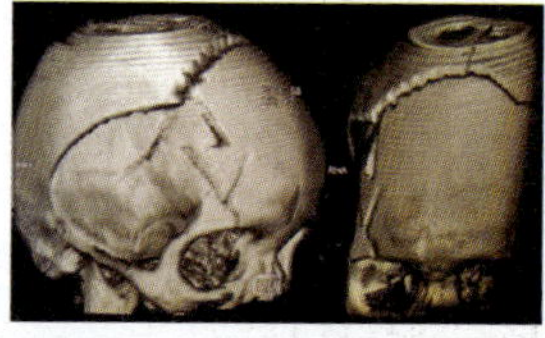

3D reconstruction of CT brain showing communited skull fracture.

Epidural (Extradural) Hematoma

- Epidural hematoma (EDH) is accumulation of blood between the skull bone and the dura.
- Usually results from arterial disruption (especially the **middle meningeal artery**). Rarely, a skull fracture may cross a venous sinus (superior sagittal sinus or transverse sinus).
- Mostly underlie a skull fracture.
- **Most common location** is the temporal fossa. Temporal squamosa is the thinnest part of the cranial vault.

Clinical presentation:

- EDH has classic 3-stage clinical presentations (in about 20% of patients): (i) Stage of concussion—transient loss of consciousness; (ii) Lucid interval—patient awakens; and (iii) Patient becomes lethargic and proceeds to coma stage.
- Dilated pupil and impaired or absent reaction to light on the side of lesion and contralateral hemiparesis are important localizing signs due to transtentorial uncal herniation and indicate imminent neurological deterioration.

Diagnosis:

- Noncontrast CT brain is indicated for confirmation of diagnosis.
- CT brain shows biconvex, hyperdense lesion with well-defined border, typically in temporal or temporoparietal region.

Treatment:

- Surgical evacuation of hematoma is indicated in following conditions: (i) Volume of hematoma more than 30 cm^3; (ii) GCS ≤8 with anisocoria; (iii) Presence of neurological symptoms; (iv) Midline shift >5 mm; and (v) Maximal hematoma thickness >1 cm.
- Small, asymptomatic EDH without midline shift and GCS >8 can be managed by close observation with serial CT.

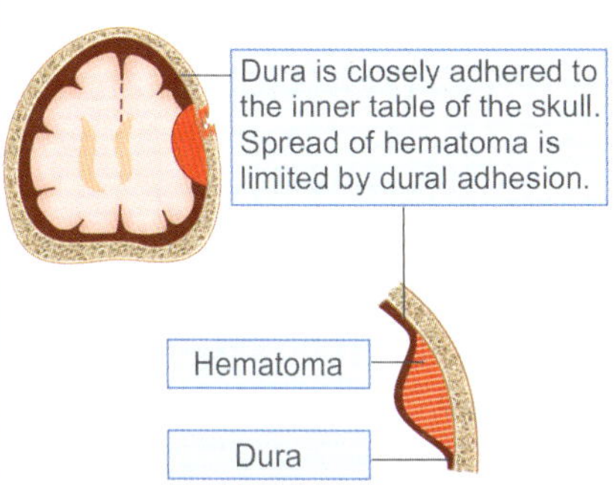

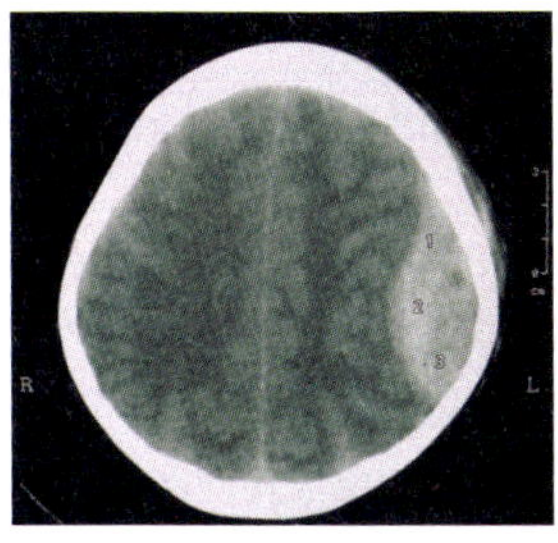

CT scan showing extradural hematoma.

Anisocoria is the difference in size of the pupil of two eyes of an individual.

- **Anisocoria is either physiological or pathological.**
- **Physiological anisocoria** (found in few percentages of population without any clinical significance) does not exceed 1 mm.

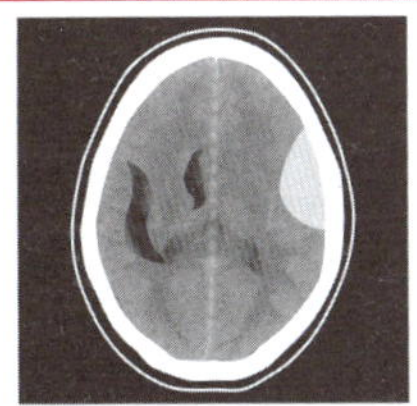

Need surgical evacuation of hematoma.

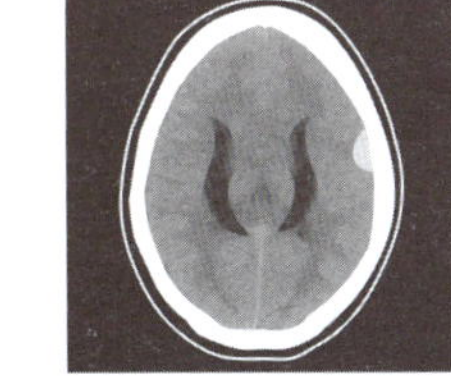

Close observation with serial CT.

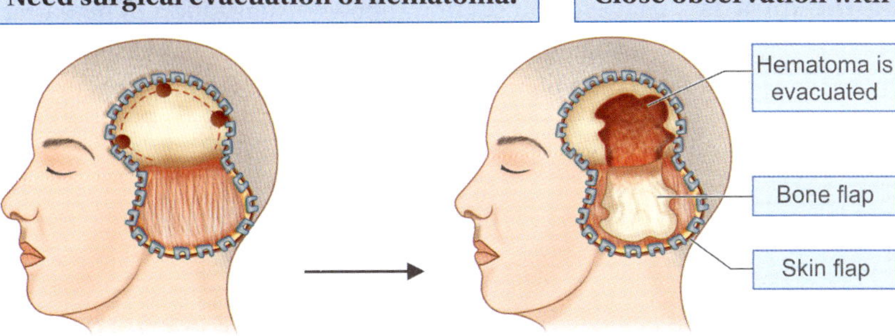

Craniotomy for EDH.

Indications of urgent CT head scan in adults after head injury (if any one of the risk factors is present):

- GCS <13 on initial assessment
- GCS <15 at 2 hours after injury on assessment in emergency department
- Suspected open or depressed skull fracture
- Any sign of basal skull fracture
- Post-traumatic seizure
- Focal neurological deficit
- More than one episode of vomiting since the head injury.

Indications of CT head scan in adults within 8 hours of head injury:

- Patient on anticoagulants
- Loss of consciousness or amnesia since the head injury with any of the risk factors: (a) Age ≥65 years; (b) A history of bleeding or clotting disorder; (c) Dangerous mechanism of injury (a pedestrian or cyclist struck by a motor vehicle, an occupant ejected from a motor vehicle or a fall from height of more than 1 meter or 5 stairs); (d) More than 30 minutes retrograde amnesia of events immediately before the head injury [as per NICE guideline].

Acute Subdural Hematoma

Acute subdural hematoma is characterized by accumulation of blood between dura mater and arachnoid mater. Subdural hematomas are more common than epidural hematomas.

Pathophysiology: Bleeding occurs due to shearing of small surface or bridging vessels of the cerebral cortex.

Clinical presentation includes altered consciousness, contralateral hemiparesis, seizure.

Diagnosis: Noncontrast CT brain is indicated for diagnosis. Acute subdural hematoma appears as biconcave hyperdense lesion.

Treatment

Indications of evacuation of hematoma in subdural hematoma: (i) Acute SDH with thickness >1 cm regardless of GCS score; (ii) Acute SDH with midline shift >5 mm regardless of GCS score; and (iii) GCS ≤8 with acute SDH <1 cm and midline shift <5 mm but GCS decreases by 2 points between the time of injury and hospital admission or pupils are asymmetric or fixed and dilated.

The longer the interval of development of hematoma and surgical intervention, more the deterioration of the patient's condition due to secondary effects.

So, quick decision making and opening the dura is necessary for better outcome.

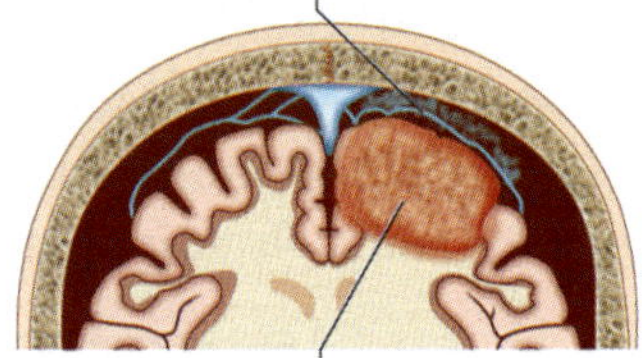

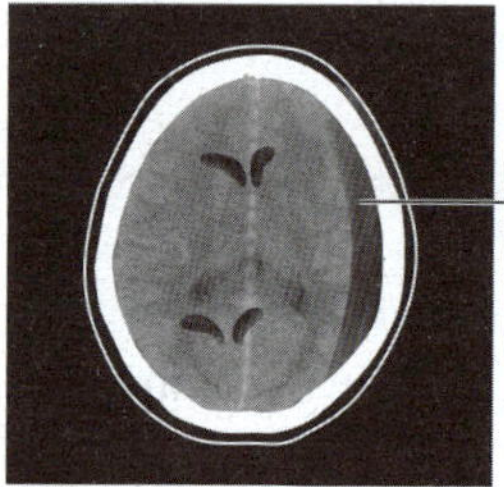

A large craniotomy flap is planned because besides evacuation of subdural hematoma, underlying cerebral hemorrhagic contusions and intracerebral hematomas have to be evacuated.

Frontotemporoparietal flap is preferred for better exposure.

Further steps includes—evacuation of clot, gentle lavage and suction (allows visualization of bleeding bridging veins), coagulation of bleeding vessels, evacuation of hematoma and necrotic brain parenchyma.

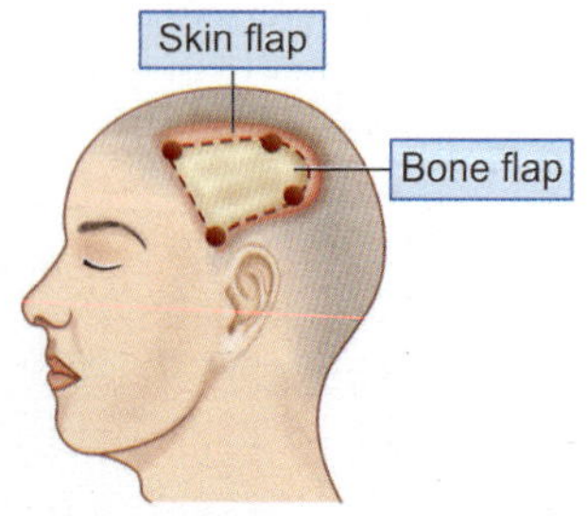

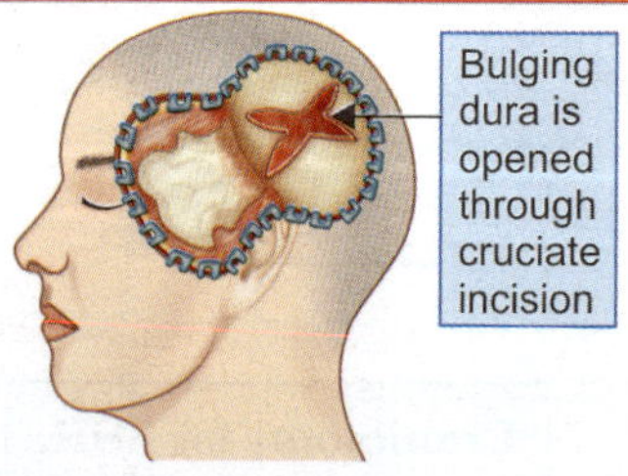

Chronic Subdural Hematoma (CSDH)

Chronic subdural hematoma most commonly develops in the elderly patients following a minor trauma.

Risk factors: (i) Older age group; (ii) Coagulation disorders; (iii) Alcoholism; (iv) Low CSF pressure (after shunt or fistula); and (v) Use of anticoagulants and antiplatelet agents.

Clinical presentations include altered consciousness, headache, seizure, and contralateral hemiparesis.

Diagnosis: Noncontrast CT brain is indicated for diagnosis. In the acute phase, the hematoma appears hyperdense without any midline shift. After 2–3 weeks (chronic phase), the hematoma appears hypodense with midline shift.

Treatment:

- Chronic SDH thicker than 1 cm and all symptomatic chronic SDH must be surgically drained.
- Small hematomas particularly associated with antiplatelet agents may be managed conservatively.

Follow-up CT scan in immediate postoperative period and after 1 month is essential to document resolution.

Pathophysiology of CSDH

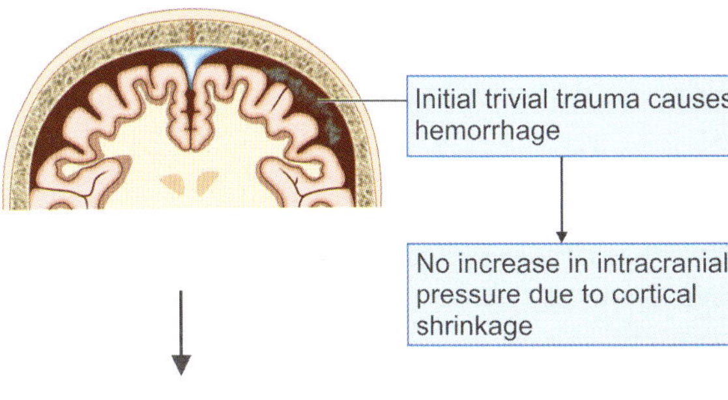

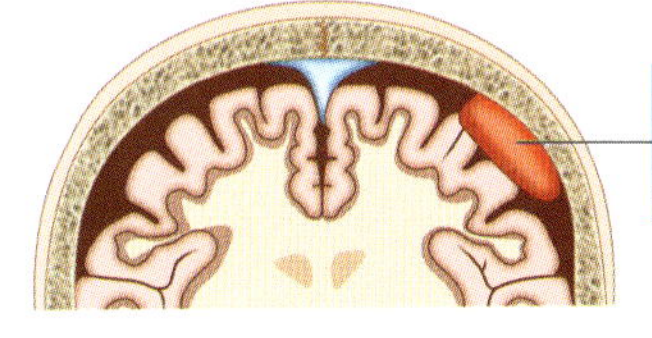

Membrane grows out from the dura to encapsulate the hematoma

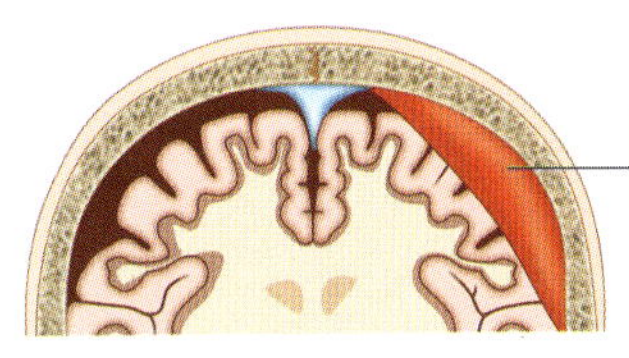

Hematoma liquefies and expands significantly

Contusions and Intracerebral Hematoma

Contusions most commonly occur in frontal and temporal lobes but may develop in any part of the brain.

Areas of contusions may change into intracerebral hematoma or a coalescent contusion with mass effect.

Diagnosis: Noncontrast CT scan is diagnostic. **In patients with contusions, repeat CT scanning within 24 hours of initial CT scan is indicated to detect any changes over time (from contusion to hematoma).**

Treatment: *Indications of surgical decompression:* (i) Midline shift >0.3 cm; (ii) Volume of hematoma >50 cm^3; (iii) Progressive deterioration of sensorium; (iv) Progressive focal neurological deficit; and (v) Increased ICP.

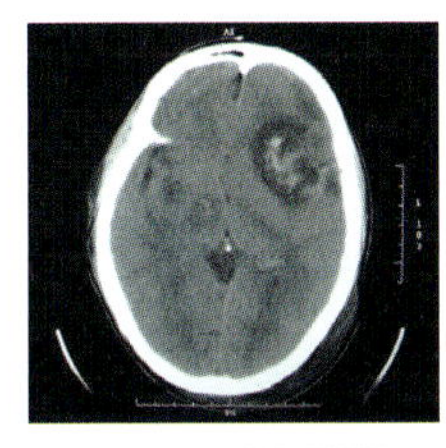

Contusion

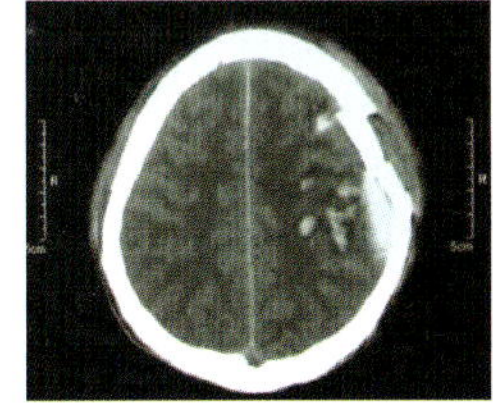

Intracerebral hematoma

Contusions and intracerebral hematomas are commonly found **frontal and temporal lobes** because these areas suffer major shear strains during acceleration-deceleration injury.

Diffuse Axonal Injury (DAI)

As a result of shearing following deceleration, **disruption of axons develops especially at the gray-white matter interface.** DAI commonly affects the white matter tracts of corpus callosum and brainstem. Macroscopically, punctate hemorrhages may seen in corpus callosum and superior cerebellar peduncle. Microscopically, retraction balls and microglial clusters are seen diffusely in the white matter. Patient may present with mild coma to death.

Diagnosis: CT has low sensitivity in detecting DAI. **MRI, specifically diffuse tensor imaging (DTI), is the imaging modality of choice.**

Treatment is primarily focused on preventing secondary injuries.

Classification of Head Injuries (based on Severity)

Mild Traumatic Brain Injury	Moderate Traumatic Brain Injury	Severe Traumatic Brain Injury
GCS 13–15	GCS 9–12	GCS 3–8

Glasgow coma scale (GCS)—Original scale	
Eye Opening (E)	
Spontaneous	4
To speech	3
To pain	2
None	1
Verbal Response (V)	
Oriented	5
Confused conversation	4
Inappropiate words	3
Incomprehensible sounds	2
None	1
Best Motor Response (M)	
Obeys commands	6
Localizes pain	5
Flexion withdrawal to pain	4
Abnormal flexion (decorticate)	3
Extension (decerebrate)	2
None (Flaccid)	1

GCS score = E + V + M
Best possible score: 15; **worst possible score:** 3
Expressed as GCS score: 3/15, 10/15, 15/15.

Glasgow coma scale (GCS)—Revised scale	
Eye Opening (E)	
Spontaneous	4
To sound	3
To pressure	2
None	1
Non-testable	NT
Verbal Response (V)	
Oriented	5
Confused	4
Words	3
Sounds	2
None	1
Non-testable	NT
Best Motor Response (M)	
Obeys commands	6
Localizing	5
Normal flexion	4
Abnormal flexion	3
Extension	2
None	1
Non-testable	NT

Assessment of severity of TBI is done by

Level of Consciousness

- Assessed by GCS scoring
- GCS score is an indicator of prognosis and have predictive value regarding neurosurgical intervention

Localizing Signs

- Pupil is assessed by: (i) Size; (ii) Equality; and (iii) Reaction to light
- Dilated pupil and asymmetry >1mm are important localizing signs.
- Asymmetric movement in response to painful stimulus-suggestive of focal lesion.

Imaging

Noncontrast CT scan brain

During assessment of neurological status using GCS score, following factors must be considered: (i) Factors that may depress neurological function [effects of alcohol or illicit drugs, use of sedatives, paralytics (for intubation), atropine (for cardiac resuscitation) in prehospital setting, hypoxia, hypotension, hypothermia]; (ii) Presence of any spinal injury; (iii) Hearing deficit, if any; and (iv) Language barrier.

Pupillary Examination in Traumatic Brain Injury Patient

Assessment of pupil size and equality:

- Size is measured as the width or diameter of each pupil in millimeters by a standardized pupil gauze (Normal diameter is between 2 and 5 mm with average pupil measuring 3.5 mm).
- Assessment for anisocoria (causes of anisocoria in trauma—compression of third cranial nerve due to uncal herniation into the tentorial notch, damage of Edinger-Westphal nucleus in the midbrain, direct orbital trauma).

Assessment of pupillary shape:

- The shape of the pupil may be round, oval- or irregular (normal pupil is roundshaped).
- Oval-shaped pupil is indicative of early compression of cranial nerve III due raised ICP.

Reactivity to light:

- Reactivity to light is described as brisk, sluggish, or nonreactive (normal pupillary response to light is brisk).
- A sluggish or nonreactive papillary response is suggestive of increased intracranial pressure.

Worse prognostic outcome in traumatic brain injury is related to:

(i) Bilaterally dilated pupils; (ii) Absent pupillary light reflex; (iii) Initial GCS score <9; (iv) Hypotension <90 mm Hg with hypoxemia; (v) Abnormal CT scan (extensive tSAH, compression or obliteration of basal cisterns); (vi) Persistent ICP >20 mm Hg; (vii) Elevated ICP during the first 24 hours; and (viii) Extremes of age (>60 years and <2 years).

Importance of Resuscitative Measures in TBI

- In TBI, the total trauma effect is the combination of primary injury and subsequent secondary injuries.
- Primary injury is the anatomic and physiologic disruption of brain itself. Secondary injury is the sequela of primary injury and resulting from cerebral edema, increased ICP, hypoperfusion, hypoxemia.
- *Hypoperfusion and hypoxemia are the most significant factors* lead to poor neurologic outcome.
- Systolic BP ≥100 mm Hg for patients 50–69 years or at ≥110 mm Hg or higher for patients 15–49 years or older than 70 years, adequate oxygenation and ventilation (pulse oximetry ≥95%), PaO_2 ≥100 mm Hg, $PaCO_2$ (35–45 mm Hg), maintaining ICP (5–15 mm Hg) are the basic goals of resuscitation.

Medical Therapies for Traumatic Brain Injury (TBI)

Fluid and electrolytes

Following should be avoided in TBI patients: (i) Hypovolemia; (ii) Fluid overload; (iii) Glucose-containing IV fluids (hyperglycemia causes further injury to brain); (iv) Hyponatremia (associated with brain edema); and (v) Hypotonic fluid. Ringer lactate or normal saline is the recommended IV fluid in TBI patients.

Hyperventilation

Hyperventilation prevents secondary injury by reducing $PaCO_2$ and causing cerebral vasoconstriction. $PaCO_2$ should be kept at approximately 35 mm Hg. Prophylactic hyperventilation ($PaCO_2$ <25 mm Hg) is not recommended [ATLS Protocol, 10th Edn].

Mannitol

Mannitol is particularly used when patient under observation develops localizing sign (e.g., dilated pupil, hemiparesis) or becomes unconscious. In hypovolemic patient (systolic BP <90 mm Hg), mannitol should be avoided because it causes further cerebral ischemia.

Anticoagulant reversal

Anticoagulant reversal is required in patients on anticoagulants or antiplatelets.

Anticonvulsants

- Prophylactic use of phenytoin is not recommended for late post-traumatic seizures. Phenytoin is recommended to decrease the incidence of early post-traumatic seizure (within 7 days of injury).
- Acute seizures are managed with phenytoin (loading dose is 1 gm IV not faster than 50 mg/min followed by maintenance dose of 100 mg/8 hours) or fosphenytoin. Continuous seizure should be controlled as soon as possible because seizure for more than 30 minutes may cause secondary brain injury.

Post-traumatic Seizure (PTS)

PTS is classified into: (i) Immediate PTS (within 24 hours of injury); (ii) Early PTS (within the first-week post-injury); and (iii) Late PTS (after one week post-injury).

Risk factors for post-traumatic seizure: (i) GCS <10; (ii) Depressed skull fracture; (iii) Cortical contusion; (iv) Subdural, epidural, or intracerebral hematoma; (v) Penetrating injury; and (vi) Seizure within 24 hours of injury. Prophylactic anticonvulsants (e.g., Phenytoin, Levetiracetam) can reduce the risk of early PTS.

Management of Intracranial Hypertension

Intracranial pressure (ICP) monitoring is indicated in: (i) Patients with severe TBI (GCS 3–8); (ii) Abnormal CT scan; (iii) Normal CT scan with two or more of the criteria—(a) Age >40 years; (b) Systolic blood pressure <90 mm Hg; and (c) Unilateral or bilateral abnormal motor posturing.

Measures to control intracranial hypertension: (i) Elevation of the head of the bed; (ii) Mannitol; (iii) Barbiturates (effective for reducing ICP refractory to other measures); (iv) Ventriculostomy (drainage of CSF); and (v) Surgical evacuation of hematoma.

- **Judicious use of anticonvulsants** is necessary because it delays brain recovery.
- **Mannitol and barbiturates should not be used in the presence of hypotension or hypovolemia.**
- **Steroid has no beneficial role** in management of intracranial hypertension.

Maxillofacial Trauma

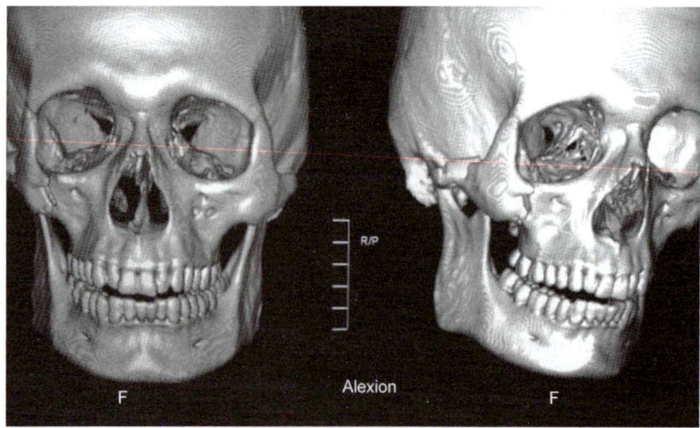

3D reconstruction of CT face showing fracture maxilla and zygomatic bone.

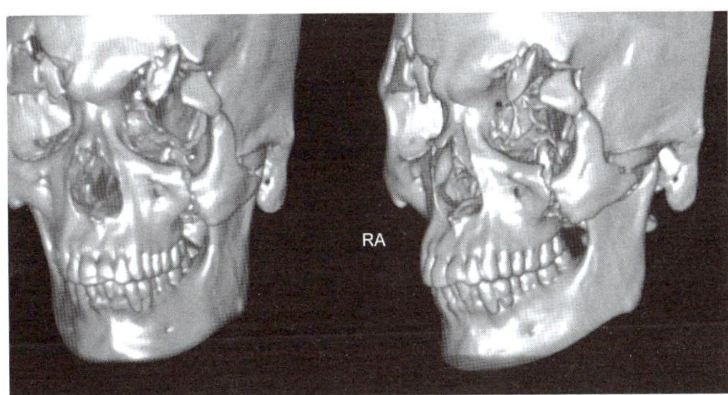

3D reconstruction of CT face showing comminuted fracture of facial bone.

Types of Injuries

Soft-tissue injuries

Bony injuries

- Fracture of mandible
- Fracture of maxilla
- Fracture of zygoma
- Fracture of nasal bone

Others

- Facial nerve injury
- Parotid duct injury
- Injury of lacrimal apparatus

- Maxillofacial injuries (particularly bony injuries) are usually not life-threatening injuries except **midfacial injuries which have a potential to develop airway obstruction**.
- Orotracheal intubation is difficult or impossible and **nasotracheal intubation is contraindicated in midfacial injuries.**
- Therefore **surgical airway** is indicated during initial resuscitation.

Principles of Treatment in Maxillofacial Injuries

- Proper cleansing of wound (to avoid pigmented scars)
- Accurate apposition of tissues in layers with fine sutures.
- Sutures ideally should be removed after 3 days to prevent additional scarring, but wound must be supported with adhesive skin tape for another 5–10 days.

Examination of the Injuries

Face must be examined from the front. Examination of the **soft tissues of face** by gentle palpation, followed by **examination of bony structures** and then **intraoral examination**.

Intraoral Examination

Intraoral examination includes examination of cheek, tongue and floor of the mouth.

Examination is to done to look for:

- Asymmetry, as a whole
- Flattening of check: Depressed zygomatic fracture
- Nasal deviation
- Intercanthal distance >3.5 cm—nasoethmoidal fracture
- Uneven pupillary level—orbital floor fracture
- Subconjunctival hemorrhage without a posterior border—orbital wall fracture
- Dental malocclusion—mandibular or maxillary fracture

Examination of Bony Structures

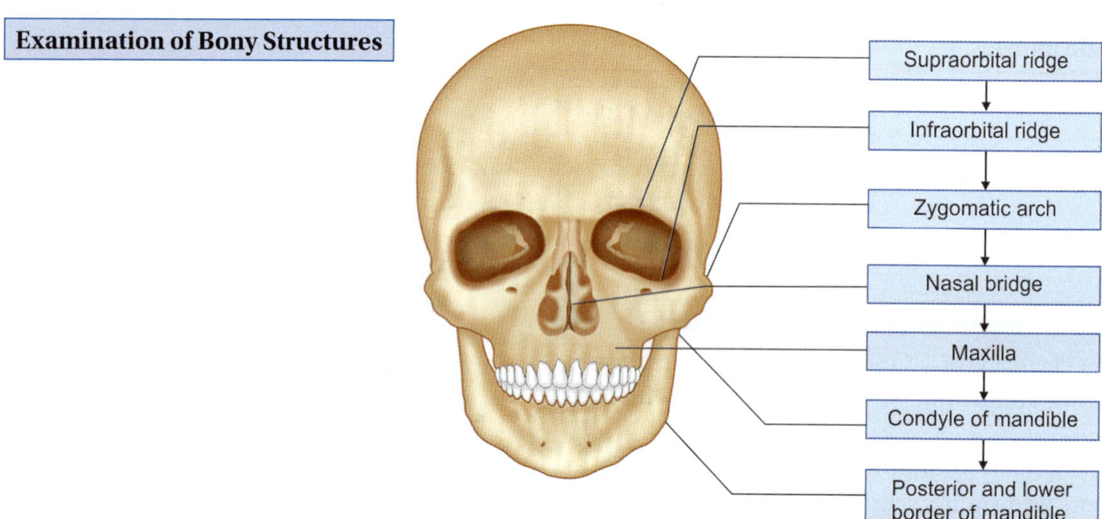

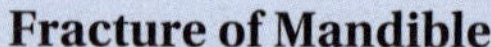

Fracture of Mandible

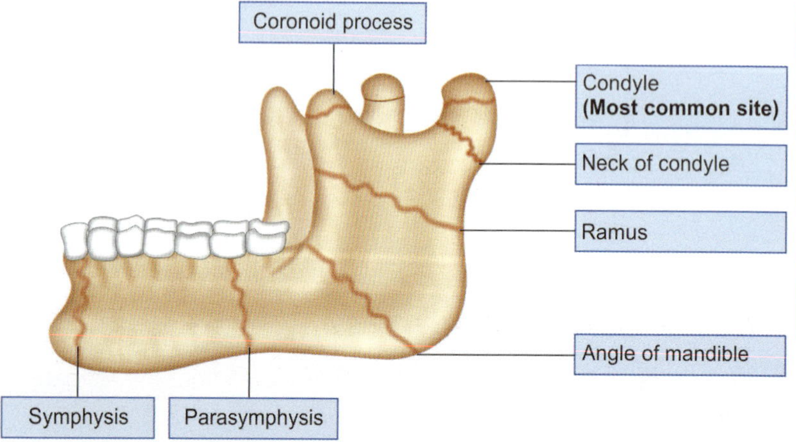

Fracture can present in any anatomical region of mandible.

- **Different imaging techniques:**
  - *Plain X-ray:* **Orthopantomogram is the radiograph of choice**.
  - Panoramic tomography
  - Helical CT
  - Treatment is reduction and fixation

Types of Fixation Methods in Fracture Mandible

Interdental eyelet wiring

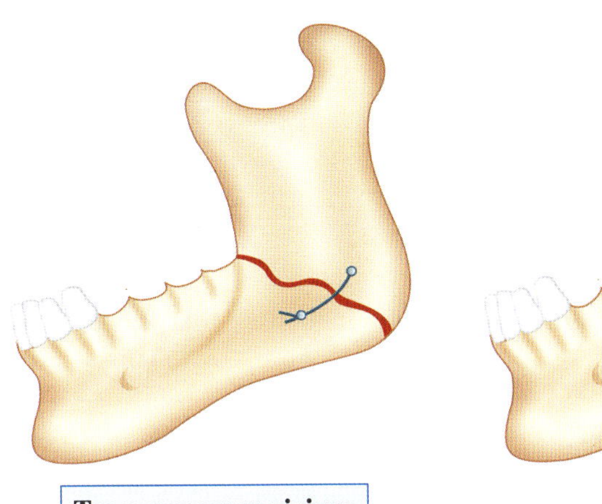

Transosseous wiring

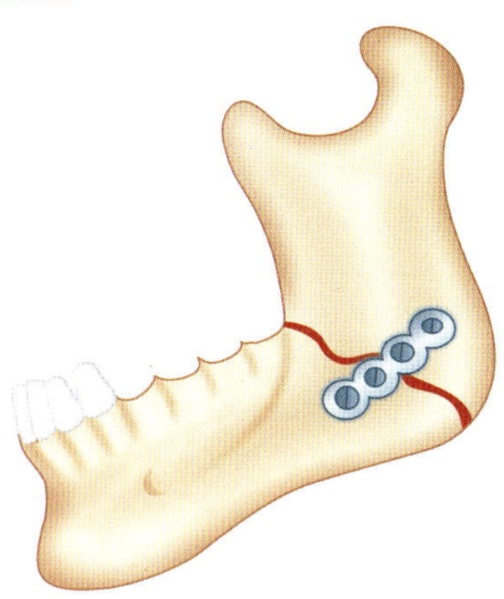

Plating

Fracture Maxilla

Le Fort classification system classifies the midface fracture according to the plane of injury.

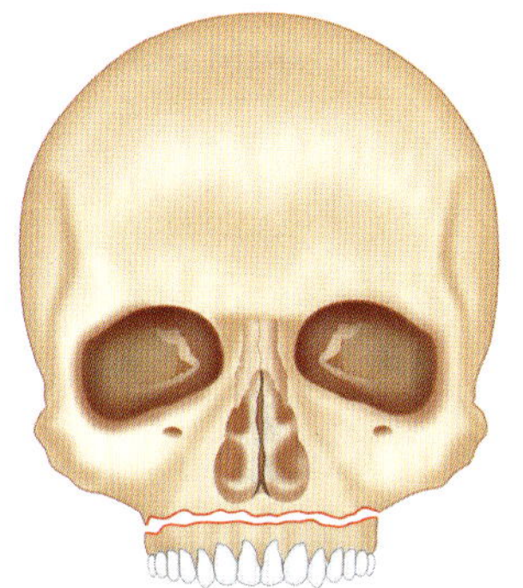

Le Fort Type I (Horizontal)

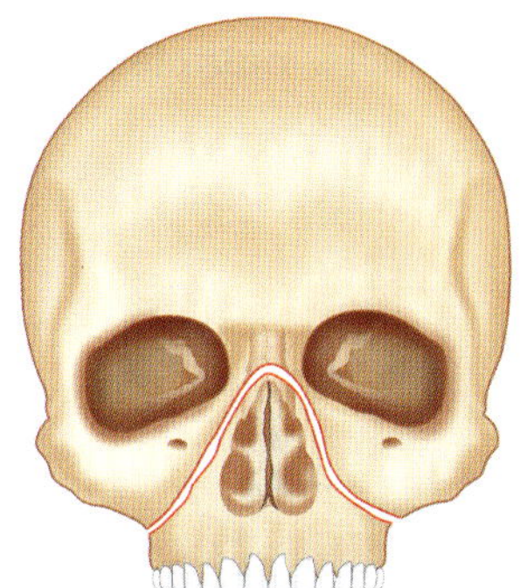

Le Fort Type II

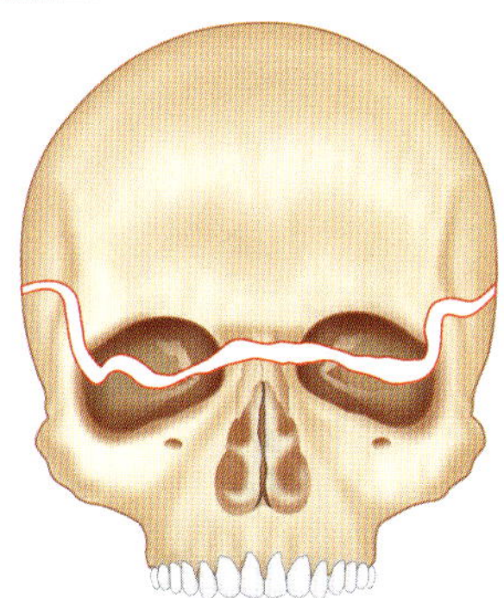

Le Fort Type III

Le Fort Type I (Horizontal)

- **Horizontal maxillary fracture**
- **Fracture line traverses through** the alveolar ridge, lateral nose, and inferior wall of the maxillary sinus, separating the teeth from the upper face.

Le Fort Type II

- **Pyramidal fracture**, where teeth form the base of the pyramid and nasofrontal suture at the apex.
- **Fracture line traverses through** the posterior alveolar ridge, lateral wall of maxillary sinuses, inferior orbital rim, and nasal bones.

Le Fort Type III

- **Craniofacial dysjunction**
- **Fracture line traverses through** nasofrontal suture, maxillofrontal suture, orbital wall, and zygomaticofrontal suture.

- **Treatment** is reduction and fixation. Different types of fixation methods are: (i) Plating; (ii) Frontal suspension; (iii) Arch bar; and (iv) Intermaxillary wiring.
- Treatment is not indicated as life-saving procedure.
- If airway is clear and antibiotic therapy is instituted, the procedure can be awaited for 24–48 hours. During this period, patient's condition can be improved, and facial edema is subsided.

Fracture Nasal Bone

- Most common fracture of face
- Without proper reduction of fracture, asymmetry and loss of normal contour may develop and also deviated nasal septum.
- Reduction is usually indicated 7–10 days of injury (facial edema is mostly subsided) and before 3 weeks (manipulation is almost impossible).

Facial Nerve Injury

- Clinical signs suggest that main division is involved.
- Primary repair (microsurgical nerve repair) is the treatment of choice.

Lacrimal Apparatus Injury

This injury may develop in Le Fort type II and III injuries. This injury should be treated by an ophthalmic surgeon.

Parotid Duct/Gland Injury

- Injury of parotid gland tissue may lead to parotid fistula if left untreated.
- Treatment is suturing the tissue in layers and a compressive dressing for 48 hours.
- If parotid duct is transected, sialogram have to performed to reveal the ductal system. Then severed ends is approximated over a fine tube using microscope.
- If expertise or proper instrument is not available, then an internal fistula can be created by suturing the gland end of the severed duct in buccal mucosa.

Neck Injuries

Neck contains **multiple vital structures** with **little anatomic protection**.

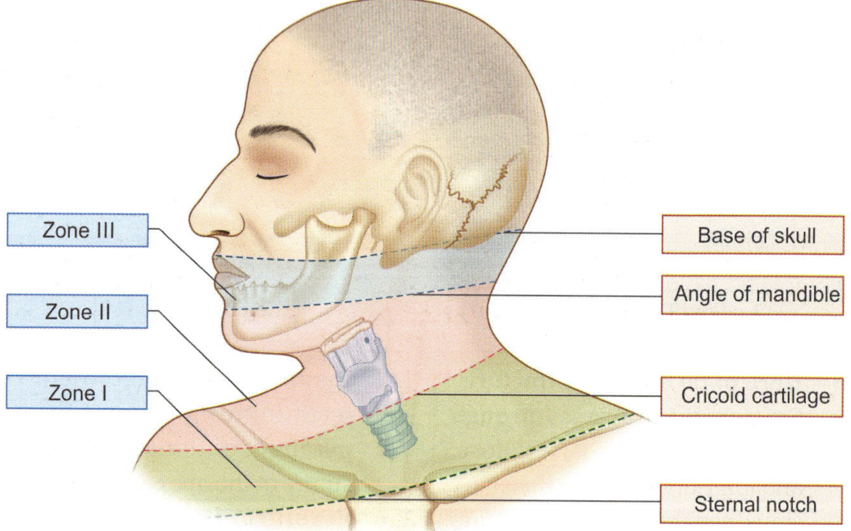

Evaluation of Penetrating Neck Injuries

- Penetrating neck injuries can be evaluated craniocaudally and anteroposteriorly.
- Craniocaudally, neck is divided into three horizontal zones—Zone I, II and III.

Major vascular (carotid arteries, subclavian arteries, jugular vein, subclavian vein), **major aerodigestive** (larynx, trachea, esophagus) structures, **thyroid, thoracic** duct—all located in the anterior triangle.

Cervical spine, spinal cord, neck musculature are all that located in the posterior triangle.

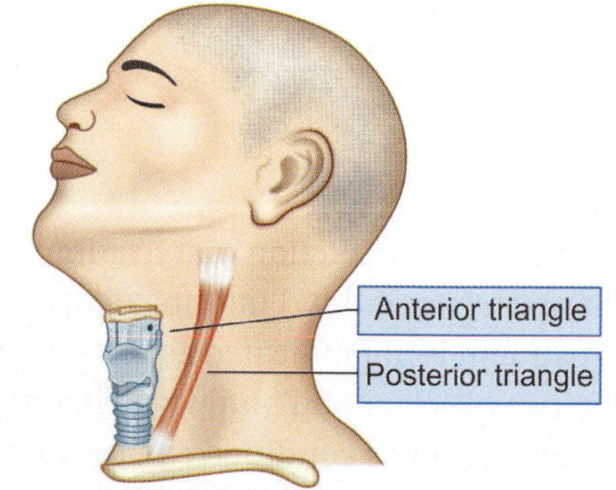

Management of Zone I Injury

- Injury in this zone carries **highest mortality** due to presence of major vessels (proximal carotid arteries, subclavian vessels, major vessels of chest).
- Management of injuries in this zone is complicated by overlying ribs, sternum, and clavicle.
- **In hemodynamically stable patients**, thorough evaluation is done by: (i) Angiography of great vessels; (ii) Contrast esophagogram; (iii) Esophagoscopy; (iv) Bronchoscopy; and (v) Thin slice CT scan of neck.
- **In unstable patients**, patient should be taken directly to the operation theater. Exploration of such a wound will require simultaneous access to both neck and mediastinum. So, a median sternotomy is also needed. Surgery should be performed by an experienced vascular surgeon.

Management of Zone II Injury

- Injuries in this zone are clinically apparent with significant hematoma or frank external hemorrhage.
- Vascular control is relatively easy.
- Stab and gunshot wounds are most commonly situated in this zone.
- Two school of thoughts regarding treatment approach (selective approach or mandatory exploration) where no suspicious clinical findings are present.

Suspicious clinical findings: (i) Significant external hemorrhage; (ii) Large or expanding hematoma; (iii) Voice changes; (iv) Dysphagia; and (v) Crepitus in neck.

In **selective approach**, exploration is done after extensive evaluation: (i) Angiography (color flow Doppler imaging is an reliable and safer alternative to angiography); (ii) Esophagoscopy; (iii) Esophagography; and (iv) Helical CT with IV contrast.

Management of Zone III Injury

- Exposure is much more difficult in this zone.
- Radiographic vascular imaging (carotid and vertebral angiography) is essential before surgical exploration in stable patients.
- Patient with evidence of vascular injury or injury to the aerodigestive tract must require surgical repair.

Principles of Neck Exploration

- Goal of neck exploration is to explore the structures of the neck.
- In case of unilateral injury, oblique incision along the anterior border of sternocleidomastoid.
- If bilateral exploration is necessary, modified collar-type incision along the sternocleidomastoid of both sides is required.
- **Intraoperative endoscopy is a very useful modality during surgical exploration.**

Management of Vascular Injuries

- Vascular injuries are common in penetrating wounds, not in blunt injuries.
- Hemostasis is primarily maintained by digital occlusion and then proximal and distal control by vascular clamps.
- Arterial injuries should be debrided and repaired primarily, if possible.
- Temporary intraluminal shunt may be considered to preserve cerebral perfusion during repair.
- Simple closure of a linear defect in common carotid or internal carotid can be simply sutured but a vein patch is preferable to prevent stenosis. If primary repair is not possible due to loss of length, an interposition graft should be used. Injuries of the proximal internal carotid can be treated by transposition procedure.
- Major injuries to the external carotid can be safely ligated, but the **surgeon must be sure that this is not the internal carotid artery**.

- Subclavian artery injuries are preferably managed by primary repair, but ligation is also safe.
- Venous injuries are best managed by ligation (Chance of air embolism must be kept in mind and can be prevented by lowering the patient's head).
- An injured internal jugular vein can be ligated if contralateral **vein is patent**.

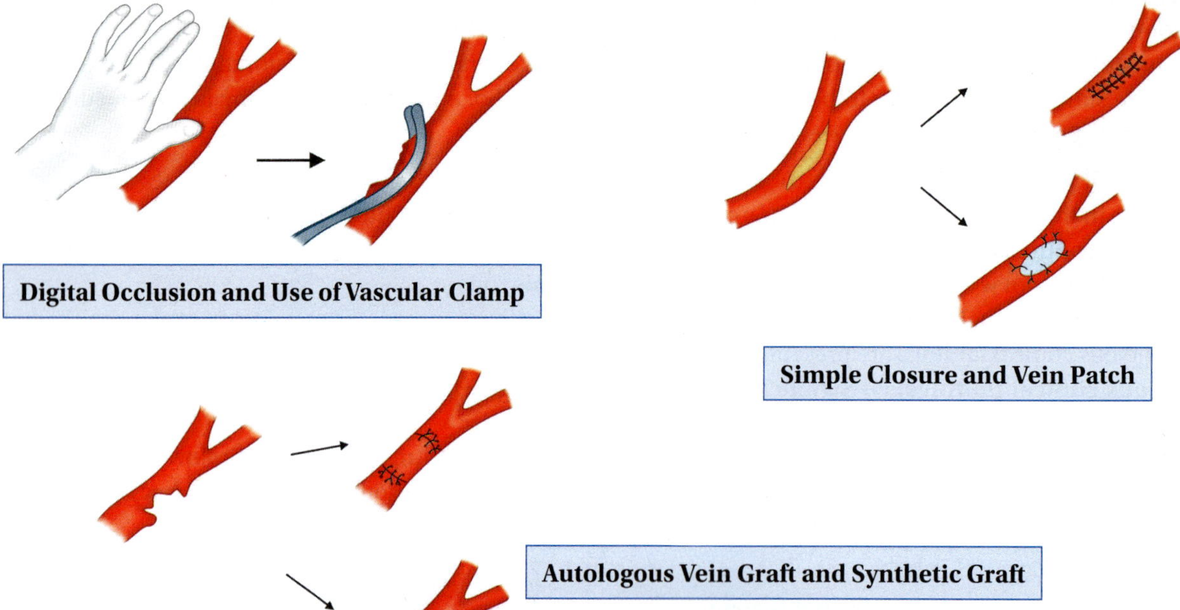

Digital Occlusion and Use of Vascular Clamp

Simple Closure and Vein Patch

Autologous Vein Graft and Synthetic Graft

Major nerve injuries are managed by primary repair.
Thoracic duct injury is best managed by ligation.
Management of airway injuries:

- Formal tracheostomy should be planned below the injury site rather than insertion of a tracheostomy tube through the injury opening.
- Laryngeal injuries are treated by repair of mucosal lacerations and repair of cartilagineous structures through the perichondrium using synthetic absorbable suture.
- Simple lacerations of trachea can be repaired by primary repair. Trachea can be mobilized for a sufficient length (about the breadth of two tracheal rings).
- Loss of large area of trachea need complex reconstructive procedures.

Management of esophageal injuries:

- If injury is diagnosed within 12 hours, primary repair with drain placement is the ideal treatment.
- If injury is more than 12 hours old, cervical esophagostomy followed by complex reconstruction later.

Clothesline Injury

- It is a special type of neck injury occurs typically when a two-wheeler rider encounters a fixed, taut and sharp object (e.g., glass-coated kite-line) stretching across its path horizontally.
- It is a life-threatening laryngeal injury characterized by cricotracheal separation.
- Most of the patients present with respiratory distress. This injury may be associated with pneumothorax and bilateral vocal cord paralysis (due to stretching or tearing of recurrent laryngeal nerves).
- Emergency tracheostomy is indicated (tracheostomy is technically difficult in this type of injury as larynx is retracted upward and trachea is retracted behind the sternum). Tracheal repair should be done in OT setup after workup (Direct laryngoscopy, esophagoscopy).
- If injury of the recurrent laryngeal nerve is present, primary repair is warranted if appropriate instruments and expertise are available.

Spinal Injury

- Most of the spinal injuries are due to road traffic accidents and fall from height. A few percentages of spinal injuries are due to gunshot injuries.
- **Spinal injuries with or without neurological injuries must be suspected in patients with multiple injuries.**

Mechanisms of Injury

Vertical compression: Burst fracture

Objects falling on head or jumping from a height.

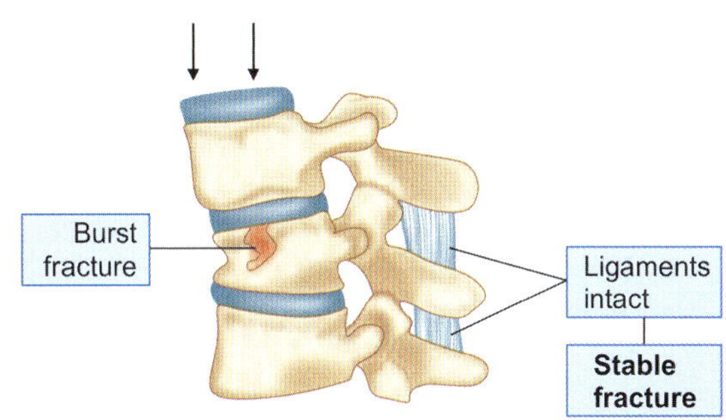

Hinge injury: Wedge fracture

Object falling on back or blow to the forehead.

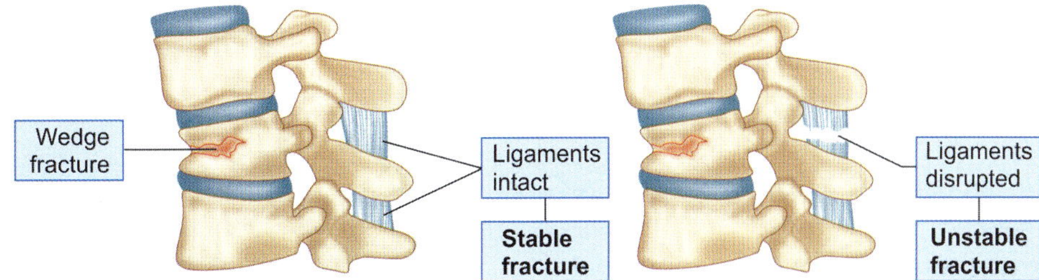

Hyperextension Injury

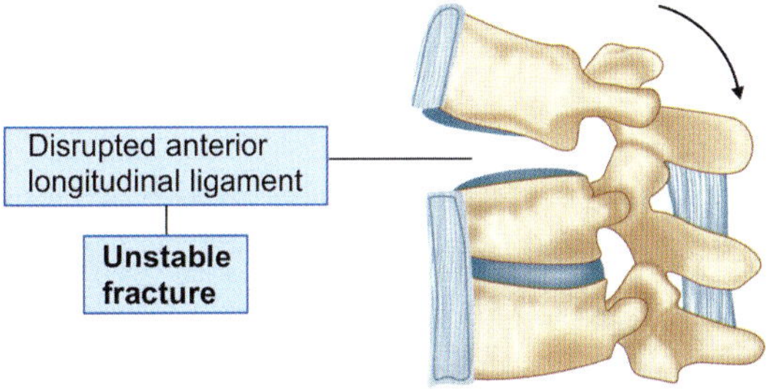

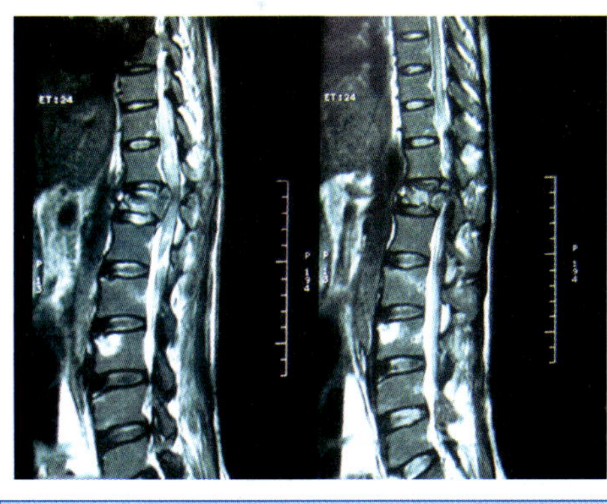

MRI Spine showing vertebral fracture

Shearing Injury

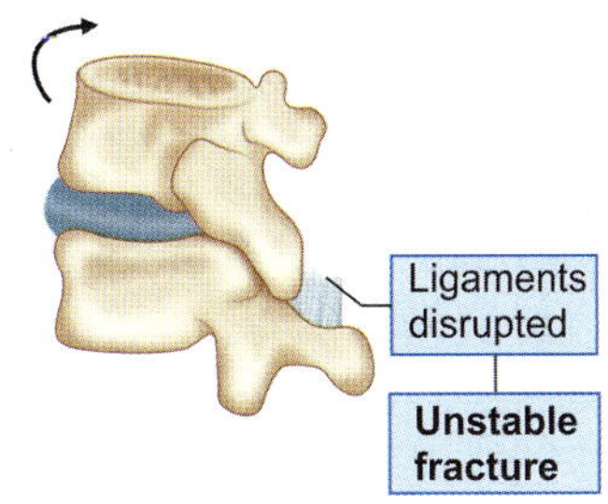

Spinal injuries should be suspected in every trauma patient.

High index of suspicion in:

- Major trauma
- Minor trauma with neurological symptoms
- Injury in RTA, fall from height or diving injuries
- If preexisting spinal diseases such as rheumatoid arthritis, osteoporosis, ankylosing spondylitis are present.

Mechanisms of Cord Injury

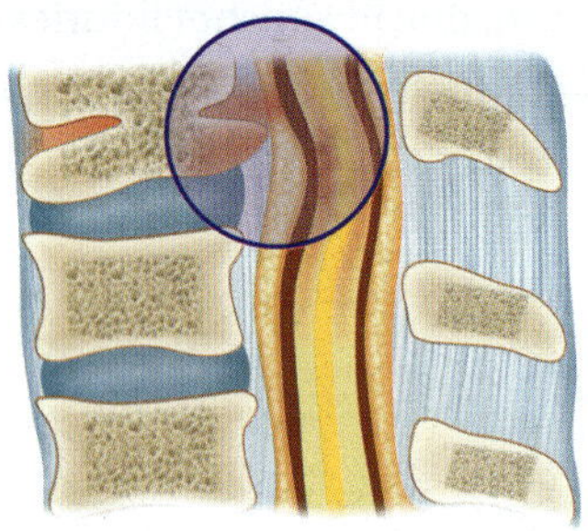

Cord compression by bony fragments.

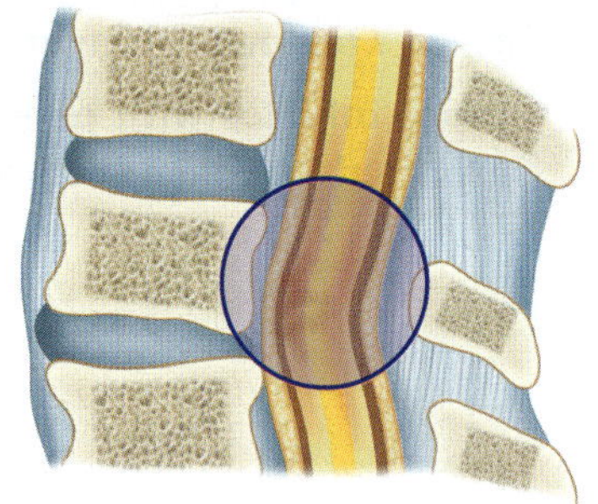

Rotational injury causing stretch injury of cord.

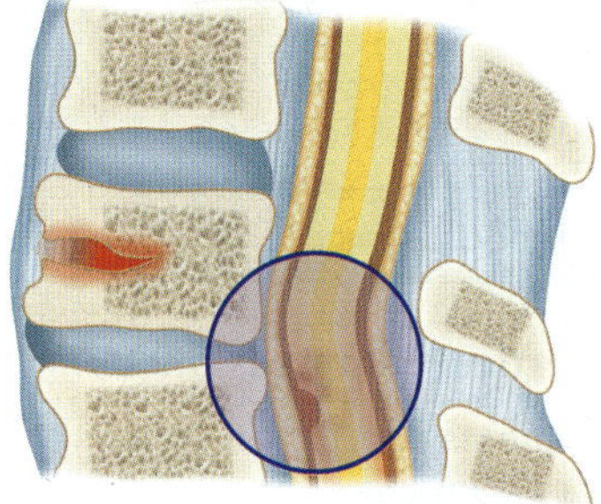

Intervertebral fragments compressing spinal cord or anterior spinal artery.

Initial Management of Spinal Injury

Spinal immobilization: Initially manual immobilization by keeping the head and neck of the patient in neutral position.

Airway: Fiberoptic intubation is preferred because less manipulation is required.

Patient with injuries above C3 are often completely apneic: Early intubation at the site of injury is necessary.

High cervical spine injuries can cause ventilatory decompensation due to loss of phrenic nerve function (C3–C5) and intercostal muscle function (thoracic root).

Circulation: If physiologic effects of shock are not reversed with fluid resuscitation alone, neurogenic shock must be suspected.

Excessive fluid administration can compromise respiratory function and increases spinal cord edema.

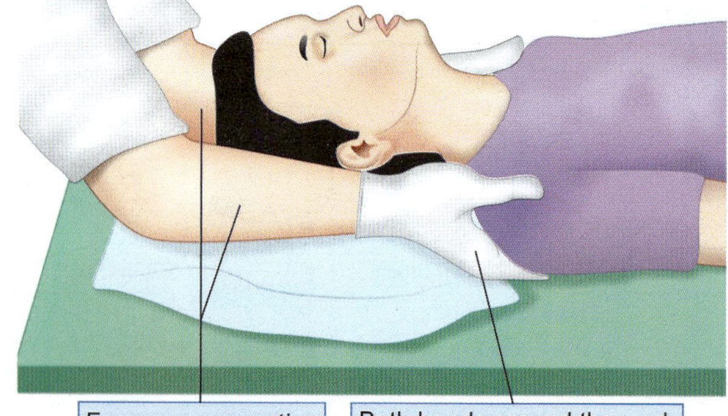

Cervical spinal injury should be suspected if:

- Flaccid areflexia
- Ability to flex but not to extend the elbow
- Hypotension with bradycardia
- Diaphragmatic breathing
- Painless urinary retention
- Priapism
- Diminished anal tone

Examination of the Patient

Examination of the Spine

- Tenderness
- Step-deformity
- Widening of interspinous spaces
- Prominence of spinous processes

For documentation of findings of motor and sensory examination, **the International Standards for Neurological Classification of Spinal Cord Injury worksheet** can be used.

Neurological Examination

Motor function of key muscles

The strength of key muscles are tested on both sides and graded on a 6-point scale (0–5).

Sensory function of all major nerve roots

Sensation is assessed by light touch and pinprick

Assessment of low spinal cord reflexes

- Anal sphincter tone
- Anal cutaneous reflex (anal sphincter contraction in response to scratching the perianal skin)
- Bulbocavernosus reflex (contraction of bulbocavernosus muscle in response to squeezing the glans penis)

Types of Spinal Cord Injury (Based on Severity of Neurological Deficit)

Incomplete Injury

- Some motor or sensory function below the level of injury
- Signs of incomplete injury are any sensation or voluntary movement in the lower extremities, sacral sparing, voluntary anal sphincter contraction, voluntary toe flexion.
- Most of the patients will improve with time.
- Restoration of spinal canal anatomy and decompression of spinal cord may lead to improved outcome.

Complete Injury

- No motor or sensory function below the level of injury.
- Very little hope of recovery.
- Restoration of spinal canal anatomy and decompression of spinal cord do not improve the outcome.

Different Patterns of Incomplete Spinal Cord Injury

- Anterior cord syndrome
- Brown-Séquard syndrome
- Central cord syndrome
- Cauda equina syndrome

Anterior Cord Syndrome

- This syndrome most commonly occurs **following cord ischemia due to injury of an anterior spinal artery**.
- Characterized by **damage of spinothalamic tract and corticospinal tract**.
- **Clinically presentation** includes paraplegia and bilateral loss of pain and temperature sensation.
- Position, vibration, and deep pressure sense are intact as **dorsal column is intact**.
- This syndrome is associated with **poorest prognosis** among the incomplete spinal cord injuries.

Corticospinal tract

Lateral spinothalamic tract

Anterior spinal artery

Brown-Séquard Syndrome

- This syndrome commonly occurs following penetrating trauma due to **hemisection of the cord**.
- **Clinical presentation** includes ipsilateral motor weakness (due to damage of corticospinal tract) and loss of position sense (due to damage of dorsal column) associated with contralateral loss of pain and temperature sensation.
- Chance of **some recovery**.

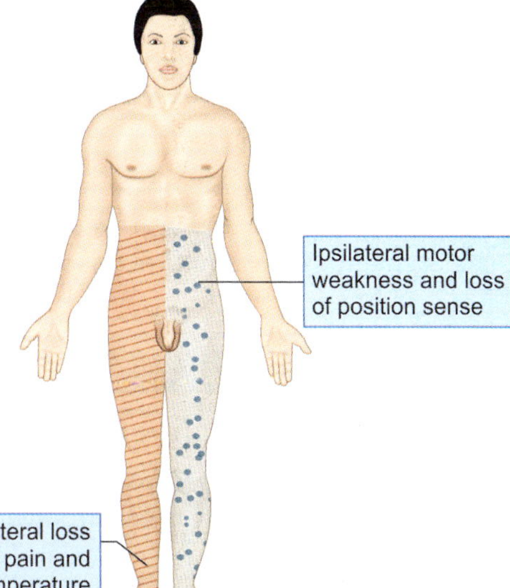

Central Cord Syndrome

- This syndrome typically occurs following hyperextension injury in patients with cervical canal stenosis.
- Blood flow in the spinal arteries is interfered resulting in hypoperfusion of the cord at watershed line.
- Clinical presentation includes loss of motor function more in upper extremities than in lower extremities, with some degree of sensory loss.
- This syndrome is associated with better prognosis than other incomplete cord injuries.

Hypoperfusion of the cord at watershed line (central part of the cord)

Cauda Equina Syndrome

This syndrome is characterized by loss of motor sensory control of urinary bladder, impotence, fecal incontinence, and sensory deficit over the 'saddle' area.

Evaluation of Spinal Injury

Radiographic Evaluation

X-ray: Decision of radiographic evaluation can be taken based on Canadian C-Spine rule or NEXUS criteria.

Standard views for cervical spine X-ray are: (i) Anteroposterior view; (ii) Lateral view; and (iii) Open-mouth odontoid view. Additional views are: (i) Swimmer's view (to visualize C7 and C7–T1 junction); (ii) Oblique view (to demonstrate facet fractures or dislocations); and (iii) Flexion-extension view (neck pain and normal X-ray).

MDCT (occiput to T1 with sagittal and coronal reconstruction) is indicated if: (i) Lower cervical spine is not adequately visualized; (ii) Areas suspicious for injury is identified in X-ray; (iii) As initial screening modality for thoracic and lumbar spine assessment; and (iv) Suspected fractures of posterior elements (pedicles, lamina, spinous processes).

MRI is indicated if: (i) Neck pain and normal X-ray findings and (ii) Suspected paraspinal ligamentous and soft-tissue injuries, spinal epidural hematoma, traumatic herniated disk.

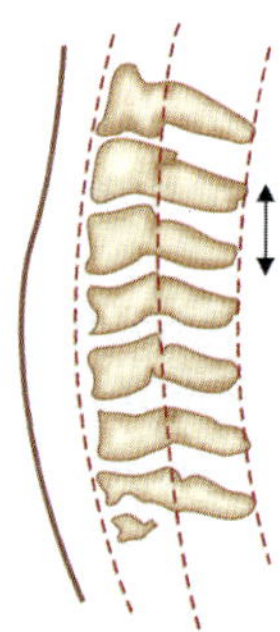

Lateral view: Most informative

Lateral view detects subluxations, compression fractures, and chance fractures.

Management of Spinal Injury

Supportive management

Mechanical ventilation is indicated for upper cervical cord injuries. A mean BP of 85–90 mm Hg should be maintained for first 7 days after injury to ensure adequate perfusion of the injured spinal cord.

Medical management

There is insufficient evidence to recommend the use of intravenous methylprednisolone in spinal cord injury.

Fluid management

Neurogenic shock is usually not responded with fluid administration alone, vasopressor therapy (phenylephrine, dopamine, norepinephrine) is needed.

Surgical management

If neurological function in incomplete cord injury is progressively deteriorating, operative decompression is indicated.

Rehabilitation

- Skin care
- Two hourly turning prevent bedsores
- Use of air or waterbed
- Patient should be trained for intermittent self-catheterization.
- Physiotherapy (to prevent flexion contracture)
- Patient with high risk of DVT require prophylaxis with LMW heparin and/or pneumatic compression stockings
- Patient education of daily living and job retraining
- Emotional support

Prognosis

- Injury above C3 require immediate ventilatory support (at the place of injury)
- Injury above C7 usually dependant on others
- Sparing of C7 segment provides a degree of independence.
- Injury in thoracolumbar region regains full degree of independence overtime.

Thoracic Trauma

Rib Fracture

- Most common injury following blunt chest trauma.
- **Ribs (4–10)** are more prone to fracture.
- **The upper ribs (1–3)** are less prone to fracture due to protective barrier formed by scapula, humerus, and clavicle along with their muscular attachments.

Types of Rib Fracture

- Isolated rib fracture
- Multiple rib fracture
- Rib fracture with flail segment
- First rib fracture.

Multiple rib fractures in young patient indicate greater transfer of force than in older patients.

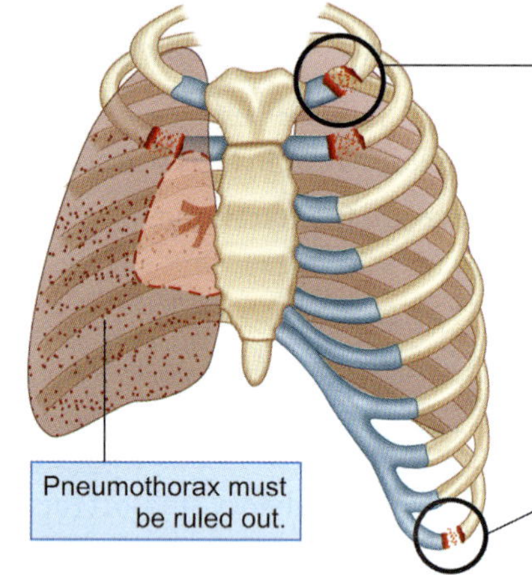

- **First rib fracture—**underlying significant chest injury, injury to heart, great vessels may be present.
- Contrast-enhanced CT is indicated to rule out these injuries.

Pneumothorax must be ruled out.

Fracture of 8th to 12th rib
Injury to spleen, liver, and kidney should be suspected.

Rib fracture in older patients is associated with more risk of pneumonia.

Clinical presentation

Patients with rib fractures are commonly present with localized pain, tenderness, palpable, or visible deformity.

Investigations

Chest X-ray is indicated to detect rib fractures and to rule out other associated injuries (e.g. pneumothorax, hemothorax). CT scan is particularly indicated if cardiac injury or injury to great vessels are suspected. CT scan is also helpful to detect occult hemothorax or pneumothorax, minimal aortic injuries.

Treatment

Adequate analgesia is an important part of management to prevent complications like atelectasis and pneumonia. Systemic analgesics, intercostal block, epidural anesthesia are effective for pain management.

Strapping the chest wall with adhesive tape, use of elastic bandage, rib belts, and external splints are contraindicated, because it interferes with adequate ventilation.

Flail chest: A flail chest develops when a segment of the chest wall does not maintain bony continuity with the rest of the thoracic cage.

- This condition develops if two or more adjacent ribs fractured in two or more areas **(lateral flail segment)** or costochondral separation from the thoracic cage **(anterior flail segment)**.
- Mechanical ventilation may be required to maintain adequate ventilation.

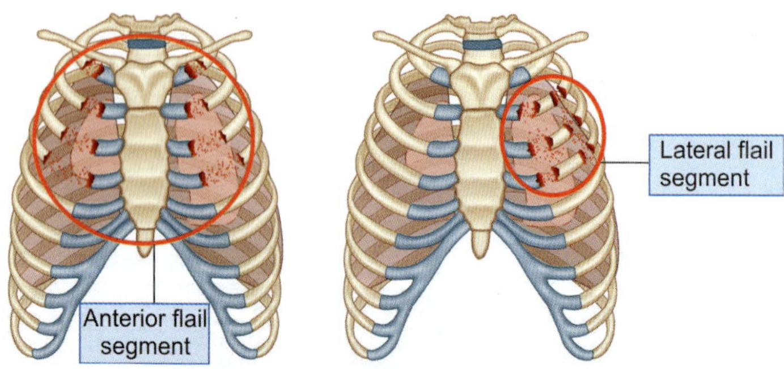

Paradoxical movement is seen in flail segment.

Sternal Fracture

- Sternal fracture occurs due to impact with steering wheel or seatbelt in deceleration injury.
- Patient complains of chest pain particularly over the sternum and crepitus is often found.
- Chest X-ray and lateral sternal X-ray are necessary for confirmation of fracture. Usually transverse fracture is found in sternum.

Underlying myocardial contusion, myocardial rupture, esophageal perforation, tracheobronchial injuries must be suspected.

- These underlying injuries need to be excluded with proper investigations (e.g., constant ECG monitoring, serial cardiac enzyme estimation).
- For stable fracture, analgesia is the treatment. For unstable chest wall and debilitating chest pain, open reduction and internal fixation is indicated.

Life-threatening Thoracic Injuries

- Airway obstruction
- Tracheobronchial tree injury
- Tension pneumothorax
- Open pneumothorax
- Massive hemothorax
- Cardiac tamponade

Potentially Life-threatening Thoracic Injuries

- Simple pneumothorax
- Hemothorax
- Flail chest
- Pulmonary contusion
- Blunt cardiac injury
- Traumatic aortic disruption
- Traumatic diaphragmatic injury
- Blunt esophageal rupture

Pneumothorax

- Simple pneumothorax
- Tension pneumothorax
- Open pneumothorax

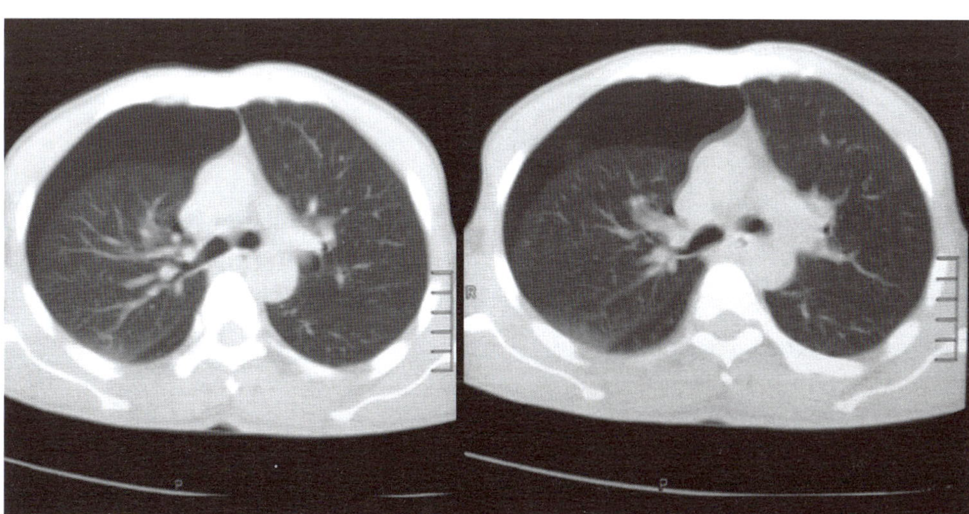

CT thorax showing right-sided pneumothorax.

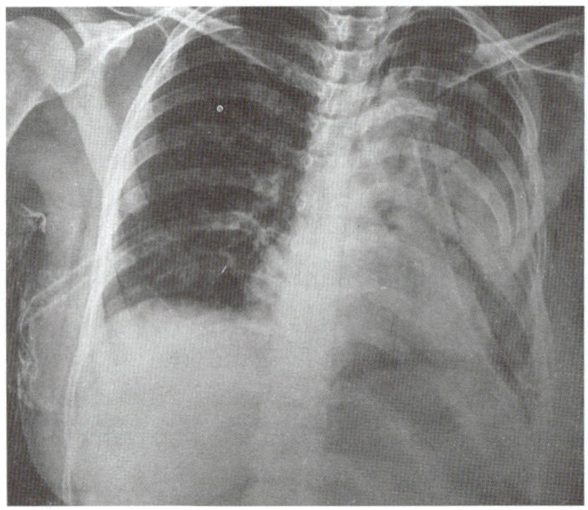

Chest X-ray showing fracture ribs, pneumothorax on right side and hemothorax on left side and chest drain in both sides.

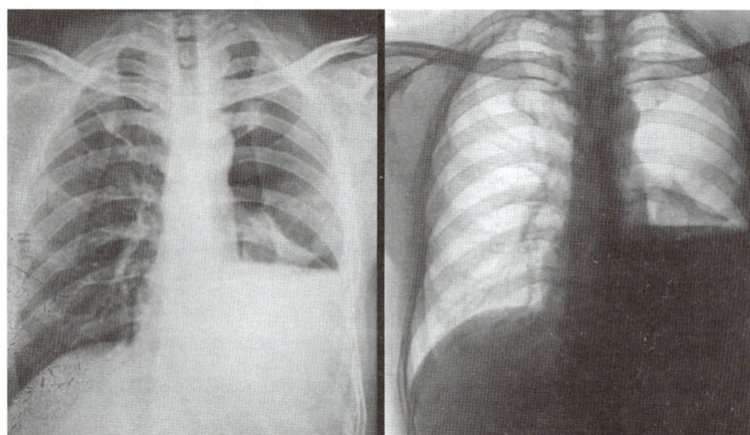

Chest X-ray showing hydropneumothorax.

Simple Pneumothorax

Air leakage following lung laceration is the most common cause of simple pneumothorax after blunt trauma. Penetrating injuries also cause pneumothorax.

On clinical examination, decreased chest expansion of affected side, percussion note is hyperresonant and diminished breath sound on affected side.

Diagnosis: Chest X-ray is indicated to confirm the diagnosis. Typical chest X-ray features: (i) Visible lung edge with absent lung markings beyond and (ii) Deep sulcus sign (hemidiaphragm on the affected side is deeper in the midline than expected).

Treatment: The ideal management is tube thoracostomy. Small, 'subclinical' pneumothorax may be closely observed and needs intervention if patient become symptomatic or pneumothorax is expanding.

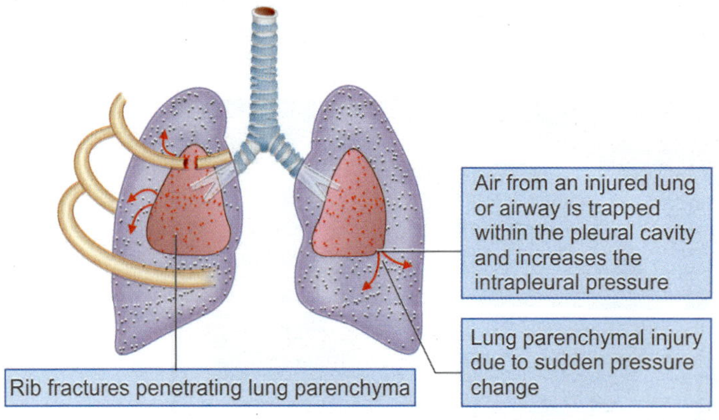

Patients having simple pneumothorax should not undergo general anesthesia or positive pressure ventilation before tube thoracostomy.

Tension Pneumothorax

Pathophysiology: Tear in the visceral pleura following trauma acts as a valve resulting in air leakage into the pleural cavity but no means of escape. The mediastinum is shifted to the opposite side resulting in compression of opposite lung and decreased venous return.

Tension pneumothorax may develop if patient with simple pneumothorax is undergone positive-pressure ventilation or patient with open pneumothorax is treated with occlusive dressings on the defect secured on four sides.

Clinical presentation: Tension pneumothorax should be suspected if a trauma patient presents with respiratory distress along with distended neck vein, deviated trachea, hyperresonant note on percussion, absent or diminished breath sound and hypotension. **Obstructive shock** may develop.

Diagnosis: If tension pneumothorax is diagnosed clinically, treatment should not be delayed. Both chest X-ray and eFAST can detect this pathology.

Treatment: Tension pneumothorax needs immediate decompression by **needle thoracocentesis** (placement of large bore needle or large over-the-needle catheter in 2nd intercostal space along midclavicular line). Successful needle decompression converts tension pneumothorax to a simple pneumothorax. If needle decompression is not successful, **finger thoracostomy** is another option. Then, **tube thoracostomy** is done for definitive management.

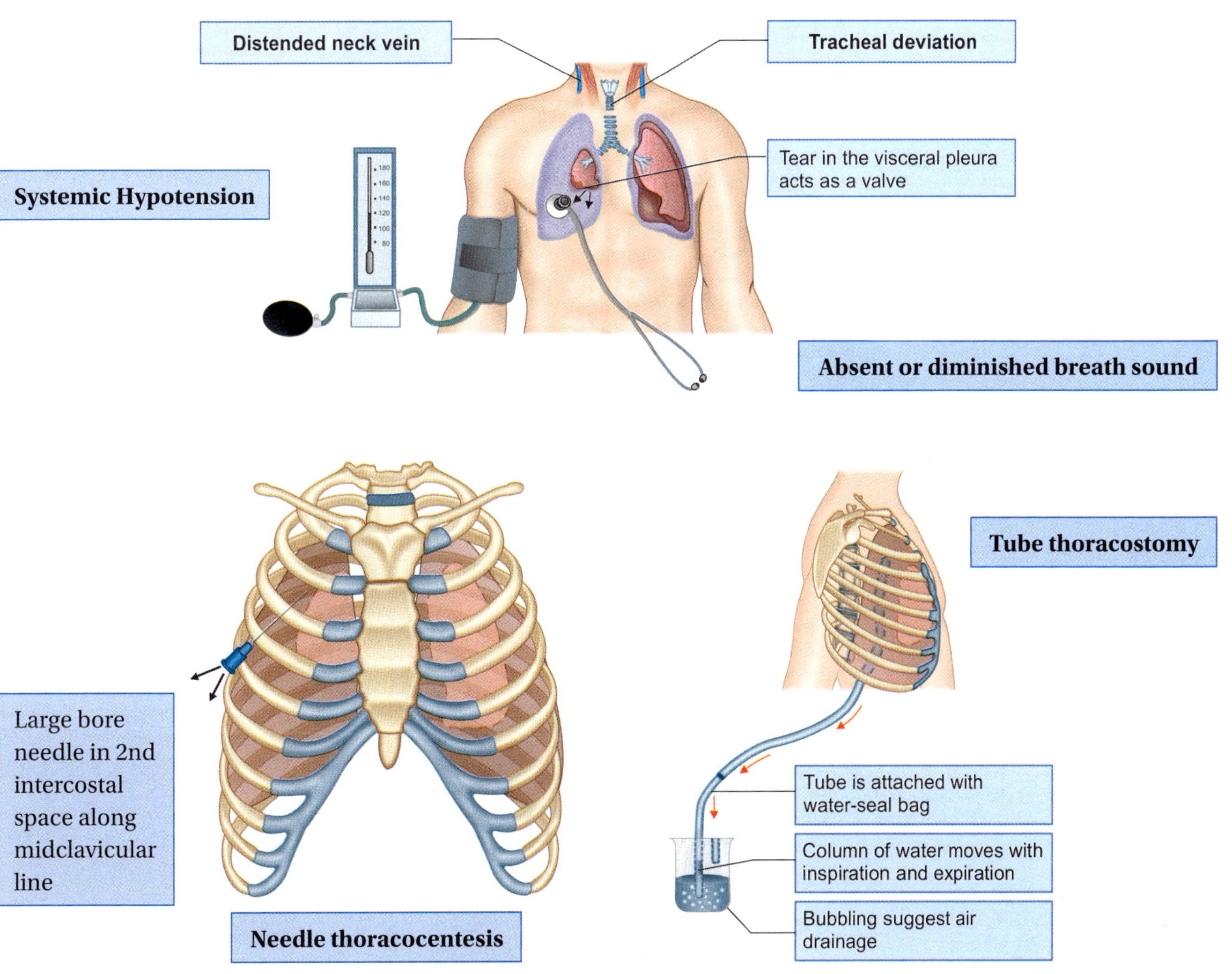

Open Pneumothorax

- **Pathophysiology:** Large chest (two-thirds of diameter of trachea) wound that remain open may develop open pneumothorax because air movement occurs through the defect instead of trachea, resulting in impaired ventilation.
- **Clinical presentation:** Patient commonly presents with difficulty in breathing, noisy movement of air through the chest wound, diminished breath sound.
- **Treatment:** Immediate treatment is sealing the wound with occlusive sterile dressing taped on three sides. Tube thoracostomy should be done away from the wound. After tube thoracostomy, surgical closure of the wound is done.

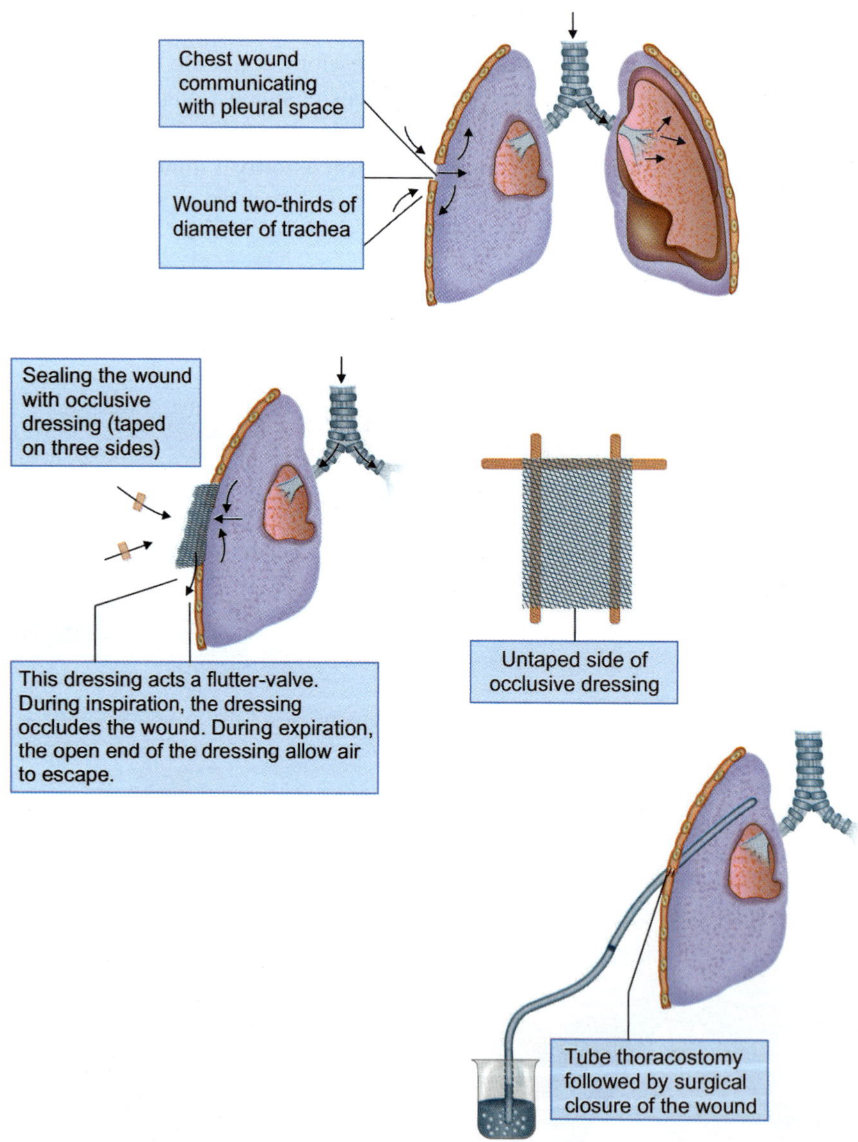

Hemothorax

Hemothorax is accumulation of blood in the pleural cavity.

Pathophysiology: Both blunt trauma and penetrating trauma can cause hemothorax. Laceration of lung, intercostal vessels or internal mammary artery are commonly responsible for formation of hemothorax.

Clinical presentation: On clinical examination, dull percussion note and diminished breath sound are found.

Diagnosis: Chest X-ray is indicated for diagnosis. Obliteration of costophrenic angle or blurring of the hemidiaphragm contour is the characteristic chest X-ray finding.

Treatment: Tube thoracostomy (with 28–32 French chest tube) is the treatment. Thoracotomy is indicated if more than 1500 mL of blood is drained immediately after tube thoracostomy or drainage of more than 200 mL/hour for 2–4 hours.

Massive Hemothorax

Massive hemothorax is accumulation of more than 1500 mL of blood in the pleural cavity. It commonly develops due to laceration of systemic or hilar vessels following penetrating trauma.

Clinical presentation: Patients commonly present with features of hypovolemic shock along with dull percussion note and absent breath sound on affected side. Distended neck vein may be present if mediastinal shift develops.

Treatment: Tube thoracostomy along with restoration of blood volume is the initial management. Thoracotomy is often required for massive hemothorax.

Thoracotomy must be considered in penetrating wounds in 'the mediastinal box' (anterior chest wound medial to the nipple line and posterior wounds medial to the scapula).

Chest Drain

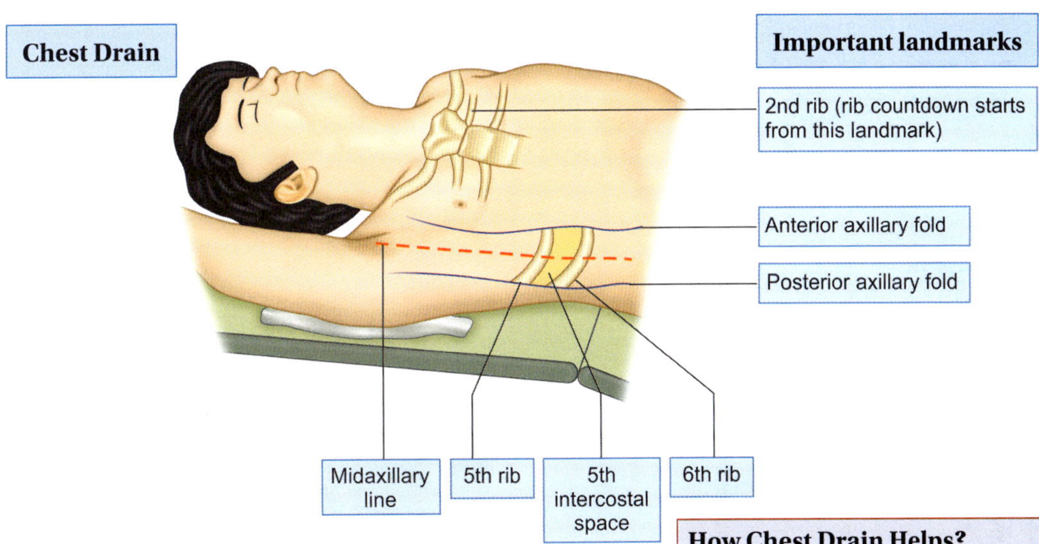

How Chest Drain Helps?

- Prevents development of tension pneumothorax from simple pneumothorax.
- Allows re-expansion of the lung. This expanded lung compresses the injured vessels and reduces further hemorrhage.
- Allows the mediastinal structures to return to the midline and relieve compression of contralateral lung.
- Prevents further development of empyema thoracis.

Indications of Chest Drain

- Traumatic pneumothorax
- Traumatic hemopneumothorax or hemothorax
- Empyema thoracis
- Secondary spontaneous pneumothorax
- Malignant pleural effusion
- After thoracotomy, cardiac surgery

Technique of Chest Drain Insertion

- Skin is cleaned with povidone-iodine solution and covered with sterile drapes.
- Skin, soft tissue and intercostal muscle at the site of insertion is infiltrated with local anesthetic (about 10 mL of 1% lignocaine).
- A 2–3 cm transverse incision is made in the 5th intercostal space, along the midaxillary line, close to upper border of the lower rib (in the 'safe triangle'). This approach prevents chance of damage of neurovascular bundles because neurovascular bundles are present at the lower border of the ribs.
- Using a large curved hemostat, the soft tissue is dissected, parietal pleura is punctured.
- Finger is introduced into the pleural space to ensure that pleural cavity has been entered and no viscera is adhered to the chest wall.
- Chest drain tube is inserted using the hemostat and is directed superiorly and posteriorly for pneumothorax and basally for fluid. Tube is connected with a water-seal drainage bag.

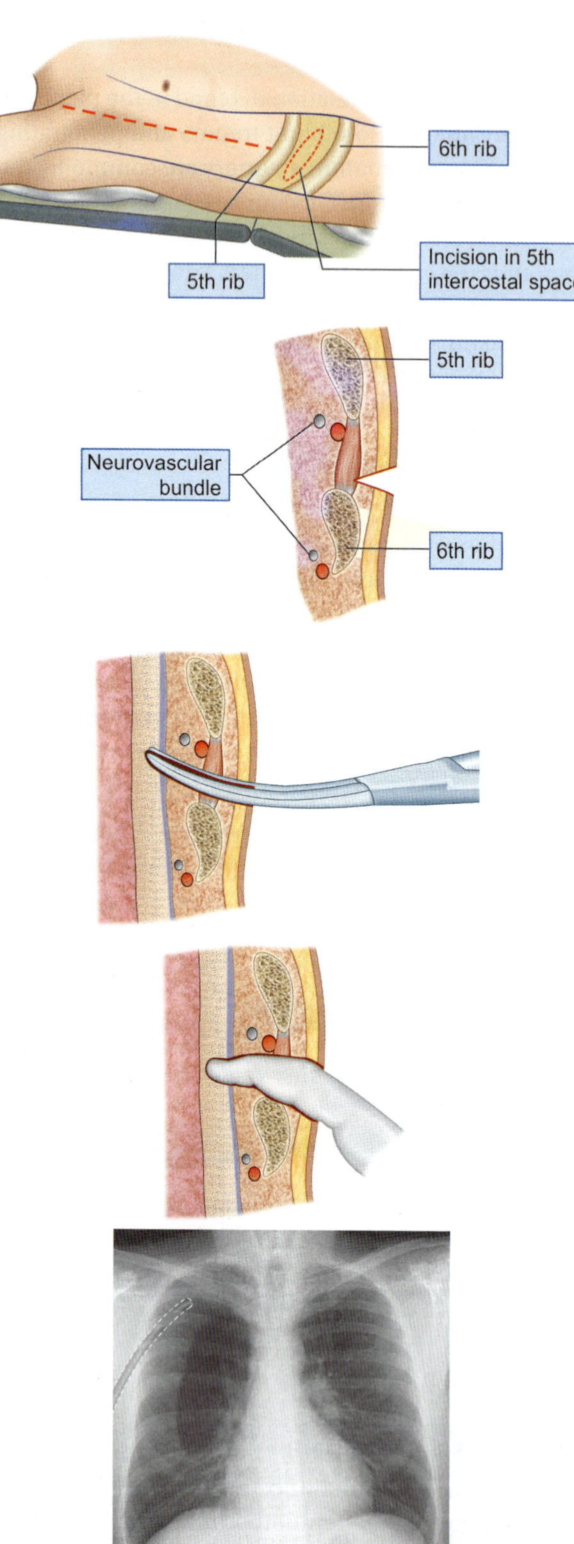

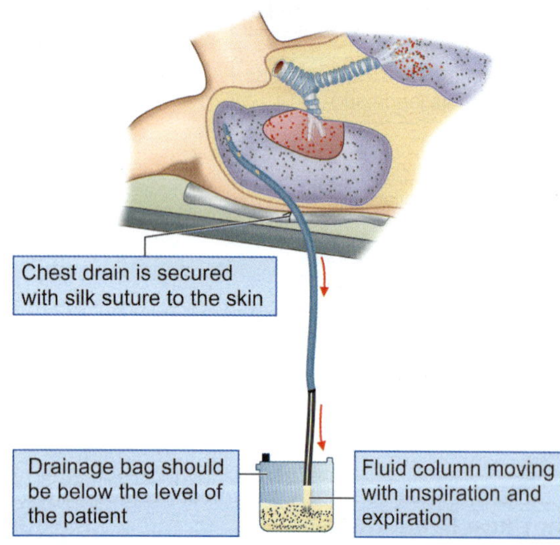

Important Facts about Chest Drain

Safe triangle: This area is bounded by anterior border of latissimus dorsi, lateral border of pectoralis major, a line superior to the horizontal level of the nipple, and an apex below the axilla. Positioning of chest drain in this area reduces the risk of injury to internal mammary artery and breast tissue.

Chest X-ray should be done after chest drain insertion to confirm proper placement of tube.

- **Small bore chest drains** are recommended for pneumothorax. **Large bore drains** (28–30 French) are recommended for hemothorax.
- For pneumothorax, **tip of the chest drain tube** should be aimed apically. For drainage of fluid (blood or effusion), tip should be aimed basally. However, any position of the tip (apical or basal) can drain the air or fluid satisfactorily.
- '*Purse string*' sutures should not be used for wound closure as it is more painful and cosmetically unacceptable.
- **The respiratory swing of fluid in chest tube** confirms tube patency and position of the tube in the pleural cavity.
- **Monitoring should be done to ensure** that the water-seal drainage system should be below the level of the patient, always upright and adequate water in the system.
- **Chest drain should be removed** while the patient performs Valsalva's maneuver.

Pulmonary Parenchymal Injury

- This injury is associated with both blunt and penetrating thoracic trauma.
- In patients with flail chest, pulmonary parenchymal injury must be ruled out because about 2/3rd of patients have parenchymal injury.
- Many of these patients are associated with pneumothorax and hemothorax.
- These patients have adequate perfusion but compromised ventilation. This ventilation-perfusion mismatch results in severe hypoxemia.

Clinical presentation includes: (i) Copious thin, blood-tinged secretions; (ii) Chest pain; (iii) Labored respiration; (iv) Restlessness; (v) Dyspnea; (vi) Tachypnea; and (vii) Cyanosis. Respiratory failure usually develops over time, if not treated.

Investigation: Chest X-ray in initial stage appears as patchy opacifications. It becomes more prominent with time and progress to diffuse opacification (suggestive of acute respiratory distress syndrome).

Treatment: Tube thoracostomy is indicated for drainage of air and blood and for monitoring of continuous air leakage.

Severe contusions often require intubation and mechanical ventilatory support.

Laceration with persistent air leak may require exploration by thoracotomy, followed by over sewing or stapling of wound or wedge/lobar resection or tractotomy (opening up the missile trajectory).

Tracheobronchial Injuries

Blunt injuries of the airway are due to compression of the airway between the sternum and the vertebral column in high velocity RTA. **About 80% of injuries are located within 1 inch (2.54 cm) from the carina**. Penetrating injuries may occur at any location.

Clinical presentation: Patients present with pneumothorax, pneumomediastinum, hemoptysis, and massive subcutaneous emphysema.

Suspect major airway injury when continuing bubbling of gas through the water-seal chest drain or lung fails to re-expand after chest drain insertion.

Treatment:

- Upper tracheal injuries require median sternotomy.
- Distal tracheal or right bronchial injuries are approached through right thoracotomy. Left bronchial injuries are approached via left thoracotomy.
- In most of the cases, debridement followed by primary repair is indicated. Complex reconstructive procedures are rarely needed.

Blunt Cardiac Injury

- Blunt cardiac injury should be suspected in all patients of high velocity RTA with chest trauma.
- Injuries vary from myocardial contusion to rupture of cardiac chamber or valves.
- **Right ventricle is most frequently involved chamber** due to its close proximity to the sternum.
- Patients may present with varying presentations from unexplained sinus tachycardia to cardiogenic shock.
- ECG is the primary investigation **(a normal ECG excludes significant BCI.)** ECG abnormality (sinus tachycardia, ST changes, T-wave changes, supraventricular and ventricular arrhythmias, RBBB) warrants for continuous ECG monitoring for 24 hours.
- In unstable patient, transthoracic echocardiogram should be performed to rule out valvular or myocardial rupture. Cardiac enzymes have no specific role in diagnosis.
- Arrhythmias are treated according to the standard management protocol.
- Patient with frank myocardial or valvular rupture require immediate operative repair.

Penetrating Cardiac Injury

- Pericardial tamponade must be suspected if patients with penetrating injury present with: (1) Muffled heart sound; (2) Distended neck vein; (3) Shock—**Beck's triad**.
- Tension pneumothorax must be excluded.
- Stable patient must undergo echocardiography (transesophageal).
- Hemodynamically unstable patients should be taken to operating room for emergency thoracotomy. The operative approach is via median sternotomy. Atrial and ventricular wounds are repaired with monofilament sutures. Care must be taken to avoid injury to coronary arteries.

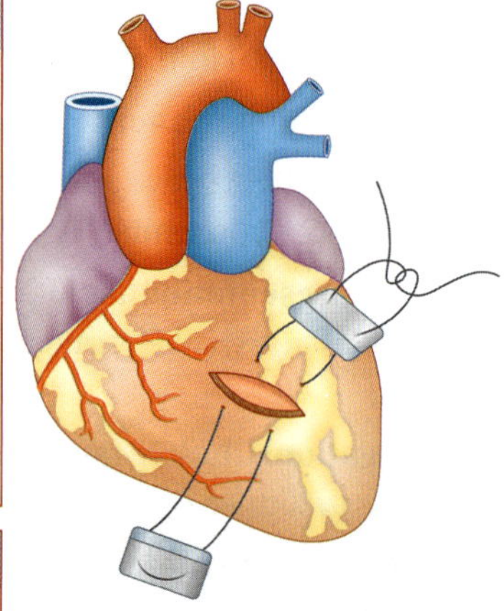

Closure of wound using buttressed sutures and avoiding coronary vessels

Pericardial Tamponade

- Blood from injured great vessel, cardiac chamber, coronary or pericardial vessel accumulated in the pericardial sac and restricts diastolic filling.
- Penetrating injuries most commonly cause cardiac tamponade, blunt trauma also may be responsible.
- The classical clinical triad of Beck's triad, pulsus paradoxus, Kussmaul's sign (i.e., a rise in venous pressure with inspiration when breathing spontaneously) not always present. Left-sided tension pneumothorax must be excluded because of similarity in clinical presentations.
- FAST is a rapid and accurate modality for detection of cardiac tamponade. If FAST is equivocal, echocardiography is indicated for diagnosis.
- After diagnosis, emergency thoracotomy or sternotomy should be considered for definitive management. If emergency thoracotomy is not feasible, subxiphoid pericardiocentesis (using over-the-needle catheter or flexible catheter) is indicated.

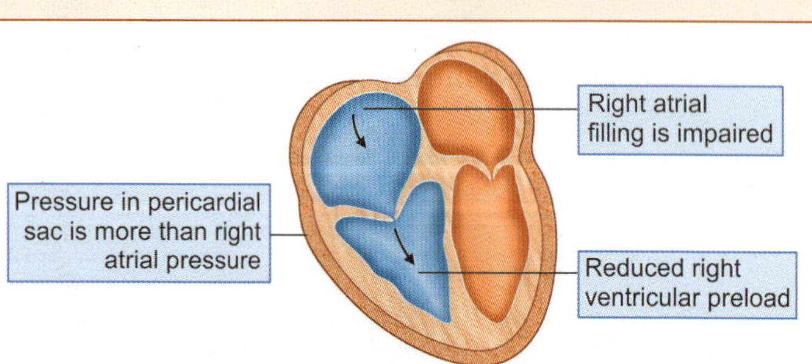

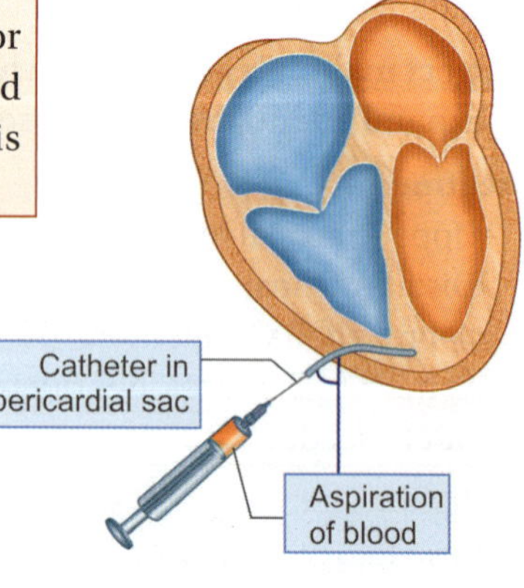

Great Vessel Injury

In Blunt Trauma

- The **descending thoracic aorta just below the origin of the left subclavian artery is the vulnerable area of the aorta for rupture** in deceleration injury (collision of vehicles or fall from great height), as it is tethered by the ligamentum arteriosum.
- Complete transection causes immediate death, only patient with partial disruption may arrive trauma center.
- **In erect chest X-ray**, findings like widened mediastinum, obscured aortic knob, opacification of aortopulmonary window, warrants further investigation.
- **Helical contrast-enhanced CT of the chest is the investigation of choice.** If interpretation is inconclusive, then four vessel arteriography is indicated.
- The injury is repaired (primary anastomosis or prosthetic interposition graft) via left anterolateral thoracotomy. Endovascular repair is another treatment option.

In Penetrating Trauma

- In stable patients, aortography, endoscopy, contrast swallow study, echocardiography, and helical CT of chest are indicated for complete evaluation.
- In unstable patient, urgent thoracotomy is indicated.
- Operative approach depends on the vessel injured (median sternotomy/left anterolateral thoracotomy)
- Primary repair should be performed for aortic and vena caval injuries. Brachiocephalic and innominate venous injuries can be ligated.

Esophageal Injuries

- Most of the esophageal trauma occurs due to penetrating injuries, rarely due to blunt trauma (esophagus is well-protected in the posterior mediastinum).

All transmediastinal gunshot wounds or stab wounds near the posterior midline should be evaluated to exclude esophageal injury.

- Esophageal injuries warrant early recognition as delay in diagnosis increases morbidity and mortality.
- Esophagoscopy and gastrograffin swallow study can detect all injuries.
- Operative approach is determined by the location of injury. The type of surgical approach is determined by the age of injury.

Right thoracotomy is the best approach for thoracic esophagus. Left thoracotomy is a better option for distal esophagus.

If injury is recognized within 24 hours, debridement, primary repair (buttressed with a vascularized flap, e.g., pleural or pericardial or fundoplication) and drain placement (near the repair) is the treatment.

If after 24 hours, then cervical esophagostomy and distal feeding access.

Diaphragmatic Injury

- Diaphragmatic injuries are most often caused by penetrating injuries.
- Diaphragmatic injury must be suspected, if the entry wound is below the nipple and above the costal margins.
- In most of the time, diagnosis is made during exploratory laparotomy. Chest X-ray or CT sometimes detect this injury.
- After blunt trauma, left-sided injuries are more common (right-sided diaphragm is protected by the liver). Patient presented with respiratory distress after severe blow to the abdomen.
- Chest X-ray demonstrates visceral herniation (in right, liver and in left, stomach, and colon).

In blunt trauma, large radial tears develop through which visceral herniation develops. In penetrating trauma, small perforations develop that ultimately lead to development of diaphragmatic hernia over years.

- Smaller defects are repaired with synthetic monofilament sutures (interrupted horizontal mattress).
- Larger defects require the use of prosthetic material.

Care should be taken in the central tendon area during repair to avoid inadvertent cardiac injury.

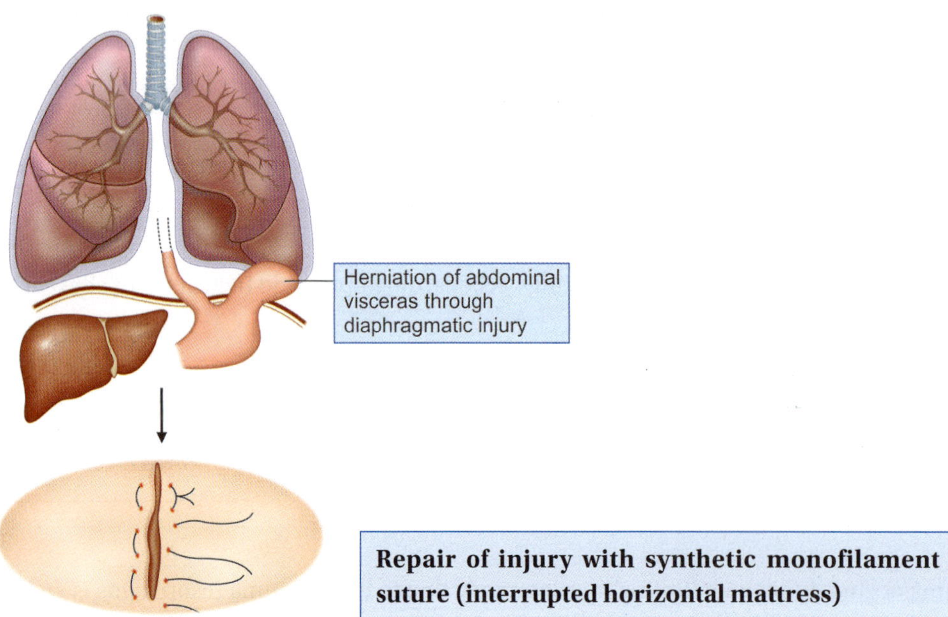

Repair of injury with synthetic monofilament suture (interrupted horizontal mattress)

Thoracic Damage Control Surgery (TDCS)

A concept of damage control surgery for life-threatening thoracic trauma.

The basic principles of TDCS are: (i) Control of hemorrhage and (ii) Maintenance of ventilation/oxygenation by relieving intrathoracic positive pressure.

Thoracic damage control techniques are: (i) Emergency thoracotomy and resuscitation; (ii) Chest drainage; (iii) Pulmonary tractotomy; (iv) Pulmonary hilar twist; (v) Temporary damage control thoracic closure; and (vi) Endovascular approach of thoracic vascular injury.

Abdominal Injuries

Abdominal Trauma

Due to blunt trauma

- Due to rapid deceleration or due to use of seat-belt (compression against vertebral column)
- Organs most commonly injured are spleen, liver, and small bowel. Pancreas, kidneys, and mesentery are also at high risk.

Due to penetrating trauma

- Abdominal organs most commonly injured in stab wound are liver, small bowel, diaphragm, and colon.
- Organs commonly injured in gunshot wound are small bowel, colon, liver, and abdominal vessels.

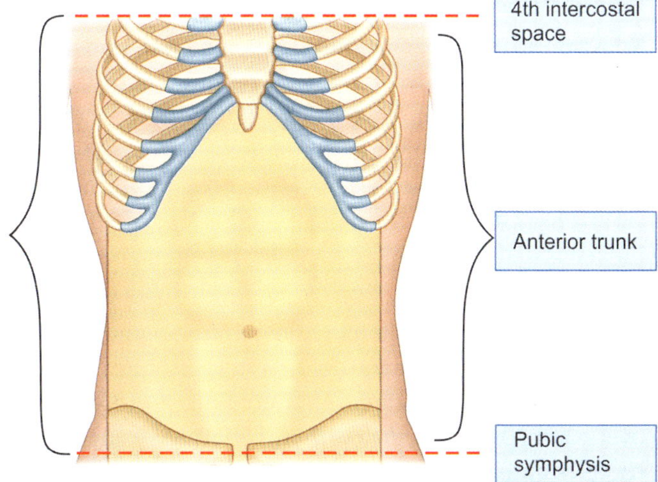

Approach to the Patient

- Is it **penetrating trauma** or **blunt trauma?**
- If penetrating trauma, is it **gunshot (GSW) wound or stab wound**?
- If gunshot wound, is it **anterior truncal GSW** or **GSW to the back and flank**?
- Entry/exit wound in anterior truncal zone suggests peritoneal penetration.

Anterior Abdomen
The anatomical area of abdomen between the costal margins superiorly, the inguinal ligaments and symphysis pubis inferiorly, anterior axillary lines laterally.

The Flank
The anatomical area between the anterior and posterior axillary lines from 6th intercostal space to the iliac crest.

The Back
The area posterior to the posterior axillary lines from the tip of the scapula to the iliac crests.

Thoracoabdomen
The anatomical area inferior to the nipple line anteriorly, infrascapular line posteriorly, and superior to the costal margins.

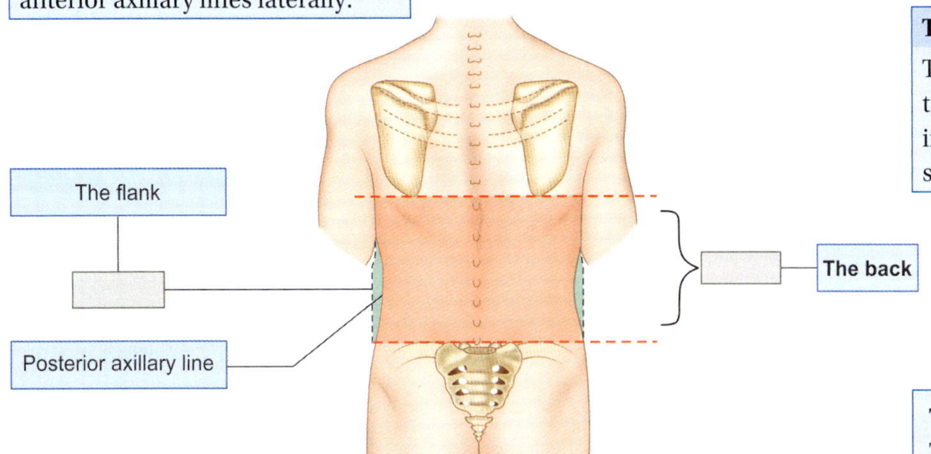

The Pelvic Cavity
The area surrounded by pelvic bones.

Assessment and Principles of Management of Penetrating Injuries

The type of penetrating injuries (e.g., stab wounds, low-energy gunshot wound, high-energy gunshot wound) and anatomic location of injuries are the major determinants in evaluation and management.

Gunshot wounds in anterior abdomen are better managed by exploratory laparotomy. A few gunshot wound in flank or back may be managed conservatively if no indications of emergency laparotomy are present.

Conservative management have some role in stab wounds if indications of urgent laparotomy are absent.

Stab wound in anterior abdomen: Nonoperative management may be considered if patient is hemodynamically stable without signs of peritonitis or evisceration. Diagnostic workup includes: (i) Serial physical examinations over a 24-hr period (with or without serial FAST); (ii) Diagnostic peritoneal lavage; (iii) CT scan; and (iv) Diagnostic laparoscopy. If no peritoneal breach is detected on local wound exploration, patient can be discharged.

Stab wound in flank or back: Nonoperative management may be considered if indications of urgent laparotomy are absent. Diagnostic workup includes: (i) Serial physical examinations over a 24-hr period (with or without serial FAST); (ii) Double- or triple-contrast CT scan; and (iii) Diagnostic peritoneal lavage. CT scan is particularly indicated to detect occult retroperitoneal colonic, duodenal; and and urinary tract injuries.

Nonoperative management in gunshot wound is a emerging concept and may be considered if patient is hemodynamically stable with no signs of peritonitis and CT evidence of tangential trajectory and absence of Intra-abdominal injury.

Indications of laparotomy in penetrating abdominal wound:

- Hemodynamically unstable patient
- Transperitoneal trajectory in gunshot wound
- Signs of peritonitis are present.
- Evisceration
- Bleeding from stomach, rectum, or genitourinary tract
- Free air, retroperitoneal air, rupture of hemidiaphragm, intraperitoneal bladder injury, renal pedicle injury detected in imaging.
- Aspiration of gastrointestinal contents, vegetable, or bile from diagnostic peritoneal lavage, or aspiration of 10 mL or more blood in hemodynamically unstable patient.

In obese patients, nonoperative management option should be judiciously considered because of low sensitivity of physical examination, imaging, and DPL.

In concussive and blast injuries, intraperitoneal injuries may develop without any external injuries or peritoneal penetration.

High-energy gunshot injuries may cause Intra-abdominal injuries by blast effect without peritoneal penetration.

Patients (intoxicated, psychiatric illness) in whom serial physical examinations are not reliable, nonoperative management should not be considered.

Assessment and Principles of Management of Blunt Trauma

History

- Mechanism of injury (road traffic accident or fall from height or others).
- If RTA, then type of collision (frontal impact, rear impact, lateral impact, or rollover), patient's position in the vehicle, condition of other occupants, type of restraints, condition of airbags.
- If fall from height, then height is an important factor.

Physical Examination

Examination of the abdomen should be done in a systematic manner: Inspection, auscultation, percussion, and palpation, followed by examination of pelvis, perineum, and urethra. Rectal and vaginal examination should be considered, if indicated. If intra-abdominal injury is suspected, **FAST, CT, Diagnostic peritoneal lavage (DPL)** are useful diagnostic studies to detect those injuries. Among these, FAST can be performed rapidly at the bedside and can determine whether laparotomy is required or not.

Blunt Trauma

- **Hemodynamically stable** → **FAST**
  - No fluid in peritoneal cavity → **Repeat FAST** → No fluid → Investigations to rule out hollow viscus injuries, if indicated
  - Fluid in peritoneal cavity → **CECT abdomen** →
    - Free air in peritoneal cavity or retroperitoneum
    - Grade IV and V injury of liver spleen, kidney
    - Ruptured hemidiaphragm
    - Contrast extravasation

    → **Laparotomy**
- **Hemodynamically unstable** → **FAST (in the resuscitation room)** → Fluid in peritoneal cavity → **Urgent laparotomy**

FAST (Focused Assessment with Sonography for Trauma)

- The ideal modality for immediate evaluation of blunt trauma abdomen.
- **The goal of FAST examination** is the detection of abnormal collections of intraperitoneal fluid, not to identify or stage solid organ injury or hollow viscus injury.
- Abdomen is examined through four sonographic windows– subxiphoid, RUQ, LUQ, and pelvis.
- FAST helps to detect which cavity have to be opened first in thoracoabdominal injuries.
- FAST can identify pericardial fluid also and helps to diagnose hemopneumothorax.
- Most surgeons recommend an initial scan in RUQ as more than half of the positive FAST examination will reveal fluid in this area.
- **eFAST (extended FAST)** includes additional evaluation of anterior and lateral pleural space to detect pneumothorax and hemothorax.

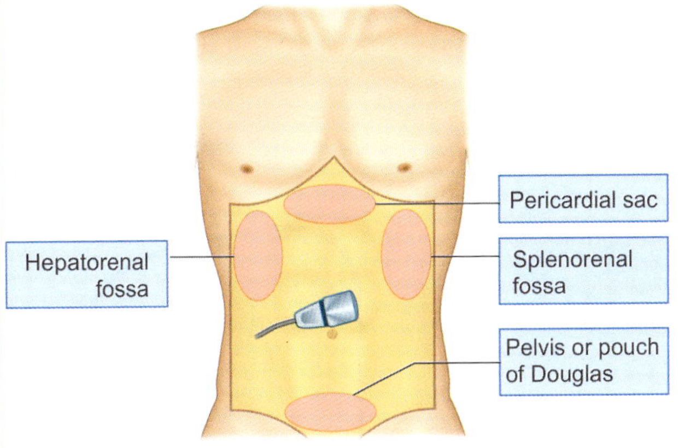

Advantages: (i) Rapid; (ii) Noninvasive; (iii) Can be performed in the resuscitation room; (iv) Operative decision making; and (v) Repeatable.

Disadvantages: (i) Operator dependent and (ii) Obesity can limit visibility.

Diagnostic Peritoneal Lavage

This modality is only indicated when FAST or CT is not available, because this technique is invasive and needs surgical expertise.

Techniques of DPL are: (i) Open infraumbilical approach and (ii) Closed (Seldinger) infraumbilical approach. An open supraumbilical approach is particularly indicated in patients with pelvic fracture and patients with advanced pregnancy.

Advantages: (i) Rapid; (ii) Operative decision making; (iii) Can be performed in the resuscitation room; and (iv) Bowel injury can be detected.

Disadvantages: (i) Invasive; (ii) Procedure cannot be repeated; and (iii) Interferes with further FAST or CT findings.

Contraindications: (i) Previous abdominal surgery; (ii) Morbid obesity; and (iii) Uncorrected coagulopathy.

Gastric and urinary decompression must be done before DPL.

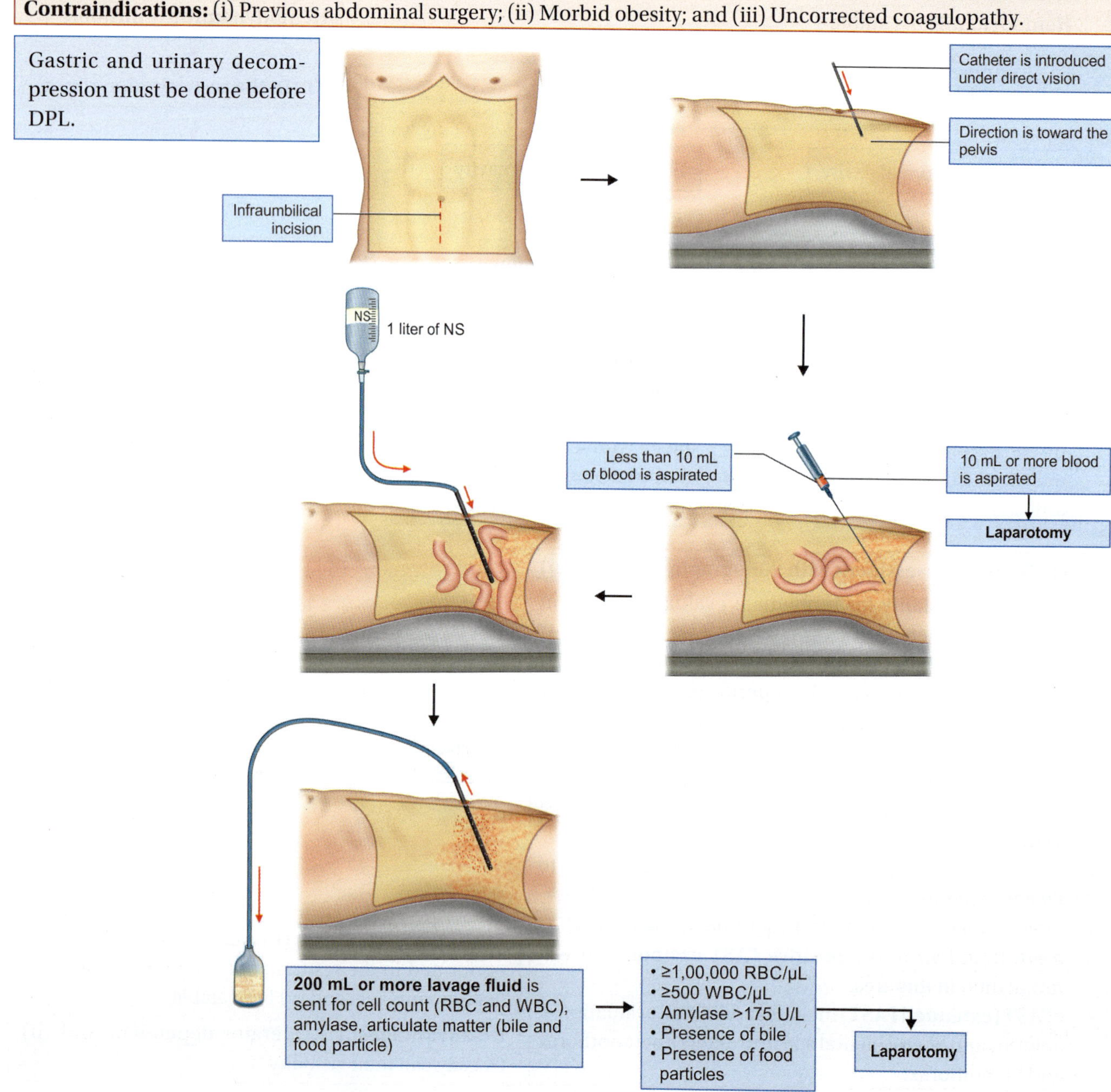

Abdominal CT

- It is indicated to evaluate a hemodynamically stable patient with blunt trauma abdomen in whom urgent exploratory laparotomy is not indicated.
- CT can detect solid organ injury and as well as grading of injury, which is useful for decision making regarding nonoperative management.
- This imaging modality is very much useful for detecting retroperitoneal injuries, but is not so reliable regarding diagnosis of hollow viscus injury.
- Multislice spiral CT is helpful regarding nonoperative management of stab wound in anterior abdomen.
- **Advantages:** (i) Noninvasive; (ii) Detection of injury in particular organ along with grading of injury; and (iii) Can detect free air and retroperitoneal air; (iv) Useful for assessment of retroperitoneal structures; and (v) Repeatable.
- **Disadvantages:** (i) Time consuming; (ii) To be shifted from resuscitation area to CT console (iii) Radiation and contrast exposure.
- **Contraindications:** (i) Uncooperative patient and (ii) Allergy to contrast agents.

Presence of free fluid in abdomen without solid organ injury in CT scan: Think of mesenteric/intestinal/bladder injury ⇒ Exploratory laparotomy is warranted.

Contrast extravasation in CT with even minor hepatic/splenic injuries ⇒ Exploratory laparotomy is indicated.

CT Findings Suggestive of Bowel Injury in Blunt Trauma Abdomen

- Free peritoneal fluid without solid organ injury
- Oral contrast extravasation
- Bowel wall hematoma
- Intraperitoneal air without pneumothorax
- Bowel wall thickening
- Mesenteric stranding

Plain X-ray

- An **AP chest X-ray** is recommended for hemodynamically stable blunt trauma patients and penetrating trauma patients (injury is above umbilicus) to rule out pneumothorax and hemothorax.
- A chest X-ray can detect ruptured hemidiaphragm (abdominal visceras in chest cavity).
- An **AP pelvic X-ray** is indicated in hemodynamically unstable blunt trauma patients with pelvic pain and tenderness.

Contrast Studies

- Contrast studies are only indicated when specific injuries are suspected.
- Urethrography, CT cystography, GI contrast study are indicated depending on the suspected organ involvement, where FAST, CT, or DPL are not informative.

Diagnostic Laparoscopy

This modality is helpful to evaluate peritoneal breach in hemodynamically stable penetrating trauma patients and to detect diaphragmatic injuries.

Management of Specific Injuries

Abdominal Wall Injuries

- Lacerated wounds are commonly present in blunt trauma. Early debridement is indicated to avoid complication like necrotizing fasciitis.
- Irrigation and debridement of entry and exit wound is necessary to remove foreign bodies, necrotic tissues.
- Large abdominal wall defects require reconstruction with prosthetic material (e.g., polypropylene mesh) or myocutaneous flap.

Stomach Injuries

- Stomach injuries are commonly developing following penetrating trauma. Injuries due to blunt trauma is rare due to partial protection by rib cage.
- Gastric injury should be suspected if: (i) Penetrating injury in upper abdomen and (ii) Ryle's tube aspirate contains blood.
- During intraoperative evaluation, the following sites must be thoroughly searched: (i) Esophagogastric junction; (ii) Posterior fundus; (iii) Posterior gastric wall; and (iv) Lesser curvature (within the mesentery).
- Penetrating wounds are managed by debridement of wound edges and primary closure in two layers).
- Injuries in both nerve of Latarjet or both vagi must be treated with a drainage procedure.
- If distal antrum or pylorus is injured, then Billroth I or II procedure is indicated.
- If there is major tissue loss, gastric resection followed by reconstruction is the best surgical option.

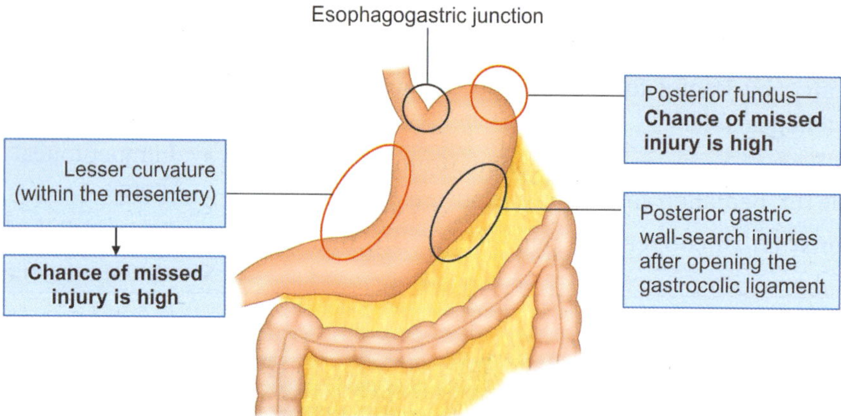

Gallbladder and Extrahepatic Bile Duct Injury

- Gallbladder injury is commonly caused by penetrating trauma, whereas extrahepatic biliary tree injury (EHBTI) is commonly associated with blunt trauma. Isolated EHBTI is extremely rare, commonly associated with injuries of liver, pancreas, duodenum.
- Nonoperative management (NOM) is the treatment of choice in hemodynamically stable patients with gallbladder hematomas without perforation.
- Laceration, avulsion or perforation of gallbladder is best managed by cholecystectomy.
- If CBD injury with minimal tissue loss, repair of wound with 4–0 or 5–0 absorbable suture along with T-tube placement is the best surgical option.
- Roux-en-Y choledochojejunostomy is recommended, if CBD is transected or significant tissue loss.

Management of traumatic injury to extrahepatic duct is technically challenging, because:

- Associated injury of adjacent structures (portal vein, hepatic artery and vena cava) are often present.
- Ducts are of normal size and normal wall thickness, so repair or anastomosis is technically difficult.

Duodenal Injury

Penetrating trauma is the most common cause of duodenal injury in adults, whereas blunt trauma commonly causes duodenal injury in pediatric population.

Why duodenal injuries are often missed:

- Injuries are often within the retroperitoneal part of duodenum.
- Duodenal contents are neutral pH, so clinical presentations are not obvious initially.
- Less bacterial load in duodenum, so in initial stage, peritonitis do not develop.

Duodenal injuries are either duodenal hematoma or duodenal perforation.

Duodenal hematoma:

- Intramural hematoma can be diagnosed with CT or upper GI gastrograffin study **(coiled spring or stocked coin sign)**.
- Treatment is prolonged nasogastric decompression and nutritional support (either TPN or enteral nutrition distal to the injury).
- If patient not responding to conservative management (obstruction not resolving) or CT shows persisting hematoma, even after 2 weeks; surgical intervention is indicated.

Duodenal perforation:

- CT scan with IV contrast is essential for diagnosis of duodeno-pancreatic injuries.
- Primary repair of duodenal injuries should be considered regardless of grade of injury. Primary repair along with pyloric exclusion with or without gastrojejunostomy may be considered for patients with AAST grade III, IV, and V duodenal injuries. In grade IV injuries, the management of bile duct injuries also to be considered.
- If pancreaticoduodenectomy is indicated, then it should be considered as a part of damage control technique and staged reconstruction after patient becomes stable.

Duodenal injury is suspected peroperatively, if:

- Retroperitoneal crepitus is present.
- Retroperitoneal bile staining
- Retroperitoneal hematoma

AAST Duodenal Injury Scale

Grade I Hematoma—single portion of duodenum
Laceration—partial thickness, no perforation
Grade II Hematoma—more than one portion
Laceration—Disruption <50% of circumference
Grade III Laceration —
Disruption 50–75% of circumference of D2
Disruption 50–100% of circumference of D1, D3, D4
Grade IV Laceration—Disruption >75% of circumference of D2 involving ampulla or distal common bile duct
Grade V Laceration—Massive disruption of duodenopancreatic complex
Vascular—Devascularization of duodenum.

Pyloric Exclusion Procedure

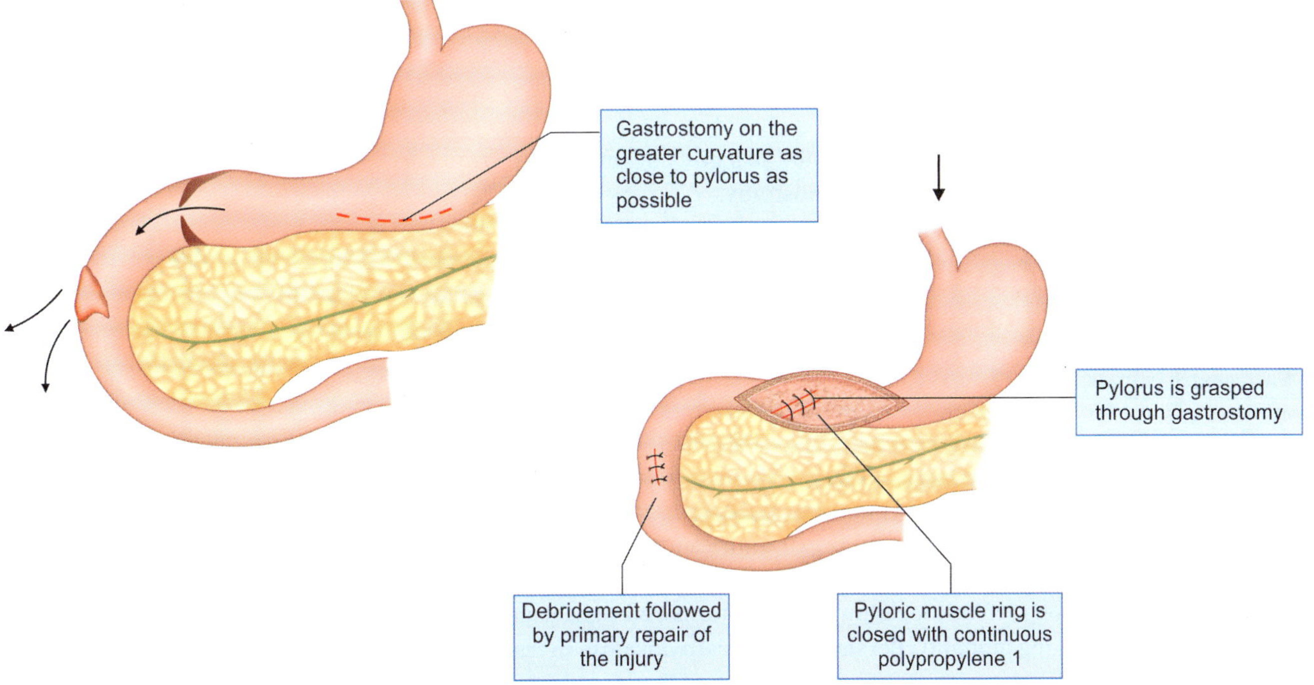

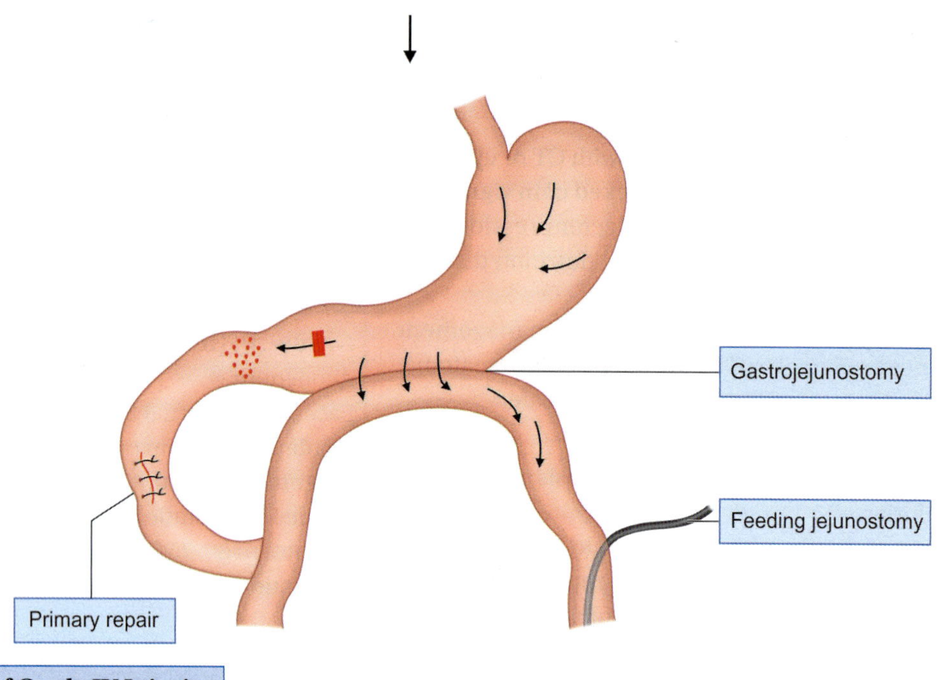

Management of Grade IV Injuries

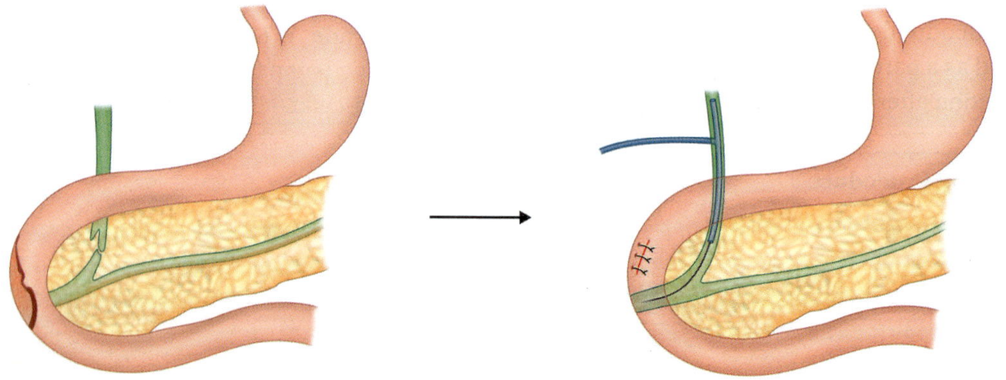

If duodenal injuries with tissue loss is distal to the papilla of Vater and proximal to the superior mesenteric vessels. It is best managed by Roux-en-Y duodenojejunostomy.

Management of Grade V injuries

Pancreaticoduodenectomy is the only option. In a trauma setting, the morbidity and mortality of this procedure is high. Trauma Whipple is a emerging concept in damage control surgery settings.

Pancreatic Injuries

- Pancreatic injuries are rare in both adult and pediatric population and accounts for about 10–20% of all abdominal injuries. Most of the injuries are due to penetrating trauma. Direct blow or seatbelt injury may cause pancreatic disruption due to compression of pancreas against vertebral column.
- Major vascular injuries and/or solid organ injuries are usually associated with pancreatic injury. Concomitant duodenal-pancreatic injuries are also common.
- Because of its retropancreatic location, the symptoms and signs usually appear lately.
- **CT** is the best imaging modality. **Persistent hyperamylasemia in trauma setting** is highly suggestive of pancreatic injuries. Upper GI gastrograffin study—**'Widening of Duodenal C Loop'** finding is highly suggestive.

Management is determined by: (i) Location of injury and (ii) Injury to the main pancreatic duct or not.

For these assessments, intraoperative assessment is the best method. For intraoperative assessment, adequate exploration is required. For adequate exploration, proper maneuvers are necessary.

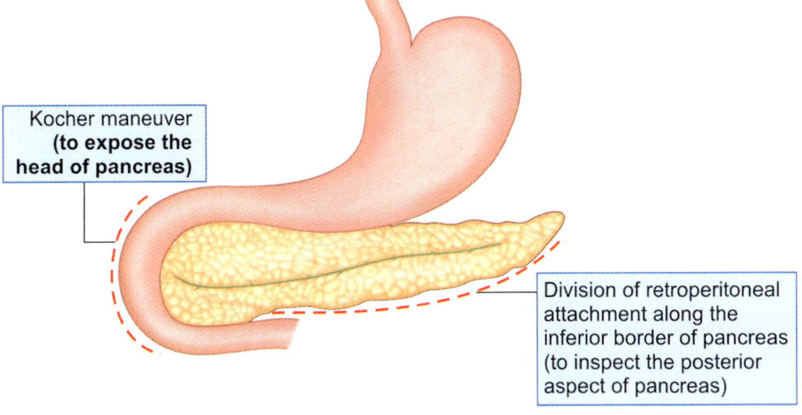

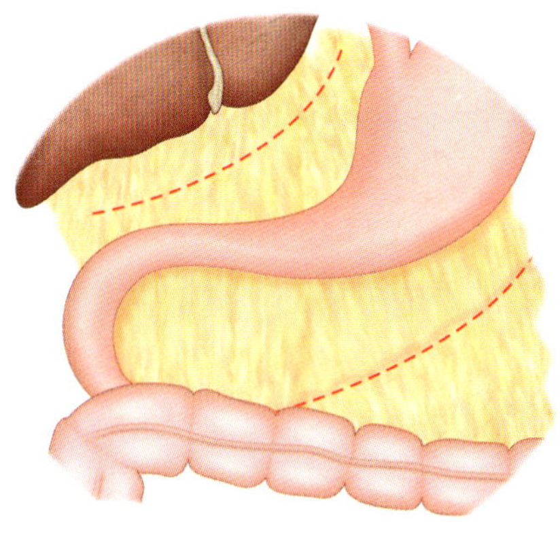

Opening of gastrohepatic and gastrocolic ligaments **(to inspect the body and tail of pancreas)**

For grade I and II injuries, debridement with drain placement (closed suction drain) is sufficient.

AAST Pancreatic Injury Scale

Grade I: Hematoma—Minor contusion without duct injury
Laceration—Superficial laceration without duct injury

Grade II: Hematoma—Major contusion without duct injury or tissue loss
Laceration—Major laceration without duct injury or tissue loss

Grade III: Laceration—Distal (left of the superior mesenteric vessels) transection or parenchymal injury with duct injury

Grade IV: Laceration—Proximal (right of the superior mesenteric vessels) transection or parenchymal injury involving the ampulla

Grade V: Laceration—Massive disruption of pancreatic head

Management of Grade III Injuries

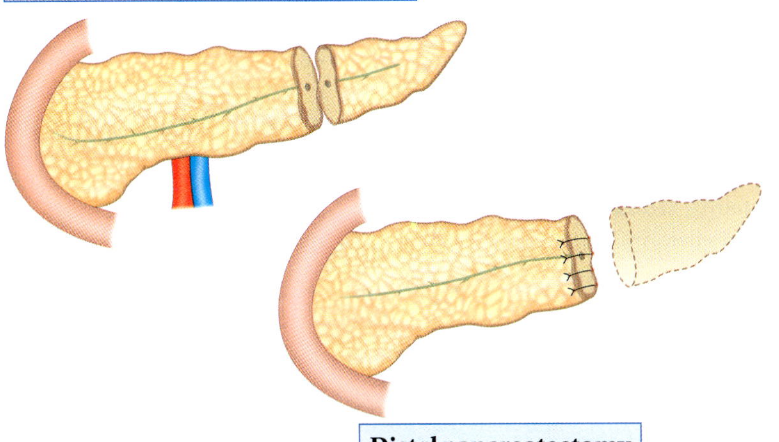

Distal pancreatectomy

Management of Grade IV Injuries

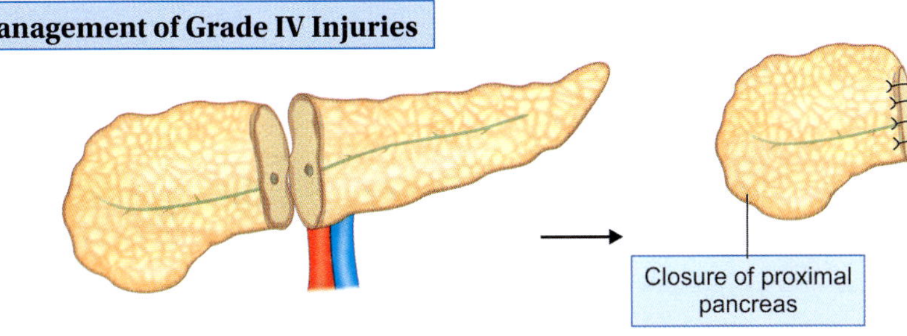

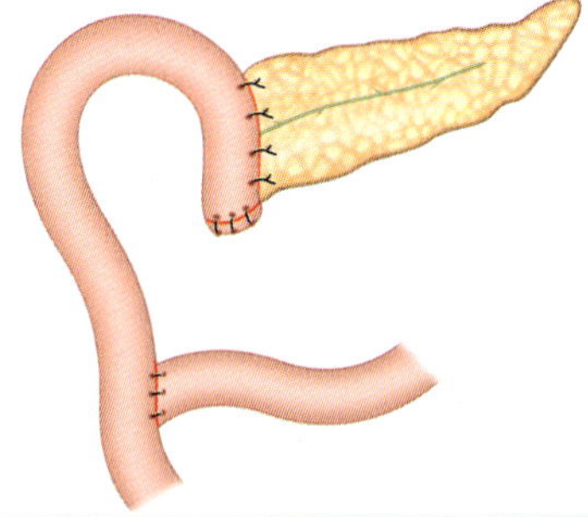

Roux-en-Y pancreaticojejunostomy

Management of Grade V Injuries

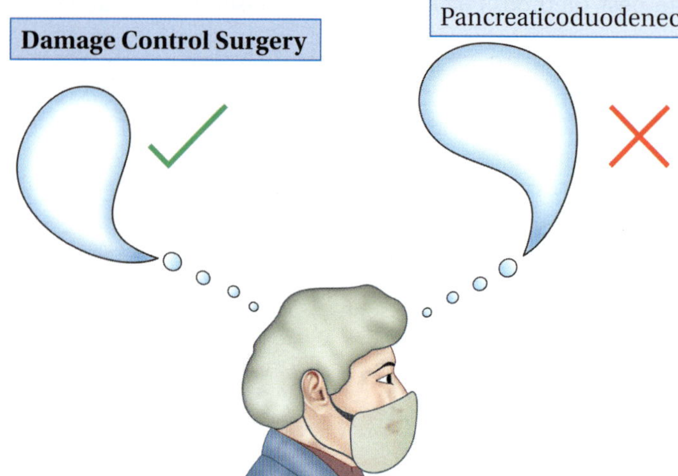

Trauma Whipple

Indication: Complete disruption of the pancreato-duodenal complex with or without bleeding from IVC or portal vein.

Principles:

- The procedure should be done in a staged manner—resection and hemostasis during the initial surgical procedure and reconstruction 24–48 hours later in a resuscitated patient.
- Gallbladder is preserved for cholecystoentero-stomy during reconstruction.
- Meticulous dissection of uncinate process is not indicated.
- Pancreatogastrostomy is preferred over pancreatojejunostomy.
- If pancreatoenteric anastomosis is not feasible due to soft, friable pancreas, distal pancreatic stump is oversewn.

Small Bowel Injuries

- Small bowel is the most common organ injured after penetrating abdominal trauma.
- **Different mechanisms of blunt trauma causing small bowel injuries are:** (i) Crush injury; (between vertebral bodies and steering wheel); (ii) Deceleration injury (shearing force at the fixed point, e.g., ligament of Treitz, ileocecal junction); and (iii) Closed loop rupture (due to sudden increase of Intra-abdominal pressure).

Small injury should be suspected if: (i) Presence of 'seatbelt sign'; (ii) Blunt trauma with signs of peritoneal irritation; (iii) All gunshot injuries in anterior abdomen; and (iv) Stab injuries with peritoneal breach.

Small bowel injury is detected by: (i) CT abdomen with oral and IV contrast; (ii) Chest X-ray; and (iii) DPL (where CT facility is not available).

After exploration of abdomen, careful examination of the entire small intestine (from ligament of Treitz to ileocecal junction) should be done. All mesenteric hematomas (adjacent to mesentery-intestinal junction must be explored because of possibility of small bowel injuries.

Seatbelt Syndrome

A group of injuries occur during motor vehicle accidents due to the impact of seatbelt on passenger's torso.

This syndrome includes:

(i) Seatbelt sign; (ii) Bowel perforation; and (iii) Fracture of lumbar spine.

"Seatbelt sign": Bruised skin in the distribution of seatbelt across the abdomen. Patient's with 'seatbelt sign' is commonly associated with injuries of small intestine, mesentery.

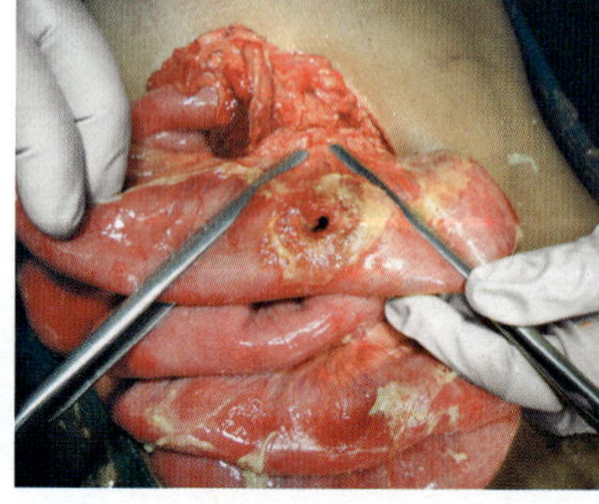

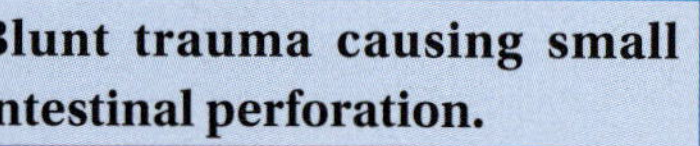
Blunt trauma causing small intestinal perforation.

Small injuries are managed by **primary repair**

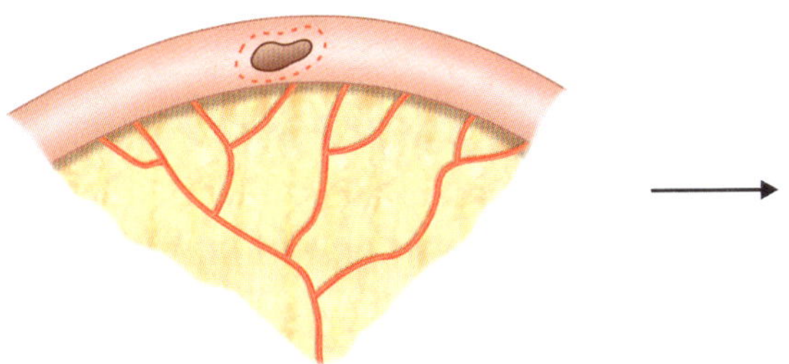

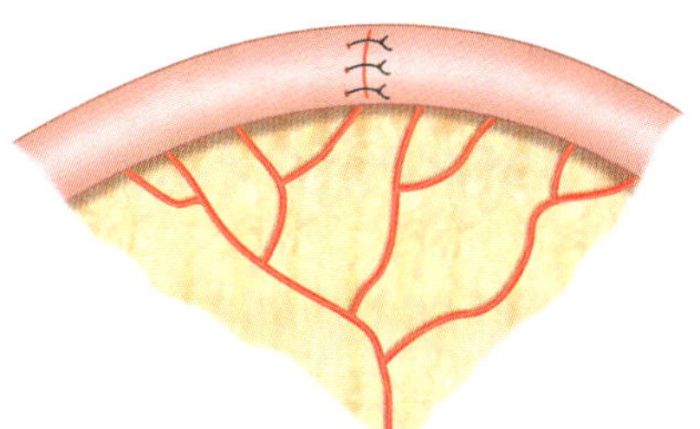

Contraindications of primary repair:
- >50% disruption of bowel circumference
- Mesenteric devascularization.

If two adjacent perforations are present, injuries can be connected and repaired in a transverse direction.

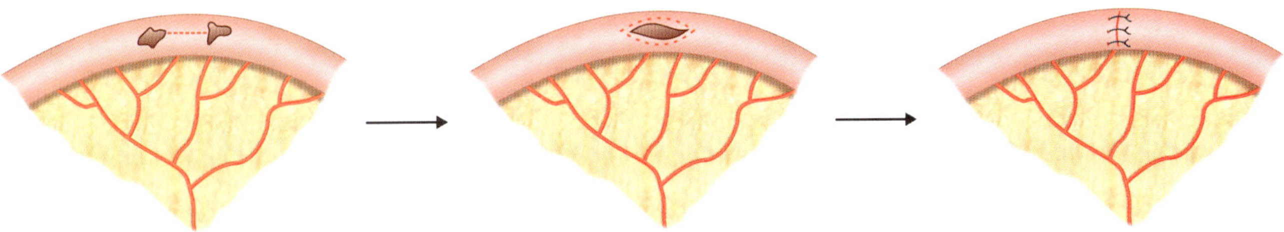

If extensive laceration, multiple laceration in a short segment, or devascularized segment is present, then resection of that segment followed by end-to-end anastomosis is indicated.

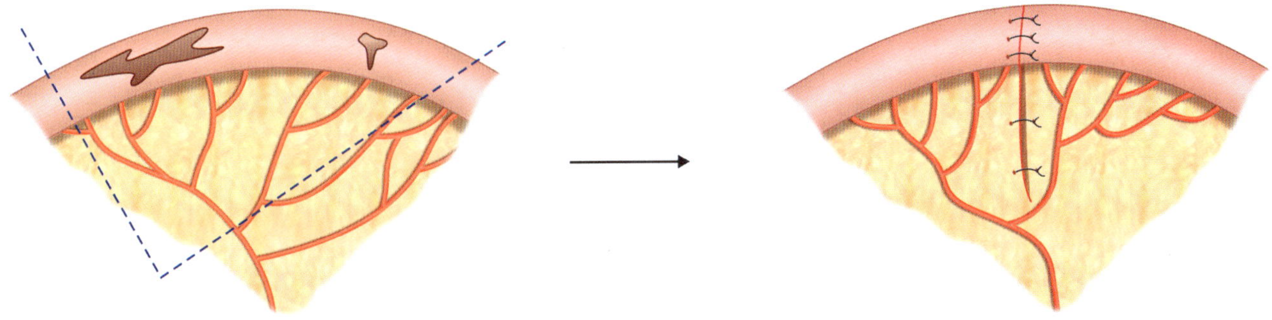

Colon Injuries

- Colon injuries are most commonly caused by penetrating trauma. Blunt trauma rarely causes colonic injuries. Most of the colonic injuries are detected following exploratory laparotomy after penetrating wound, particularly after gunshot wound in anterior abdomen.
- Triple contrast (oral, IV and rectal) CT scan is indicated in stab wound in back or flank to exclude bowel injuries.
- **Methods of treating colonic injuries are:** (i) Primary repair; (ii) Resection anastomosis; and (iii) Stoma.
- **Primary repair or resection anastomosis is the treatment of choice if:** (i) Laparotomy within 4–6 hours; (ii) Patient is not in shock; (iii) Absence of gross contamination of peritoneal cavity; and (iv) Absence of colonic vascular injury.

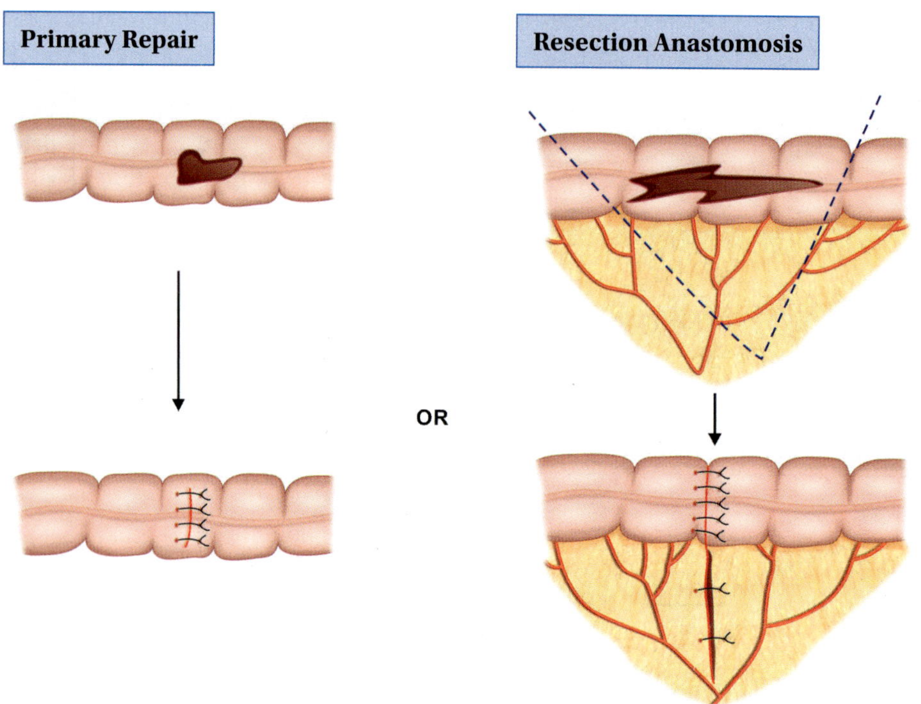

Stoma is the safe option if primary repair or resection anastomosis is not considered as safe.

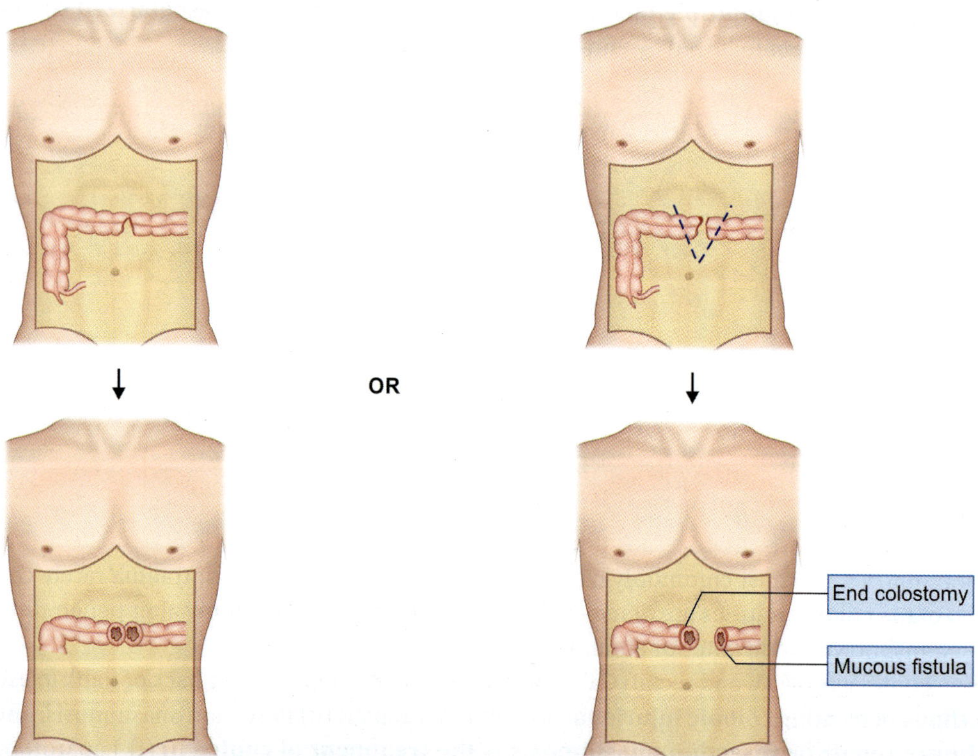

Injured colon is exteriorized as loop colostomy.

Rectal Injuries

- Most of the rectal injuries are penetrating injuries, particularly from gunshot wounds.
- Rectal injury should be suspected if transpelvic gunshot wounds or penetrating injury to the lower abdomen and buttock.
- Presence of blood in digital rectal examination is suggestive of rectal injury.
- In proctoscopy and rigid proctosigmoidoscopy, hematoma, contusion, or gross blood is indicative of rectal injury.
- **If diagnosis in doubt**, soluble contrast enema is indicated. **If still in doubt**, then patient should be treated as they do have an injury.
- Rectal injuries may be **intraperitoneal** or **extraperitoneal**.

Management of Intraperitoneal Rectal Injury

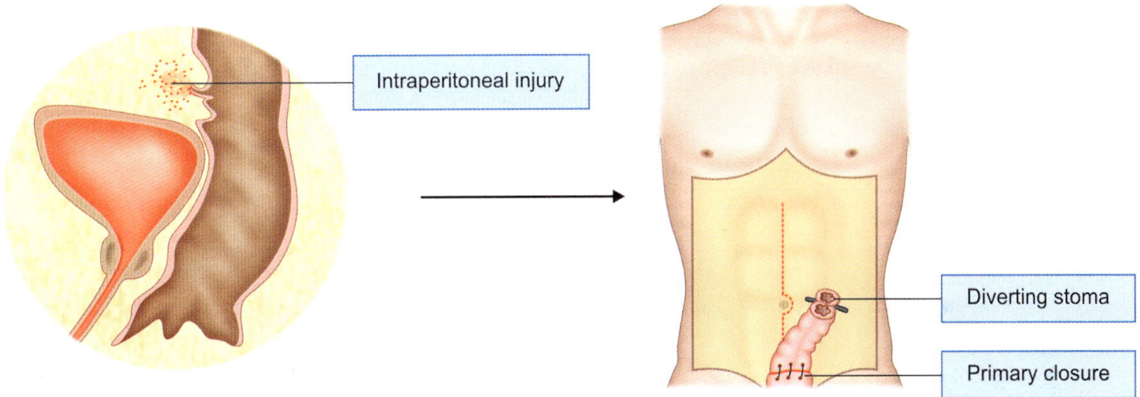

If intraperitoneal injuries are so extensive, that primary repair is not feasible, then resection of the injured part of rectum followed by Hartmann procedure is the best surgical option.

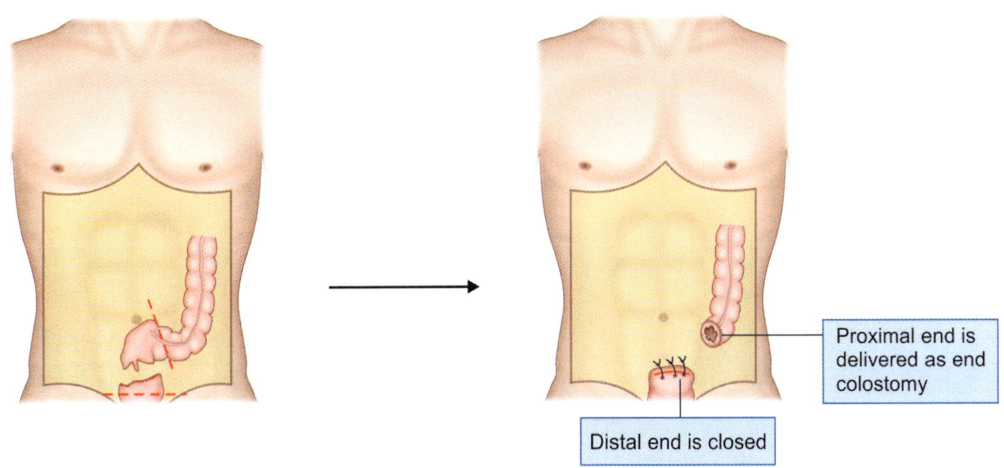

Management of Extraperitoneal Rectal Injury

Access to extraperitoneal injuries are technically difficult. During management, 3 Ds should be considered: **(i) Diversion; (ii) Drainage; and (iii) Distal washout**.

Diversion

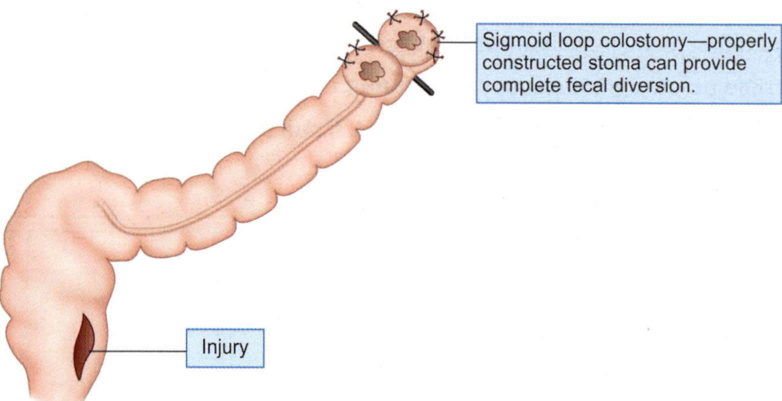

Drainage

Presacral drain (Penrose/closed suction) prevents fecal contamination of perirectal space.

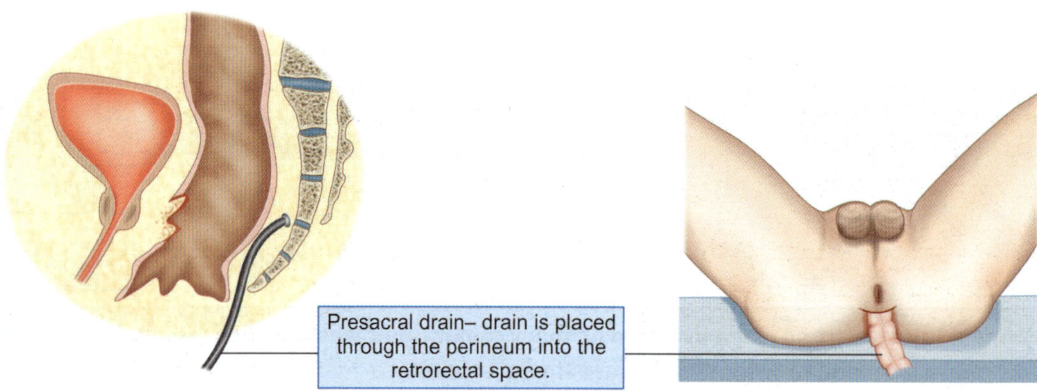

Distal Washout

Washout of distal rectal stump decreases the incidence of pelvic abscess, rectal fistula, and sepsis.

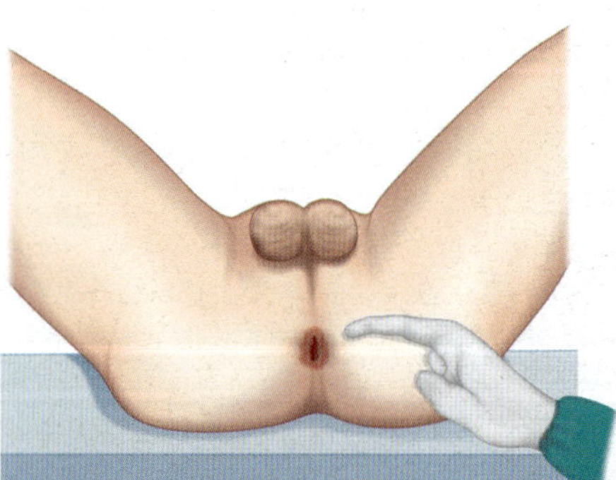

Anus should be mechanically dilated

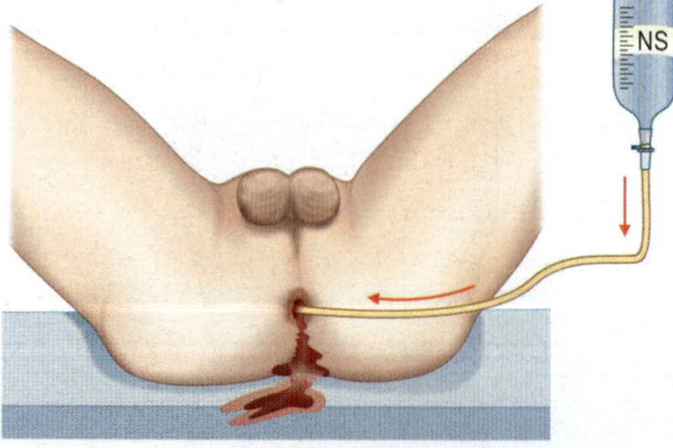

Irrigation fluid should be isotonic

Liver Injury

- Liver is one of the commonly injured organs in blunt trauma abdomen. Penetrating trauma, particularly high-energy gunshot injuries are responsible for life-threatening liver injuries.
- Most of the minor or moderate injuries (AAST grade I, II, and III) are managed by **Nonoperative management (NOM)**. A selected group of patients with severe injuries (AAST grade IV and V) are also candidates for NOM after development of multimodal approaches (e.g., EVTM).

In pediatric population, NOM is the optimal management for liver trauma.

- **The decision making of NOM vs. operative management** depends on patient's hemodynamic status, grade of injury, associated injuries.
- **Abdominal CT with IV contrast** is indicated for detection and grading of liver injuries.

Nonoperative Management (NOM) in Blunt Liver Trauma

- NOM should be the treatment of choice for all **hemodynamically stable** minor (AAST I-II), moderate (AAST III), severe (AAST IV-V) injuries in the absence of other intra-abdominal injuries requiring surgery.
- In patients considered **transient responders** with moderate (AAST III) and severe (AAST IV-V) injuries, NOM should be considered only if facility of immediate availability of trained surgeons, operating rooms, continuous monitoring ideally in an ICU setting, access to angiography, angioembolization, blood and blood products are available.
- **Angiography with embolization** may be considered in hemodynamically stable patient with arterial blush on CT scan.

  CT scan is recommended during follow-up after NOM if there is clinical suspicion of complications (e.g., re-bleeding, intrahepatic abscess, biliary complications)
- **NOM should not be considered if patient is hemodynamically unstable, or features of peritonitis are present.**

Complications after NOM in blunt liver trauma: (i) Bile leakage; (ii) Intrahepatic abscess; (iii) Perihepatic abscess; (iv) Re-bleeding; (v) Biloma; (vi) Biliary peritonitis; and (vii) Hepatic artery pseudo-aneurysm.

EVTM (EndoVascular Resuscitation and Trauma Management)

A new and rapidly evolving concept in trauma management. It is a multidisciplinary team approach for gaining hemodynamic control in unstable exsanguinating patients.

Elements of EVTM are: (i) Vascular access; (ii) REBOA (Resuscitative Endovascular Balloon Occlusion of the aorta); (iii) Embolization; and (iv) Placement of endograft.

AAST Liver Trauma Grading

Grade I Hematoma—Subcapsular <10% surface
Laceration—Capsular tear <1 cm parenchymal depth

Grade II Hematoma—Subcapsular 10–50% surface area; intraparenchymal, <10 cm diameter
Laceration—1–3 cm parenchymal depth, <10 cm in length

Grade III Hematoma—Subcapsular >50% surface area or expanding, ruptured subcapsular or parenchymal hematoma. Intraparenchymal hematoma >10 cm
Laceration >3 cm parenchymal depth

Grade IV Laceration—Parenchymal disruption 25–75% of hepatic lobe

Grade V Laceration—Parenchymal disruption involving >75% of hepatic lobe
Vascular—Juxtavenous hepatic injuries, i.e., retrohepatic vena cava/central major hepatic veins

Grade VI Hepatic avulsion

Advance one grade for multiple injuries up to grade III.

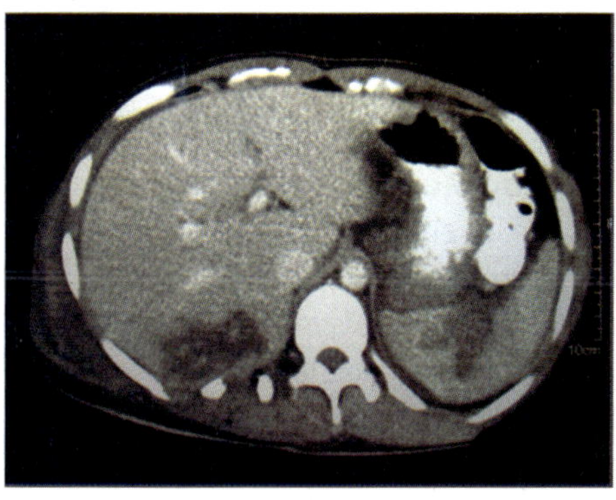

Contrast CT showing liver trauma.

Nonoperative Management (NOM) in Penetrating Liver Trauma

- NOM can be safely considered in stab wound and low-energy penetrating wounds, if patient is hemodynamically stable, no evisceration or impalement and absence of any intra-abdominal injury that warrant surgery.
- Angioembolization may be considered in arterial bleeding in hemodynamically stable patient.
- **NOM should not be considered if:** (i) High-energy gunshot wound; (ii) In CT, bullet trajectory close to hollow viscus with surrounding hematoma.

Role of Angioembolization in Liver Trauma

- In hemodynamically stable patients with arterial blush in CT scan
- Persistent arterial bleeding after non-hemostatic or damage control procedures.
- For treatment of post-traumatic hepatic artery pseudo-aneurysm.

Operative Management in Liver Trauma

Indications of operative management: (i) Hemodynamically unstable and nonresponder patients; (ii) High-energy gunshot wounds and other ballistic injuries; (iii) Presence of evisceration and or impalement; (iv) Patient with features of peritonitis; (v) CT scan showing free intra- or retroperitoneal air; and (vi) CT scan showing bullet trajectory close to hollow viscus with surrounding hematoma.

Principles of operative management:

- The primary aim of operative intervention is to control hemorrhage and bile leak. For control of hemorrhage, generous exposure is required. For exposure, division of triangular ligament, superior and inferior coronary ligament may be required.
- Minor bleeding can be controlled by: (i) Electrosurgery; (ii) Argon beam coagulation; (iii) Bipolar devices; (iv) Simple suturing of liver parenchyma or suturing over omentoplasty; and (v) Topical hemostatic agents.
- For major bleeding, approaches are: (i) Manual compression; (ii) Perihepatic packing; (iii) Ligation or repair of vessels (Repair for hepatic artery proper and portal vein); (iv) Pringle maneuver; (v) Balloon tamponade; (vi) Hepatic vascular exclusion with shunting; (vii) Hepatic debridement and finger fracture; and (viii) Resuscitative endovascular balloon occlusion of the aorta (REBOA)/Resuscitative endovascular balloon occlusion of the vena cava (REBOVC).
- 'Open abdomen' approach should be considered if any risk of development of abdominal compartment syndrome or 'second look' operation is indicated after damage control surgery.

Perihepatic Packing

- Perihepatic packing is strategically placing of laparotomy pads above and below the bleeding parenchyma. Additional pads are placed between the liver, diaphragm, and anterior abdominal wall.
- Perihepatic packing is most effective for venous injuries. It is particularly effective for control of hemorrhage from right lobe, not so effective for left lobe.

Complications: (i) Hypotension due to vena caval compression and (ii) Decreased tidal volume and functional residual capacity due to cephalad displacement of diaphragm.

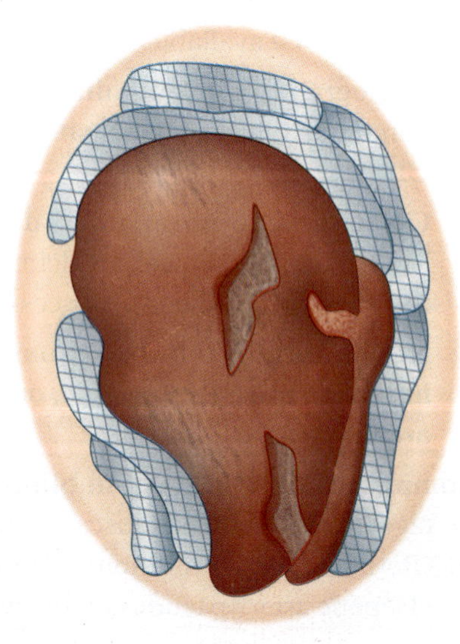

Inflow Occlusion by Pringle maneuver

- If bleeding is not controlled by perihepatic packing, inflow occlusion is the most appropriate measure.
- **Vascular clamp or Rummel tourniquet** is applied around the porta hepatis (Lower blade is within **the foramen of Winslow), thereby portal triad** is occluded.
- If bleeding stops after clamping, it can be interpreted that the injury is in the portal vein or hepatic artery.
- If bleeding continues after clamping, an injury to the hepatic veins or retrohepatic vena cava is suspected.
- **Duration of clamping is important** because liver cannot tolerate warm ischemia for more than 1 hour.

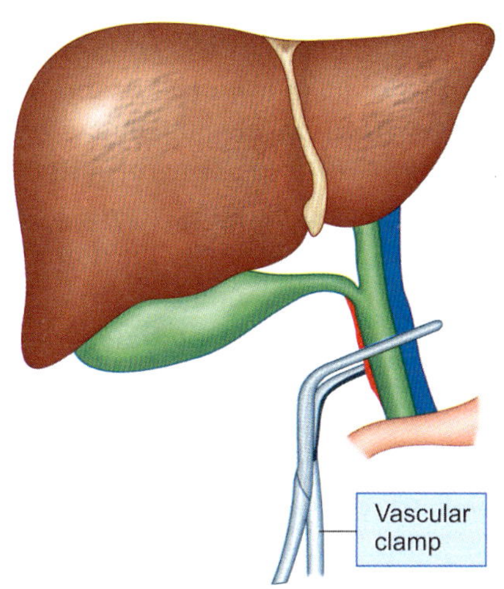

Options for Outflow Control

If major bleeding is not controlled by perihepatic packing and Pringle maneuver, outflow control should be seriously considered.

Options for achieving outflow control are: (i) Atriocaval shunt and (ii) Complete hepatic vascular occlusion.

Treatment Options for Control of Minor Bleeding

- Raw surface oozing can be controlled by **electrosurgery, Argon beam coagulation** or **topical hemostatic agents** (microcrystalline collagen, oxidized cellulose).
- Persistently bleeding lacerations can also be controlled by **interrupted horizontal mattress** sutures parallel to the edge of laceration using No. O-chromic in large curved blunt needle.
- **Omentum** can also be used to fill large defects over which sutures can be given.
- Deep liver lacerations should not be simply closed due risk of abscess formation and hemobilia. By finger fracture technique, the lacerations are extended to expose the **bleeding vessels and ducts and then these structures are ligated**.
- If multiple superficial lacerations are present, wrapping of each lobe by the **absorbable mesh** is a useful technique.

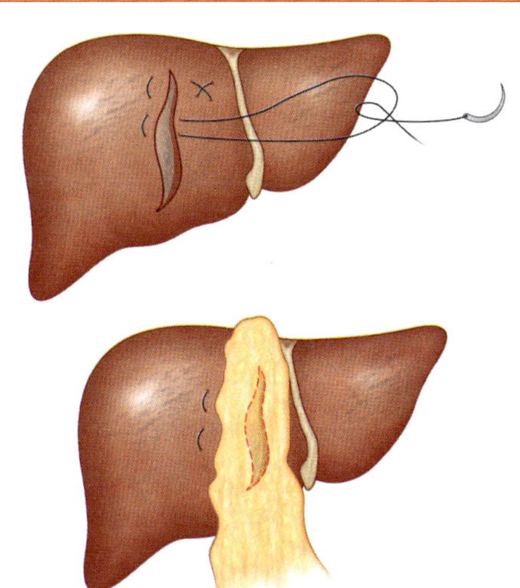

Omentum is a rich source of macrophage, thereby it fills dead space with viable tissue.

Splenic Injuries

- Splenic injuries are among the commonly occurring trauma-related injuries. Management of splenic injuries ranges from Nonoperative management, splenorrhaphy, partial splenectomy to splenectomy. The management **focuses on restoration of hemostasis with preservation of spleen, if possible,** particularly in pediatric patients. The decision of optimal management is based on physiology of the patient, grading of splenic injury and other associated injuries.
- **CT scan with IV contrast** is the gold standard diagnostic modality in hemodynamically stable or stabilized adult and pediatric patients to define the anatomy of injury and grading.

Nonoperative Management (NOM) in Splenic Trauma

- **NOM can be considered if:** (i) Patient is hemodynamically stable; (ii) Absence of other organ injuries that warrant surgical intervention; (iii) Absence of peritonitis, bowel evisceration or impalement; and (iv) Facility of intensive care facility, always available operating room are present.
- NOM is recommended as **first-line treatment for hemodynamically-stable pediatric patients in isolated blunt splenic trauma.**
- CT scan with IV contrast is indicated before considering NOM.
- **NOM should not be considered in:** (i) Penetrating injury in pediatric patient and (ii) Suspected hollow viscus injuries.
- **In NOM,** patient should be monitored in ICU for 48–72 hours with continuous monitoring of vital signs and serial abdominal examination and serial hematocrit estimation. If patient become stable, patient must be shifted to intermediate care unit and clinical monitoring must be continued. On discharge, patient is advised to avoid intense physical activity and contact sports for 3 months. During NOM, if patient developing hemodynamic unstability and falling hematocrit, surgery have to be considered.
- **Angioembolization** may be considered in hemodynamically stable patient with arterial blush in CT.

Operative Management in Splenic Trauma

Indications:

- Patient with hemodynamic instability and/or features of peritonitis or bowel evisceration.
- Hemodynamically stable AAST grade III-V injuries where facility of intensive monitoring, always available operating room and/or angioembolization facility is not available.
- During NOM, significant drop in hematocrit or continuous transfusion is required or angioembolization becomes unsuccessful.

Different surgical options: (i) Splenorrhaphy; (ii) Partial splenectomy; and (iii) Splenectomy. In pediatric patients, splenic preservation should be attempted, whenever possible.

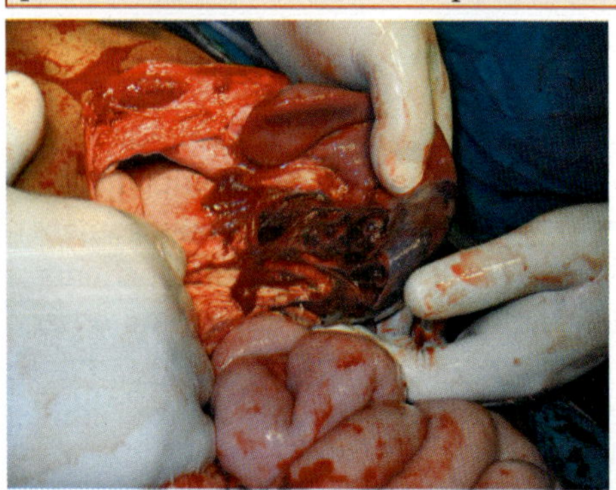

Operative picture of splenic trauma.

AAST Splenic Trauma Grading

Grade I Hematoma—Subcapsular, <10% surface area

Laceration—Capsular tear, <1 cm parenchymal depth

Grade II Hematoma—Subcapsular, 10–50% surface area

Intraparenchymal, <5 cm diameter

Laceration—1–3 cm parenchymal depth not involving a parenchymal vessel

Grade III Hematoma—Subcapsular, >50% surface area or expanding

Ruptured subcapsular or parenchymal hematoma

Intraparenchymal hematoma >5 cm

Laceration >3 cm parenchymal depth or involving trabecular vessels

Grade IV Laceration—Laceration of segmental or hilar vessels producing major devascularization (>25% of spleen)

Grade V Laceration—Completely shattered spleen

Vascular—Hilar vascular injury which devascularized spleen.

Pediatric patients are good candidates for NOM in splenic trauma because:

- Splenic capsule is thicker in children, less prone to severe injury
- Low incidence of delayed bleeding
- Spleen in children more likely to fracture parallel to splenic arterial distribution following trauma, that leads to less blood loss from splenic parenchyma.
- More efficient contraction and retraction of splenic arterioles.

Role of Angioembolization in Splenic Trauma

- Hemodynamically stable and rapid responder patients with AAST grade III-V with contrast blush in CT.
- Management of post-traumatic splenic pseudoaneurysm.

Small Capsular Laceration

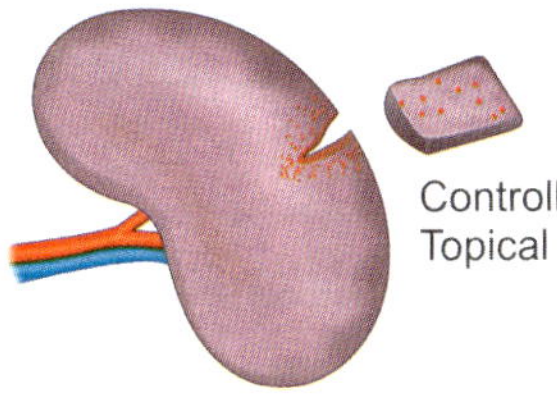

Controlled by
Topical hemostatic agent

Deeper Laceration

Repair by **horizontal mattress sutures** (2-0 sorbable)

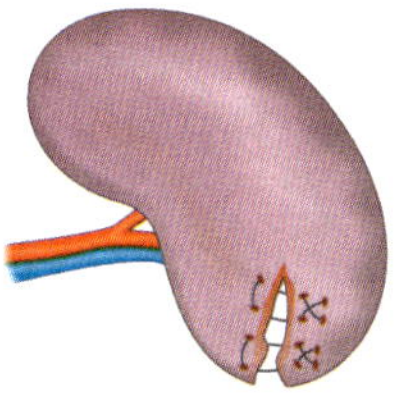

Covering the injury by the **omentum**

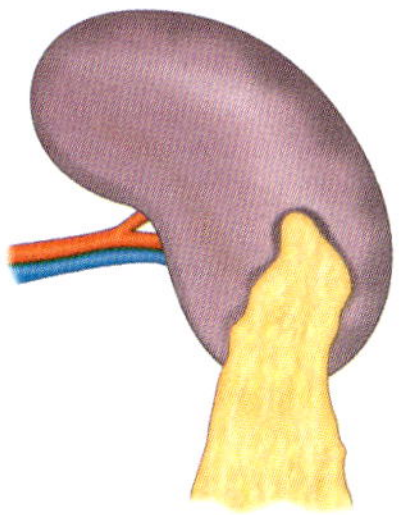

Wrapping the injured part of spleen with **vicryl mesh**

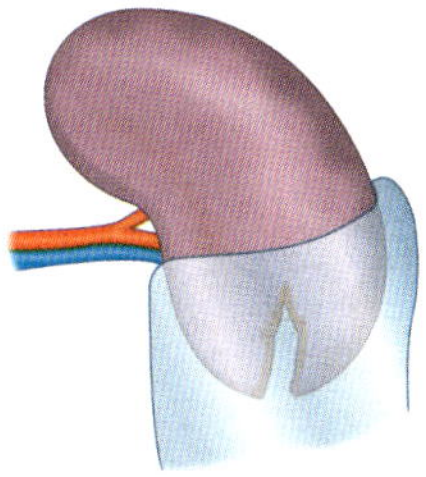

Major Laceration Involving Superior or Inferior Pole

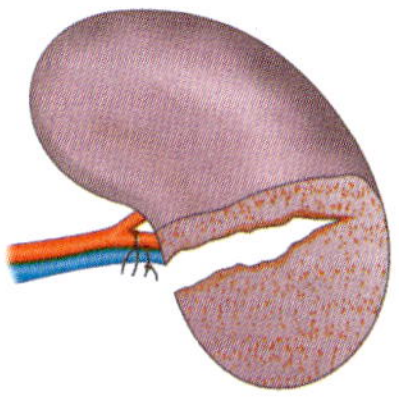

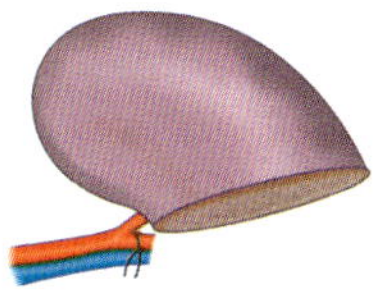

Partial splenectomy

Shattered Spleen

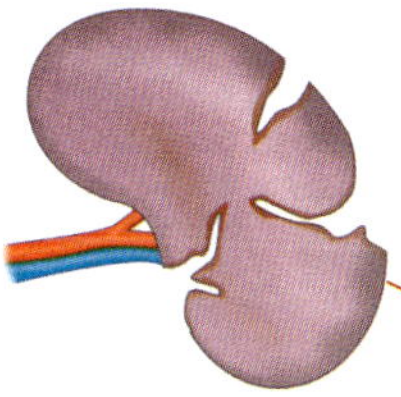

Injury Involving the Hilum or Central Area of Spleen

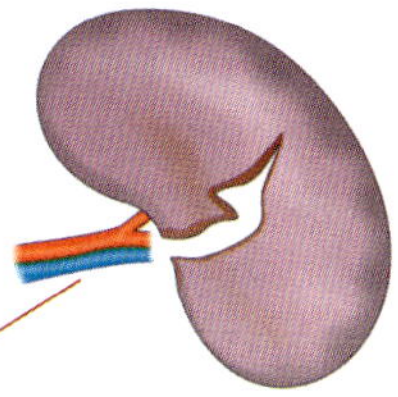

Splenic autologous transplantation has no proven role in reduction of morbidity or mortality in post-splenectomy period.

Splenectomy

Laparoscopic splenectomy in the trauma setting is not recommended.

Hemodynamically Unstable Adult Patient

On admission, systolic blood pressure <90 mm Hg, or >90 mm Hg but requiring bolus infusions/transfusions and/or vasopressor drugs and/or admission base excess >–5 mmol/L and/or shock index >1, and/or transfusion requirement of at least 4–6 units of PRBC within the first 24 hours **(Adapted from WSES Guideline)**.

Blood pressure <90 mm Hg and heart rate >120 bpm, with evidence of skin vasoconstriction (cool, clammy, decreased capillary refill), altered level of consciousness and/or shortness of breath (**as per ATLS Guideline, 9th Edition**).

Rapid Responders

- These group of patients quickly respond to initial fluid bolus and become hemodynamically stable.
- Further fluid bolus or blood administration are usually not required.

Transient Responders

- These group of patients respond to initial fluid bolus, but showing failure to respond once maintenance fluid is initiated.
- Blood transfusion is indicated in these group of patients.
- Surgical management or angioembolization have to considered for control of ongoing hemorrhage.

Nonresponders

- These group of patients do not respond to initial fluid bolus and blood transfusion.
- Immediate surgical intervention or angioembolization should be considered to control the exsanguinating hemorrhage.

Hard Signs of Arterial Injury

- External arterial bleeding
- Rapidly expanding hematoma
- Palpable thrill
- Audible bruit.

Presence of hard signs warrant immediate surgical intervention.

Soft Signs of Arterial Injury

- History of arterial bleeding at the scene
- Proximity of penetrating/blunt injury to major artery
- Diminished unilateral distal pulse
- Small nonpulsatile hematoma.

Presence of soft signs mandate further evaluation.

Following arteries should be repaired:

(i) Aorta; (ii) Carotid artery; (iii) Innominate artery; (iv) Brachial artery; (v) Hepatic artery proper; (vi) Superior mesenteric artery; (vii) Renal artery; (viii) Common iliac artery; (ix) Femoral artery; and (x) Popliteal artery

Following veins should be repaired:

(i) Superior vena cava; (ii) Suprarenal vena cava; (iii) Superior mesenteric vein; and (iv) Popliteal vein

Retroperitoneal Injuries

Retroperitoneal injuries present with frank Intra-abdominal hemorrhage or retroperitoneal hematoma due to injury of major retroperitoneal vessels or their abdominal branches.

All zone I hematomas following blunt and penetrating injuries warrant operative exploration:

- These hematomas are caused by injuries to supra- or infrarenal aorta, celiac axis, proximal SMA, proximal renal artery, and IVC.
- Proximal and distal control of the involved vessel should be obtained prior to exploration of hematoma.

Zone III hematomas are usually due to pelvic fractures:

- These hematomas should not be explored unless iliac vessel injury is suspected.
- For temporary control of hemorrhage, pelvic binder around the pelvis is helpful.
- Pelvic angiography with selective embolization is the intervention of choice where pelvic fractures are the suspected source of ongoing hemorrhage.

Zone II hemotomas are suggestive of injury to renal artery, vein or renal parenchyma:

- Unless the hematoma is rapidly expanding, pulsatile or ruptured, it should not be explored.
- CT is necessary to assess the function of kidneys.
- If exploration of the hematoma is required, nephrectomy (total or partial) is indicated for a shattered kidney.

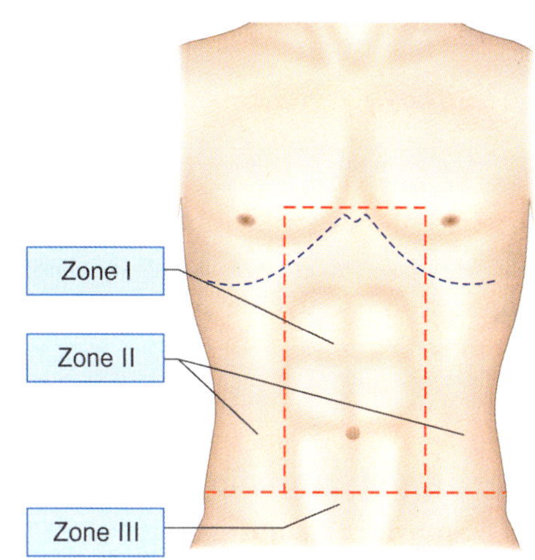

Zone I (Midline retroperitoneum): Extends from the aortic hiatus to sacral promontory.

Zone II: Extends on either side from the renal hilum to the pericolic gutters.

Zone III (Pelvic retroperitoneum): Encompasses the pelvis.

For exploration of retroperitoneal hematoma, proximal control of the aorta at the level of the diaphragm along with right-sided medial visceral rotation **(Cattell-Braasch maneuver)** or left-sided medial visceral rotation **(Mattox maneuver)** is necessary.

Cattell-Braasch maneuver: A right-sided medial visceral rotation to expose the entire inframesocolic retroperitoneal organs including intra-abdominal IVC, right renal pedicle and right iliac artery and vein, duodenum and head of the pancreas. Extended Kocher's maneuver is a part of Cattell-Braasch maneuver. The two areas of retroperitoneum that are inaccessible after this maneuver are retrohepatic IVC and suprarenal aorta.

Mattox maneuver: A left medial visceral rotation to expose the abdominal aorta along with the celiac axis, the superior mesenteric artery, the left renal pedicle, and the left iliac artery and vein. Retrohepatic IVC and suprarenal aorta are accessible after Mattox maneuver.

Management of vascular injuries: Vena cava, iliac veins, SMV, portal vein, renal veins should be repaired. Aorta, iliac arteries, common hepatic artery, SMA, renal artery must be repaired. Left gastric artery, splenic artery may be ligated. If ligation of splenic artery is needed, then splenectomy have to be done.

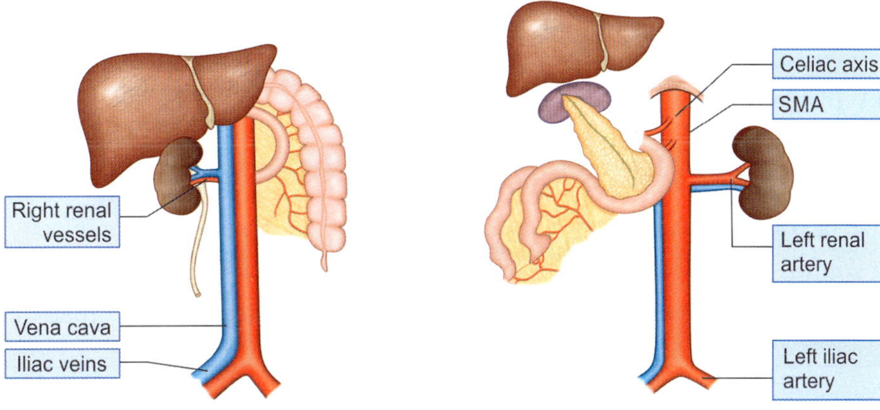

Genitourinary Injuries

Renal Injuries

- The kidneys are the **most commonly injured genitourinary organ**. Kidney is vulnerable to deceleration injuries because it is fixed only by renal pelvis and the vascular pedicle. **In pediatric population**, kidney is a commonly injured organ following blunt abdominal trauma.
- Flank ecchymosis, fractured lower ribs, penetrating injury of flank or lower chest along with gross or microscopic hematuria are **suggestive of renal injury**.
- **CT scan with IV contrast** is the most preferred imaging modality in patients with suspected kidney injuries.
- **Treatment:** Nonoperative approach can be considered in hemodynamically stable patients with upto grade III injuries. Injuries of the parenchymal collecting system often resolve spontaneously. If renal pelvis or proximal ureteral avulsion is suspected, urgent endoscopic or open surgical intervention is indicated.
- **Indications of surgical explorations in renal trauma:** (i) Continuing hemodynamic instability and unresponsiveness to aggressive resuscitation; (ii) Grade V vascular injuries; and (iii) Expanding or pulsatile peri-renal hematoma, identified during peroperative period.
- **Different surgical options are:** (i) Renal preservation techniques; (ii)Partial nephrectomy; and (iii) Nephrectomy.
- **Renal preservation techniques** are indicated in solitary or bilateral kidney injuries. Different renal preservation techniques are: (i) Renorrhaphy (mattress sutures through the parenchyma); (ii) Use of hemostatic agents (i.e., combined acellular matrix and fibrin sealants); and (iii) Absorbable mesh kidney bags.
- **Early complications of renal injury:** (i) Bleeding; (ii) Perinephric abscess; (iii) Urinary fistula; (iv) Hypertension; (v) Urinary extravasation; and (vi) Urinoma.
- **Delayed complications of renal injury:** (i) Retroperitoneal bleeding; (ii) Hydronephrosis; (iii) Chronic pyelonephritis; (iv) Hypertension; (v) Arteriovenous fistula; and (vi) Pseudoaneurysms.

Kidney is commonly injured in pediatric age group due to:

- Thinner abdominal muscles
- Incomplete ossification of ribs
- Larger kidney
- Less perirenal fat

AAST Grading of Renal Injuries

Grade I

Contusion: Microscopic or gross hematuria

Hematoma: Subcapsular, nonexpanding without parenchymal laceration

Grade II

Hematoma: Nonexpanding perirenal hematoma confined to renal retroperitoneum.

Laceration: <1 cm parenchymal depth of renal cortex without urinary extravasation.

Grade III

Laceration: >1 cm parenchymal depth of renal cortex without collecting system rupture or urinary extravasation.

Grade IV

Laceration: Parenchymal laceration extending through cortex, medulla, and collecting system.

Vascular: Main renal or venous injury with contained hemorrhage.

Grade V

Laceration: Completely shattered kidney.

Vascular: Avulsion of renal hilum, kidney is devascularized.

Principles of Surgical Exploration in Renal Trauma

- Approach should be **transperitoneal** so that other Intra-abdominal organs can be examined.
- **Early vascular control** before opening Gerota's fascia can decrease renal tissue loss.
- **The goal of operative exploration** of injured kidney is to control the bleeding first, repair the injury (if possible) and then perirenal drainage.

Renorrhaphy

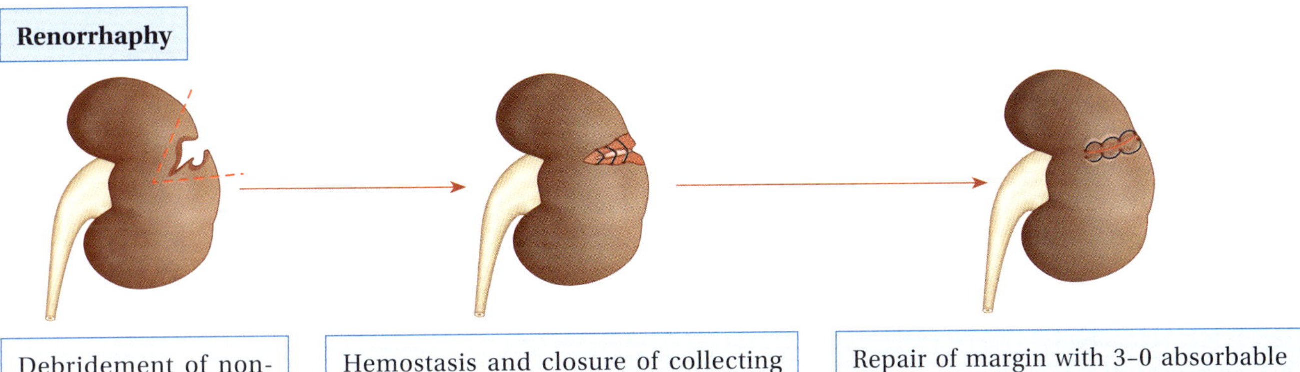

Debridement of non-viable tissue.

Hemostasis and closure of collecting system.

Repair of margin with 3-0 absorbable suture and gelfoam bolster.

Partial Nephrectomy

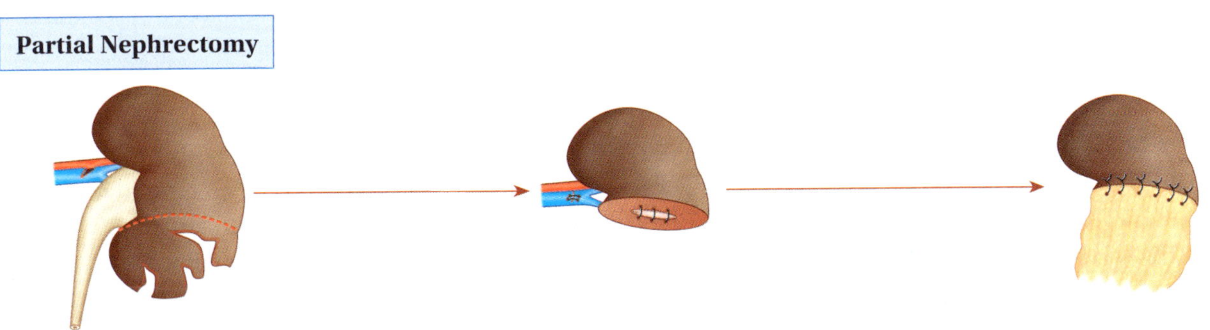

Sharp removal of non-viable tissue.

Water-tight closure of collecting system along with repair of renal artery or vein with 5-0 suture.

Coverage of open parenchyma with omental pedicle flap.

Nephrectomy

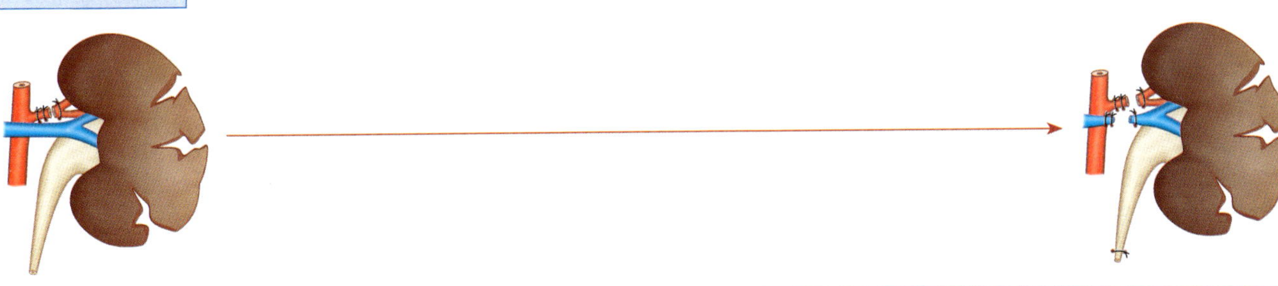

Nephrectomy is indicated in extensive renal injuries in a hemodynamically unstable patient (provided the contralateral kidney is normal).

Ureteral Trauma

Iatrogenic trauma (gynecologic, urologic, colorectal surgeries) is the most common cause of ureteral injury. Blunt trauma and penetrating trauma may also cause ureteral injuries.

Ureteral injuries should be suspected: (i) After rapid deceleration injuries and (ii) Trajectory of the high velocity gunshot wound is near the pathway of ureter.

CT with IV contrast with 10 min delayed image should be performed to exclude ureteral injury.

CT findings suggestive of ureteral injury are contrast extravasation and lack of contrast distal to the suspected injury site.

Treatment: In hemodynamically stable patient, laceration injuries are repaired at the time of laparotomy.

In unstable patient, principles of damage control surgery should be followed. At the time of initial laparotomy, ligation of the ureter followed by placement of percutaneous nephrostomy tube is to be done. Definitive repairs have to planned whenever patient's condition improve.

Ureteral injuries proximal to the iliac vessels are managed by spatulated, tension-free primary ureteral repair over a ureteral stent. If anastomosis is not technically feasible, ureteral reimplantation is done by bladder psoas hitch or Boari bladder flap. **Ureteral injuries distal to the iliac vessels** are treated by tension-free reimplantation (with psoas hitch or flap).

Risk factors for iatrogenic trauma:
- Prior surgery or irradiation
- Advanced malignancy
- Endometriosis
- Anatomical abnormalities
- Major hemorrhage

Iatrogenic trauma can occur by several mechanisms:
- Ligation with suture
- Crushing by hemostatic forceps
- Partial or complete transection
- Thermal injury.

Preventive measures to avoid iatrogenic ureteral trauma:
- Prophylactic preoperative insertion of ureteral stent
- Visual identification of the ureters during peroperative period and careful intraoperative dissection.

Principles of repair of ureteral injury:
- **Mobilization of ureter** 1 cm away to avoid delicate vascular plexus
- Debridement of devitalized tissue
- **Spatulation** of both ends
- **Watertight mucosa-to-mucosa anastomosis** with absorbable sutures
- **Internal stenting**
- Placement of external drain
- Isolation of injury with peritoneum or omentum.

Mobilization of Ureter

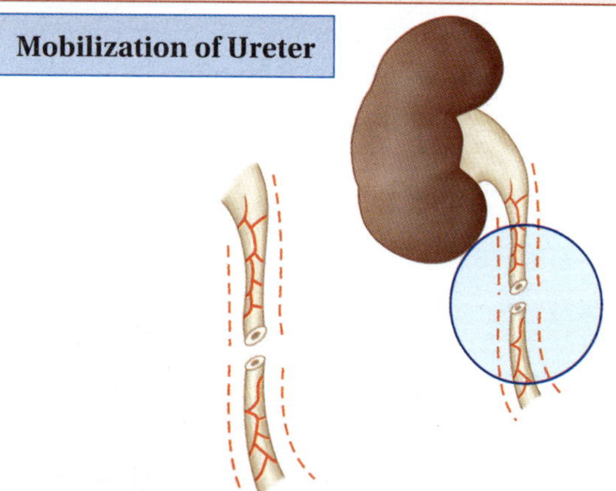

Spatulated, tension free, stented, and watertight anastomosis.

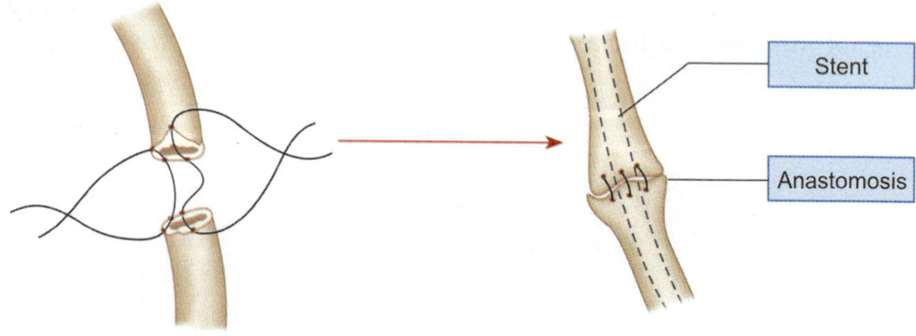

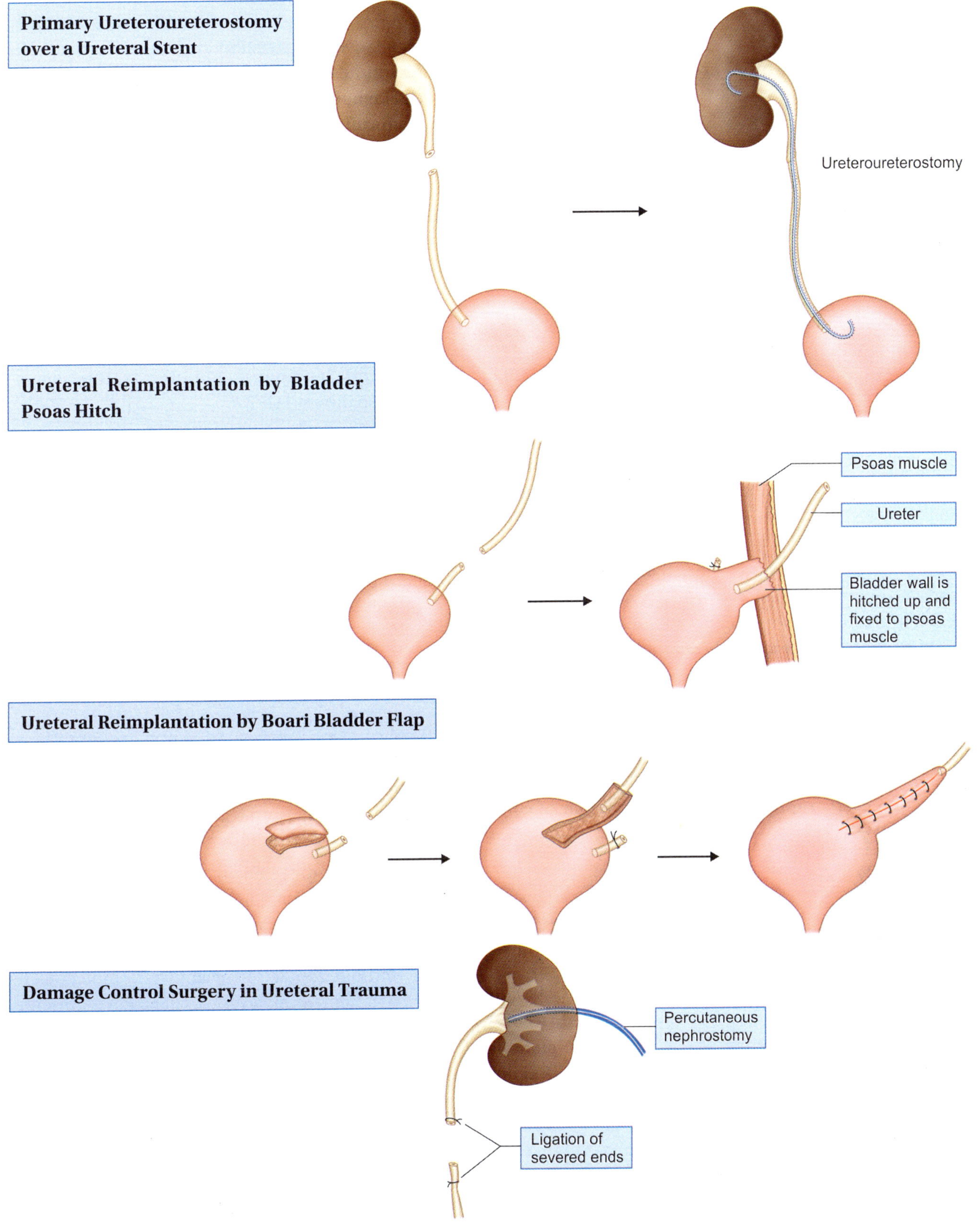
Primary Ureteroureterostomy over a Ureteral Stent
Ureteroureterostomy
Ureteral Reimplantation by Bladder Psoas Hitch
Psoas muscle
Ureter
Bladder wall is hitched up and fixed to psoas muscle
Ureteral Reimplantation by Boari Bladder Flap
Damage Control Surgery in Ureteral Trauma
Percutaneous nephrostomy
Ligation of severed ends

Bladder Injuries

Most of the bladder injuries are extraperitoneal, rest of the injuries are intraperitoneal. A few percentages of patients sustain both extraperitoneal and intraperitoneal injuries.

Mechanisms of extraperitoneal bladder injury: (i) Distortion of pelvic ring, with shearing of contralateral bladder wall near the bladder base and (ii) Direct injury by sharp bony fragments.

Mechanisms of intraperitoneal bladder injury: (i) Sudden increase in intravesical pressure of a distended bladder due to blow to pelvis or lower abdomen; (ii) Penetrating injuries; and (iii) Blast injuries.

Gross hematuria is the most reliable clinical presentation for suspecting bladder injury. Other clinical presentations are inability to void, suprapubic tenderness, and lower abdominal bruising.

CT cystography is the investigation of choice to detect bladder injury. If CT cystography facility is not available, plain film cystography is indicated. In plain film cystography, post-void film can detect lateral and posterior injuries.

Treatment

Uncomplicated extraperitoneal bladder injuries are managed by urethral Foley's catheter drainage (catheter should be left in situ for 2–3 weeks). For complicated extraperitoneal bladder injuries (e.g., exposed bony spicules in bladder lumen, concurrent lacerated injury in rectum or vagina, associated bladder neck injuries), surgical repair is indicated.

Intraperitoneal bladder injuries are managed by two-layer repair with absorbable sutures. During repair, integrity of the bladder neck and ureteral orifices should be confirmed.

Follow-up cystography is indicated after repair of complex injuries.

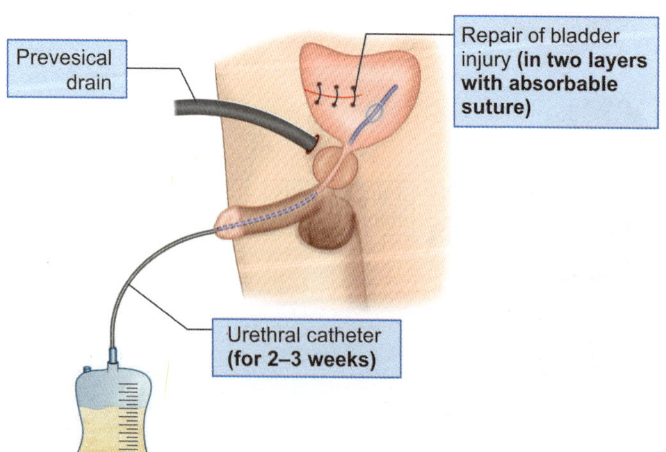

External iatrogenic bladder trauma occurs during:

- Cesarean section
- Radical hysterectomy
- Vaginal hysterectomy
- Abdominal hysterectomy
- Laparoscopic inguinal hernia repair

Signs of external iatrogenic bladder injury are:

- Extravasation of urine
- Clear fluid in surgical field
- Appearance of bladder catheter.

Internal iatrogenic bladder trauma may develop during TURB.

Preventive measures to avoid iatrogenic bladder injury:

- Emptying of bladder by **catheterization** before surgery
- Intraoperatively, **palpation of the balloon of the catheter** to identify bladder.
- **During TURB** for tumors of the lateral wall of urinary bladder, obturator nerve block or GA with adequate muscle relaxation may decrease the chance of bladder injury during TURB.

Management of Iatrogenic Bladder Injury

- If iatrogenic bladder trauma is recognized intraoperatively, the injury should be primarily closed.
- If injury detected in postoperative period, surgical repair is indicated for intraperitoneal injuries. In extraperitoneal injuries, exploration with drainage of the collection with or without repair of the injury is indicated if symptomatic extravesical collection is present.

Urethral Injuries

Urethral injuries are classified into: (i) Injuries to the **posterior urethra** (at or above the membranous urethra) and (ii) Injuries to the **anterior urethra** (penile or bulbar urethra).

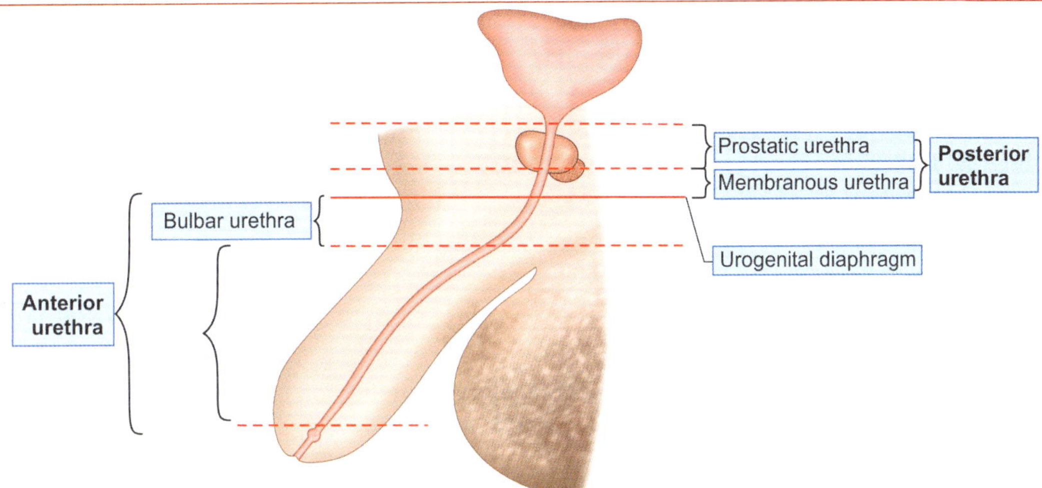

Causes of Urethral Injury

- Iatrogenic
- Blunt trauma (bulbar urethra is commonly injured by straddle injuries)
- Pelvic fracture (causes posterior urethral injuries)
- Insertion of foreign bodies
- Penetrating injuries

Posterior urethral injuries are almost exclusively associated with pelvic fractures.

Urethral injuries are rare in females, if it develops, often caused by pelvic fracture, and commonly associated with rectal or vaginal injuries.

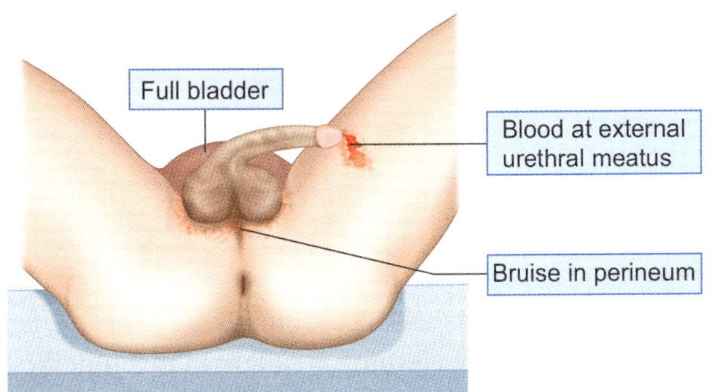

Suspect urethral injury, if:
Blood is at the external meatus
Bruise in the perineum
Bladder full
Bogginess of pelvis.

Iatrogenic Causes of Urethral Injury

- Transurethral catheterization (most of the catheter-induced stricture develop in bulbar urethra)
- Transurethral procedures (e.g., urethral dilation, TURP)
- Radical cystectomy
- Cystectomy

Clinical Presentations Suggestive of Urethral Injury

- Blood at the urethral meatus (most common presentation)
- Inability to urinate
- Perineal or genital ecchymosis
- High-riding prostate and pelvic bogginess on digital rectal examination.

Clinical findings suggestive of urethral injury in female:

- Blood at the vaginal introitus
- Hematuria
- Vaginal laceration
- Urethrorrhagia
- Labial swelling
- Urinary retention

Injury to Bulbar Urethra

- **Most common type** of urethral injury
- Most commonly associated with **straddle injuries** (e.g., accident in loose manhole cover, bicycle accident, gymnasium accident)
- Hematoma following injury is contained by Colles' fascia and patient presents with perineal hematoma.

Injury to Posterior Urethra

- Posterior urethral injuries are almost exclusively associated with **pelvic fracture**.
- **'Straddle fracture'** is associated with high risk of posterior urethral injuries
- **Pelvic fracture urethral injury (PFUI)** is associated with increased incidence of urethral stricture and erectile dysfunction.

Injury to Penile Urethra

- Uncommon type of urethral injury
- This injury commonly develops following penetrating trauma.
- Hematoma following injury is contained by Buck's fascia and dissect along the penile shaft.

Staging of Urethral Injuries Based on Retrograde Urethrography (According to 2004 Consensus Panel on Urethral Trauma)

Anterior urethra

- Partial disruption
- Complete disruption

Posterior urethra

- Stretched but intact
- Partial disruption
- Complete disruption
- Complex (involves bladder neck/ rectum)

Investigations

Retrograde urethrography is the investigation of choice for evaluation of male urethral injury. In suspected female urethral injury, urethroscopy and vaginoscopy are the diagnostic modalities of choice.

Treatment

Straddle injuries of the anterior urethra are initially treated with suprapubic cystostomy. Retrograde urethrogram and/or voiding cysto-urethrogram is recommended to define the site and extent of stricture. For stricture, delayed urethroplasty is recommended.

In penetrating injuries of anterior urethra, immediate surgical repair is recommended.

Pelvic fracture urethral injury (PFUI) is managed by immediate supra-pubic cystostomy followed by delayed urethroplasty. In stable patient, primary endoscopic realignment of the ruptured urethra followed by delayed repair is the preferred treatment. In unstable patient, endoscopic realignment may be considered when patient becomes stable. Open posterior urethroplasty through perineal approach is the most preferred surgical option for urethral distraction injuries. During follow-up period, retrograde urethrogram and cystoscopy are indicated to detect complications (e.g., urethral stricture).

In acute setting of a partial urethral tear, **a single attempt with a well-lubricated catheter** may be attempted by an **experienced one.**

Any undue attempt of catheterization converts an incomplete tear to a complete one.

Penile Injuries

Different types of penile injuries are:

- Degloving injuries
- Zipper injuries
- Human and animal bites
- Strangulation injuries
- Fracture of penis.

Degloving Injuries

- Degloving injuries occur mostly due to industrial accidents where clothing is caught in machinery.
- Management includes copious irrigation of the wound to remove foreign bodies followed by **burying the denuded penile shaft in a scrotal tunnel** or **split thickness skin grafting.**

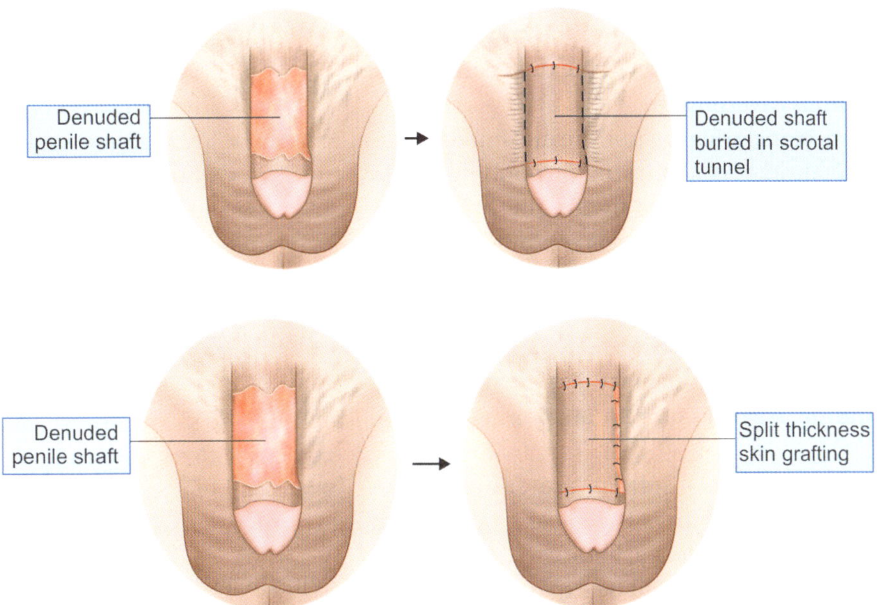

Zipper Injuries

Zipper injuries commonly occur in impatient boys and intoxicated adults.

Most commonly, the foreskin is trapped within the zipper.

Different methods of freeing the entrapped skin:

- Zipper sliding piece and adjacent skin are lubricated and single attempt to unzip.
- Cloth material connected to the zipper is incised perpendicularly between each tooth to release the lateral support of zipper.
- Cutter can be used to cut the median bar of the sliding piece, thereby upper and lower shields of the sliding device fall apart.
- After freeing the entrapped skin, it is essential to assess the injury and then treated accordingly.

Animal and Human Bites

Dog bite is the most common type of bite injury.

Management includes: (i) Copius irrigation of the wound with normal saline; (ii) Debridement (if needed); and (iii) Primary closure after infiltrating Rabies immunoglobulin.

Strangulation Injuries

- Strangulation injuries in children may be caused by accidentally placed thread, rubber band.
- In adults, string, metal constricting device are used for sexual gratification or to prolong erection, that can cause strangulation injuries.
- String, thread, rubber band can be incised without much difficulty. Removal of metal constricting device is technically challenging. Plier can be used to cut the metallic ring. "String technique" is also an effective technique.

String Technique

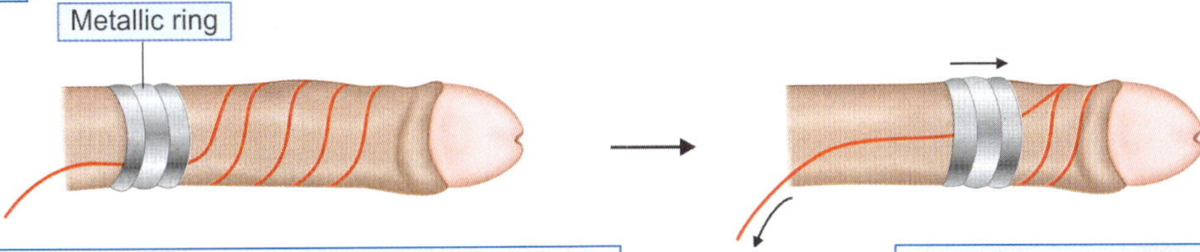

Thick silk or umbilical tape is passed proximally under the strangulating object and wrapped the penis distal to the strangulating object.

Unwinding the tape from proximal end will displace the object distally.

Fracture of Penis

- Fracture of penis involves disruption of the tunica albuginea with rupture of corpus cavernosum.
- Fracture typically occurs during vigorous sexual intercourse.
- Patient commonly describes a cracking or popping sound followed by pain, detumescence and swelling of shaft.
- If Buck's fascia is intact, the hematoma is contained between the skin and tunica, resulting in eggplant deformity.
- If Buck's fascia is disrupted, hematoma is extended to the scrotum, perineum, and suprapubic regions. The penis is often deviated to the side opposite the tunical tear.
- **Urethral evaluation is necessary in all penile fracture patients.**
- Typical history and clinical findings are sufficient for diagnosis. **MRI is indicated if** there is clinical suspicion but absence of typical history and clinical findings.
- All suspected penile fractures should be explored as early as possible.
- Conservative management of penile fracture is not recommended because of increased risk of complications, i.e., penile curvature, impotence, missed urethral disruption, and penile abscess.

Causes of Penile Fracture

- Sexual intercourse
- Forced flexion (taqaandan)
- Masturbation
- Rolling over

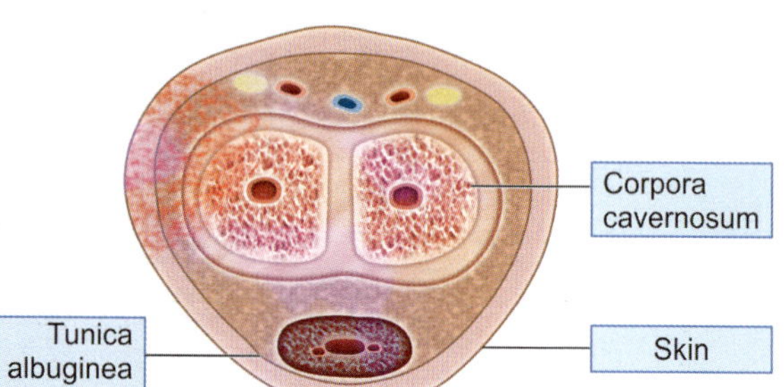

For repair of penile fracture, the conventional surgical approach is through a **circumferential incision proximal to the coronal sulcus.** Longitudinal incisions on the area of fracture or ventral longitudinal approaches are newer approaches.

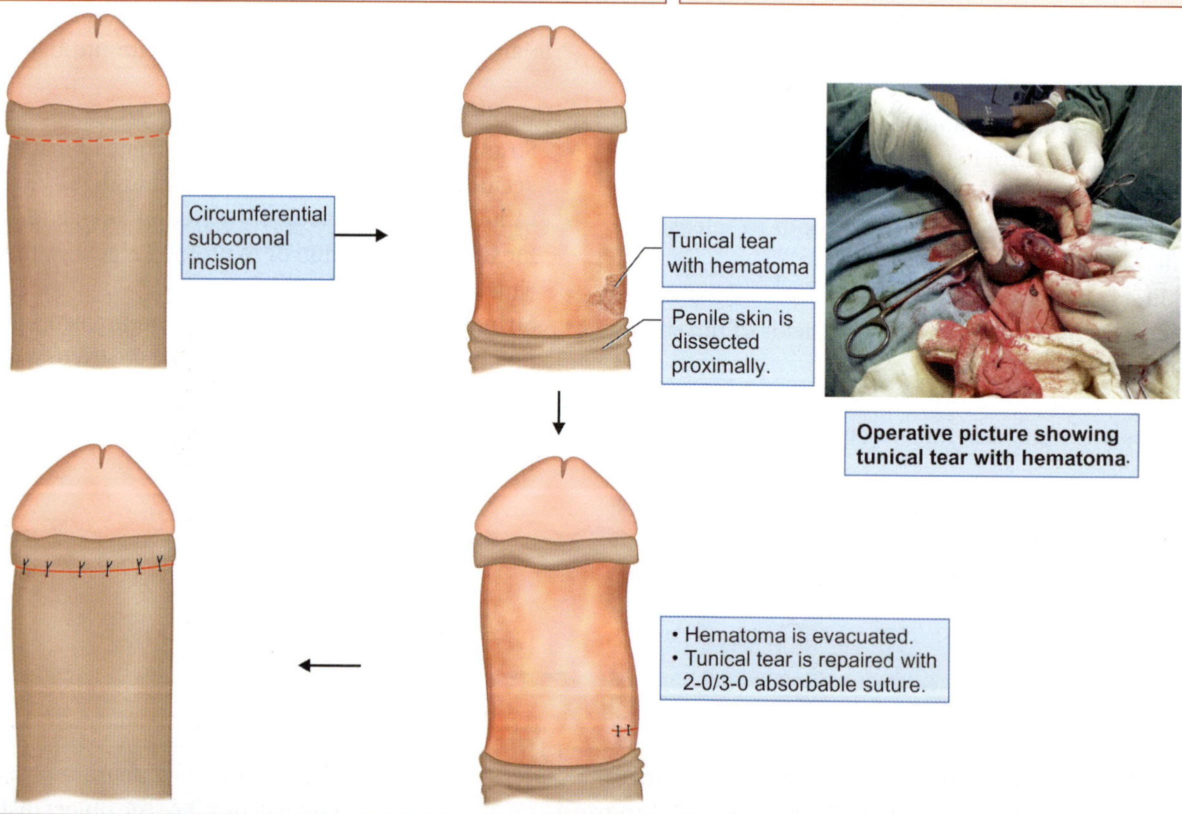

Operative picture showing tunical tear with hematoma.

Deep corporal ligation or excessive debridement of cavernosal tissue must be avoided.

Testicular Injury

- Testicular injury mostly occurs due to blunt trauma (assault, contact sports, motor vehicle accidents)
- Patients present with swelling and ecchymosis.
- USG with Doppler is helpful to assess the integrity as well as vascularity of testis.
- Even small defects in the tunica must be repaired (with absorbable suture).

Rupture of testis must be suspected in every case of blunt scrotal injury.

Salvaging the testis should be attempted, if possible.

Scrotal Injury

Blunt trauma to the scrotum may cause:
(i) Scrotal hematoma; (ii) Hematocele; (iii) Testicular rupture; and (iv) Testicular dislocation.

- Upto 50% scrotal skin loss can be managed by **primary repair**.
- More extensive skin loss warrants placement of testis in **thigh pouches** or wrapping with wet dressing until reconstruction.
- **Meshed split-thickness skin grafting** is indicated for scrotal reconstruction.

Damage Control Surgery

- The concept of 'damage control surgery' is developed to cut-off the vicious cycle of **coagulopathy, hypothermia,** and **metabolic acidosis** resulting from persistent bleeding.
- 'Damage control' should be considered if: **pH <7.2, core temperature <34°C, shock, coagulopathy.**
- **Goal of** 'damage control surgery' is to restore the normal physiology rather than normal anatomy.
- **DCS is divided into 4 phases:** (i) Phase 0 (Pretheater phase); (ii) Phase I (Initial operation); (iii) Phase II (Secondary resuscitation); and (iv) Phase III (Re-operation).

Phase 0 (Pretheater Phase)
Elements of this phase are: (a) Rapid sequence Induction (RSI) of anesthesia and intubation; (b) Early rewarming; and (c) Expedient transport to the operating theater.

Phase I (Initial Operation)

Elements of this phase are:

- Hemorrhage control
- Limitation of contamination (in abdomen)
- Packing of oozing spaces of pleural cavity, abdominal cavity, liver, spleen, retroperitoneum
- Temporary intravascular shunting or ligation of arteries or veins) in abdomen and extremities
- Temporary closure of incisions in abdomen, chest, extremity by towel clip, vacuum-assisted device, silo.

Principles of Damage Control Laparotomy

- Instrument trays consisting of laparotomy set, instruments for chest and vascular surgery, adequate laparotomy pads.
- No leads or tubings should be present on anterior or lateral chest wall (median sternotomy, resuscitative left thoracotomy, and bilateral tube thoracostomy may be necessary).
- Patient is prepped from chin to midthigh and lateral chest wall.
- Incision is vertical midline extending from the xiphoid process to symphysis pubis.
- On entering the peritoneal cavity, first step is hemorrhage control. Damage control principles are to be followed according to type of organ injured and type of injuries.
- Secondly, limitation of contamination by controlling spillage of intestinal contents or urine.
- Temporary closure of incision.

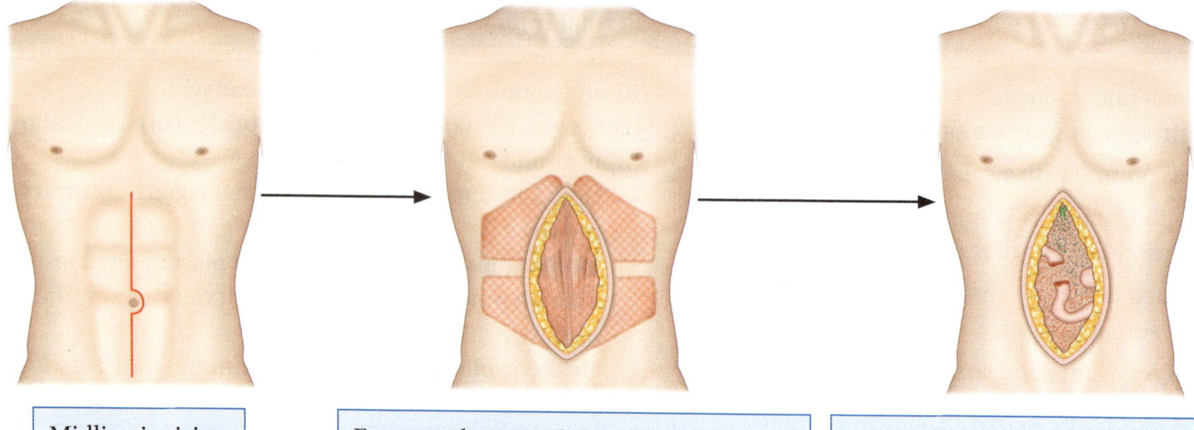

Midline incision

Four quadrant packing, then sequential removal of packing, then control of hemorrhage in particular quadrant.

- Attention is then focused to find out spillage of intestinal contents, bile, or urine.
- No anastomosis, no stoma
- Only drain placement

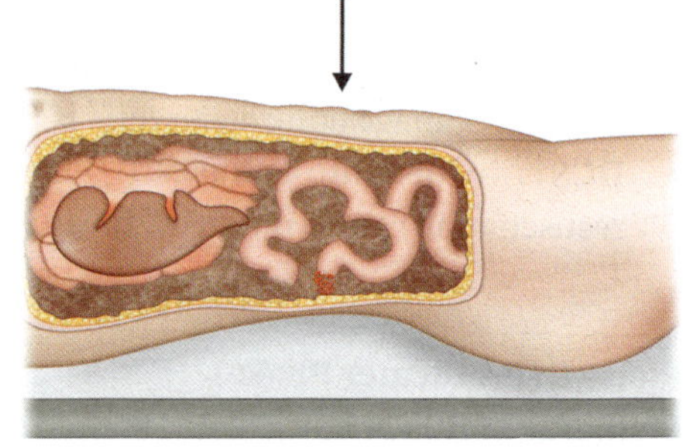

- Laparotomy pads are reinserted.
- No primary fascial closure.
- Temporary closure of incision (Vaccum-assisted closure, Bogota bag, skin closure with towel clips)

Phase II (Secondary Resuscitation)

Elements of this phase are:

- Patient is shifted to ICU from operation theater and focus is given to **correct hypothermia, coagulopathy, and acidosis**. Resuscitation should be continued until physiological parameters are within acceptable range. Hypothermia can be prevented by elevating room temperature, using warm blankets, transfusion of prewarmed IV fluids and blood. Coagulopathy is managed by rapid infusion of FFP, cryoprecipitate, and platelets. Recombinant factor VIIa is also helpful. Reversal of hemodynamic instability corrects the metabolic acidosis.
- **Monitoring of intra-abdominal pressure** for early detection of abdominal compartment syndrome (ACS).
- Taking decision of **timing of re-operation**.

Phase III (Reoperation)

- **Elements of this phase are planned re-exploration and definitive repair,** usually after 48–72 hours after initial operation and optimal secondary resuscitation.
- Early re-operation is indicated in specific conditions (e.g., ongoing transfusion requirements, persistent acidosis despite normal coagulation parameters and core temperature, development of ACS, shunt occlusion in ischemic limb).

Principles of Reoperation

- Copious irrigation of normal saline into packs and then gentle removal (to avoid clot disruption or further visceral damage).
- Thorough re-examination to find any missed injuries.
- Any bleeding is controlled, vascular repair is done, intestinal continuity is restored.
- Complex reconstructions and high-risk anastomoses are better avoided.
- Standard fascial closure must be attempted.
- An abdominal X-ray should be arranged to ensure that all packs have been removed.

Intra-abdominal Hypertension (IAH) and Abdominal Compartment Syndrome (ACS)

Intra-abdominal hypertension (IAH) is defined as sustained Intra-abdominal pressure (IAP) ≥12 mm Hg

Abdominal compartment syndrome (ACS) is defined as sustained IAP >20 mm Hg associated with new organ dysfunction or failure.

Risk Factors for Development of ACS

Related to abdominal collections of fluid, air, or blood:

- Abdominal infection (pancreatitis, peritonitis, abscess)
- Hemoperitoneum
- Major trauma
- Liver dysfunction with ascites

Related to increased Intra-abdominal contents:

- Ileus
- Intraperitoneal or retroperitoneal tumor
- Damage control laparotomy
- Colonic pseudo-obstruction

Related to diminished abdominal wall compliance:

- Burns with abdominal eschars
- Correction of large hernias, gastroschisis, omphalocele
- Abdominal wall bleeding or rectus-sheath hematoma

Medical Treatment Options to Reduce IAP

Improve abdominal wall compliance:

- Sedation and analgesia
- Neuromuscular blockade
- Avoid head of bed >30°

Evacuate intraluminal contents:

- Nasogastric decompression
- Rectal decompression
- Gastro-/colo-prokinetic agents

Evacuate abdominal fluid collections:

- Paracentesis
- Percutaneous drainage

Correct positive fluid balance:

- Avoid excessive fluid resuscitation
- Diuretics
- Colloids/hypertonic fluids
- Hemodialysis/ultrafiltration

Organ support:

- Optimize ventilation, alveolar recruitment

IAP should be monitored every 4 hours during the medical management of IAH.

If abdominal compartment syndrome develops, surgical abdominal decompression should be strongly considered.

(**Adapted from guidelines of the World Society of the Abdominal Compartment Syndrome**).

- **Normal IAP** is 5–7 mm Hg
- **The reference standard** for intermittent IAP measurements is via the urinary bladder with a maximal instillation volume of 25 mL of sterile saline.
- **IAP should be expressed** in mm Hg and measured at end-expiration in the supine position after ensuring that abdominal muscle contractions are absent and with the transducer zeroed at the level of the midaxillary line.

Grading of IAH:

Grade I, IAP 12–15 mm Hg

Grade II, IAP 16–20 mm Hg

Grade III, IAP 21–25 mm Hg

Grade IV, IAP >25 mm Hg

Complications of Increased IAP

- Decreased cardiac output and venous return.
- Reduction in blood flow to liver, kidneys, and intestines.
- Diaphragms are displaced to thoracic side, leading to decreased thoracic volume.
- Elevation of CVP, pulmonary capillary wedge pressure, right atrial pressure.

Timing of Intervention in Different Compartmental Syndromes

Immediate decompression: Thoracic compartment syndrome (due to tension pneumothorax), Mediastinal compartment syndrome (due to cardiac tamponade), Orbital compartment syndrome (due to trauma, retrobulbar hemorrhage).

Early decompression (within 3–12 hours from diagnosis): Extremity compartment syndrome (due to trauma, crush injuries, full thickness burn), abdominal compartment syndrome, compartment syndrome in brain (refractory elevated intracranial pressure).

Open Abdomen

Open abdomen (OA) is defined as intentional decision to leave the fascial edges of the abdomen un-approximated after laparotomy to decrease the risk of development of IAH/ACS or to facilitate re-exploration.

Indications:

Trauma patients: (i) Persistent hypotension, acidosis (pH <7.2), hypothermia (temperature <34°C); (ii) In 'Damage control surgery'; (iii) Post-traumatic bowel injuries where re-evaluation of bowel perfusion is indicated; and (iv) Extreme visceral or retroperitoneal swelling.

Non-trauma patients: (i) In vascular emergencies, e.g., ruptured abdominal aortic aneurysm; (ii) In severe peritonitis with sepsis, where a second-look surgery is indicated; and (iii) In severe acute pancreatitis, if step-up conservative management is not effective, surgical decompression and open abdomen approach may be indicated.

Complications of open abdomen: (i) Enteroatmospheric fistula; (ii) Frozen abdomen; (iii) Intra-abdominal abscess; and (iv) Ventral hernia.

Management includes: (i) Damage control resuscitation; (ii) Serial measurement of IAP (particularly in patients at risk of ACS); (iii) Temporary abdominal closure; (iv) Nutritional support (to manage the hypermetabolic state); (v) Re-exploration; (vi) Definitive closure; and (vii) Management of complications.

Delayed decompression (after 12 hours from diagnosis): Extremity compartment syndrome, brain (refractory elevated intracranial pressure).

Prophylactic decompression: In extremity (following vascular injuries, revascularized acute limb ischemia), in brain (following post-traumatic intracranial hematoma, in ischemic and hemorrhagic strokes).

Open Abdomen Classification (Bjork Classification 2016)

1A Clean open abdomen (OA) without adherence between bowel and abdominal wall or fixity

B Contaminated OA without adherence/fixity

C Enteric leak, no fixation

2A Clean OA developing adherence/fixity

B Contaminated OA developing adherence/fixity

C Enteric leak, developing fixation

3A Clean, frozen abdomen

B Contaminated, frozen abdomen

4 Established enteroatmospheric fistula, frozen abdomen

Techniques of Temporary Abdominal Closure

- Skin only closure (skin staples, towel clips or sutures)
- 'Bogota' bag (sterile 3 liter saline bag is shaped and sutured to fascial edges)
- Negative pressure wound therapy with a dynamic component (mesh-mediated fascial traction or dynamic sutures)
- Negative pressure wound therapy without a dynamic component (Barker's VAC)
- Opsite Sandwich technique (Polyethylene sheet, Opsite dressings, abdominal packs, two suction drains, and wall suction)
- Absorbable mesh (e.g., vicryl mesh)

Negative pressure wound therapy with continuous fascial traction is the preferred technique of temporary abdominal closure.

Techniques of Definitive Abdominal Closure

Non-mesh mediated techniques:

- Primary fascial closure
- Component separation technique
- Planned ventral hernia (only skin graft or skin closure)—indicated in presence of enteroatmospheric fistula.

Mesh-mediated techniques:

- Non-crosslinked biologic mesh in sublay position
- Crosslinked biologic mesh in fascial-bridge position
- NPWT in combination with biologic mesh

Case 1

History and Physical Examination

A 28-year-old male patient presented with history of road-traffic accident about 8 hours back. Patient was initially treated in local hospital and then referred to higher center. Patient complained of pain abdomen without any other symptoms. Patient had no history of unconscious, vomiting, convulsion, and bleeding from ear. No history of respiratory difficulty.

Physical examination

- Patient alert; conscious; cooperative; GCS 15/15
- Pulse 116/min; BP 90/62 mm Hg; Respiratory rate 18/min
- Abdomen soft, bruise marks present over the left hypochondrium and left lower chest wall
- Chest auscultation revealed no obvious abnormality.

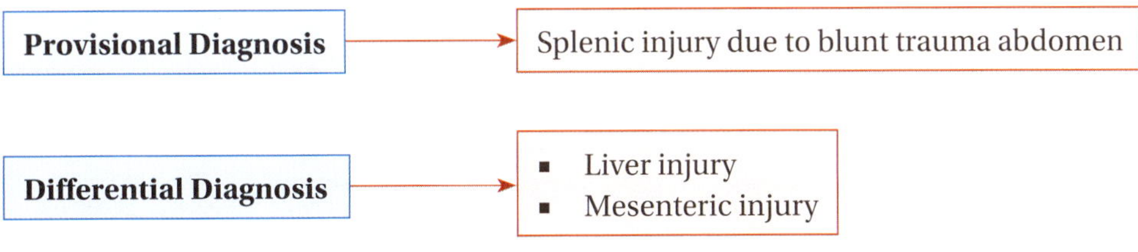

Investigations

FAST revealed moderate amount of free fluid in the peritoneal cavity. Chest X-ray revealed no evidence of hemothorax or pneumothorax.

Discussion

Young male patient presented with history of RTA with clinical features suggestive of hypovolemic shock. Bruise marks in left hypochondrium and left lower chest wall indicative of splenic injury. FAST confirmed the presence of blood in the peritoneal cavity. Chest X-ray excluded any hemothorax or pneumothorax. Decision of urgent laparotomy was taken based on the response of the patient to fluid resuscitation.

Management Algorithm

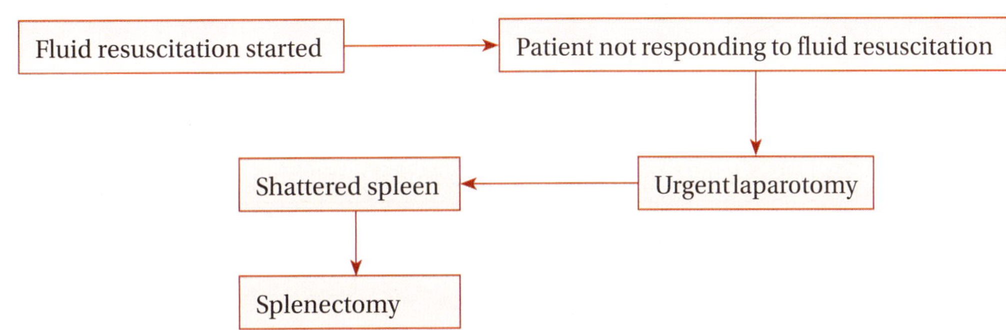

Case 2

History and Physical Examination

An 18-year-old male patient presented in the surgical emergency with a history of injury in the head by a cricket bat about 3 hours back. Patient complained nausea and pain over the site of trauma. Patient had no history of unconsciousness or convulsion. Patient had two episodes of vomiting.

Physical examination

- GCS 13/15; Pulse 62/min; BP 108/76 mm Hg
- *Pupil:* Bilateral equal, reacting to light
- On palpation, lacerated scalp with depression of the right parietal bone noted
- No neuromuscular deficit
- *Chest:* Normal vesicular breath sound

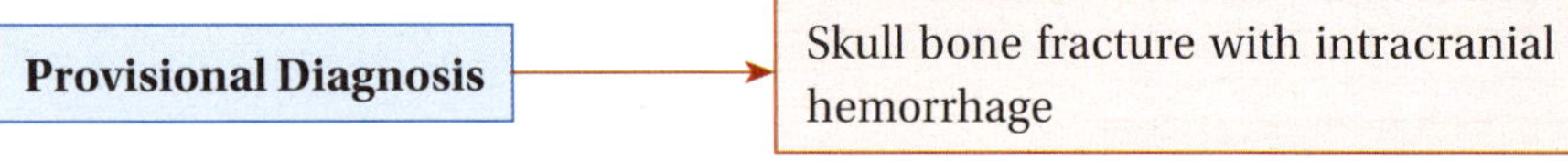

Investigations

Noncontrast CT brain revealed extradural hematoma in the right parietal region along with undepressed fracture of the parietal bone. The midline shift was 3 mm.

Discussion

A young male patient presented with history of head injury by an blunt object. Clinical examination revealed GCS 13/15 and scalp laceration along with depressed parietal bone. Noncontrast CT brain revealed EDH with undepressed parietal bone fracture along with midline shift of 3 mm. As patient's GCS was 13/15, skull fracture was undepressed and EDH with midline shift of only 3 mm, surgical management was not planned.

Management Algorithm

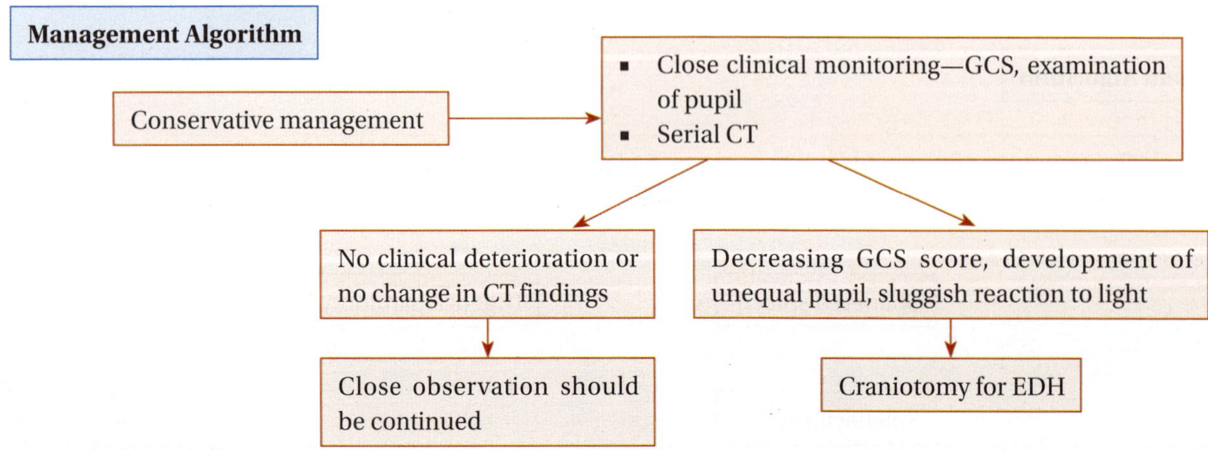

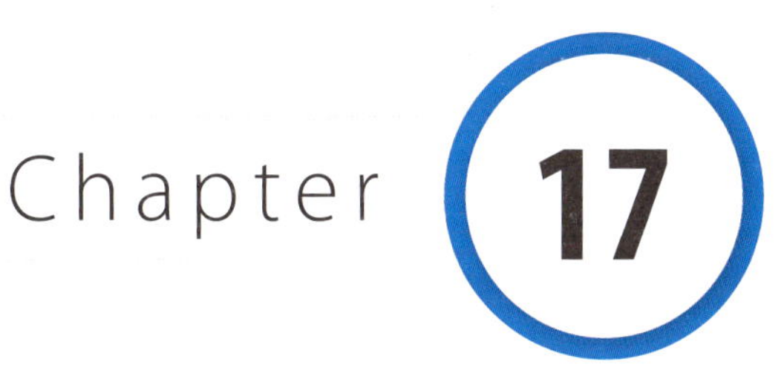

Chapter 17

Burn

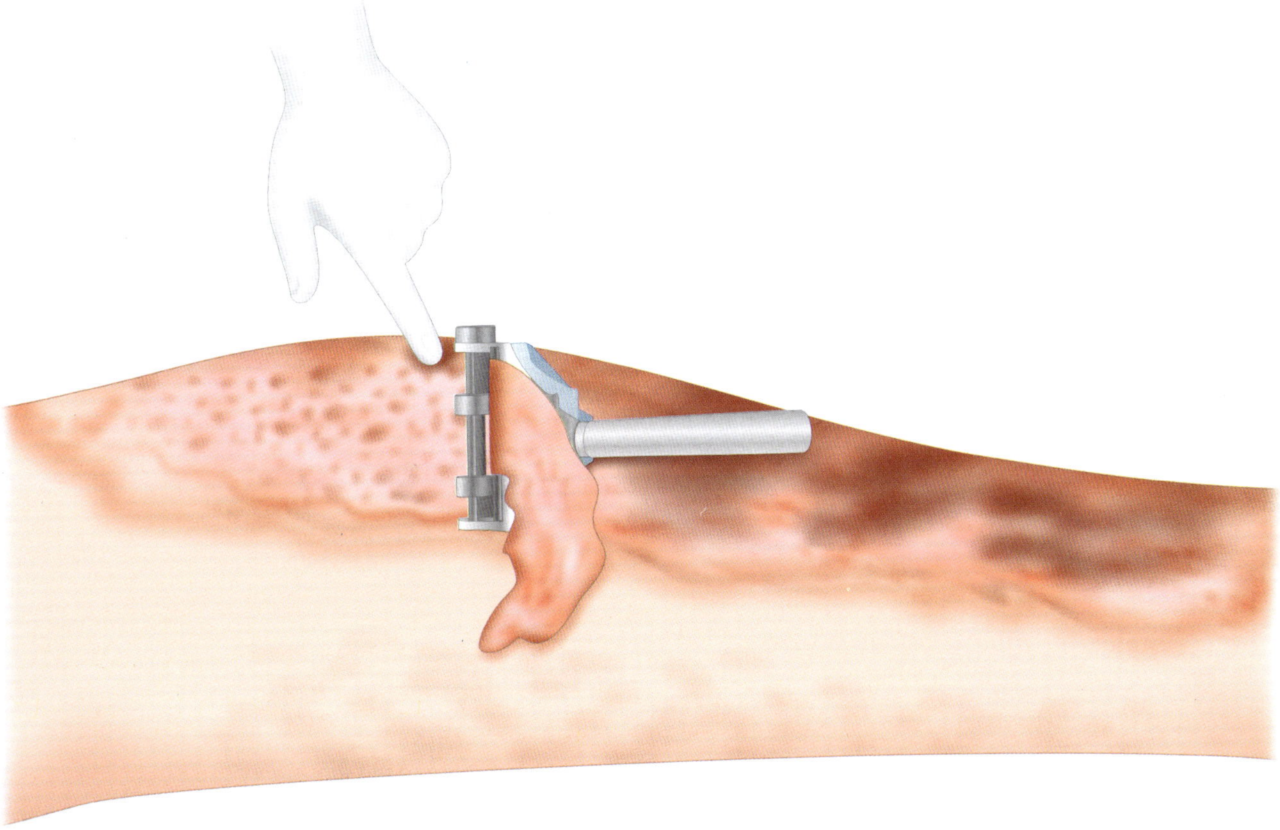

Important Topics

- Mechanisms of Burn Injury
- Management of Burn Injury
- Systemic Changes in Burn
- Electric Burn
- Chemical Burn
- Late Complications of Burn

'Clinical science has as good a claim to the name and rights and self subsistence of a science as any other department of biology.'

James Paget (1814–1899)
British Surgeon and Physiologist

Mechanisms of Burn Injury

Burn injury implies injury of skin and its contents by thermal, electrical, chemical energies or its combinations.

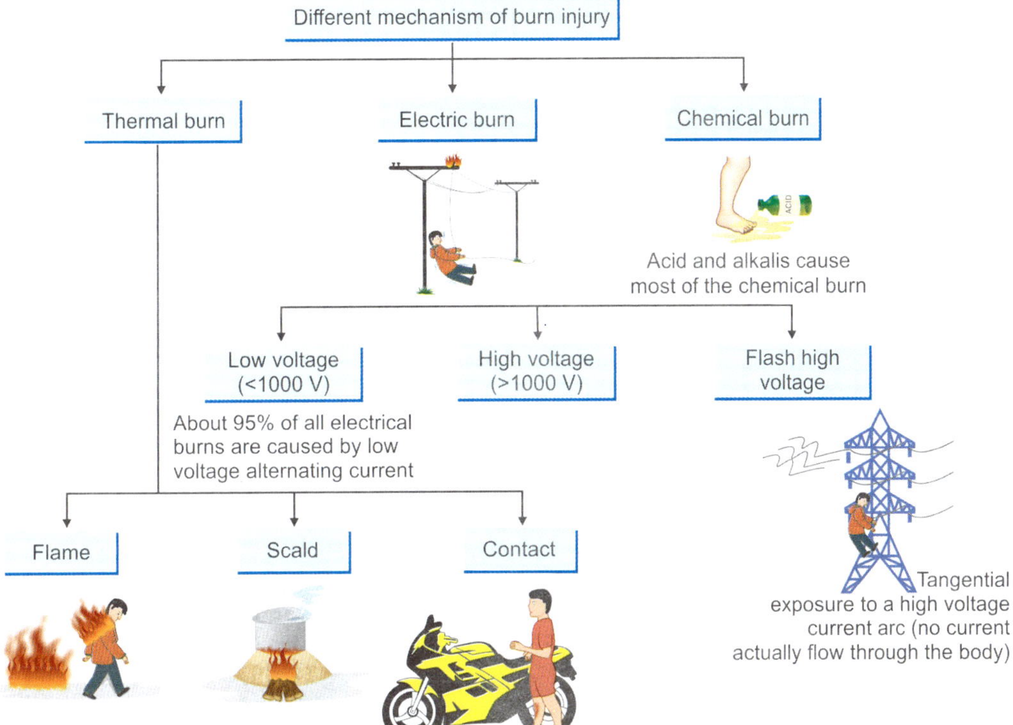

Flame burn

- Ignition of clothing during cooking
- Improper use of stoves
- Use of open fires at night of winter season
- Smoking related (smoking in the mosquito net)

Scald

- Scald from hot water—most commonly
- Thick soup, hot oil, sauces also cause scald.
- Tar and Asphalt burn are a special kind of scald

Contact burn

- Contact with hot metals, plastic, hot coals
- In motor vehicle accidents, contact with hot engine parts
- The exhaust pipe of motorcycle cause a characteristic burn in the medial aspect of lower leg

Exposed areas of skin tend to be burned less deeply than clothed areas, because clothing retains the heat as well as the hot liquid for longer period.

Immersion scald burns are usually deep burns, spill scald burns are not so deep.

Criteria for referring to a specialized burn unit (Adapted from Wound International guideline)

- >10% TBSA in children and >15% TBSA in adults
- Full thickness burn in any age group and any percentage of TBSA
- Deep dermal burns >5% TBSA in adults and all deep dermal burns in children
- All chemical and electrical burns; exposure to ionizing radiation; high-pressure steam injury; suspected nonaccidental injury
- Age <10 or >49 years
- Burn in face, hands, genitals or perineum
- Burn in any flexural surface such as neck, axilla, front of the elbows or back of the knee
- Circumferential deep burns in any age group
- Burn with a suspicion of inhalation injury
- Burn with associated injuries (fractures, head injury or crush injury)
- Burn patients who require social, emotional or long-term rehabilitation.

Management of Burn Injury

At the Scene

- Burned patients must be removed from the source of injury.
- All burned clothes are removed as soon as possible.
- Rings, watches, jewelery, diaper must be removed as it retain heat and produce a tourniquet like effect when edema develops.
- Room temperature water can be poured in the wound to reduce the depth of burn.
- **Iced water should not be used:** Causes systemic hypothermia and further thermal damage due to cutaneous vasoconstriction.
- Patient must be covered with a clean blanket to limit hypothermia. Pediatric patients are at high risk of hypothermia.
- **Inhalation injury is always suspected** and 100% oxygen should be given by facemask.
- Emergency medical personnel should start IV fluid administration with lactated ringer solution
- In high voltage electrical injuries or carbon monoxide poisoning, CPR may be warranted.
- If patient is unconscious or in respiratory distress, endotracheal intubation should be performed (if facility and expertise is available).

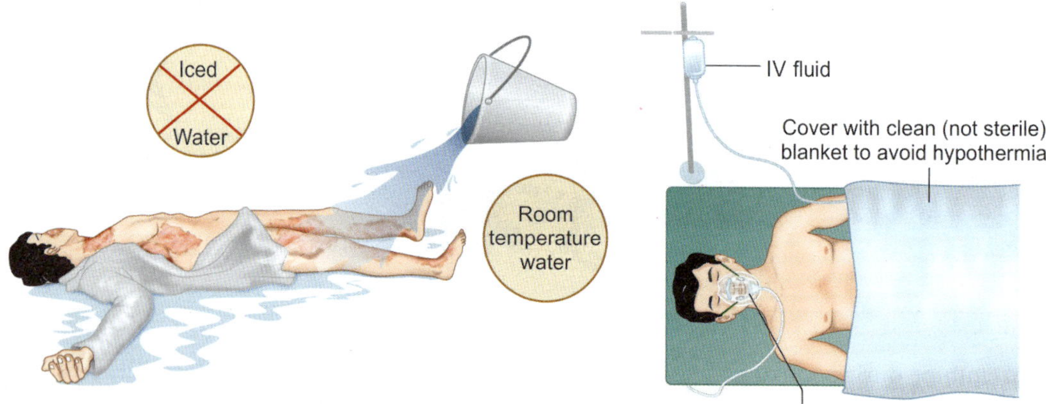

In the Emergency

- All burn patients must be assessed by **primary survey** and **secondary survey**.
- Burned patients should be evaluated and treated as patients of **polytrauma** because of associated injuries secondary to explosion, fall or escape attempts.
- **Primary survey includes:** (i) Airway management; (ii) Breathing and ventilation; (iii) Circulation; (iv) Disability; and (v) Exposure.
- **Airway management:** Early endotracheal intubation is indicated in: (i) Symptomatic inhalation injury; (ii) Thermal injury to the face, neck, oropharynx; and (iii) Symptoms and signs of impending airway compromise.
- The decision of intubation should be made early to avoid difficult intubation or intubation failure.
- Emergency tracheostomy is indicated if there is intubation failure.
- Management of compromised airway: (i) Jaw-thrust maneuver; (ii) Chin lift; (iii) Endotracheal intubation; and (iv) Tracheostomy.

Symptoms and Signs of Impending Airway Compromise

- Singed facial hair
- Carbonaceous sputum
- Soot in or around the mouth
- Hoarseness
- Stridor
- Wheezing.

Inhalation injury is suspected if:

- History of burn injury in a closed space
- Carbonaceous sputum
- Hoarseness
- Wheeze
- Diminished consciousness
- Presence of soot in the oral cavity.

Breathing

- Rhonchi or crepitation suggest inhalation injury or aspiration.
- Severely burned patients may develop early respiratory failure. Circumferential burns in trunk and neck may impair respirations

Circulation

- Burn causes both hypovolemic and distributive shock-due to release of inflammatory mediators.
- Due to fluid shift from intravascular compartment to the interstitial spaces.
- Due to evaporative fluid loss from the injury site.

Disability

Associated injuries, substance use, inhalation injury must be considered during assessment.

Exposure

All clothes should be removed to prevent further injury from the burnt clothes and to assess the BSA involved. Burn area must be irrigated with normal saline to remove burned residues.

Secondary Survey

Secondary survey includes estimation of percentage of burn and assessment of depth of burn.

Estimation of percentage of burn (% TBSA):

- **Wallace's "rule of nines":** (i) A quick and effective method for assessment in adults; (ii) Not so accurate; and (iii) Tends to overestimate TBSA.
- **Lund-Browder chart:** For infants and children.
- **"Rule of the palm":** (i) Indicated for smaller and odd-shaped burn; (ii) Palmar surface of the patient's hand including the digits is 1% TBSA; and (iii) Not accurate for medium sized burn.

Superficial or first-degree burn should not be calculated within the TBSA calculation.

Assessment of depth of burn:

- Depth of burn is the primary determinant of patient's functional and cosmetic outcome.
- According to depth, burn injury is divided into—first degree, second degree, third degree, and fourth degree.
- When nonoperative treatment is the main approach, accurate assessment of depth of burn is of little importance.
- When operative treatment is the main approach, accurate assessment of depth is crucial.
- Clinical assessment by an experienced surgeon is accurate in most of the cases. Other methods of assessment are: (i) Ultrasound; (ii) Laser Doppler; (iii) Thermography; and (iv) Light reflectance method.

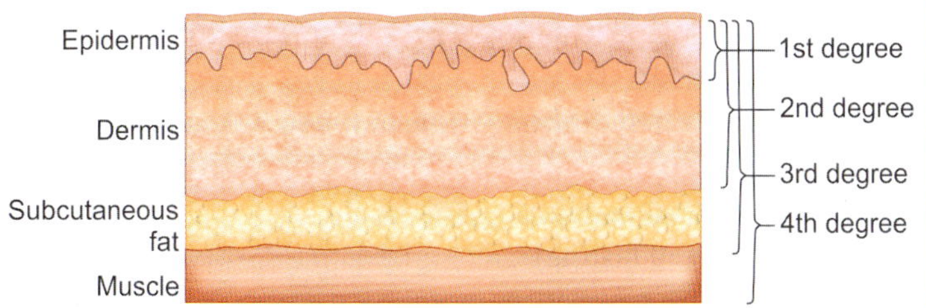

Importance of Estimation of %TBSA

- To take decision whether patient will be transferred to specialized burn center or not
- To calculate the amount of fluid for resuscitation.
- To calculate the calorie requirements.

Wallace's "Rule of Nines"

- Head (anterior and posterior): 9%
- Anterior trunk: 18%
- Back: 18%
- Each upper extremity: 9%
- Each lower extremity: 18%
- Perineum and genitalia: 1%
- 'Rule of nines' is accurate for adults, but not for pediatric patients. Infants and children have a proportionally greater BSA in the head and neck and less in the lower extremities.

First degree

- Limited to epidermis
- Painful burn
- No blisters
- Spontaneous healing after 3–4 days

Second degree

- Limited to dermis
- Painful burn
- Blister develops.

Third degree

- All layers of skin and its appendages, sensory fibers for touch, pain, temperature and pressure and damaged
- Painless burn.

Fourth degree

Also involve fascia, muscle and bone.

Zones of Burn Wound

Zone of Coagulation/Necrosis

- At the center of the wound
- No tissue perfusion
- Irreversible tissue damage due to coagulation necrosis

Zone of Stasis

- Surrounding the zone of coagulation
- Decreased tissue perfusion
- Release of mediators
- Tissue repair may happen

Zone of Hyperemia

- At the periphery of the wound
- Good tissue perfusion
- Chance of tissue repair is maximum.

Treatment

Treatment of Inhalation Injury [adapted from ISBI guideline]

- Moderate elevation of the head of bed (facilitates venous and lymphatic drainage)
- Supplemental oxygen by mask
- Airway must be cleared of secretions and debris by suctioning
- Endotracheal intubation (if symptoms and signs of airway obstruction are present)
- Treatment of CO poisoning: (i) Administration of 100% oxygen, preferably by a non-rebreathing mask, at a rate of 8–15 L/min, for at least 6 hour (100% oxygen shortens the half-life of COHb from 4 hour to 40–60 min) and (ii) Intubation and mechanical ventilation may be indicated (as per level of consciousness)
- Treatment of HCN poisoning: (i) High-flow oxygen and (ii) Immediate administration of hydroxycobalamin (hydroxycobalamin binds to cyanide).

Components of Inhalation Injury

- Obstruction of the upper airway (due to edema in first 24–48 hours)
- Injury of the lower airway (by combustion products in smoke)
- Carbon monoxide (CO) and hydrogen cyanide (HCN) poisoning.

Treatment of Burn Injuries

(i) Oxygen supplementation; (ii) Fluid resuscitation; (iii) Tetanus immunization; (iv) Analgesia; (v) Stress ulcer prophylaxis; (vi) Cleansing of burn wound; (vii) Burn wound dressing; (viii) Management of sepsis; (ix) Escharotomy; (x) Management of blisters; (xi) Surgical management of burn wound; (xii) Nutritional support; and (xiii) Rehabilitation.

Fluid Resuscitation

Principles of fluid resuscitation (adapted from ISBI guideline):

- Early initiation of appropriate resuscitation
- Both over and under-resuscitation should be avoided (over-resuscitation can result in compartment syndrome of extremities and abdomen, airway compromise and under-resuscitation can result in hypoperfusion, renal failure).
- Patients with inhalation injuries, electrical burns, and delayed resuscitation need additional fluid.
- Patients with burn <30% TBSA can be resuscitated by oral fluid.
- Pediatric patients require more fluid comparable to those of adults (due to increase in body surface area-to-weight ratio).
- Resuscitation formulas serve as a guide, resuscitation should be titrated to obtain urine output 0.3–0.5 mL/kg/hour in adults and 1.0 mL/kg/hour in children.
- A source of glucose should be added to resuscitation fluid as well as maintenance fluid in pediatric patients (in pediatric population, glycogen stores deplete after 12–14 hours of fasting).

Access for fluid resuscitation:

(i) Peripheral intravenous access; (ii) Central venous access; and (iii) Intraosseous access (in pediatric patients). Central venous access should be used when peripheral access is not feasible.

Type of fluid and amount of fluid:

- For the first 24 hours, **Ringer lactate** is the IV fluid of choice. Amount of fluid is calculated by **modified Parkland formula. The formula is:** Total calculated volume of RL for 24 hours = [4 × body wt (in kg) × % BSA] mL
- Half of the calculated volume is given in the first 8 hours, rest half is given in the next 16 hours.
- The time is calculated from the time of injury, not from when patient is attended. Prehospital fluid resuscitation volume must be subtracted from the total estimated volume.
- Formula is for a near accurate estimation of fluid, more or less fluid is further determined according to urine output (30–50 mL/hours).
- **Role of colloid:** For first 24 hours postburn period, colloid infusion increases mortality, rather than beneficial. After 24 hours, colloid may be used to decrease the total volume of crystalloids, thereby minimizing the cardiopulmonary and electrolyte related complications.

Monitoring urine output:

- Catheterization (with Foley's catheter) is indicated to monitor urine output (reliable index of adequate resuscitation).
- Urine output 1 mL/kg/hour in children (≤30 kg) and 0.5 mL/kg/hour in adults is indicative of adequate fluid resuscitation.

Tetanus Prophylaxis

- Tetanus immunization is indicated because burn is a tetanus—prone wound.
- Immunization within 5 years—no prophylaxis
- Immunization within 10 years—booster dose of tetanus toxoid.
- Unknown immunization status—tetanus immunoglobulin (250 IU) + Tetanus toxoid.

Site of toxoid and immunoglobulin injection should not be in same arm

Analgesia

- During shock phase, opioid analgesics should be given intravenously.
- IV opioid analgesics should be given in small doses to avoid hypotension, respiratory depression.

Stress Ulcer Prophylaxis

By H_2 blockers or proton pump inhibitors.

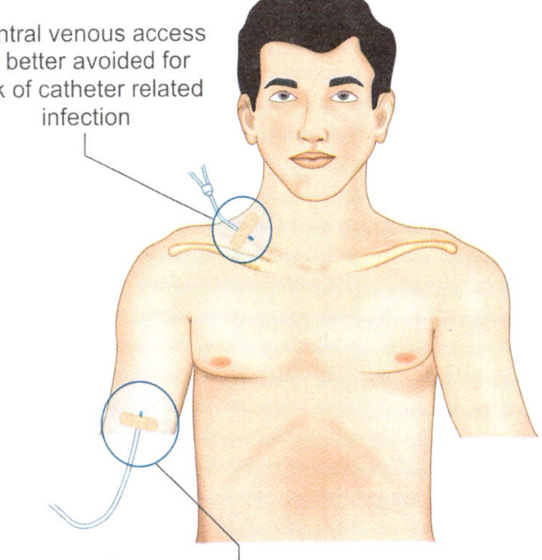

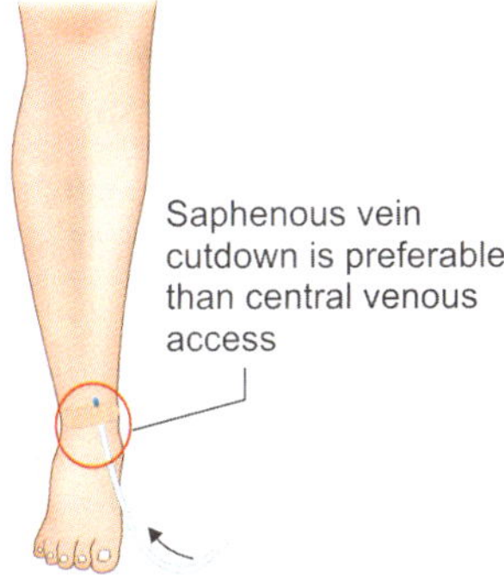

Other Formulas for Calculation of Fluid

- Brooke formula
- Modified Brooke formula
- Galveston formula—for pediatric patients.

Opioid analgesics in intramuscular route should not be given in shock phase, because of variable absorption due to peripheral vasoconstriction. Injected opioid analgesics form a pool at the site of injection.

When resuscitation becomes adequate, there is sudden pooling of the drug in the circulation, leading to hypotension, oversedation and particularly respiratory depression.

Cleansing of Burn Wound

- Wound cleansing is indicated to remove foreign bodies, wound debris, excess exudates, microorganisms (in case of infected wound), superficial slough.
- For clean wounds, cleansing should be gentle so not to injure the deeper layers of the epidermis
- In infected wounds, aggressive cleansing is indicated
- The cleansing should be either mechanical or surgical
- Cleansing wound with antiseptic/antimicrobial solution after mechanical or surgical cleansing is indicated particularly in infected wound.

Escharotomy

Escharotomy nullifies the tourniquet effect of any eschar that affects distal perfusion.

Indications:

- Circumferential or near circumferential eschar of the extremities compromising the circulation distal to it.
- Eschar on the trunk or neck compromises aeration and breathing
- Circumferential or near circumferential abdominal eschar causing intra-abdominal hypertension or abdominal compartment syndrome.

Principles of escharotomy:

- Escharotomy should be done at least 72 hours after burn injury.
- Systemic causes of distal hypoperfusion (e.g., hypovolemia, decreased cardiac output) should be ruled out before considering escharotomy.
- Escharotomy should be done whenever indicated, without delay.
- The length and depth of escharotomies should be adequate.
- Incision should not be too deep to damage nerves or tendons.
- In limb, incisions are longitudinal and in the mid-axial lines (medial and lateral). In hands and feet, incisions are on the dorsum.
- In trunk, incisions are along the anterior axillary lines with bilateral subcostal and subclavicular extensions.
- The extent of the incision in the eschar should range from normal skin to normal skin, if possible, to ensure decompression. If not possible, from joint above to joint below.
- Depth of incision should be at the level of upper subcutaneous fat.

Escharotomy is done either by scalpel or by electrosurgery without any anesthesia (general anesthesia for infants and young children) and can be performed at bedside.

Management of Blisters

- **Leaving blisters intact:** In small vesicles not impending to rupture or not interfering movements or dressing.
- **Deroofing of blister:** Large blisters impede the mobility of the patient or wall of the blisters thin and likely to rupture.
- **Snip open the vesicle:** Large blisters impending to rupture or impedes movement or dressing.
- **Blisters on the palm of the hand should be left intact unless they restrict movements.**
- **Small blisters overlying superficial burns** is better to leave intact because the blisters offer protection of the underlying dermis and permit healing in a sterile environment.
- **Blisters overlying larger areas of burn** is better to debride because the blister fluid contains inflammatory mediators that impairs local microcirculation.

Assessment of distal perfusion by:

- Capillary filling in the nail beds
- Doppler flowmetry
- Pulse oximetry

Adequate escharotomy is indicated by:

- Bulging of the subcutaneous fat from the base of the incision
- Absence of fibrous bands in the incision
- Profuse exudation of edema fluid from the wound.

Complications of Escharotomy

- Inadequate length and depth
- Bleeding
- Injury to neurovascular bundles.

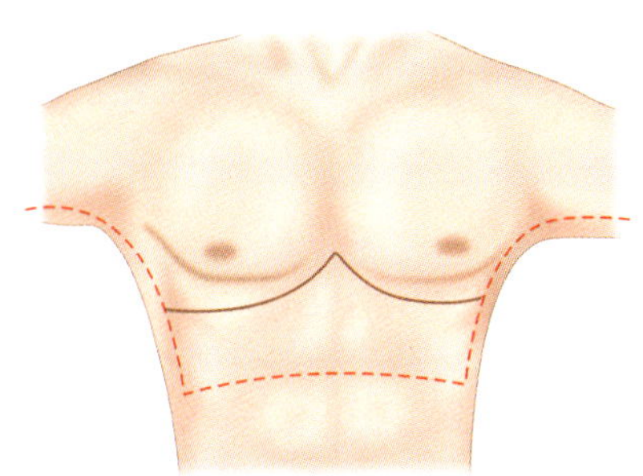

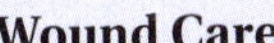

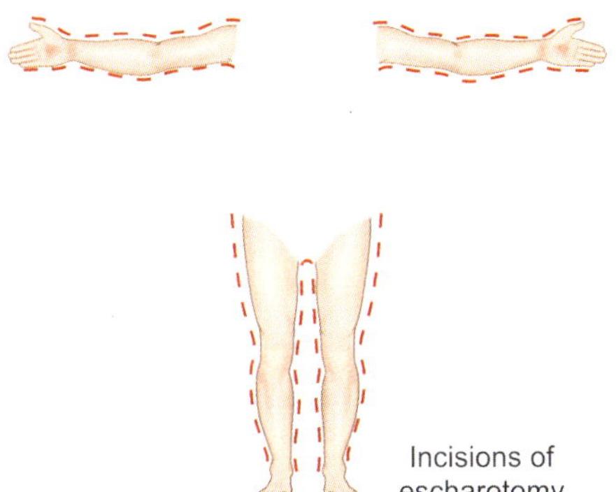

Incisions of escharotomy

Wound Care

Wound care includes: (i) Wound dressing; (ii) Application of topical antimicrobials; and (iii) Surgical management of burn wound.

Wound dressing

Superficial epidermal burn: Aloe vera gel or moisturizing cream

Superficial dermal burn:

- Moderate to high exuding wound—Absorbent dressing, e.g., foams, alginates, CMC, hydrocolloid
- Low exuding wound—Silicone wound contact layer
- Contaminated wound—Silver sulfadiazine or silver-impregnated dressings

Deep dermal burn:

- Sloughy wound—Hydrogels or honey
- Moderate to high exuding wound—Foams, alginates
- Contaminated wound—Silver sulfadiazine or silver-impregnated dressings.

Topical antimicrobials

- Topical antimicrobials are not indicated for superficial epidermal burn, but indicated for superficial dermal burn and deep dermal burn.
- Commonly used topical antimicrobials for burn wound are—Silver sulfadiazine, Mafenide acetate, Bacitracin

Silver Sulfadiazine

- Most commonly used topical antimicrobial.
- Broad spectrum coverage (gram-positive and gram-negative bacteria, fungus).
- Painless application.
- Transient leukopenia after 3–5 days. It resolves spontaneously. No need of cessation of application.

Mafenide Acetate

- Broad spectrum activity (due to sulfa moiety)
- Particularly effective against resistant pseudomonas, enterococcus species.
- Can penetrate eschar **[Silver sulfadiazine can't]**
- Carbonic anhydrase inhibitory property, so it may cause metabolic acidosis.

Advantages of Wound Dressing

- Protect the damaged epithelium
- Minimizes bacterial and fungal colonization
- Reduce evaporative heat loss
- Gives comfort in a painful wound.

Closed dressing

- Closed dressing is indicated if early excision (tangential excision and grafting) is planned
- Closed dressing maintains soft eschar, that is helpful for tangential excision
- Prolongs the contact of antimicrobial agent with the eschar.

Open dressing

- It is the most cost-effective method of burn care, particularly in low resource settings
- Indicated when early excision is not feasible
- Enhances early eschar separation and facilitates piecemeal excision
- Allows regular assessment of wound
- In facial burn in children and in perineal burns
- Risk of infection is more in comparison to closed method.

Semi-open dressing

- Is indicated in isolated back burns, in face and perineum
- Topical antimicrobials are applied to the wound and covered with gauze with/without bandage.

Surgical Management of Burn Wound

Surgical management is indicated in deep second and third degree burns because dead burned tissue serves as a nidus for infection and inflammation. Excision should be performed as early as possible after the patient is stabilized. Usually within a week of injury. Different types of surgical management are: (i) Early tangential excision and grafting; (ii) Debridement with dressing and subsequent delayed grafting; and (iii) Fascial excision and grafting.

Early tangential excision and skin grafting

- Tangential removal of thin slices of burned tissue until a viable bed appears (visible capillary bleeding).
- Excision is performed by humbly knife or power driven (nitrogen) dermatome.
- Each excision should be limited to <20% BSA or not more than 2 hours operating time.

Advantages: (i) Enhanced recovery; (ii) Less chance of infection; and (iii) Improved long-term outcome.

Disadvantages: (i) Bleeding; (ii) Possibility of progression to burn necrosis; and (iii) Needs surgical expertise to assess adequate depth of excision.

Fascial excision and skin grafting

- Excision of the burned tissue including subcutaneous fat up to the level of investing fascia
- Particularly indicated for deep, large full thickness burns.
- Excision is performed by electrocautery.
- Assures a viable bed for grafting.
- Leaves a permanent cosmetic defect.
- More chance of injury to neuromuscular structures.

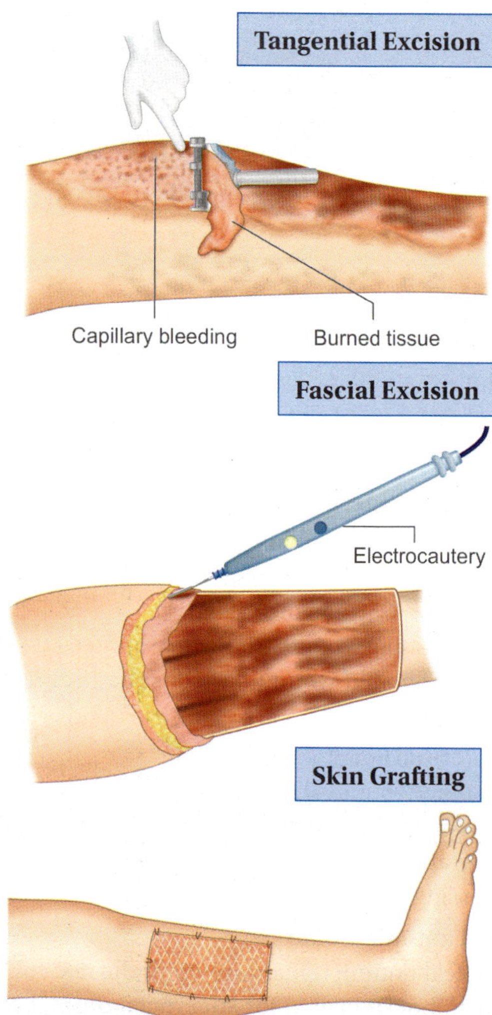

Skin Grafting

Skin grafting is indicated after surgical management of burn wound. Skin graft may be split-thickness or full-thickness and meshed or nonmeshed.

Donor sites for split-thickness skin graft: (i) Thigh; (ii) Buttock; and (iii) Scalp.

Donor sites for full-thickness skin graft: (i) Inguinal crease; (ii) Postauricular region; and (iii) Supraclavicular area.

Sites where nonmeshed skin grafts are indicated: (i) Face; (ii) Neck; and (iii) Hand.

If burn area is small and donor area is adequate—Non-meshed graft or meshed graft with narrow ratio (≤2:1). If burn area is large and donor area is limited—Widely expanded graft (4:1).

Meek Micrografting Technique

A recently emerged technique of burn coverage by skin graft, particularly for larger burn area with limited donor sites.

Characteristic features: (i) Large expansion ratio, upto 1:9, is possible; (ii) Any small skin fragments can be used; (iii) Uniform epithelialization; and (iv) Excellent graft take.

Skin Substitutes

Human cadaveric allograft (i) Glycerol-preserved allograft; and (ii) Cryopreserved allograft

Xenograft: Porcine skin allograft

Permanent skin substitutes: (i) Integra (Dermal substitute); (ii) Alloderm (Dermal substitute); (iii) Novosorb (Dermal substitute); (iv) Apligraft (Epidermal substitute); and (v) PermaDerm (Dermo-epidermal substitute).

Nutritional Support

- Hypermetabolism and increased nitrogen loss start immediately after burn injury in response to injury irrespective of etiology.
- Nutritional support is needed to prevent protein-calorie malnutrition and maintain organ function.

Calculation of calorie requirements:

By using Long's modification of Harris-Benedict equation (for burn >40% TBSA), in burn <40%- Curreri formula.

Compositions of nutritional supplement:

- Protein—1–2 g/kg/day
- Carbohydrate—7 g/kg/day
- Fat—additional fat has little support to prevent malnutrition.
- All vitamins (fat-soluble and water-soluble) must be supplemented.
- Vitamin C has particular role in wound healing by participating in collagen synthesis (1000 mg of vitamin C daily is the recommended dose).
- Mineral and trace element supplementation may be needed.
- Zinc deficiency is documented in burn patients. So, emperic zinc supplementation is indicated following major burn.
- Ideal nutritional regime: High protein, high carbohydrate, low fat along with vitamins (particularly vitamin C), minerals (particularly zinc), glutamine, trace element supplementation.

Routes of administration

- Total Enteral Nutrition (TEN)—Early enteral nutrition through enteric tube is the preferred approach.
- Total Parenteral Nutrition (TPN)—TPN is indicated only when patient cannot tolerate enteral feeding.

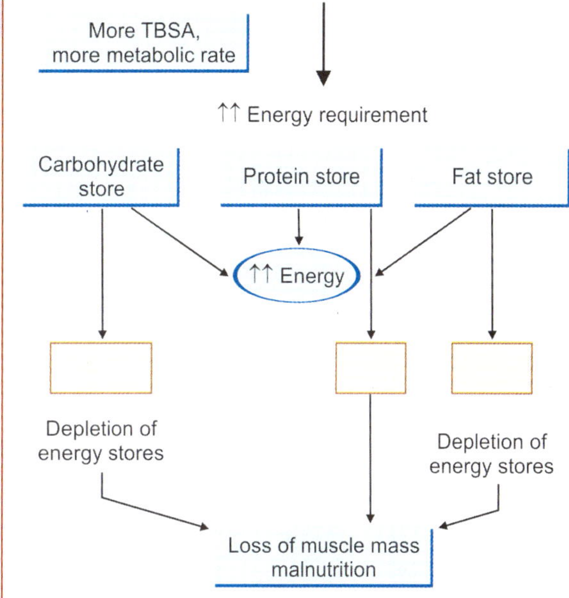

Advantages of Early Enteral Feeding

- Maintain gut mucosal thickness and control of permeability
- Stimulation of gut-associated lymphatic tissue (GALT) and other immune factors (e.g., IgA)
- Decreases bacterial translocation
- Enteral nutrition enhances splanchnic perfusion and decrease Curling's ulcer formation.

Management of Sepsis

- TBSA of burn is related with the incidence of infection. <20% TBSA is rarely associated with life-threatening sepsis. Children are more susceptible than adults for any given size of burn.
- Prophylactic systemic antibiotics are not ideally indicated, as they only lead to increased bacterial resistance.
- Hypotension, decreasing urine output, feeding intolerance, falling platelet count are all suggestive of sepsis.

Rehabilitation

Care of the skin of burn scar

- Prolonged exposure to sun should be avoided. If exposure is inevitable (in face and hands), UV screening agents should be used.
- Creams and lotions can be used to prevent drying and cracking.

Hypertrophic scar and keloid

Can be minimized by the use of pressure garments for about 1 year (till the scar matures)

Management of Postburn Pruritus

- **Pharmacologic treatment:** (i) Oral antihistaminics; (ii) Gabapentin; and (iii) Topical antihistaminics.
- **Non-pharmacologic treatment:** (i) Emollients and moisturizers; (ii) Silicon gel; (iii) Scar massage; (iv) Pulsed dye laser; and (v) Transcutaneous electrical nerve stimulation.

Systemic Changes in Burn

Increased Vascular Permeability

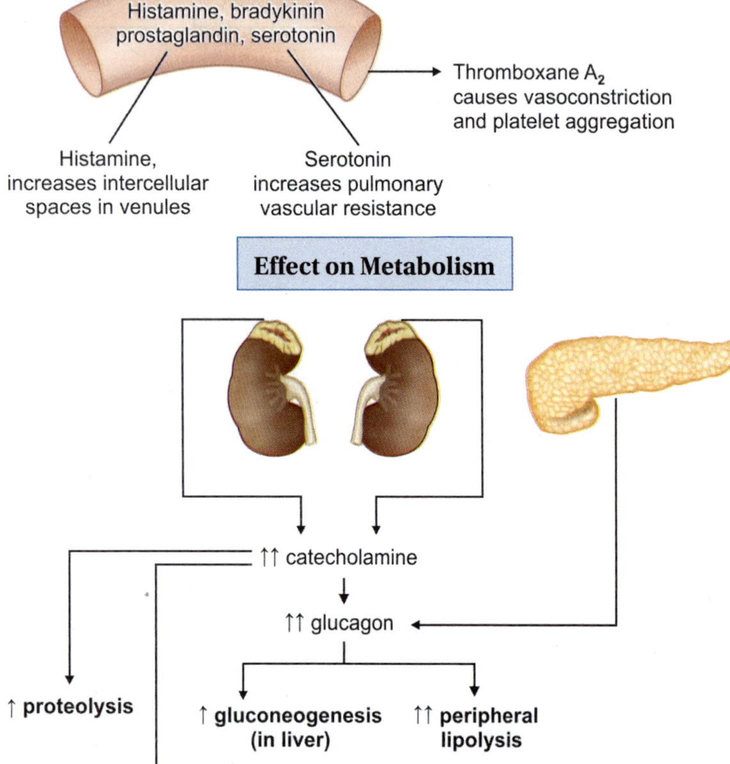

Effect on Renal System

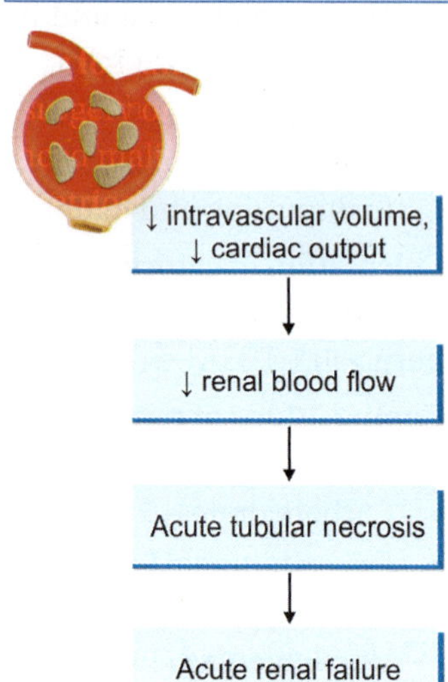

Effect on GI System

- Mucosal atrophy
- Decreased absorption of glucose, amino acid and fatty acid
- Increased permeability to macromolecules.

Effect on Immune System

- Diminished macrophage production
- Impairment of functions of neutrophils (e.g., diapedesis, chemotaxis and phagocytosis)
- Function of helper T-cell, cytotoxic T-cell are decreased.

Electric Burn

Severity of electric burn injury depends on:

Voltage: Low (<1,000 V) or high (>1,000 V)

Tissue resistance: Tissues with higher resistance (bone > fat > tendon > skin) are more damaged than tissues with less resistance (blood and nerve).

Types of current:

- Alternating current causes repetitive, tetanic muscle contraction.
- Direct current causes single muscle contraction, throwing the person away from the electricity.
- Flexors are stronger than extensors, so the hand basically grips the electrical source, causing longer electrical exposure.

Pathway through the body:

- Current passing through the heart or brainstem causes ventricular fibrillation or apnea
- Current passing through the muscle causes rhabdomyolysis, leads to myoglobinuria
- Thrombosis frequently develops, leads to local tissue necrosis.

Duration of contact

Three types of electrical injury:

1. Injury from current flow
2. Arc or flash injury
3. Flame injury from the ignition of clothings.

Management of electric burn:

Care at the site of injury:

- ABC evaluation and support should be initiated accordingly
- CPR should be started according to advanced cardiac life support protocol (if pulses are not palpable)
- Other life-threatening injuries (injuries due to fall from height, due to tetanic contractions) should be searched.

Definite care:

- Fingers, hands, forearms, feet, lower legs have more chance of damage than trunk, chest or abdomen (smaller the area through which electricity passes, more intense heat production and less dissipation into surrounding tissue).
- High voltage electric injury may cause cardiac damage (myocardial contusion, infarction or conduction defect). If no dysrhythmia is found in ECG during initial evaluation, the likelihood of further development is rare.
- Rhabdomyolysis may develop after electrical injury. Following rhabdomyolysis, myoglobin is released from injured cells. Precipitation of myoglobin in the renal tubules can cause ARF.
- If clinical features are suggestive of ARF, mannitol infusion and infusion of sodium bicarbonate is indicated.
- Every patient must have neurologic examination, because nervous system is very much sensitive to electrical energy.
- Delayed transverse myelitis, anterior spinal artery syndrome may cause functional impairment.
- Cataract may develop after high-voltage electrical injury, usually within 1-2 years.

Wound management

- Careful monitoring for compartment syndrome—if compartment pressure ≥30 mm Hg or clinical features are suggestive, then early escharotomy and fasciotomy is indicated.
- Clinical findings suggestive of progressive median or ulnar nerve deficit warrants decompression at the wrist.
- Definite surgical procedures (excision and grafting) must be considered, if indicated.

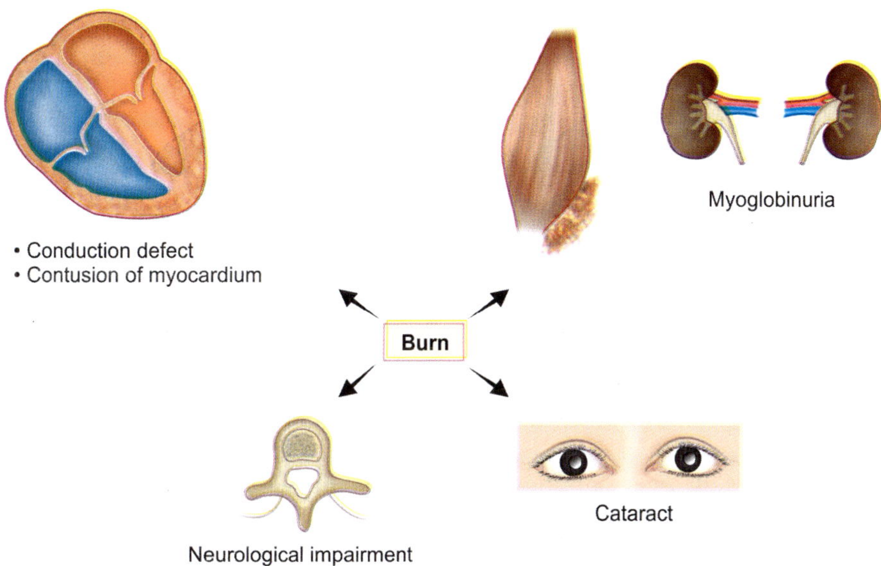

Chemical Burn

- Most chemical burns are accidental.
- Strong acids and alkalis cause most of the chemical burns. These burns are typically associated with industrial accidents, assaults, improper use of household cleaners.

Care of the burn:

- All involved clothing should be removed.
- Dry powders must be brushed before irrigation.
- Irrigating the area for at least 15 minutes under a stream of tepid water dilutes the chemical.
- If chemical composition is known (acid/alkali), surface pH is checked, continue the irrigation still pH is reached the physiologic range (7–7.5).
- Resuscitation is guided according to involved TBSA.
- After resuscitation, operative debridement must be done. After debridement, wound are dressed with antimicrobial agents or skin substitutes.
- In acid injury, injuries may be more superficial than they appear; the reverse is true in case of alkali injury.
- Attempts to neutralize alkali with weak acids should not be attempted (heat released by neutralization reaction causes further injury)]

Hydrofluoric acid burn:

- This burn is managed differently from other acid burns due to its chemical properties.
- Hydrofluoric acid produces dehydration and corrosion of tissues by free hydrogen ions. Fluoride ion complexes with calcium and magnesium causing hypocalcemia, resulting in life-threatening arrhythmias.
- Burned area is irrigated with clean water and 2.5% calcium gluconate gel. The gel is changed every 15 minutes. If pain is not relieved after several applications of gel or symptoms recur, intradermal injection of 10% calcium gluconate or intraarterial injection of calcium gluconate or both (in affected extremity) should be considered.
- All patients must be admitted for cardiac monitoring, particularly for prolongation of QT interval. Serum Mg^{2+}, K^+ are closely monitored.

Late Complications of Burn

Keloid and hypertrophic scar:

- Can be limited by pressure garments
- If keloid develops, intrakeloidal triamcinolone is helpful.

Scar contracture:

- In localized linear contracture, Y-V plasty.
- In broad contracture, release of contracture followed by skin grafting.

Heterotopic ossification:

- Calcification may develop in muscle and surrounding soft tissue of the joint in large full thickness burns.
- Upper extremity is most commonly affected.

Marjolin's ulcer:

- Chronic breakdown of a healed burn scar—Marjolin's ulcer should be in differential diagnosis
- Squamous cell carcinoma is the most common type of malignancy that may develop.
- Wide local excision is the treatment.

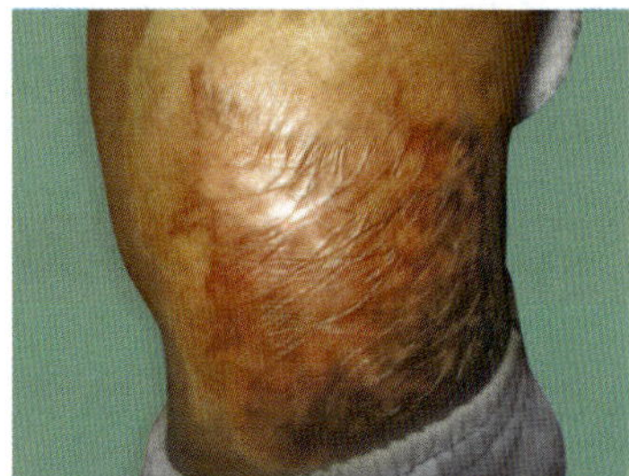

Hypertrophic scar

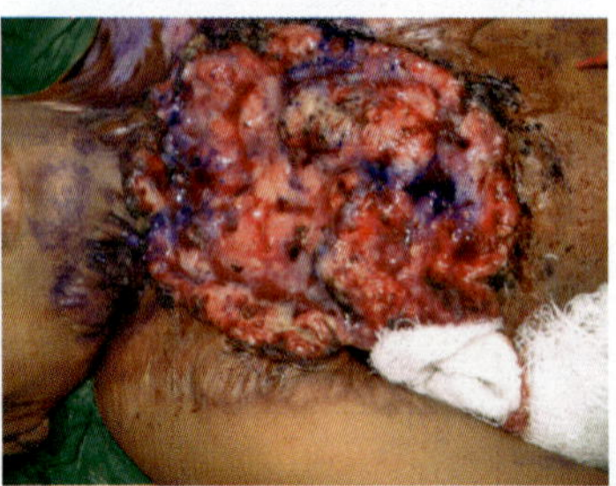

Marjolin's ulcer

Case 1

History and Physical Examination

A 26-year-old female patient admitted in the surgical emergency sustaining flame burn injury during cooking. The incident happened about 6 hours back, patient initially treated in primary health care facility and then referred to tertiary care center with burn care facility. No history of comorbidities.

Physical Examination

- Patient alert, conscious, cooperative
- Pulse: 116/min, BP: 100/68 mm Hg, Respiratory rate: 20/min
- Burn injury involving part of the face, both upper limbs, part of chest: about 35% TBSA of varying degree
- Auscultation of chest: No obvious abnormality
- Urine output: 200 mL in last 5 hours, high-colored.

Investigations

- In the initial phase of burn, most of the laboratory parameters were within normal limit.
- On the 3rd day, Hb: 10.5 gm%, Total WBC count: 8,500/cumm, Serum creatinine: 1.2 mg/dL, Na^+: 128 mEq/L, K^+: 3.2 mmol/L
- On 5th day—Hb: 9.2 gm%, Total WBC count: 17,000/cumm, Serum sodium and potassium within normal range.

Discussion

A young female patient (estimated body weight 62 kg) sustained 35% burn injury without any inhalation injury. On admission, urine output was diminished because of delay in initiating proper fluid management from the time of injury. Initial fluid management in the tertiary care center started according to body weight and percentage of burn injury. In the initial period of burn, patient developed hypokalemia and hyponatremia. On the 5th day, TC WBC raised to 17,000/cumm.

Management Algorithm

Fluid Resuscitation

Ringer lactate in first 24 hours = (62 × 35 × 4) mL = 8,680 mL 4,340 mL (9 bottles) in first 8 hours and 9 bottles in next 16 hours. Time was calculated from the time of injury.

- Catheterization
- Moist oxygen inhalation
- Tetanus immunization
- Analgesia with opioid analgesics

→ After 24 hours, fluid management initiated based on urine output.

→ On 5th day, parenteral antibiotic therapy coverage against gram-negative aerobes started.

Case 2

History and Physical Examination

A 23-year-old male patient by occupation plumber presented in the surgical emergency with high-voltage electrical injury while carrying long pipes for construction of deep tube well. Patient presented with deep burns in the face, both hands and feet.

Physical Examination

- Patient conscious, alert, cooperative
- Deep burn with charring of tissues involving the face, hands and both foot (about 25% of TBSA)
- Pulse: 100/min with regular rhythm, BP: 100/76 mm Hg, Respiratory rate: 20/min, Chest: clear.

Management Algorithm

- Fluid resuscitation started based on weight and TBSA
- Catheterization (besides assessment of fluid resuscitation, myoglobinuria can also be detected)
- ECG monitoring
- Pain management

→

- No arrhythmia detected in ECG monitoring
- Urine output adequate, no myoglobinuria

↓

Patient died after about 7 hours of injury (most likely due to neurogenic shock).

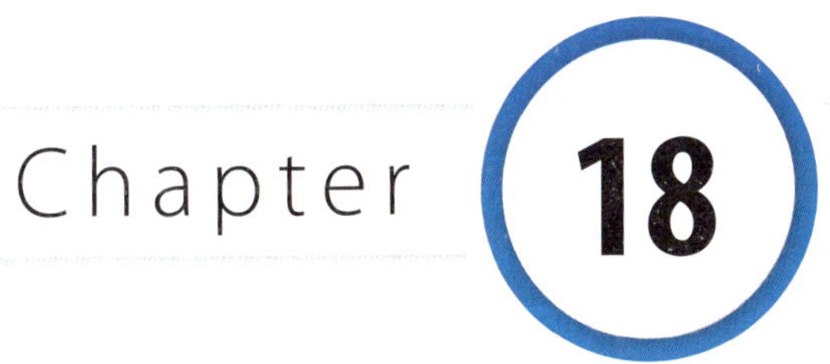

Arterial, Venous, and Lymphatic Diseases

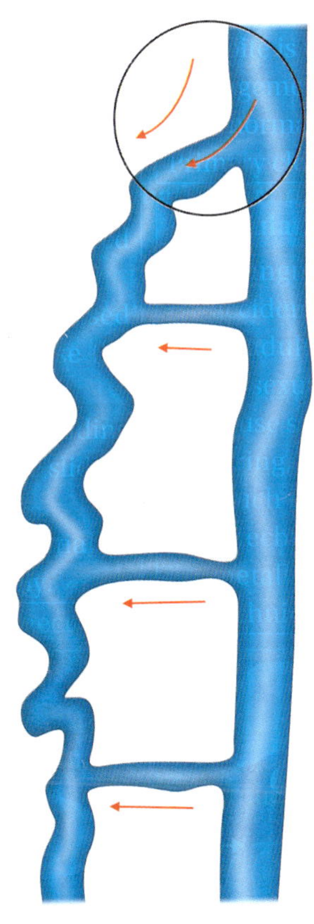

Important Topics

- Arterial Occlusive Diseases
- Aneurysmal Vascular Disease
- Aortic Dissection
- Vascular Trauma
- Superficial Thrombophlebitis
- Deep Vein Thrombosis
- Venous Insufficiency
- Lymphangitis
- Lymphedema
- Tumor of the Lymphatics

'Where observation is concerned, chance favours only the prepared mind.'

Louis Pasteur (1822–1895)
French Microbiologist

Diseases of Arteries

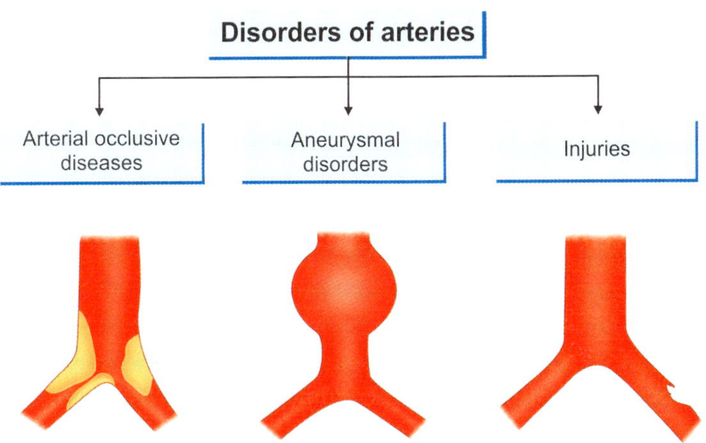

Arterial Occlusive Diseases

Majority of arterial occlusive diseases are secondary to atherosclerotic changes of the intimal layer. Adverse events occur due to impaired circulation in the vital end organs (brain, heart, abdominal viscera) and extremities.

Peripheral arterial occlusive disease:

- Peripheral arterial occlusive disease is stenosis or occlusion of aorta or the arteries of the limb. It is classified into four categories based on presentation: (i) Asymptomatic; (ii) Claudication; (iii) Critical limb ischemia; and (iv) Acute limb ischemia.
- Atherosclerosis is the major cause of PAD in patients of ≥40 years old.

Risk factors for PAD:

Hypercholesterolemia: Increased level of serum cholesterol and LDL cholesterol **(bad cholesterol)**—associated with increased risk. HDL cholesterol **(good cholesterol)**—associated with decreased risk

Smoking:

- Increased morbidity and mortality from coronary, cerebral and peripheral vascular diseases.
- Direct toxic effect of tobacco metabolites on the vascular endothelium.

Diabetes mellitus:

- Induces hypercholesterolemia
- Increases the risk of myocardial infarction, stroke and gangrene of lower extremities.

Hypertension: Independent risk factor for coronary atherosclerosis.

Other risk factors:

- Advanced age
- Male gender
- Hypertriglyceridemia
- Hyperhomocysteinemia
- Sedentary lifestyle
- Family history.

Other Causes of Occlusion

- Thrombosis
- Embolism
- Vasculitis
- Trauma
- Fibromuscular dysplasia

Atherosclerosis

- **A complex, chronic inflammatory process that primarily affects the intimal layer,** predilections for some locations and sparing others, characterized by plaque (atheroma) formation.
- Lesions progress through a well-characterized stages before the development of clinical manifestations.
- Growth of plaque does not follow a regular fashion, rather intermittent periods of relative quiescence followed by periods of rapid evolution.

- **LDL** has critical role in delivering cholesterol to peripheral tissues.
- **HDL** mobilizes cholesterol from developing and already existed atheromas and transports it to liver for excretion.

Pathophysiology of Atheroma

Numerous hypotheses have been proposed, but the **response to injury hypothesis** is the most accepted one. This **'response to injury'** hypothesis views the atherosclerosis as a chronic inflammatory response of the arterial wall to endothelial injury.

Stages of Atheroma Development

1. **Endothelial injury**

Endothelial injury is either due to mechanical injury (shear stress, turbulence, stasis) or toxic injury. Toxic injury is due to-cigarette smoke, homocysteine, infectious agent (cytomegalovirus, herpes virus).

Plaques tend to occur at the bifurcation or bends: (i) Infrarenal abdominal aorta; (ii) Carotid bifurcation; (iii) Iliofemoral arteries (especially superficial femoral artery); and (iv) Popliteal arteries.

2. **Circulating monocytes attach to the damaged endothelium**

3. **Smooth muscle recruitment + Macrophage activation and recruitment**

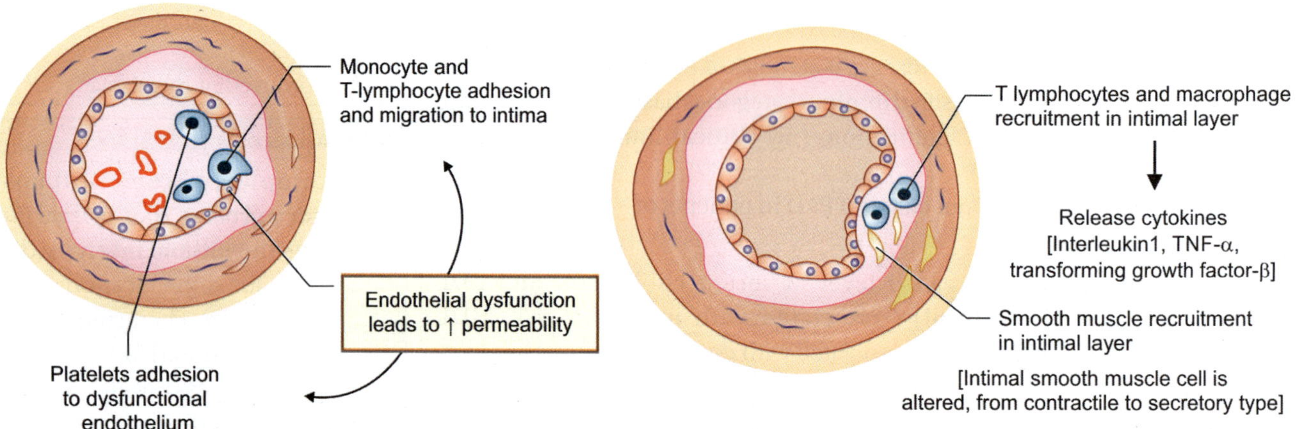

4. **Macrophages and smooth muscle cells (SMCs) engulf lipid**

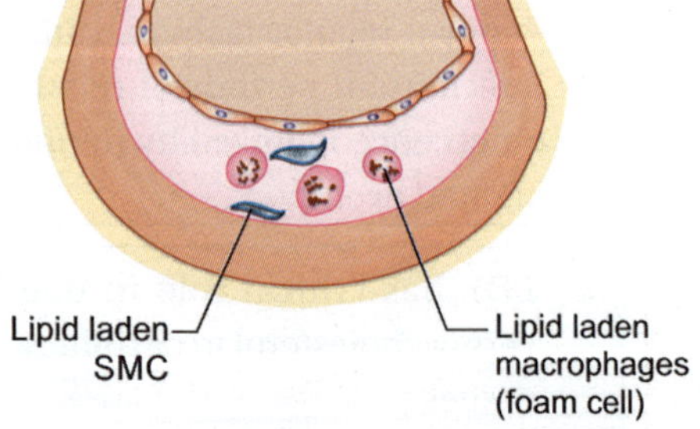

The initial lesion that can be seen is the **'fatty streak'** consists of lipid-laden macrophages overlying lipid-laden smooth muscle cells.

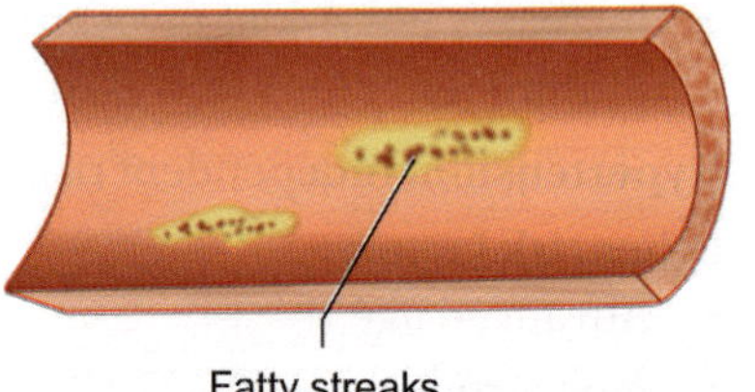

5. **Some foam cells die as a result of apoptosis, forming the lipid rich center (necrotic core) and some foam cells release cytokines and growth factors. Further recruitment of SMCs and their elaboration of extracellular matrix finally converts a accumulation of foam cells and SMCs to a atherosclerotic plaques.**

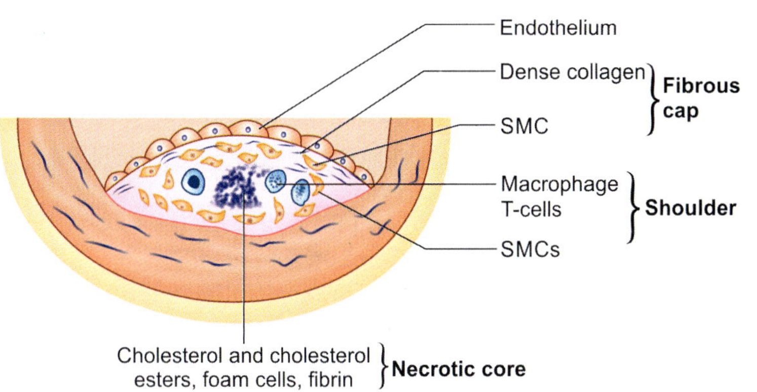

Atherosclerotic plaque made up of three areas:
1. Fibrous cap
2. Shoulder
3. Necrotic core

Atherosclerotic plaque contains three types of components:
1. **Cellular component:** SMC, macrophage, T-cells.
2. **Extracellular matrix:** Collagen, elastic fibers, proteoglycans.
3. **Lipid**

Complications of atherosclerotic plaques.

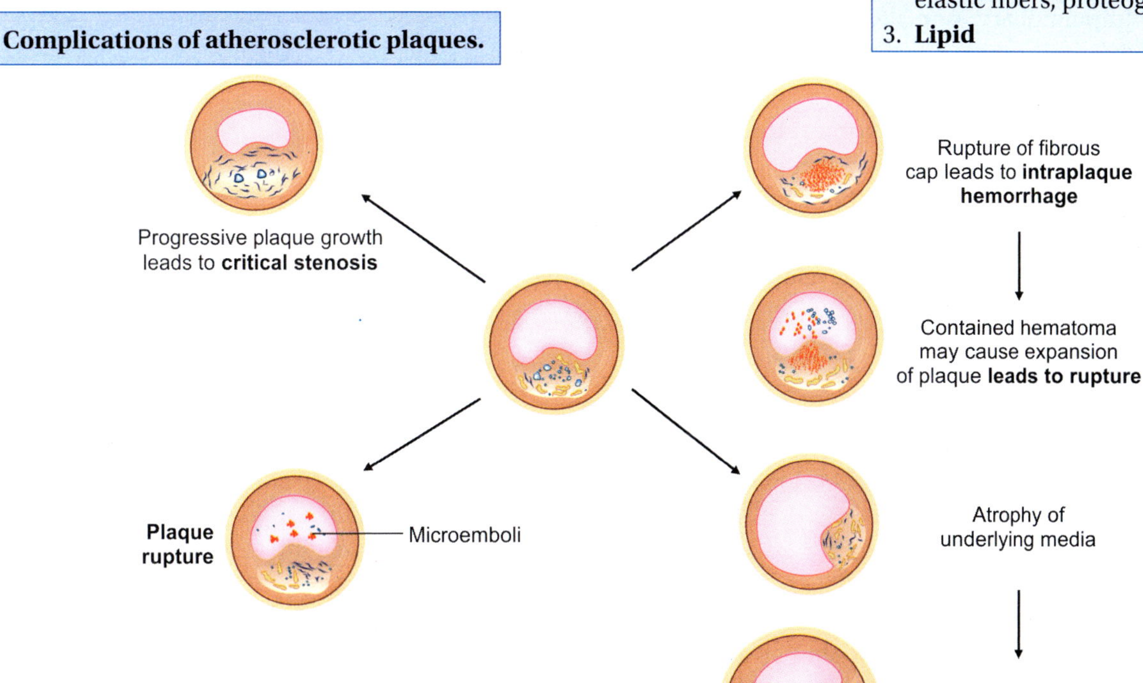

Acute Arterial Occlusion of the Extremities

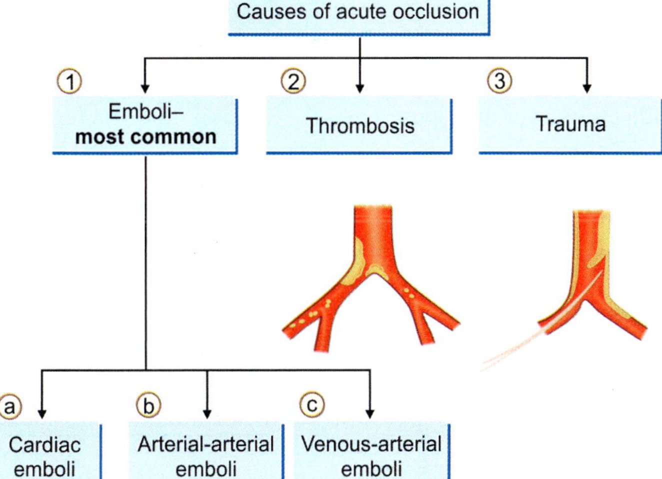

Cerebral infarction develops after 4–8 minutes of ischemia.

Myocardial infarction develops after 15–20 minutes of ischemia.

Emboli

Cardiac emboli: About 80% of arterial emboli are cardiac in origin.

Arterial-arterial emboli:
- Emboli arising from ulcerated atheroma, unstable atheroma, disrupted plaque, from aneurysm cause distal obstruction and ischemia.
- Aortic aneurysms contain thrombi, but rarely embolize.
- Femoral and popliteal aneurysms frequently embolize.

Venous-arterial emboli:
- Due to intracardiac shunt (e.g., patent foramen ovale)
- Due to intrapulmonary AV malformations (in Osler-Weber-Rendu syndrome)

Thrombosis:
- Acute thrombosis usually develops over a pre-existing atherosclerosis.
- Acute thrombosis also develops in the setting of sepsis and hypercoagulable states (e.g., hyperhomocysteinemia, antithrombin III deficiency, antiphospholipid antibody, protein C deficiency).

Trauma: Stenosis or occlusion may develop after an intimal flap or arterial wall hematoma.

Sources of Cardiac Emboli

- Atrial fibrillation (thrombi in atrial appendages)—most common source
- Ventricular mural thrombus (as a complication of AMI)—second most common source
- Vegetations (in bacterial or fungal endocarditis)
- Prosthetic valve
- Atrial myxoma

Clinical Features

Symptoms of acute occlusion depend on the location, duration, and severity of the obstruction.

Presentation includes six Ps:

1. **Pain:**
   - Most common symptom.
   - Sudden onset severe ischemic pain in extremity in a previously asymptomatic patient-**highly suggestive of embolic occlusion.**
2. **Pallor:**
   - Cold, pale extremity with no sign of cutaneous blood flow.
   - Absence of distal pulses can indicate the site of occlusion.
3. **Pulselessness:** Absence of peripheral pulse
4. **Paresthesia:** Light touch sensation is absent?—beginning of irreversible ischemia.
5. **Paralysis:** Onset of motor paralysis indicates impending gangrene—warrants urgent revascularization.
6. **Poikilothermy:** Inability to thermoregulate.

'Blue toe' Syndrome

- Diffuse microembolization causes painful, bluish discoloration of toes with cutaneous gangrene, livedo reticularis. Peripheral pulses are present.
- It may also affect renal and mesenteric circulations leads to progressive renal failure and intestinal infarction.

Acute Limb Ischemia (ALI)

Acute (<2 weeks), severe hypoperfusion of limb characterized by these features: pain, pallor, pulselessness, poikilothermia (cold), paresthesia, and paralysis.

(Adapted from AHA/ACC guideline)

Categories of Acute Limb Ischemia (ALI)

I. Viable limbs that are not immediately threatened.
IIa. Marginally threatened and salvageable, if promptly treated.
IIb. Immediately threatened limbs that require immediate revascularization if salvage is to be accomplished.
III. Irreversibly damaged limbs, resultant major tissue loss or permanent nerve damage is inevitable.

Assessment of ALI

Assessment includes: (i) Duration of symptoms; (ii) Motor and sensory deficit severity; and (iii) Doppler study of arterial and venous system

Acute embolic or **acute thrombotic occlusion** in extremity can be differentiated by history taking and clinical examination in most of the cases.

Treatment

- Once a diagnosis of acute arterial occlusion (due to emboli/thrombus) is made, immediate anticoagulation by IV heparin (preferably unfractionated heparin) should be started to slow the propagation of the thrombus and allows some time to assess the status of collateral circulation and preparation for surgical intervention.
- For category I ALI, revascularization should be performed on an urgent basis (within 6–24 hours).
- For category IIa and IIb ALI, revascularization should be performed emergently (within 6 hours).
- For category III ALI, amputation should be performed as the index procedure.
- Catheter-based thrombolysis is the most preferred revascularization procedure.

In embolic occlusion: Balloon embolectomy is the preferred procedure.

Acute Embolic Occlusion

- Presence of risk factors (e.g., atrial fibrillation, recent AMI, prosthetic heart valve)
- Normal contralateral extremity
- No history of intermittent claudication.

Acute Thrombotic Occlusion

- No risk factors for embolism
- Contralateral extremity is also diseased
- History of intermittent claudication.

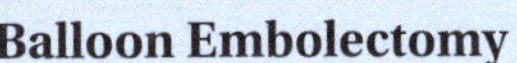

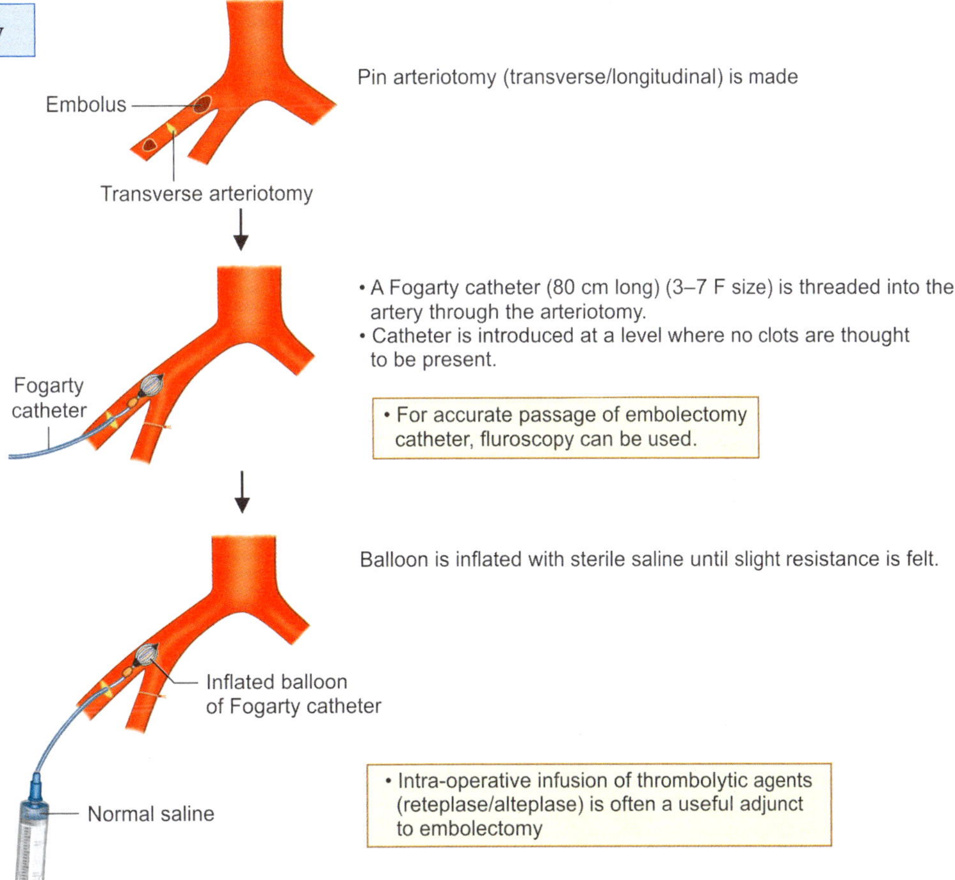

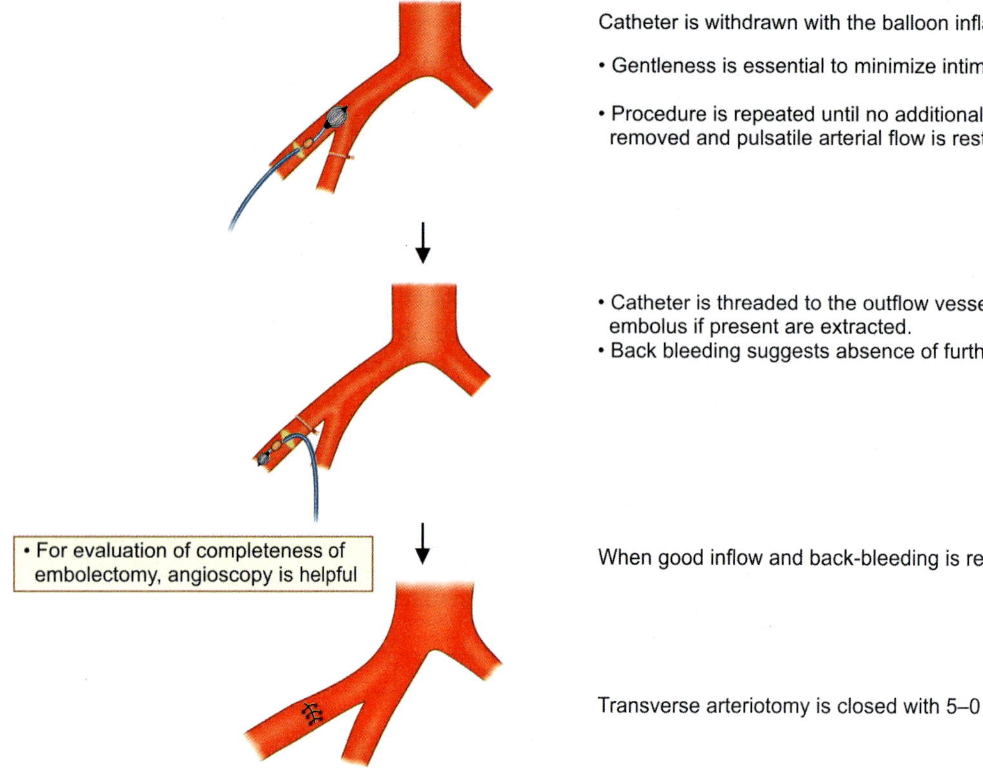

- **Transesophageal Echocardiography** is indicated to find source of cardiac emboli.
- **CT of descending thoracic and abdominal aorta** is indicated to find aortic thrombus.

Acute Thrombotic Occlusion

Arteriogram is indicated to determine: (i) Site of thrombotic occlusion; (ii) Degree of occlusion; (iii) Short or long segment involvement; and (iv) Status of inflow and outflow vessels.

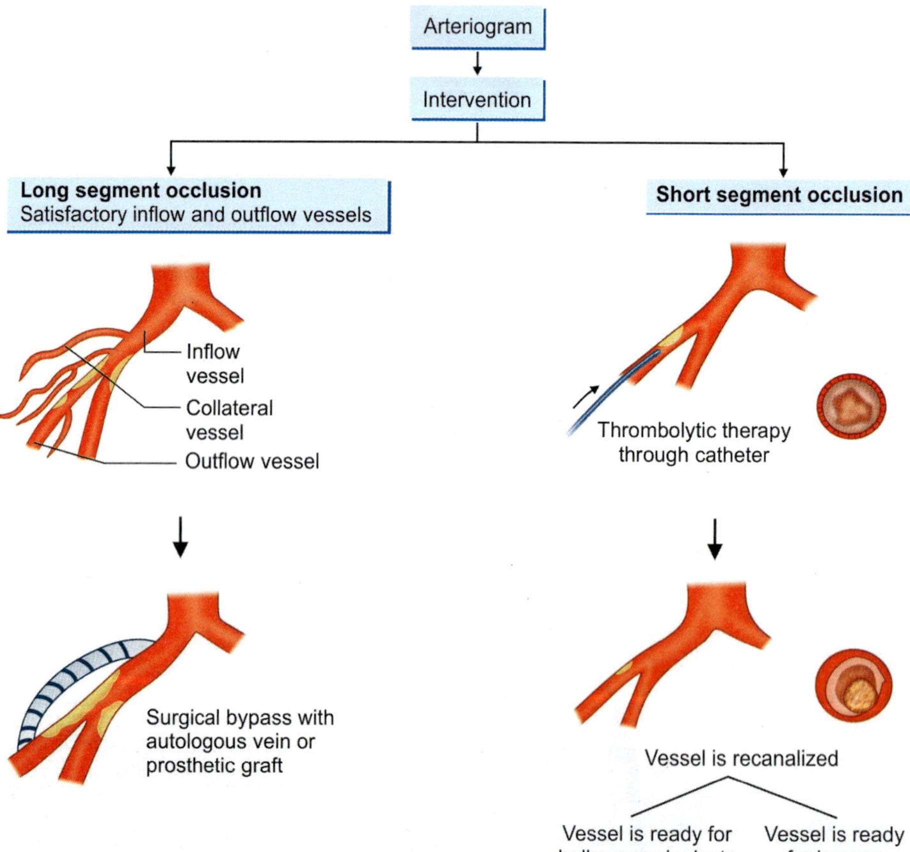

Thrombolytic Therapy

- Reteplase, alteplase are the thrombolytic agents.
- Fresher the thrombus, more the chance of successful thrombolysis.
- During thrombolysis, patient is monitored in ICU. Thrombin time, fibrinogen level, fibrinogen degradation product should be measured.
- PTT and CBC must be evaluated to assess the risk of hemorrhage.
- Duration of therapy between 4–16 hours.
- Repeat arteriography is done after 6–18 hours to evaluate the result.

Thrombolytic therapy is contraindicated in patients with increased risk of hemorrhage (e.g., traumatic occlusion, recent surgery, intracranial tumors, pregnancy).

Traumatic Occlusion

- Operative exploration should be done if limb is ischemic/arteriogram shows intimal flap/hematoma
- Proximal and distal control of the injured artery must be taken
- End-to-end anastomosis/graft placement (autologous vein graft) is done
- Completion angiogram is indicated to document the distal flow.

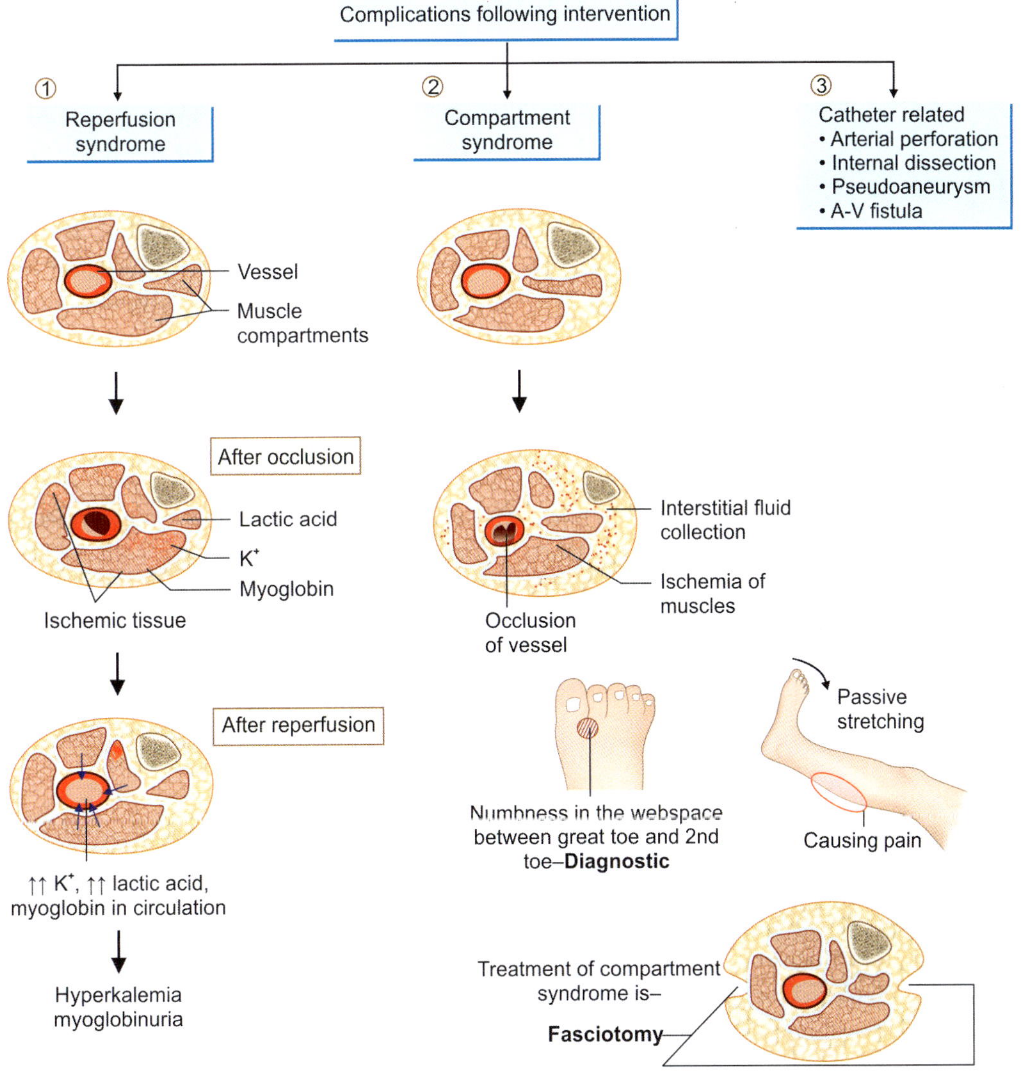

Chronic Occlusive Disease of the Extremities

- Lower extremities are more commonly affected by chronic occlusive disease of the arteries.
- Lower extremity chronic occlusive disease is subdivided into three anatomic sections:
  - **Aortoiliac** (inflow disease): Involves the infrarenal aorta, common iliac and external iliac arteries.
  - **Femoral-popliteal** (outflow disease): Involves the common femoral, superficial femoral and popliteal arteries.
  - **Tibial-peroneal** (runoff disease): Involves distal to popliteal artery.

Clinical Presentation

Intermittent claudication

- Most common symptom
- Defined as pain, ache, cramp or sense of fatigue in the muscles, brought on by walking, gradually progresses until the patient is compelled to stop walking.
- Site of claudication is distal to the site of occlusive lesion.
- In femoropopliteal and tibial-peroneal occlusive disease, intermittent claudication develops in calf region.
- Claudication less commonly occurs in the upper limb. If pain develops, is brought on by activities like writing or manual work.

Claudication: Fatigue, discomfort, cramping, or pain of vascular origin in the muscles of the lower extremities that is consistently induced by exercise and consistently relieved by rest (within 10 minutes).

(Adapted from AHA/ACC guideline)

Claudication distance: The distance walked at the onset of claudication pain.

Absolute claudication distance: The distance at which pain is so severe that patient is compelled to stop walking.

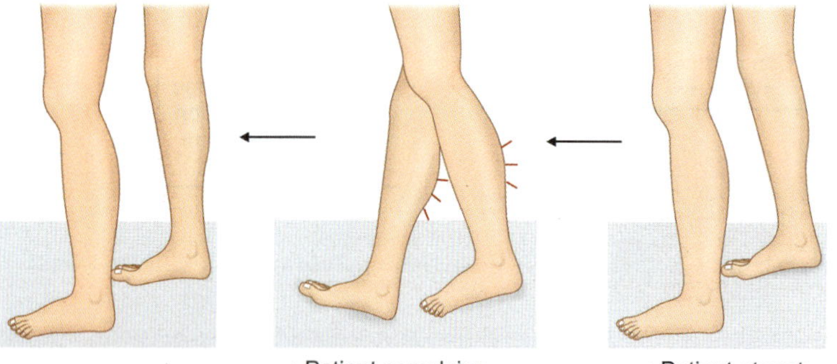

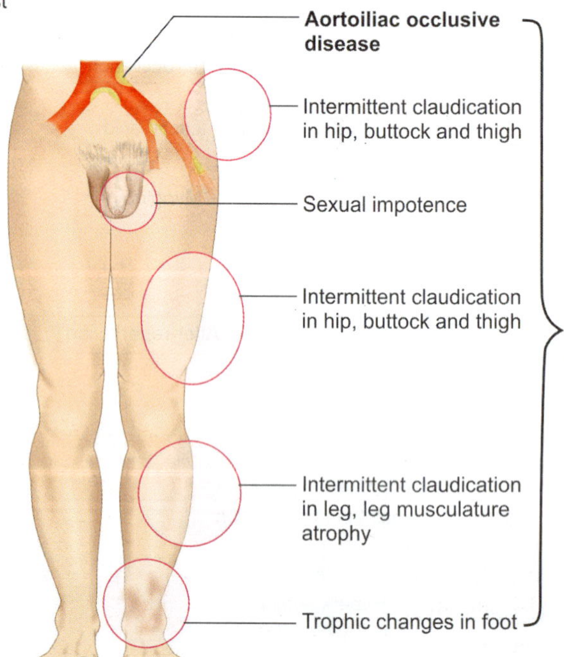

Critical Limb Ischemia (CLI)

A condition characterized by chronic (≥2 weeks) ischemic rest pain, nonhealing wound/ulcers, or gangrene in one or both legs attributable to objectively proven arterial occlusive disease.

Classification Systems in Peripheral Artery Disease

- **Fontaine classification:** This system is based on clinical symptoms only, typically used for clinical research.
- **Rutherford classification:** This system is based on clinical symptoms, Doppler findings, ABI and pulse volume recordings.

Rest pain

- Severe burning pain usually confined to the forefoot.
- Pain aggravated by elevation of the extremity or in horizontal position.
- Patient can obtain same relief by hanging the leg over the side of the bed (Gravity helps the delivery of arterial blood).
- Rest pain usually preceded by claudication.

Numbness and paresthesia

Common symptom in severe ischemia.

Erectile dysfunction

If arterial flow is obstructed in both hypogastric arteries.

Clinical Examination

Arterial pulsation

Arterial pulsation is absent or diminished distal to obstruction.

Bruit

- Systolic bruit is produced due to turbulence just proximal to the stenotic segment.
- After total occlusion, usually bruit disappear.

Disappearing pulse

When peripheral pulses are apparently normal, after exercising the patient to the point of claudication, the palpable pulses become disappear. After taking a few minutes of rest, the pulse reappears.

Skin temperature

Decreased temperature is best detected by palpation of dorsum of patient's foot with the back of examiner's hand.

Color changes

- Blanching of limb on elevation and purple discoloration on dependency indicates advanced ischemia.
- The angle of elevation at which blanching appears gives a rough estimations of degree of ischemia.
- The more it takes time to return of skin color on dependency, the more severe is the obstruction.

Integumentary changes

- Loss of hair in foot
- Thickening of toenails
- Atrophy of skin and subcutaneous tissue

Atrophy

Gradual development of soft tissue and muscle atrophy in the ischemic area.

Ulceration and gangrene

- Ischemic ulcers are very painful, develop on the dorsum of feet, on the skin, around the malleoli.
- Margin of ulcer is punched out, base is devoid of granulation tissue.
- Usually, dry gangrene develops. The blackened, mummified skin and tissues have a characteristic appearance.

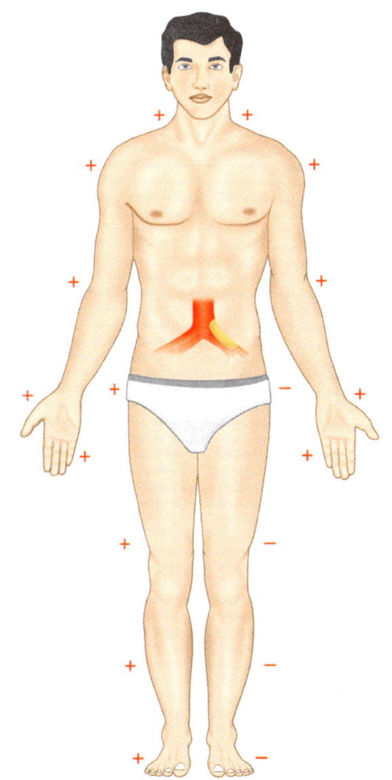

Absence of **dorsalis pedis pulse** is less reliable than posterior tibial pulse because dorsalis pedis artery pulse may not be palpable in a significant percentage of healthy individuals.

Arterial Occlusive Disease of the Upper Extremities

- An uncommon disease in comparison to occlusive disease of the lower extremities.
- Most commonly affected vessel—Proximal subclavian artery > axillary artery > brachial artery.
- Typically present with arm claudication, ischemic or necrotic changes in fingers and hands.
- Most of the patients with subclavian artery occlusion are asymptomatic.

Subclavian Steal Syndrome

Pathophysiology

If obstruction in subclavian artery develops proximal to the origin of vertebral artery, posterior cerebral circulation may be impaired due to retrograde flow from ipsilateral vertebral artery.

Clinical manifestations include drop attacks, ataxia, sensory loss, and diplopia.

Investigations

Noninvasive modalities: (i) Ankle-Brachial Index (ABI); (ii) Segmental limb pressure measurement; (iii) Duplex scanning; (iv) CT angiography (CTA); (v) MR angiography (MRA); and (vi) Digital subtraction angiography (DSA).

Invasive modalities: Conventional angiography.

Ankle-Brachial Index (ABI):

- A quick screening test, calculated by measuring blood pressure at arms (brachial arteries) and ankles (dorsalis pedis and posterior tibial arteries) in the supine position by Doppler device.
- ABI ≤0.90 is suggestive of PAD
- ABI 0.91–0.99—may possibly have PAD and should undergo exercise ABI, if clinical suspicion is significant.
- ABI >1.40—noncompressible, commonly associated with diabetes mellitus and/or advanced chronic kidney disease.
- When patients with suspected PAD having ABI >1.40, toe-brachial index (TBI) should be measured. TBI ≤0.70 is diagnostic of PAD.
- Exercise treadmill ABI testing is indicated in patients with suspected PAD when resting ABI is normal or borderline. This investigation can differentiate claudication from pseudoclaudication.

Duplex scan, CT angiography or MR angiography is indicated if revascularization is planned and PAD is confirmed by ABI or TBI. If these imaging modalities cannot provide useful findings, then invasive angiography is indicated.

Duplex scan: This imaging modality is a combination of **B-mode ultrasound** and **Doppler ultrasound**. In Doppler waveform, triphasic signal is normal whereas biphasic and monophasic signals are considered abnormal.

Management of Subclavian Arterial Occlusion

- Carotid-subclavian bypass (using prosthetic graft)—if ipsilateral common carotid is patent
- Subclavian-subclavian bypass—if ipsilateral common carotid carotid is occluded.

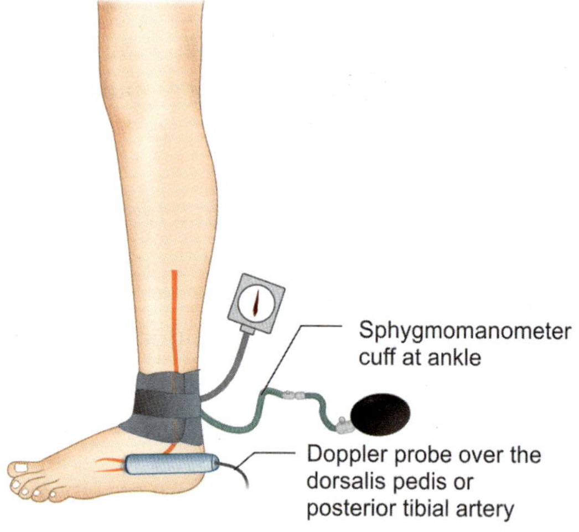

- **B-mode ultrasound** creates grey-scale anatomic image of vessels.
- **Doppler ultrasound** creates image of the moving structures in the vessels.
- **Triphasic waveform:** Peak systole, reverse diastolic flow and forward diastolic flow.

Treatment

- **Objectives of treatment in PAD are:** (i) Relief of symptoms; (ii) Prevention of limb loss; (iii) To prevent further progression of disease process; and (iv) To reduce the risk of associated cardiovascular events (e.g., AMI).
- **Different treatment options include:** (i) Conservative; (ii) Endovascular; and (iii) Surgery.

Conservative Management

Risk Factor Modification

- **Cessation of smoking:** By counseling and adjunctive drug therapy.
    - Smoking cessation reduces risk of cardiovascular ischemic events, limb-related events, bypass graft failure, amputation and death in PAD patients. A comprehensive smoking cessation program (counseling and pharmacologic therapy with varenicline, bupropion, nicotine replacement therapy) is helpful for cessation of smoking.
- **Control of hypertension:**
    - Goal 130/85 mm Hg
    - ACE inhibitors and β-blockers help to reduce mortality associated with cardiovascular events.
    - Antihypertensive therapy reduces the risk of MI, stroke, heart failure, and cardiovascular death.
- **Cholesterol (LDL cholesterol) reduction:**
  Goal <100 mg/dL: By treating with statins. Statin therapy reduces the 4-year adverse limb-related events (i.e., worsening claudication, new CLI, new ischemic amputation) also improve pain-free walking time.
- **Control of diabetes:**
    - Aggressive control of diabetes is associated with slowing of progression of atherosclerotic disorder. Control of diabetes decreases the risk of adverse outcomes (i.e., progression to CLI, amputation, death).
    - Goal—Glycosylated Hb 7%.

Exercise Rehabilitation

- Unsupervised walking to supervised exercise on a treadmill, all significantly improves walking ability.
- Exercise for ≥30 minutes and ≥3 times a weeks are most effective.

Foot Care

- Feet should be inspected and washed daily.
- Well fitting and protective shoes are advised.
- Toe nails should be trimmed carefully.
- Even minor foot infections and injuries should be treated aggressively.
- Avoid amateur chiropody.
- Avoid excessive drying by applying moisturizing creams.
- Educating the patient to understand the importance of foot care.

Pharmacotherapy

Cilostazol:

- A type III phosphodiesterase inhibitor.
- Inhibits platelet aggregation, increases vasodilation, inhibits smooth muscle proliferation, lowers HDL cholesterol and triglyceride.
- Cilostazol is effective to improve claudication symptoms and increase walking distance.
- At least 3 months should be continued before making decision about efficiency.
- Contraindicated in CHF.

Antiplatelet therapy (aspirin or clopidogrel):

- Antiplatelet therapy with aspirin alone (75–325 mg/d) or clopidogrel alone (75 mg/d) reduces the risk of MI, stroke and vascular death in symptomatic PAD patients
- Clopidogrel is more effective but much more expensive.

Endovascular Therapy

Indications:

- For disabling, progressive, severe symptoms of intermittent claudication despite medical therapy.
- In patient with critical limb ischemia.

Different types of endovascular therapies:

Percutaneous transluminal angioplasty: Dilation of a stenotic arterial segment using inflatable balloon catheter. When balloon inflates, it stretches the media and adventitia, fractures the plaque, thereby widens the lumen.

Stenting:

Indications: Angioplasty failure, Eccentric stenotic lesions, recanalized iliac occlusion, ulcerated emboligenic lesion.

Types: (i) Balloon-expandable (Palmaz type) and (ii) Self-expanding (Wallstent type).

In aortoiliac occlusive disease, balloon angioplasty and stent placement produce excellent long-term patency. In infrainguinal occlusive disease, balloon angioplasty and stenting produce poorer results than surgical bypass.

Atherectomy: A endovascular procedure where plaque is removed by shaving with a cutting or rotating catheter.

Surgery

- All patients undergoing surgery warrants preoperative cardiac risk assessment.
- All patients undergoing surgery need angiographic evaluation of the symptomatic arterial segment.
- Screening for carotid disease must be performed (history of stroke, TA and carotid auscultation).
- Patient with angina, prior AMI, ventricular ectopic, heart failure, diabetes are at increased risk.
- Surgical options depend on location and extent of obstruction and general medical condition of the patient.

Aortoiliac Occlusive Disease

Aortobifemoral bypass

- Treatment of choice in low-risk point with diffuse aortoiliac occlusion and stenoses.
- Knitted dacron graft is used for bypass.

Axillobifemoral bypass

Preferred procedure for high-risk point with short life expectancy (<5 years).

Femorofemoral, ilioiliac, and iliofemoral bypass

Choice for high-risk point with unilateral iliac disease.

Aortoiliac endarterectomy

May indicated in points with disease localized to distal aorta and common iliac vessels.

Femoral, Popliteal and Tibial Occlusive Disease

Autogenous vein bypass graft

- Great saphenous vein is the vein of choice
- Short saphenous vein or arm vein are the suitable alternatives.

PTFE graft and cryopreserved vein graft

- When autogenous vein not available
- Cryopreserved vein graft is useful in a setting of infected field.

Endarterectomy

May be indicated where autogenous vein unavailability or in the pressure of infected field.

Amputation

- Indicated for patients with gangrene or persistent painful limb not amenable to vascular reconstruction
- Length of the limb should be preserved as safely possible
- Level of amputation is determined by clinical judgement.

Thromboangiitis Obliterans (Buerger's Disease)

Buerger's disease is inflammatory occlusive disease involving small and medial sized arteries and veins of extremities. Most frequently develop in men **<40 years with history of smoking**.

Clinical Presentation

Clinical triad of: 1. Claudication of affected extremity, 2. Raynaud's phenomenon, 3. Migratory superficial thrombophlebitis.

- Arteriography is helpful to make the diagnosis, but pathological examination is necessary for confirmation of diagnosis.
- No specific treatment except abstinence from smoking.

Smoking cessation: (i) Improves ulcer healing; (ii) Improves patency and limb salvage rates in those patients who are candidates for surgical revascularization; and (iii) reduces the incidence of amputation.

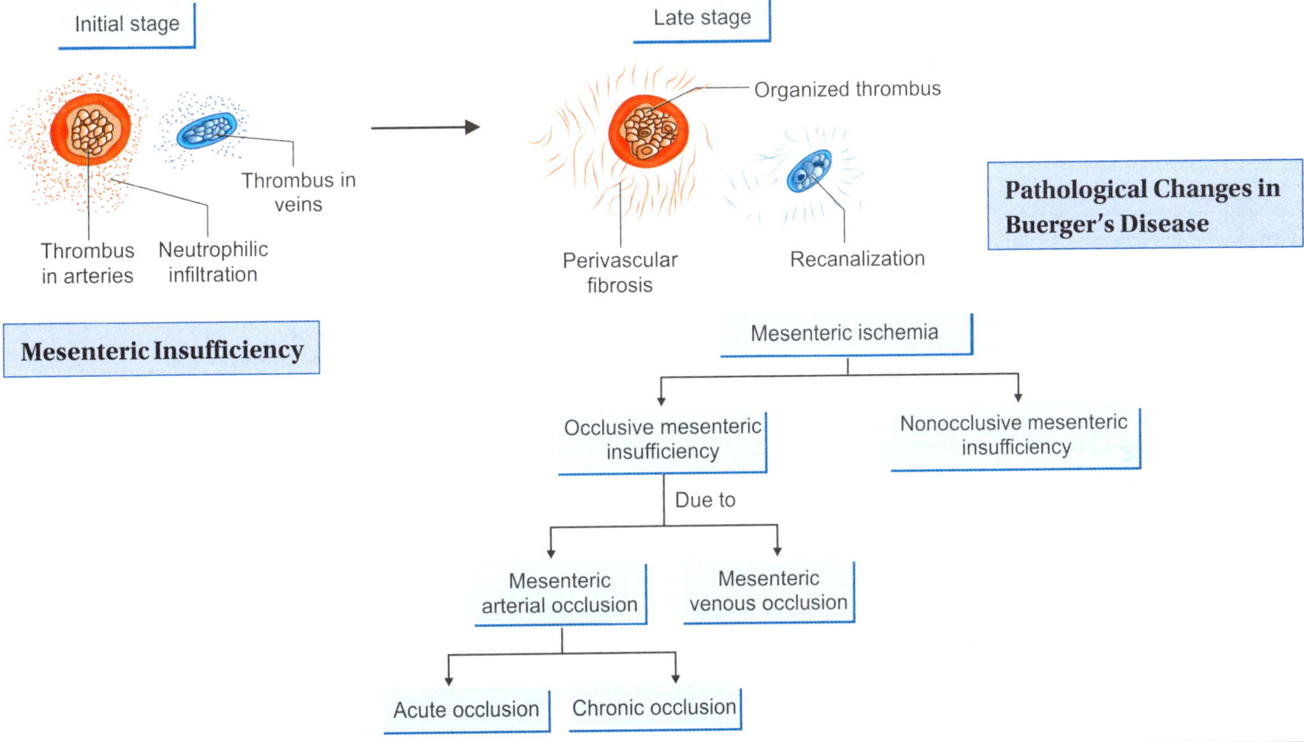

Acute Mesenteric Arterial Occlusion

- Mostly due to cardiogenic embolus. Embolus usually lodge at the segment of superior mesenteric artery from where middle colic and jejunal branches arise.
- **Risk factors are:** (i) Atrial fibrillation; (ii) Recent myocardial infarction; (iii) Endocarditis; (iv) Previous history of embolic disease; and (v) Left ventricular aneurysm.
- Sudden onset severe abdominal pain centered in the periumbilical region. The **pain is out-of proportion to the degree of abdominal tenderness**. In advanced stage, patient may present with features of peritonitis.
- Laboratory examination reveals elevated WBC count, metabolic acidosis.
- Plain radiograph shows fluid-filled bowel loops with bowel wall edema.
- The mainstay of diagnosis is angiography of mesenteric vessels. Helical CT can detect the proximal mesenteric thrombosis.
- Early management is crucial for a acceptable outcome, but early management depends **on high index of suspicion**.
- Surgery should not be delayed if patient has enough clinical evidence.

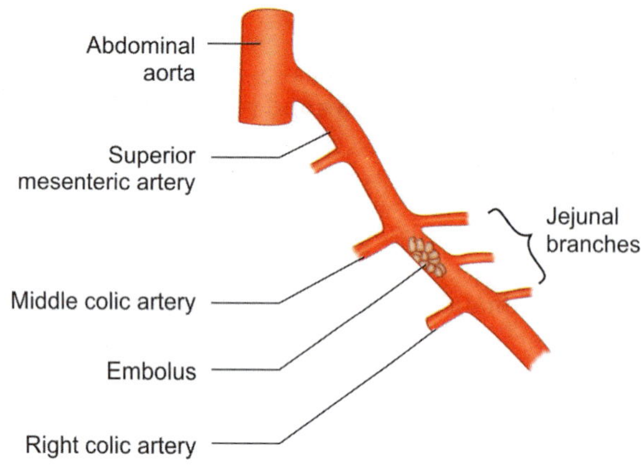

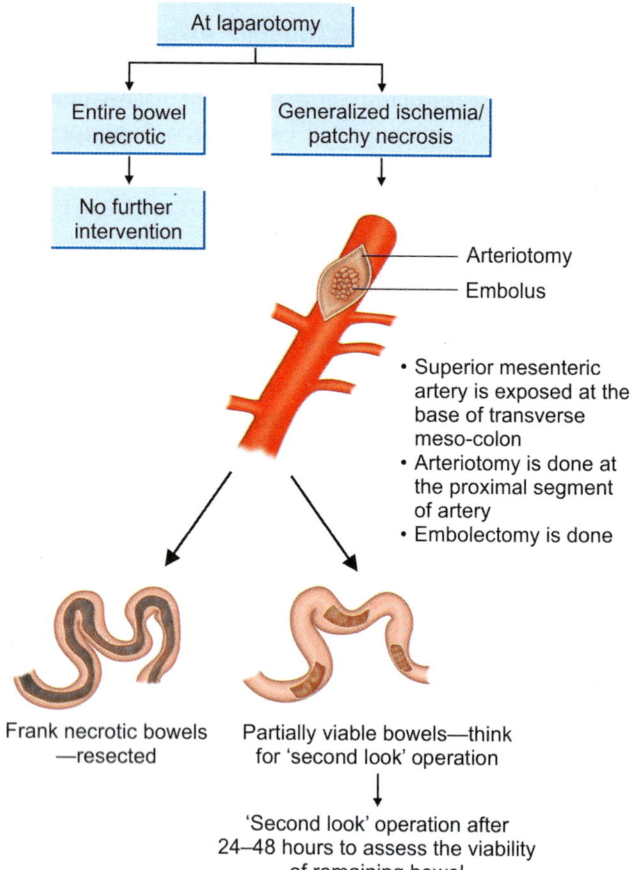

Computed tomography angiography (CTA) is the most appropriate imaging modality in any patient with suspected acute mesenteric ischemia.

Superior mesenteric artery is particularly affected because of its relatively large diameter and low takeoff angle from the aorta.

CTA findings suggestive of irreversible ischemia: (i) Intestinal dilatation; (ii) Reduced or absent visceral enhancement; (iii) Pneumatosis intestinalis; and (iv) Portal venous gas.

Chronic Mesenteric Arterial Occlusion

- Diffuse atherosclerosis involving the aorta and proximal superior mesenteric artery. Abundant collaterals develop in the period of chronic occlusion.
- **Clinical presentation:** Abdominal main begins within an hour after eating and abating within 4 hours—**Intestinal angina.**
- Patients also present with significant weight loss due to decreased absorption of nutrients and decreased food intake due to pain.
- **Diagnosis** mainly depends on classical history and exclusion of other diagnosis (e.g., chronic pancreatitis, gastric ulcer and malignancy).
  Abdominal bruit present in about 75% of cases.
  Duplex Doppler can detect occlusion of proximal SMA and celiac artery in most of the patients.
  For definite diagnosis, arteriography is indicated.
- **Treatment options are:** (i) Endovascular (balloon angioplasty or stenting); (ii) Endarterectomy; and (iii) Bypass grafting.

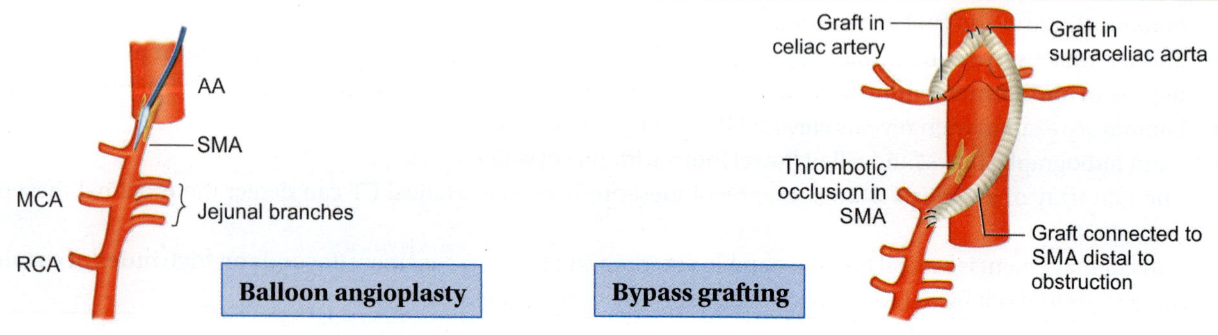

Mesenteric Venous Occlusion

- **Venous occlusion may develop in various clinical conditions:** (i) Cirrhosis with portal hypertension; (ii) Inflammatory and infective conditions (peritonitis, IBD and intra-abdominal abscess); (iii) Hypercoagulable states (DVT, neoplasm, antithrombin III and proteins deficiency); and (iv) After splenectomy.
- **Clinical presentation:** Patients present with vague abdominal pain. Clinical findings are often equivocal.
- **Diagnosis:** CT and arteriography reveals lack of prompt filling of the portal system.
- **Treatment** consists of hemodynamic support, anticoagulation and close observation.
  If peritonitis develops, then exploratory laparotomy is indicated.
  Surgical thrombectomy is not so beneficial.
- Prognosis is good because abundant collateral venous outflow develops.

Nonocclusive Mesenteric Insufficiency

- Usually associated in patient with sepsis and cardiovascular compromised state resulting in vasoconstriction of mesenteric vascular bed.
- **Clinical presentation:** Diffuse abdominal pain with out of proportional tenderness.
- **Classic arteriographic findings:** (i) Absent large vessel occlusion; (ii) Focal vasospasm with 'beading' of the major mesenteric branches; and (iii) Pruned tree appearance to the distal vasculature.
- **Treatment:** Fluid resuscitation, antibiotics, withdrawal of vasoconstrictors, infusion of papaverine into the SMA, angiographic monitoring of vasospasm are the basic components of management.
  Surgery is indicated only when peritonitis develops.
- Prognosis is not good.

Non-occlusive mesenteric ischemia should be suspected in any critically ill patients with multiple organ dysfunction requiring vasopressor support, presenting with abdominal pain or distension.

Aneurysmal Vascular Disease

Aneurysm–derived from the Greek Work 'aneurysma,' means 'widening.'
Aneurysm is permanent and irreversible localized dilation of arteries, at least 50% increase in diameter.

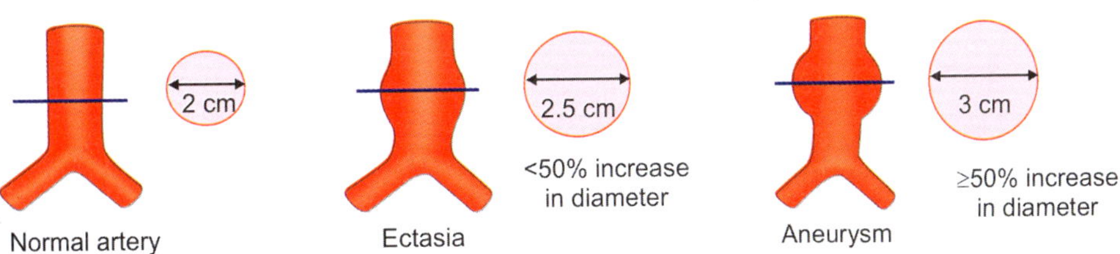

Types of Aneurysm

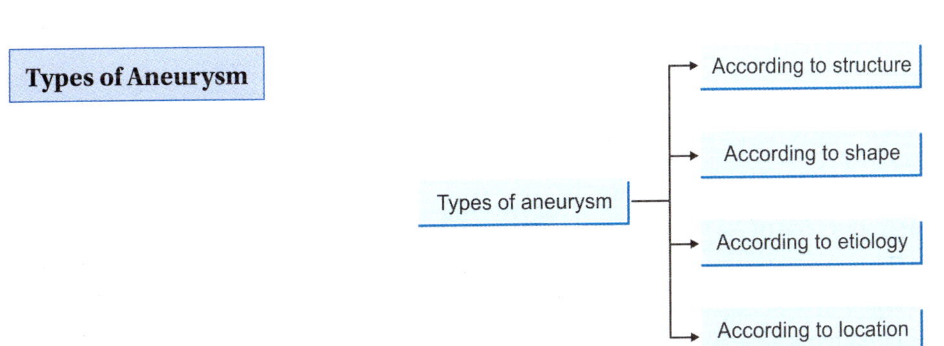

According to Structure

True aneurysm: Involves all three layers of the arterial wall. *Example:* (i) Aortic aneurysm (most common); (ii) Iliac artery aneurysm; and (iii) Popliteal artery aneurysm.

Pseudoaneurysm: Lined by adventitia only or by fibrous capsule. *Example:* (i) Following iatrogenic injury during arterial catheterization and (ii) Following arterial graft anastomotic disruption.

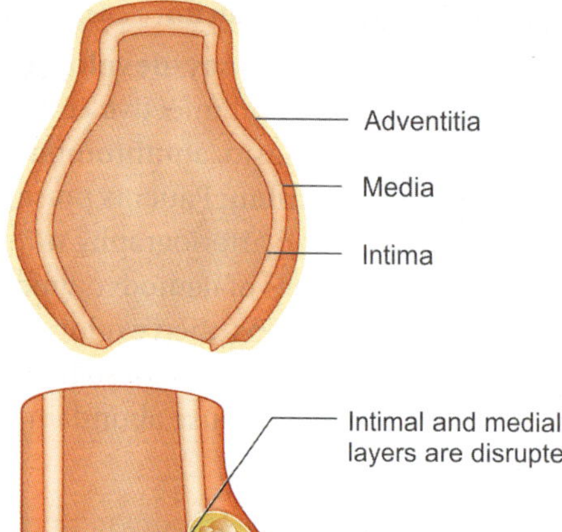

According to Shape

Fusiform: Entire circumference of a segment of vessel.

Saccular: Part of circumference of vessel.

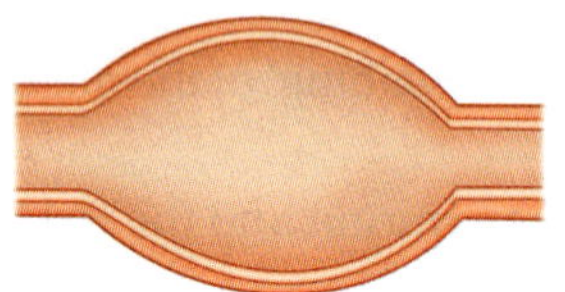

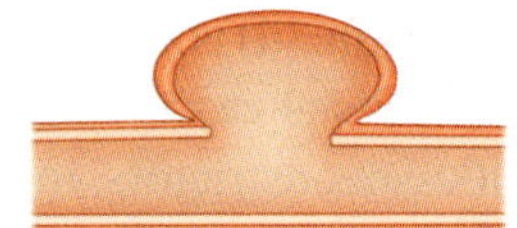

According to Location

- Aortic
- Peripheral
- Splanchnic
- Cerebral

According to Etiology

Degenerative, e.g., Atherosclerotic
- In Marfan's syndrome and Ehler-Danlos syndrome type IV.

Inflammatory, e.g., Mycotic aneurysm
- In syphilis, tuberculosis.

Congenital, e.g., Berry aneurysm.

Dissecting: Classically seen in arch of aorta in (Marfan's syndrome)

Width of the aneurysm is the predicting factor of rupture.

Abdominal Aortic Aneurysms (AAAs)

- Most common type of aneurysm
- Five times more common in males.

Risk factors:

Age: Prevalence increases with age

Atherosclerosis: Associated with increased risk

Black race: Negative risk factor

Cigarette smoking: 8:1 preponderance of aneurysm in smokers

Chlamydia pneumoniae infection: About 55% of AAAs show *C. pneumoniae* by immunohistochemistry

COPD: Associated with increased risk

Diabetes mellitus: Inverse relationship between DM and AAA

Family history: 1st degree relatives of patients have a 11 fold increase in relative risk to develop AAA.

Pathophysiology

- About 90% of AAAs are degenerative in origin
- Pathogenesis is multifactorial
- Genetic factor is also responsible:
  - Familial clustering in about 15–25%
  - Inherited as either autosomal dominant or autosomal recessive or X chromosome linked.

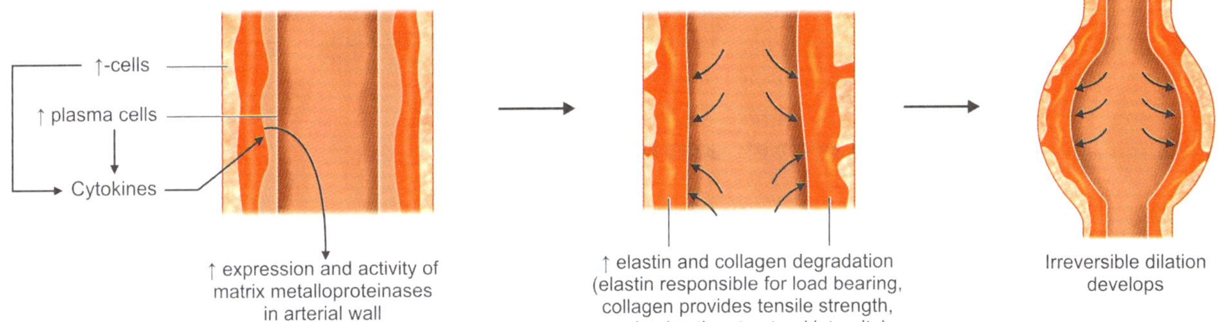

- About 90% of AAAs are degenerative in origin.
- **Aortic aneurysms are most commonly located in infrarenal aorta**. Other locations are—juxtarenal, pararenal, and suprarenal.

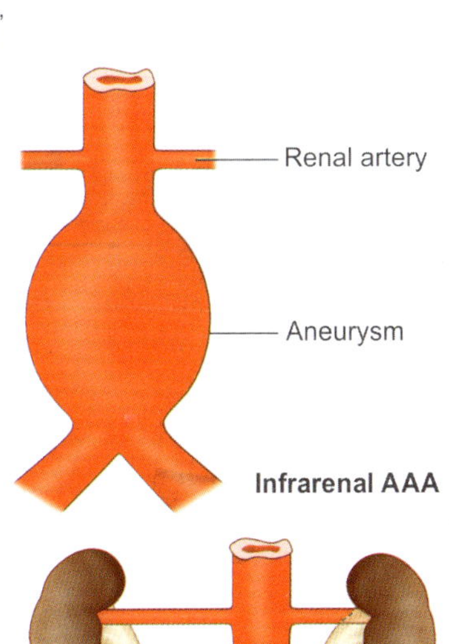

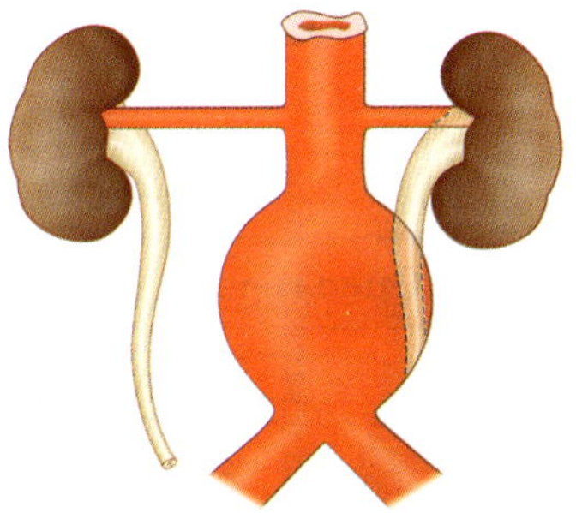

Clinical Presentation

Asymptomatic

Detected during clinical examination for nonrelated symptoms. The aneurysm presents as nontender, pulsatile mass palpable just above and left side of umbilicus.

Pressure Symptoms

- Compression of ureter
- Compression of adjacent bowel—causing chronic abdominal pain, early satiety
- Compression of spine—causing deep back pain.

Thrombosis and Embolism

Rupture into the retroperitoneal space or peritoneal cavity: Severe abdominal pain with shock.

Fistula: Aortoiliac fistula, aortocaval fistula and aortoenteric fistula. Patients aortoiliac or aortocaval fistula present with Unilateral or bilateral lower extremity edema, high output congestive heart failure, continuous abdominal bruit or palpable thrill. Aortoenteric fistula patient presents with shock and massive GI bleeding.

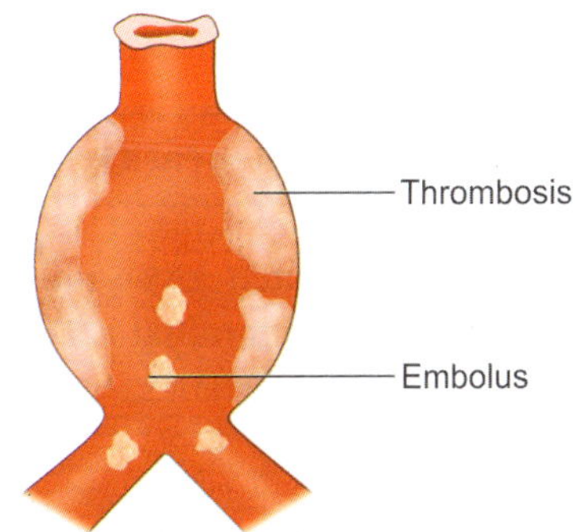

Investigations

Plain X-ray of Abdomen

- 'Eggshell' pattern of calcification
- Negative findings does not exclude the diagnosis.

Ultrasound of Abdomen
- Most widely used noninvasive test for AAAs
- Helpful to delineate structural details of the vessel wall, presence of atherosclerotic plaques.
- Can accurately measure the size of aneurysm in both directions (longitudinal and cross-sectional).

CT Scan
- Most accurate test for AAAs
- Can identify proximal and distal extent of the aneurysm
- Can identify occlusive or aneurismal disease in renal, visceral and iliac arteries
- Size of the aortic lumen, location of mural thrombus, presence of calcific disease can be well delineated
- Can also identify dissecting aneurysm, if present.

Three-dimensional CT angiography: Optimal imaging modality when planning for AAA repair.
Three-dimensional MR angiography: It is indicated in patients with renal insufficiency is being planned for AAA repair.

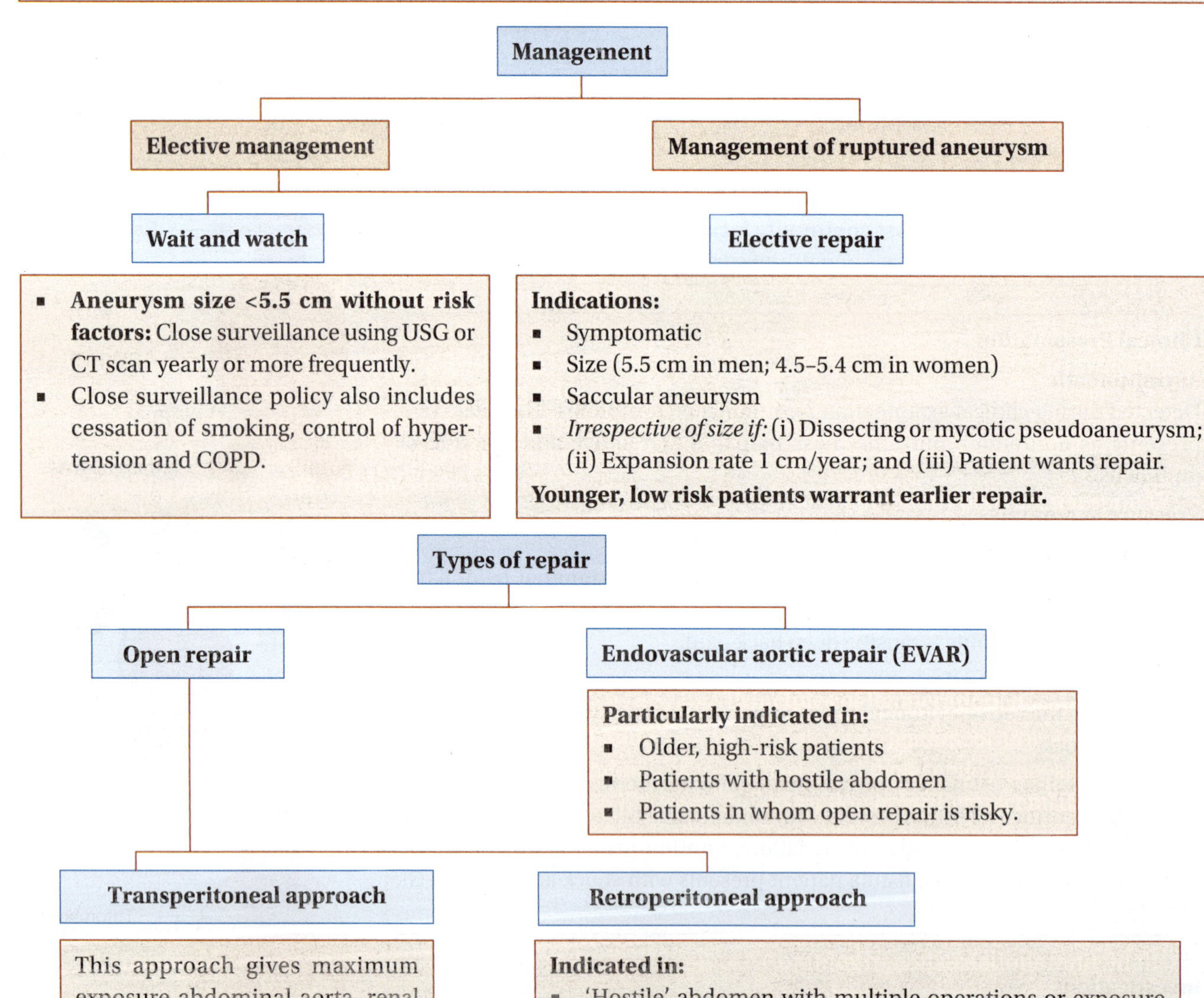

Endovascular Aortic Aneurysm Repair

- An endovascular stent graft excludes the aneurysm from blood flow.
- Insertion of the stent is done through cannulation of both femoral arteries.

Criteria to be assessed before stent insertion

- Length and diameter of nondilated infrarenal aorta (neck of aneurysm).
- Angle between neck and aneurysm.
- Presence or absence of intraluminal thrombus.
- Shape of the aortic neck.

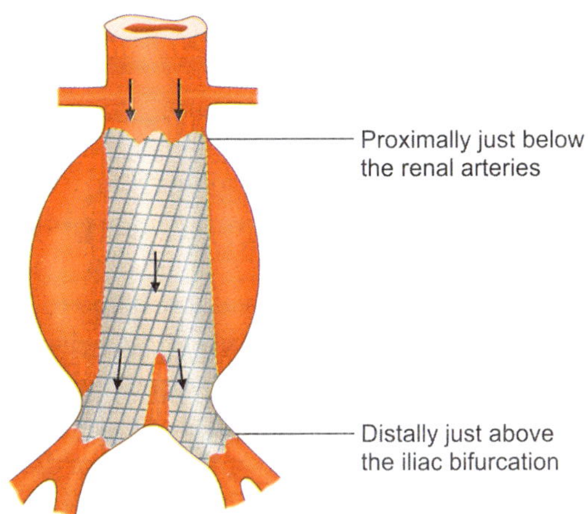

Management of Ruptured Abdominal Aortic Aneurysm

- Vigorous resuscitation with crystalloids, colloid, blood. Resuscitation is better done in the operating room rather than emergency ward.
- Exploration through transperitoneal approach.
- First priority is to control the hemorrhage by gaining proximal control of aorta at the supraceliac level through the lesser omentum.
- After control of bleeding, rest of the maneuvers are similar to electric repair.

Popliteal Artery Aneurysm

- Most common peripheral aneurysm.
- Patients are mostly male (about 97%).
- *Indications for intervention:* All symptomatic patients, size >2 cm, thrombus in aneurysm, angiographic evidence of distal embolization.
- Reconstruction with a saphenous vein graft is the gold standard method of repair.

Recognition of popliteal artery aneurysm and its intervention is important because of the risk of limb loss.

Femoral Artery Aneurysm

- Second most common peripheral artery aneurysm
- Mostly associated with aortoiliac aneurysm
- True aneurysms are always degenerative atherosclerotic aneurysms
- False aneurysms develop following catheterization, disruption of graft-artery anastomosis
- True aneurysms >2 cm—Elective repair
- Surgical treatment includes resection and replacement with prosthetic graft.

Splenic Artery Aneurysm

- Most common visceral artery aneurysm
- Most are saccular type.
- Most are caused by degenerative atherosclerosis.
- Mostly females are affected.
- Percutaneous embolization of splenic artery is the preferred treatment.

Diseases Associated with Increased Incidence of Visceral Artery Aneurysm

- Marfan syndrome
- Ehler-Danlos syndrome
- Fibromuscular dysplasia
- α_1-antitrypsin deficiency
- Polyarteritis nodosa
- Scleroderma

Renal Artery Aneurysm

- Most are saccular, mostly present at the bifurcation of primary or secondary branches.
- Medial fibroplasia is the most common cause of true aneurysm.
- Spontaneous or traumatic dissection is the most common cause of false aneurysm.
- If aneurysm ruptures in pregnant woman, fetal mortality 75%, maternal mortality 50%, so aneurysm >2 cm in women of childbearing age warrants repair.
- Treatment includes reconstruction with a patch or bypass and treatment of underlying renovascular hypertension.

Aortic Dissection

- Most common catastrophic event of the aorta.
- The initiating event is a primary intimal tear with secondary dissection into the media.
- The tear in the intima allows blood to flow from the true lumen to a newly formed channel (false lumen) by dissecting the aortic wall.
- The initial tear after occurs along the right lateral wall of the ascending aorta or descending thoracic aorta just below the ligamentum arteriosum.

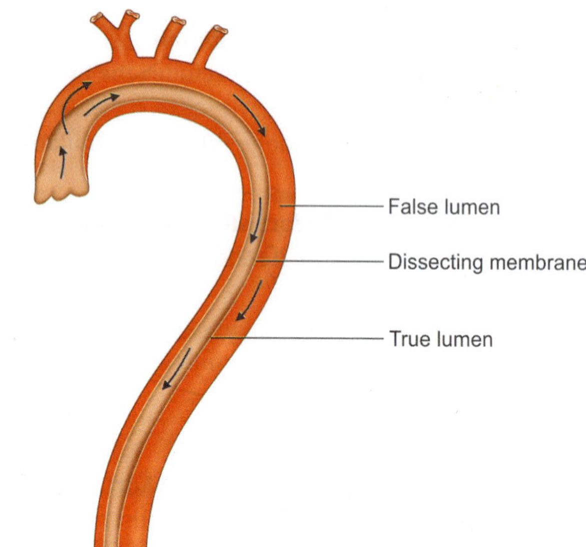

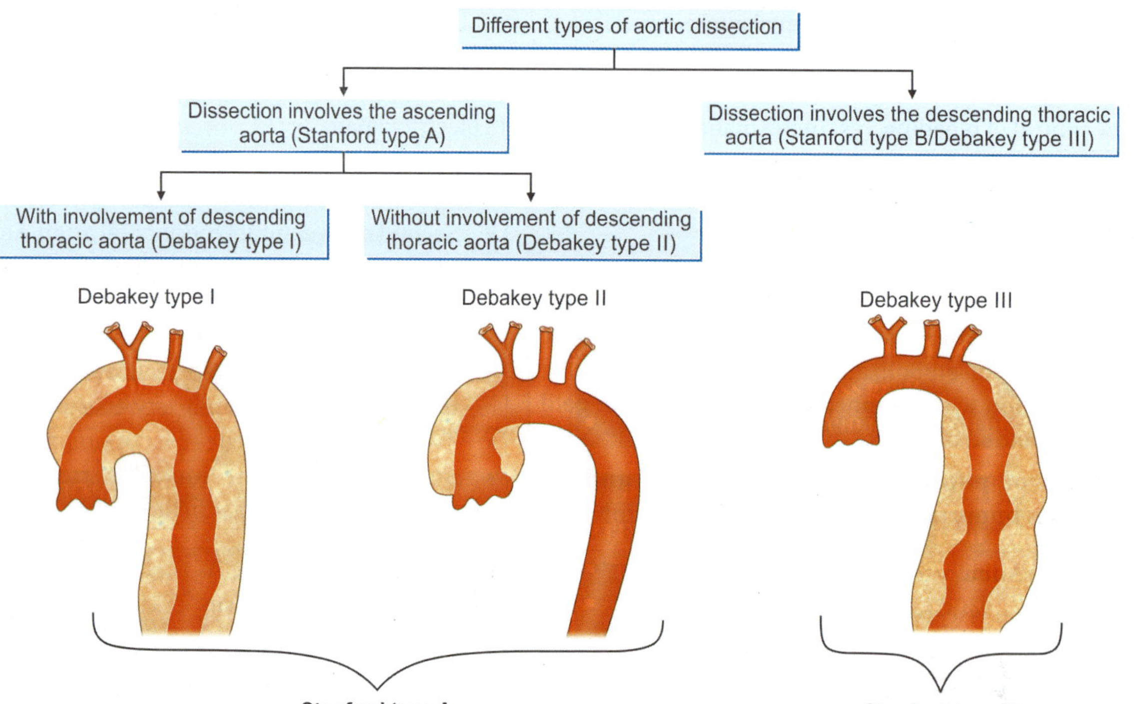

Predisposing Factors

- Systemic hypertension
- Cystic medial necrosis
- Marfan syndrome
- Ehler-Danlos syndrome
- Inflammatory aortitis (e.g., Takayasu's arteritis, giant cell arteritis)
- Congenital valve anomalies (e.g., bicuspid valve)
- Trauma (during cardiac catheterization)
- Pregnancy (increased risk during 3rd trimester).

Clinical Presentation

- Abrupt onset excruciating chest pain-classically described as 'tearing', associated with diaphoresis.
- Location of pain depends on according to the aortic segment involved.
- Site of dissection and acuteness of dissection (acute dissection <14 days, chronic dissection ≥14 days) have important clinical implications.

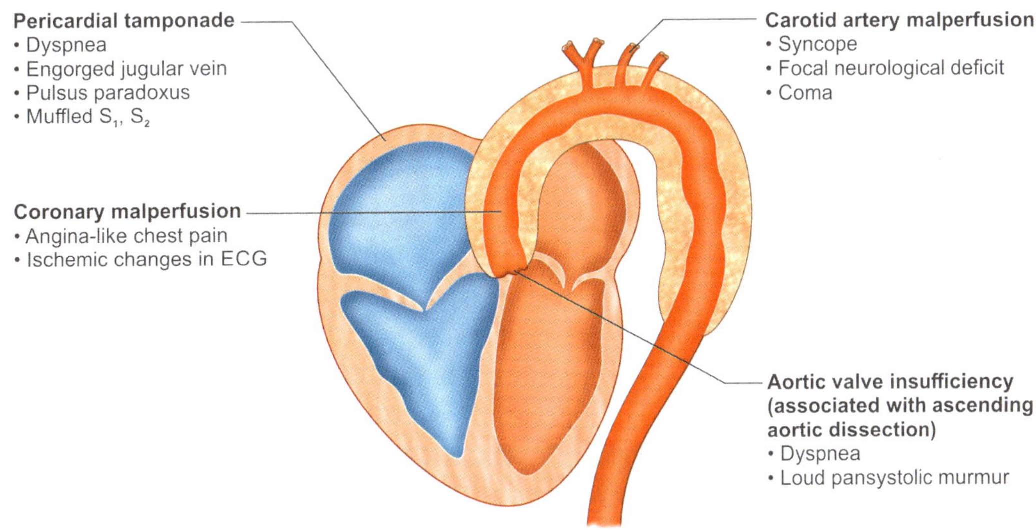

Diagnosis

Once the diagnosis of aortic dissection is considered, contrast CT is the investigation of choice. Double-lumen aorta is the classic finding in CT. If CT facility not available, then transthoracic or transesophageal echocardiography is indicated.

Treatment

Whenever clinical suspicion of dissection (any type, any location), pharmacologic therapy and 'Antihypertensive therapy' (β-blockers, vasodilators, calcium-channel blockers, and ACE inhibitors) should be started.

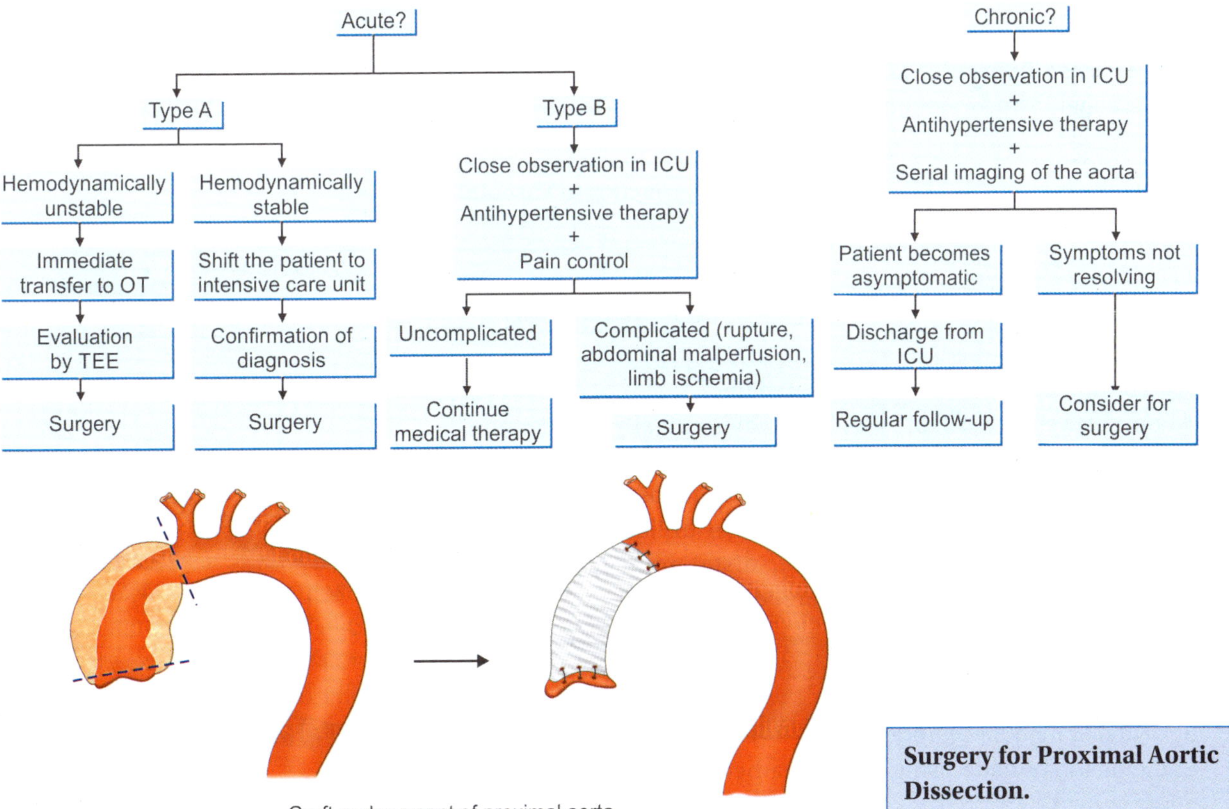

Graft replacement of proximal aorta

Surgery for Proximal Aortic Dissection.

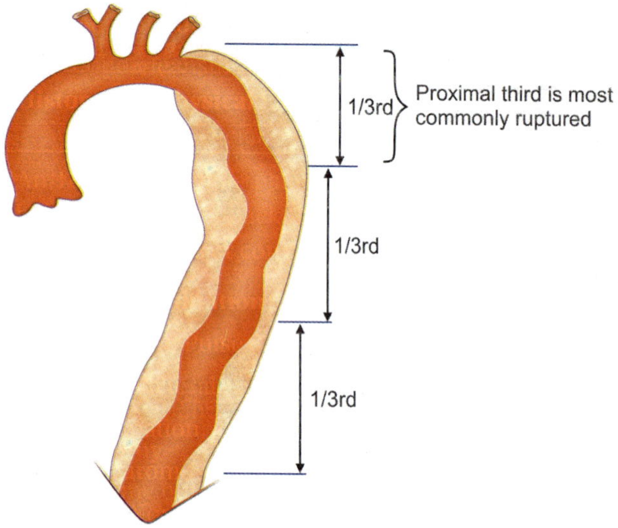

1/3rd
Proximal third is most commonly ruptured
1/3rd
1/3rd

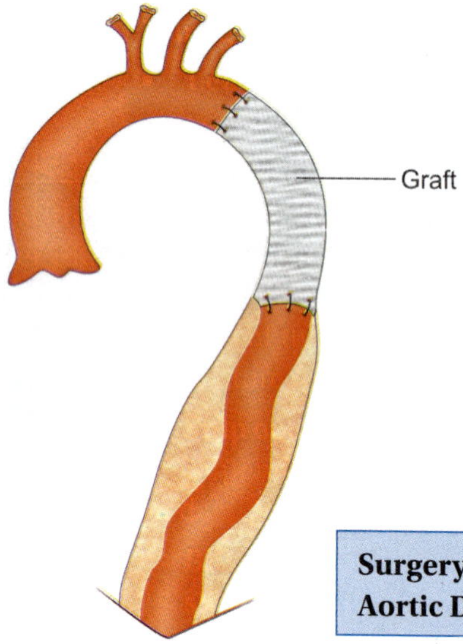

Graft

Surgery for Distal Aortic Dissection

Vascular Trauma

Different types of vascular trauma

- Laceration of vessel
- Transection of vessel
- Intimal disruption only
- Almost full thickness injury

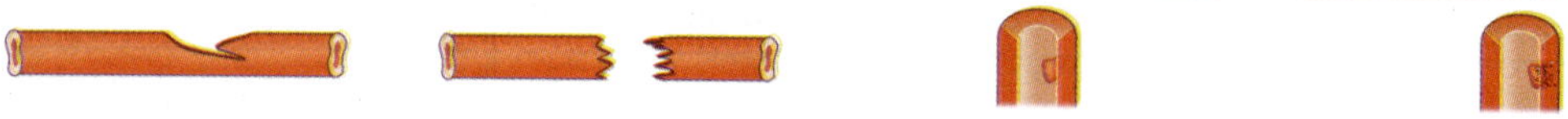

Consequences of vascular trauma: (i) Exsanguinating hemorrhage; (ii) Spasm of severed ends of arteries; (iii) Pseudoaneurysm formation; and (iv) Arterio-venous fistula.

Different Approaches to Vascular Injuries

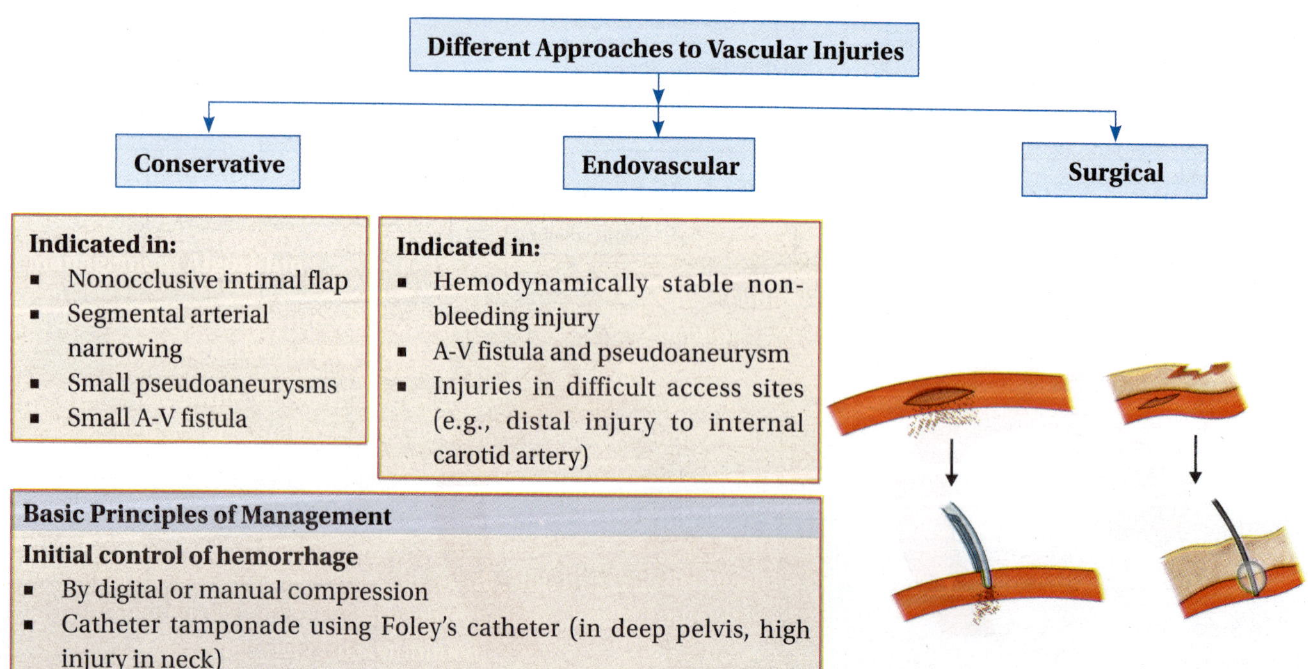

Conservative

Indicated in:
- Nonocclusive intimal flap
- Segmental arterial narrowing
- Small pseudoaneurysms
- Small A-V fistula

Endovascular

Indicated in:
- Hemodynamically stable non-bleeding injury
- A-V fistula and pseudoaneurysm
- Injuries in difficult access sites (e.g., distal injury to internal carotid artery)

Surgical

Basic Principles of Management

Initial control of hemorrhage
- By digital or manual compression
- Catheter tamponade using Foley's catheter (in deep pelvis, high injury in neck)

Proper Exposure

- In neck—by vascular exposure technique
- In chest—by choosing appropriate thoracotomy incision
- In abdomen—by appropriate operative maneuvers (e.g., Mattox maneuver, Cattell-Braasch maneuver)

Proximal Control of Bleeding Vessel

Selection of appropriate repair technique (ligation/suturing/shunt insertion/reconstruction)

Damage Control Approach

Ligation?

Suturing?

Shunt insertion?

Reconstruction?

Graft

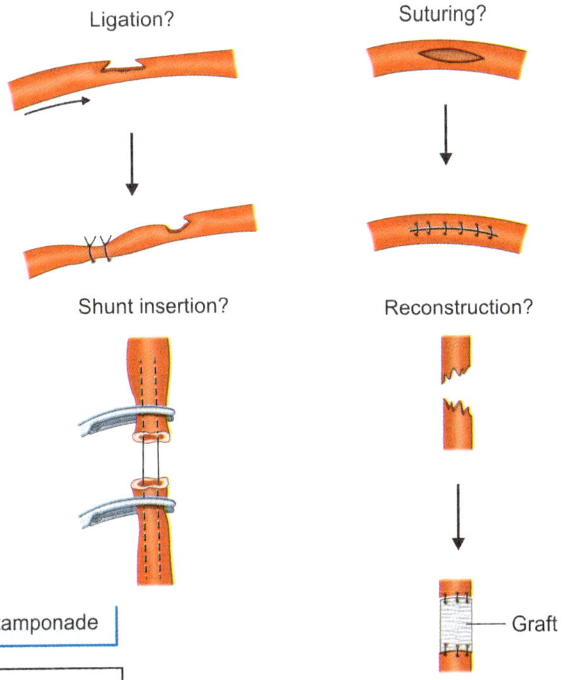

Temporary control of hemorrhage by ligation or balloon tamponade

Ligation of injured vessel

(External carotid, celiac axis, internal iliac arteries)

Temporary intra-arterial shunt

(To maintain distal perfusion about 50% of normal flow)

If patient becomes stable

Plan for complex reconstruction

Damage Control Approach

Venous Diseases

Superficial Thrombophlebitis

- Superficial thrombophlebitis is characterized by inflammatory reaction and thrombi formation in superficial veins.
- Appear spontaneously in patient with varicose veins, in pregnancy, in Buerger's disease, after IV therapy, after localized trauma.
- **Clinical presentations** include erythema, indurations, tenderness along the course of affected vein.
- Duplex scan is the **diagnostic modality of choice**.
- **Treatment** is indicated: (i) To relieve symptoms; (ii) To prevent extension of thrombus along the superficial veins; and (iii) To prevent thromboembolic complications.

NSAIDs, elevation of the limb, local application of heat are the primary treatment. Anticoagulant therapy is indicated if thrombophlebitis involving close to saphenofemoral or saphenopopliteal junction or patient is at increased risk of DVT. Surgery (ligation of vein at the junction) is indicated if progressive proximal extension of thrombus.

Thrombophlebitis Migrans

- Thrombophlebitis migrans is migratory superficial thrombophlebitis associated with abdominal malignancy.
- This type of superficial thrombophlebitis is most commonly associated with pancreatic cancer (Trousseau's syndrome).

Deep Vein Thrombosis

Deep vein thrombosis (DVT) and **pulmonary embolism** are the two most clinically significant manifestations of **venous-thrombo-embolism**.

Pathophysiology of DVT

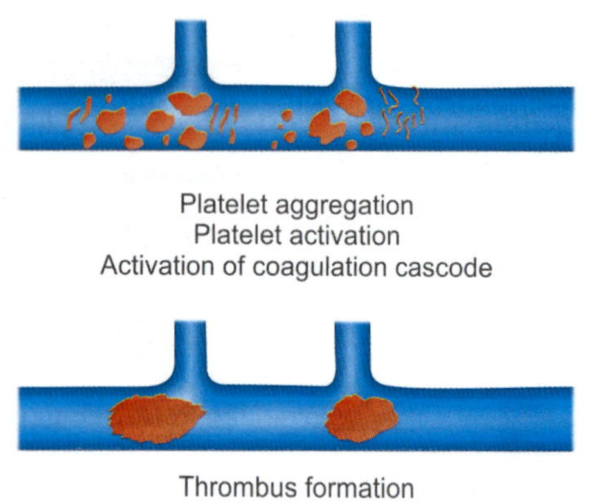

Stasis of blood flow—due to immobility, debilitating conditions

Virchow's Triad

Hypercoagulable State
- Factor V Leiden mutation
- Protein C deficiency
- Protein S deficiency
- Antithrombin III deficiency
- Surgery
- Hyperhomocysteinemia
- Myeloproliferative disorders
- Malignancy (lung, colon, stomach, and breast)
- Chemotherapy (cyclophosphamide, methotrexate, and 5-FU).

Endothelial Damage

Due to:
- Trauma
- Venous cannulation
- Transvenous pacing
- Chemotherapy (bleomycin, vincristine, and doxorubicin)

Risk Factors

- **Immobilization due to:** (i) Postoperative convalescence; (ii) AMI; (iii) CHF; and (iv) CVA.
- Hypercoagulable states
- **Surgery:** (i) Orthopedic (particularly hip and knee surgery); (ii) Abdominal; and (iii) Genitourinary.
- **Trauma:** Fractures of spine, pelvis, femur and tibia.
- Malignancy (pancreas, stomach, lung and breast)
- Pregnancy
- Estrogen (as replacement or as contraceptive)
- Venulitis (Buerger's disease, Behçet's disease, homocystinuria)
- History of DVT

Diagnosis

For diagnosis, a high index of suspicion is needed:
- Symptoms and signs are not so helpful, as half of the patients are asymptomatic, particularly patients with calf thrombi.
- **Homan's sign** (calf pain on passive dorsiflexion of ankle) is not so reliable for clinical diagnosis.
- **Duplex ultrasound:** This imaging modality can detect the occluded venous segments and can also demonstrate flow pattern. **Lack of vein compressibility** is the main criteria for diagnosis.
- **Magnetic resonance venography** is particularly indicated to detect thrombosis of iliac veins and IVC.

Outcomes of DVT

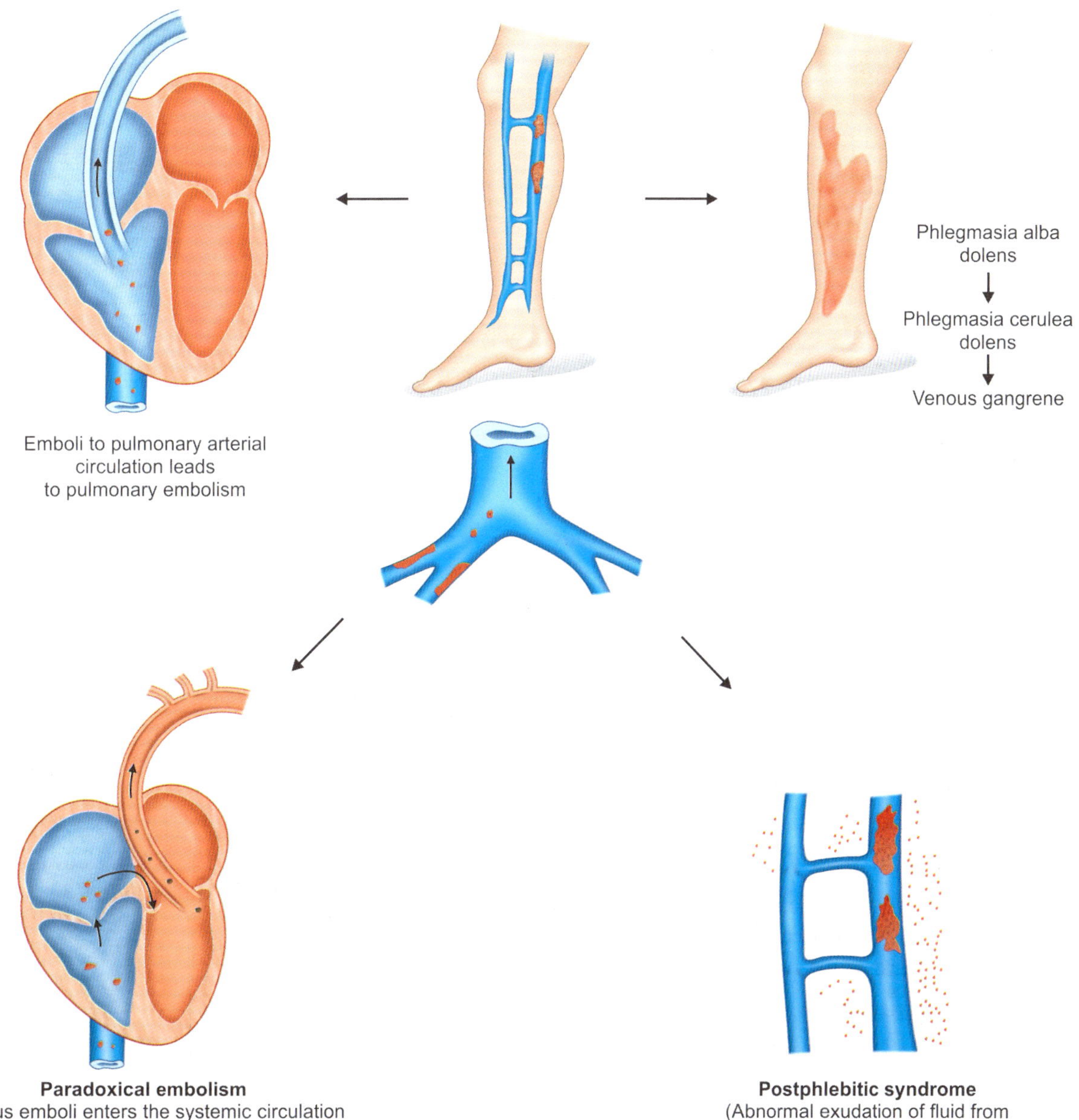

Emboli to pulmonary arterial circulation leads to pulmonary embolism

Paradoxical embolism
(Venous emboli enters the systemic circulation through patent foramen ovale or ASD)

Postphlebitic syndrome
(Abnormal exudation of fluid from veins due to damage of valves)

Phlegmasia Alba Dolens

Also known as "milk leg", characterized by massively swollen leg, pitting edema and blanching.

Phlegmasia Cerulean Dolens

Characterized by swollen, blue painful limb. The prompt diagnosis is important because early and aggressive therapy can prevent the development of venous gangrene.

Prophylaxis

The goal of DVT prophylaxis is to prevent the morbidity and mortality of venous thromboembolism

Potential candidates of prophylaxis:

- Elderly patient undergoing major abdominal (particularly cancer surgery) or major orthopedic surgery (e.g., hip replacement).
- Patient with major trauma.
- Prolonged immobility (>3 days).

Types of DVT prophylaxis

Pharmacological prophylaxis

- Low dose unfractionated heparin (5,000 U SC BID)
- Low molecular weight heparin (LMWH)—30 mg SC BID
- Fondaparinux

Mechanical prophylaxis

- Intermittent pneumatic compression (IPC)
- Elastic stockings
- Inferior vena cava (IVC) filter.

Advantages of LMWH

- Longer half-life
- Higher bioavailability
- More predictable anticoagulant response
- No laboratory monitoring is necessary (PTT is unaffected)
- No contraindication in head injury and other traumas.

Fondaparinux

- A new class of synthetic pentasaccharide anticoagulant.
- It inhibits the action of factor Xa but does not inhibit thrombin.
- It does not interact with platelets.
- Longer half-life than heparin.
- Dosing—2.5 mg SC OD

Thromboprophylaxis for General and Abdominal-pelvic Surgery Patients

Very low-risk for VTE (<0.5%)—Rogers score <7, Caprini score 0

Only early ambulation is recommended, no specific pharmacologic or mechanical prophylaxis.

Low-risk for VTE (nearly 1.5%)—Rogers score 7–10, Caprini score 1–2

Mechanical prophylaxis, preferably with intermittent pneumatic compression, over no prophylaxis is suggested.

Moderate risk for VTE (nearly 3%)—Rogers score >10, Caprini score 3–4, not at high-risk of bleeding

LMWH, LDUH, or mechanical prophylaxis, preferably with IPC, over no prophylaxis, is suggested.

Moderated risk for VTE (nearly 3%) with high-risk for major bleeding

Mechanical prophylaxis, preferably with IPC, over no prophylaxis, is suggested.

High-risk for VTE (nearly 6%)—Caprini score ≥5, not at high-risk for major bleeding

LMWH or LDUH is recommended over no prophylaxis. Addition of mechanical prophylaxis with elastic stockings or IPC is suggested.

High-risk for VTE (nearly 6%), not at high-risk for major bleeding, LMWH and unfractionated heparin are contraindicated

Low-dose aspirin, fondaparinux, or mechanical prophylaxis, preferably with IPC , over no prophylaxis, is suggested.

(Adapted from ACCP guideline)

Treatment of DVT

Treatment is necessary: (i) To prevent morbidity and mortality associated with pulmonary embolism; (ii) To prevent the postphlebitic syndrome; (iii) To decrease the recurrence rate; and (iv) To limit further thrombosis.

Different Treatment Options

① Antithrombotics

② Thrombolytics
- Only indication is if phlegmasia develops

③ IVC filters
- Indicated to whom antithrombotic therapy is contraindicated or failure of anticoagulation
- Filters filter the emboli while allowing venous blood flow through IVC

④ Thrombectomy
- Indicated in phlegmasia cerulea dolens and impending venous gangrene

Antithrombotics:

Unfractionated heparin
80 U/kg—bolus dose
↓
15 U/kg—infusion
[PTT should be checked after 6 hours. Dosing must be adjusted to maintain PPT at 60–80 seconds]

Warfarin
Is started on the same day (INR must be 2.5–3.0)

LMWH
Can be administered as an outpatient basis along with warfarin
(LMWH prevent clot propagation, warfarin protects against recurrent thrombosis)

Venous Insufficiency

Types of primary venous insufficiency

① Telengiectasias
- Small intradermal dilated vein
- <1 mm in diameter

② Reticular vein
- Subcutaneous dilated veins that enter the tributaries of main axial vein
- Nonpalpable subdermal vein <4 mm

③ Varicose vein
- Tortuous, dilated, superficial veins in the lower limb, along the anatomical distribution of great saphenous and short saphenous vein
- Dilated, palpable subcutaneous vein >4 mm in diameter

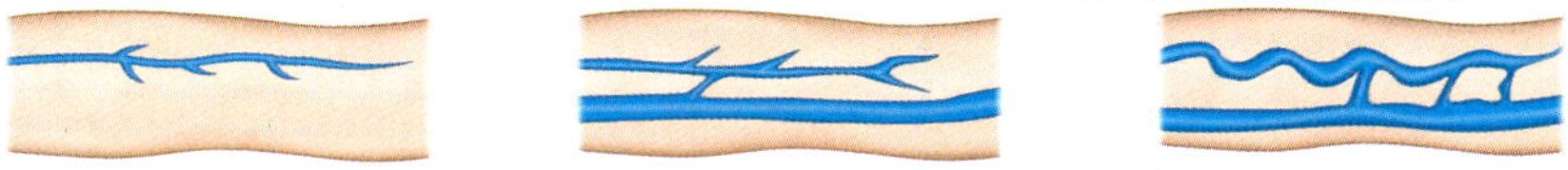

Risk Factors
- Occupation (prolonged standing)
- Positive family history
- Gender (female sex)
- Obesity
- History of DVT
- Chronic constipation
- Multiparity.

3-factors maintain normal venous return, failure of any one factor or more cause varicose vein:
- Valvular competence
- Patency of veins
- Calf muscle pump.

All varicose veins result from **venous hypertension** caused by flooding of venous blood in low pressure superficial venous system.

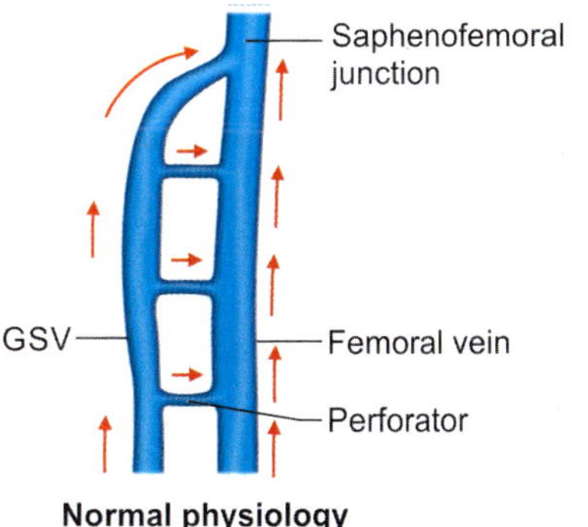

Normal physiology

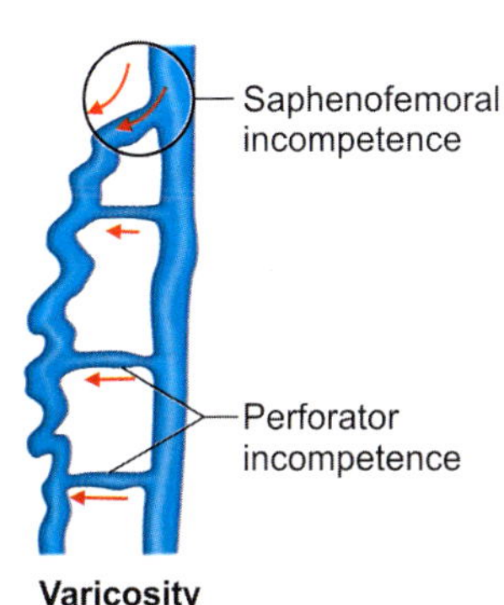

Varicosity

- Venous valves are bicuspid valves.
- The great saphenous vein has at least 6 valves (ranges between 4–25) and short saphenous vein has a median of 7–10 valves (ranges between 4–13).

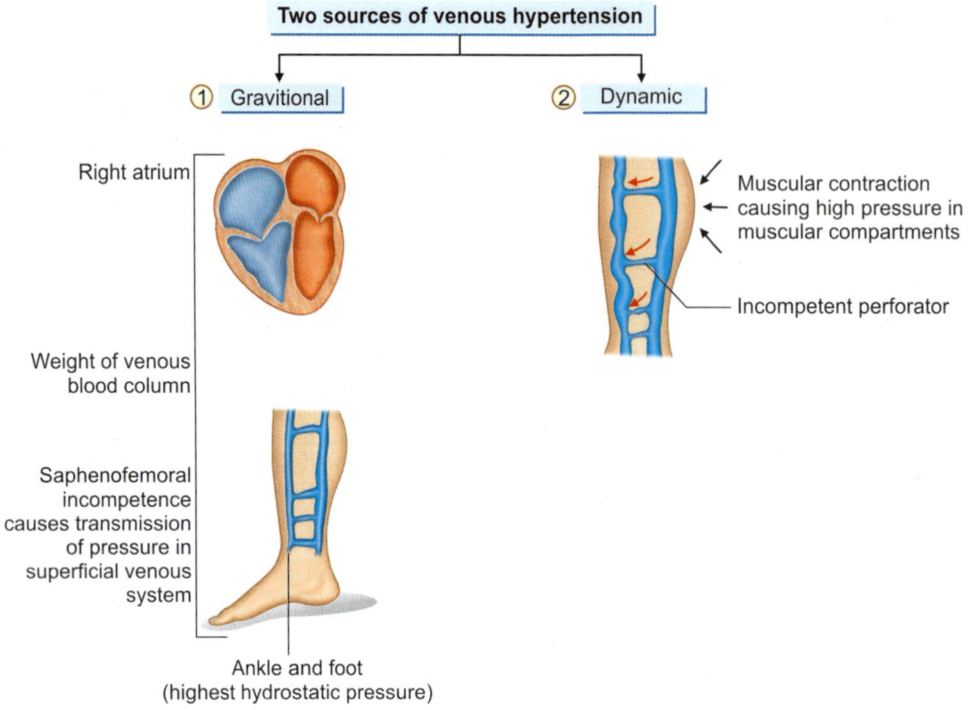

Clinical Presentation

- Venous prominences and tortuosity along the course of great saphenous or short saphenous vein or their tributaries
- Heaviness of leg
- Swollen leg
- Ankle flare (corona phlebectatica).
- Pale area around ankle (atrophie blanche).
- Blackening and deformity around ankle (lipodermatosclerosis/champagne bottle leg)
- Eczema
- Ulceration in the gaiter area (over the medial malleolus).
- Venous claudication (pain during and after exercise that is relieved with rest and leg elevation) may present in patients with previous DVT.

Clinical Examination

Examination in the standing and lying down position

Examination and assessment of:

- GSV territory, SSV territory or both involvement
- Saphenofemoral incompetency
- Saphenopopliteal incompetency
- Perforator incompetency
- Searching for complications—eczema, blackening, ulceration, bleeding
- Palpation of arterial pulses.
- Ankle mobility (patients with advanced disease often have decreased mobility)

Clinical Methods

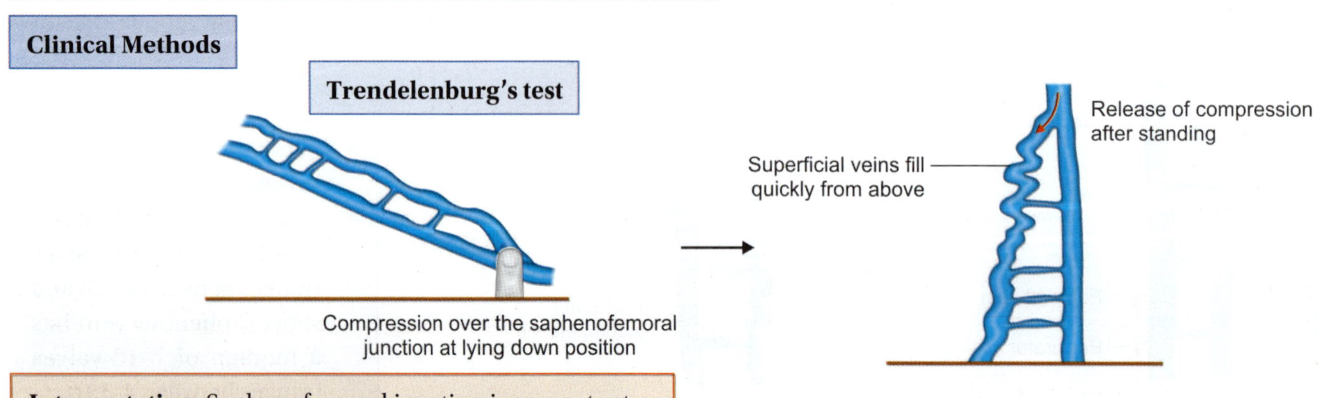

Interpretation: Saphenofemoral junction incompetent

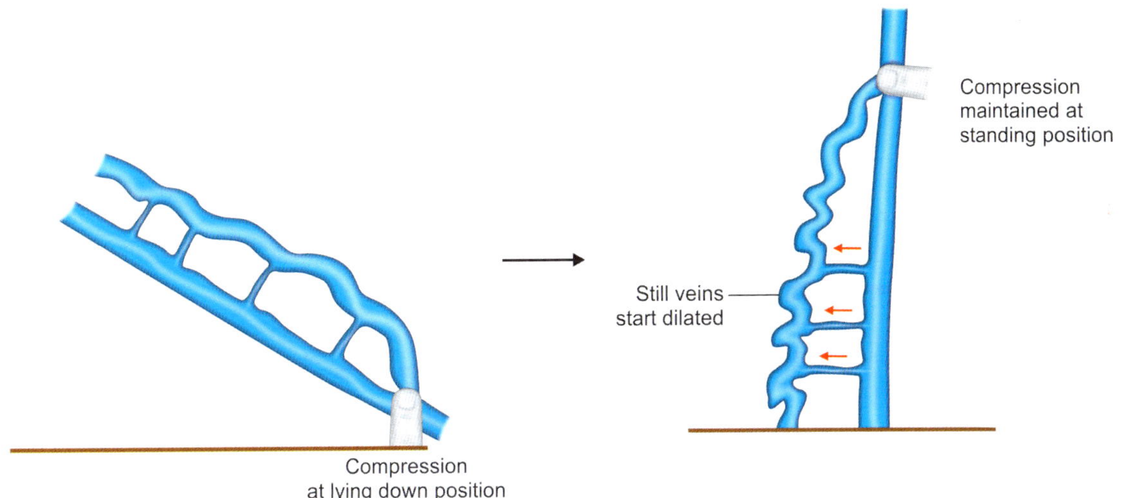

Interpretation: Perforator incompetence

Ochsner–Mahorner Test (Multiple Tourniquet Test)

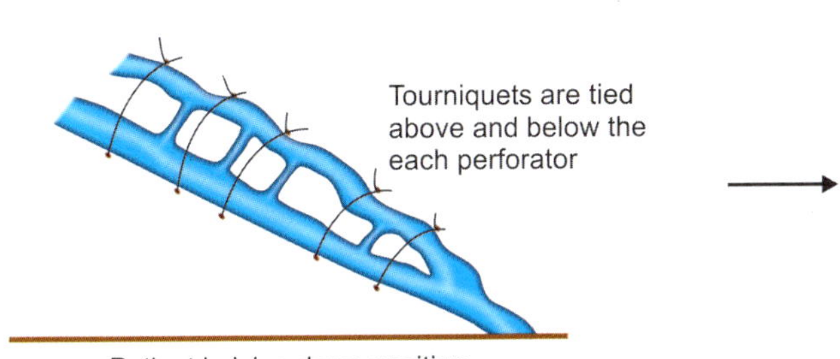

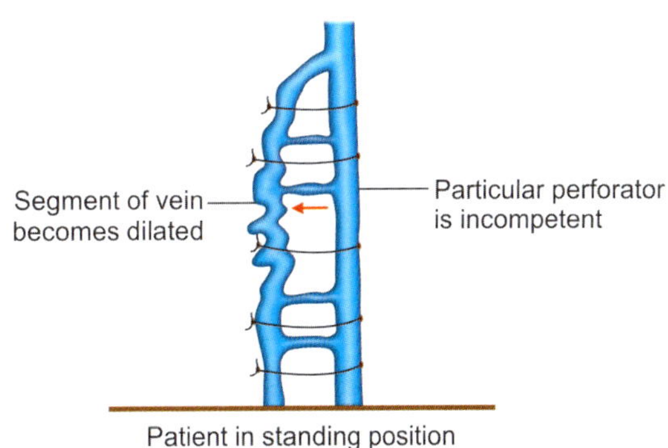

Schwartz test

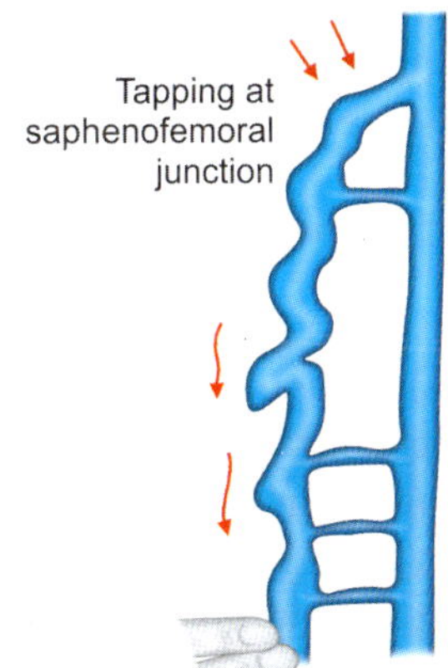

Fegan's test

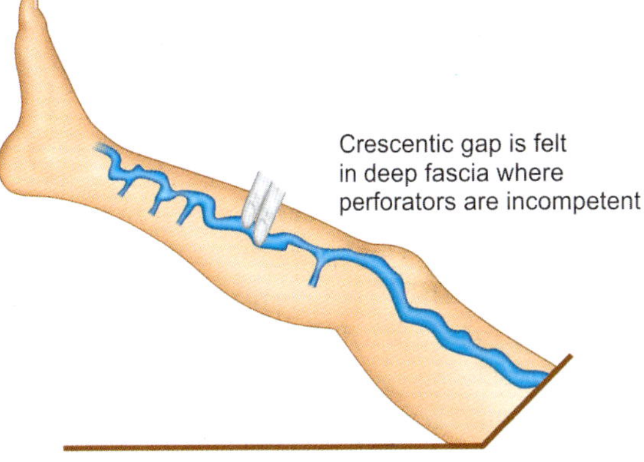

Modified Perthe's Test

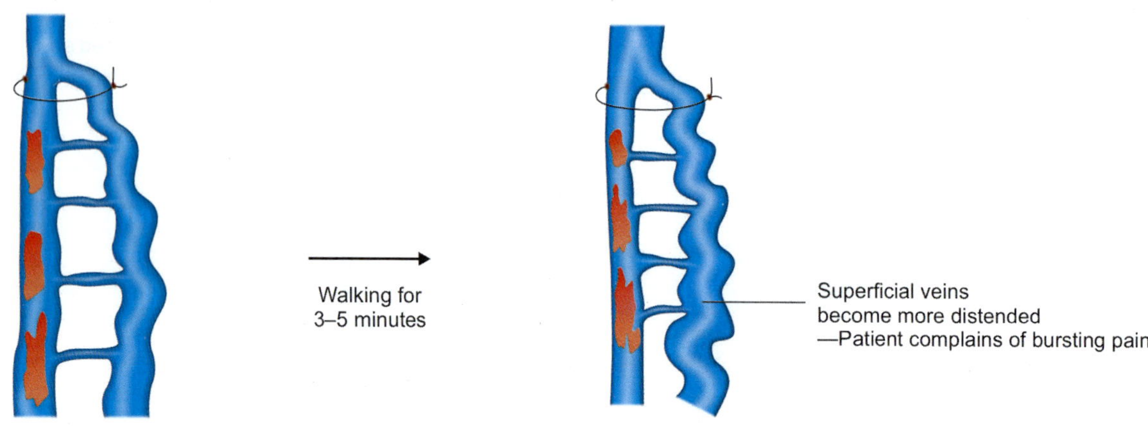

Interpretation: Deep vein is occluded by thrombus.

CEAP (Clinical, etiological, anatomical, and pathophysiological) classification system is most commonly used grading system for chronic venous disorders.

Clinical (C)

- **C_0:** No visible or palpable veins
- **C_1:** Telangiectasias or reticular veins
- **C_2:** Varicose vein
- **C_3:** Varicose vein with edema
- **C_{4a}:** Pigmentation and/or eczema
- **C_{4b}:** Lipodermatosclerosis and/or atrophie blanche
- **C_5:** Healed venous ulcer
- **C_6:** Active venous ulcer

Etiological (E)

- **E_c:** Congenital
- **E_p:** Primary
- **E_s:** Secondary (post-thrombotic)

Anatomical (A)

- **A_s:** Superficial veins
- **A_p:** Perforator veins
- **A_d:** Deep veins

Pathophysiological (P)

- **P_r:** Reflux
- **P_o:** Obstruction
- **$P_{r,o}$:** Reflux and obstruction

Different formats of CEAP classification: (i) Basic CEAP classification (used for routine clinical practice); (ii) Comprehensive CEAP classification (used as research tool); and (iii) Revised format of CEAP classification. Basic CEAP classification along with revised Venous Clinical Severity Score (VCSS) is recommended in routine clinical practice.

The revised VCSS is the best available instrument for qualitative assessment of improvement and changes in severity of chronic venous disease during follow-up.

Diagnosis

- **Duplex scanning of the venous system** is the initial diagnostic modality for all patients with suspected chronic venous disorders. Duplex scanning provides following informations: (i) Status of GSV; (ii) Status of SFJ (competent or incompetent); (iii) Status of SSV; (iv) Status and location of SPJ (competent or incompetent)—SPJ is very much inconstant in location; (v) Status of deep veins; and (vi) Location and status (competent or incompetent) of leg and thigh perforators.
- **Air plethysmography** is particularly indicated in patients with advanced CVD (CEAP C_3-C_6) if duplex scanning cannot provide information regarding pathophysiology.
- Advanced imaging modalities (e.g., **CT or MR venography**) is rarely indicated for simple varicose vein.

Treatment

All symptomatic primary varicose veins should be intervened. All varicose veins with complications must be intervened.

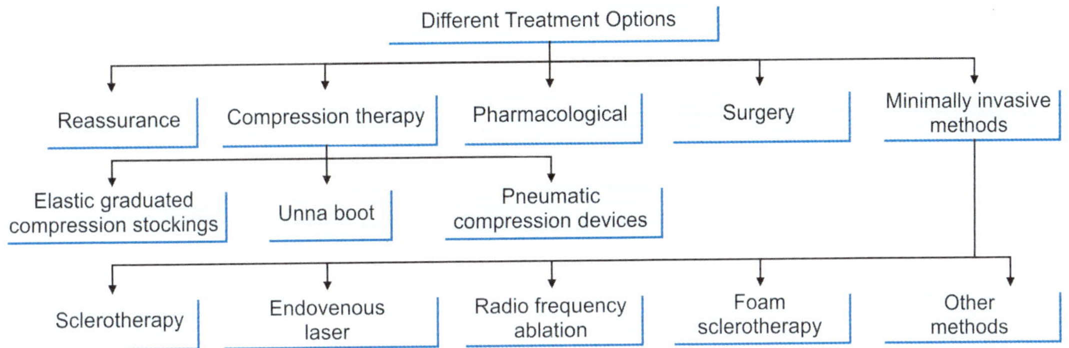

Compression Therapy

Compression therapy is the most commonly used treatment for varicose veins. Compression therapy decreases the ambulatory venous hypertension in patients with CVD.

Compression therapy is indicated in:

- Post-thrombotic syndrome varicose veins
- Patient with minimal symptoms
- Not fit or unwilling to surgery
- After surgery, sclerotherapy and endovenous laser.

Elastic graduated compression stockings is the most commonly used compression therapy method.

Types of compression stockings:

- Class I—Pressure 18–21 mm Hg
- Class II—Pressure 26–34 mm Hg
- Class III—Pressure >34 mm Hg.
  - Class II stockings is used for uncomplicated varicose vein.
  - Class III stockings is used for complicated varicose vein.

Contraindications: (i) Suspected or diagnosed peripheral arterial disease; (ii) Severe peripheral neuropathy; and (iii) Congestive cardiac failure.

Complications: (i) Skin breakdown and (ii) Frank necrosis.

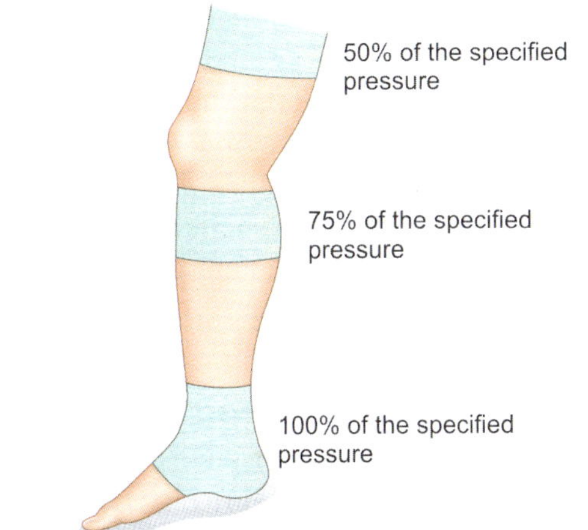

Other forms of ambulatory compression methods are:

- Multilayer elastic wraps
- Elastic and nonelastic bandages
- Unna boot.

Noncompliance is due to discomfort, skin irritation, difficulty in donning and cost.

Pharmacotherapy

- Indicated in early stage of varicose veins, in association with compression therapy.
- Commonly used phlebotropic drugs:
  - **Micronized purified flavonoid fraction:** Acts by—(i) Improving RBC rheology; (ii) Anti-inflammatory property; (iii) Protective effect on venous valve; and (iv) Protective effect on venous wall.
  - **Calcium dobesilate:** Acts by—(i) Increasing venous tone and (ii) Antiedema and capillary protection effects.
  - **Diosmin:** Acts by—(i) Profibrinolytic action and (ii) Anti-inflammatory property.
  - **Rutin and troxerutin:** Acts by—(i) Improving RBC rheology and (ii) Protective effect on venous wall.

Sclerotherapy

Indicated in: Telengiectasias, reticular veins and small varicose veins.

Mechanism of action of sclerotherapy: Sclerosing agents cause destruction of venous endothelium resulting in exposure of subendothelial collagen fibers, ultimately formation of fibrotic obstruction.

Types of sclerotherapy are: (i) Liquid sclerotherapy and (ii) Foam sclerotherapy. Delivery of the sclerosing agent as a foam prolongs the time of contact and increases the effect of sclerosing agent.

Sclerosing agents are: (i) Polidocanol; (ii) Sodium tetradecyl sulfate (STS); and (iii) Sodium morrhuate. Polidocanol is the most commonly used sclerosing agent.

Foam Sclerotherapy

- This method is the least invasive of the endovenous ablation techniques.
- The most popular technique is Tessari method. This method uses a three-way stopcock connected with two syringes, 1 part solution of STS or polidocanol to 4 or 5 parts of air. Mixing the sclerosing agent with air using two syringes and pushing the mixture from one syringe into other atleast 20 times to make a smooth, consistent foam. The foam must be used within 60 seconds of production.
- Not ≥20 mL foam should be injected at one sitting. Multiple sitting may be required for maximum success.

Complications of sclerotherapy: (i) Matting; (ii) Pigmentation; (iii) Skin urticaria; and (iv) Pain.

Rare complications are: Thrombophlebitis, nerve injury (saphenous, sural), inadvertent arterial injection of the sclerosant, visual disturbances.

Varicose vein <8 mm

- Sodium tetradecyl sulphate 0.5–3%
- Polidaconol 1–3%

Reticular veins 2–4 mm

- Sodium tetradecyl sulphate 0.25–0.5%
- Polidaconol 0.6–1.0%

Telengiectasia 0.1–2.0 mm

- Sodium tetradecyl sulphate 0.125–0.255%
- Polidaconol 0.25–0.6%

25–30 needle is used for sclerotherapy

- No single injection dose exceeds 0.1 mL
- Multiple injections may required
- Pressure dressings must be kept for 72 hours after sclerosant injection.

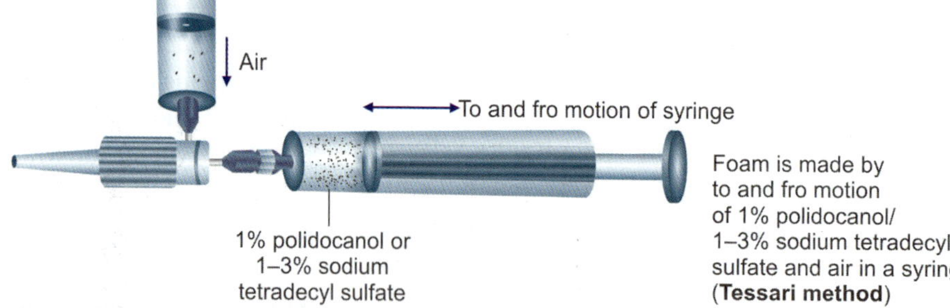

Endovenous Thermal Ablations (Laser and Radiofrequency Ablation)

These techniques are preferred over open surgery in the treatment of incompetent saphenous vein due to less pain and morbidity.

Mechanism of action of thermal ablation: Direct thermal injury causes destruction of endothelium, collagen denaturation of tunica media resulting in fibrotic and thrombotic occlusion of the vein.

Contraindications of endovenous thermal ablation: (i) Vein size (<2 mm and >15 mm); (ii) History of superficial thrombophlebitis resulting in partially obstructed saphenous vein; (iii) Tortuous GSV on duplex study; (iv) Aneurysmal dilations of the SFJ; (v) Uncorrectable coagulopathy; (vi) Immobility; and (vii) Pregnancy.

Complications of endovenous thermal ablation: (i) Thrombophlebitis; (ii) Ecchymosis; (iii) Skin pigmentation; (iv) Paresthesia; and (v) Proximal thrombus extension.

Surgery

Surgery is indicated in: (i) Varicosities >4 mm; (ii) Varicosity with complications; and (iii) Refractory to pharmacological therapy or compression therapy.

Trendelenburg's Operation

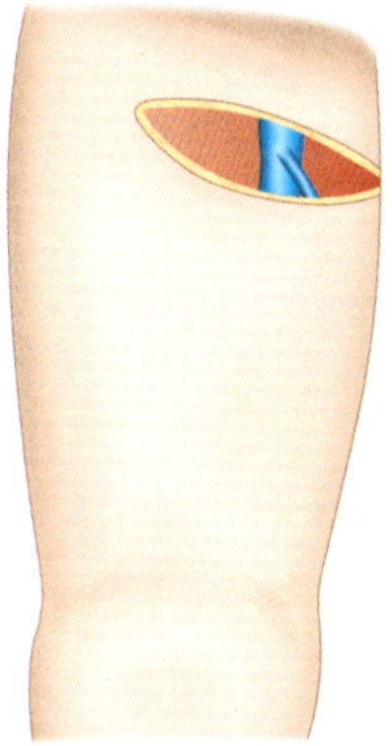

Identification of GSV and saphenofemoral junction

Femoral vein
Superficial epigastric vein
Superficial external pudendal vein
Superficial circumflex iliac vein
Great saphenous vein

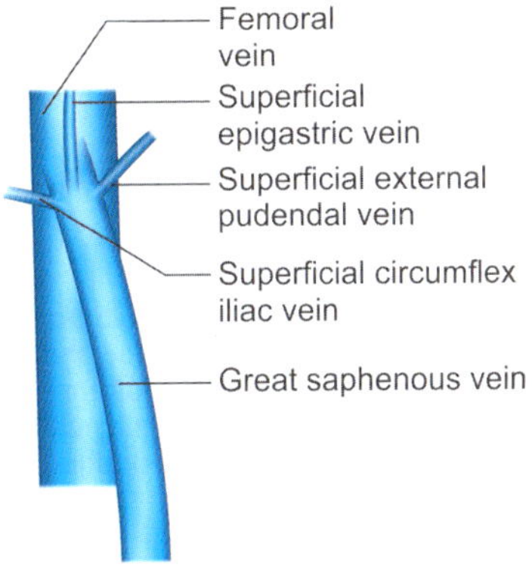

Identification of tributaries of GSV

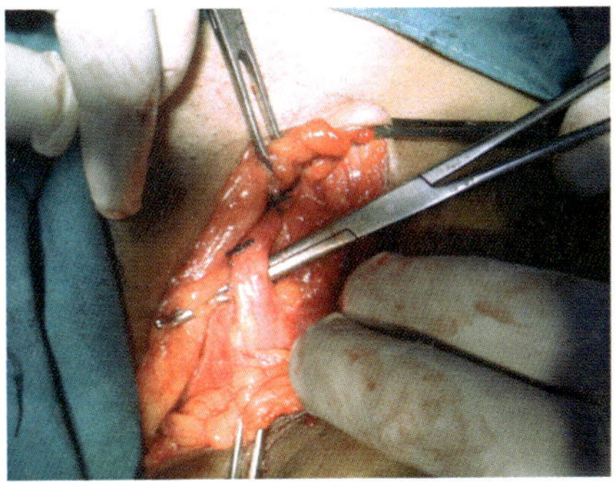

Operative picture showing GSV along with ligated tributaries

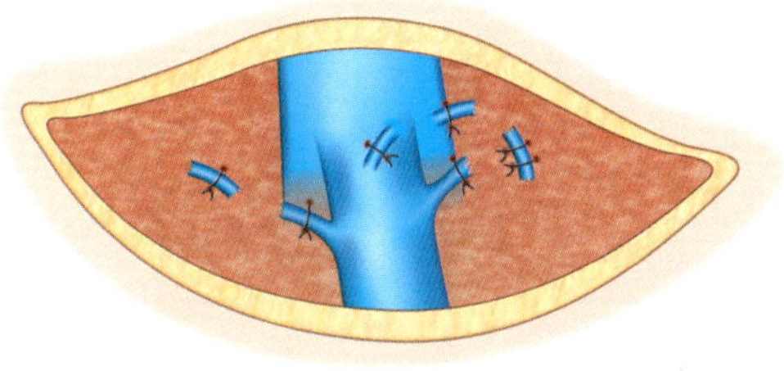

Ligation of tributaries

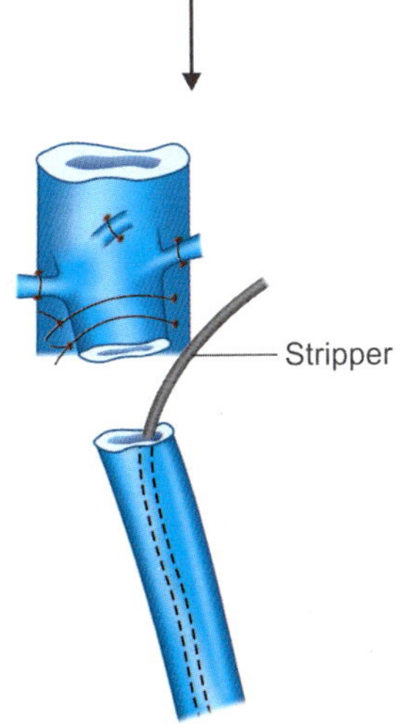

Ligation of saphenofemoral junction

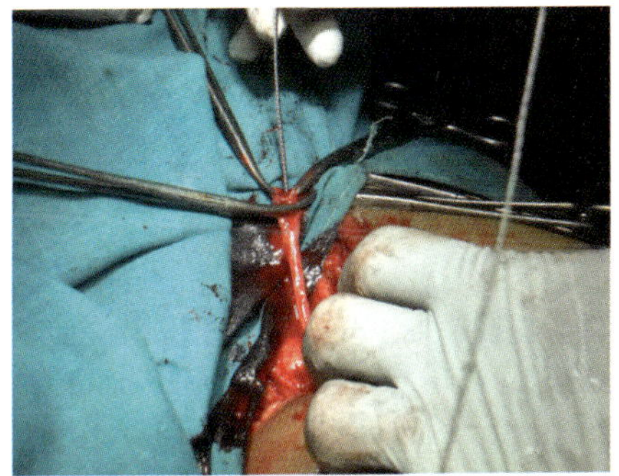

Stripper is introduced through the separated end of GSV

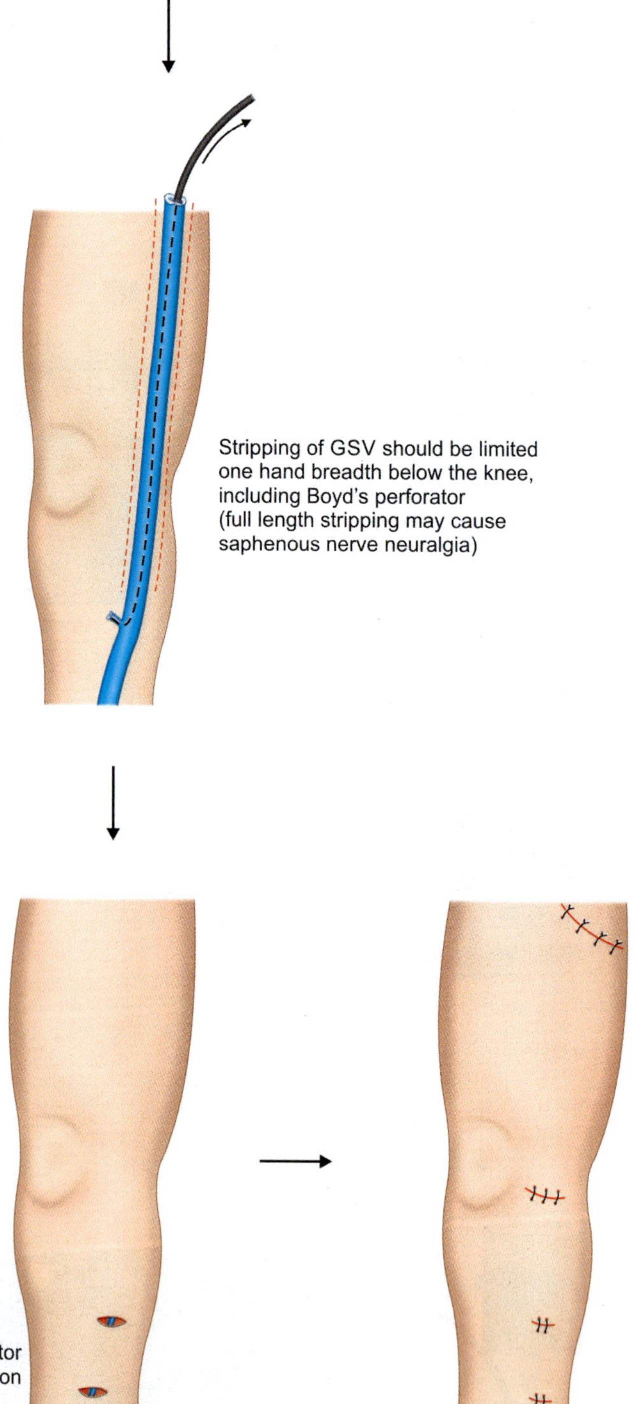

SEPS (Subfascial Endoscopic Perforator Ligation)

- In SEPS, balloon dissection and CO_2 insufflation (30 mm Hg) are used along with pneumatic thigh tourniquet. Occlusion of the perforators are done by endoscopic clips or harmonic scalpel. Complications are wound infection and saphenous neuralgia.
- In presence of lipodermatosclerosis, lack of space in subfascial area leads to difficulty in introduction of endoscope and visualisation of perforators.

Venous Leg Ulcer

A venous ulcer is an open skin lesion of the leg or foot that occurs in an area affected by venous hypertension. [Adapted from SVS/AVF guideline]

Workup of venous leg ulcer includes:

- Documentation of site, area, depth, wound edge, wound base, presence of any discharge or infection
- Venous duplex US of the lower extremity (includes direct visualization of superficial, deep, and perforator veins; compressibility; phasic venous flow with or without augmentation maneuvers; documentation of venous reflux with measurement of valve closure time)
- Measurement of ankle-brachial index.

Management of venous leg ulcer:

- Cleaning of the ulcer with neutral, nonirritating solution
- *Debridement:* Surgical/hydrosurgical/ultrasonic/enzymatic/biologic. Among them, surgical debridement is superior.
- Ulcer with clinical evidence of infection should be treated with systemic antibiotics based on culture-sensitivity report.
- Dressing should be done with dressing substances with high absorptive capabilities (e.g., foams, alginates).
- *Compression therapy:* Graduated compression elastic stockings or Four-layer bandage (4LB).
- To reduce dermatitis underneath compression stockings, skin lubricants can be used. Topical steroids are indicated for ulcer associated dermatitis.
- Wound biopsy is indicated if ulcer is not improving with standard ulcer care and compression therapy for 4–6 weeks.
- Apligraf (an allogenic bilayer cellular therapy) has shown improved outcomes in venous ulcers that are not responding to conventional management for 4–6 weeks.
- In patient with venous leg ulcer (C6) and incompetent superficial veins that have axial reflux directed to the bed of the ulcer, ablation of the incompetent veins (by USG-guided sclerotherapy or endovenous thermal ablation) are indicated in addition to standard compression therapy.

Four-layer bandage is multicomponent bandage consisting of four components: (i) Orthopedic wool; (ii) Crepe bandage; (iii) elastic bandage; and (iv) Elastic cohesive bandage.

Compression bandages or stockings are contraindicated if ankle-brachial index is 0.5 or less or if absolute ankle pressure is ≤60 mm Hg (suggestive of underlying arterial occlusive disease).

Causes of Nonvenous Leg Ulcer

Vascular cause: (i) Peripheral arterial occlusive disease; (ii) Thromboangiitis obliterans; (iii) Lymphedema; (iv) Diabetes mellitus; and (v) Vasculitis.

Neurologic cause: (i) Diabetic neuropathy; (ii) Alcoholic peripheral neuropathy; (iii) Poliomyelitis; and (iv) Spina bifida.

Hematologic cause: (i) Sickle cell anemia; (ii) Thalassemia; and (iii) Polycythemia vera.

Metabolic cause: (i) Diabetes mellitus and (ii) Gout.

Malignant cause: (i) Squamous cell carcinoma (Marjolin's ulcer) and (ii) Angiosarcoma.

Autoimmune disorders: (i) Rheumatoid arthritis; (ii) Polyarteritis nodosa; and (iii) Systemic lupus erythematosus.

Medications: (i) Hydroxyurea and (ii) Methotrexate.

Diseases of Lymphatic System

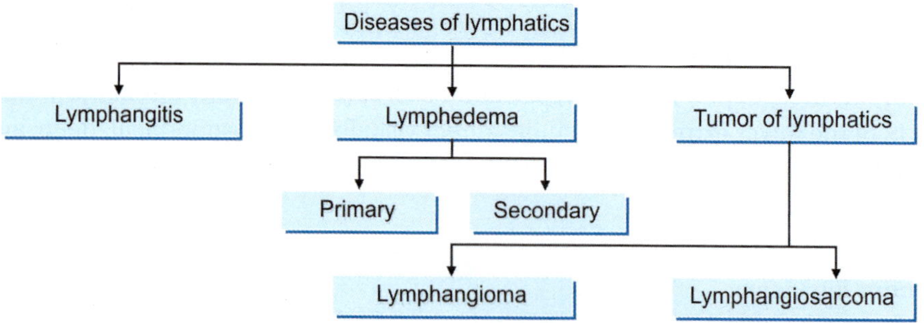

Acute Lymphangitis

- Acute inflammation of the lymphatics when an area infected by pyogenic bacteria (specially, streptococci and *Staph. aureus*), drained by the lymphatic system.
- Affected lymphatics are dilated and filled with exudate of neutrophils and monocytes.
- **Clinically**, lymphangitis is manifestated by red painful subcutaneous streaks (inflammed lymphatics) with tender, enlarged draining lymph nodes (acute lymphadenitis).

Treatment:

- Rest of the affected part (to reduce lymphatic drainage)
- Elevation (to reduce swelling)
- Intravenous antibiotic (to treat the primary infection)

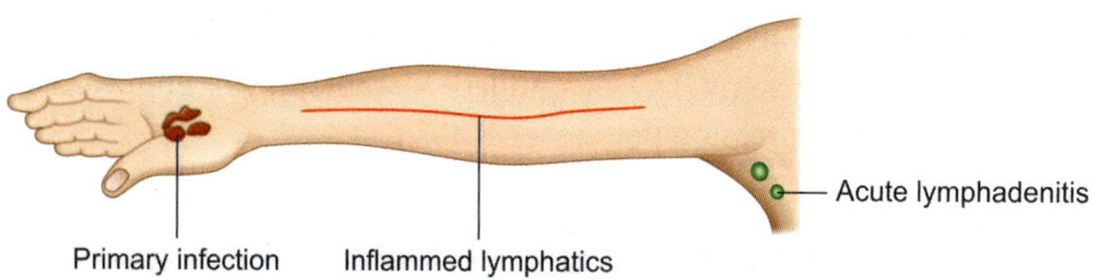

Lymphedema

Pathophysiology

Lymphedema is the end result of improper lymphatic outflow due to aplasia, hypoplasia, hyperplasia, primary decreased lymphatic contractility or inflammatory obliteration.

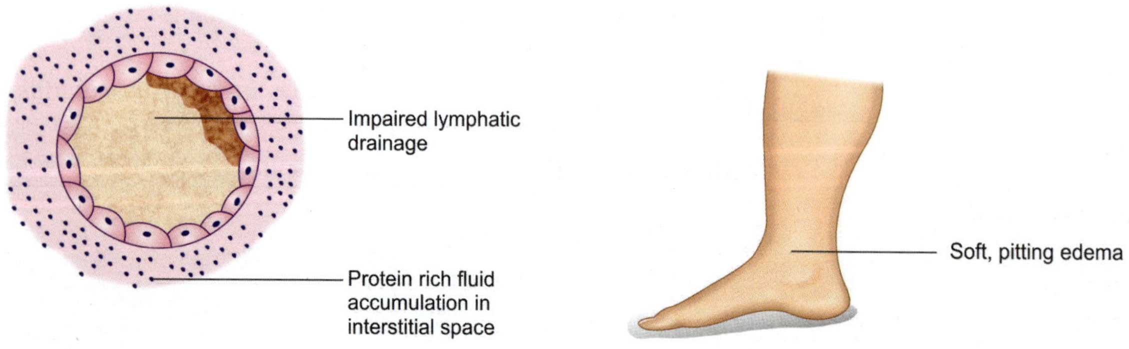

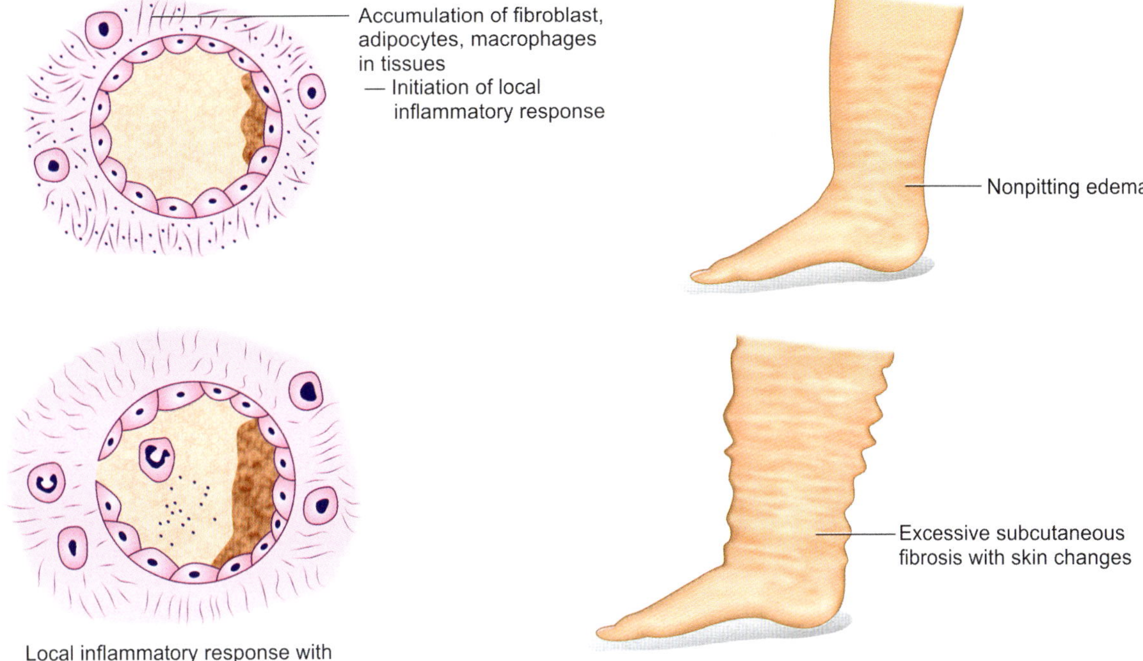

Local inflammatory response with recurrent episodes of infection

Classification of Lymphedema

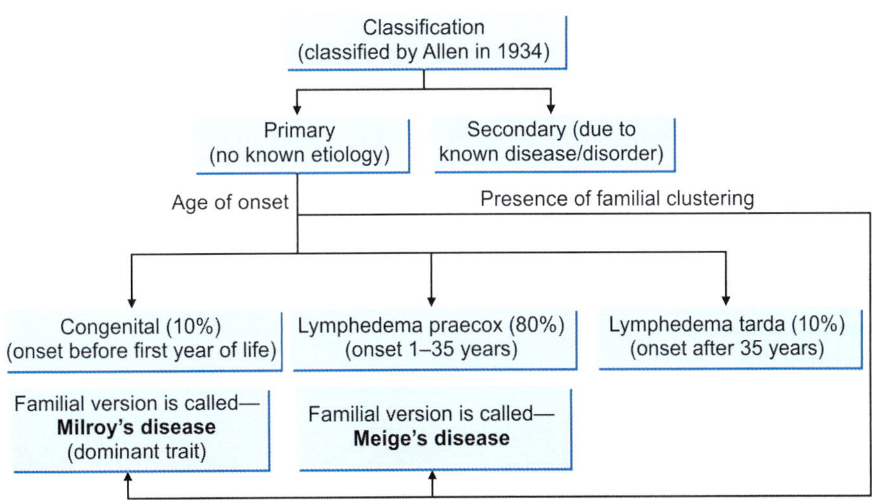

- Secondary lymphedema is more common than primary lymphedema.
- Most common form of primary lymphedema is **lymphedema praecox**.
- Most common form of secondary lymphedema worldwide is **filarial lymphedema**.
- In developed countries, common causes of secondary lymphedema are tumor invasion, resection or ablation of regional lymph nodes by surgery, radiation therapy.

Mutations Associated with Primary Lymphoedema

- FOXC2 (lymphoedema-distichiasis syndrome)
- VEGFR-3 (Milroy's disease)
- SOX18 (Hypotrichosis-lymphoedema-telengiectasia syndrome)

Clinical Presentation

- Lymphedema characteristically involves the foot.
- Contour of the ankle is lost due to filling of submalleolar depression. '**buffalo hump**' forms on the dorsum of the foot. Toes appear 'square'.
- Skin over the edema cannot be pinched due to subcutaneous fibrosis **(Stemmer's sign)**.
- In early cases, pitting edema. In advanced stage, nonpitting edema due to fibrosis and dermal thickening.
- In advanced stage, chronic eczema, fungal infection of skin (dermatophytosis) and nail (onychomycosis), fissuring, verrucae, papillae are seen.
- Ulcer may develop after a minor trauma.
- Chylous ascites, chylothorax, chyluria, chylorrhea (discharge of lymph from skin vesicles) suggest lymphangiectasia and chylous reflux.
- **Lymphangiosarcoma should be suspected if ulceration, nonhealing bruise, purple-red nodules are present.**

International Society of Lymphology (ISL) Lymphoedema Staging

Stage 0: A subclinical state where swelling is not evident despite impaired lymph transport.

Stage I: Accumulation of tissue fluid that subsides with limb elevation. The oedema may be pitting at this stage.

Stage II: Limb elevation alone rarely reduces swelling and pitting is manifested.

Late stage II: There may or may not be pitting as tissue fibrosis is more evident

Stage III: The tissue is hard (fibrotic) and pitting is absent. Skin changes such as thickening, hyperpigmentation, increased skin folds, fat deposits and warty overgrowths develop.

Assessment of Lymphedema

Assessment of limb volume by: (i) Circumferential limb measurement; (ii) Water displacement method; (iii) Perometry; and (iv) Bioimpedance.

Skin condition assessment: Dryness, fungal infection, hyperkeratosis, lymphangiectasia, papillomatosis, ulcers, etc.

Assessment of peripheral arterial status: By ankle-brachial index (ABI) or Toe-brachial index (TBI).

Functional assessment: Range of joint movement, wearing or removing underwear/compression garments/bandaging, ability to lift leg, etc.

Psychosocial assessment: Any depression, alteration of body image, problems with sexual or social relationship.

Primary Lymphedema

Lymphedema Congenita (10%)

- Onset before 1st year of life
- More common in males
- More commonly bilateral and involving the whole leg
- The familial version is called the 'Milroy's disease'
- This type may be associated with disorders like yellow nail syndrome and Pierre-Robin syndrome.

Lymphedema Praecox (80%)

- Onset from 1–35 years of age
- More common in females, peak incidence shortly after menarche
- More commonly unilateral
- Only extends upto the knee
- Familial version is called "Meige's disease".

Lymphedema Tarda (10%)

- Onset after 35 years of age
- Patient must be investigated for malignancy of the pelvic organs, prostate and external genitalia.

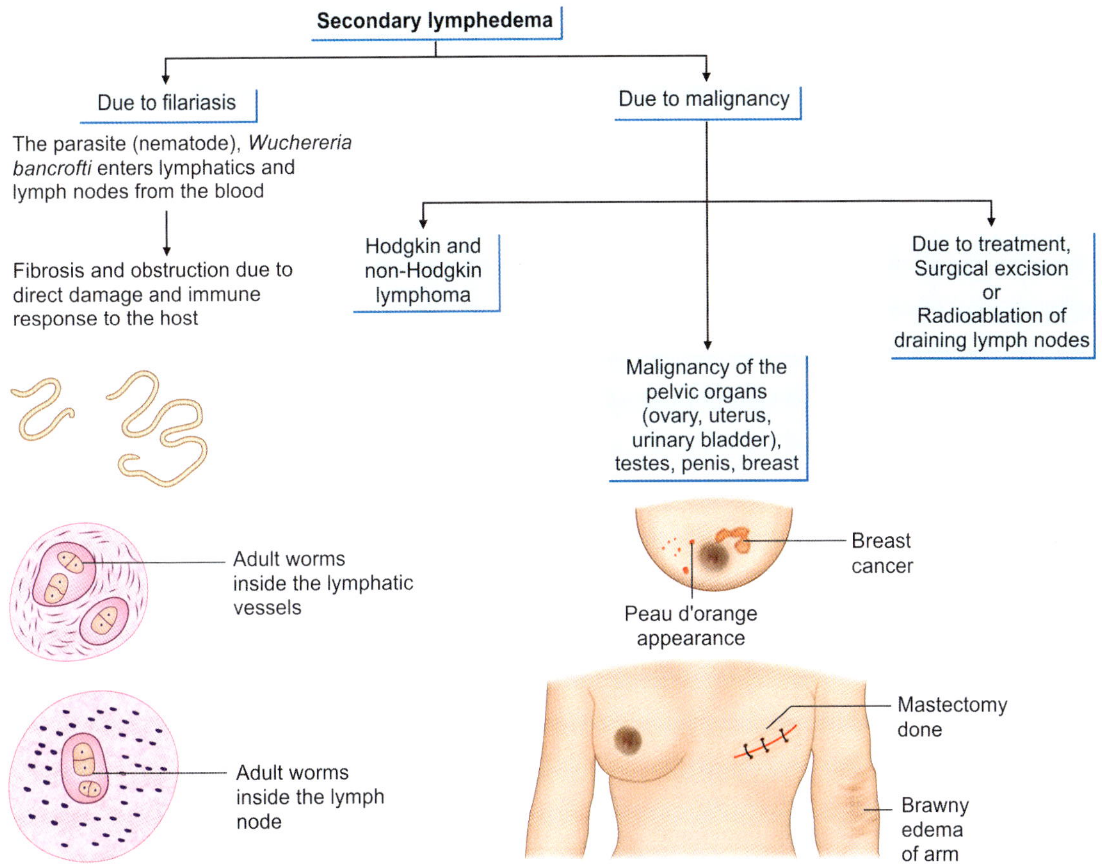

Risk Factors for Upper Limb Lymphedema

- Axillary lymph node dissection
- Postoperative axillary radiotherapy
- Trauma in 'at risk' arm (venepuncture, IM injection, BP measurement)
- Taxane chemotherapy
- Arterio-venous shunt for dialysis.

Risk Factors for Lower Limb Lymphedema

- Filariasis
- Inguinal lymph node dissection
- Postoperative pelvic radiotherapy
- Abdominal tumors compressing lymphatic vessels
- Post-thrombotic syndrome.

Diagnosis

- **Lymphoscintigraphy** is the investigation of choice for primary lymphedema. This modality is almost 100% specific to differentiate lymphedema from other causes of limb swelling.
- **CT or MRI** can detect any mass obstructing the lymphatic channels. MRI can differentiate lymphedema from chronic venous edema and lipedema.
- **Lymphangiography** is indicated when surgery is planned for lymphedema.

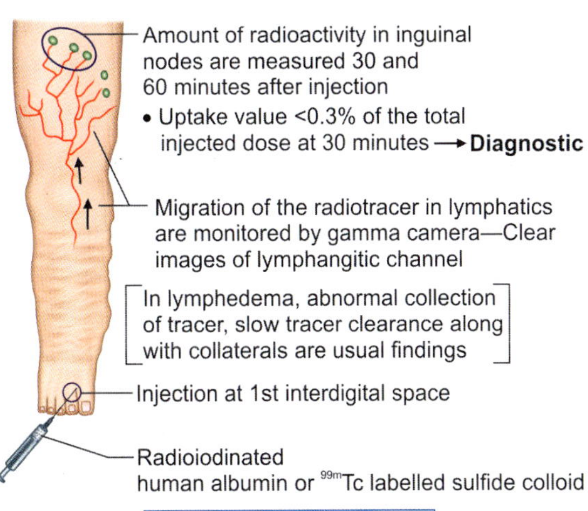

Lymphoscintigraphy

Management

Principles of management:

- To increase the lymphatic and venous flow
- To reduce the volume of limb
- To improve the consistency of subcutaneous tissue
- Maintaining skin care and to look for any complications
- To avoid conditions that increase lymphoedema.

Treatment options:

General measures

- Patients must be educated about skin care and avoidance of injures
- Patients must be instructed to attend his/her physician whenever there is early signs of infection
- Infections must be aggressively treated with appropriate antibiotics
- Eczema requires treatment with steroid.

Compression garment

- **Indicated for** initial management of mild lower limb and upper limb lymphoedema (ISL stage I) with intact resilient skin and no or minimal shape distortion of limbs.
- Can be used for lymphoedema of head-neck, trunk, breast or genitalia.
- Also indicated for transition and long-term management of upper limb and lower limb lymphoedema.

Criteria suitable for using compression garment: (i) Intact, resilient skin; (ii) Minimal shape distortion; (iii) Absent or minimal pitting edema; and (iv) Can tolerate or manage.

Contraindications to compression garment: (i) ABI <0.5 in lower limb; (ii) Extensive ulceration; (iii) Presence of lymphorrhoea; and (iv) Severe peripheral neuropathy.

Multi-layer inelastic lymphoedema bandaging (MLLB)

This technique uses inelastic bandages that produce high working pressures and lower resting pressures (elastic bandages produce sustained compression with minimal variation during movement)

Indications: (i) In presence of skin changes, e.g., hyperkeratosis, papillomatosis, ulceration; (ii) In presence of lymphorrhoea; (iii) In distorted limb; and (iv) Limb with extensive skin folds.

Components of MLLB: (i) Skin care; (ii) Finger or toe bandaging; (iii) Tubular bandage; (iv) Soft synthetic wool or foam roll or sheet; (v) Dense foam; (vi) Inelastic bandages; and (vii) Tape.

Contraindications to MLLB: (i) ABI <0.5; (ii) Severe peripheral neuropathy; and (iii) Uncontrolled heart failure.

Modified MLLB

Modified MLLB includes skin care, exercise/movement, elevation, simple lymphatic drainage, psychosocial support along with MLLB.

Indicated in ISL stage II or late stage II lymphoedema, in cancer-related lymphoedema.

Manual lymphatic drainage (MLD) and simple lymphatic drainage (SLD)

Indications: (i) Lymphoedema at the root of a limb and (ii) Trunk and midline oedema (e.g., head-neck, chest, breast, back, abdomen, and genitalia).

Contraindications: (i) Acute cellulitis/erysipelas; (ii) Cirrhosis with ascites; (iii) Unstable angina; and (iv) Severe cardiac insufficiency.

SLD is a simplified version of MLD that patient or caregivers can easily learn and apply.

Intermittent pneumatic compression (IPC)

An electrical air compression pump attached to an inflatable plastic garment, placed over the diseased limb.

Surgery

- Only about 10% of the patients need surgical intervention.
- Surgery may be considered in patients with stage II and stage III lymphedema with severe functional impairment or recurrent episodes of lymphangitis.
- Surgical interventions are either reconstructive or excisional. Reconstructive surgical options include: (i) Lymphovenous anastomoses; (ii) Lymphatic or venous vessel grafting; and (iii) Lymph node transplantation. Excisional surgical options include: (i) Homan's operation and (ii) Charles operation.

Chylothorax

- Chylous pleural effusion.
- Due to thoracic duct trauma or advanced malignancy with lymphatic metastasis.
- Presence of chylomicron in pleural fluid and triglyceride >110 mg/dL in pleural fluid—**Diagnostic**.
- Tube thoracostomy and medium-chain-triglyceride rich diet are the initial treatment.
- In patient with thoracic duct injury, if effusion persists for more than 1 week, ligation of the thoracic duct should be done using video-assisted thoracoscopy.
- Pleurodesis is the last option.

Chylous Ascites

- **Causes are:** (i) Congenital lymphatic abnormality and (ii) Malignancy involving abdominal lymph nodes
- Presence of chylomicron and triglyceride level >110 mg/dL in ascitic fluid is diagnostic
- Treatment is abdominal poracentesis and medium-chain triglyceride rich diet
- In duct injury, if chylous ascites not responds after 2 weeks duct must be ligated.

Chyluria

- Filaria is the most common cause. Other causes are: Ascariasis, tumor, and tuberculosis.
- Presents as painless passage of milky white urine, particularly after a fatty meal
- IVU/Lymphangiography demonstrate the presence of lymphourinary fistula
- Treatment is low fat diet, plenty of fluid to prevent clot, ligation of involved lymphatic channel.

Tumor of the Lymphatics

Lymphangioma

- Benign vascular lesion with lymphatic differentiation.
- **Two types:** (i) Capillary lymphangioma and (ii) Cavernous lymphangioma or cystic hygroma.
- Most of the lymphangiomas (cystic hygromas) present at birth.
- Treatment is surgical excision.

Lymphangiosarcoma

- Develops as a complication of long-standing lymphedema.
- Originally described in post-mastectomy lymphedema (Stewart-Treves syndrome).
- Clinically presents as gradually increasing edema, appearance of subcutaneous nodules.
- Treatment is wide excision.
- Prognosis is poor.

Case 1

History and Physical Examination

A 55-year-old male patient presented in the surgical OPD with painful blackish discoloration of left great toe for last 2 weeks and pain in the left foot for last 1 month. Patient also complained of pain in the left calf on walking for last 6 months and relieved on taking rest. For the last 1 month, patient complained of continuous pain in the left foot. No pain or blackish discoloration of right foot or leg. Patient was a chronic smoker for last 25 years. Patient was on oral antidiabetics and antihypertensives. No significant past history or family history.

Physical Examination

Pulse: 88/min; BP: 144/92 mm Hg

Black eschar measuring 2.5 cm × 2.2 cm in the plantar aspect of left great toe. The eschar was non-tender. Sensory function of the left foot was normal. On the left lower limb, pulsations of the arteria dorsalis pedis and posterior tibial artery were absent. Pulsation of the arteries of right lower limb were present.

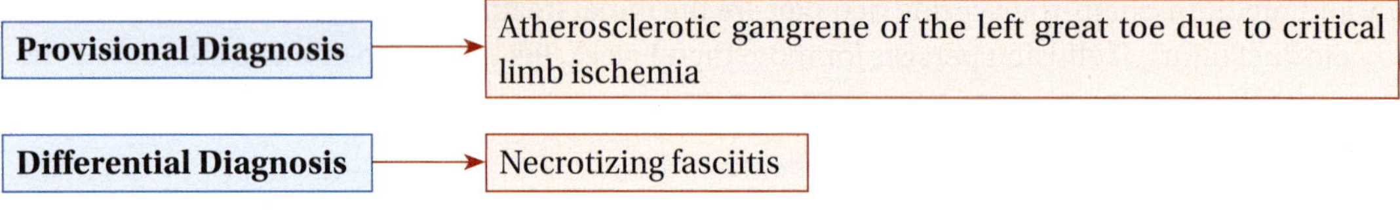

Investigations

- Ankle brachial index (ABI): 0.3
- Blood sugar and lipid profile were within normal range
- Duplex Doppler USG of the arterial system of the both lower limbs revealed gross atherosclerotic changes with biphasic flow pattern in left ADP and ATA. Rest of the arteries of the lower limb revealed triphasic flow pattern. Mild atherosclerotic changes in right lower limb arteries with triphasic flow pattern.

Discussion

A 55-year-old male patient, smoker, diabetic, hypertensive presented with clinical features suggestive of occlusive peripheral arterial diseases of the lower extremities. The gangrenous changes in left great toe was suggestive of critical limb ischemia. ABI was also suggestive of CLI. Doppler USG revealed the level of occlusion.

Management Algorithm

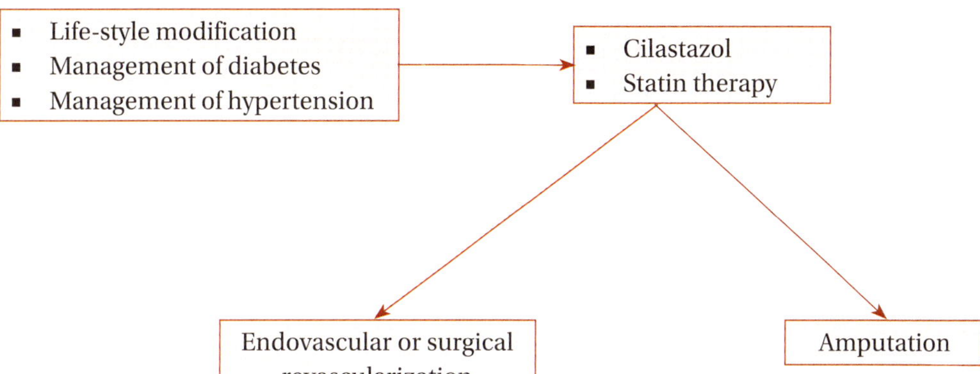

Case 2

History and Physical Examination

A 43-year-old male patient presented with heaviness of left leg along with venous prominences in the medial aspect of left leg and thigh for last 4 months. Patient also complained of skin changes in the left ankle region for 2 months. No obvious symptoms present in the right leg. Patient was by occupation security guard for last 4 years. No history of diabetes or hypertension.

Physical Examination

Examination of the left lower limb: Tortous venous prominences along the course of great saphenous vein (GSV) along with eczematous changes in the ankle region and a healed ulcer scar mark just above the medial malleolus. Clinical examination also revealed saphenofemoral incompetence along with multiple perforator incompetence. Examination of the right lower limb revealed no abnormality.

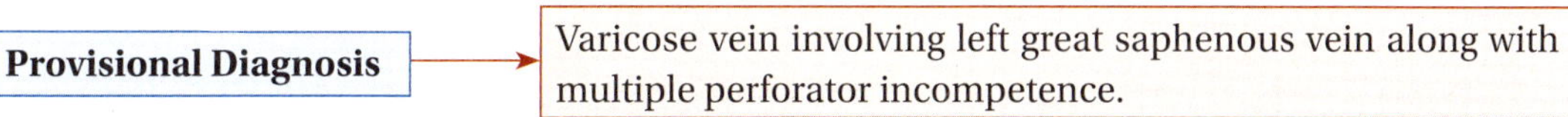

Investigations

Doppler USG of venous system of both lower limb revealed left sapheno-femoral junction (SFJ) incompetence along with incompetence of perforators (below knee medial lower third and mid third). Right SFJ was competent. Sapheno-popliteal junction (SPJ) competent on both sides. Deep veins were normal.

Discussion

A middle aged male patient presented with heaviness of leg along with venous prominence in his left leg. Clinical examination revealed varicosities affecting left GSV along with evidence of healed venous ulcer. Doppler USG revealed the SFJ incompetency along with perforator incompetency in multiple levels with no evidence of deep venous thrombosis. Surgery was planned. During the period of preparation for surgery, treatment was started with phlebotropic drugs and elastic stockings.

Management Algorithm

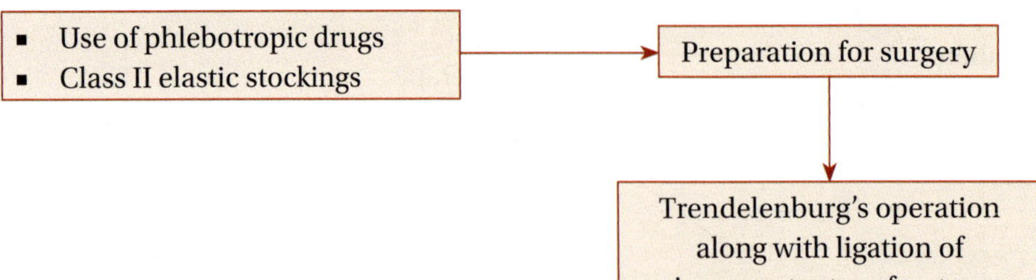

Chapter 19

Hernia

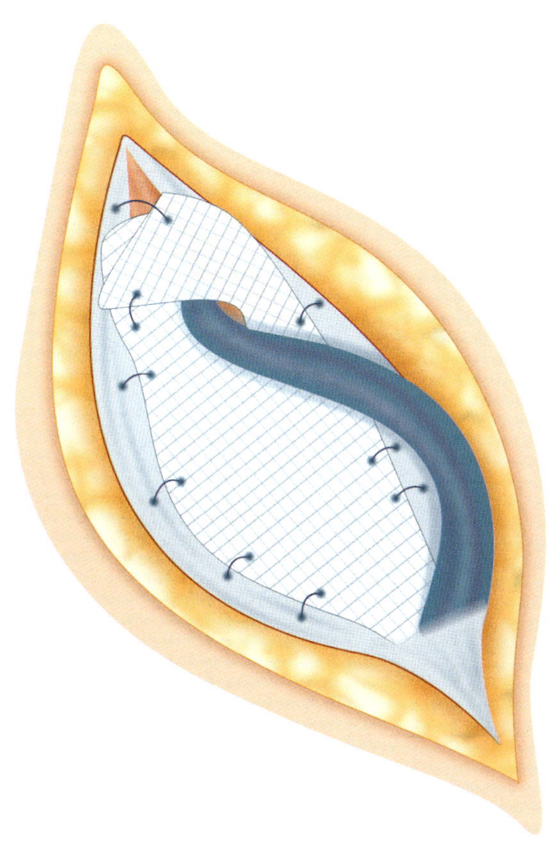

Important Topics

- Types of Hernia
- Anatomy of the Groin
- Classification of Groin Hernia
- Inguinal Hernia
- Femoral Hernia
- Umbilical Hernia
- Epigastric Hernia
- Incisional Hernia
- Spigelian Hernia
- Lumbar Hernia
- Obturator Hernia
- Sciatic Hernia
- Perineal Hernia
- Interparietal Hernia
- Parastomal Hernia
- Internal Hernia
- Trocar Site Hernia
- Mesh

'The history of science, like the history of all human ideas, is a history of irresponsible dreams, of obstinacy and of error. But science is one of the very few human activities—perhaps the only one— in which errors are systemically criticized and fairly often, in time, corrected. This is why we can say that, in science, we often learn from our mistakes, ...'

Karl Raimund Popper (1902–1994)
Austrian born British Philosopher of Science

Hernia

The word 'hernia' derived from Latin word meaning 'a rupture.'

Hernia is an abnormal protrusion of an organ or tissue through a defect in its surrounding wall.

Hernia can occur in various sites, but it develops most commonly through the abdominal wall.

Pathophysiology

Hernia may develop through the **normal weak areas** due to anatomical configurations (e.g., deep inguinal ring, femoral ring, linea alba), **congenital weakness** (e.g., connective tissue disorders) or **acquired weakness** (e.g., operative scar).

Connective Tissue Disorders Associated with Hernia Development

- Osteogenesis imperfecta
- Ehler–Danlos syndrome
- Marfan syndrome

Composition of Hernia

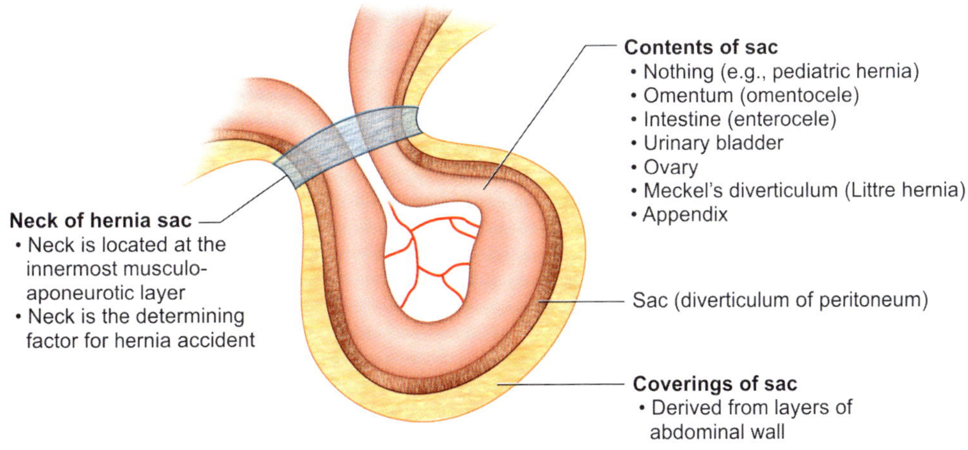

Types of Hernia

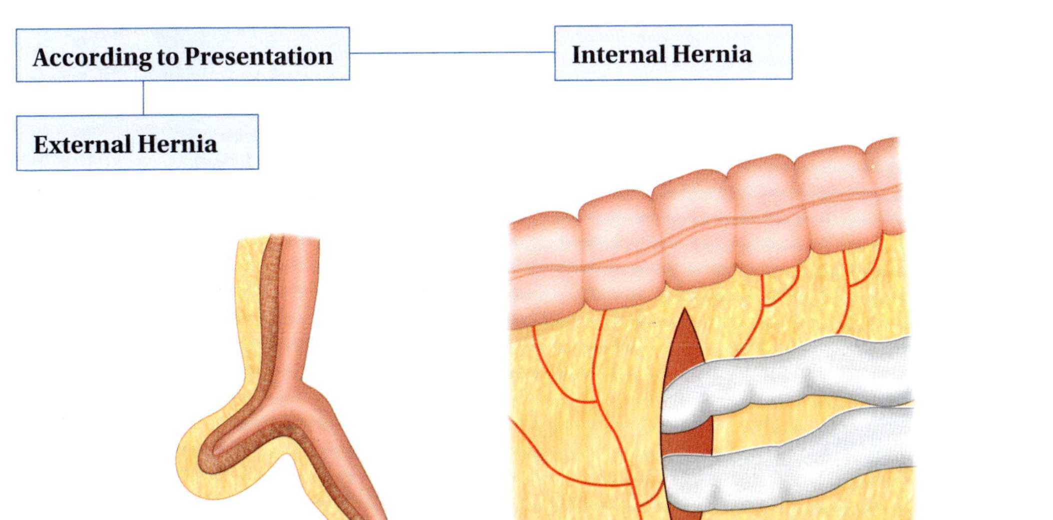

According to Site

Inguinal Hernia

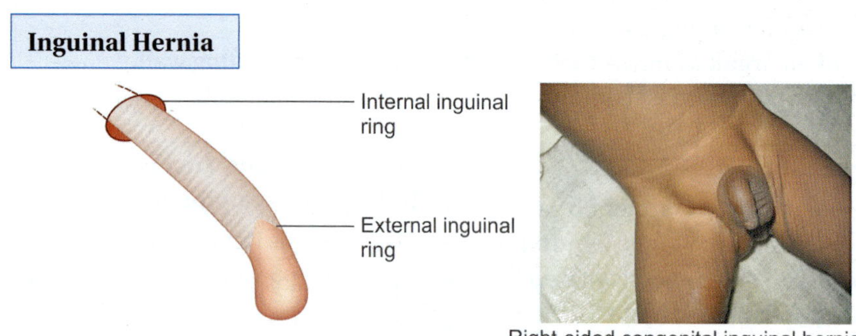

Right-sided congenital inguinal hernia

Femoral Hernia

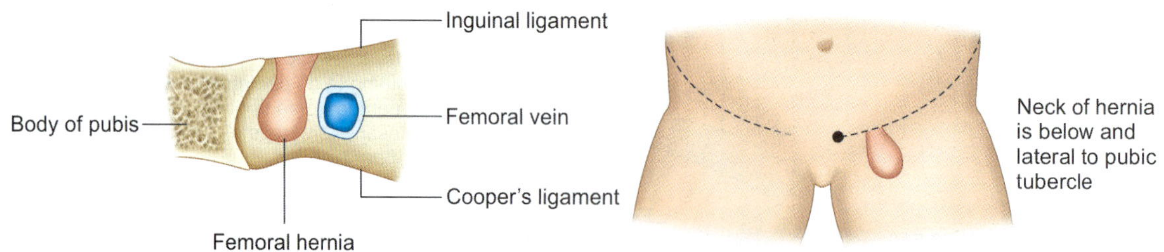

Umbilical Hernia

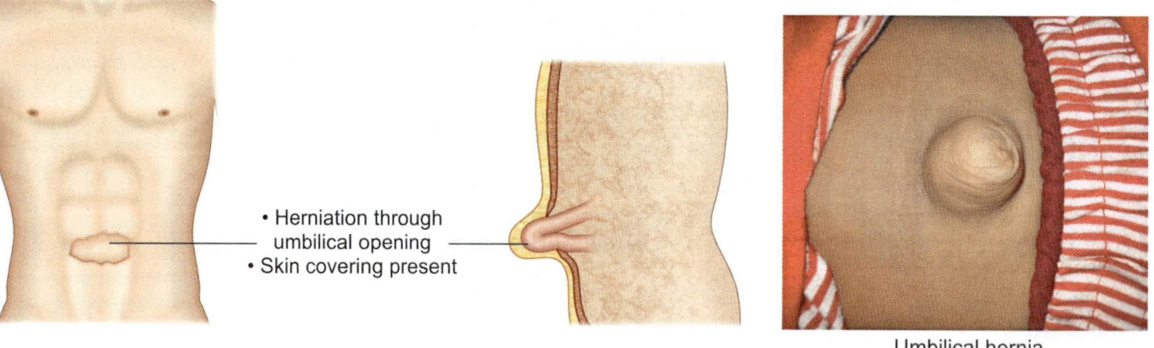

Umbilical hernia

Epigastric Hernia

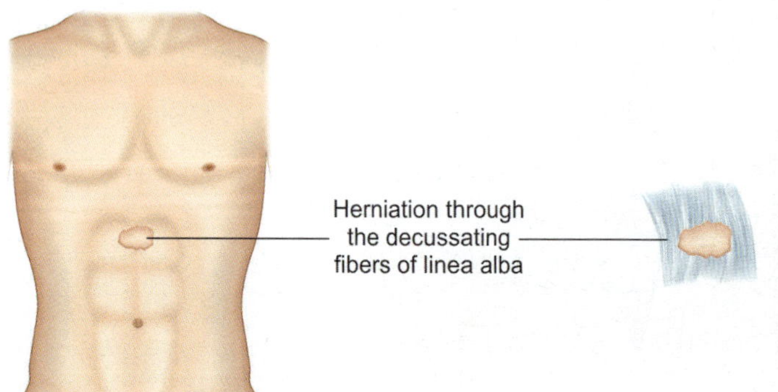

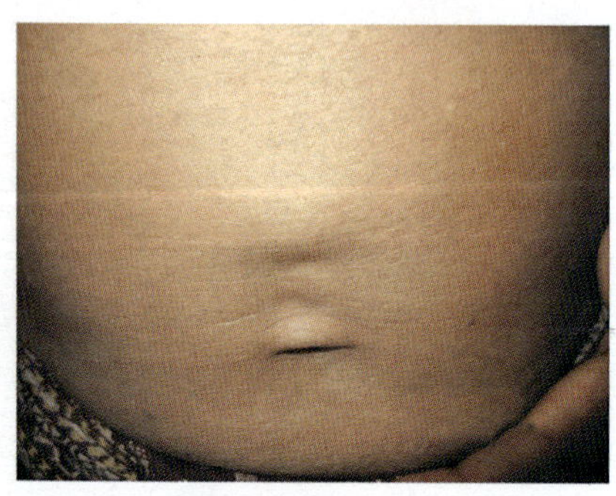
Epigastric hernia

Incisional Hernia

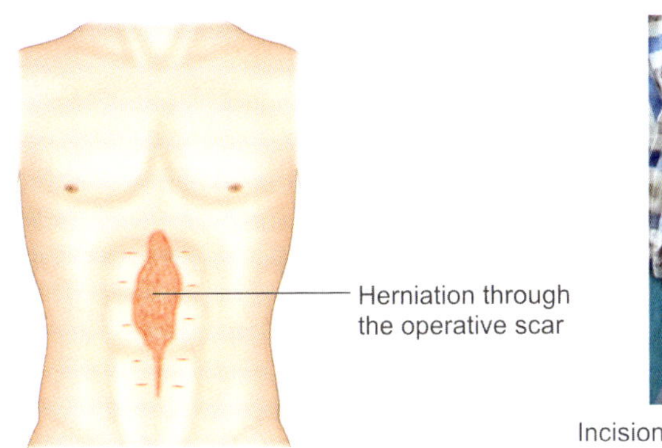

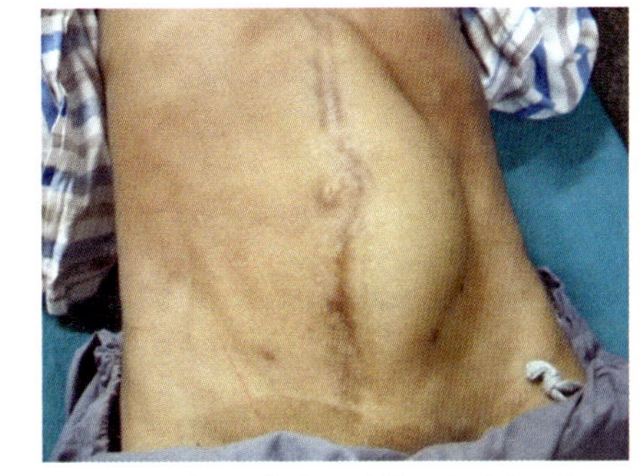

Incisional hernia through the midline incisional scar

Obturator Hernia

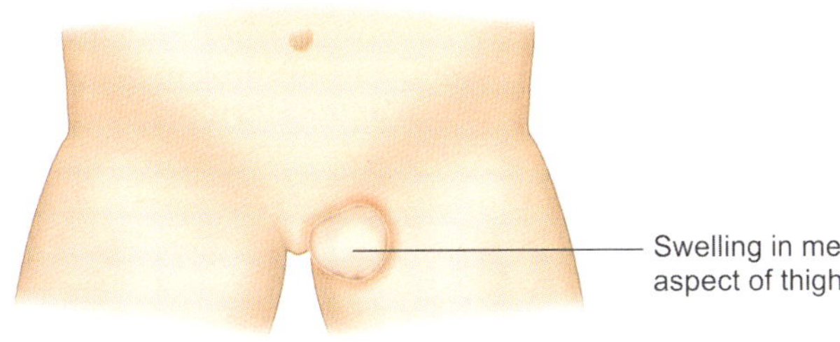

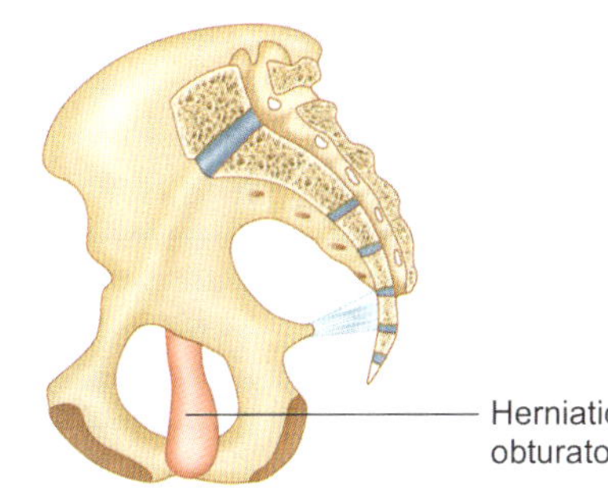

Spigelian Hernia

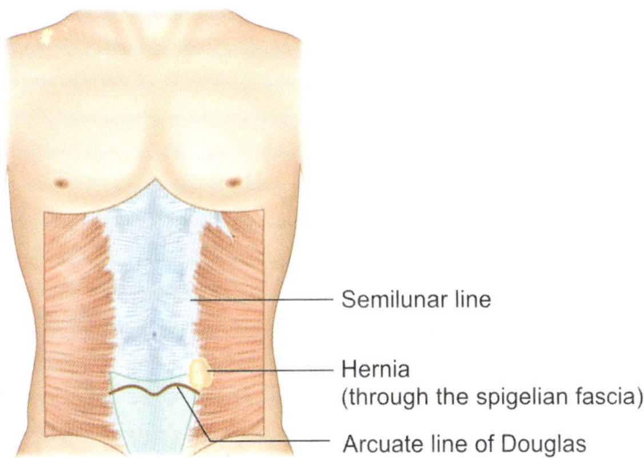

Lumbar Hernia

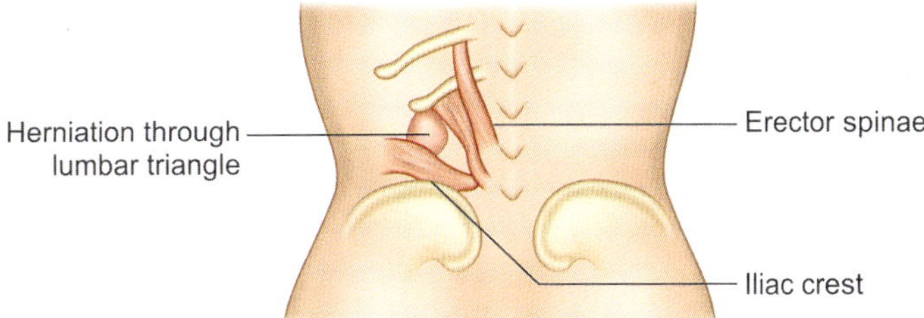

Sciatic Hernia

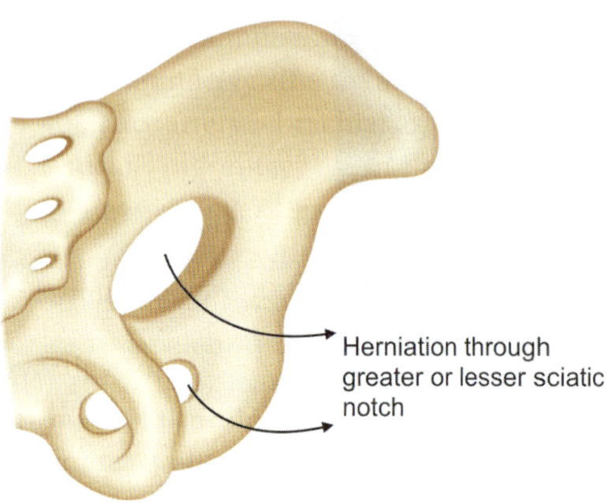

Perineal Hernia

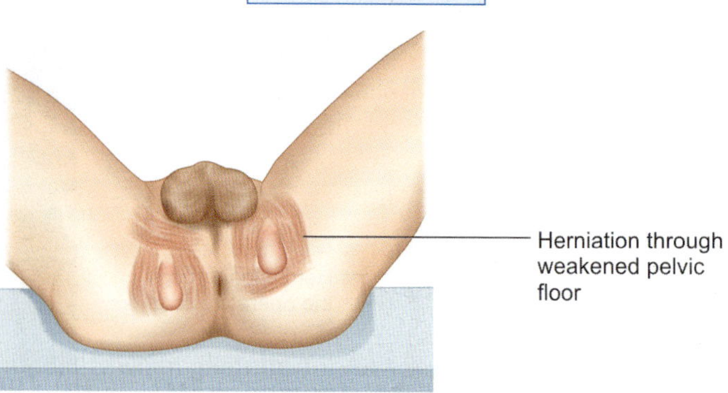

According to Complications

Irreducible (Incarcerated) Hernia

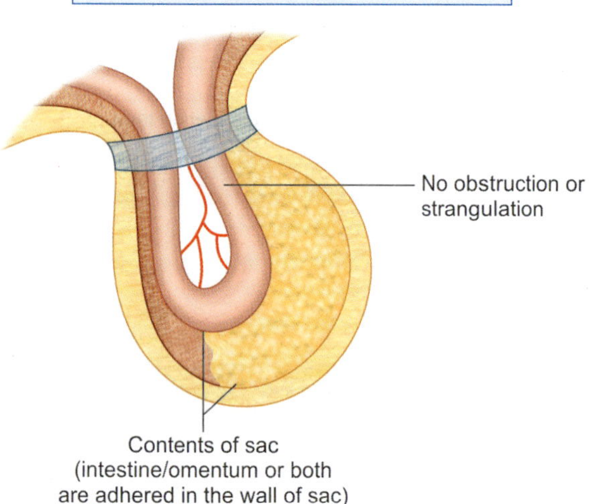

Obstructed Hernia

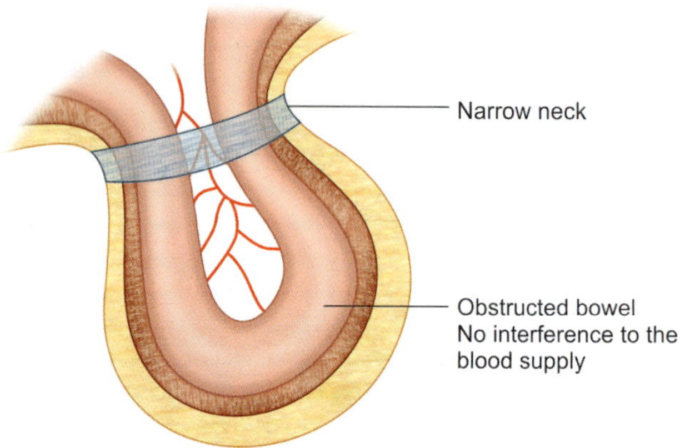

Strangulated Hernia

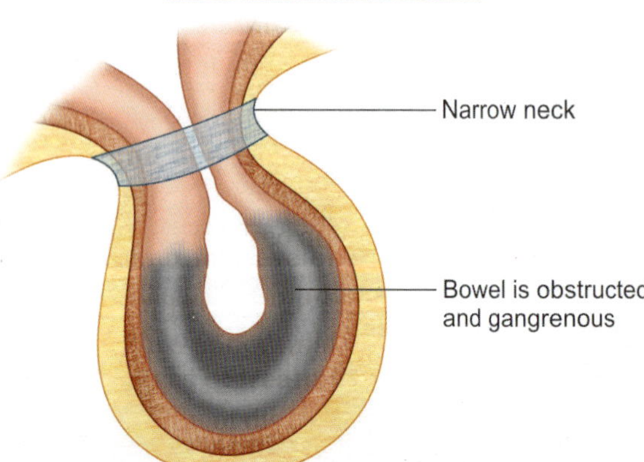

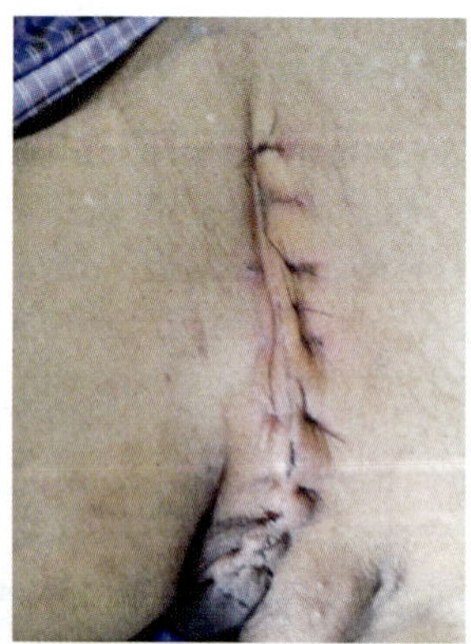

Management for obstructed or strangulated hernia (note the extension of incision up to the root of the scrotum).

Anatomy of the Groin

- Anatomy is to be understood according to the surgeon's approach to hernia repair.
- When surgeon is operating through an **open approach**, anatomy is to be considered from **skin to the peritoneal cavity**.
- When surgeon is operating through a **laparoscopic approach**, one should consider anatomy from **peritoneal cavity to the skin**.
- Surgeon must know the anatomy to select the most suitable approach for repair, to lower the recurrence rate and to avoid the complications.

Anatomical Landmarks for Open Groin Hernia Repair

Groin Hernia

Groin hernia is herniation through the inguinal or femoral canal.

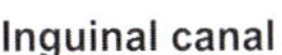

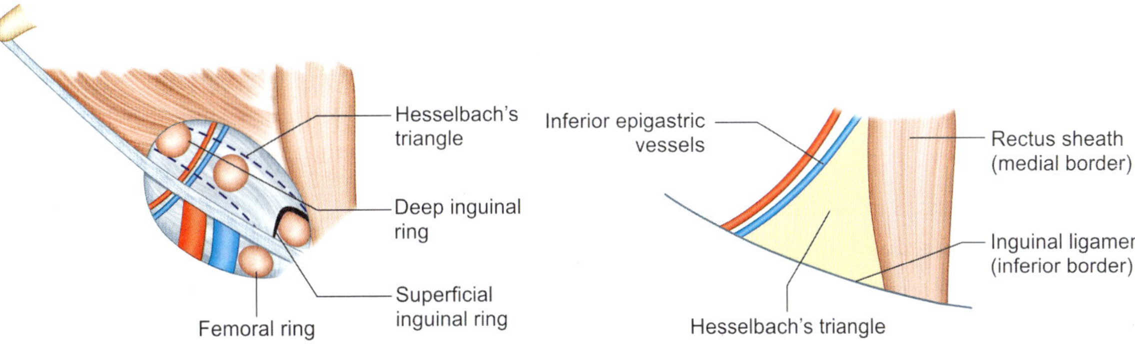

Myopectineal Orifice of Fruchaud

- According to Fruchaud, all groin hernias (indirect, direct and femoral) arise due to a common anatomic defect rather than an isolated cause for each one.
- His concept was that, all groin hernias are **due to failure of the transversalis fascia over myopectineal orifice to retain the peritoneum**.
- **The myopectineal orifice is surrounded:**
  - **Superiorly**, by internal oblique and transversus abdominis
  - **Inferiorly**, by Cooper's ligament
  - **Medially**, by lateral border of rectus muscle and sheath
  - **Laterally**, by Iliopsoas muscle
- The **inguinal ligament and iliopubic tract** divide the myopectineal orifice of Fruchaud into **superior and inferior compartment**.

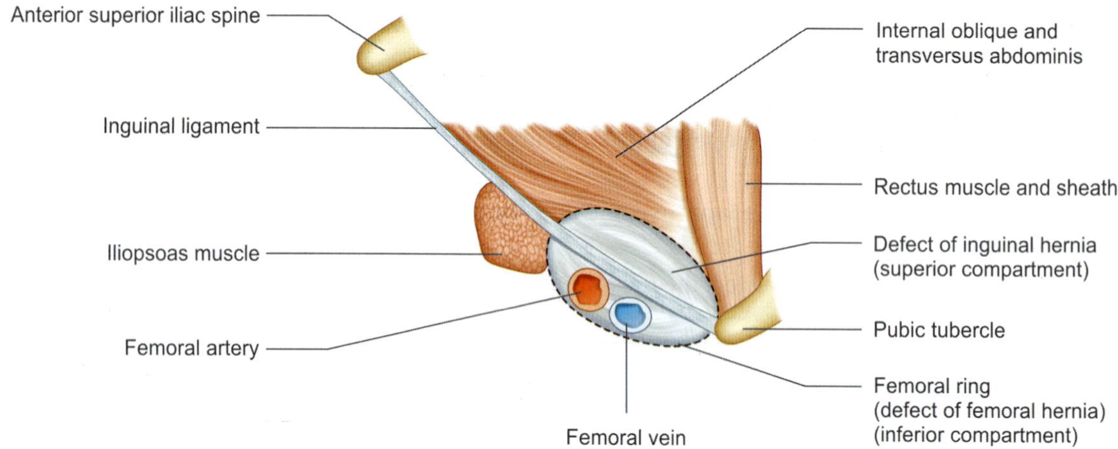

Anatomical Landmarks for Laparoscopic Inguinal Hernia Repair

Peritoneal Landmarks

Five peritoneal folds:
- Median umbilical fold-1
- Medial umbilical fold-2
- Lateral umbilical fold-2

Three flat fossa:
- Fossa lateralis
- Fossa medialis
- Fossa vesicalis

Preperitoneal Space Landmarks

- Transversalis fascia
- Vessels (Inferior epigastric vessels, Iliac vessels, Corona mortis)
- Vas deferens
- Nerves (Genitofemoral nerve, lateral femoral cutaneous nerve)
- Iliopubic tract
- Cooper's ligament
- Preperitoneal retropubic space
- The space of Bogros

Median umbilical fold:
- Present in the midline
- It is the obliterated urachus.
- It extends from urinary bladder to the umbilicus.

Paired medial umbilical fold:
- One on either side of median umbilical ligament
- It is the obliterated umbilical artery.
- Landmark for lateral extension of urinary bladder
- Most prominent landmark.

Paired lateral umbilical fold:
- Present lateral to the medial umbilical fold on each side
- Contains inferior epigastric vessels.
- Any hernia lateral to lateral umbilical fold is indirect hernia and medial to this fold is direct hernia.

Transversalis Fascia

- A bilaminar structure with strong anterior layer and deep membranous layer (extraperitoneal fascia)
- The deep membranous layer divides the preperitoneal space into visceral and parietal compartment
- The parietal compartment contains the epigastric vessels and numerous tributaries. Genitofemoral and lateral femoral cutaneous nerves also run within this compartment.
- Dissection along this plane may cause troublesome bleeding.
- Visceral compartment is avascular. It is the right plane for dissection as well as mesh placement.

Inferior Epigastric Vessels

- Most important landmark in myopectineal orifice
- Any hernia lateral to these vessels is indirect hernia and medial to these vessels is direct hernia

Fossa lateralis:
- Located in between the lateral umbilical ligament and the iliopubic tract
- Corresponds to origin of indirect inguinal hernia

Fossa medialis:
- Located between the lateral and medial umbilical ligament, inferiorly limited by iliopubic tract
- Corresponds to origin of direct inguinal hernia

Fossa vesicalis:
- Located medial to the medial umbilical ligament and cranial to the iliopubic tract, pubic bone, and urinary bladder
- Corresponds to the origin of supravesical hernia

Areas of Concern

The triangle of doom:
- A triangular area bound by vas deferens, the testicular vessels and the peritoneal fold
- External iliac artery and vein are present in this area

The triangle of pain:
- A triangular area, lateral to the 'Triangle of doom', is bound by the iliopubic tract, the testicular vessels and the peritoneal fold.
- This area (from lateral to medial) includes the lateral femoral cutaneous nerve, the femoral branch of the genitofemoral nerve and the femoral nerve.

Iliac vessels:
- Located at the bottom of the pelvis and in the middle of the preperitoneal space
- These vessels are accompanied by fatty tissue, lymph nodes, and overdissection may lead to bleeding, lymphatic leakage.

Corona mortis ("Crown of death"):
- A vascular connection between the inferior epigastric and obturator vessels, visualized about 5 cm away from the pubic symphysis, arching over Cooper's ligament
- This variant found in 20–30% of patients
- If corona mortis vessels are injured during dissection, significant hemorrhage may occur due to dual supply and hemostasis is also difficult because they may retract into the obturator canal.
- Surgeons must alert during dissection and fixation on Cooper's ligament.

Iliopubic tract:
- An important landmark in the groin
- It divides the groin in an upper and lower part
- Below the tract, dissection must be meticulous to avoid injury to vessels, cord and nerves (Trapezoid of disasters)
- Above the tract, epigastric vessels only pose any risk.

Cooper's ligament:
- It is a white, shiny tendinous tissue
- "Corona mortis" may arch over this ligament
- Mesh and tacks are fixed to this ligament.

Nyhus Classification of Groin Hernia

Type I: Indirect inguinal hernia
- Internal inguinal ring normal

Type II: Indirect inguinal hernia
- Internal inguinal ring dilated
- Posterior wall intact

Type III: Posterior wall defect
- Direct inguinal hernia
- Indirect inguinal hernia—Internal ring dilated and medially encroaching the transversalis fascia
- Femoral hernia

Type IV: Recurrent hernia
- Direct
- Indirect
- Femoral
- Combined

EHS Groin Hernia Classification System

EHS groin classification system	Primary/Recurrent				
	0	1	2	3	X
Lateral (L)					
Medial (M)					
Femoral (F)					

0 = No hernia detectable; **1** = <1.5 cm (one finger); **2** = <3 cm (two fingers); **3** = >3 cm (more than two fingers); **X** = not investigated

L = Lateral/indirect hernia; **M** = medial/direct hernia; **F** = Femoral hernia

Inguinal Hernia

- In both male and female, inguinal hernias are the most common type of hernia
- Men are 25 times more likely to develop groin hernia
- Anatomically inguinal hernia is classified into indirect and direct inguinal hernia. **Indirect hernia** is protrusion of hernia sac through the deep inguinal ring, lateral to the inferior epigastric vessels. **Direct hernia** is protrusion of hernia sac through Hesselbach's triangle, medial to inferior epigastric vessels.
- Among inguinal hernias, about 75% are indirect and rest are direct hernias
- **Bilateral hernias** are commonly direct hernias than indirect hernias
- The prevalence of hernias as well as likelihood of strangulation increases with age
- Among all strangulated hernias, most are indirect inguinal hernias.

Both indirect and femoral hernias commonly occur in right side due to:

- Delayed obliteration of processus vaginalis
- Tamponading effect of sigmoid colon on the left femoral canal

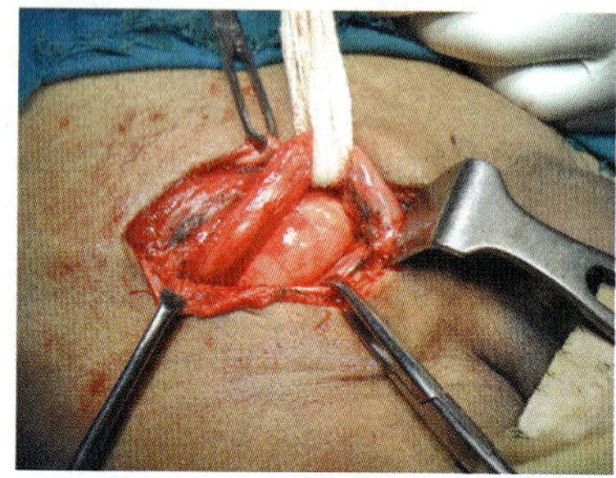

Direct Inguinal Hernia

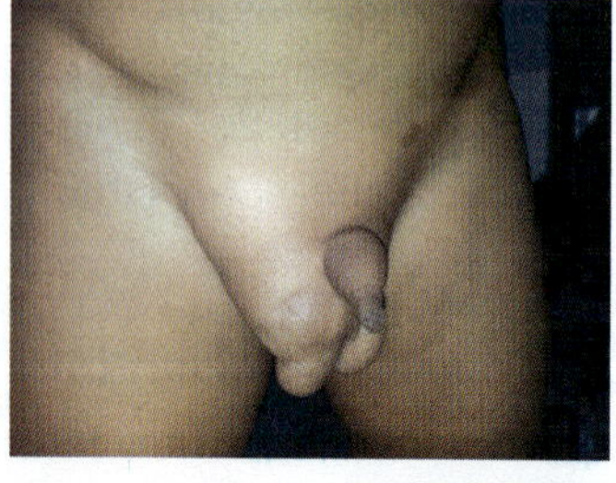

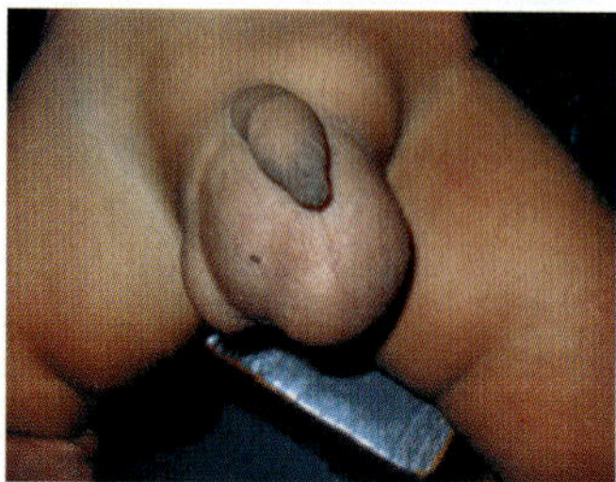

Congenital Inguinal Hernia

Pathophysiology

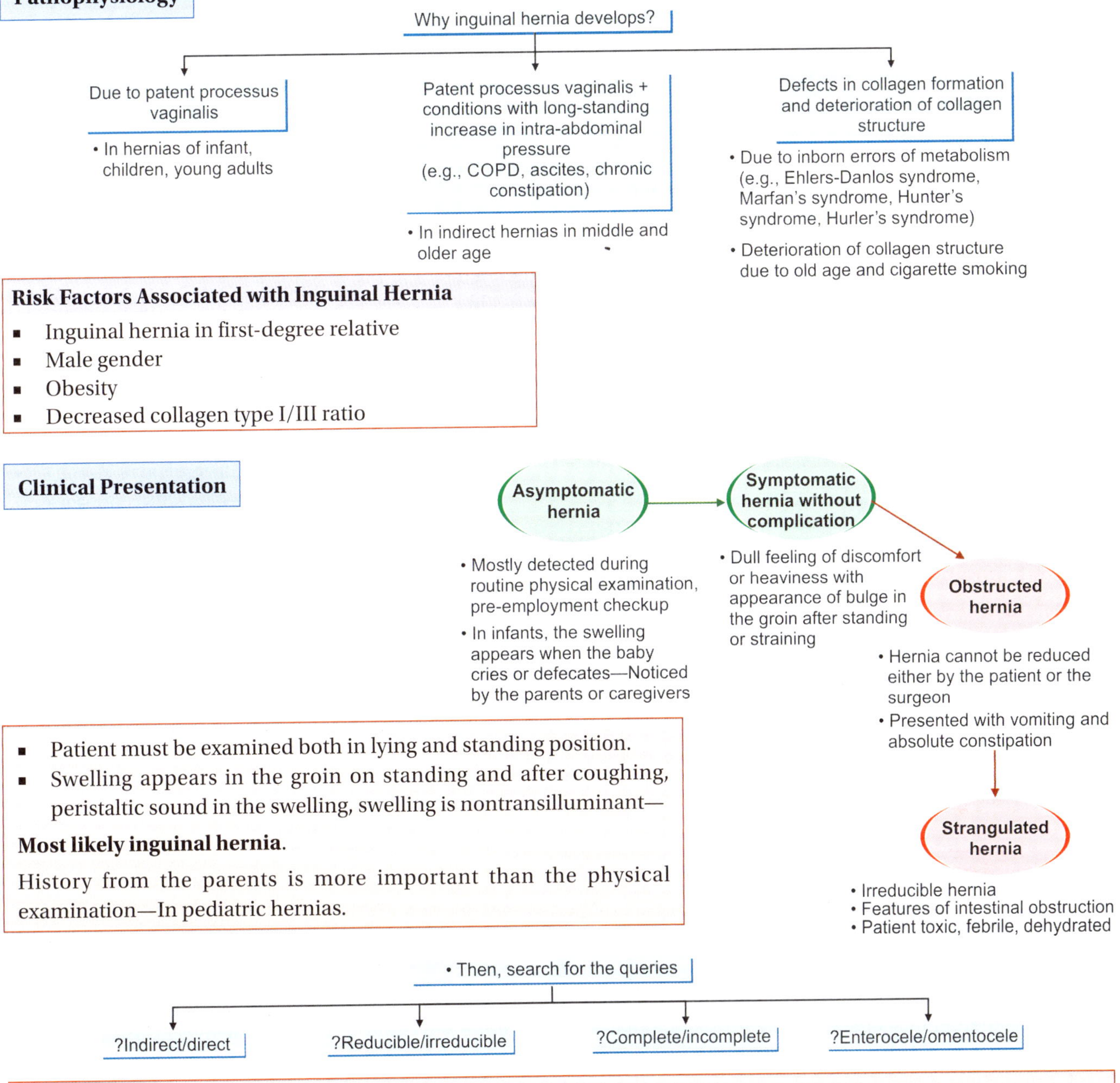

Risk Factors Associated with Inguinal Hernia

- Inguinal hernia in first-degree relative
- Male gender
- Obesity
- Decreased collagen type I/III ratio

Clinical Presentation

- Patient must be examined both in lying and standing position.
- Swelling appears in the groin on standing and after coughing, peristaltic sound in the swelling, swelling is nontransilluminant—

Most likely inguinal hernia.

History from the parents is more important than the physical examination—In pediatric hernias.

- A hernia that descends into the scrotum—**almost certainly an indirect inguinal hernia.**
- Groin swelling moving lateral to medial in the inguinal region after coughing—**Most likely indirect inguinal hernia.**
- On straining, swelling (symmetric, circular) near the external ring appears from deep to superficial—**Most likely direct inguinal hernia.**
- When reducing the hernia, a gurgling sound is audible—**Most likely an enterocele.**
- A patient who is used to reduce the swelling manually now cannot do it and surgeon cannot reduce the hernia by 'Taxis'—**It is an irreducible hernia.**

The distinction between indirect and direct inguinal hernia cannot be done accurately by clinical examination always and it is not essential to differentiate because hernia repair is approached in a same way regardless of type of hernia.

Diagnosis

- Appearance of swelling in groin after standing or coughing, presence of cough impulse, gurgling sound during reduction—these clinical findings are highly suggestive of inguinal hernia, in most cases. No need of further investigation for confirmation.
- According to patient, swelling appears in the groin after straining, but not present on clinical examination—Standing or ambulatory for a period sometimes makes the undiagnosed hernia to become visible. **Repeat examination at another time** is also helpful for diagnosis.
- Combined clinical examination and ultrasound is recommended as most suitable for diagnosis of vague groin swelling and possible occult hernia (asymptomatic hernia not detected by clinical examination). This combined modality is also helpful to detect recurrent inguinal hernia.
- If clinical suspicion of hernia but USG is inconclusive, **dynamic MRI or CT** can be considered.

Treatment

Symptomatic inguinal hernias should be electively repaired unless specific contraindications present.

"Watchful waiting" policy may be followed in asymptomatic or minimally symptomatic male inguinal hernia patients since their risk of hernia-related emergencies is low. **The lower morbidity of elective hernia repair has to be weighed against the higher morbidity of emergency surgery for obstructed or strangulated hernia.**

- If patient has associated **significant prostatic hyperplasia, chronic cough**, it should be treated before the hernia repair.

Causes of Inguinal Swelling

- Inguinal hernia
- Inguinal lymphadenopathy
- Undescended testis
- Encysted hydrocele of the cord
- Round ligament varicosities

Causes of Inguino-scrotal Swelling

- Inguinal hernia
- Varicocele
- Infantile hydrocele
- Encysted hydrocele of the cord

Causes of Femoral Swelling

- Femoral hernia
- Lymphadenopathy
- Ectopic testis
- Saphena varix

In **pregnant women** with groin swelling, **round ligament varicosities** should be excluded because clinical presentation is almost similar to hernia.

Principles of Hernia Repair

- Open inguinal hernia repair includes elimination of hernia sac (herniotomy) and strengthening of the floor of the inguinal canal (herniorrhaphy or hernioplasty). Only herniotomy is indicated in pediatric hernia and hernia in young adults.
- **Antibiotic prophylaxis** is not recommended in open mesh repair in average risk patients in low-risk environment and in laparoendoscopic repair in any patient in any risk environment (International Guidelines for Groin Hernia Management, 2018)
- **Regional anesthesia** is preferred by most of the surgeons for open inguinal hernia repair. **Local anesthesia** is recommended for open repair of inguinal hernia if surgical team is experienced in this techniques. For laparo-endoscopic repair, **general anesthesia** is recommended.
- **Mesh-based repair (hernioplasty)** is recommended for repair of inguinal hernia due to less risk of recurrence.
- **For bilateral inguinal hernia**, laparoendoscopic repair is recommended provided expertise and instrumentation is available.
- **Non-mesh repair (primary tissue repair)** may be considered if mesh is not available or patient not willing to mesh use. **Shouldice technique** is recommended for non-mesh repair.
- **For recurrent inguinal hernia**, laparoendoscopic repair is recommended after failed anterior tissue or mesh-repair. If recurrence develops after a posterior repair, anterior mesh-repair is recommended.

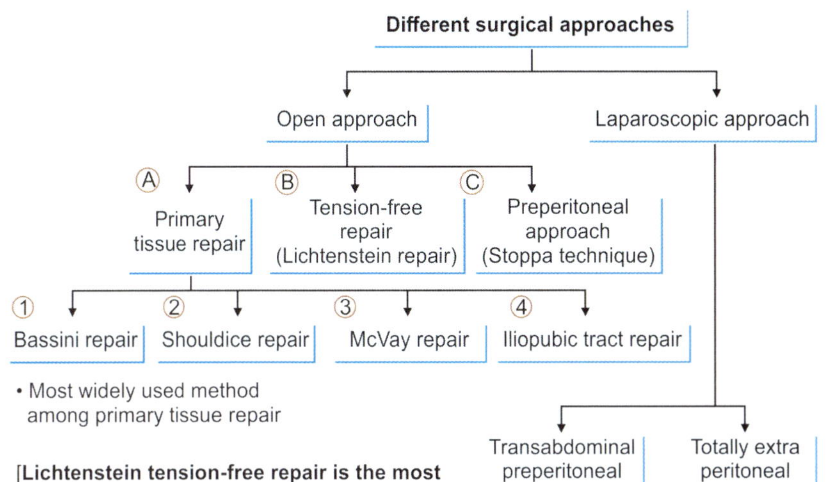

[Lichtenstein tension-free repair is the most common approach for inguinal hernia repair]

Other Surgical Approaches

- **Primary tissue repair**
    - Desarda technique
- **Mesh-based repair**
    - Prolene Hernia System
    - Trabucco technique

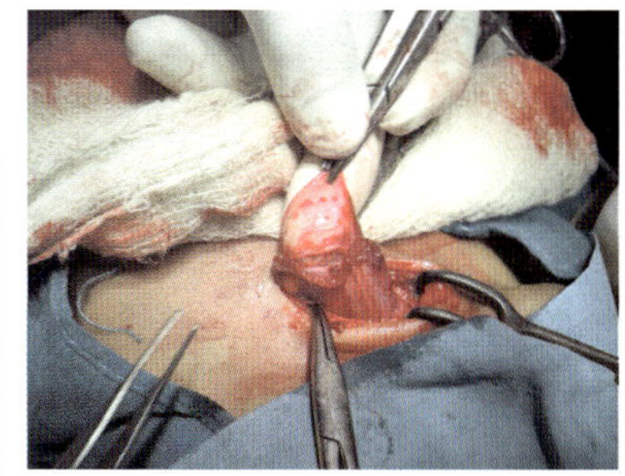

Treatment of Hernia Sac

- In indirect herina, the sac (*pearly white structure* lying on outer side of cord) is dissected from the cord structures (pampiniform plexus, vas deferens) and cremasteric muscle
- During dissection of sac, care must be taken to avoid injury to vas, spermatic artery and pampiniform plexus
- Large indirect sac extending upto the scrotum should not be dissected beyond the pubic tubercle due to increased risk of ischemic orchitis
- Sac is opened, to look for any hernia contents (intestine or omentum)
- Contents are reduced, sac is dissected upto the neck (extraperitoneal fat is seen and inferior epigastric vessels on the medial side). Sac is ligated at the neck with absorbable suture.
- **Direct sacs** should not be opened or ligated but must be freed from transversalis fibers.
- **In preperitoneal approach**, sac is reduced but not ligated
- **In sliding hernia**, sac is opened but no attempt should be made to dissect the contents from the sac, then the sac is inverted.
- *Mobilizing the testis into the inguinal canal should be avoided to minimize the risk of testicular ischemic injury.*
- *In female patients, it is better to avoid division of the round ligament in open repair.*

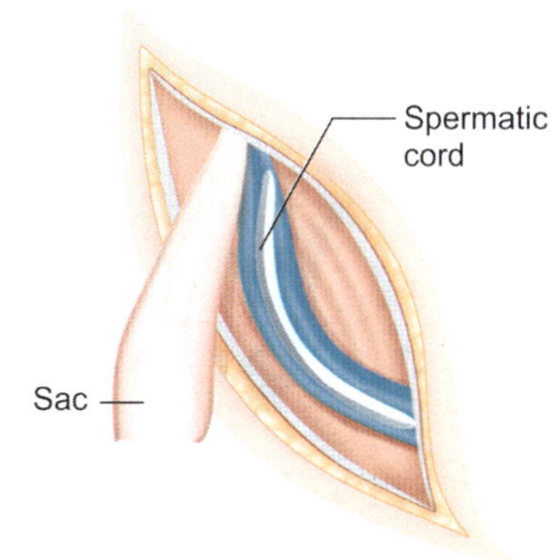

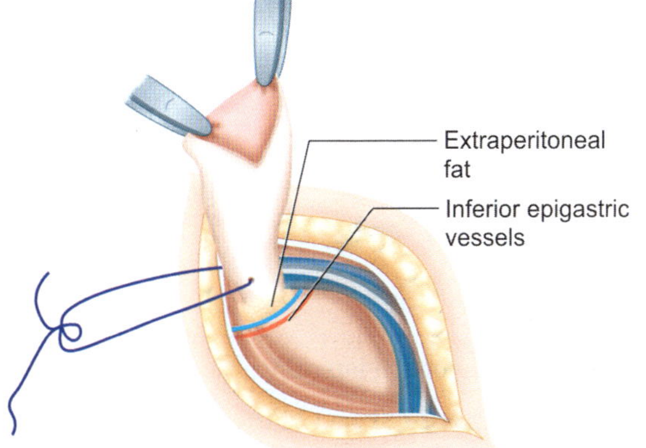

Opening of sac.

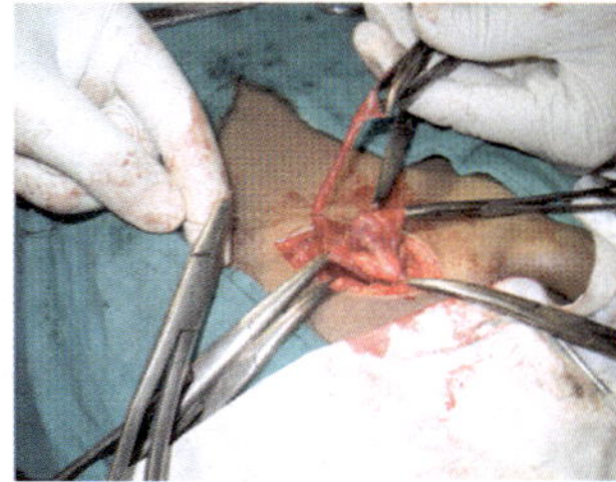

Ligation of sac.

Reconstruction of Inguinal Floor

Techniques of reconstruction or strengthening of inguinal floor includes primary tissue repair and mesh-based repair.

Primary tissue-based repair includes: (i) Modified Bassini repair; (ii) Shouldice repair; (iii) Desarda technique; (iv) McVay repair; and (v) Iliopubic tract repair.

Mesh-based repair includes: (i) Lichtenstein tension-free repair; (ii) Plug-and-patch technique; (iii) Open preperitoneal approach; and (iv) Laparoendoscopic approach (TEP and TAPP)

Open Preperitoneal Approach

Preperitoneal approach through anterior dissection

- Rives' technique
- Transinguinal preperitoneal repair (TIPP)
- Onstep technique

Preperitoneal approach through posterior dissection

- Transrectus preperitoneal approach (TREPP)
- Ugahary technique
- Kugel technique
- Wantz technique

Rives' technique is the most commonly performed open pre-peritoneal approach.

Modified Bassini repair: Conjoint tendon is approximated to the inguinal ligament with the help of nonabsorbable suture (polypropylene)

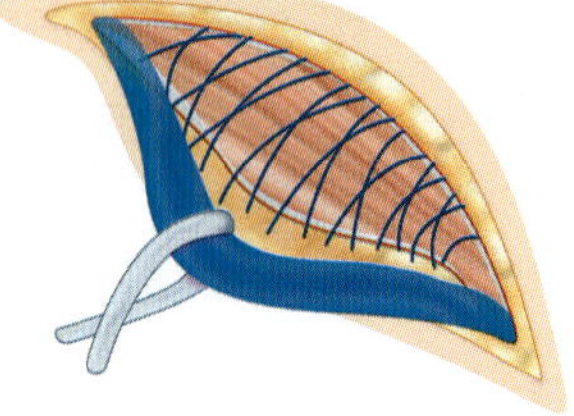

Shouldice Repair

A multilayer repair of the posterior wall of the inguinal canal by continuous running suture technique.

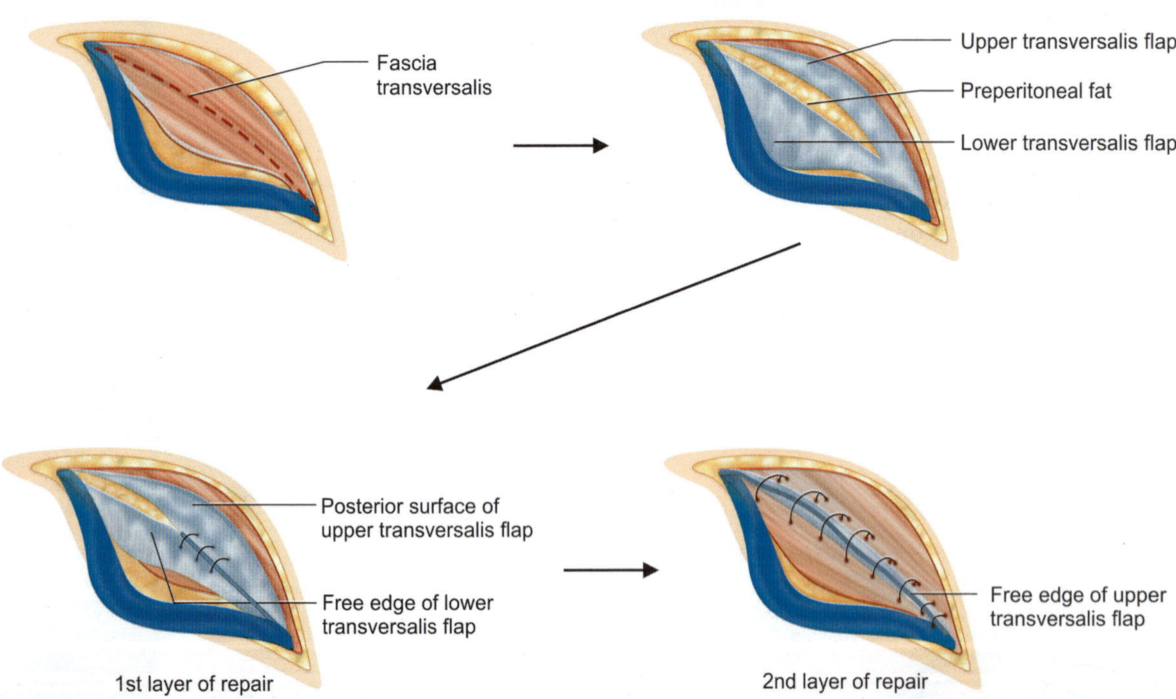

- The 3rd layer brings together the conjoint tendon medially with the inguinal ligament laterally.
- The 4th layer brings together the anterior rectus sheath medially with the posterior aspect of the external oblique aponeurosis laterally.

McVay (Cooper's ligament) Repair

- **Is the only technique that repairs both inguinal and femoral hernias.**
- Edge of transversus abdominis is approximated to Cooper's ligament with nonabsorbable sutures.

Iliopubic Tract Repair

Transversus abdominis aponeurotic arch is approximated to the iliopubic tract with nonabsorbable interrupted sutures.

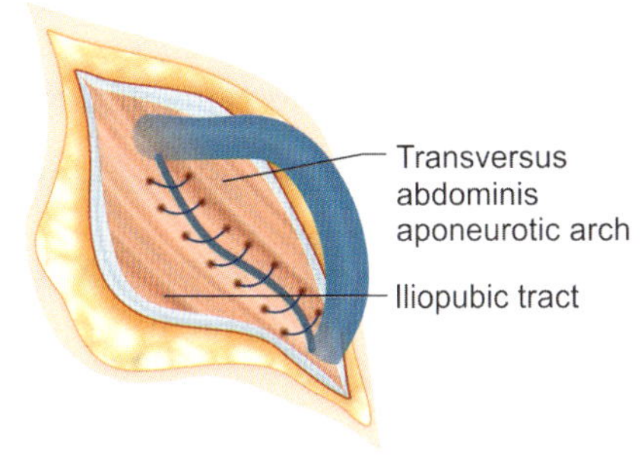

Desarda Repair

This repair is done **using a flap of the external oblique aponeurosis** sutured to the inguinal ligament below and to the aponeurotic part of the internal oblique above.

Lichtenstein Repair

- The Lichtenstein repair is **onlay placement of a flat mesh**. A piece of polypropylene mesh is placed over the floor of inguinal canal.
- Mesh is sutured to the fascia overlying the pubic tubercle, inferiorly; conjoint tendon, medially; inguinal ligament, laterally.
- Mesh is slit at the level of internal ring, the two limbs are crossed around the spermatic cord, thus creating a new internal ring.

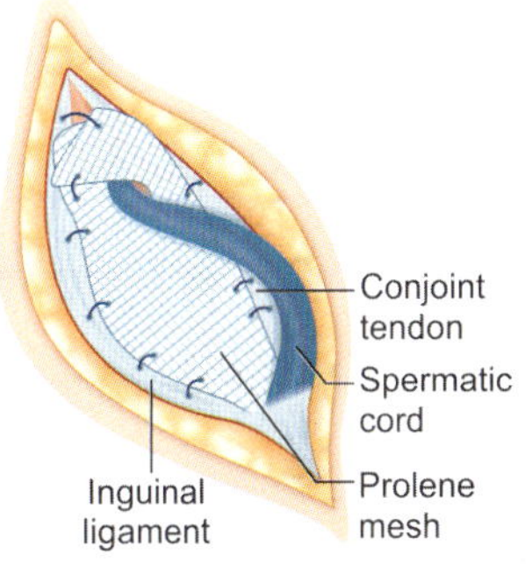

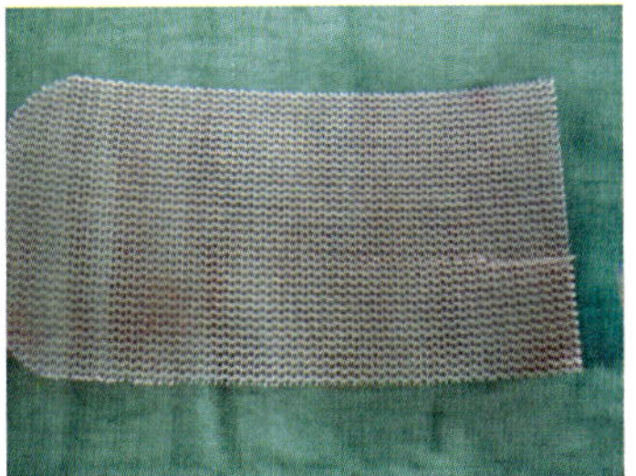

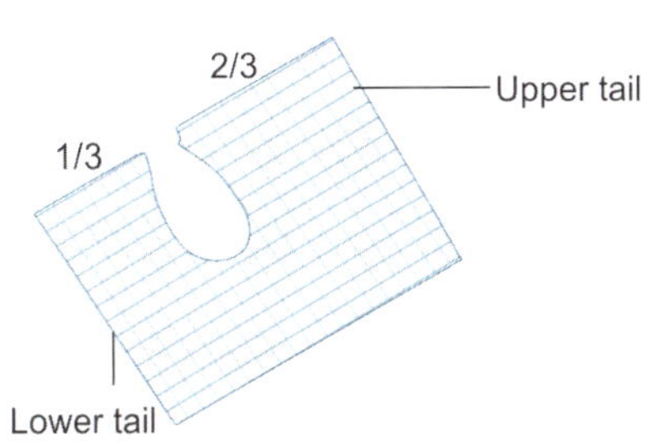

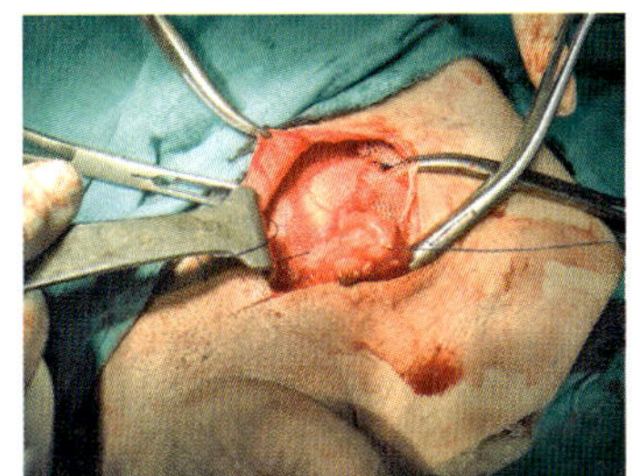

Plug-and-patch (Rutkow-Robbins) Repair

A mesh plug in the form of 'upside down umbrella' or 'cone' is snugly placed in the internal ring.

Bilayer Mesh Repair

Onlay patch is placed in the inguinal floor, underlay patch is placed in the preperitoneal space.

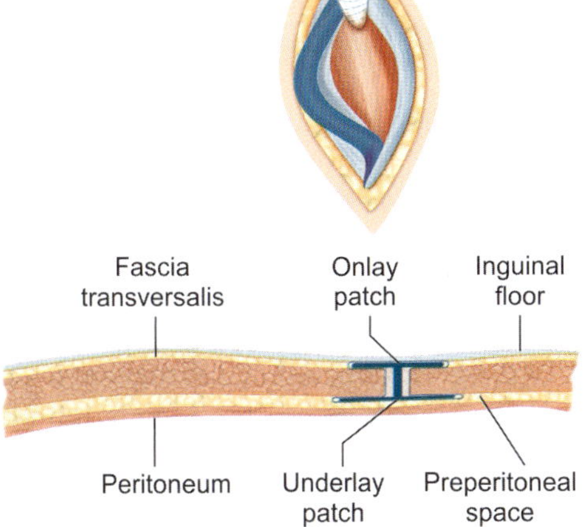

Both plug-and-patch technique and bilayer mesh repair are not recommended because of excessive use of foreign body material, need to explore both anterior and posterior planes and more cost.

Open Preperitoneal Approach

- This approach is based on the principle that the repair fixes the hernia defect in the space between hernial contents and hernia defect.
- Large mesh is placed in the preperitoneal space to cover the inguinal floor and myopectineal orifice.
- Indicated in recurrent inguinal hernia, sliding hernia, bilateral hernia.

Complications of Open Inguinal Hernia Repair

- Surgical site infection
- Seroma
- Hematoma
- Injury to the vas deferens
- Prosthetic complications
- Chronic postoperative inguinal pain (CPIP)
- Recurrence

Laparoendoscopic Approach

- This approach is based on the principle of preperitoneal approach.
- **Two techniques:** (i) TAPP (Transabdominal pre-peritoneal and (ii) TEP (Totally extraperitoneal). In both techniques, initial access is different but the final target is same (preperitoneal space).
- Particularly indicated in bilateral and recurrent inguinal hernias.

TAPP and TEP have comparable outcomes, so the choice of the technique should be based on the surgeon's expertise and experience.

In TAPP repair, the preperitoneal space is accessed after entering into the peritoneal cavity.

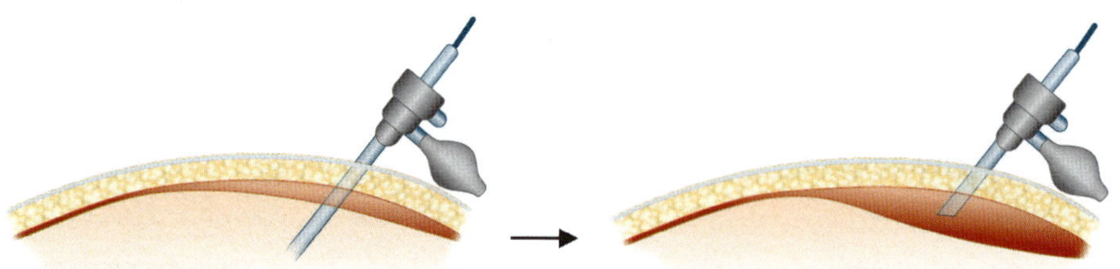

In TEP repair, the preperitoneal space is created using a balloon dissector.

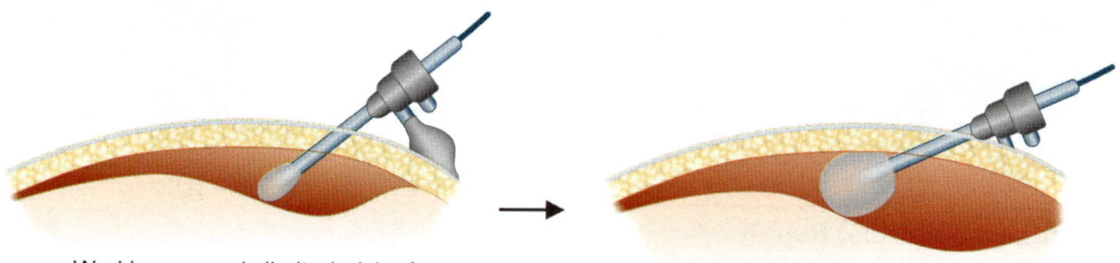

Recommendations of International Guidelines for Groin Hernia Management, 2018 Regarding Mesh

- HerniaSurge recommends large pore (1–1.5 mm) monofilament synthetic flat meshes with a burst strength of 16 Nm^2 and consisting of a minimum tensile strength in all directions (including subsequent tearing force) of 16 N/cm^2.
- Mesh fixation is recommended in patients with large direct hernias (M3-EHS classification) undergoing TAPP or TEP to reduce recurrence risk.

Complications of Laparoscopic Hernia Repair

(i) Vascular injuries (during access to the peritoneal cavity in TAAP, during dissection); (ii) Bowel injury; (iii) Bladder injury; (iv) Nerve entrapment or injury (commonly affected nerves are lateral femoral cutaneous nerve, genitofemoral nerve); (v) Migration of mesh; (vi) Mesh infection; (vii) Ischemic orchitis; (viii) Testicular swelling; (ix) Groin pain; and (x) Recurrence

Sliding Inguinal Hernia (Hernia-en-glissade)

- A type of indirect inguinal hernia where the posterior wall of the sac is formed by the sliding visceras.
- On the right side, the cecum is most commonly involved; on the left side, the sigmoid colon; and on either side, part of urinary bladder.
- Exclusively found in males, most of them are present in the left side.
- After dissecting the sac from the cord, the sliding hernial sac can be reduced by series of inverting sutures (Bevan technique) and then reconstruction of the posterior wall of the inguinal canal.
- Very large sliding hernia can be treated by entering the peritoneum through a separate incision, pulling the bowel back into the abdomen, fixing it to the posterior abdominal wall and then reconstruction of floor of the canal.
- **It should be suspected in any large inguinal hernia that cannot be completely reduced.**
- **It is essential to identify the condition early in the operation otherwise inadvertent injury to the bowel or bladder may occur.**
- **No attempt should be made to dissect the sliding viscera free from peritoneum, it may cause fistula or peritonitis due to devascularization.**

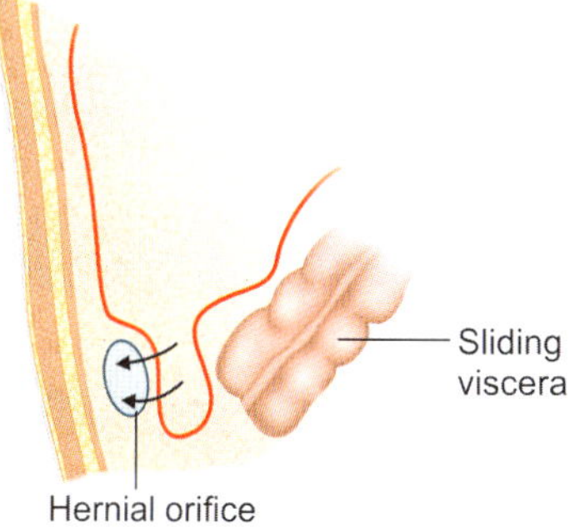

Sliding inguinal hernia.

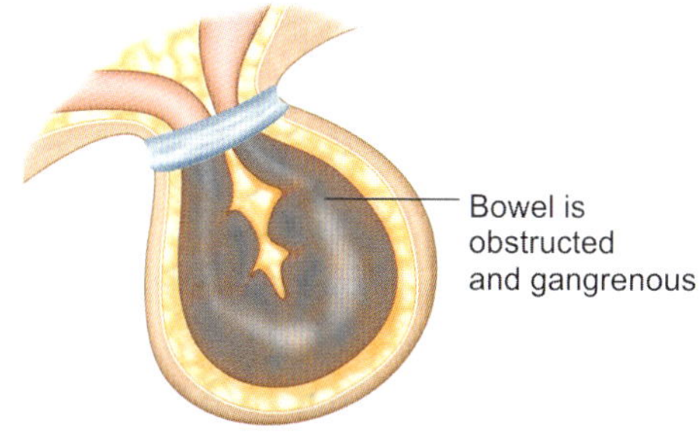

Strangulated inguinal hernia.

Strangulated Inguinal Hernia

- Indirect inguinal hernias are more commonly strangulated than direct hernias.
- The risk of strangulation is highest in the first months to years after the initial presentation.
- Usually, the small intestine is involved in strangulation. Large intestine rarely becomes involved.
- Treatment is resuscitation with IV fluids, nasosgastric suction, parenteral antibiotics followed by emergency hernia repair. Emergency hernia repair includes resection of gangrenous gut followed by primary repair or mesh repair.
- If gross enteric spillage is absent, emergent prosthetic repair with synthetic mesh can be performed (without any increase in 30-day wound-related morbidity). If strangulated hernia with bowel necrosis and/or gross enteric spillage during intestinal resection or peritonitis from bowel perforation, primary tissue repair is recommended when defect is small (<3 cm); when tissue repair is not feasible, biological mesh may be used (adapted from WSES Guideline).

Inguinodynia (Chronic Postoperative Inguinal Pain)

- Inguinodynia is pain or discomfort impacting daily activities lasting more than 3 months after surgery.
- Risk factors include: (i) Young age; (ii) Female gender; (iii) High preoperative pain; (iv) Early high postoperative pain; (v) Recurrent hernia; and (vi) Open repair.
- Nerves commonly injured are ilioinguinal, iliohypogastric, and genital branch of genitofemoral nerves. Nerve injury may occur from traction, electrosurgery, suture, or mesh entrapment.
- Pragmatic resection of the ilioinguinal nerve and/or the iliohypogastric nerve is recommended, if iatrogenic nerve injury occurs or if the nerve (s) interfere (s) with mesh position.
- Neurectomy (selective or triple) with or without mesh removal may be considered.

Risk Factors for Recurrence

- Direct inguinal hernia
- Female gender
- Poor surgical technique
- Sliding hernia
- Obesity

Femoral Hernia

- Protrusion of extraperitoneal fat or abdominal contents through the femoral canal.
- Most of the patients are 60–80 years old female patients.
- More common in women than men
- Femoral hernia may present with intermittent groin bulge or tender groin lump.
- On clinical examination, rounded bulge appears in the upper thigh just below the inguinal ligament, below and lateral to the pubic tubercle.
- *Elective mesh repair* is recommended for femoral hernia. *'Wait and Watch' policy* should not be followed because chance of strangulation is high.
- Femoral hernia can be repaired by **open** *or laparoendoscopic approach.*
- Femoral hernia can be repaired by different surgical approaches, but all approaches **follow the same principles:** (i) Complete excision of hernial sac; (ii) Inspection of the contents; and (iii) Mesh-based or suture repair of the defect in femoral canal.
- *Different surgical approaches for open femoral hernia repair:* (i) Lothessein's transinguinal approach; (ii) Lockwood's infra-inguinal approach; and (iii) McEvedy high approach.

Lothessein's Transinguinal Approach

- Incision is similar to inguinal hernia, but closer to the inguinal ligament.
- Fascia transversalis is incised along the line of incision.

Sac is identified and after opening it, is excised.

Femoral ring is obliterated by suturing the inguinal ligament to the Cooper's ligament.

Posterior wall of the inguinal canal must be reconstructed as it has been weakened by exposure.

It is a preferred approach for complicated femoral hernia because of better exposure of femoral ring and easier handling of strangulated contents.

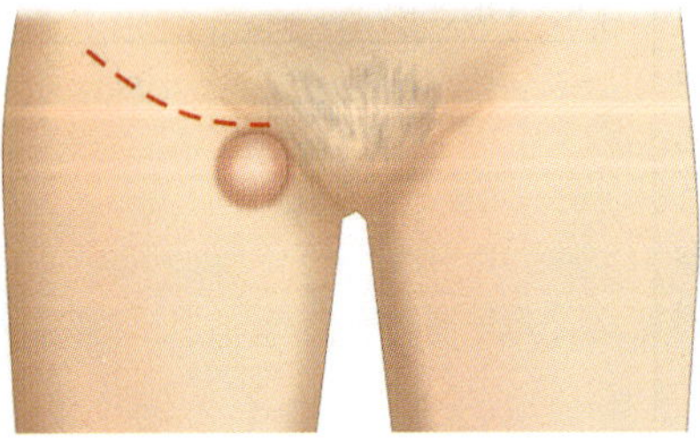

- ***Femoral canal*** is surrounded by bone and ligaments on three sides.
- ***The narrowness of the sac*** **and the *rigidity of femoral ring*** make it most likely to be strangulated.

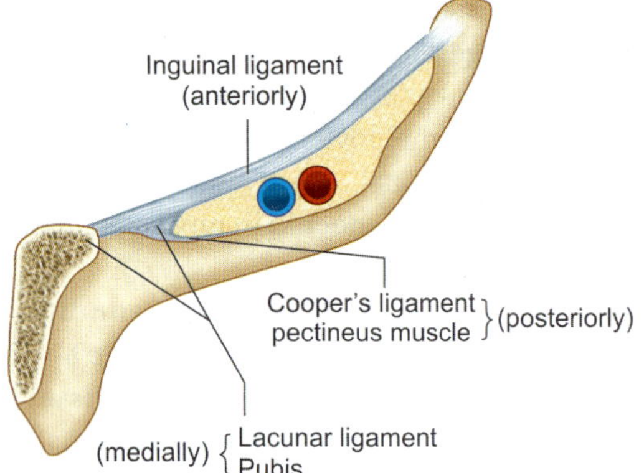

Boundaries of Femoral Canal

The inguinal ligament anterosuperiorly; Cooper's ligament and pectineus muscle posteriorly; junction of iliopubic tract and Cooper's ligament medially, the femoral vein laterally.

- An elderly female patient presenting with small bowel obstruction, but no history of abdominal surgery—**Think of occult femoral hernia**.
- Tender femoral hernia without features of intestinal obstruction—**Think of Richter's hernia**.

Variants of Femoral Hernia

Hesselbach's hernia—lateral to femoral vessels

Velpeau's hernia—superficial to femoral vessels (prevascular)

Serafini's hernia—deep to the femoral vessels (retrovascular)

Laugier's hernia—through the lacunar ligament

Cloquet's hernia—through the pectineal fascia

Lockwood's Infra-inguinal Approach

- An easy surgical approach for ***uncomplicated femoral hernia repair***.
- Incision is 1 cm below and parallel to the inguinal ligament
- Risk of abnormal branch of obturator artery is high in comparison to other approaches.

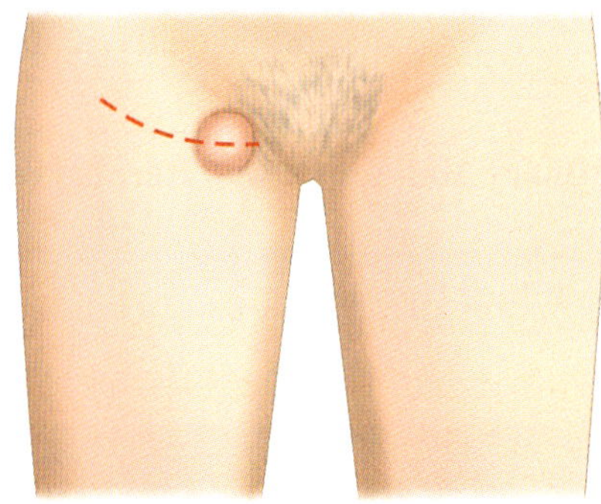

McEvedy's High Approach

- It is the best surgical approach for complicated femoral hernia repair.
- A vertical incision is made in the lower abdomen at the lateral edge of rectus abdominis.
- This incision provides good access to the preperitoneal space.

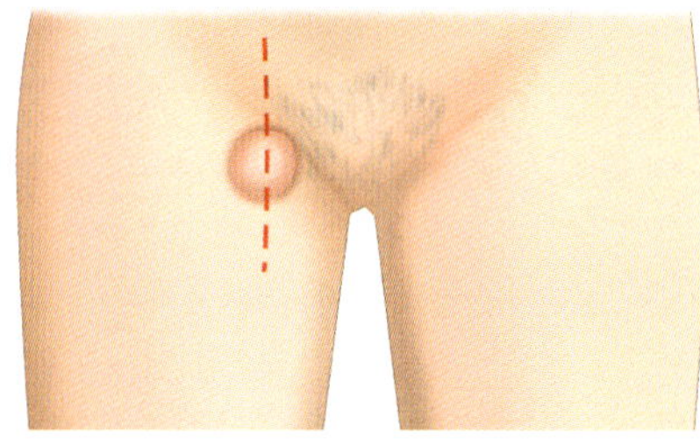

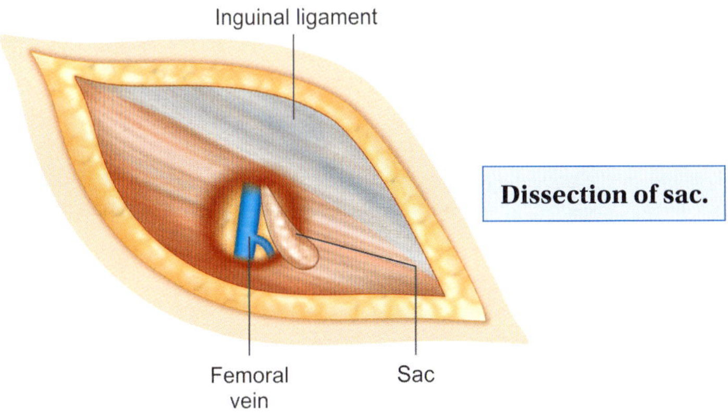

Dissection of sac.

- During repair, laterally **femoral vein** and medially **bladder** must be protected.
- Surgeon must aware about the presence of **aberrant obturator artery** (originates from inferior epigastric artery)
- During **placement of medial suture**, aberrant obturator artery, if present, may be injured.

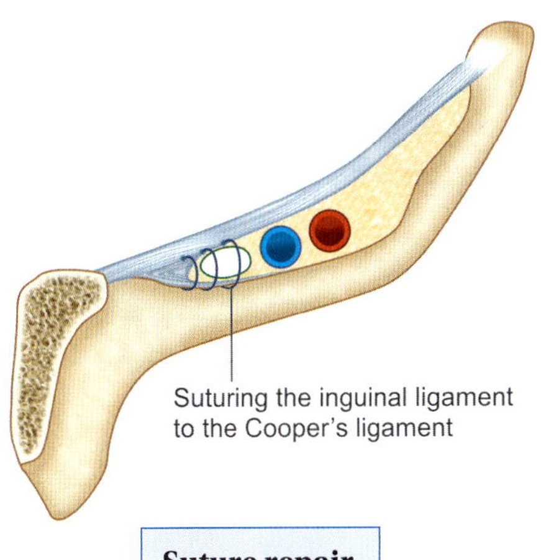

Suture repair.

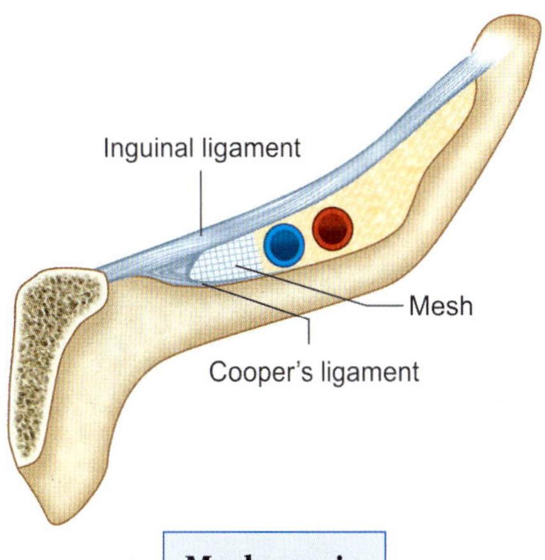

Mesh repair.

Abdominal Wall Hernia — Incisional Abdominal Wall Hernia

Primary Abdominal Wall Hernia (Ventral Hernia)

Umbilical Hernia

'A primary hernia with the defect located in the midline within the umbilical ring.' (EHS guideline)

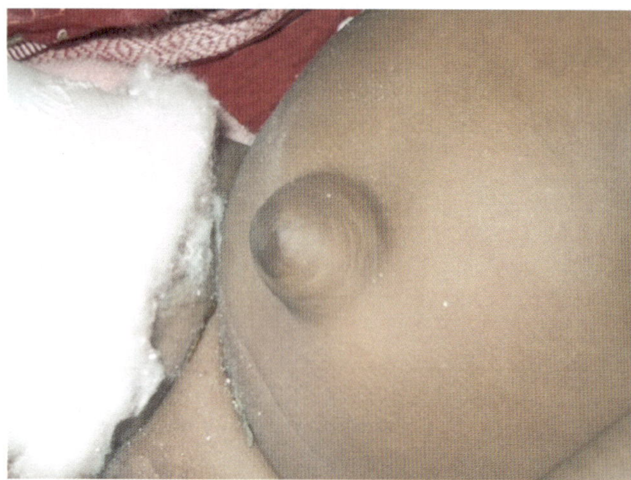
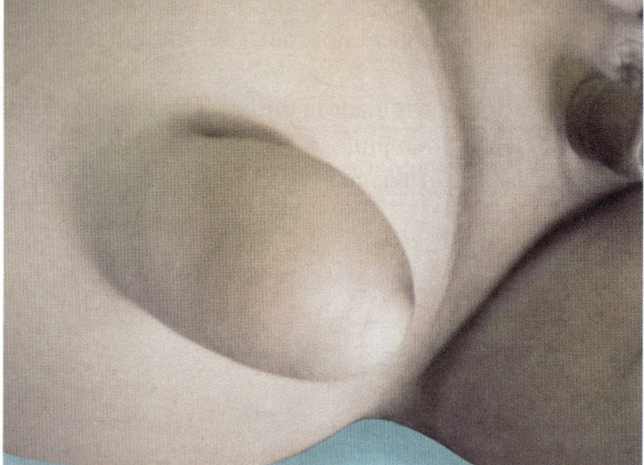

Congenital umbilical hernia.

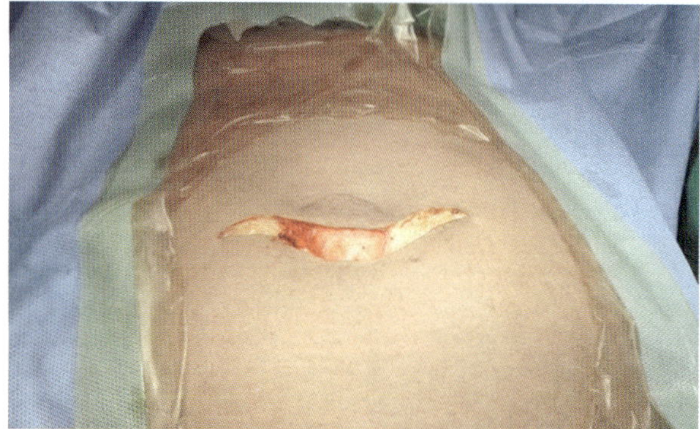

Incision for umbilical hernia repair.

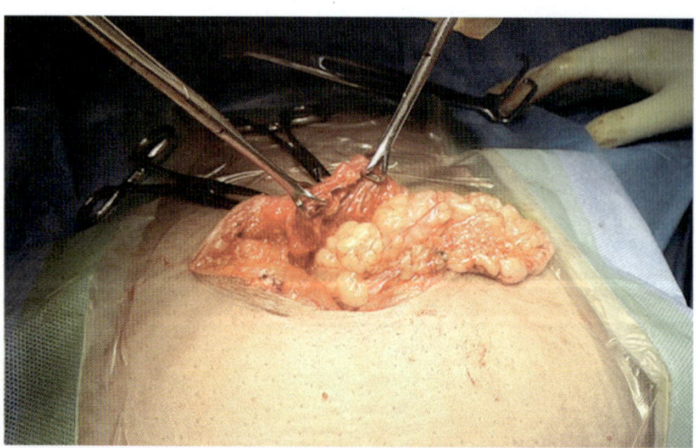

Umbilical hernia sac and its content.

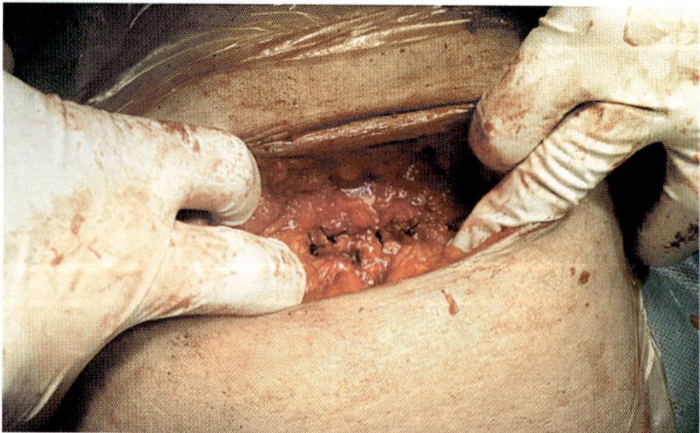

Anatomical repair of umbilical hernia.

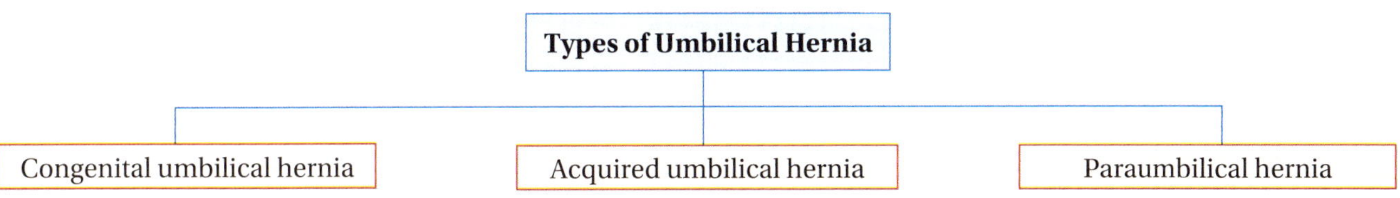

EHS Classification for Primary Abdominal Wall Hernias

EHS primary abdominal wall hernia classification		Diameter (cm)	Small (<2 cm)	Medium (≥2–4 cm)	Large (≥4 cm)
Midline	Epigastric				
	Umbilical				
Lateral	Spigelian				
	Lumbar				

Congenital umbilical hernia develops when umbilical scar fail to develop or weak.

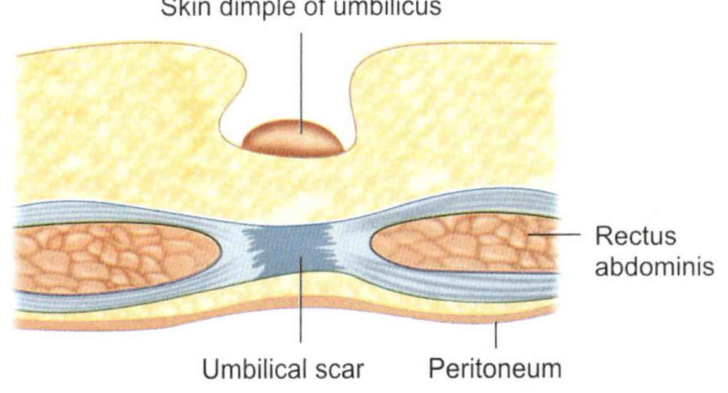

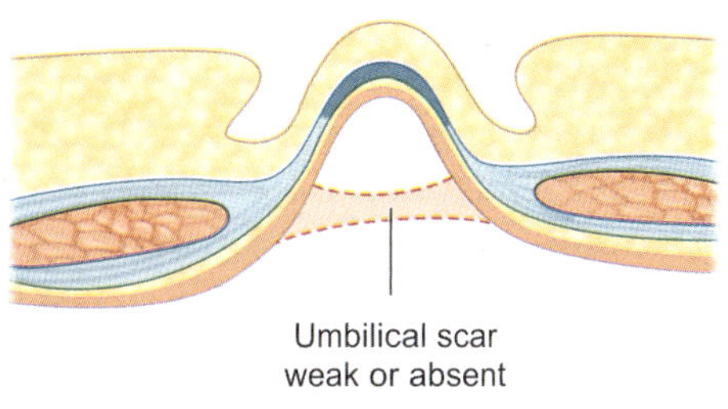

Acquired umbilical hernia develops when umbilical scar is stretched by raised intra-abdominal pressure.

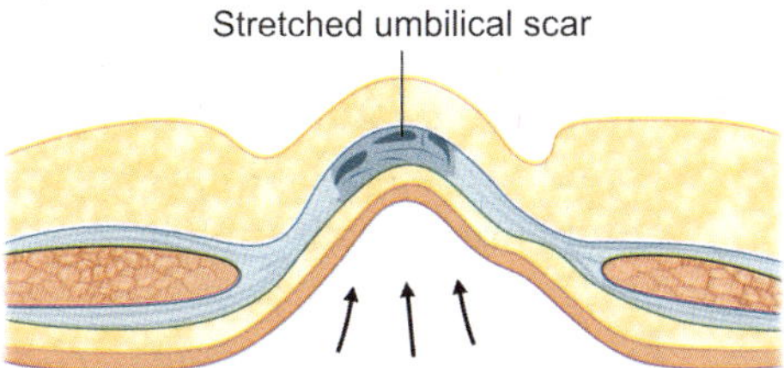

Paraumbilical hernia develops just above or just below the umbilicus.

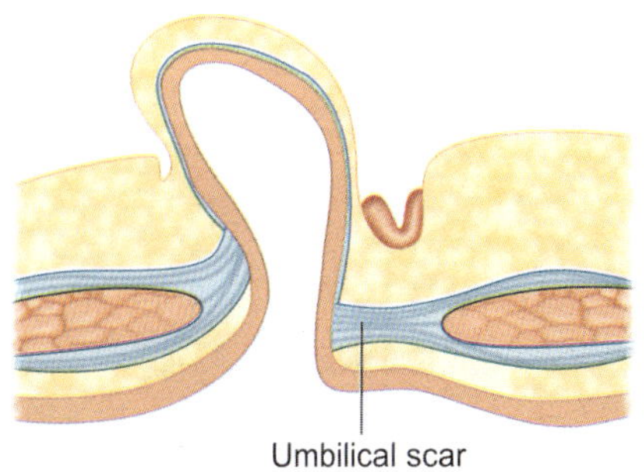

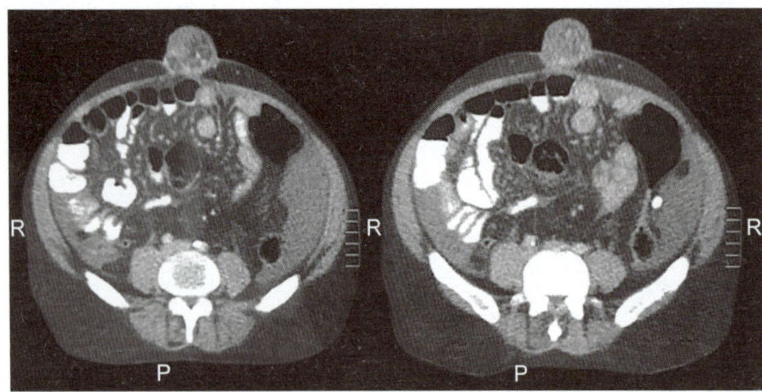

CT scan showing acquired umbilical hernia.

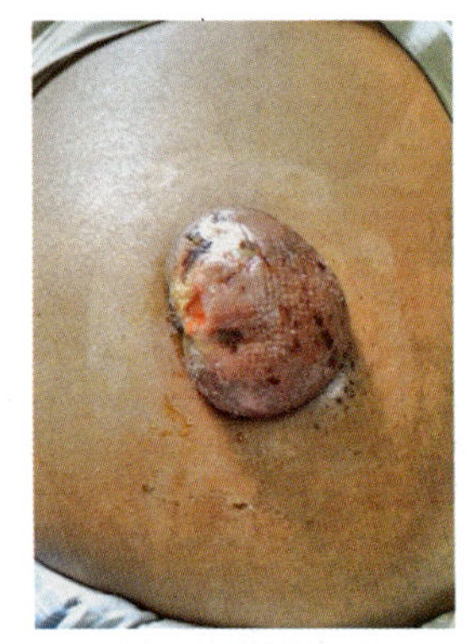
Acquired umbilical hernia in a patient with ascites (note the skin changes).

- **Umbilical hernia in infants and children** are congenital umbilical hernia.
- Usually, **spontaneous closure of congenital umbilical hernia** occurs by the age of 2 years. If defect persists even after 5 years, surgery is to be considered.
- In adults, umbilical hernias are acquired. Acquired umbilical hernias are more common in women, usually associated with pregnancy, obesity, and ascites.
- **Umbilical hernia is commonly diagnosed by clinical examination only**. Ultrasound or CT is indicated if clinical findings are inconclusive.
- **Surgical options for umbilical hernia repair are:** (i) Sutured repair and (ii) Mesh repair.

Surgical Principles of Umbilical Hernia Repair

- **For small umbilical hernia** (defect diameter 0–1 cm), sutured repair with a nonabsorbable or slowly absorbable suture is preferred.
- **For medium-sized hernia** (diameter >1 ≤ 4 cm), open mesh repair (a flat mesh in the preperitoneal space with a mesh overlap of 3 cm) is preferred. Laparoscopic repair (preperitoneal or retromuscular mesh placement) may be considered for multiple defects or in patients with high risk of wound infection.
- **For large umbilical hernias**, laparoscopic repair is preferred. Laparoscopic IPOM (Classical IPOM or 'IPOM plus') is the most used technique nowadays.
- **Elective surgery for umbilical and epigastric hernias should be postponed** until after last pregnancy (because pregnancy after hernia repair increases the chance of recurrence), if hernia is reducible. If surgery cannot be postponed until after the last pregnancy, sutured repair is suggested (mesh repair is associated with increased risk of chronic pain) [EHS guideline 2020].

Classical IPOM repair: Intraperitoneal mesh placement for bridging the defect. **Complications:** (i) Higher seroma formation and infection and (ii) Bulging of the non-closed defect mimic recurrence.

IPOM plus: Closure of the defect followed by intraperitoneal mesh placement. **Advantages:** (i) Less recurrence; (ii) Less seroma formation; and (iii) Less bulging.

Newly Emerging Laparo-enodoscopic Approaches

Subcutaneous onlay laparoscopic approach (SCOLA): An effective approach for umbilical hernia associated with concomitant diastasis recti.

Endoscopic-assisted linea alba reconstruction (ELAR): A new operative approach for diastasis recti and concomitant umbilical, trocar or epigastric hernia.

Mini- or Less-open Sublay Operation (MILOS) and **Endoscopic-assisted MILOS (eMILOS)**: For repair of primary umbilical and epigastric hernia.

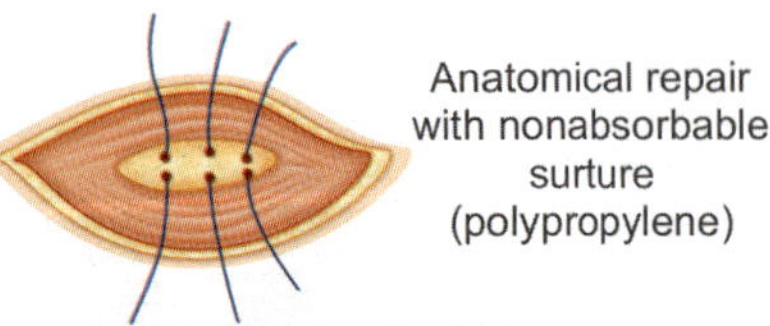

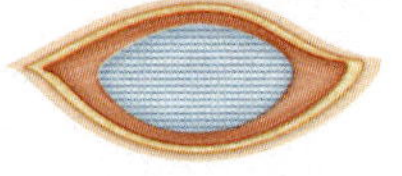

Epigastric Hernia

- **Epigastric hernia (Fatty hernia of the linea alba)** occurs through a defect in the linea alba anywhere between the xiphoid process and the umbilicus.
- This defect develops due to **weakened decussating fibers of linea alba** associated with increased intra-abdominal pressure or chronic strain in abdominal wall.
- In most cases, the hernia contains **preperitoneal fat only** and no sac. If sac presents, it usually contains omentum and rarely intestine.
- Middle-aged male persons are mostly affected.
- Multiple epigastric hernia may be present. **Failure to recognize the other hernial defects is the cause of 'recurrence'**.
- In most cases, epigastric hernias are asymptomatic. It is better felt than it can be seen. In symptomatic cases, it is felt as a small, soft, reducible, mildly tender mass **in the midline anywhere between xiphoid and umbilicus**. This mass becomes more prominent with standing and Valsalva maneuver.
- Most of the epigastric hernias are diagnosed by clinical examination. Imaging (USG or CT) is only indicated if clinical findings are inconclusive.
- All symptomatic hernias must be treated by **sutured repair or mesh repair**.

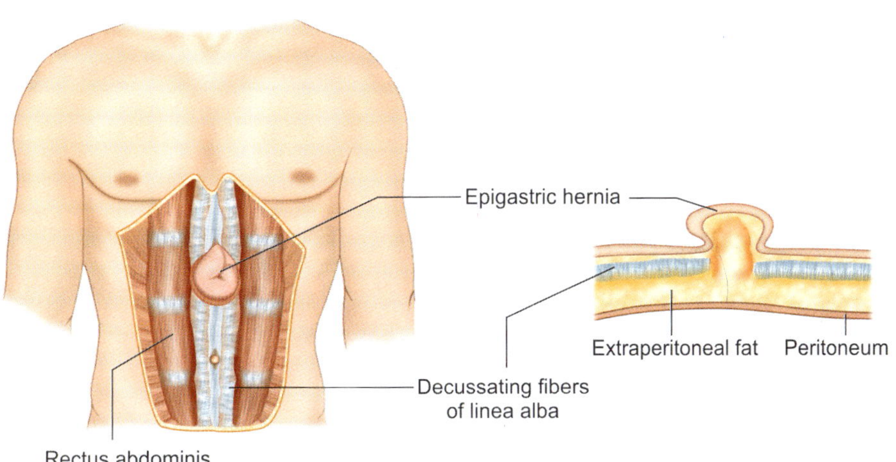

Principles of Epigastric Hernia Repair

For small epigastric hernia, sutured repair with a non-absorbable or slowly absorbable suture is preferred.

For medium-sized hernia, open mesh repair is preferred. A flat mesh in the preperitoneal space with a mesh overlap of 3 cm. Laparoscopic repair (preperitoneal or retromuscular mesh placement) may be considered for multiple defects or in patients with high risk of wound infection.

For large umbilical and epigastric hernias, laparoscopic repair is preferred. Laparoscopic IPOM (Classical IPOM or 'IPOM plus') is the most used technique nowadays.

- In epigastric and umbilical hernia patients with **compromised liver function** (cirrhosis and/or ascites), open onlay or preperitoneal mesh repair is the safe treatment option. Sutured repair has high recurrence rate.
- Elective surgery for umbilical and epigastric hernias should be postponed until after last pregnancy (because pregnancy after hernia repair increases the chance of recurrence), if hernia is reducible. If surgery cannot be postponed until after the last pregnancy, sutured repair is suggested (mesh repair is associated with increased risk of chronic pain) [EHS Guideline 2020].
- **Newly emerged laparoendoscopic approaches for epigastric hernia are:** (i) Endoscopic-assisted linea alba reconstruction (ELAR); (ii) ELAR plus (for diastasis recti and concomitant ventral hernia); and (iii) eMILOS.

Incisional Hernia

Definition of incisional hernia: Any abdominal wall gap with or without a bulge in the area of a postoperative scar perceptible or palpable by clinical examination or imaging (EHS guideline).

- Develops at previous incision as a result of improper healing of fascial tissues.

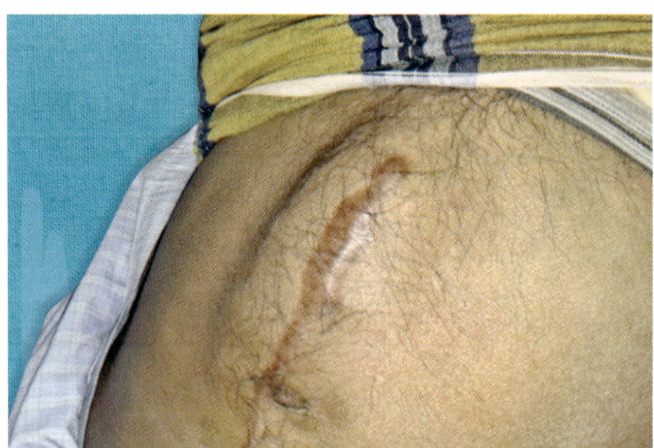

Incisional hernia in midline incision.

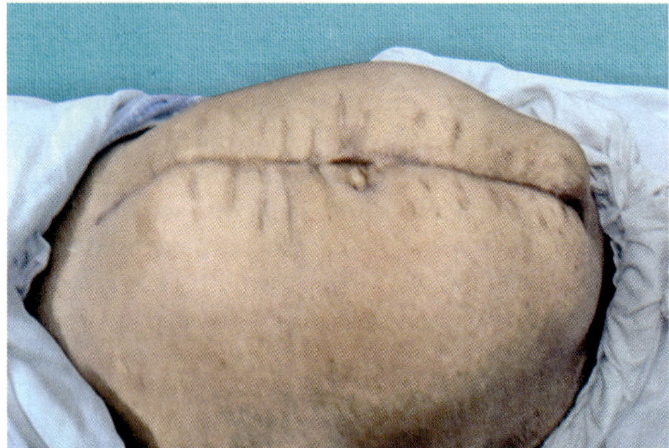

Incisional hernia (common in midline incision).

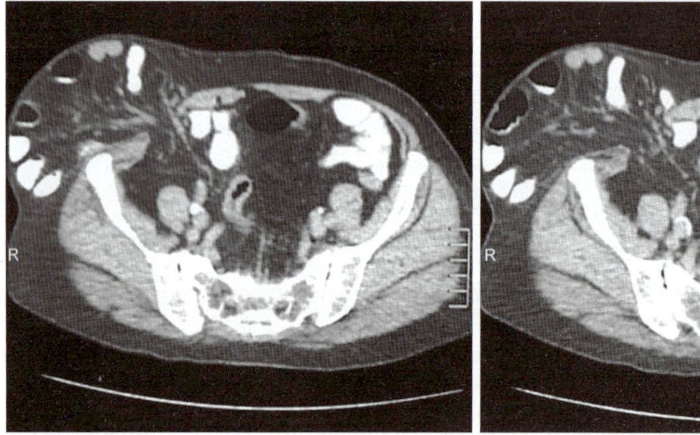

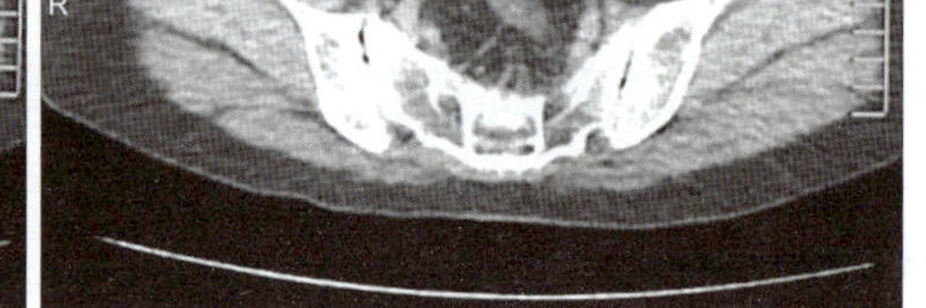

CT scan showing incisional hernia (clear delineation of hernial defect along with hernial content).

Factors Responsible for Development of Incisional Hernia

Patient-related factors

- Advanced age
- Ascites
- Anemia
- Corticosteroid use
- Cancer (malignancy)
- Cytotoxic drugs
- C vitamin deficiency
- Cigarette smoking
- Debilitated state (malnutrition)
- Diabetes mellitus
- Jaundice
- Obesity
- Surgical site infection
- Uremia

Operative factors

- **Types of surgery** (elective/emergency)—emergency surgery is associated with higher risk.
- **Types of incision**—Midline and paramedian incisions are associated with more risk.
- **Techniques of closure**—inadequate fascial bites, increased tension of fascial edges, excessive tight closure, placement of drain or stoma in primary operative wound are associated with increased risk.
- **Type and length of suture material**—suture-to-wound length ratio greater than 4:1 is associated with less risk.

For elective midline incision, use of a slowly absorbable monofilament suture in a single layer aponeurotic closure technique without separate closure of the peritoneum and using a small bites technique (5 mm from midline and 5 mm apart) with a suture-to-wound length ratio atleast 4: 1 is the current recommended method of fascial closure.

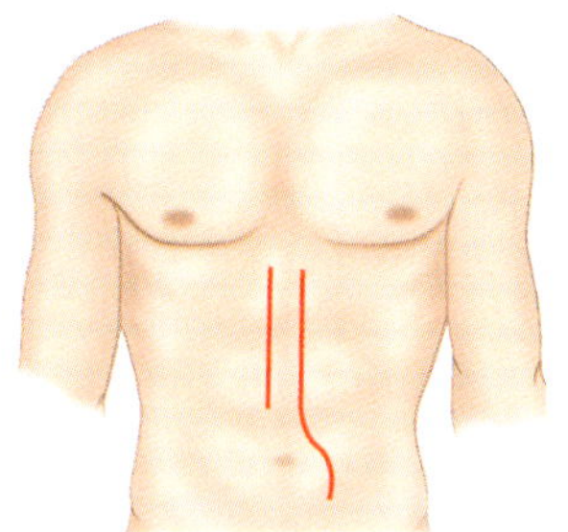
Increased risk in midline, paramedian incision

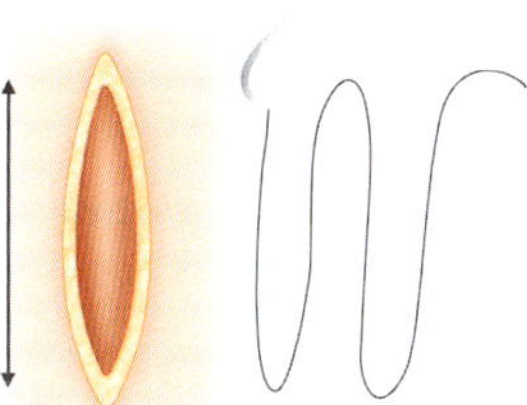

Ideal suture-to-wound length ratio—4:1 or more

Clinical Presentation

- Appearance of swelling over the operative scar on straining.
- In large hernias, skin may become pressure necrosed leading to ulceration.
- On examination, the entire length of incision must be inspected and palpated carefully, as multiple defects may be present.

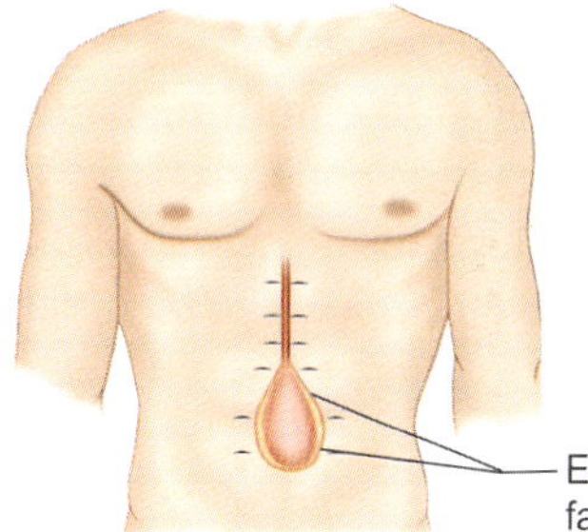

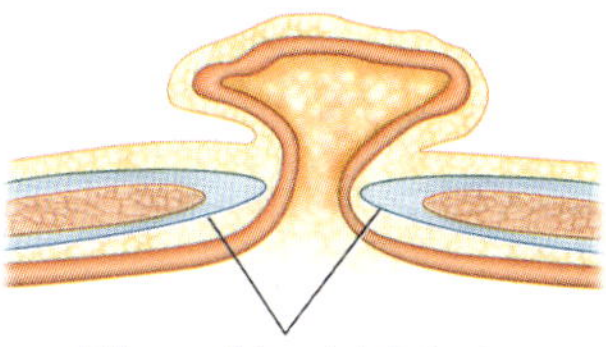

EHS Incisional Hernia Classification			
Midline	Subxiphoidal	M1	
	Epigastric	M2	
	Umbilical	M3	
	Infraumbilical	M4	
	Suprapubic	M5	
Lateral	Subcostal	L1	
	Flank	L2	
	Iliac	L3	
	Lumbar	L4	
Recurrent incisional hernia		Yes	No

Length:	cm	**Width:**	cm
Width (cm)	W1 <4 cm	W2 ≥4–10 cm	W3 ≥10 cm

The abdomen was divided into a **midline zone** and **lateral zone.** The borders of the midline zone are—*Cranial:* The xiphoid; *Caudal:* The pubic bone; *Lateral:* The lateral margin of the rectus sheath. All incisional hernias between the lateral margins of both rectus muscle sheaths are classified as midline hernias. *The borders of the lateral zone are: Cranial:* The costal margin; *Caudal:* The inguinal region; *Medially:* The lateral margin of the rectus sheath; *Laterally:* The lumbar region.

The 5 M zones are:

M1: Subxiphoidal (from the xiphoid till 3 cm caudally)

M2: Epigastric (from 3 cm below the xiphoid till 3 cm above the umbilicus)

M3: Umbilical (from 3 cm above till 3 cm below the umbilicus)

M4: Infraumbilical (from 3 cm below the umbilicus till 3 cm above the pubis)

M5: Suprapubic (from pubic bone till 3 cm cranially)

The four L zones on each side are defined as:

L1: Subcostal (between the costal margin and a horizontal line 3 cm above the umbilicus)

L2: Flank (lateral to the rectus sheath in the area 3 cm above and below the umbilicus)

L3: Iliac (between a horizontal line 3 cm below the umbilicus and the inguinal region)

L4: Lumbar (laterodorsal of the anterior axillary line)

- **The width of the hernia defect** is the greatest horizontal distance in cm between the lateral margins of the hernia defect on both sides.
- **The length of the hernia defect** is the greatest vertical distance in cm between the most cranial and the most caudal margin of the hernia defect.
- **In multiple hernia defects**, the width is measured between the most laterally located margins of the most lateral defect on that side.

Diagnosis

CT is the preferred imaging modality for diagnosis as well as proper evaluation of incisional hernia.

Role of CT:

- CT scan is helpful for preoperative planning as well as predict need for complex abdominal wall repair techniques.
- CT is also useful to detect occult hernias, multiple defects, differentiating incarcerated hernias from abdominal wall neoplasms.
- CT is helpful to assess the anatomic details of incisional hernia when the defect cannot be palpated in certain situations (e.g., obese patients, acute or chronic incarceration).

Diagnosis

Indications for surgery:

- Relief of symptoms (e.g., generalized pain)
- Incarceration
- Overlying skin problems
- Cosmesis

Different approaches of incisional hernia repair are: (i) Open repair and (ii) Laparoscopic repair

Different open repair techniques are: (i) Suture repair; (ii) Sublay repair; (iii) Onlay repair; (iv) Open IPOM; and (v) Open component separation

Different laparoscopic repair techniques are: (i) Laparoscopic IPOM; (ii) Endoscopic component separation (ECS); and (iii) Laparoscopic preperitoneal repair (TEP and TAAP)

Mesh reinforcement is recommended for all ventral hernia repairs (diameter >1 cm) in a clean case. [IEHS guideline 2019]. Sublay mesh placement is preferred because of less recurrence and surgical site infection than onlay or inlay mesh placement.

Different Techniques of Open Component Separation

- Anterior component separation
- Perforator-sparing anterior component separation
- Posterior component separation
- Transversus abdominis release (TAR)
- Posterior component separation with transversus abdominis release (PCS-TAR).

In laparoscopic ventral and incisional hernia repair the mesh area-to-defect ratio should be at least 16:1 (the radius of the mesh should be at least four times the radius of the defect.

In open incisional hernia, mesh overlap of 4–5 cm is recommended.

Sutured Repair

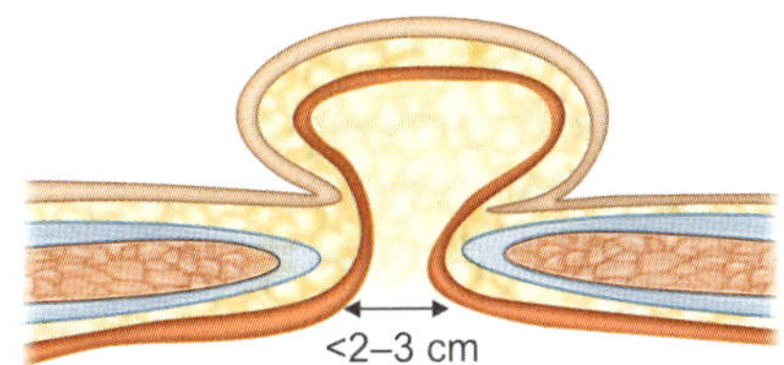

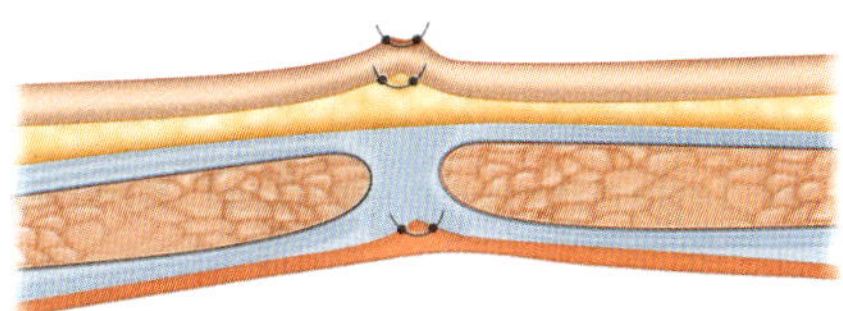

Different Techniques of Mesh Placement

- Prefascial plane above the linea alba (Onlay)
- Fixing the mesh to the borders of the repair (Inlay plug)
- Between the rectus muscle and posterior rectus sheath (Retrorectus)
- Between the posterior rectus sheath and the peritoneum (Preperitoneal)
- Intraperitoneal

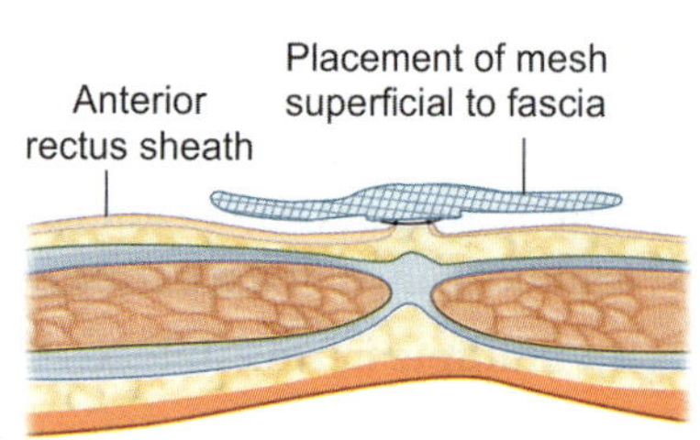

Onlay Technique

This technique of mesh placement is discouraged due to following disadvantages: (i) Increased chance of infection; (ii) Increased chance of seroma formation; and (iii) High risk of recurrence.

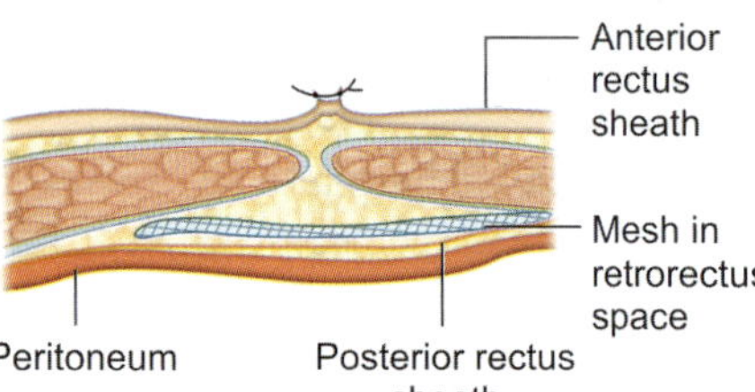

Retrorectus placement of mesh.

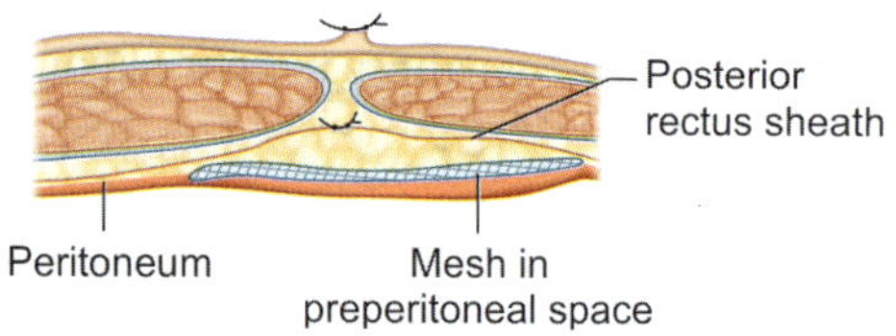

Preperitoneal placement of mesh

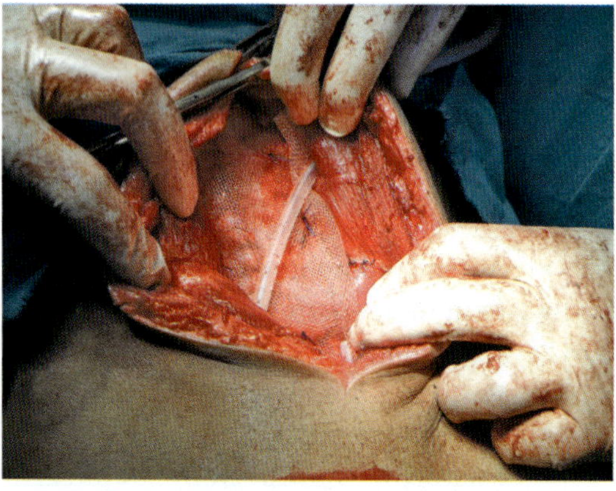

Laparoscopic incisional hernia repair.

Different laparoscopic repair techniques are: (i) Laparoscopic IPOM and IPOM-plus; (ii) Endoscopic component separation (ECS); and (iii) Laparoscopic preperitoneal repair (TEP and TAAP)

Contraindications of laparoscopic ventral hernia repair: (i) Loss of domain (in case of massive hernia sac containing greater than 30% of the abdominal contents and possibly some of the solid organs); (ii) Abdominal skin graft (overlying the hernia defect); (iii) Need to remove previously placed prosthetic mesh; (iv) Small defect but large hernia sac; (v) Incarcerated hernia; and (vi) Active enterocutaneous fistula [Adapted from SAGES Guideline].

Factors associated with technical difficulties of laparoscopic ventral hernia repair: (i) Hernia defect >10 cm in diameter; (ii) Incarcerated hernia; (iii) Recurrent hernia; (iv) Hernias with small defect but large hernia sac; (v) Hernias in unusual locations (i.e., subxiphoid, suprapubic, flank); and (vi) Distended bowel.

Complications of laparoscopic ventral hernia repair: (i) Seroma; (ii) Tissue eventration; (iii) Mesh eventration; (iv) Recurrence; and (v) Pseudorecurrence.

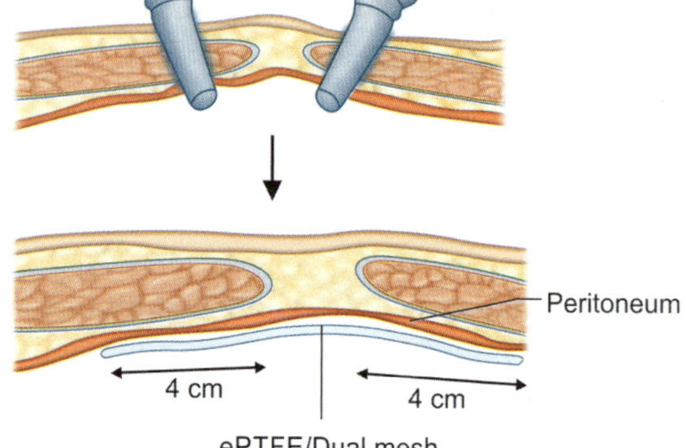

Mesh for intraperitoneal use in repair of incisional hernia: (i) ePTFE (expanded polytetrafluoroethylene)—Dual mesh; (ii) Composite mesh with absorbable-coated barrier; (iii) Composite mesh with permanent coated barrier; and (iv) Biologic mesh.

Prosthesis-related factors associated with lower recurrence: (i) Sublay mesh placement; (ii) Large prosthesis defect size ratio; (iii) Prosthesis reaches lateral-to-rectus muscles; and (iv) Overlap from defect edges >5 cm.

Component Separation Technique

- This technique involves myofasciocutaneous medialization to reconstruct the abdominal wall for larger abdominal wall defects not amenable to traditional open or laparoscopic mesh repair.
- Component separation technique is indicated for large complex incisional hernias.
- Different techniques of component separation techniques: (i) Anterior component separation (ACS); (ii) Perforator-sparing anterior component separation; (iii) Posterior component separation (PCS); (iv) Transversus abdominis release (TAR); (v) Posterior component separation with transversus abdominis release (PCS-TAR); (vi) Endoscopic component separation; and (vii) Robot-assisted PCS with TAR.
- Component separation technique (CST) is done with or without mesh reinforcement. CST without mesh is associated with high recurrence rate.
- *Complications:* (i) Soft tissue necrosis; (ii) Bulging of the lateral abdominal wall; and (iii) Morgagni hernia (following TAR).

Anterior Component Separation (ACS)

This is the most commonly used component separation technique.

This technique includes: (i) Midline scar excision; (ii) Dissection of the hernial sac; (iii) Skin flap mobilization by dissecting the skin and subcutaneous tissue from the anterior rectus sheath from the costal margin to the inguinal ligament and laterally to the anterior axillary line; (iv) A vertical incision 1–2 cm lateral to the semilunar line from the costal margin to just above the inguinal ligament and division of the muscle fibers; (v) Separation of the external oblique complex from the internal oblique aponeurosis by blunt dissection; and (vi) Midline fascial closure with monofilament suture.

Open ACS is associated with high surgical site occurrence rate.

Posterior Component Separation (PCS)

This technique includes: (i) Midline scar excision; (ii) Dissection of the hernial sac; (iii) Incision at the most medial border of the posterior rectus sheath from the xiphoid process to the arcuate line; (iv) Both blunt and sharp dissection of posterior rectus sheath from the rectus abdominis from the medial border to the lateral border of the muscle, cranially up to the subxiphoid space and caudally up to the space of Retzius; and (v) Approximation of posterior rectus sheath in midline with running suture.

Classic PCS and PCS-TAR are associated with better outcomes in comparison to classic and modified ACS.

Transversus Abdominis Release (TAR)

This technique is basically ***a type of posterior component separation.*** TAR technique includes: (i) Retrorectus dissection and release of posterior rectus sheath from rectus abdominis; (ii) Incision on posterior rectus sheath 1 cm medial to the perforating vessels; (iii) Exposure and division of the transversus abdominis; (iv) Separation of the muscle from underlying transversalis fascia; and (v) Reapproximation of posterior rectus sheath at midline with running monofilament suture.

Spigelian Hernia

- Spigelian hernia is protrusion through a defect in the **Spigelian fascia or aponeurosis.**
- This hernia may be congenital or acquired (e.g., as a complication of chronic ambulatory peritoneal dialysis).
- Most commonly located in the '**Spigelian hernia belt**' (a 6-cm wide zone above the interspinal line).
- **This hernia may present as** local discomfort or appearance of swelling adjacent to iliac crest on standing.
- **Diagnosis** is made by clinical examination and USG or CT.
- **Risk of strangulation is higher** due to sharp fascial margin around the defect.
- **Treatment** is mesh repair by open approach (preperitoneal mesh placement) or laparoscopic approach (TEP, IPOM, TAPP).

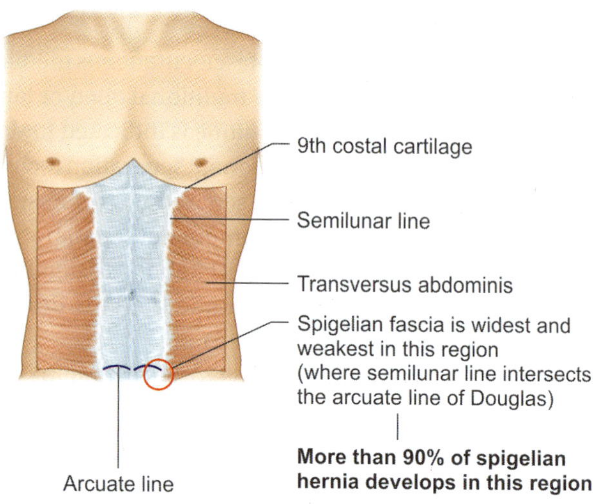

Spigelian aponeurosis: The aponeuroses of the transverse abdominal muscle limited by the semilunar line laterally and lateral edge of the rectus muscle medially.

Lumbar Hernia

Lumbar hernia is protrusion through a parietal wall defect (lumbar triangle) in the lumbar region. Lumbar region is divided into two well-defined areas of weakness:

Superior Lumbar Triangle

- Inverted triangle
- Greater surface area
- Deeper and more constant
- Not penetrated by neurovascular bundles
- Lumbar hernia is more common.

Inferior Lumbar Triangle

- Upright triangle
- Lesser surface area
- More superficial and less constant
- Penetrated by neurovascular bundles
- Lumbar hernia is less common.

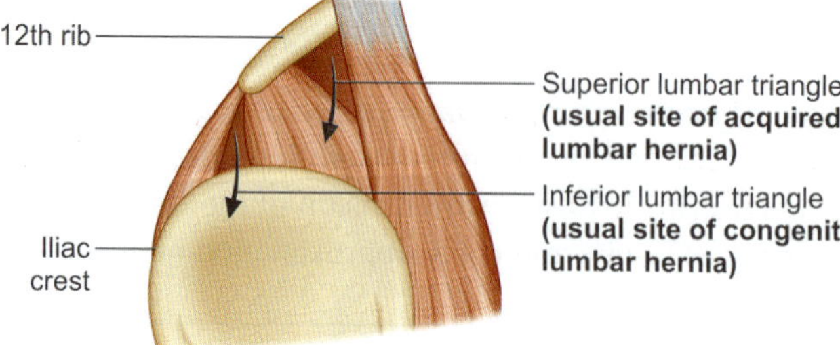

Boundaries of Superior Lumbar Triangle (Grynfelt-Lesshaft triangle)

Superiorly 12th rib, anterolaterally the internal oblique muscle, posteromedially, the quadratus lumborum. Roof is formed by the latissimus dorsi and floor is formed by the aponeurosis of the transversus muscle.

Boundaries of Inferior Lumbar Triangle (Petit triangle)

Inferiorly iliac crest, anterolaterally the external oblique muscle, posteromedially the latissimus dorsi. Floor is formed by the lumbodorsal fascia and transversalis muscle.

Classification of Lumbar Hernia

Anatomical Classification of Lumbar Hernia

Superior Lumbar Hernia (Grynfelt-Lesshaft Hernia)

Herniation of abdominal contents through the superior lumbar triangle. This hernia is more common than inferior lumbar hernia (because superior lumbar triangle has more area of weakness and not penetrated by neurovascular bundles).

Inferior Lumbar Hernia (Petit Hernia)

Herniation of abdominal contents through the inferior lumbar triangle. Congenital lumbar hernia and traumatic lumbar hernia are usually this type of hernia.

Clinical Presentation

- Most of the patients are male in their fifth or sixth decades.
- Patients usually present with small or diffuse swelling in the lumbar region. Swelling is usually soft, become more prominent on coughing or bearing down.

Strangulation is rare, because three boundaries of the defect are soft and muscular.

Differential diagnosis: (i) Lipoma; (ii) Cold abscess; (iii) Pseudo-hernia; and (iv) Hematoma.

Diagnosis

CT or MRI is indicated to confirm the diagnosis, and to assess the location of defect.

Treatment

Treatment is repair of hernia by an open approach with preperitoneal mesh placement or by laparoscopic approach with preperitoneal or intraperitoneal mesh placement.

Etiological Classification of Lumbar Hernia

Congenital Lumbar Hernia

A rare congenital anomaly, usually unilateral, commonly associated with lumbocostovertrebral syndrome. Other associated anomalies are VACTERL syndrome (vertebral anomalies, anal atresia, cardiac defects, tracheoesophageal fistulas, renal anomalies, limb defects), congenital diaphragmatic hernia, atrial septal defects.

Primary Acquired Hernia

More common than secondary acquired lumbar hernias (about 75%) and confined to the boundaries of the superior or inferior lumbar triangles. Risk factors for development are: (i) Advanced age; (ii) Obesity; (iii) Chronic debilitating disease; (iv) Wound infection; (v) Rapid weight loss; and (vi) Postoperative sepsis.

Secondary Acquired Lumbar Hernias

These hernias usually extend beyond the margin of lumbar triangles. These hernias are either traumatic (following blunt trauma) or postsurgical etiology (open nephrectomy, adrenalectomy, repair of abdominal aortic aneurysm, iliac bone harvesting). Traumatic lumbar hernia usually develop after severe blunt abdominal trauma and seatbelt injuries and commonly through the inferior lumbar triangle.

Acquired lumbar hernia are more common (about 80%) than congenital lumbar hernia.

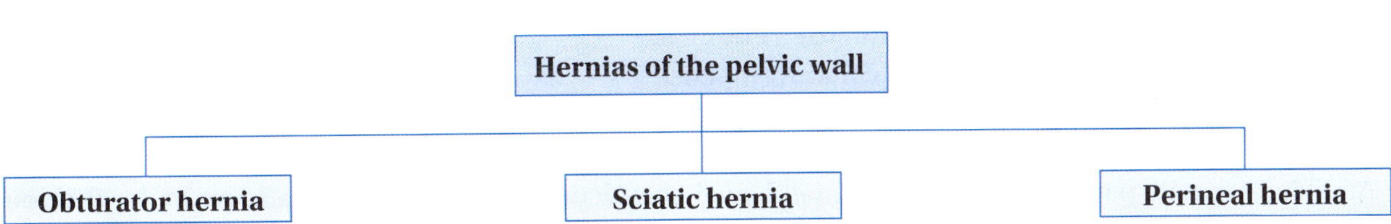

Obturator Hernia

- Obturator hernia is herniation of preperitoneal fatty tissue or intra-abdominal organs through the **obturator canal.**
- This hernia (the little old lady's hernia) commonly develops in thin, **elderly females**. This hernia is 6–9 times **more common in females due to**: (i) Wider pelvis; (ii) Horizontally inclined obturator canal; and (iii) Greater transverse diameter of the obturator canal.
- Mostly, obturator hernias develop on the **right side** (left obturator foramen is covered by the sigmoid colon)

Risk factors for development of hernia: (i) Thin body habitus; (ii) Multiparity; and (iii) Emaciation

Clinical presentation: (i) Acute small intestinal obstruction—most common presentation; (ii) *The Howship-Romberg sign:* This sign is pathognomonic but found only in 15–50% patients; (iii) History of recurrent intestinal obstruction; (iv) Palpable, tender mass in groin rarely noted upon a rectal or vaginal examination; and (v) The Hannington-Kiff sign (Absent adductor reflex). This sign is more specific but less commonly found in these patients.

- These hernias are at **increased risk of strangulation, particularly Richter type**.

Diagnostic modalities include USG, Contrast herniography, CT scan but among them CT abdomen and pelvis is the most sensitive and accurate imaging modality.

Treatment is surgery. In emergency setting, the approach is exploratory laparotomy (through a low midline incision) followed by suture repair or mesh repair of hernia. Other open approaches are lower midline extraperitoneal and anterior thigh exposure. If the diagnosis is established before surgery and no features of strangulation, laparoscopic TEP approach may be appropriate.

The Howship-Romberg sign—pain in the medial thigh elicited by extension, abduction, and medial rotation of the ipsilateral lower extremity (due to compression of the obturator nerve between the canal and the sac).

The Hannington-Kiff sign (Absent adductor reflex) is elicited by percussion over the medial thigh 5 cm above the knee joint. Positive sign means absence of muscular contraction.

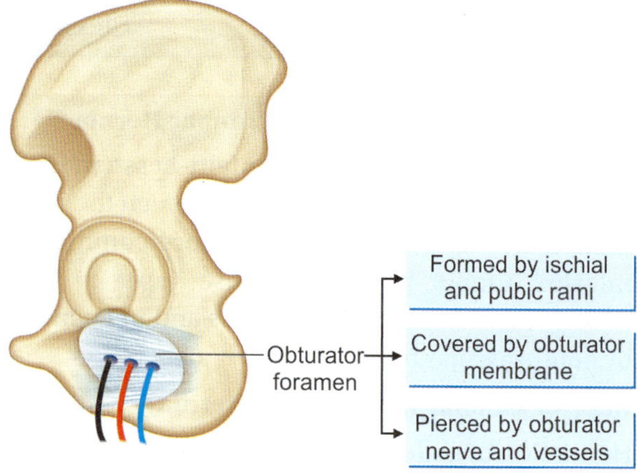

Obturator canal is a fibro-osseous tunnel about 2–3 cm in length and 1 cm in width, in the superior aspect of the obturator foramen.

Obturator foramen is formed by the superior pubic ramus superiorly, the body and inferior pubic ramus interiorly, and the ramus and body of the ischium inferiorly.

Obturator foramen is shielded by the obturator membrane.

The obturator nerve, artery and vein pass through the obturator canal after piercing the obturator membrane. Besides the obturator neurovascular bundle, this canal contains fat which prevents herniation of abdominal visceras.

Course of the Hernial Sac

Most commonly, the sac follows the anterior division of the obturator nerve below the pectineus muscle and above the obturator externus muscle.

The sac may follow the posterior division of the obturator nerve between the upper and middle fascicule of the obturator externus muscle.

- An elderly female patient presents with small bowel obstruction—**obturator hernia must be in differential diagnosis.**
- Elderly female patient with history of pain in medial thigh or history of recurrent episodes of intestinal obstruction—**obturator hernia should be suspected.**

Sciatic Hernia

Sciatic hernia is a rare type of pelvic floor hernia characterized by herniation of abdominal visceras **through the greater or lesser sciatic foramen**.

Three types of sciatic hernia are: (i) Suprapiriform (superior to piriformis muscle); (ii) Infrapiriform (inferior to piriformis); and (iii) Hernia below the sacrospinous ligament (through lesser sciatic foramen)

Contents of hernia may be ovary, fallopian tube, ureter, bladder, small and large intestine.

Most of the patients are female (due to wider pelvis and larger sciatic foramen).

Clinical presentation: (i) Acute or chronic pain in the pelvis, buttock or thigh; (ii) Sciatica (due to compression of the sciatic nerve by the hernia sac); (iii) Bulge in the gluteal area more pronounced on standing; (iv) Acute intestinal obstruction; and (v) Ureteric obstruction (in ureteric sciatic hernia)

Clinical diagnosis is difficult because of large gluteal muscles overlapping the sciatic foramen.

Diagnostic modalities are CT scan, MRI, herniography, however, CT is the imaging modality of choice.

Treatment is mesh repair of hernia by open (transabdominal or transgluteal) or laparoscopic approach (transabdominal extraperitoneal repair).

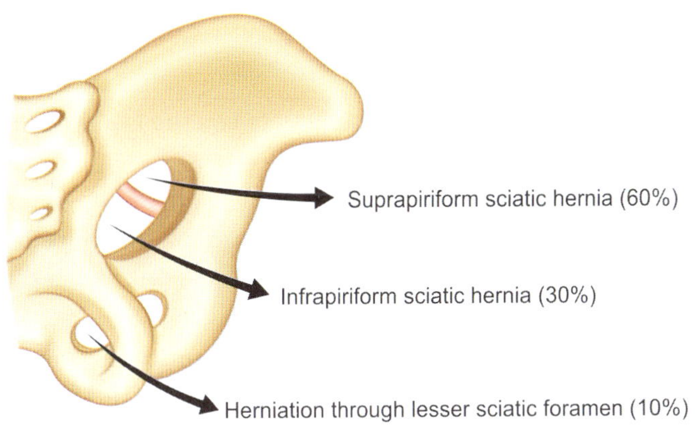

Ureteric sciatic hernia

Herniation of the pelvic ureter through the greater or lesser sciatic foramen leading to obstructive uropathy.

"Curlicue ureter" sign in excretory or retrograde urogram is found in ureteric sciatic hernia.

Perineal hernia (Ischiorectal Hernia, Pudendal Hernia)

Herniation of intraperitoneal or extraperitoneal contents into the perineum through a congenital or acquired defect in the pelvic diaphragm.

Types of Perineal Hernia

According to Etiology

Congenital—rare type of perineal hernia

Primary acquired perineal hernia—develops commonly in middle-aged multiparous women.

Secondary acquired perineal hernia—more common, usually develops following abdominoperineal resection (APR), hysterectomy, pelvic exenteration.

According to Location of Defect

Anterior perineal hernia—develops only in females, occur through triangle-shaped urogenital diaphragm.

Posterior perineal hernia—develops in both males and females, occur through the levator ani muscle or in between the levator ani and the coccygeus muscle.

Clinical Presentation

Typical clinical presentation of anterior perineal hernia is a palpable mass in the posterior aspect of labia.

In posterior perineal hernia, the typical symptom is unilateral soft, reducible mass in the perineal area, between the anus and the ischial tuberosity.

Diagnosis

CT or pelvic MRI is the imaging modality of choice for diagnosis as well as for assessment of the defect.

Treatment

Treatment is surgical management by: (i) Open suture repair or mesh repair (abdominal or perineal approach) and (ii) Laparoscopic transabdominal mesh repair.

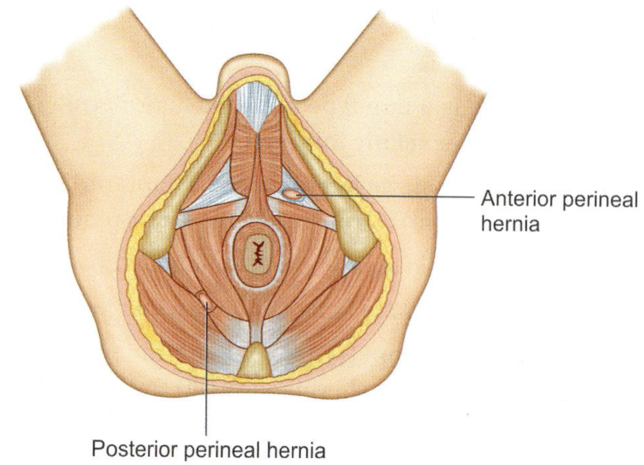

Perineal hernias must be differentiated from more common cystocele or rectocele.

Interparietal Hernia

Interparietal hernias are a group of rare hernias which are located in the inguinal region between the layers of the abdominal parietes.

Anatomically, interparietal hernias are classified into: (1) **Properitoneal**—hernia sac lies between the peritoneum and the transversalis fascia; (2) **Interstitial**—hernia sac lies between the transversalis fascia and the transversalis, internal oblique, or external oblique muscles; and (3) **Superficial**—hernia sac lies between the aponeurosis of the external oblique and the integument.

Properitoneal hernia: This hernia may be classified as: (i) Inguinoproperitoneal hernia—as a diverticulum from a pre-existing inguinal hernia; (ii) Cruroproperitoneal hernia—as an outpouching of a femoral hernia; and (iii) Simple properitoneal hernia—independent of inguinal or femoral canals. Incidence is more common in men. Right side is more commonly involved. Most of the patients present with features of acute intestinal obstruction.

Interstitial hernia: The hernia sac may present in any of the following positions: (i) Between the transversalis muscle and fascia; (ii) Between the transversalis and internal oblique muscles; (iii) Between the fibers of the internal oblique muscle; and (iv) Between the internal and external oblique muscles (most common type of interstitial hernia). Incidence is more common in men. Most of the patients present with features of acute intestinal obstruction.

Superficial hernia: In inguinosuperficial hernia, the sac descends into the inguinal canal, then through the external inguinal ring, and spreads out between the aponeurosis of the external oblique and the skin. In inguinofemoral hernia, sac descends over Poupart's ligament and then lie directly over the femoral opening between the deep fascia of the thigh and the skin. Incidence is more common in men. Patients present with features of acute intestinal obstruction.

Treatment: Urgent surgical intervention is indicated as most of the interparietal hernias present as incarcerated or strangulated hernias. The surgeon must remember that the strangulation may be at the internal ring, the neck of the interstitial diverticulum or sac, or the external ring.

Parastomal Hernia

Definition of parastomal hernia: Parastomal hernia is an abnormal protrusion of the contents of the abdominal cavity through the abdominal wall defect created during placement of a colostomy, ileostomy, or ileal conduit stoma. [Adapted from EHS Guideline]

Classification of parastomal hernia:

Type I: Parastomal hernia (PH) ≤5 cm without concomitant incisional hernia (cIH)

Type II: PH ≤5 cm with cIH

Type III: PH >5 cm without cIH

Type IV: PH>5 cm with cIH

EHS Grid for Classification of Parastomal Hernia

EHS Parastomal Hernia Classification

		Small ≤5 cm	**Large** >5 cm
Concomitant incisional hernia?	No	I	III
	Yes	II	IV

P: primary parastomal hernia
R: recurrence after PH treatment

P ☐ R ☐

Parastomal hernia is commonly associated with end colostomy, loop colostomy, and loop ileostomy.

Diagnosis: Most of the cases, parastomal hernia is diagnosed clinically (in supine or erect position using Valsalva maneuver. USG or CT is indicated when there is diagnostic dilemma (to differentiate between parastomal hernia and stoma prolapse). Intrastomal 3D USG is an emerging imaging modality for confirmation of diagnosis.

Management: During creation of elective permanent end colostomy, use of prophylactic synthetic non-absorbable mesh reduces the incidence of parastomal hernia.

Methods of parastomal hernia repair are: (i) Suture repair; (ii) Stoma relocation; and (iii) Mesh repair. Mesh repair techniques are either open mesh repair or laparoscopic mesh repair.

Laparoscopic Mesh Repair Techniques

- **Laparoscopic keyhole repair** (placement of a mesh with a central hole or slit around the bowel loop forming the stoma)
- **Laparoscopic modified Sugarbaker technique** (the mesh covers the bowel loop, which lies in a side-to-side fashion onto the abdominal wall)
- **Sandwich technique** (combination of these two techniques)

Open Mesh Repair Techniques

- **Onlay** (fixation onto the fascia of anterior rectus sheath and the aponeurosis of the external oblique muscle)
- **Retromuscular** (dorsally to the rectus muscle and anteriorly to the posterior rectus sheath)
- **Intraperitoneal** (intra-abdominal fixation onto the peritoneum)
- **Sugarbaker**
- **Keyhole**

The hybrid parastomal endoscopic re-do (HyPER) technique is a combination of open and laparoscopic repair using a funnel-shaped mesh.

Internal Hernia

Internal hernias are defined as protrusion of a viscus or part of viscus through a normal or abnormal peritoneal or mesenteric aperture within the confines of the peritoneal cavity.

Types of Internal Hernia

Based on Location (as described by Meyers)

- Paraduodenal (53%)
- Pericecal (13%)
- Foramen of Winslow (8%)
- Transmesenteric and transmesocolic (8%)
- Intersigmoid (6%)
- Retroanastomotic (5%)
- Paravesical (7%).

Based on the Type of Hernia Orifice (Doishita et al.)

Normal foramen

- Foramen of Winslow hernia

Unusual peritoneal fossa or recess into retroperitoneum

- Pericecal hernia
- Intersigmoid hernia
- Most types of pelvic internal hernia (except for broad ligament hernia)

Abnormal opening in a mesentery or peritoneal ligament

- Small bowel mesentery-related hernia
- Greater omentum-related hernia
- Most types of lesser sac hernia (except for Foramen of Winslow hernia)
- Transverse mesocolon-related hernia
- Transmesosigmoid and intramesosigmoid hernia
- Falciform ligament hernia
- Broad ligament hernia
- Roux-en-Y anastomosis-related hernia

Pericecal Hernia (Congenital or Acquired, Abnormal Aperture)

- In these hernias, bowel loops, particularly an ileal segment, herniated into the right paracolic gutter through a congenital or acquired defect in the cecal mesentery.
- Four kinds of pericecal recesses have been defined: Superior ileocecal recess, inferior ileocecal recess, retrocecal recess, and paracolic sulci.

Through all these recesses, herniation may occur **but the presentation and management are same.**

Paraduodenal Hernia (Congenital, Normal Aperture Subtype)

- **Most common type of internal hernia** (as per older literature)
- They are entrapments of the small intestine into a congenital paraduodenal fossa.
- More common in men (3:1)
- Two subtypes are present: (i) Left paraduodenal hernia and (ii) Right paraduodenal hernia.

Left paraduodenal hernia:

- These hernias are three times more common than right paraduodenal hernias.
- They occur when intestine prolapsed through the *fossa of Landzert,* an unusual congenital peritoneal fossa behind the descending mesocolon.

Right paraduodenal hernia:

- They occur when bowel herniates through the *Waldeyer's fossa* (or mesentericoparietal fossa), a congenital defect in the first part of the jejunal mesentery.
- These hernias mostly associated with nonrotation of small bowel.

Foramen of Winslow Hernia (Congenital, Normal Aperture)

- **Most common type of "lesser sac hernia"**
- In these hernias, viscera enter the lesser sac through ***the foramen of Winslow***. In most of the cases, the herniated viscera are small intestine; the terminal ileum, cecum and ascending colon are herniated in about 25–30% of patients
- **Risk factors** for development of this type of hernia include an enlarged foramen of Winslow, an abnormally long small-bowel mesentery, persistence of the ascending mesocolon, an enlarged right hepatic lobe (such as Riedel's lobe).

Transmesenteric Hernia (In children: Congenital, Abnormal Aperture; In Adult: Acquired, Abnormal Aperture)

- Occurs in presence of congenital or acquired defect in small bowel mesentery, usually close to the ligament of Treitz or terminal ileum.
- In children, it is the most common type of internal hernia.
- In adults, this type of hernia usually related to prior abdominal surgery, especially Roux-en-Y anastomosis
- Three types: (i) Transmesocolic (most common)—after laparoscopic Roux-en-Y gastric bypass; (ii) Jejunojejunostomy mesenteric; and (iii) Peterson type.

Sigmoid Mesocolon-related Hernia (Type 1—Congenital, Normal Aperture; Type 2 and 3—Acquired, Abnormal Aperture)

- Three types of sigmoid-related hernia are present—Type 1 (intersigmoid type); Type 2 (transmesosigmoid type); Type 3 (intramesosigmoid type)
- **Intersigmoid type** is the most common one, develops when bowel, commonly ileum, herniates into the intersigmoid fossa (formed between two adjacent sigmoid segments and their respective mesenteries).
- **Transmesosigmoid type** develops when small bowel herniates through a complete defect involving both layers of the sigmoid mesocolon.
- **Intramesosigmoid type** is the least common one, develops when bowel herniates within the sigmoid mesocolon.

Retroanastomotic Hernia (Acquired, Abnormal Aperture)

- This hernia occurs when small bowel loops herniated posteriorly through a defect related to Roux-en-Y anastomosis.
- More commonly associated with antecolic form of surgery
- Develops most commonly during the first postoperative month.

Trocar Site Hernia

Classification

Trocar site hernias are of 3 types: (i) Early-onset type; (ii) Late-onset type; and (iii) Special type [Tonouchi, et al.].

Early-onset type is characterized by: (a) Dehiscence of the anterior fascial plane, posterior fascial plane, and peritoneum and (b) Presents as small bowel obstruction as in Richter's hernia.

Late-onset type is characterized by dehiscence of anterior and posterior fascial planes while hernia sac is constituted by the peritoneum.

Special type is characterized by: (a) Dehiscence of the whole abdominal wall and (b) Develops immediately after surgery.

Predisposing factors:

Technical factors:

- Trocar size (risk is more if trocar size 10 mm or more)
- Trocar location (more incidence is in umbilical trocar site)
- Improper closure of fascial defect
- Enlargement of port site to retrieve specimen
- Sudden withdrawal of cannula (may cause suction effect leads to entrapment of omentum or bowel in port site)

Patient-related factors:

- Obesity
- Port-site wound infection
- Diabetes mellitus

Diagnosis: In early-onset type, CT abdomen is useful to locate the site of incarceration. The special type can be diagnosed without any imaging modalities.

Prevention:

- All trocar sites 10 mm or more should be closed.
- Sudden withdrawal of cannula should be avoided.
- Closure should be done under direct vision.
- Peritoneum should be incorporated into the fascial closure.
- Use of 10–12 mm nonbladed trocar in nonmidline port sites above the arcuate line.

Treatment: Hernia repair is indicated once the diagnosis is certain.

Mesh

Based on porosity (by Klinge et al.):

Class I: Large pore meshes (characterized by a textile porosity of >60% or an effective porosity of >0%): (Ia) Monofilament; (Ib) Multifilament; and (Ic) Mixed structure or polymer.

Class II: Small pore meshes (characterized by a textile porosity of <60% and without any effective porosity): (IIa) Monofilament; (IIb) Multifilament; and (IIc) Mixed structure or polymer

Class III: Meshes with special features (e.g., meshes with special surface coatings, composite meshes or covered meshes) for intraperitoneal use

Class IV: Meshes with films, i.e., meshes with submicronic pores or without any porosity

Class V: 3D meshes, i.e., meshes or devices which are pre-shaped, different from the routine flat mesh

Class VI: Biologicals; these were further subgrouped as nonabsorbable or absorbable, as well as synthetic or biological depending on the source: (VIa) Noncross-linked; (VIb) Cross-linked; and (VIc) Special features.

Based on composition and design:

1. **Non-absorbable synthetic meshes:** (i) Polypropylene; (ii) Polytetrafluoroethylene (PTFE); (iii) Polyester; and (iv) ePTFE.
2. **Non-absorbable synthetic-coated mesh:** (i) Titanium-coated mesh; (ii) Polypropylene covered by oxidized collagen; (iii) Polypropylene covered by absorbable hydrogel barrier; and (iv) Polypropylene covered by Omega-3 fatty acid
3. **Absorbable synthetic mesh:** (i) Polyglactin 910 (Vicryl mesh); (ii) Polyglycolic acid (67%) + Trimethylene carbonate (33%); and (iii) Poly-4-hydroxybutyrate (P4HB)
4. **Biologic mesh:** (i) Acellular human cadaveric dermis; (ii) Acellular porcine dermis; (iii) Porcine small intestinal submucosa; and (iv) Bovine pericardium
5. **Mesh with special design:** (i) Three-dimensional mesh (3D mesh); (ii) Mesh with an positioning system; and (iii) Self-fixating mesh with microgrip technology.

Complications: (i) Mesh erosion; (ii) Mesh migration; (iii) Mesh shrinkage; and (iv) Mesh infection.

Mesh fixation methods: Tacks, staples, self-fixing, fibrin sealants, glues, and sutures.

Named Hernias

1. **Amyand's hernia:** Inguinal hernia-containing appendix
2. **Bochdalek hernia:** It is a congenital diaphragmatic hernia through the posterolateral diaphragmatic defect. It is the most common type of congenital diaphragmatic hernia.
3. **Canal of Nuck hernia:** Herniation through canal of Nuck (a peritoneal fold extending to labia majora, analogous to processus vaginalis in males)
4. **Cloquet's hernia:** Femoral hernia developing through the pectineal fascia
5. **De Garengeot hernia:** Femoral hernia containing appendix
6. **Grynfeltt-Lesshaft hernia:** Also called superior lumbar hernia
7. **Hesselbach's hernia:** Femoral hernia developing lateral to the femoral vessels
8. **Laugier's hernia:** Femoral hernia developing through the lacunar ligament
9. **Littre hernia:** Hernia containing Meckel diverticulum.
10. **Maydl's hernia (hernia in "W"):** A type of incarcerated inguinal hernia where hernial sac contains a double loop of intestine. In this 'W' shaped bowel loop, the apex of the 'W' becomes gangrenous.
11. **Morgagni hernia:** It is a congenital diaphragmatic hernia through the foramen of Morgagni.
12. **Pantaloon hernia (Romberg hernia or Saddle bag hernia):** Type of inguinal hernia where both direct and indirect hernial sacs are present.
13. **Petersen hernia:** It is a type of internal hernia that occurs after Roux-en-Y reconstruction, through the Petersen's space.
14. **Petit hernia:** Also called inferior lumbar hernia
15. **Richter hernia (Partial enterocele):** Protrusion of the antimesenteric wall of the bowel through the hernial orifice without compromising the entire lumen
16. **Serafini hernia:** Femoral hernia developing deep to the femoral vessels (retrovascular)
17. **Spigelian hernia:** Herniation between the muscles of anterior abdominal wall along the semilunar line
18. **Velpeau hernia:** Femoral hernia developing superficial to the femoral vessels (prevascular).

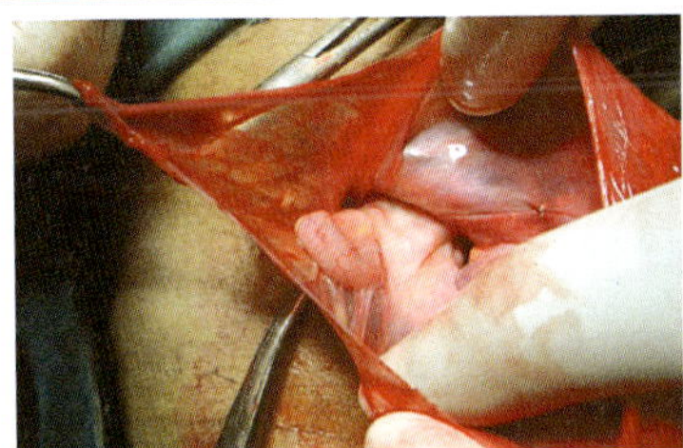

Amyand's hernia.

Case 1

History and Physical Examination

A 55-year-old male patient presented with swelling in both groin appeared on straining and standing for last 6 months. The swelling disappeared on lying down position. Patient had also history suggestive of bladder outlet obstruction for last 7 months. No history of chronic cough or chronic constipation. Patient was diabetic and on oral hypoglycemic for last 6 years.

Physical Examination

- No obvious findings in general examination
- Local examination of inguinoscrotal region—cough impulse present on both side, swelling was reducible. On deep ring occlusion test, hernia swelling appeared medial to the compressing finger on both side, suggestive of direct inguinal hernia. Both testes appeared normal. External genitalia appeared normal.

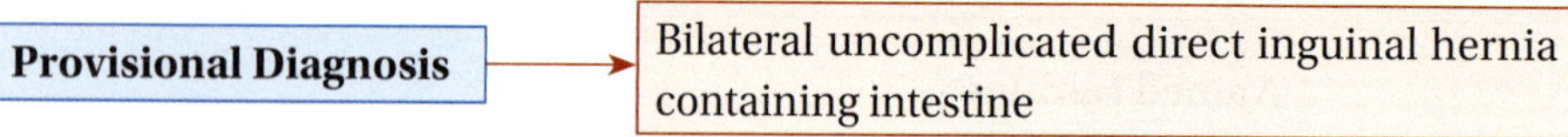

Provisional Diagnosis

→ Bilateral uncomplicated direct inguinal hernia containing intestine

Investigations

No imaging was required as no doubt in clinical diagnosis. USG of KUB and prostate was indicated to exclude prostatomegaly and to know the residual volume of urine. USG revealed prostate volume 30 cc and residual volume of urine 80 cc. Laboratory and other investigations were done as preoperative workup.

Discussion

History and clinical findings were suggestive of bilateral direct inguinal hernia. History of bladder outlet obstruction was also present but residual volume of urine was not significant. As there was no uncertainty in clinical diagnosis, no further investigation was not done to confirm the diagnosis. Bilateral open hernioplasty was planned. TAAP could not be planned due to unavailability of instrumentation.

Management Algorithm

Preoperative workup → Stoppa procedure

Case 2

History and Physical Examination

A 36-year-old male patient presented with pain and swelling over the operative scar site in upper abdomen that was not reduced for last 24 hours along with vomiting, absolute constipation and abdominal distension. For the last 2 years, patient complained a swelling over the operative scar site appeared on straining and disappeared on lying down position. Patient did not consult with any physician as no obvious symptoms were present. Patient had a history suggestive of laparotomy for peptic perforation about 4 years back but no documents available. Patient was alcoholic for about 8 years but stopped drinking after laparotomy. No history of smoking. No history of diabetes or hypertension.

Physical Examination

Patient alert, conscious, cooperative

Pulse: 110/min, BP: 92/68 mmHg, Respiratory rate: 22/min

Examination of abdomen: Abdomen distended, diffuse tenderness all over the abdomen, irreducible swelling over the midline scar, IPS—absent

Digital rectal examination: Rectum empty.

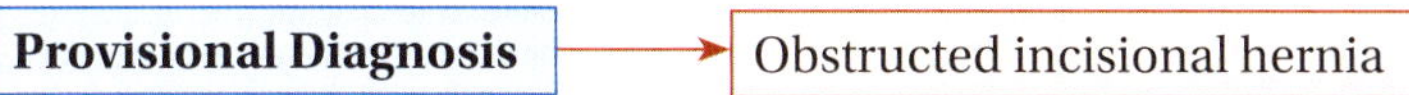

Provisional Diagnosis → Obstructed incisional hernia

Investigations

Straight X-ray abdomen: Multiple air-fluid levels suggestive of intestinal obstruction

Hb: 11.8 gm%; *Total leukocyte count:* 9000/cumm; *Blood sugar (Random):* 102 mg/dL;

Serum creatinine: 1.2 mg/dL.

Discussion

History of laparotomy 4 years back followed by appearance of swelling (appeared on straining and disappeared on lying down) over the operative scar was suggestive of incisional hernia. History of pain and irreducibility for last 24 hours along with clinical features of acute intestinal obstruction were suggestive of obstructed incisional hernia. X-ray abdomen revealed acute intestinal obstruction. Emergency laparotomy was planned after proper resuscitation.

Management Algorithm

- Fluid resuscitation
- Nasogastric decompression by Ryle's tube catheterization
- Parenteral antibiotics

→

Exploratory laparotomy:
Loops of small intestine obstructed, no gangrenous changes

↓

Mesh repair of incisional hernia—mesh placed in retrorectus plane.

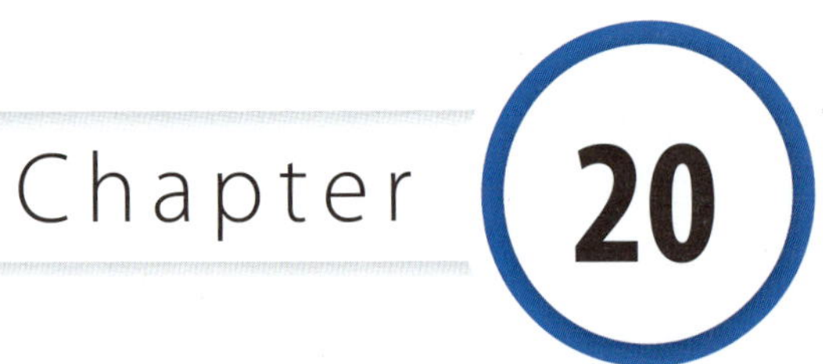

Diseases of Testes, Scrotum, and Penis

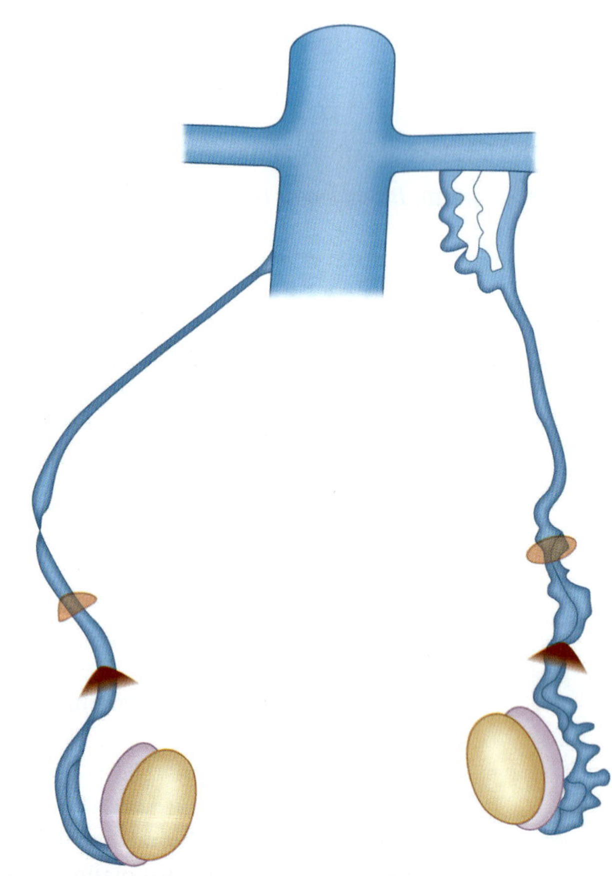

Important Topics

- Undescended Testis
- Torsion of Testis
- Acute Epididymitis
- Varicocele
- Hydrocele
- Other Scrotal Diseases
- Phimosis
- Paraphimosis

'Science can never be a closed book. It is like a tree, ever growing, ever reaching new heights. Occasionally, the lower branches, no longer giving nourishment to the tree, slough off. We should not be ashamed to change our methods; rather we should be ashamed to do so.'

Charles Value Chapin (1856–1941)
American Physician and Public Health Officer

Undescended Testis

Cryptorchidism or undescended testis

Failure of a testis to descend into a scrotal position

Congenital cryptorchidism
Testes that are extrascrotal from the time of birth

Acquired cryptorchidism
Testes that are intrascrotal at birth but later shifted to extrascrotal position

Ascending
From intrascrotal to extrascrotal position spontaneously at some time after birth

Entrapped
From intrascrotal to extrascrotal position after inguinal surgery

Congenital Cryptorchidism

- Found in 3% of full-term male newborns and 30% of preterm newborns
- More prevalent in preterm, small for gestational age, low birth weight, and twin neonates. About 70–77% of undescended testes will spontaneously descend, by 3 months of age
- By the age of 1 year, incidence of spontaneous descent become 1%.
- Risk is 6.9-fold if brothers is affected, risk is 4.6 fold if father is affected.

Possible Sites of Cryptorchid Testis

- Canalicular (within the inguinal canal)
- At superficial inguinal ring
- Prescrotal (above or at the scrotal inlet)
- Abdominal (proximal to the internal inguinal ring, near the urinary bladder, kidney, iliac vessels)

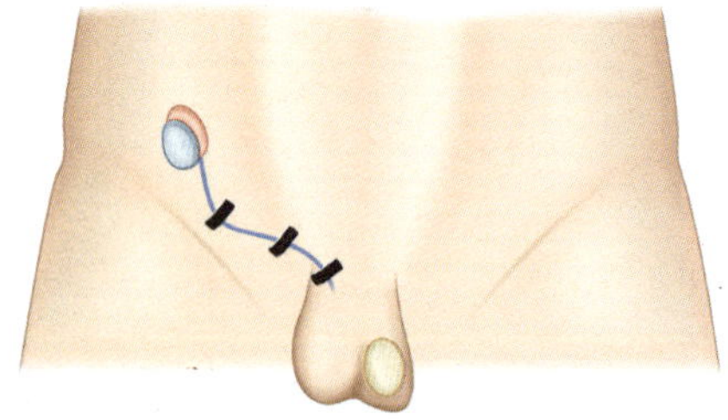

Descent is arrested anywhere in its path of its descent.

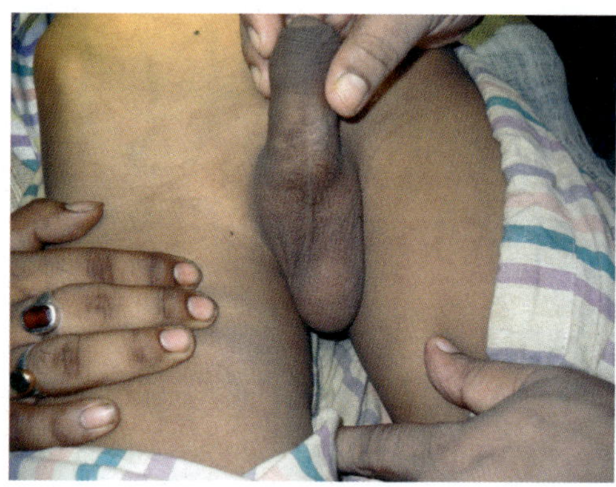

Right sided undescended testis.

Ectopic Testis

- Testis descends along the normal pathway upto external ring. Then, it deviates on an ectopic location.
- Ectopic testis is fully developed.

Possible Sites of Ectopic Testis

- Superficial inguinal pouch (distal and lateral to the superficial inguinal ring, between Scarpa's fascia and external oblique fascia)
- Femoral
- Prepubic
- Peripenile
- Perineum
- Contralateral scrotum (crossed ectopia)
- Perirenal

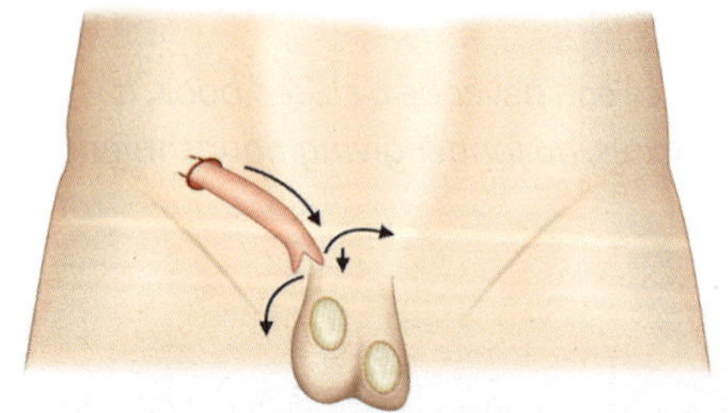

Deviation to different ectopic locations.

Retractile Testis

Testis that moves easily out of scrotal position, but can be manually replaced in scrotal position easily.

Predisposing factors: (i) Hyperactive cremasteric reflex; (ii) Short patent processus vaginalis; and (iii) Entrapping adhesions.

To differentiate undescended from retractile testes: Manipulation of a extrascrotal testis into the scrotum and maintained into that position for 30 seconds (to fatigue cremasteric muscle), then release, if it remains in place, it is retractile testis and if it immediately retracts to an extrascrotal position, it is undescended testis.

Treatment: Boys with retractile testis should be monitored yearly, up to puberty or till the testis no longer retractible.

Recurrent cryptorchidism: Testes that was undescended at birth, descended spontaneously, and then become extrascrotal subsequently.

Vanishing testis: Testis was developed at initial phase but disappeared at some point of development (may be due to spermatic cord torsion or vascular accident). Unilateral absent testis is termed as Monorchia and bilateral absent testes is termed as Anorchia.

Peeping testis: In nonpalpable testes during laparoscopic exploration, after insufflation of the abdomen, the testis moves through the internal ring and can be palpated.

Testicular Descent

Adjacent to metanephros

Transabdominal descent

Internal ring

Transinguinal descent

External ring

Extracanalicular descent

Scrotum

Testicular descent is divided into three phases:

1. **After 23rd weeks of gestation:** Testis descends to just inside the internal ring
2. **After 28th weeks of gestation:** Testis travels through the inguinal canal alongside and posterior to processus vaginalis
3. **After 28th weeks of gestation:** From external ring to the scrotum.

Factors Responsible for Testicular Descent

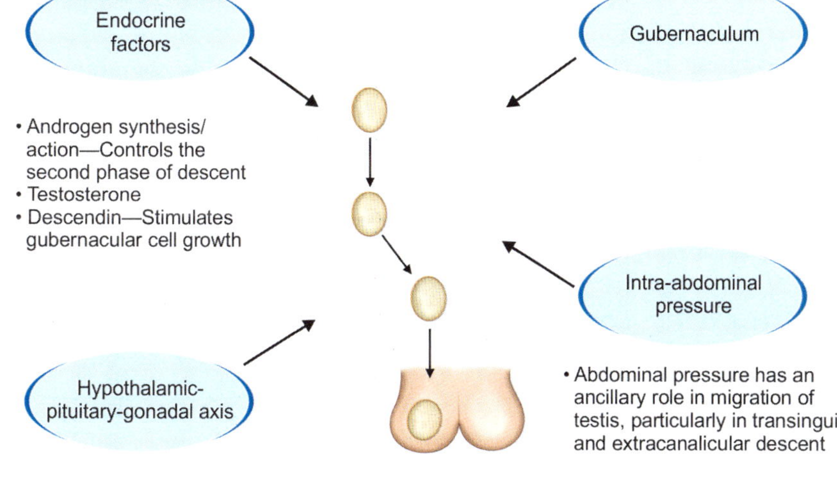

Syndromes Associated with Cryptorchidism

- Persistent Müllerian duct syndrome
- Klinefelter syndrome
- Down syndrome
- Prune belly syndrome

Histological Changes in Cryptorchid Testes

Changes started between 1–2 years of age.

Changes:
- Decreased numbers of Leydig cells
- Degenerated Sertoli cells
- Delayed disappearance of gonocytes
- Delayed appearance of adult dark (Ad) spermatogonia
- Developmental failure of primary spermatocytes
- Decreased number of total germ cell counts.

Hypoplasia of the Leydig cells–earliest postnatal histological abnormality.

Complications

Infertility: Paternity is almost 90% in unilateral cryptorchidism, 35–65% in bilateral cryptorchidism.

Neoplasia: Men with persisting or treated cryptorchidism have a relative risk of 3.6 for developing testicular cancer (seminoma); no increase in risk in men with history of spontaneous descent.

[Most common tumor in cryptorchid testis is seminoma]

Hernia: Patent processus vaginalis is found in more than 90% of patients.

Torsion of testis: Increased susceptibility is due to developmental anatomic abnormality between the testis and its mesentery.

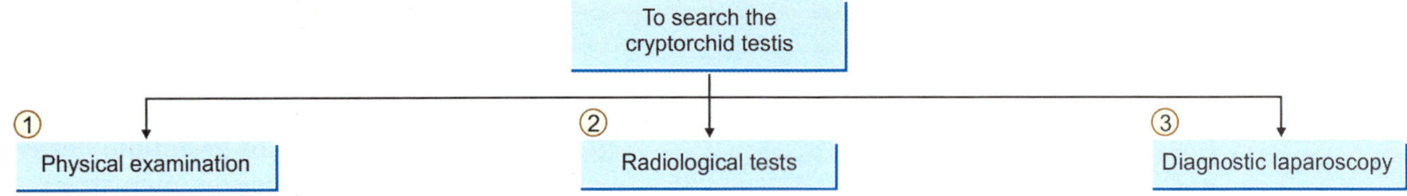

Methods of examination of testes in infants: Infants in supine position with legs gently frog-legged or sitting on the lap of the parent, then gentle downward pressure from the anterior superior iliac spine to the scrotum along the path of inguinal canal with counter palpation with the opposite hand.

In older children, the baby have to examined in either upright cross-legged or supine position. Complete examination of the groin, perineum, femoral region, contralateral hemiscrotum (to exclude transverse testicular ectopia), pubic area is necessary to classify testis as palpable or nonpalpable.

In prepubertal boys with nonpalpable testes, examine under anesthesia is recommended to assess whether testis is palpable or not.

In laparoscopic exploration, search for testis is done from the level of kidney to the internal ring.

- **If testis is identified** and anatomy appropriate for salvage, then primary orchidopexy or Fowler Stephens orchidopexy (one stage/two stage) is planned, if not appropriate for salvage, then orchiectomy.
- **If testis is not identified**, exploration should be continued to identify the testicular vessels. If the vessels end blindly in the retroperitoneum, exploration can be terminated or may be explored distal to the internal ring.
- If vessels entering the inguinal ring, then inguinal canal or scrotum should be explored. If any nubbin (vanishing testis) is present, it should be sent for histopathological examination.

Other clinical findings that have to be searched:
- Is scrotum underdeveloped or not
- Is any penile malformations present (hypospadias, micropenis)
- Any paratesticular abnormalities, any hernia or hydrocele in contralateral side.

When testis becomes nonpalpable:
- Intra-abdominal testis
- Absent (vanishing testis)
- Atrophic testis
- Missed on clinical examination.

Role of Imaging in Undescended Testis

Both USG and MRI have limited accuracy in diagnosis of nonpalpable testes and therefore not recommended for management of nonpalpable testes. MRI may be helpful to locate abdominal ectopic testis that cannot be detected by diagnostic laparoscopy.

A newborn with male phallus and bilateral nonpalpable gonads is potentially a genetic female (46XX) with congenital adrenal hyperplasia until proven otherwise. These patients may present with shock, hyponatremia, and hyperkalemia. Serum electrolyte estimation, hormonal profile (17-hydroxyprogesterone, LH, FSH, testosterone, androstenedione), and karyotyping is indicated.

If bilateral nonpalpable testes is without congenital adrenal hyperplasia, either bilateral abdominal testes or bilateral congenital anorchia should be suspected. Serum MIS (Mullerian Inhibiting Substance) or AMH (Anti-Mullerian Hormone), inhibin B, FSH, LH, and testosterone should be assessed for anorchia.

Treatment

- Definitive treatment should be started between 6 and 12 months of age, particularly in bilateral or unilateral intra-abdominal testis (to preserve most of the testicular tissues).
- Child presenting after this time period also must be treated by orchiopexy to prevent further testicular impairment (spermatogenic as well as endocrinal) and to attain the scrotal position for easy palpation (early detection is possible if any malignant transformation). **Orchiopexy does not reduce the risk of development of cancer.**
- Orchiectomy is indicated only for postpubescent patients, particularly for abdominal testis or difficult to mobilize with contralateral normally descended testis.

Benefits of Orchidopexy

- Optimization of testicular function (spermatogenic and endocrinal)
- Early diagnosis of testicular malignancy (if any malignant transformation)
- Less risk of testicular torsion
- Psychological

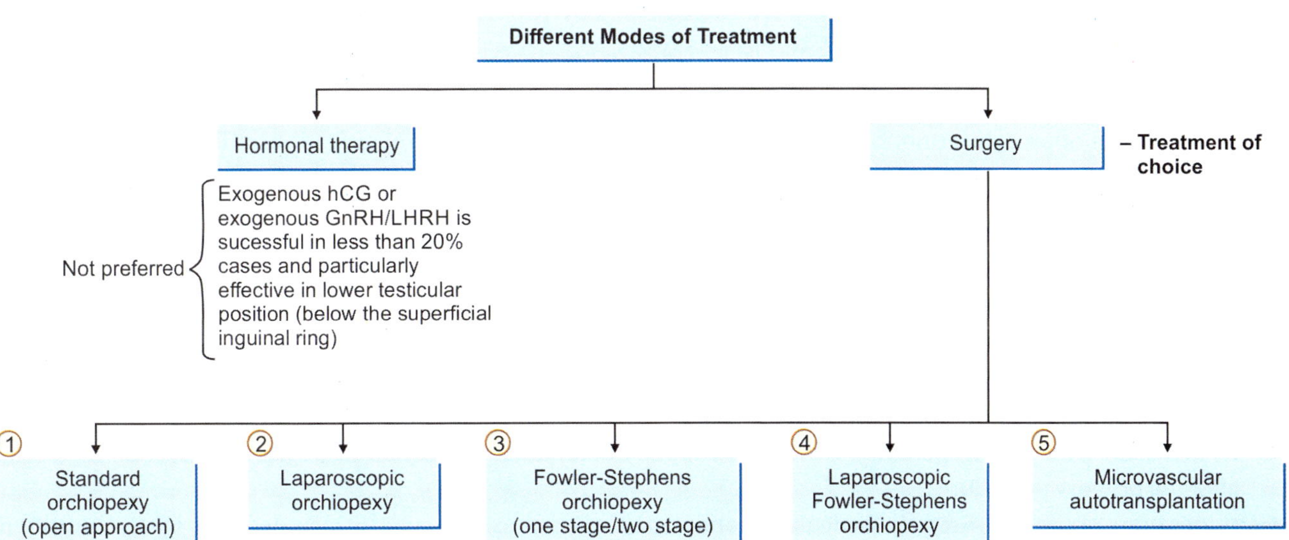

Standard Orchiopexy (Open Approach)

Standard Two-incision (Inguinal and Scrotal) Approach

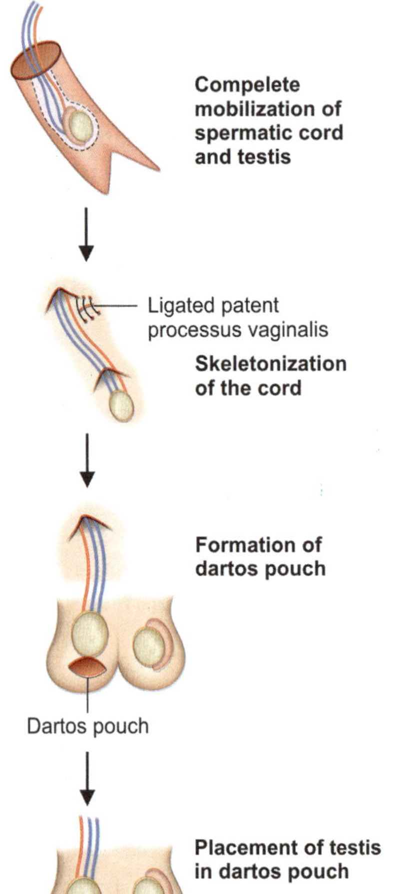

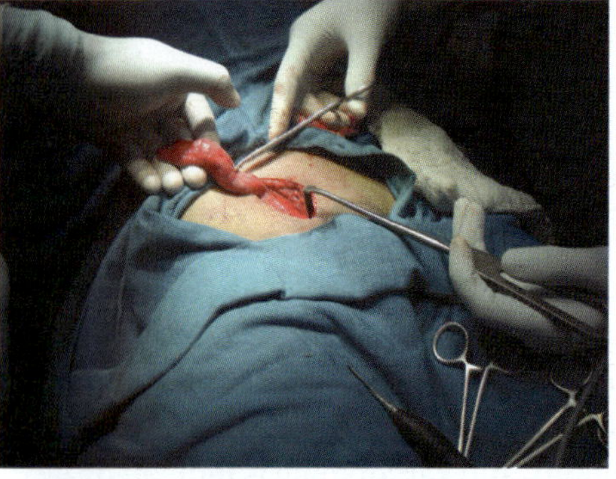

Operative Picture Showing Complete Mobilization of Spermatic Cord and Testis

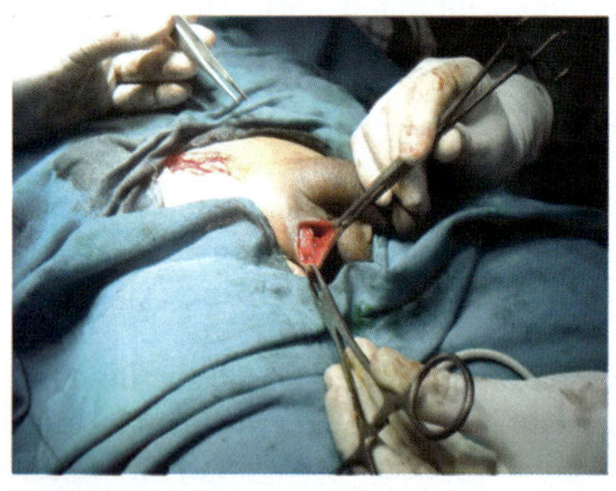

Placement of Testis in Dartos Pouch

Primary Single Incision Scrotal Approach

Another approach for low lying (distal to the external inguinal ring) palpable testes.

- **Different incisions for transscrotal orchidopexy are:** (i) Bianchi incision; (ii) Midline scrotal approach; and (iii) Transverse low scrotal approach.
- **Advantages:** (i) Less operative time; (ii) Enhanced recovery; and (iii) Better cosmesis

Laparoscopic Orchidopexy

A useful surgical approach for nonpalpable undescended testes. In this approach, mobilization of the spermatic cord structures can be done under vision. Laparoscopic approach is also indicated for rare conditions, e.g., bilateral undescended testes, polyorchidism, transverse testicular ectopia.

Fowler-Stephens Orchidopexy

- Fowler-Stephens orchidopexy (one-stage or two-stage) is indicated for high intra-abdominal testes. This orchidopexy is now commonly performed laparoscopically.
- **In one-stage procedure**, spermatic vessels are clipped by laparoscopic approach followed by testicular mobilization (open or laparoscopic approach) in the same sitting. During dissection, collateral vessels between the spermatic vessels and the vas should be preserved.
- **In two-stage procedure**, spermatic vessels are clipped in the initial stage, then testicular mobilization 6 months after the primary procedure.

Complications of orchidopexy: (i) Testicular atrophy; (ii) Testicular ascent; and (iii) Vas deferens injury. **Modified Prentiss maneuver:** A method of testicular rerouting to gain adequate length for orchiopexy in high inguinal undescended testes (HIUT).

Torsion of the Testis (Torsion of the Spermatic Cord)

Torsion of the testis is one of the common causes of **acute scrotum** and a **true surgical emergency**.

Predisposing Factors

- Bell-clapper deformity (abnormal proximal fixation of tunica vaginalis on the cord)—this deformity allows the testis to rotate and swing freely within the tunical vaginalis just like a 'clapper' inside the 'bell'
- Cryptorchidism

Pathophysiology

- When there is sudden contraction of cremasteric muscle (following trauma, athletic activity, physical activity) or even at sleep, twisting of the spermatic cord happens. This results in venous congestion with subsequent decrease in arterial flow to the testis that leads to necrosis.
- Spiral attachment of cremaster onto the cord favors rotation around a vertical axis (as much as 360°)

Clinical Presentation

- Most of the patients are around puberty, but torsion may develop at any age.
- Patients most commonly present with acute onset severe unilateral scrotal pain with nausea and vomiting. Clinical findings include **generalized testicular tenderness, high lie of the testis, absent cremasteric reflex**, thickening of the cord, scrotal edema.

Diagnosis

- If history and clinical findings are strongly suggestive of testicular torsion, patient should be referred for immediate surgical exploration. Imaging should not be planned in this scenario because imaging related delay decreases the testicular salvage rates and also chance of false-negative report.
- In pediatric patients (3 months to 18 years of age), **TWIST (Testicular Workup for Ischemia and Suspected Torsion), a clinically validated scoring system**, has been shown to have high positive predictive values.
- **US duplex Doppler** of the bilateral scrotum and inguinal area is the most appropriate imaging modality in suspected testicular torsion.

Management

- **If there is any doubt about diagnosis, the scrotum should be explored urgently.**
- On exploration, testis with good or marginal viability must be preserved and after detorsion, it must be placed in dartos pouch and fixed with fine, nonreactive, nonabsorbable suture.
- If necrotic testis is found, orchidectomy should be done.
- **Contralateral hemiscrotum must be explored and the testis must be fixed to reduce the risk of metachronous torsion.**

Causes of Acute Scrotum

- Torsion of testis
- Torsion of the appendix testis and epididymis
- Acute epididymitis
- Acute epididymo-orchitis
- Mumps orchitis
- Scrotal hematoma
- Incarcerated hernia
- Idiopathic scrotal edema
- Scrotal fat necrosis.

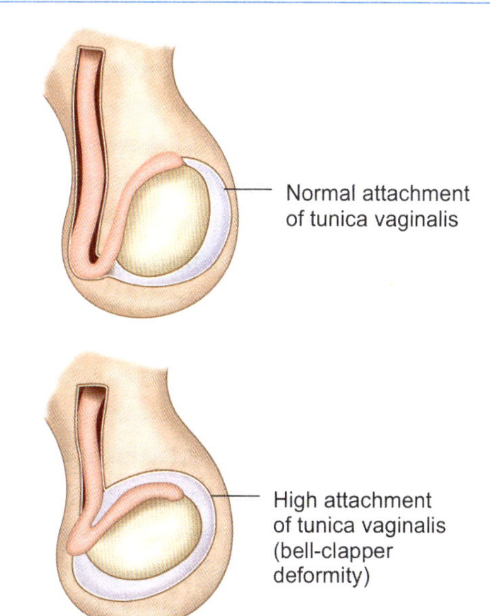

Cremasteric Reflex (Genitofemoral Reflex Arc)

- A superficial reflex in males. This reflex normally present after 2 years of age.
- This is elicited by scratching the inner thigh, causes elevation of the ipsilateral testis.
- The female counterpart of this reflex is Geigel reflex.

Two most important determinants of testicular salvage rate are:

(i) Time interval between onset of symptoms and detorsion.
(ii) Degree of cord twisting. If torsion is more than 360°, testis becomes non-viable within few hours (≥4 hours) of onset of torsion.

TWIST Scoring System.

Criteria	Score
Testicular swelling	2
Hard testes	2
Absent cremasteric reflex	1
Nausea or vomiting	1
High riding testicle	1

- **Score 0-2:** Low-risk—100% negative predictive value for torsion; no USG or urological consultation required.
- **Score 3-4:** Intermediate-risk—USG warranted.
- **Score 5 or above:** High-risk—100% positive predictive value for torsion
- USG not required, urgent urological consultation and surgery required to salvage testicle.

Indications of Orchiectomy (Orchidectomy)

- **Unilateral simple orchiectomy**—for testicular torsion, trauma when testicular salvage is impossible; in postpubescent patients, particularly for abdominal testis or difficult to mobilize with contralateral normally descended testis.
- **Bilateral subcapsular orchiectomy**—in hormonally-responsive metastatic prostate cancer patients who like to avoid medical androgen deprivation therapy
- **Radical orchiectomy**—in suspected testicular cancer.
- **Bilateral simple orchiectomy**—in sex reassignment surgery.

Testicular Prosthesis

- Testicular prosthesis is a silicone implant, inflatable with normal saline, available in various sizes, i.e., Extra small, Small, Medium, and Large.
- The prosthesis can be implanted via scrotal, high-scrotal, and inguinal incision into the subdartos pouch.
- Complications are pain, discomfort, infection, extrusion, migration, implant deflation, fibrosis.

Torsion of the Appendix Testis and Epididymis

- **The most common cause of acute scrotum in prepubertal boys is appendage torsion** (torsion of the appendix testis and epididymis). This condition most commonly occurs in prepubertal age group (7–12 years), but may occur at any age.
- **Clinical presentations** are almost similar to torsion of testis or acute epididymo-orchitis. Pathognomonic **"blue dot sign"** (blue or purple discoloration at the upper pole of testis visible through stretched scrotal skin) is not so common. Other clinical findings include palpable nodule with localized tenderness at the upper pole of testis and intact cremasteric reflex. As the condition progresses, scrotal erythema and edema develops along with tenderness of testis and epididymis.
- **Color Doppler USG** rarely detects appendage torsion but shows hyperperfusion of the epididymis.
- **Treatment** includes scrotal support, ice pack, anti-inflammatory agents. Surgery is indicated only if testicular torsion cannot be excluded or if pain is prolonged or recurrent.

- **Appendix testis** is a vestigial remnant of the mullerian duct, present on the upper pole of the testis or in the groove between testis and epididymis.
- **Appendix epididymis** is a vestigial remnant of the wolffian duct, present along the caput.

Acute Epididymitis

- Acute epididymitis is the most common cause of acute scrotal pain. It is commonly seen in patients 19 to 25 years of age.
- **Causative organisms:** (i) Sexually transmitted infections (e.g., *Chlamydia trachomatis, N. gonorrhoeae, M. genitalium*) and (ii) Enteric organisms (e.g., *Escherichia coli*)
- **Risk factors:** (i) Anal intercourse; (ii) Abnormalities of the lower urinary tract; and (iii) Urinary tract instrumentation, prostate biopsy
- **Clinical presentation:** Patients commonly present with gradual onset unilateral scrotal pain. History of urinary tract infection, urethral discharge, sexual activity, voiding difficulty may be present. Clinical findings include palpable swelling and tenderness of the epididymis, tender, and swollen spermatic cord. The pain may be relieved with the elevation of the testis **(Prehn's sign)**. As the condition progresses, scrotum becomes swollen and erythematous. Cremasteric reflex should be intact.
- **Diagnosis:** (i) Culture and sensitivity of mid-stream urine in all patients; (ii) Urethral swab or smear for gram staining and culture if *N. gonorrhoeae* is likely; (iii) Nucleic acid amplification test (NAAT) on first-voided urine for C. trachomatis and *N. gonorrhoeae* in patients with suspected sexually transmitted infections (STI); and (iv) Color Doppler USG should be done if any suspicion of testicular torsion.
- **Treatment:** (i) Scrotal support; (ii) Ice pack; (iii) Anti-inflammatory agents; and (iv) Antibiotics
- **Choice of antibiotics: (i) Patients with low risk of gonorrhoeae**—Doxycycline 200 mg initial dose then 100 mg twice daily for 10–14 days plus antibiotic active against Enterobacteriaceae for 10–14 days; **(ii) Patients with high risk of gonorrheal acute epididymitis**—Ceftriaxone 500 mg intramuscularly single dose plus Doxycycline 200 mg initial dose, then 100 mg twice daily for 10–14 days; and **(iii) Non-sexually active patients**—Fluoroquinolones (e.g., Levofloxacin 500 mg once daily for 10–14 days)

Varicocele

- Varicocele is abnormal dilation and tortuosity of internal spermatic veins in the pampiniform plexus of the spermatic cord. Most of the varicoceles are on left-side. Tall, thin men with pendulous scrotum are more frequently develop varicocele.
- **Pathophysiology:** Factors likely to be responsible are increased venous pressure in left renal vein, collateral venous anastomoses, incompetent valve at the junction of left internal spermatic vein and left renal vein. Genetic factors may also play some role.
- **Clinical presentation:** Most of the varicoceles are asymptomatic, detected during routine clinical examination or by the patient during self-examination. Clinical examination should be done in **both standing and supine position, with and without Valsalva maneuver.** Varicocele is typically described as painless compressible mass (consistency of a **"bag of worms"**) above the testis. Varicocele is not palpable when the patient is in supine position. If the veins do not decompress, retroperitoneal pathology or previous varicocele repair should be suspected. **Testicular volume should be assessed to detect testicular hypotrophy.**
- **Treatment:** Indications of surgery are: (i) Unilateral or bilateral varicocele with objective evidence of testicular hypotrophy; (ii) Varicocele with abnormal semen analysis findings; (iii) Symptomatic varicocele; and (iv) Bilateral palpable varicocele.

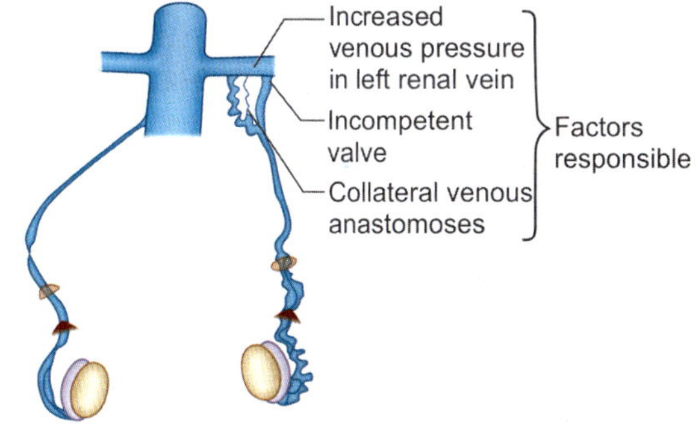

Clinical Grading of Varicocele

- **Grade 0 (subclinical)**—nonpalpable and visualized only by color Doppler USG
- **Grade 1**—palpable only with Valsalva maneuver
- **Grade 2**—easily palpable but not visible
- **Grade 3**—Easily visible

Measurement of Testicular Volume

- Prader orchidometer
- Takihara orchidometer
- Ultrasound

Testicular hypotrophy—Testis that is smaller by 2 mL or 20% to other testis.

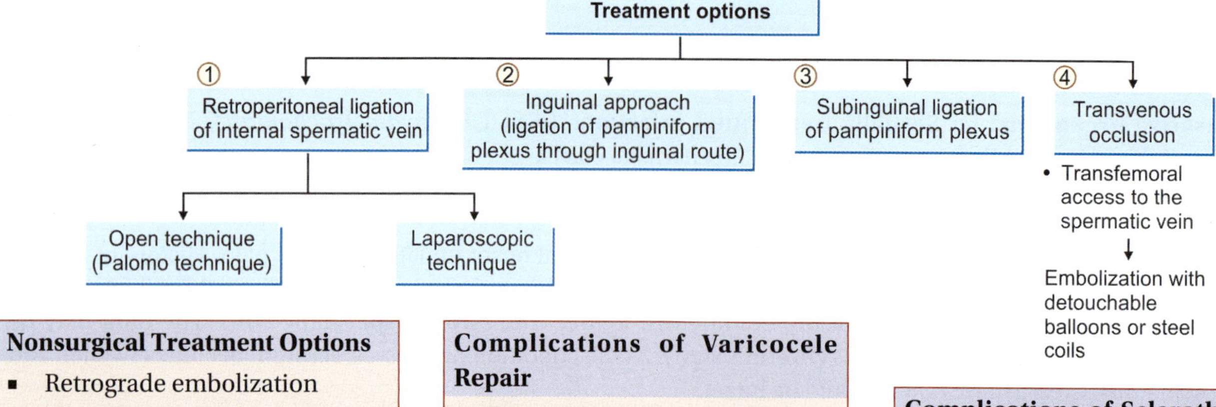

Nonsurgical Treatment Options

- Retrograde embolization
- Antegrade sclerotherapy
- Retrograde sclerotherapy

Complications of Varicocele Repair

- Recurrence
- Hydrocele
- Injury to the genitofemoral nerve

Complications of Sclerotherapy and Embolization

- Thrombophlebitis
- Venous perforation
- Retroperitoneal hemorrhage
- Migration of coils

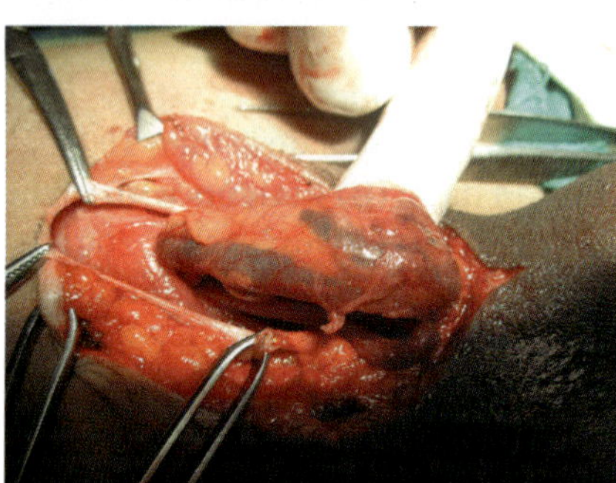

Inguinal Approach of Varicocele Repair

Hydrocele

Abnormal collection of fluid in tunica or processus vaginalis.

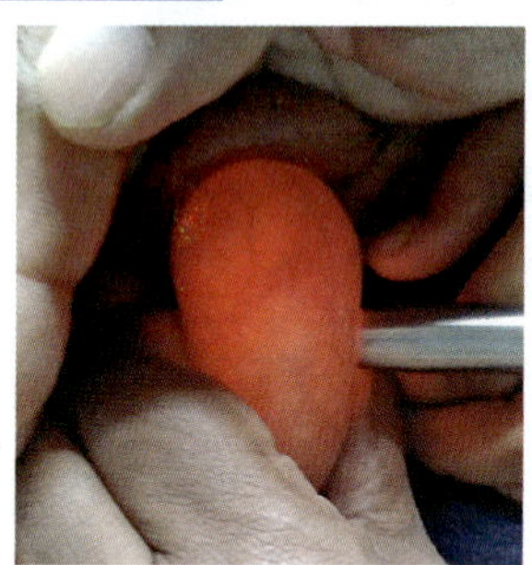

Congenital hydrocele—a transilluminant scrotal swelling.

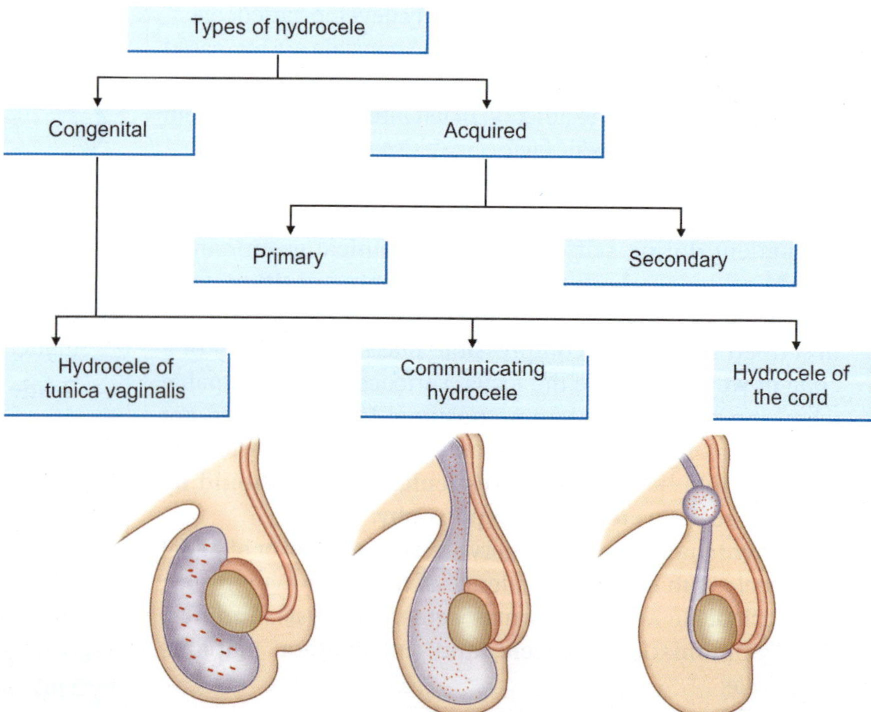

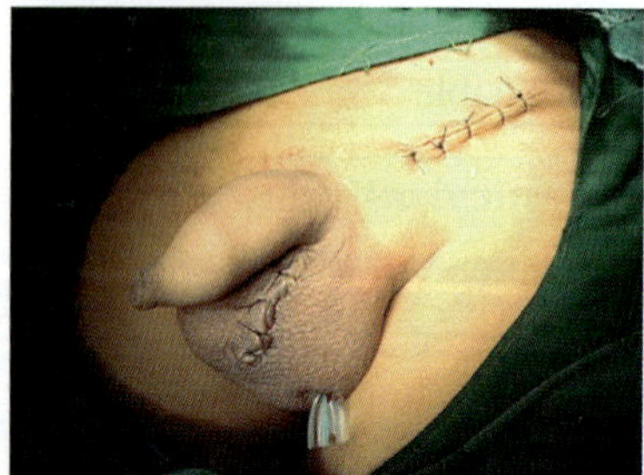

Surgical approach for congenital hydrocele.

Hydrocele of Tunica Vaginalis

- It develops due to delayed closure of processus vaginalis
- Fluid is trapped within the tunica vaginalis only
- Commonly seen at birth
- Tense, nontender pure scrotal swelling with positive transillumination test
- Most of them resolve within 2 years of life
- If surgical intervention is indicated it must be intervened through an inguinal approach

Communicating Hydrocele

- Persistence of processus vaginalis allows peritoneal fluid to communicate with the tunica vaginalis
- Classic description is that, the swelling is smaller in the morning and becomes more prominent as day progresses
- Communication is too small to allow herniation of intra-abdominal contents
- Most communicating hydroceles close spontaneously by 1 year of age
- All persistent communicating hydroceles must be explored through inguinal incision

Hydrocele of the Cord

- Due to segmental closure of processus vaginalis
- Manifested as painless groin swelling contiguous with the cord structures
- Can be palpated at any position just above the testis to superficial inguinal ring
- Swelling moves downwards and becomes less mobile when testis is pulled downwards
- Exploration must be done through inguinal approach. Ligation of the processus vaginalis at internal ring and excision or unroofing of the cyst is the treatment

Hydrocele of the Canal of Nuck

- It is the female counterpart of the hydrocele of the cord in males. Hydrocele of the canal of Nuck develops due to failure of obliteration of canal of Nuck.
- **There are three types of hydrocele of canal of Nuck:** (i) Encysted hydrocele (no communication with the peritoneal cavity); (ii) Hydrocele with persistent communication between peritoneal cavity and hydrocele; and (iii) Hour-glass type (constriction at deep inguinal ring so that proximal part is retroperitoneal and distal part is in the inguinal canal)
- **Clinical presentation:** Patient presents with painless irreducible translucent inguinolabial swelling.
- **Diagnosis:** USG or MRI is helpful for diagnosis but most of the patients are finally diagnosed after surgical exploration.
- **Treatment:** Surgical exploration followed by careful isolation of the cyst from the round ligament, excision of the cyst and high ligation of the hernial sac.

Canal of Nuck

- A pouch of parietal peritoneum accompanies the round ligament of uterus in the inguinal canal.
- It is analogs to processus vaginalis in males.

Hydrocele Fluid

- Amber colored
- Sterile
- Contains albumin and fibrinogen

Primary Vaginal Hydrocele

- Primary vaginal hydrocele is abnormal serous fluid collection between the parietal and visceral layer of tunica vaginalis. It is the most common cause of painless scrotal swelling. This hydrocele most commonly develops in middle aged or elderly men.
- **Pathophysiology:** Primary vaginal hydrocele develops due to defective absorption of fluid in tunica vaginalis (imbalance between secretion by mesothelial cells and absorption of fluid by lymphatics)
- **Clinical presentation:** Patients present with gradual onset painless scrotal swelling. Clinical examination reveals nontender scrotal swelling, 'get above the swelling' present, fluctuation and transillumination positive, testis cannot be felt separately.
- **Diagnosis:** Imaging is not indicated if the diagnosis of primary hydrocele is confirmed by history and clinical findings. Imaging is indicated if any suspicion of secondary hydrocele or other pathologies.
- **Treatment:** Surgery is the treatment of choice.

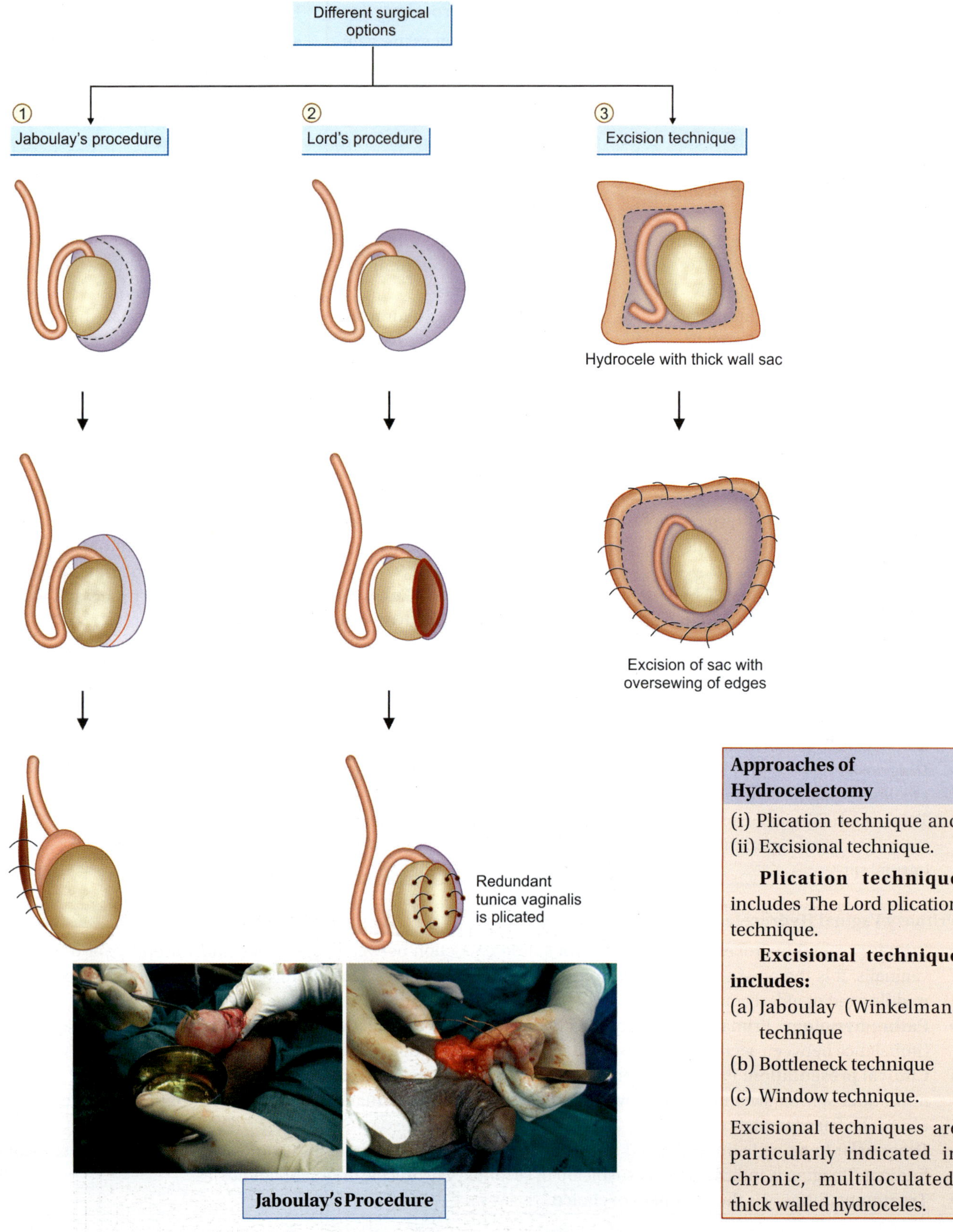

Approaches of Hydrocelectomy

(i) Plication technique and
(ii) Excisional technique.

Plication technique includes The Lord plication technique.

Excisional technique includes:

(a) Jaboulay (Winkelman) technique
(b) Bottleneck technique
(c) Window technique.

Excisional techniques are particularly indicated in chronic, multiloculated, thick walled hydroceles.

Secondary hydrocele is due to:

- Lymphatic filariasis
- Epididymoorchitis
- Testicular tumor
- Trauma
- After varicocelectomy

Filarial Hydrocele

- Filarial hydrocele is the most common urological complication of lymphatic filariasis.
- **Pathophysiology:** Adult worms (***W. bancrofti***) causes mechanical blockage of lymphatic channels, initiating immune reactions, resulting in dilation of scrotal lymphatics and accumulation of fluid in tunica vaginalis. **Endosymbiont Wolbachia** is likely to be responsible for the production of lymphangiogenic factors like VEGF-C by the endothelial cells.
- **Diagnosis:** (i) Detection of microfilaria in blood or hydrocele fluid and (ii) USG of scrotum (Filarial dance sign)
- **Treatment:** The treatment of choice is hydrocelectomy. Doxycycline may be beneficial in the early stage of the disease.

Urological Complications of Lymphatic Filariasis

- **Hydrocele**
- Chylocele
- Chyluria
- **Lymph scrotum**
- Genital lymphedema

Filarial Dance Sign

In 2D B-mode USG, the twirling motion of microfilariae are detected in dilated scrotal lymphatic channels. It is a characteristic sign of scrotal filariasis.

Lymph Scrotum (Superficial Scrotal Lymphangiomatosis)

- It is the most crippling complication of lymphatic filariasis.
- Characterized by presence of multiple lymphatic vesicles on the surface of scrotum. The scrotal skin becomes thickened, spongy, and porous.
- Patients present with continuous dripping of milky fluid from 'blisters' on scrotal skin.
- Treatment is complete scrotectomy followed by mesh skin grafting.

Primary Hydrocele

- Develops due to defective absorption of fluid
- Moderate to large in size
- Tense cystic hydrocele
- Testis is not palpable separately
- Transillumination positive
- Treatment is surgery

Secondary Hydrocele

- Due to increased production of fluid
- Small in size
- Lax hydrocele
- Testis is palpable
- Transillumination negative
- Treatment of underlying cause with or without surgery

A young patient with lax hydrocele—testicular tumor should be excluded before any surgical intervention.

Hematocele

- Accumulation of blood within the tunica vaginalis
- Develops following trauma, surgery, neoplasm
- Clinically presents as scrotal swelling with transillumination test negative
- Diagnosis is made by USG
- Treatment is evacuation of hematoma.

Pyocele

- Pyocele is collection of pus within the tunica vaginalis
- Develops following acute epididymo-orchitis, hematocele, rupture of testicular abscess
- USG is the imaging modality of choice for diagnosis
- Treatment is surgical drainage with broad-spectrum antibiotics

Chylocele

- Collection of chylous fluid within the tunica vaginalis
- Develops as a complication of lymphatic filariasis due to rupture of lymphatic vessels into tunica vaginalis
- Treatment is rest and aspiration of chylous fluid.

Other Scrotal Swellings

Epididymal Cyst

- Cystic degeneration of epididymis
- Usually both epididymis are involved
- Contains crystal-clear fluid, therefore brilliantly transilluminant
- If cyst causing symptoms, then only it should be excised.

Cyst of Testicular Appendage

- Usually unilateral
- Globular swelling at the superior pole
- Liable to torsion, so early intervention is indicated.

Spermatocele

- Unilocular retention cyst contains spermatozoa
- Always present in the head of epididymis
- Clinically palpable as a soft, cystic lesion, above and behind the upper pole of testis
- If it becomes larger, patient may feel it as a **'third testis'**
- Smaller ones need observation. Larger ones need to be aspirated or excised.

Other Scrotal Diseases

Fournier's Gangrene

Fournier's gangrene is a **severe type of necrotizing soft tissue infection** involving the genital area and or perineum. The **Colles' fascia** (superficial fascia of the perineum) is continuous with the **Scarpa's fascia** (fascia of the anterior abdominal wall), **Buck's fascia** (deep fascia of the penis) and **Dartos fascia** (fascia of the scrotum). Therefore, infection may spread to the abdominal wall, thigh, perirectal, and gluteal spaces. The dartos layer acts as a barrier to the spread of necrotizing fasciitis to the deeper structures of the scrotum (testis is not involved).

Precipitating factors: (i) Procedures in the perineal or periurethral area (e.g., urethral dilatation, sclerotherapy of hemorrhoids); (ii) Diabetes mellitus; and (iii) Immunocompromised state.

Organisms most commonly responsible—*Staphylococcus*, hemolytic *Streptococcus*, *E. coli*, *C. welchii*.

Fournier's gangrene severity index (FGSI) is a scoring system for predicting outcome. This includes temperature, heart rate, respiratory rate, serum sodium, potassium, creatinine, leukocyte count, hematocrit, and bicarbonate at admission. Score ranges from 0–14. A FGSI score >9 is a sensitive and specific mortality predictor.

Treatment is **early and aggressive surgical debridement.** Multiple surgical debridement is often indicated. Use of fecal diversion tube along with negative pressure wound therapy is an effective way for isolation of wound from fecal contamination. Diverting colostomy is the last option if other options are not available.

Sebaceous Cyst in Scrotum

Scrotum is a common site for sebaceous cyst. Treatment is excision of cyst if cyst is single. If multiple cysts involve a part of scrotal skin, that part of skin is excised along with cysts.

Carcinoma of Scrotum

Also called "chimney sweeper's cancer" or "mule-spinner's cancer". Workers using tar and shale oil are at more risk. Carcinoma starts as a wart or ulcer. Treatment is wide excision ± bilateral inguinal block dissection upto external iliac group of lymph nodes.

Scrotal Fat Necrosis

The patient is commonly in prepuberty age group, with history of recent cold exposure (usually after swimming). Bilateral intrascrotal masses caudal to the testes are palpable.

Acute Idiopathic Scrotal Edema

A rare and self-limiting condition, commonly found in children. It is a diagnosis of exclusion.

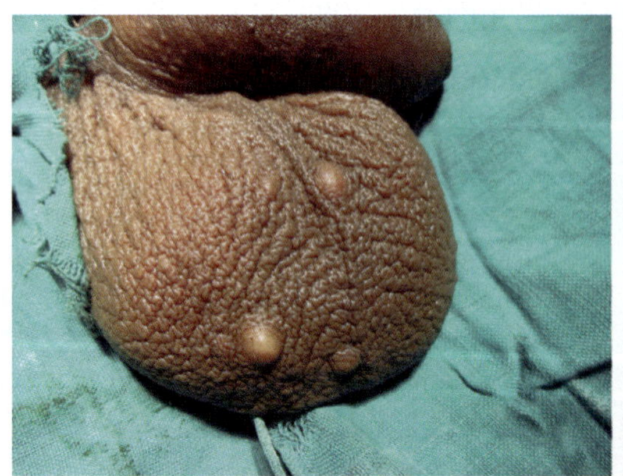

Sebaceous cyst in scrotum.

Characteristic Features of Scrotal Skin

- Presence of rugosity (due to underlying attachment to dartos muscle)
- Elastic
- Deeply pigmented
- Temperature regulatory capability (helpful for spermatogenesis)
- Highly vascular.

Indications of Scrotectomy (Partial/Total)

- Fournier's gangrene
- Filarial scrotum
- Postradiation lymphedema
- Hidradinitis suppurativa
- Penoscrotal paget disease
- Scrotal violation during assessment or treatment of testicular malignancy.

Methods of Reconstruction Following Scrotectomy

- Primary closure with remaining scrotal skin
- Fasciocutaneous flaps(from superomedial or anterolateral thigh)
- Meshed split-thickness skin graft.

Phimosis

Phimosis is inability to retract the foreskin over the glans penis. Phimosis is either physiologic or pathologic.

Physiologic phimosis: In physiologic phimosis, the foreskin is nonretractile due to natural adhesion between prepuce and glans (preputial glanular adhesion). Accumulation of epithelial debris and intermittent penile erection gradually make the foreskin more retractable. By the age of 3 years, 90% of the foreskin are retractable. A 6- to 8-week course of topical corticosteroids to the preputial outlet twice daily loosens the phimotic ring in most of the patients.

Pathologic phimosis: In pathologic phimosis, the foreskin is nonretractile due to circumferential scarring of the preputial orifice. Causes of pathologic phimosis are recurrent episodes of balanitis or balanoposthitis, balanitis xerotica obliterans.

Complications of phimosis: (i) Recurrent urinary tract infection; (ii) Balanitis; (iii) Balanoposthitis; (iv) Paraphimosis; and (v) Penile carcinoma.

Indications of circumcision: (i) Phimosis after age 7 years resistant to topical corticosteroid; (ii) Phimosis with ballooning of foreskin or recurrent balanitis; (iii) Recurrent urinary tract infection; (iv) Paraphimosis; (v) Prior to radiotherapy for carcinoma penis (to expose the glans penis); (vi) In suspected penile growth (to expose the glans for incisional biopsy); and (vii) Religious reasons—in muslims and jews.

Complications of circumcision: (i) Hematoma; (ii) Hyperesthesia of glans; (iii) Removal of too much skin; (iv) Insufficient removal of skin; (v) Wound infection; and (vi) Injury of the glans.

Circumcision should not be performed:

- In neonates with hypospadias
- Chordee without hypospadias
- Dorsal hood deformity
- Webbed penis
- Micropenis
- Neonate with large hydrocele or hernia.

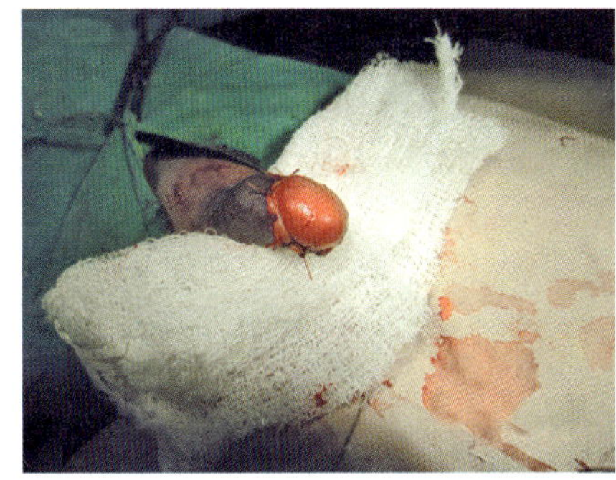

After Circumcision

"Evaluation of current evidence indicates that the health benefits of newborn male circumcision outweigh the risks; furthermore, the benefits of newborn male circumcision justify access to this procedure for families who choose it. Specific benefits from male circumcision were identified for the prevention of urinary tract infections, acquisition of HIV, transmission of some sexually transmitted infections, and penile cancer."

—**[American Academy of Pediatrics Task force on Circumcision 2012]**

Methods of Neonatal Circumcision

- Classical surgical method
- Circumcision clamps—Gomco, Plastibell, and Mogen.

Paraphimosis

- Develops when a tight prepuce is retracted beyond the corona that cannot be reduced to its normal position.
- Arterial supply to glans may be compromised, so emergency reduction must be done.
- Manual compression of edematous foreskin followed by forceful reduction of foreskin is successful in most of the cases.
- If reduction fails, then the constriction ring is incised or circumcision have to be done.
- If manual reduction is successful, patient must be informed about the necessity of circumcision, but that procedure is better to be deferred till swelling subsides.

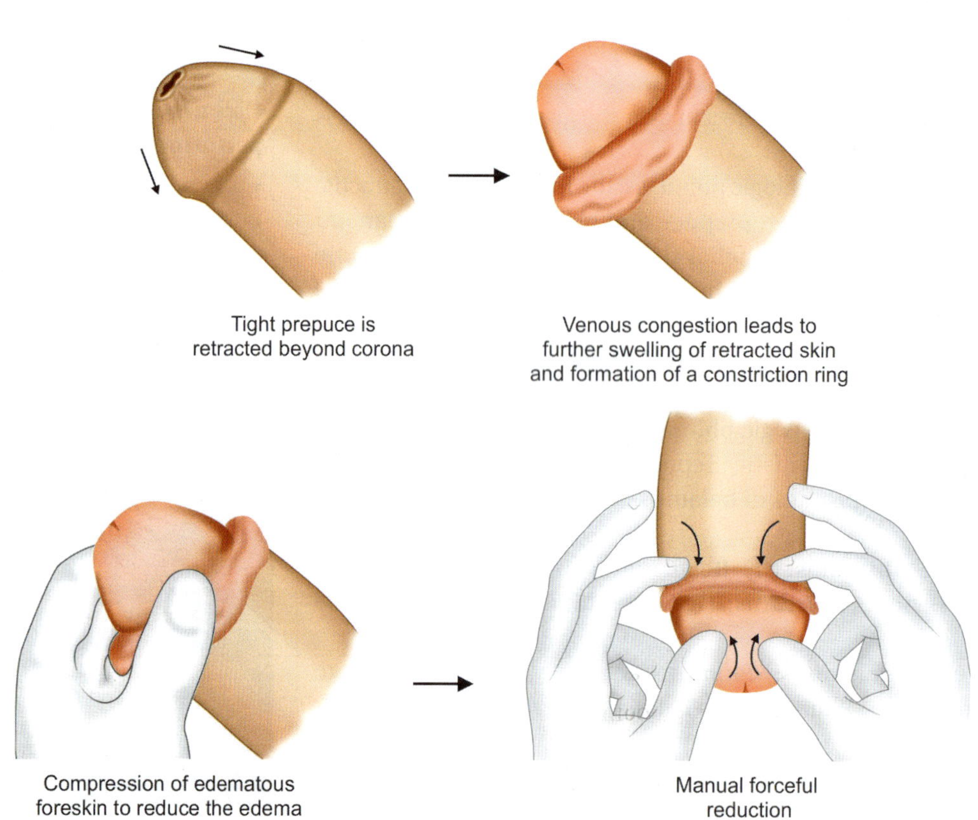

Case 1

History and Physical Examination

A mother of 3-year-old male baby complained that she noticed that the right scrotum of her baby was bigger than the left one. On further enquiry, she told that the right scrotal swelling became more prominent at the end of the day and less prominent in the morning. No other complaints related to other scrotum or external genitalia. No history of premature birth.

Physical Examination

No relevant clinical findings except mild swelling of the right scrotum.

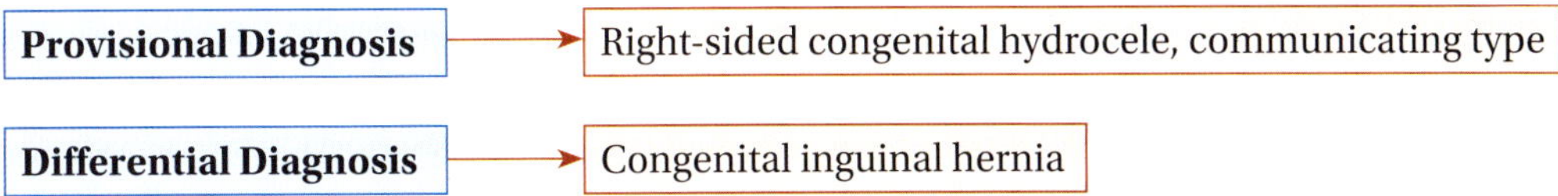

Investigations

No investigations were done for confirmation of diagnosis as there was no uncertainty in clinical diagnosis. Laboratory investigations and imaging were done as preoperative workup.

Discussion

The classic history from the baby's mother was suggestive of congenital hydrocele. No further investigations were required for confirmation of diagnosis. Exploration through inguinal incision was planned.

Management Algorithm

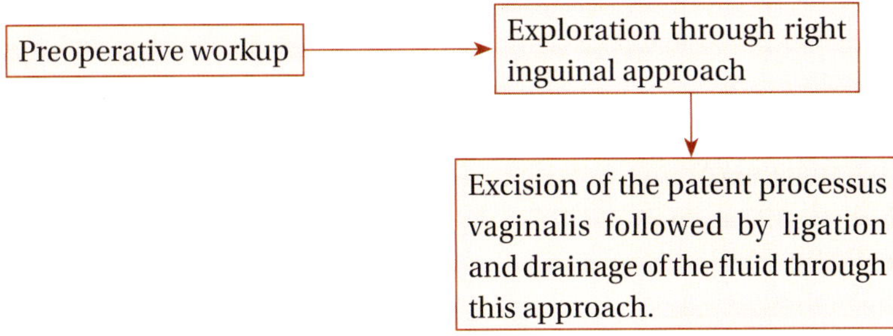

Case 2

History and Physical Examination

A 16-year-old boy presented in the surgical emergency with acute onset severe pain in the right scrotum for last 4 hours along with nausea. Patient had no history of scrotal pain in the recent past. No history of trauma.

Physical Examination

- Pulse:100/min
- Tenderness of the right testis with high lie of the testis, absent cremasteric reflex. Left testis was normal.
- TWIST scoring done, score was 3.

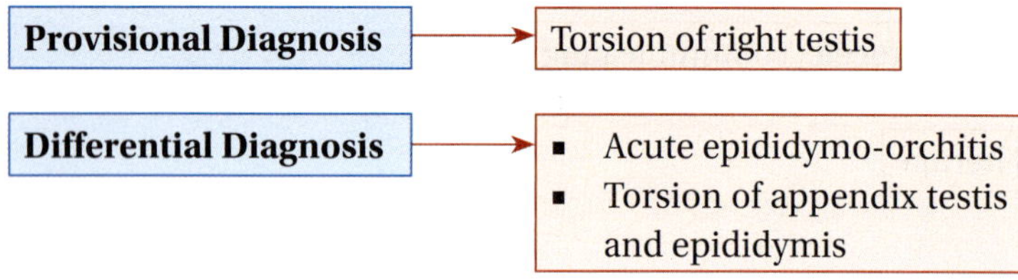

Investigations

Doppler USG revealed hypoechoic right testis with diminished vascularity and twisting of the spermatic cord. Left testis appeared normal.

Discussion

Acute onset severe unilateral scrotal pain in a pubertal boy was highly suggestive of testicular torsion. Clinical findings were also suggestive of torsion. As TWIST score was 3, Doppler USG was performed before definitive intervention. Doppler USG confirmed the diagnosis of right testicular torsion. Urgent exploration was planned to salvage the right testis.

Management Algorithm

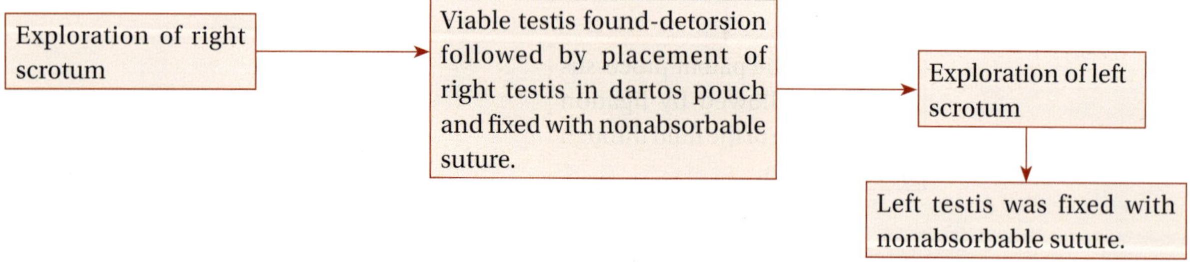

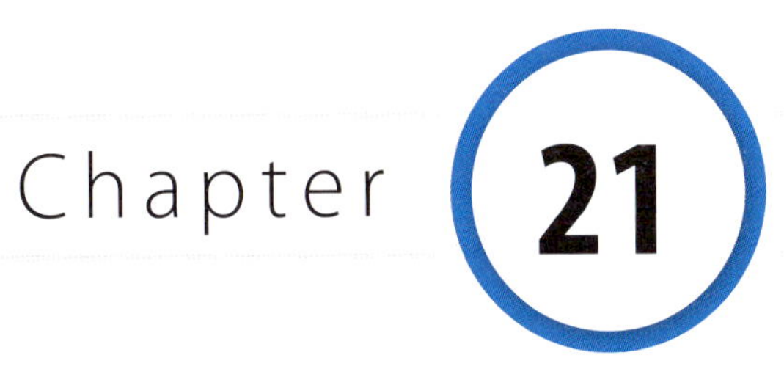

Diseases of the Esophagus

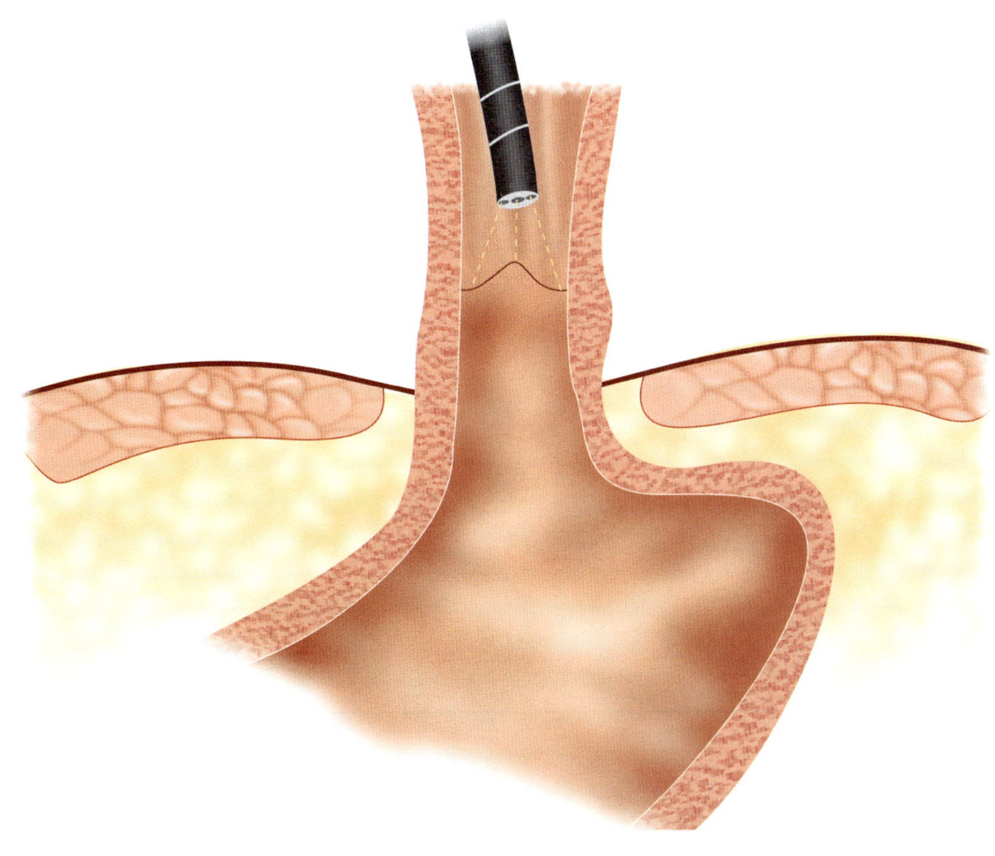

Important Topics

- Hiatal Hernia
- Gastroesophageal Reflux Disease
- Achalasia
- Other Motility Disorders of Esophagus
- Esophageal Diverticulum
- Esophageal Perforation
- Stricture of Esophagus
- Caustic Injury of Esophagus
- Foreign Body Ingestion
- Barrett Esophagus
- Esophageal Carcinoma
- Esophageal Stenting

'Everything should be made as simple as possible, but not simpler.'

Hiatal Hernia

- Hiatus hernia develops when a lax or defective phrenoesophageal membrane allows herniation of stomach through the esophageal hiatus of the diaphragm.
- Most commonly develop in women of 5th and 6th decades.
- Most of the hiatal hernias are acquired.

Types of Hiatal Hernia

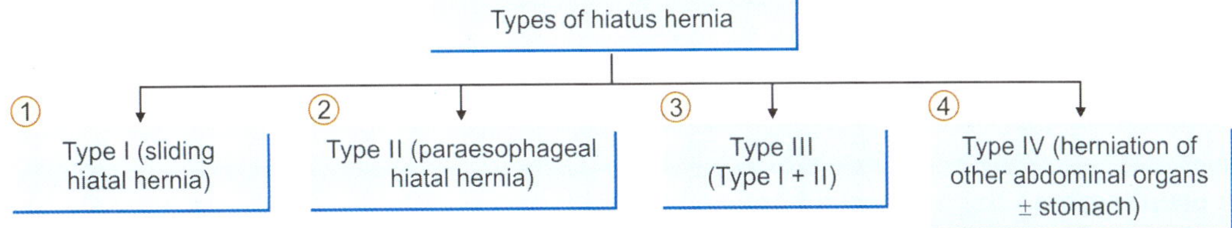

Paraesophageal Hernia

Type II, III and IV hiatal hernias are termed as paraesophageal hernia. **In paraesophageal hernia, fundus is located above the gastroesophageal junction**. Type II is also termed as **"true" paraesophageal hernia**. Paraesophageal hernia is a true hernia with hernial sac. Type III is the most common type of paraesophageal hernia. Paraesophageal hernias most commonly herniated through the left anterior part of the esophageal hiatus.

Giant paraesophageal hernia: It is a type of paraesophageal hernia where at least half of the stomach is in the mediastinum or in endoscopy, hernia is 6 cm or more.

Type I Hiatal Hernia (Sliding Hiatal Hernia)

- Phrenoesophageal ligament is intact but lax.
- Gastroesophageal junction is above the diaphragm.

Most common type of hiatal hernia.

Type II Hiatal Hernia

- This hernia is also termed as "rolling" hiatal hernia.
- Focal defect in phrenoesophageal Ligament (defect in anterior and lateral to esophagus)
- Fundus herniates in the mediastinum anterior to the esophagus with normally positioned GE junction.

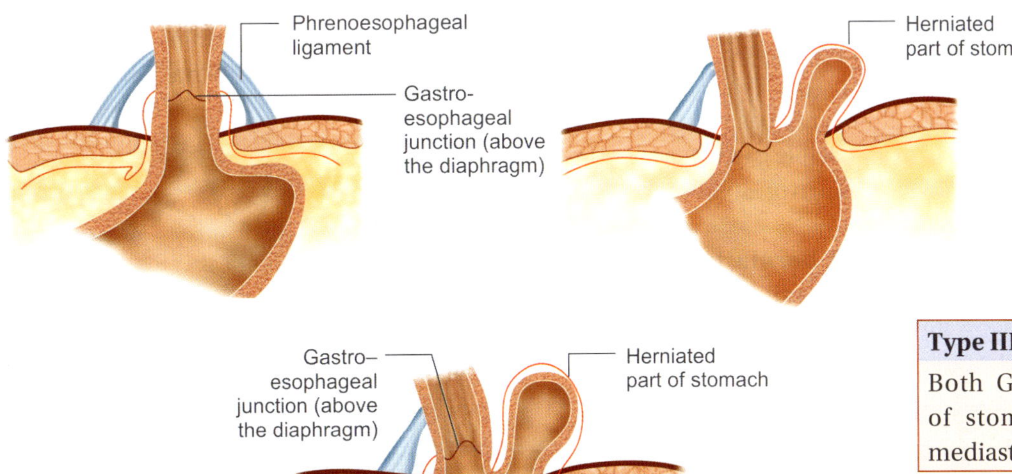

Type III Hiatal Hernia

Both GE junction and fundus of stomach herniate into the mediastinum.

Type IV Hiatal Hernia

Herniation of stomach and other abdominal organs into the mediastinum.

Clinical Presentation

- Patient with sliding hiatal hernia presents with symptoms related to gastroesophageal reflux (heartburn, regurgitation, dysphagia).
- Type I and III hernias present with postprandial pain or bloating, early satiety, difficulty in breathing during food intake, dysphagia.
- The herniated gastric part is susceptible to volvulus (organoaxial), obstruction, infarction.
- About one third of patients with paraesophageal hernia become anemic, due to recurrent bleeding from ischemic longitudinal ulcers in the mucosa of herniated stomach **(Cameron ulcer)**.

Diagnosis

- **Barium esophagram**—the most useful imaging modality to identify anatomy and location of paraesophageal hernia. This imaging modality gives information about the extent of hernia, location of gastroesophageal junction and type of hernia. It also gives functional information by assessing gastric emptying and evidence of gastroesophageal reflux.
- **Endoscopy:** Fiberoptic esophagoscopy is also a useful modality for diagnosis and classification of hiatal hernia.
- **Manometry** is not mandatory for evaluation of para-esophageal hernia.
- Presence of air-fluid level in the posterior mediastinum in lateral view of chest X-ray—**hiatal hernia must be in the differential diagnosis.**

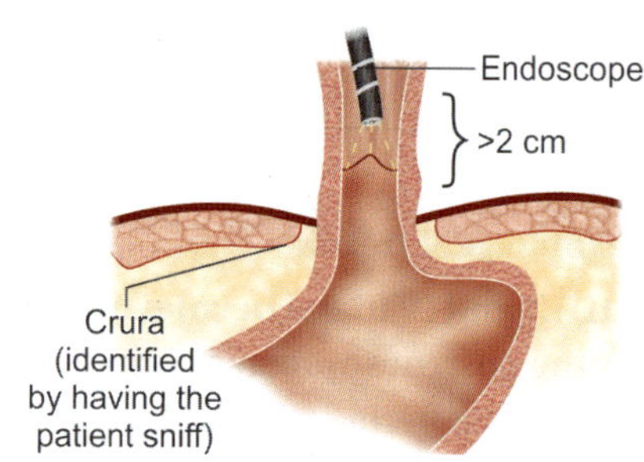

Identification of pouch lined with gastric rugal folds at least 2 cm proximal to the crura—**Type I hiatal hernia.**

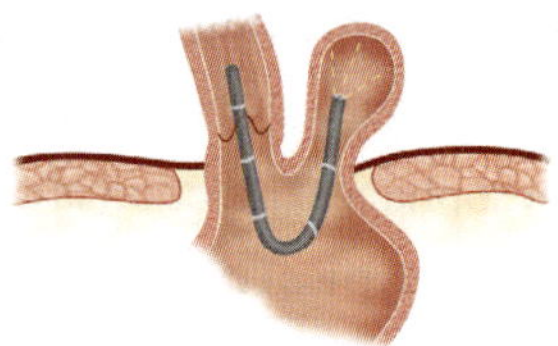

On retroversion of the scope, a separate orifice adjacent to gastroesophageal junction identified and where gastric rugal folds ascend—**Type II hiatal hernia.**

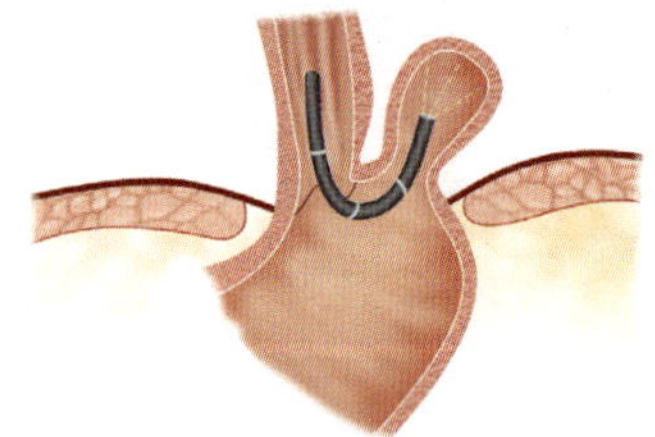

The scope is entering the pouch through a separate orifice proximal to the crura—**Type III hiatal hernia.**

Treatment

- **Asymptomatic sliding hernia**—no treatment required; **Asymptomatic paraesophageal hernia—**watchful waiting.
- **Indications of surgery:** (i) Symptomatic sliding hernia; (ii) Symptomatic paraesophageal hiatal hernia; (iii) Paraesophageal hernia with acute gastric volvulus, incarceration or strangulation; and (iv) Hiatal hernia detected during operations like Roux-en-Y gastric bypass, sleeve gastrectomy, placement of adjustable gastric bands.
- **Surgical approaches:** (i) Abdominal (open or laparoscopic) and (ii) Thoracic.
- **Surgical repair of paraesophageal hernia includes:** (i) Dissection of hernial sac(away from mediastinal structures); (ii) Returning the herniated fundus and GE junction to infradiaphragmatic position; (iii) Primary sutured crural repair with or without reinforcement by mesh (on-lay fashion); and (iv) Fundoplication (Nissen or Partial).

- **Mesh reinforcement decreases short term recurrence.**
- **Fundoplication** helps to prevent development of **GERD symptoms** after paraesophageal hernia repair. After hiatal repair, the length of the intra-**abdominal esophagus should be atleast 2–3 cm.**

Gastroesophageal Reflux Disease (GERD)

Definition of GERD: As per Montreal consensus, "a condition which develops when the reflux of contents causes troublesome symptoms and/or complications". [Symptoms are "troublesome" if they adversely affected an individual's wellbeing].

Pathophysiology

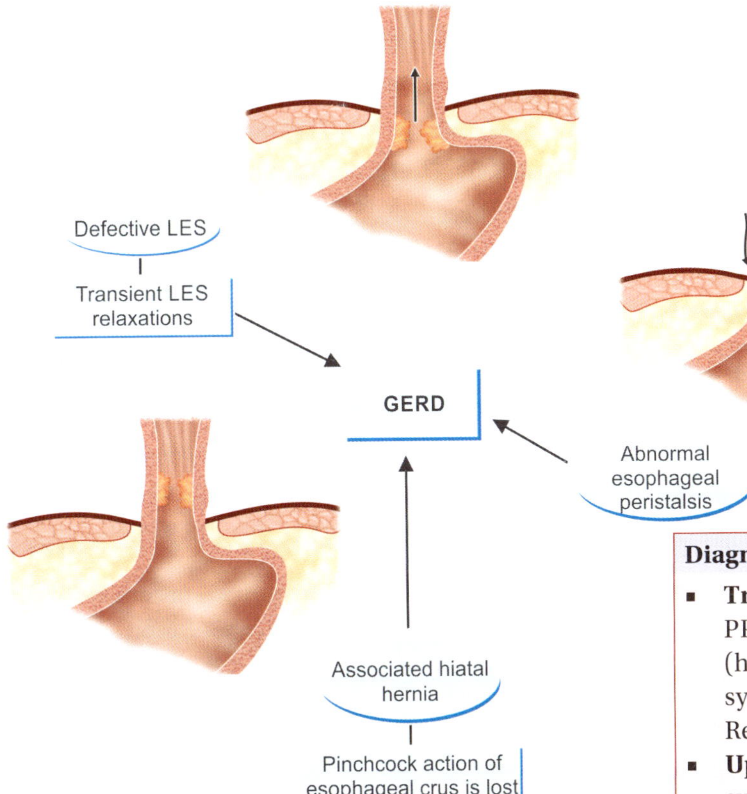

Clinical Presentation

- **Typical symptoms**: Heartburn, regurgitation, dysphagia. Heartburn is the most common symptom of GERD.

  Substernal or epigastric burning pain that is aggravated in lying down position and promptly relieved after taking antacids—the classic presentation.
- **Atypical symptoms:** Dyspepsia, epigastric pain, nausea, bloating
- **Extraesophageal symptoms:** Chest pain, chronic cough, throat clearing, asthma, laryngitis, pharyngitis.
- **Complications:** (i) Peptic stricture; (ii) Barrett's esophagus; and (iii) Adenocarcinoma of esophagus.

- **Heartburn** is substernal burning sensation arising from the epigastrium upto the neck.
- **Regurgitation** is effortless return of gastric contents toward the mouth accompanied by acid or bitter taste.

Diagnosis

- **Trial of PPI therapy:** An 8-week trial of empiric PPI therapy in patients with classic symptoms (heartburn, regurgitation) without any alarming symptoms is a practical approach for diagnosis. Response to therapy is diagnostic of GERD.
- **Upper GI endoscopy:** Indicated in: (i) Classic GERD symptoms that are persistent or progressive despite 8-week PPI therapy; (ii) Dysphagia or odynophagia; (iii) Patients presenting with alarming symtoms (GI bleeding, weight loss); and (iv) Patients with multiple risk factors for Barrett's esophagus. PPI should be stopped for atleast 2 weeks before diagnostic endoscopy.

  In endoscopy, LA grade B, C and D erosive esophagitis or Barrett's esophagus segment >3 cm with intestinal metaplasia on biopsy is diagnostic of GERD.
- **Ambulatory reflux monitoring (pH or impedance pH):** Reflux monitoring is indicated if normal endoscopy finding or LA grade A. Abnormal findings in reflux monitoring is diagnostic of GERD.
- **Esophageal impedance measurement:** Measurment of mucosal impedance during endoscopy by catheter-based balloon lined by sensors. This is a useful adjunct to endoscopy in diagnosis.

Esophageal manometry and contrast study are not recommended for diagnosis.

Ambulatory Reflux Monitoring

Methods of reflux testing: (i) Wireless telemetry capsule attached to esophageal mucosa during endoscopy (monitoring can be continues for 48–96 hours) and (ii) Transnasal catheter-based testing (monitoring can be continued for 24 hours).

- Several informations are collected (e.g. total no. of reflux episodes, largest episode of reflux, extent of reflux in upright and supine position). **DeMeester score** is calculated based on the results of reflux testing.

Esophageal Manometry

- High-resolution esophageal manometry is indicated when surgery is planned.
- Can define the location and function of LES and helps to exclude other esophageal motility disorders.
- Can also assess the status of esophageal contractility and peristatic wave progression, so that Surgeon can choose the best antireflux procedure.

Newer developments of high-resolution manometry (HRM): (i) Physiologic assessment of EG junction morphology and (ii) Provocative testing with multiple rapid swallows or rapid drink challenge.

DeMeester score: It is a composite score to categorize GERD according to severity and comprised of six variables: (i) total esophageal acid exposure time; (ii) Upright acid exposure time; (iii) Supine acid exposure time; (iv) Number of episodes of reflux; (v) Number of reflux episodes lasting more than 5 minutes; and (vi) The duration of the longest reflux episode.

Los Angeles (LA) classification of Esophagitis (Based on Endoscopic Assessment of Reflux Esophagitis)

- **Grade A:** One (or more) mucosal break no longer than 5 mm that does not extend between the tops of two mucosal folds.
- **Grade B:** One (or more) mucosal break more than 5 mm long that does not extend between the tops of two mucosal folds.
- **Grade C:** One (or more) mucosal break that is continuous between the tops of two or more mucosal folds but which involve less than 75% of the circumference.
- **Grade D:** One (or more) mucosal break which involves at least 75% of the esophageal circumference.

Treatment

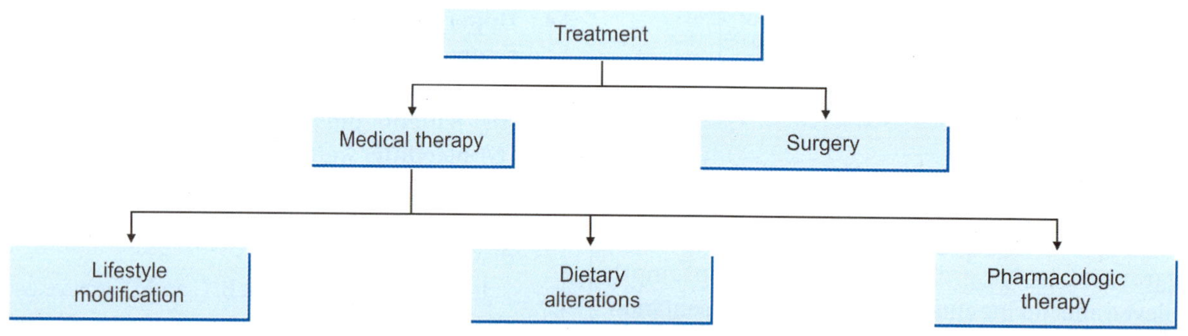

- Tobacco and alcohol cessation
- Elevation of the head of the bed
- Lying left-side down at night
- Avoidance of late-night meals and bedtime snacks
- Avoidance of eating before going to sleep
- Weight loss for obese patients

- Avoidance of food that potentially aggravate symptoms (coffee, chocolate, citrus and spicy food, carbonated beverages, foods with high fat content)
- Smaller amount more frequent meals

- Proton pump inhibitors
- H_2-blockers

Surgical Management

Indications of antireflux surgery: (i) GERD along with complications (e.g., Barrett esophagus, stricture); (ii) Presence of extraesophageal manifestations (e.g., chronic cough, laryngitis, asthma); (iii) Failed medical therapy (inadequate symptom control, side effects of medications); and (iv) Patient's choice.

Surgical approaches for GERD

- Transabdominal
  - **Nissen fundoplication**
    - Most commonly performed surgical procedure for GERD
    - 360° fundic wrap around the lower esophagus through laparoscopic (preferred) or open method
    - Wrap must be short, untwisted, loose to avoid complications (inability to vomit, dysphagia)

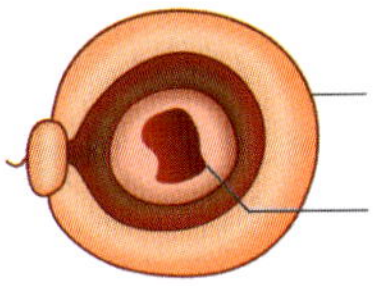

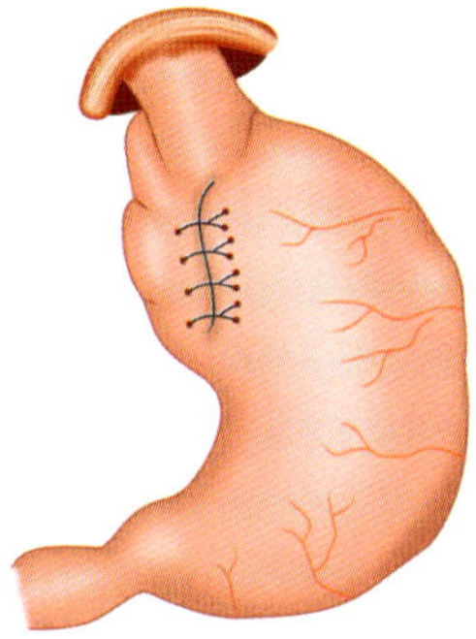

    Fundus of stomach

    Esophagus
  - **Toupet fundoplication**
    - Partial 270° fundoplication 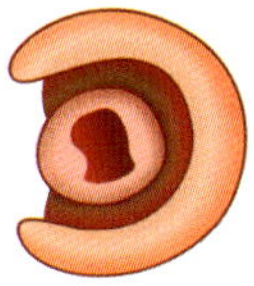
    - Edges of the fundus are sutured to the left and right lateral wall of the esophagus, and also to the right diaphragmatic pillar
  - **Lind fundoplication**
    - Partial 300° posterior fundoplication
- Transthoracic
  - Belsey mark IV fundoplication — Rarely performed nowadays
    - 270° fundoplication
    - Less dysphagia than Nissen fundoplication

    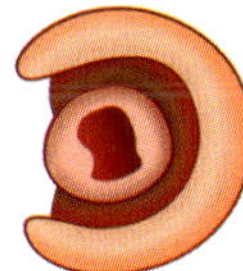
  - Nissen fundoplication
    - Result similar to transabdominal approach

- **Laparoscopic fundoplication** is associated with better early outcomes (shorter hospital stay, early return to normal activities) and no significant differences in late outcomes compared to open fundoplication.
- **Partial fundoplication** is associated with less postoperative dysphagia, less reoperations and same patient satisfaction compared to total fundoplication upto 5 years after surgery.

Shoeshine Maneuver

A maneuver done in laparoscopic Nissen fundoplication to ensure that the fundic wrap is in good position without tension and no redundant fundus lies posterior to esophagus.

Recently Developed Minimally Invasive Therapeutic Options for GERD

- **The Stretta procedure**—delivery of radiofrequency energy to the esophagogastric junction via endoscopically placed catheter. This modality acts by tissue necrosis followed by tightening of LES or by neurolysis.
- **Transoral incisionless fundoplication (TIF)**—Two devices (EsophyX and MUSE) act by this approach. EsophyX rebuilds the gastroesophageal valve mechanism by creating 210–300 degree fundoplication using full-thickness fasteners. The MUSE device (Medigus ultrasonic surgical endostapler) uses disposable endoscopic stapling device to apply transmural surgical staples under ultrasound guidance.
- **Magnetic sphincter augmentation (LINX device)**—Implant (made of interlinked titanium beads with magnetic cores) is placed around the LES by laparoscopic approach. The LINX is MRI-compatible (upto 1.5 Tesla).

Antireflux surgery is not an appropriate surgical option in certain conditions:

- Patient with morbid obesity (BMI >35)
- Strictures not responsive to dilation
- Patients with high-grade dysplasia or adenocarcinoma
- History of gastric bypass, sleeve gastrectomy or vertical banded gastroplasty

Achalasia

- Most common primary esophageal motility disorder, **characterized by** loss of effective esophageal peristalsis and failure of LES to relax, resulting in impaired esophageal emptying and gradual esophageal dilation.
- Develops equally among both sexes and in all adult age groups.
- Etiology is unknown.
- **Characteristic pathology** is loss of inhibitory neurons in the myenteric plexus of the distal esophagus and lower esophageal sphincter.

Triple-A Syndrome (Allgrove Disease)

- Achalasia
- Alacrima
- ACTH-resistant adrenal insufficiency

Pathophysiology

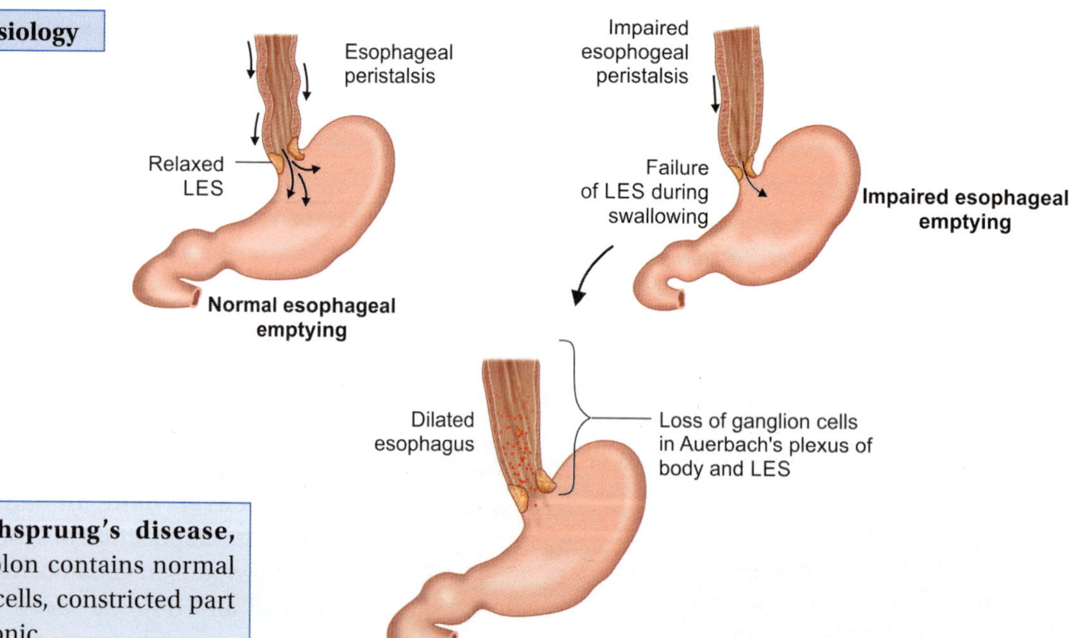

In Hirschsprung's disease, dilated colon contains normal ganglion cells, constricted part is aganglionic.

Clinical Presentation

Patients usually present with classic triad of symptoms:

1. **Dysphagia:** Progressive dysphagia (Initially with liquids and then progress to solids) is the most common symptom. Stress and cold liquids exacerbate dysphagia.
2. **Regurgitation:** Regurgitation of undigested foods with foul odor tends to regurgitate after meals and in supine position.
3. **Weight loss**

Other symptoms: Heartburn, chest pain. Pneumonia, lung abscess, bronchiectasis may develop in longstanding achalasia due to recurrent aspiration.

Eckardt symptom score is a scoring system to evaluate the symptoms and treatment response.

Diagnosis

Endoscopy: Classic endoscopic findings are dilated esophagus with retained saliva and food with a puckered and tight esophagogastric junction fails to open with insufflations. With gentle pressure, the scope can be admitted.

Endoscopy is also helpful to rule out **pseudoachalasia** and other causes of mechanical obstruction.

Barium esophagram: Classic findings in advanced disease are Dilated esophagus with a narrowed GEJ ('bird beak' appearance), lack of peristaltic waves in the body. In early stage, esophagram findings are nonspecific.

High-resolution manometry: Current gold standard diagnostic modality for achalasia. This investigation is helpful to distinguish achalasia into clinically relevant subtypes (type I, II and III).

Treatment

The goals of all treatment modalities are to relieve symptoms, improve esophageal emptying and preventing further dilation of esophagus by reducing the LES tone.

- **Treatment modalities include:** (i) Pharmacotherapy; (ii) Botulinum toxin; (iii) Pneumatic dilation; (iv) Surgical myotomy; and (v) Peroral endoscopic myotomy (POEM).
- **Pharmacotherapy:** Nitrates (e.g., isosorbide dinitrate 5 mg sublingual before meals) and Calcium channel blockers (nifedipine 10-30 mg sublingual before meals) are the commonly used medications for achalasia.

  Pharmacotherapy is the least effective treatment option for achalasia.
- **Botulinum toxin:** Injection of botulinum toxin acts by irreversible inhibition of the release of acetylcholine from presynaptic cholinergic terminals. Intrasphincteric injection (in four quadrants of LES-total dose 100 U) has short term effect (about 6 months). This therapy is particularly indicated for patients with shorter life expectancy or who are poor candidates for definitive management.

Pseudoachalasia

- Rapid onset weight loss in elderly patients with suspected achalasia-pseudoachalasia should be suspected.
- Endoscopic ultrasound or cross-sectional imaging is indicated to rule out causes of pseudoachalasia.

Time Barium Esophagram

- This technique involves intake of large bolus of barium in upright position and radiograph after 1 and 5 minutes for assessment of height of barium column.
- This is a useful imaging modality to predict response to treatment (e.g. balloon dilation, myotomy).

Manometric Subtypes of Achalasia

Type I: 100% failed peristalsis (aperistalsis) with the absence of panesophageal pressurization to more than 30 mmHg

Type II: 100% failed peristalsis (aperistalsis) with panesophageal pressurization to greater than 30 mm Hg

Type III: Spastic contractions with or without periods of panesophageal pressurization

Achalasia type II is most common followed by type I.

Functional Lumen Imaging Probe (FLIP)

A high-resolution impedance system to study the pressure geometry relationship and motor function of esophagus. Its role in diagnosis of achalasia is evolving.

Pneumatic dilation: This treatment approach acts by partial disruption of the circular muscles of LES. The dilator is placed across the LES under fluoroscopic or endoscopic guidance and dilation is performed in a controlled manner by using hand-held manometer. This approach needs repeated dilation (about 4 weeks interval).

Serial pneumatic dilation is the most effective nonsurgical treatment option.

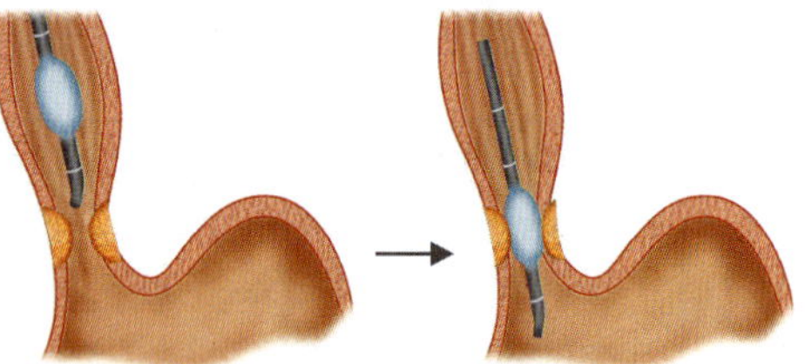

Surgical myotomy: Laparoscopic Heller myotomy with partial fundoplication (Dor or Toupet) is the surgery of choice in achalasia.

Peroral Endoscopic myotomy (POEM): This procedure is effective for all types of achalasia (particularly achalasia type III) as a primary treatment or in patients of treatment failure to Heller myotomy or pneumatic dilation.

Steps involved in POEM: (i) Endoscopic measurement of the anatomic landmarks in reference to the overtube; (ii) Saline lift and mucosotomy; (iii) Creation of submucosal tunnel across EG junction and proximal stomach; (iv) Controlled myotomy (division of circular muscles) across the EG junction (6 cm into esophagus and 2 cm below the squamocolumnar junction); and (v) Closure of mucosotomy.

Complications: (i) GERD; (ii) Mucosal injury; (iii) Pneumomediastinum; and (iv) Pneumothorax.

Esophagectomy is indicated in megaesophagus or sigmoid esophagus when other treatment modalities become unsuccessful.

Modified Heller Myotomy

Anterior myotomy
Proximal extent of myotomy [6–7 cm above GE junction]
Distal extent—Controversial 1.5 cm gastric myotomy? or 3 cm gastric myotomy?

Achalasia Dilator

- Achalasia dilator is a noncompliant, cylindrical polyethylene balloon dilator. The dilators come in three sizes (3.0, 3.5 and 4.0 cm) and used in a graded manner.
- The balloon is inflated with air and the inflated balloon is positioned across the LES for 15–60 seconds.

- Type III achalasia is less responsive to pneumatic dilation.
- **Tailored POEM or laparoscopic Heller myotomy is the preferred treatment approach for type III achalasia.**

Surgical myotomy is either original Heller myotomy (described by Ernest Heller) or modified Heller myotomy. This surgery involves division of the muscle fibers of the LES without disrupting the mucosa.

In original Heller myotomy, both anterior and posterior myotomies are performed along the GEJ through thoracotomy or laparotomy approach.

In modified Heller myotomy, only anterior myotomy is done.

Complications: (i) Mucosal perforation and (ii) GERD

Adding a fundoplication procedure after myotomy reduces the chance of GERD.

Sigmoid Esophagus

In late-stage achalasia, esophagus is severely dilated and develop tortuosity.

Third-space Endoscopy (Submucosal Endoscopy)

It is the technique of access to submucosal space using SEMF (Submucosal endoscopy with mucosal flap safety valve) technique.

Use of third-space endoscopy:

- Peroral endoscopic myotomy (POEM)—for achalasia cardia
- Gastric peroral endoscopic myotomy (G-POEM)—for refractory gastroparesis
- Peroral endoscopic myotomy for Zenker diverticulum (Z-POEM)—for Zenker diverticulum
- Submucosal tunneling endoscopic resection (STER)—for resection of subepithelial tumor
- Peroral endoscopic tunneling for restoration of esophagus (POETRE)—for esophageal stricture.

Diffuse Esophageal Spasm

Loss of normal peristaltic coordination resulting in simultaneous contraction of segments of the esophageal body.

- **Patients present** with severe spastic pain, dysphagia, regurgitation and weight loss.
- **Diagnosis** is confirmed by **esophageal manometry**. Characteristic manometric findings are spontaneous, repetitive, prolonged, high amplitude contractions.
- **Barium esophagogram** may reveal classic 'corkscrew' esophagus.
- **Mainstay of treatment is nonsurgical.**
- Pharmacologic/endoscopic + treatment of associated psychiatric disorders (depression, anxiety, etc.). Nitrates, calcium channel blockers, anticholinergics are used as pharmacologic therapy.
- **Surgery is only indicated** when patients not responding to medical treatment.
- Long esophagomyotomy (proximal extension upto the aortic arch) along with Dor (anterior, partial) fundoplication is the surgery of choice.

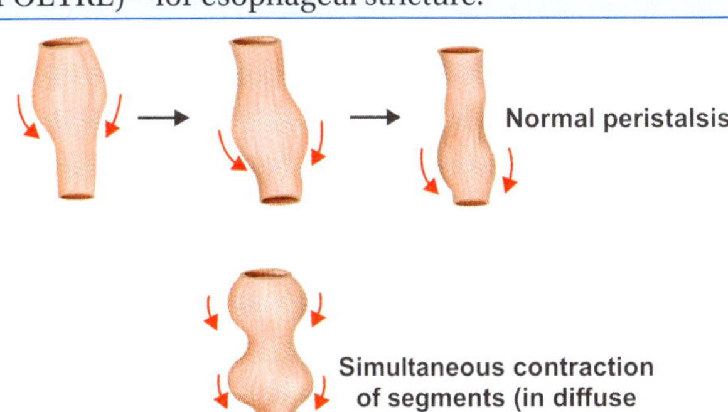

Nutcracker Esophagus

- Hypermotility disorder characterised by high amplitude (>180 mm Hg), prolonged (>6s) peristaltic contractions.
- **Patients present** with chest pain and dysphagia
- Peristaltic contractions 2 standard deviations above the normal values in manometric study is **diagnostic**
- **Treatment** is medical (Ca^{2+} channel blocker, nitrates, antispasmodics).

Esophageal Diverticula

- Diverticula are focal pouches of esophageal wall consisting of mucosa, submucosa and sometimes muscular coat.
- **Different types:**
  - **According to location:**
    - Pharyngoesophageal diverticulum [Zenker's]
    - Parabronchial [midesophageal]
    - Epiphrenic [supradiaphragmatic]
  - **According to pathophysiology:**
    - Traction diverticula (resulting from an extrinsic process)—they are true diverticula (consists of all layers of the esophageal wall)
    - Pulsion diverticula (resulting from elevated intraluminal pressure)—they are false diverticula (consists of mucosa and submucosa only).

Zenker Diverticulum

- Pharyngoesophageal or Zenker diverticulum is the most common esophageal diverticulum. **It is a pulsion diverticulum.**
- This diverticulum herniates through the **Killian's triangle**—a triangle formed by oblique fibers of the thyropharyngeus muscle and horizontal fibers of cricopharyngeus muscle.
- **Pathophysiology:** Killian triangle is exposed to high pressure due to loss of coordination during the second stage of swallowing, which leads to formation of diverticulum.
- **Clinical presentation:** Patients present with progressive cervical dysphagia, cough on recumbent position, spontaneous regurgitation of undigested food. Abnormal noise during swallowing and halitosis are also common.
- **Diagnosis:** Barium or gastrograffin swallow is the useful imaging modality for diagnosis. Esophagoscopy is indicated only when malignancy is suspected.
- **Treatment:** Treatment options are: (i) Surgical cricopharyngeal myotomy (for <2 cm diverticula); (ii) Surgical cricopharyngeal myotomy along with diverticulectomy or diverticulopexy; (iii) Endoscopic stapling diverticulostomy; (iv) Endoscopic diverticulostomy with laser or cautery; and (v) Peroral endoscopic myotomy for Zenker diverticulum (Z-POEM).

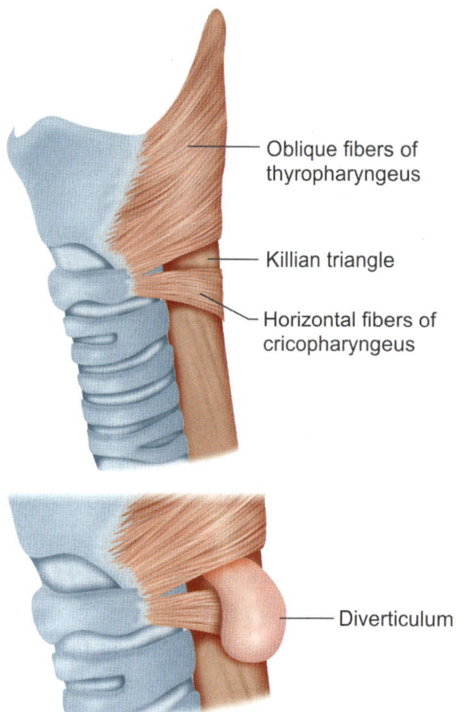

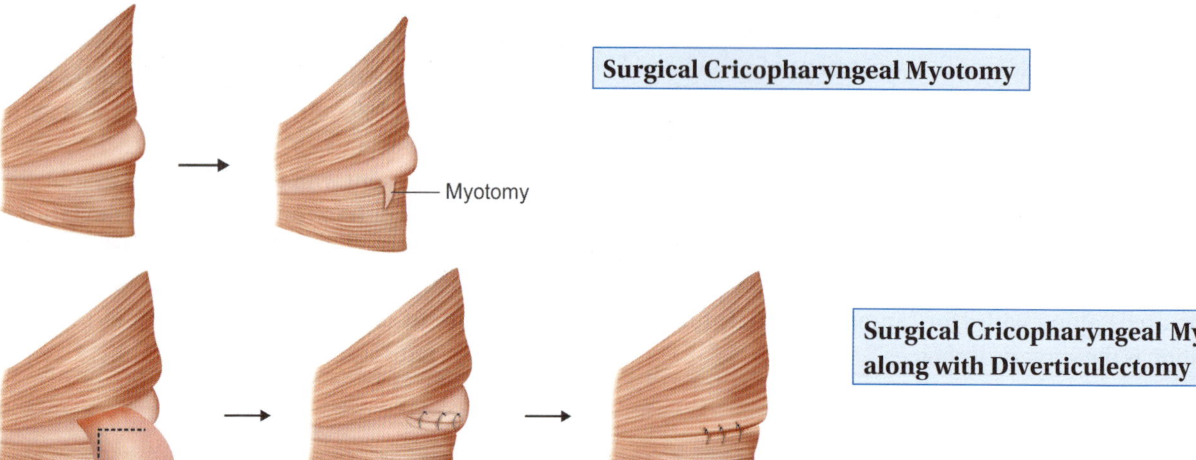

Surgical Cricopharyngeal Myotomy

Surgical Cricopharyngeal Myotomy along with Diverticulectomy

Epiphrenic Diverticulum

It is a pulsion diverticulum, typically present within the distal 10 cm of esophagus. This diverticulum commonly arises from the right side of the esophagus.

- **Pathophysiology:** Epiphrenic diverticulum develops due to high intraluminal pressure secondary to a relatively distal obstruction.
- **Clinical presentation:** Most patients are asymptomatic. The diverticulum is often diagnosed as incidental finding during workup of a motility disorder. Symptomatic patients usually present with dysphagia, regurgitation of undigested foods.
- **Diagnosis:** Contrast esophagram is essential for diagnosis, but manometric study and endoscopic examination are also indicated to assess the underlying physiology.

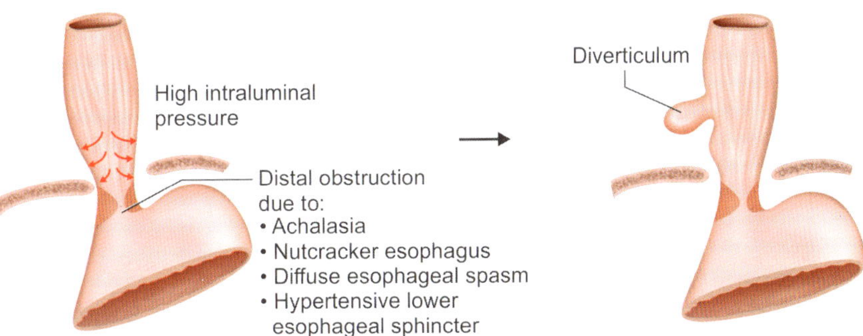

Treatment: Asymptomatic, small (<2 cm) diverticula do not need any surgical intervention. Patients with symptoms, documented motor abnormality warrants surgical intervention.

Surgical options are: (i) Diverticulectomy and esophagogastric myotomy with partial fundoplication (e.g. Belsey Mark IV fundoplication) via left posterolateral thoracotomy; (ii) Diverticulectomy with distal esophageal myotomy via VATS or VATS along with laparoscopic approach; and (iii) Diverticulectomy and esophagogastric myotomy along with fundoplication (Toupet or Dor) via laparoscopic transhiatal approach.

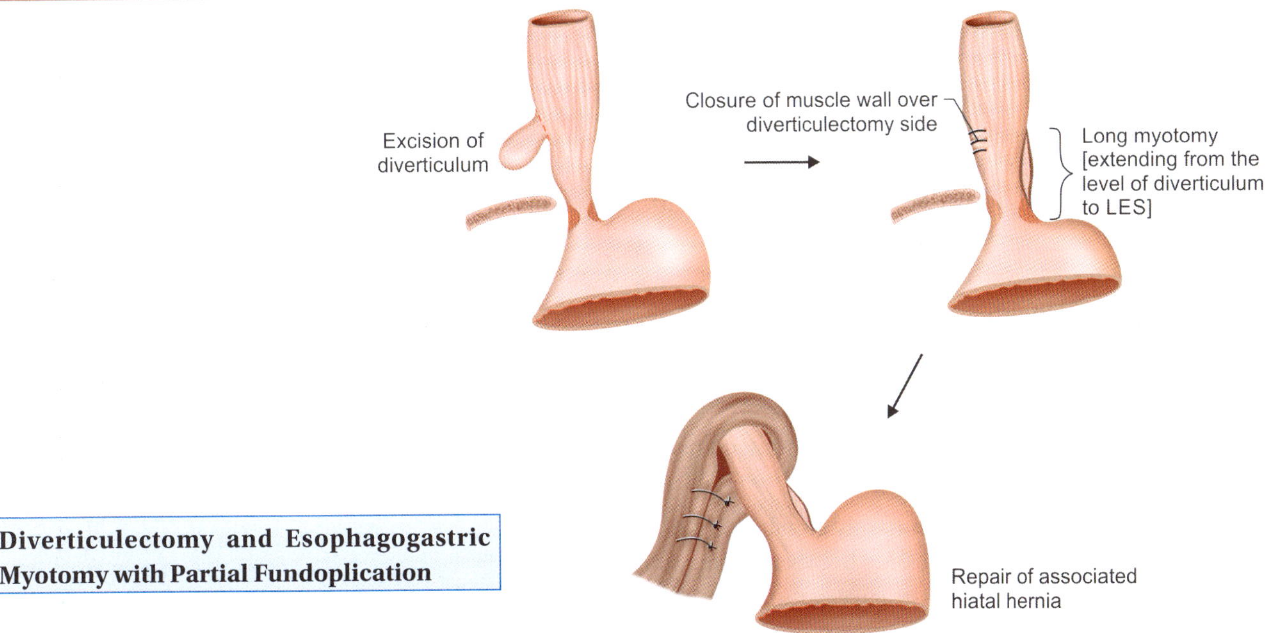

Diverticulectomy and Esophagogastric Myotomy with Partial Fundoplication

Mid-esophageal Diverticulum

Mid-esophageal diverticulum is a traction diverticula.

- **Pathophysiology:** Develops in conjunction with mediastinal granulomatous diseases (e.g. tuberculosis, sarcoidosis, histoplasmosis).
- **Clinical presentation:** Most of the patients are asymptomatic. Symptomatic patients present with intermittent dysphagia, retrosternal pain.
- **Diagnosis:** Lateral view of barium esophagogram is needed to assess the size and location of diverticula. CT is helpful to identify mediastinal structures as well as diverticula. Manometric study is required in all patients to rule out primary motor disorder.
- **Treatment:** If diverticulum <2 cm and symptomatic, watchful waiting is the preferred option. If diverticulum >2 cm or presence of symptoms, diverticulopexy is indicated.

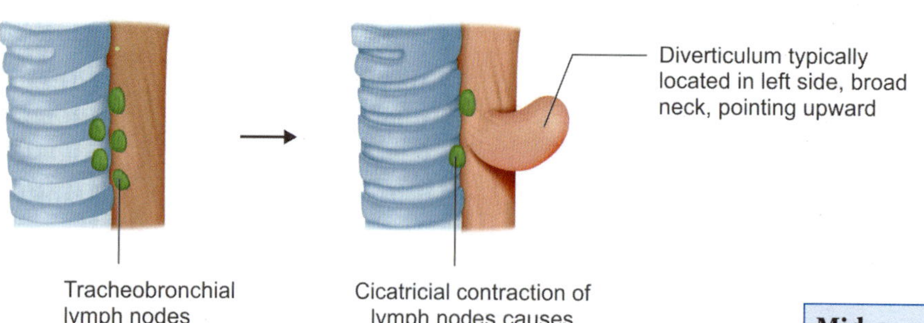

Mid-esophageal Diverticulum

Esophageal Perforation

Esophageal perforation is a life-threatening emergency.

Etiologies

Intraluminal causes:

- **Instrumentation (75%):**
  - Endoscopy
  - Dilatation for stricture
  - Sclerotherapy for varices
  - Stent insertion.
- Ingested caustic substances (Alkali)—Causes liquefaction necrosis.
- Foreign bodies—From sharp objects (e.g., fish bone), erosion due to impacted bolus.
- Barotrauma—Induced by Heimlich maneuver, forceful vomiting (Boerhaave syndrome) during childbirth
- Cancer of esophagus
- Medications—NSAIDs, etidronate, potassium chloride.

Extraluminal causes:

- Penetrating injuries, most commonly gunshot wounds
- Blunt trauma—Due to compression between sternum and spine
- Iatrogenic—During thyroidectomy, vagotomy, fundoplication.

Iatrogenic (endoscopic procedures) perforation is the most common cause of esophageal perforation.

Boerhaave Syndrome (Spontaneous Esophageal Perforation)

- Esophageal perforation develops due to abrupt increase in the intraluminal pressure of esophagus during forceful vomiting effort in the absence of relaxation of superior esophageal sphincter.
- The perforation most commonly develops on the left border of the lower third of thoracic esophagus.

Sites of Perforation

- Level of cricopharyngeus
- Gastroesophahgeal junction (common sites for iatrogenic perforation and perforation associated with Boerhaave syndrome)
- Piriform sinus (in trumpet players, singers, manual laborers)
- Killian triangle

Clinical Presentation

- Clinical presentation depends on the location of injury, size of perforation, extent of contamination of body cavities and time interval since occurrence of injury.
- Injuries in **cervical esophagus** usually present with subcutaneous emphysema in neck, dysphagia or odynophagia, pain in neck and stiffness.
- **Thoracic perforations** present with shortness of breath and retrosternal chest pain.
- **Abdominal perforations** usually present with symptoms and signs of acute abdomen.

History of recent esophageal instrumentation or vomiting along with these symptoms and signs—esophageal injury should be suspected.

Diagnosis

A high degree of suspicion is required to avoid delay in diagnosis and management. Early diagnosis can reduce the morbidity and mortality.

- **Contrast-enhanced CT and CT esophagography** is the imaging modality of choice in suspected esophageal perforation. CT is highly sensitive to detect perforation and helpful to guide initial therapy by assessing the severity of extraesophageal contamination. CT is also helpful to exclude other diagnosis (e.g., aortic dissection).
- **Contrast esophagography (gastrograffin or barium)** in upright and lateral decubitus position is also a useful imaging modality to detect perforation and provides information regarding the contamination of body cavities (mediastinum, pleural space, peritoneal cavity) and associated esophageal pathologies (e.g. stricture, tumor, motility disorder), if any.
- **Chest X-ray** in upright position can be used as an initial screening imaging in patients with suspected esophageal perforation.
- **Diagnostic flexible fiberoptic upper GI Endoscopy** is particularly useful when esophageal perforation is suspected but CT findings are equivocal. Endoscopy can accurately determine the site and size of perforation but unable to assess the degree of extraesophageal contamination. This procedure should be done by an experienced one because of increased risk of aggravating the perforation and extraesophageal contamination.

CT Findings Suggestive of Esophageal Perforation

- Pneumomediastinum
- Mediastinum fluid collection
- Subcutaneous emphysema
- Pleural effusion
- Pneumoperitoneum
- Abdominal abscess

- **Barium** is used for suspected **thoracic perforation** and **gastrograffin** for **abdominal perforation**.
- Barium is inert in chest but may cause peritonitis, gastrograffin can cause pneumonitis.

Chest X-ray Findings Suggestive of Esophageal Perforation

- Pneumomediastinum
- Mediastinal emphysema
- Mediastinal widening
- Subcutaneous emphysema
- Pneumothorax
- Pleural effusion
- Hydrothorax.

Treatment

Management options include: (i) Non-operative management; (ii) Endoscopic management; and (iii) Surgical management.

Non-operative management includes: (i) Nil per mouth; (ii) Intravenous fluids; (iii) Broad-spectrum antibiotics (coverage against aerobic and anaerobic bacteria); (iv) PPI therapy; (v) Endoscopic placement of nasogastric tube; (vi) Access for TPN; (vii) Image-guided drainage of pleural and periesophageal collections; and (viii) Drainage of pleural collections and pleural decortications by videothoracoscopy.

Endoscopic treatment: Endoscopic management is the ideal treatment option for perforations occur during an endoscopic procedure and also recognized during the procedure. Different methods are: (i) Endoluminal suturing; (ii) Endoscopic clip placement [Through-the-scope (TTS) clips or over-the-scope clips]—standard management for closure of small (<2 cm) perforations; (iii) Endoscopic vacuum therapy (EVT); and (iv) Stenting with self-expandable stents (metal or plastic)—highly effective treatment option for iatrogenic and spontaneous perforations and postoperative leaks.

Criterias for Nonoperative Management

- Absence of any symptoms and signs of sepsis
- Initiation of management within 24 hours
- Radiological evidence suggestive of perforation of cervical or thoracic esophagus, contained perforation, minimal peri-esophageal extravasation of contrast, absence of massive pleural contamination
- No previous esophageal pathology
- Round-the-clock radiological and surgical facility available.

Pittsburgh perforation severity score is used for decision making. Score ≤2 is eligible for non-operative management.

Surgical Management

Principles of surgical management:

- **Primary repair**
  The first 24 hours are the golden period for primary closure. At any time, during surgical exploration, healthy tissue bed is found, primary closure may be considered.
- **Muscle flap**
  If tissue bed is friable, severe mediastinitis—Muscle flap to be considered.
- **Exclusion? resection?**
  If primary repair not feasible or muscle flap fails—Cervical esophagostomy along with gastrostomy/feeding jejunostomy followed by delayed reconstruction.

Management of Cervical Esophagus Perforation

Surgical management includes following steps: (i) Approach through left neck incision (along the anterior border of sternocleidomastoid) or collar incision; (ii) Circumferential esophageal mobilization; (iii) Debridement of perforation; (iv) Single or double-layer, tension-free closure of perforation; (v) Buttressing of the repair with vascularized tissue (sternocleidomastoid muscle or digastric muscle); (vi) Tube drainage; and (vii) Placement of nasogastric tube and feeding jejunostomy tube

External drainage with construction of esophageal stoma- if primary repair is not feasible.

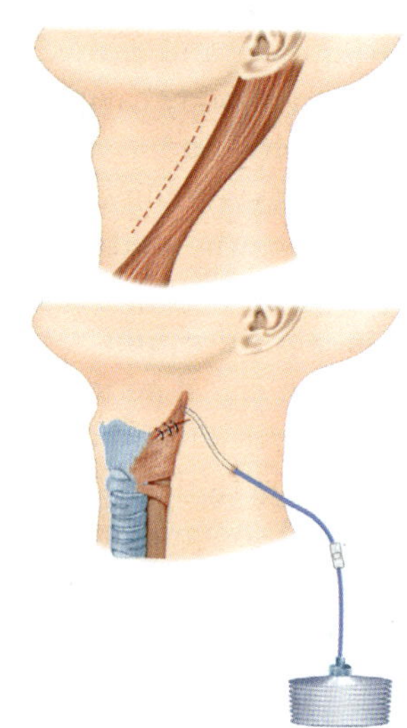

Management of Thoracic Esophagus Perforation

Surgical management includes following steps: (i) Thoracotomy or transhiatal approach via midline laparotomy; (ii) Esophageal mobilization; (iii) Debridement of perforation; (iv) Two-layer repair of perforation (separate repair of mucosa and muscle); (v) Buttressing of the repair with intercostal muscle flap, pleural or pericardiac patch; (vi) Drainage of the mediastinum and pleural cavity; and (vii) Placement of nasogastric tube and feeding jejunostomy tube.

Esophageal exclusion/diversion/resection—if primary repair is not feasible.

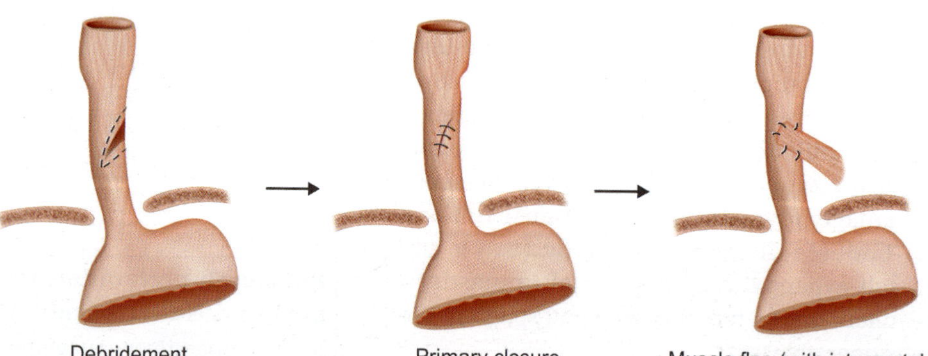

Management of Abdominal Esophagus Perforation

Surgical management includes following steps: (i) Approach by midline laparotomy; (ii) Debridement of necrotic tissues of perforation; (iii) Single or double-layer tension-free repair of perforation; (iv) Buttressing the repair with gastroplasty using gastric fundus; (v) Placement of nasogastric tube and feeding jejunostomy tube; and (vi) Placement of drainage tube in subphrenic space.

Stricture of Esophagus

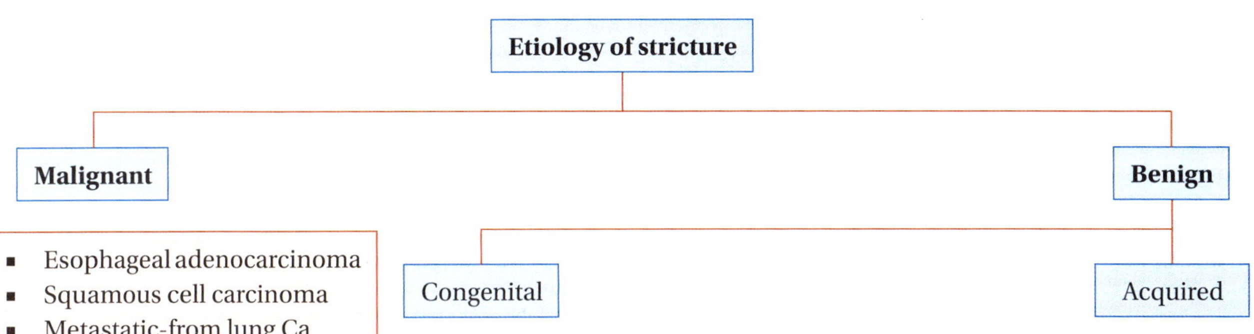

- Esophageal adenocarcinoma
- Squamous cell carcinoma
- Metastatic-from lung Ca

Due to presence of congenital web (as a result of inappropriate canalization of esophagus during development)

Classification of Benign Stricture

Simple esophageal stricture—short stricture with symmetric or concentric lumen, diameter ≥12 mm, allows easy passage for endoscope. Example: Peptic stricture, Schatzki's ring.

Complex esophageal stricture—long stricture (>2 cm), angulated or irregular, diameter <12 mm. *Example:* Post-radiation stricture, stricture after caustic injuries.

Acquired Causes of Esophageal Stricture

- GERD (peptic stricture)
- Corrosive ingestion
- Iatrogenic (after esophagectomy, sclerotherapy for varices, after radiation Therapy)
- Schatzki's ring
- Medications (potassium chloride, quinidine, ferrous sulfate, NSAIDs)
- Sarcoidosis
- Infection *(Candida albicans)*
- Eosinophilic esophagitis

Clinical Presentation

- Dysphagia to solid food is the typical presenting feature. In advanced stage, dysphagia to liquid develops.
- Odynophagia, chest pain may also present.

Diagnosis

- **Barium swallow** should be the initial investigation in patients with suspected esophageal stricture. This imaging modality can evaluate the location, number, length and severity of strictures. This modality is also helpful where standard endoscope cannot pass through the stricture.
- **Esophagoscopy** is also essential to assess the location, length, distensibility and to obtain biopsy or brushings. This diagnostic modality is essential to differentiate benign stricture from malignant stricture.

Ogilvie Dysphagia Scoring System

Score 0: No dysphagia: able to eat normal diet;
Score 1: Moderate passage: able to eat some solid foods;
Score 2: Poor passage: able to eat semi-solid foods;
Score 3: Very poor passage: able to swallow liquids only;
Score 4: No passage: unable to swallow anything.

Treatment

Different treatment modalities are: (i) Dilation; (ii) Self-expandable metal stent; (iii) Surgery; and (iv) Peroral endoscopic tunneling for restoration of esophagus (POETRE).

Stricture Dilation

Most of the strictures are amenable to dilation.

- **Esophageal dilators are of three types:** (i) Weighted push type (Maloney dilator) or bougie; (ii) Polyvinyl wire-guided bougie dilator (Savary-Gilliard); and (iii) Balloon dilator (wire-guided and TTS).
- Bougie dilators are safe and effective for simple strictures, i.e., peptic stricture. Wire-guided dilation or TTS balloon dilation is recommended for complex strictures.
- Absolute contraindication is presence of an esophageal perforation.
- **Complications of esophageal dilation:** (i) Perforation; (ii) Bleeding; and (iii) Aspiration.

Esophageal Stents

Stents (plastic stent) are particularly indicated for refractory benign strictures not responding to sequential dilation and/or corticosteroid injection. Fully covered metal stent or biodegradable stent may be used.

Surgery

Surgery is indicated for benign strictures refractory to endoscopic therapy and for malignant strictures.

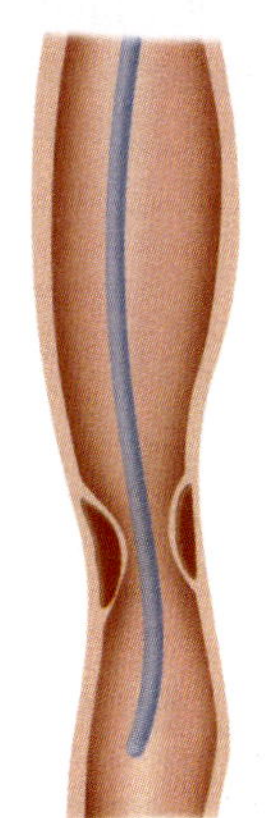

Bougies causes fracture of fibrous tissue

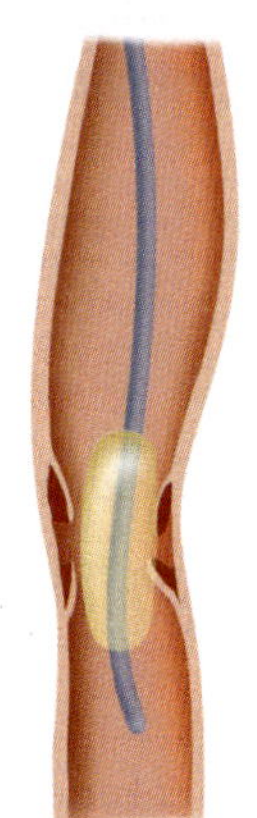

Radial stretching of fibrotic stricture

"Rule of three"

This rule is applicable for bougie dilation, not for balloon dilation. Not more than three dilations per sessions while successively increasing the diameter of dilator of 1 mm.

Refractory Stricture

Strictures that are unable to attain a luminal diameter of 14 mm over five sessions of dilation done at 2-weeks interval.

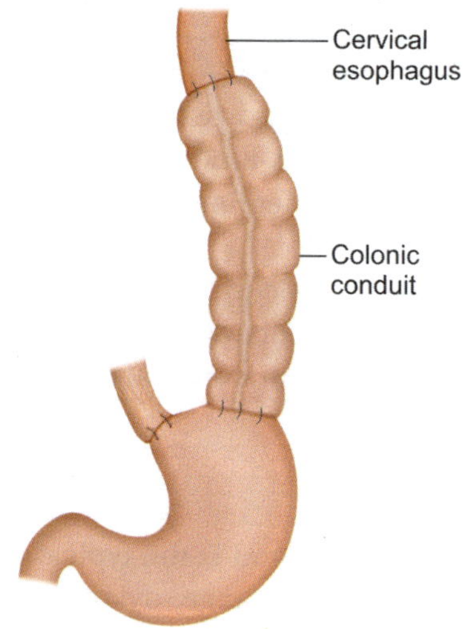

Colonic Conduit for Malignant Stricture

Caustic Injury of Esophagus

Strong acids and alkalis are responsible for most of the severe caustic injuries.

- **Substances causing caustic injuries:**
  - Alkali-containing caustic agents—Drain-cleaners, oven-cleaners, bleach, lye
  - Acid-containing caustic agents—Lysol toilet cleaners, swimming pool cleaners, anti-rust compound.
- **Severity of caustic injury depends on following factors:** (i) Acid or alkali; (ii) pH of the substance; (iii) Concentration; (iv) Amount of consumption; (v) Physical form of substance; (vi) Contact time; and (vii) Viscosity.

The injury patterns of alkaline substances: (i) Alkali causes liquefaction necrosis; (ii) Commonly causes transmural injury; and (iii) More injury to the esophagus (due to higher surface tension allows longer contact time with esophagus).

The injury patterns of acidic substances: (i) Acid causes coagulation necrosis; (ii) Less likelihood of transmural injury (acid reacts with tissue proteins to form coagulum. This coagulum prevents further spread in deeper plane); and (iii) More injury to the stomach than esophagus (pyloric spasm causes more contact time with stomach, lower surface tension allows less contact time with esophagus and protective eschar formation allows acid to bypass esophagus).

Substances with pH<2 or pH>12 can cause significant injuries.

Histopathologic Phases of Caustic Injury

- **Acute necrotic phase**—first 72 hours of injury
- **Ulcerative or granular phase**—3 days to 3 weeks. Esophagus is weakest in this phase and at increased risk of hemorrhage or perforation.
- **Cicatrization and stricturing phase**—3 weeks to 3 months. In this phase, stricture develops.

Clinical Presentation

- History includes accidental or intentional ingestion, name of the substance, amount ingested, solid or liquid, time interval between time of ingestion and time of presentation.
- Patient may present with dysphagia, odynophagia, vomiting, refusal to drink, epigastric pain, hematemesis, hoarseness, stridor.
- Hoarseness and stridor are highly suggestive of injury to the larynx and airways. Hematemesis and epigastric pain are suggestive of stomach injury. Dysphagia, odynophagia, drooling, chest pain are suggestive of esophageal injury.

Complications of Caustic Injuries

Early complication

- Perforation of esophagus or stomach

Delayed complications

- Esophageal stricture (multiple, long, irregular)
- Gastric outlet obstruction
- Carcinoma of esophagus (adenocarcinoma and squamous cell carcinoma)
- Tracheoesophageal fistula

Diagnosis

- **Contrast-enhanced CT scan of neck, thorax and abdomen** is the preferred initial diagnostic modality. CT scan should be done 3-hours after ingestion. CT scan can detect transmural injuries of the GI tract, guide the immediate management and can predict esophageal stricture formation.
- **Endoscopy** is also considered as an important diagnostic modality. It is helpful for full evaluation of esophagus but cannot accurately predict transmural necrosis. Its role in emergency situation is nowadays limited to pediatric patients (risk of transmural necrosis is less) and in patients who contrast-enhanced CT is contraindicated.
- **X-ray of chest and abdomen:** Presence of mediastinal air, pleural effusion or pneumoperitoneum are suggestive of GI perforation.
- **Contrast esophagram** has very limited role in emergency assessment in the era of high-resolution endoscopy and CT.

CT Classification of Esophageal Caustic Injuries

Grade I: Homogeneous enhancement of the esophageal wall while wall edema and mediastinal fat stranding are absent.

Grade IIa: Internal enhancement of the esophageal mucosa and hypodense aspect of the esophageal wall which appears thickened while concomitant enhancement of the outer esophageal wall may sometimes confer a "target" aspect.

Grade IIb: Fine rim of external wall enhancement, the necrotic mucosa does not enhance and fills the esophageal lumen which shows liquid density.

Grade III: Absence of post-contrast wall enhancement.

Management

- Maintenance of airway, hemodynamic stabilization
- Broad-spectrum antibiotics

Avoidance of: (i) Induced emesis (emesis causes second insult to the esophagus); (ii) Neutralizing agents (exothermic reaction causes further damage); and (iii) Ingestion of milk or activated charcoal (endoscopic evaluation is impaired due to coating of the mucosa with milk or contrast).

Management of esophageal caustic injuries as per CT evaluation (based on WSES guideline):

Grade I: Feeding can be started immediately, patient may be discharged within 24–48 hours. Risk of stricture formation is nil. Long-term followup is not indicated.

Grade IIa: Oral feeding can be started as soon as patient can swallow. Risk of stricture formation is low (<20%). Long-term followup is recommended (after 4–6 months).

Grade IIb: Total parenteral nutrition or feeding jejunostomy is indicated. Risk of stricture formation is high (>80%). Long-term followup is recommended (after 4–6 months).

Grade III (transmural necrosis): Emergency surgery

Management of complications:
Esophageal stricture:

- Endoscopic dilation (with Savary bougies or balloon dilators) is the first line of management. Dilation (preferably with Savary bougies) should be attempted 3–6 weeks after injury and interval between dilations should be between 1 and 3 weeks.
- Esophageal reconstruction (gastric conduit or colonic interposition graft) should be considered if: (i) Failure to achieve satisfactory patency after 5–7 attempts; (ii) Patient refused serial dilations; and (iii) Perforation during dilation.
- There is no clear supporting data regarding the use of intraluminal stenting.

Gastric outlet obstruction:

- Obstruction may develop after a few days up to 6 years after injury. Endoscopic balloon dilation is an effective treatment option for short strictures (<2.5 cm).
- Surgery (pyloroplasty or gastrojejunostomy) should be considered at least 3 months after injury. Gastrojejunostomy is a better surgical option.

Zarger Endoscopic Classification of Caustic Injuries

Grade 0: Normal

Grade 1: Superficial mucosal edema and erythema

Grade 2: Mucosal and submucosal ulcerations

Grade 2a: Superficial ulcerations, erosions, exudates

Grade 2b: Deep discrete or circumferential ulcerations

Grade 3: Transmural ulcerations with necrosis

Grade 3a: Focal necrosis

Grade 3b: Extensive necrosis

Grade 4: Perforations

Principles of Emergency Surgery in Caustic Injuries

- Esophagectomy with gastric preservation for isolated esophageal transmural necrosis.
- Total gastrectomy with preservation of esophagus for isolated stomach necrosis.
- Stripping esophagectomy with gastrectomy for transmural necrosis of both esophagus and stomach.
- Extended resection is indicated for necrosis of adjacent organs.
- Resection should be abandoned if massive intestinal necrosis is found at laparotomy.
- Feeding jejunostomy should be considered after the definitive surgical procedure.

Characteristic Features of Esophageal Caustic Strictures

- Long (>2 cm)
- Irregular
- Angulated
- Multiple
- Longer "remodeling time" (6 months to 3 years)

Foreign Body Ingestion

Esophageal perforation is a life-threatening emergency.

Clinical Presentation

- Foreign body ingestion is more common in **pediatric population.** In adults, **accidental foreign body ingestion** is associated with alcohol intoxication, elderly population or patients with psychiatric disorders. **Intentional foreign body ingestion** may be found in prisoners seeking secondary gain.
- **Food bolus impaction commonly develop in patients with certain esophageal pathologies.**
- Impaction, obstruction or perforation may develop at the sites of **physiological narrowing of alimentary tract** following foreign body ingestion.
- **Types of foreign bodies:**
  - Sharp, pointed objects—Fish bone, meat bone, toothpick, open safety pin, pin, and nail
  - Short, blunt objects—Coins and buttons
  - Long objects—Pen, pencil, toothbrush, dental appliance Magnets, and batteries
  - Illicit drug packets—Illicit drugs wrapped in plastic bags or latex condoms.

Clinical Presentation

- **Classic clinical presentation** of esophageal foreign body impaction is acute onset of dysphagia or inability to swallow saliva. Other clinical features are odynophagia, retrosternal pain, sore throat, foreign body sensation, retching, vomiting, drooling. Choking, stridor, dyspnea may present as a result of aspiration of saliva or tracheal compression by foreign body.
- **Clinical signs of complete esophageal obstruction:** (i) Hypersalivation and (ii) Inability to swallow liquids.
- **On clinical examination,** presence of fever, tachycardia, subcutaneous emphysema, swelling of neck or chest are highly suggestive of esophageal perforation. Clinical evaluation is also necessary to exclude small-bowel obstruction and peritonitis.

Diagnosis

- **X-ray of neck, chest and abdomen** is a useful imaging modality to assess the presence, location, shape, size and number of radiopaque objects. Biplanar radiography reduces the false-negative rate. Food bolus, fish or chicken bone, plastic, glass, wood are not readily seen in X-ray.
- **CT scan** provides better anatomic information and particularly indicated in patients with suspected perforation or other complications that may require surgery.
- **Contrast swallow (barium or gastrograffin)** is not recommended due to risk of aspiration and coating of the foreign body and mucosa interferes with endoscopic evaluation.

Sites of Physiological Narrowing

- Upper esophageal sphincter
- At the level of aortic arch and left main stem bronchus
- Lower esophageal sphincter
- Pylorus
- Duodenal sweep
- Ileocecal valve
- Anus

- **Duodenal sweep** is a physiological angulation. Objects longer than 5–6 cm cannot pass through the duodenal sweep.
- Objects diameter >2–2.5 cm cannot pass through the pylorus or ileocecal valve

Esophageal Pathologies Associated with Food Bolus Impaction

- Peptic stricture
- Eosinophilic esophagitis
- Esophageal cancer
- Achalasia
- Nutcracker esophagus
- Radiation-induced stricture
- Zenker's diverticulum

Complications of Impacted Foreign Body in Esophagus

- Perforation
- Perforation with mediastinitis
- Retropharyngeal abscess
- Aorto-esophageal fistula

Treatment

- **Most of the esophageal foreign bodies are best managed by flexible endoscopy.** The timing of endoscopic intervention depends on patient's clinical condition, size, shape and location of the foreign body and time since ingestion.
- **For esophageal food bolus impaction**, the recommended procedure is push technique (gently pushing the bolus into the stomach).
- **Other foreign bodies** need endoscopic retrieval.
- **Surgery is indicated** for irretrievable foreign body, perforation and other complications (mediastinitis, pleural empyema, aortoesophageal fistula).
- **Different surgical approaches are:** (i) Removal of foreign body by esophagotomy followed by primary closure; (ii) Thoracotomy (right or left); and (iii) Rescue esophagectomy with primary or delayed reconstruction.

  The surgical approach depends upon location of foreign body, type of complication, degree of contamination and patient's general condition.

Timing of Therapeutic Flexible Endoscopy and their Indications

Emergent endoscopy (preferably within 2 hours, at latest within 6 hours)

- Food bolus impaction with complete esophageal obstruction
- Sharp-pointed objects
- Disk battery ingestion
- Magnet ingestion

Urgent endoscopy (within 24 hours)

- Other esophageal foreign bodies without complete obstruction

Nonurgent endoscopy (within 72 hours)

- Coins in the esophagus
- Foreign body in stomach with diameter >2.5 cm
- Disk and cylindrical batteries in stomach without any signs of GI injury.

Barrett Esophagus

Definition: "Presence of at least 1 cm of metaplastic columnar epithelium that replaces the stratified squamous epithelium normally lining the distal esophagus." [adapted from ACG guideline]. It is a complication of long standing GERD. Barrett's esophagus (BE) is a premalignant condition and a major risk factor for esophageal adenocarcinoma.

Risk Factors for Barrett's Esophagus

- Long standing GERD >5 years
- Age >50 years
- Male gender
- Tobacco usage
- Central obesity
- Family history of BE.

Factors Associated with Decreased Risk of BE

- *H. pylori* infection (particularly with CagA+ strains)
- Use of NSAIDs and statins.

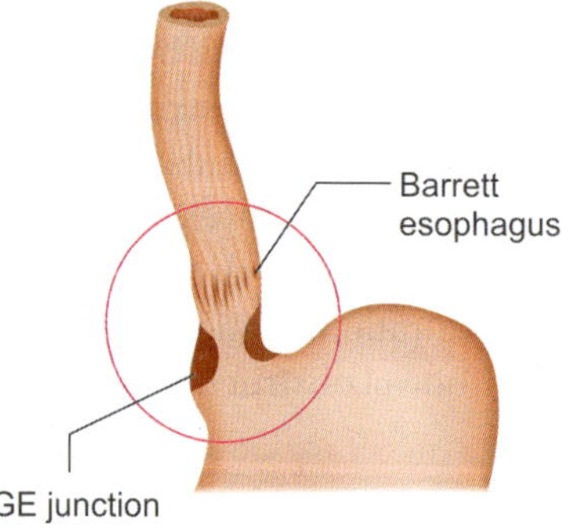

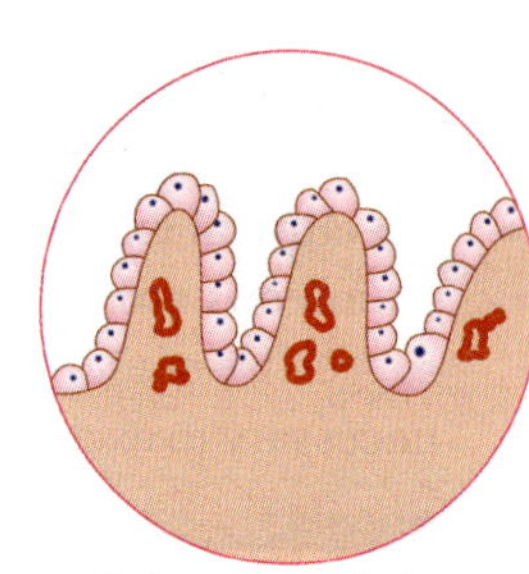

Risk Factors for the Development of Esophageal Adenocarcinoma in BE

- Advancing age
- Male gender
- Central obesity
- Longer duration of BE (>10 years)
- Long-segment Barrett.

Based on length of Barrett Epithelium, Barrett's esophagus is classified into:

- Long-segment BE (≥3 cm)
- Short-segment BE (≥1 to <3 cm)
- Ultra-short segment BE (<1 cm)

Screening for BE

Screening recommendations for Barrett's esophagus (as per ACG guidelines):

In male: Chronic (>5 years) and/or frequent (weekly or more) symptoms of gastroesophageal reflux (heartburn or acid regurgitation) along with two or more risk factors for Barrett's esophagus or esophageal adenocarcinoma [age >50 years, Caucasian race, central obesity (waist circumference >102 cm or waist-hip ratio >0.9), current or past history of smoking, confirmed family history of BE or EAC (in a first-degree relative)].

Screening for BE in females is not recommended.

Standard-definition white light endoscopy is recommended for screening of BE.

Diagnosis of BE

BE is diagnosed by recognition of extension of salmon-colored mucosa into the tubular esophagus extending ≥1 cm proximal to the gastroesophageal junction **with biopsy confirmation of intestinal metaplasia. At least 8 random biopsies** should be obtained.

Surveillance of BE

The goal of surveillance of BE is to early detection of dysplasia.

High-definition white light endoscopy is recommended for surveillance of BE. Routine use of advanced imaging techniques other than electronic chromoendoscopy is not recommended.

Endoscopic surveillance includes inspection of the Barrett segment, four-quadrant biopsies at 2 cm intervals and sampling of mucosal abnormalities with EMR.

Management of BE

- **Nondysplastic BE:** Repeat endoscopy with biopsies with interval of 3–5 years
- **Indefinite for dysplasia:** Repeat endoscopy after optimization of acid suppressive therapy for 3-6 months
- **Low-grade dysplasia and high-grade dysplasia:** Endoscopic eradication therapy.
- **Surgery is reserved for** high-grade dysplasia with nodularity or long-segment involvement.

The Prague classification: Endoscopic assessment of circumferential extent (C) and maximal extent (M) of BE segment.

Based on degree of dysplasia, BE is classified into:

- Nondysplastic
- Indefinite for dysplasia
- Low-grade dysplasia
- High-grade dysplasia

Advanced Endoscopic Imaging Techniques for Barrett's Esophagus

- Electronic chromoendoscopy
- Narrow band imaging
- Autofluorescence endoscopy
- Confocal laser endomicroscopy
- Volumetric laser endomicroscopy

WATS3D (wide-area transepithelial sampling with computer-assisted 3D analysis) is a new technique of detection of high-grade dysplasia/adenocarcinoma in patients with Barrett's esophagus. This technique includes an abrasive brush biopsy of the BE mucosa with computer-assisted pathological analysis.

Endoscopic Eradication Therapy

Endoscopic resection:

- Endoscopic mucosal resection (EMR)
- Serial radical endoscopic resection (SRER)
- Endoscopic submucosal dissection (ESD)

Endoscopic mucosal ablation:

- Radiofrequency ablation
- Photodynamic therapy
- Argon plasma coagulation
- Cryoablation

Esophageal Carcinoma

- Esophagus is a unique organ because it covers three anatomic compartments: Neck, thorax and abdomen.
- Esophageal cancer is unique among GI malignancies because it may present two distinct histopathologic varieties, squamous cell carcinoma and adenocarcinoma.
- Squamous cell carcinoma is most common in Eastern Europe and Asia. Adenocarcinoma is most common in North America and Western Europe.

Risk Factors

Tobacco and alcohol use:

- Tobacco use and alcohol consumption are independent risk factors for squamous cell carcinoma.
- Tobacco use is also a risk factor for adenocarcinoma. Quiting smoking decrease the risk of squamous cell carcinoma, but not the risk of adenocarcinoma.
- Alcohol is an independent risk factor for squamous cell carcinoma. Amount of alcohol, type of beverage have relationship with risk. No risk of adenocarcinoma in use of alcohol.

Dietary factors:

- Deficiency of vitamins (A, C, E)
- Deficiency of trace metals (zinc, molybdenum, selenium)
- Fungal contamination of foods
- Presence of nitrosamines and their precursors (nitrate, nitrite).

Esophageal disorders:

GERD: One of the strongest risk factors of adenocarcinoma

Barrett esophagus: Single most important risk factor for adenocarcinoma

Tylosis: An autosomal dominant disorder characterized by hyperkeratosis of palm, sole and esophageal papilloma.

Plummer-Vinson syndrome: Characterized by iron-deficiency anemia, glossitis, cheilitis, splenomegaly and esophageal webs. [About 10% of patient develop esophageal epidermoid carcinoma.]

Corrosive stricture: Squamous cell carcinoma may develop after lye stricture, usually 40–50 years after injury

Achalasia: 16–30 fold increased risk of developing squamous cell carcinoma.

H. pylori (particulary CagA+ strain) infection may have a protective role in development of SCC in East Asian populations.

Risk Factors for Adenocarcinoma

- Barrett esophagus (30–60 times greater risk)
- Long standing GERD
- Male gender
- High BMI (≥30 kg/m^2)
- Smoking
- Familial Barrett esophagus

Risk Factors for Squamous Cell Carcinoma

- Tobacco and alcohol consumption
- History of aerodigestive cancer
- History of caustic injury
- Diets high in N-nitrosamines and pickled vegetables
- Achalasia
- Tylosis
- Bloom syndrome
- Fanconi anemia

Hereditary cancer predisposition syndromes associated with increased risk for esophageal and esophagogastric junction cancers:

- Tylosis (focal nonepidermolytic palmoplantar keratoderma)
- Bloom syndrome
- Fanconi anemia
- Familial Barrett's esophagus.

Pathology

- Histologically, esophageal cancer is classified into **squamous cell carcinoma** and **adenocarcinoma**.
- **Squamous cell carcinoma usually affects** the upper two-thirds (cervical, upper and middle third of thoracic esophagus). **Adenocarcinoma affects the lower one-third**.
- **SCC is associated with more risk of lymphatic spread and poorer prognosis.**

Classification of Esophageal Tumors

Siewart type I: EGJ tumors with epicenter located within 1 cm to 5 cm above the anatomic EGJ

Siewart type II: True carcinoma of the cardia with tumor epicentre within 1 cm above and 2 cm below the EGJ. **Siewart type I and II tumors are treated as esophageal adenocarcinoma.**

Siewart type III: Subcardial carcinoma with tumor epicenter between 2 and 5 cm below the EGJ. **This type of tumor is treated as per guideline of gastric cancer.**

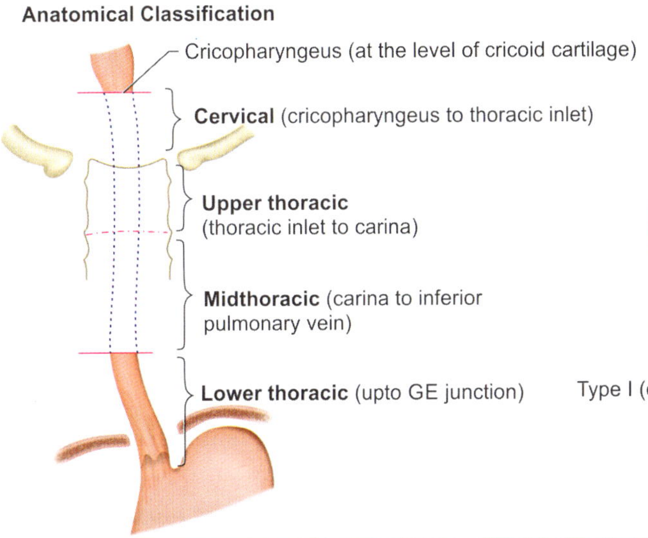

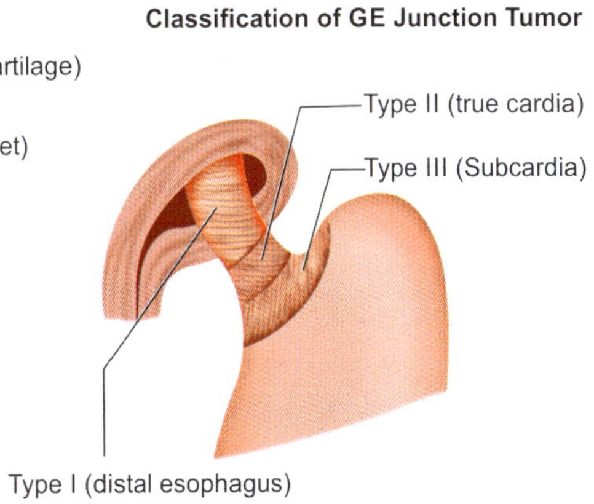

Anatomical Classification

Classification of GE Junction Tumor

Clinical Presentation

- **Most commonly present** with progressive dysphagia (initially difficulty in swallowing solids, then liquids and lastly saliva), weight loss and odynophagia.
- **Symptoms of local invasion and distant metastases**—Odynophagia, dull retrosternal pain, cough, hoarseness of voice. **Unusual presentation** include pneumonia (due to tracheoesophageal fistula), exsanguinating hemorrhage (due to aortic invasion).

Diagnosis

- **Flexible upper GI endoscopy with endoscopy guided biopsy** is the preferred initial diagnostic modality in patients with dysphagia and weight loss. Endoscopy provides information about the location, length, percentage of circumferential involvement, gross morphology of the lesion, location in relation to incisor and EGJ. Multiple biopsies (six or more) should be taken to achieve high sensitivity (96–100%).
- **Barium esophagogram (Barium swallow)** must be the initial study in any patient with dysphagia where GI endoscopy facility is not available. This imaging modality is helpful to differentiate whether the lesion is intraluminal or extraluminal the classic **'apple-core lesion'** is highly suggestive. This modality is also helpful to assess the distal extent of the when standard endoscope cannot be negotiated.
- **Endoscopic ultrasonography (EUS)** should be considered as a diagnostic tool where suspicion of esophageal carcinoma is high, but biopsy or brush cytology is inconclusive.

- **In tight malignant stricture,** standard endoscope cannot be negotiated. **Transoral or transnasal ultrathin endoscope is** helpful to assess the extent and length of the tumor. **Barium study** may also considered to assess the distal extent of the tumor.
- **Brush cytology** is also indicated in tight malignant stricture because conventional biopsy is technically not feasible.

High-resolution endoscopy and **advanced endoscopic imaging techniques** (e.g., narrow-band imaging) are useful to detect early lesions.

Staging

Staging is crucial for selecting the most appropriate treatment option. Staging is for determination of—(i) Extent of disease; (ii) Depth of esophageal wall involved; (iii) Regional lymph node status; and (iv) Presence or absence of distant metastases.

CT scan of chest, abdomen and pelvis with oral and IV contrast is indicated to evaluate the distant metastatic disease and lymph node involvement. This imaging can detect liver and lung metastases and also highly accurate for detection of aortic and tracheobronchial involvement.

Endoscopic ultrasonography (EUS) is highly accurate in both T and N staging and is superior to CT. EUS has high sensitivity for detecting lymph node metastases in comparison to CT and FDG-PET/CT. Biopsy can be taken from the tumor mass as well as from the lymph node.

FDG–PET: The accuracy in assessing regional lymph nodal status is superior than CT, but not so accurate like EUS. This imaging modality is superior to CT in detecting distant metastases. PET/CT is particularly indicated when CT and EUS reveal regional invasive tumor but no distant metastases. FDG-PT/CT is also a useful modality for evaluating response to chemo and radiotherapy.

Bronchoscopy is indicated for tumors in upper and middle esophagus to rule out involvement of membranous trachea and tracheoesophageal fistula.

HER2, MSI-H (microsatellite instability-high), dMMR (deficient mismatch repair), and PD-L1 (Programmed death-ligand 1) should be assessed in all esophageal or EGJ cancer patients if metastatic disease is documented or suspected.

Treatment

- **High-grade dysplasia and T1 disease (intramucosal carcinoma):** Endoscopic therapy.
- **Localized respectable disease (T1-2, N0):** In patients with respectable esophageal cancer (>5 cm from cricopharyngeal), esophagectomy is the primary treatment.

  In patients with cervical or cervicothoracic esophageal cancers <5 cm from the cricopharyngeal, chemoradiation is the primary treatment.
- **Locally advanced disease (T1-3, N1):** Preoperative chemoradiation (paclitaxel, carboplatin), then resection.
- **Treatment of metastatic disease (any T, any N, M1):** Palliation and targeted therapy.

Role of targeted therapy in locally advanced and metastatic cancer:

- **Trastuzumab** is indicated for HER2-positive, locally advanced or metastatic esophageal and EGJ cancers.
- **Ramucirumab (VEGFR-2 antibody)** is indicated for locally advanced gastric or EGJ adenocarcinoma refractory or progressive following first-line chemotherapy with platinum-or fluoropyrimidine-based chemotherapy.
- **Pembrolizumab (Monoclonal PD-1 antibody)** is indicated for unresectable or metastatic MSI-H or dMMR tumors that have progressed following first-line treatment. It is also indicated for recurrent, locally advanced, or metastatic PD-L1-positive (CPS ≥1) gastric or EGJ adenocarcinoma who have progressed after two or more lines of therapy.

Endoscopic therapy includes endoscopic resection and endoscopic ablation.

Techniques of endoscopic resection are EMR and ESD.

Techniques of endoscopic ablation are: (i) Radiofrequency ablation; (ii) Photodynamic therapy; (iii) Cryotherapy; and (iv) Argon plasma coagulation.

Principles of Esophagectomy

Two most common surgical approaches are: (i) Transthoracic esophagectomy and (ii) Transhiatal esophagectomy.

Transthoracic esophagectomy is either Ivor Lewis esophagectomy or McKeown esophagectomy. **Minimally invasive esophagectomy (MIE) approaches are:** (i) Minimally invasive Ivor Lewis esophagectomy and (ii) Minimally invasive McKeown esophagectomy.

At least 15 lymph nodes must be resected during esophagectomy for adequate nodal staging. Among **gastric conduit** or **colon interposition**, gastric conduit is the preferred esophageal reconstruction approach.

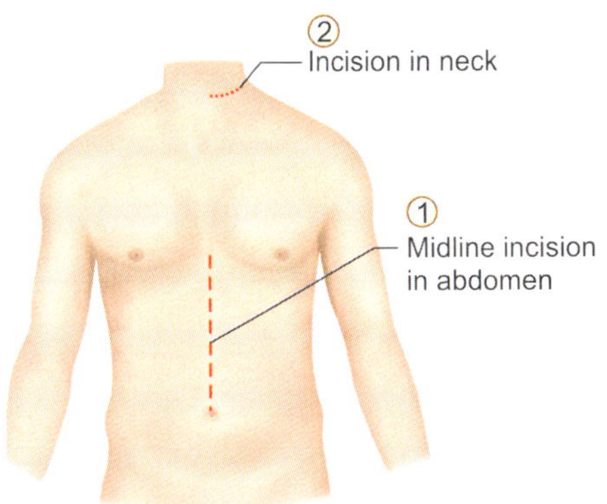

Transhiatal Esophagectomy

- This surgical approach is performed through **laparotomy** and **left cervical incision**.
- The esophagectomy and creation of gastric conduit are completed through the **abdominal incision**. Gastric conduit is exteriorized in the **cervical incision** for esophagogastric anastomosis.
- **This approach is used for tumors in any location of esophagus.**

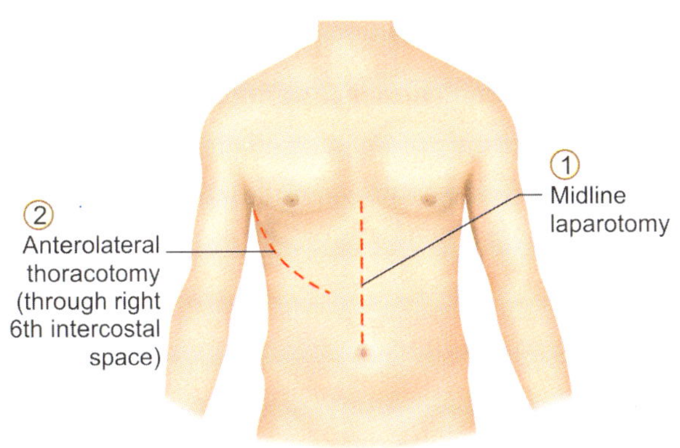

Ivor Lewis Esophagectomy

- This surgical approach is performed through **right anterolateral thoracotomy and laparotomy**.
- **Through laparotomy approach**, Lymph node dissection around celiac trunk and its branches, around porta hepatis and along the splenic artery, along lesser curvature of stomach along with creation of gastric conduit are performed.
- **Through thoracotomy approach**, lymph node dissection of peribronchial, hilar and tracheal lymph nodal basins, pulling up of gastric conduit into the thorax and upper thoracic esophagogastric anastomosis is done.

This technique is used mainly for tumors in upper thoracic esophagus.

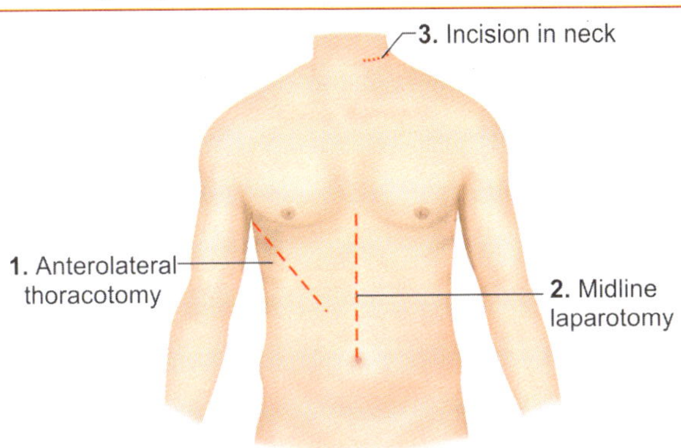

McKeown Esophagectomy

- This surgical approach is performed through **right thoracotomy** followed by **laparotomy** and **cervical anastomosis**. Thoracic esophageal mobilization, lymph node dissection is performed through **right anterolateral thoracotomy**.
- **Through laparotomy**, lymph node dissection along with creation of gastric conduit is performed.
- Esophagogastric anastomosis is done through **left neck incision**. This technique is used for tumors in any location of esophagus.

Minimally Invasive Esophagectomy

Minimally invasive esophagectomy (MIE) includes:

- **Minimally invasive Ivor Lewis esophagectomy** (laparoscopy and limited right thoracotomy)
- **Minimally invasive McKeown esophagectomy** (right thoracoscopy, limited laparotomy/laparoscopy, cervical anastomosis)
- **Relative contraindications of MIE esophagectomy:** (i) Previous abdominal surgery and (ii) Bulky tumor.

Advantages of Cervical Anastomosis

- Thoracotomy can be avoided.
- Anastomotic leakage related complications are less severe.
- Less severe symptoms of reflux.

Advantages of Thoracic Anastomosis

- Lower stricture rate.
- Lower incidence of anastomotic leakage.
- Less chance of recurrent nerve injury.

Palliative Therapy

- **Dysphagia:** Endoscopic tumor ablation, placement of self-expanding metal stent (SEMS)
- **Obstruction:** Wire-guided dilation or balloon dilation, fully or partially covered SEMS, EBRT.

  Feeding access through endoscopic or radiographic-assisted feeding jejunostomy or gastrostomy is necessary if endoscopic lumen restoration is not feasible.

Esophageal Stenting

Types of stents: (i) Self-expandable metal stent (Fully covered SEMS, partially covered SEMS and uncovered SEMS); (ii) Self-expandable plastic stent (SEPS); and (iii) Biodegradable.

Indications:

- **Benign**—(i) Refractory benign stricture; (ii) Iatrogenic perforation; (iii) Benign rupture of esophagus (Boerhaave's syndrome); (iv) Anastomotic leak; and (v) Acute variceal bleeding (refractory to medical or endoscopic therapy)
- **Malignant:** (i) Malignant tracheoesophageal fistula; (ii) Malignant bronchoesophageal fistula; and (iii) As palliative therapy in esophageal cancer.

Complications of stenting: (i) Perforation; (ii) Aspiration pneumonia; (iii) Stent migration; and (iv) Tissue in/overgrowth.

Case 1

History and Physical Examination

A 50-year-old male patient presented with dysphagia to solid foods for last 6 months. Patient was suffering from gastroesophageal reflux disease (GERD) for last 6 years and irregularly taking medications. No history of loss of appetite but weight loss in last 3 months. No history of hematemesis or melena.

Physical Examination

No significant clinical findings.

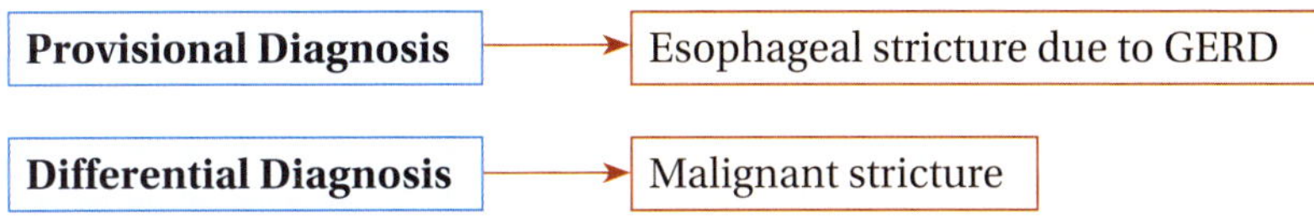

Investigations

Upper GI endoscopy revealed a short, symmetric stricture of 50% of the lumen in lower third of esophagus.

Discussion

A 50-year-old male patient presented with dysphagia to solid foods for last 6 months who had a history of GERD for 6 years. These history suggestive of peptic stricture, but malignant stricture was also a possibility. Upper GI endoscopy revealed a short, symmetric stricture that ruled out malignant stricture. Dilation with bougies was planned.

Management Algorithm

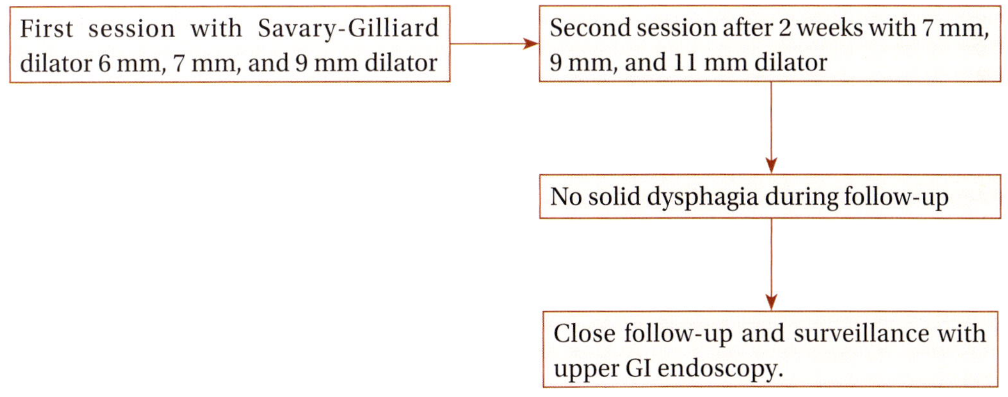

Case 2

History and Physical Examination

A 6-year-old boy admitted in the pediatric surgery emergency ward with history of ingestion of disc battery of toys about 4 hours back. No history of difficulty in swallowing or breathing difficulty.

Physical Examination

- Patient alert, conscious, cooperative
- Vital parameters were stable
- Examination of chest and abdomen were normal.

Investigations

Plain X-ray of chest and abdomen (in erect posture) revealed a round-shaped radiopaque shadow in the area of lower esophagus.

Discussion

The foreign body, disc battery remains in the lower part of esophagus after 4 hours of ingestion. This foreign body may cause esophageal erosion or even perforation by chemical injury. So, decision of urgent upper GI endoscopy and retrieval of foreign body was taken.

Management Algorithm

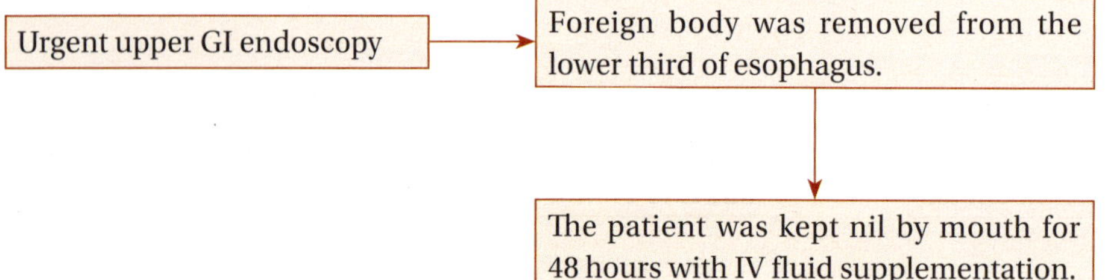

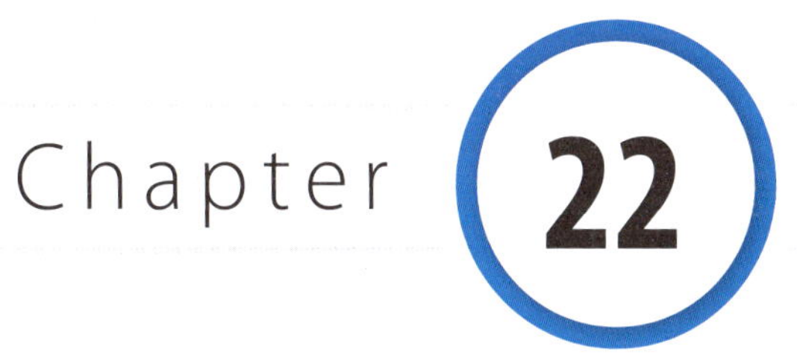

Diseases of the Salivary Gland

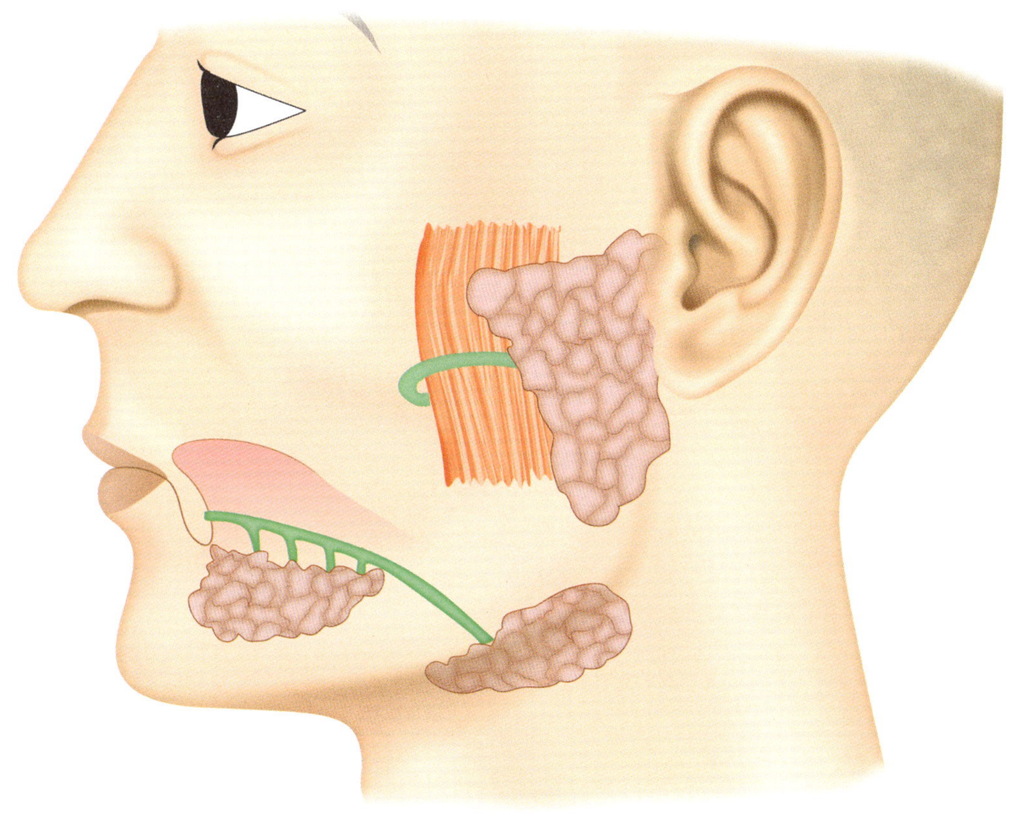

Important Topics

- Surgical Anatomy of the Salivary Glands
- Sialadenitis
- Sialolithiasis
- Ranula
- Salivary Gland Tumors
- Surgical Procedures

'Education is what remains after one has forgotten everything he learned in school.'

- **Major salivary glands consist of:** Paired parotid, submandibular and sublingual glands.
- **Minor salivary glands** are present all over the oral mucosa, mucosa of the lips, oropharynx, larynx, trachea.

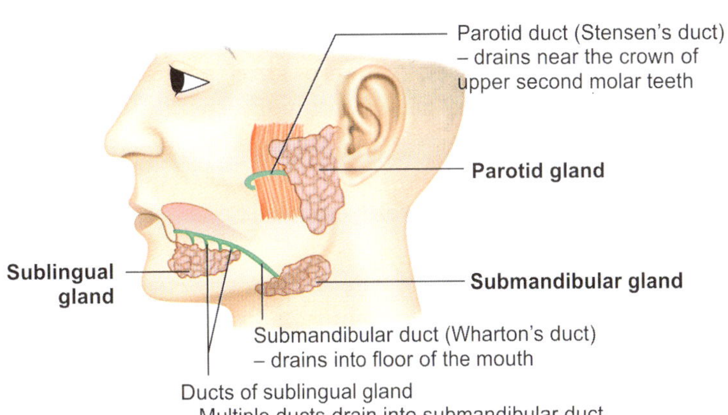

Duct of Parotid Gland (Stensen's Duct)

- Length: 5 cm
- Drains opposite the upper second molar crown.
- **Socia parotidis:** Occasional islets of parotid tissue, separated from main parotid gland, lying anteriorly just above the commencement of the parotid duct.

Duct of Submandibular Gland (Wharton's Duct)

- Length: 5 cm
- Drains in the floor of the mouth on the summit of the sublingual papilla at the side of the frenulum of the tongue.

Ducts of Sublingual Gland (Ducts of Rivinus)

- 8–20 excretory ducts drain separately onto the summit of sublingual fold.
- **The largest excretory duct called the Bartholin's duct** drains into the Wharton's duct near the sublingual caruncle.

Submandibular Triangle

Boundaries: *Anteriorly*—Anterior belly of the digastric muscle; *Superiorly*—Inferior border of the body of the mandible and mylohyoid; *Inferiorly*—Posterior belly of the digastric; *Posteriorly*—Posterior border of the submandibular gland.

Contents: (i) Submandibular gland with Wharton duct; (ii) Lingual nerve and submandibular ganglion; and (iii) Hypoglossal nerve.

Sublingual Space

Boundaries: *Anteriorly and laterally*—Mandible; *Superiorly*—Mucosa of the floor of mouth; *Inferiorly*—Mylohyoid muscle. Mylohyoid muscle separates the submandibular triangle from sublingual space.

Contents: (i) Sublingual gland; (ii) Hypoglossal nerve; and (iii) Deep part of the submandibular gland.

Diseases of the Salivary Gland
- **Inflammatory pathology**
- **Obstructive pathology**
- **Neoplastic pathology**

Most Common Site

- **Pleomorphic adenoma:** Parotid gland
- **Sialolithiasis:** Submandibular gland
- **Ranula:** Sublingual gland

Viral Sialadenitis

- Most commonly caused by **mumps virus (a paramyxovirus)**
- May affect all salivary glands but predominantly affects both **parotid glands**. Mumps parotitis commonly affects children younger than 15 years.
- **Patient commonly presents** with bilateral tender parotid swelling, otalgia, trismus
- **Diagnosis** is confirmed by viral serology
- **Complications** include orchitis, oophoritis, meningitis, encephalitis, pancreatitis, hearing loss.
- Mumps parotitis is a self-limiting disease. Treatment is mainly symptomatic (anti-inflammatory agents, adequate hydration, maintenance of oral hygiene).

Viruses Causing Sialadenitis

- Paramyxovirus (most common)
- Epstein-Barr virus
- Coxsackievirus
- Influenza A virus
- Parainfluenza virus
- HIV virus

Characteristic Features of HIV-associated Sialadenitis

- Diffuse, nontender, multiple cystic enlargement of major salivary glands
- Most commonly involved is parotid gland
- 'Swiss cheese' appearance in CT and MRI.

Acute Bacterial Sialadenitis

Acute bacterial sialadenitis most commonly affects one of the major salivary glands, most commonly the parotid. It commonly develops in medically debilitated or postoperative patients.

Pathophysiology: Stasis of the salivary flow due to dehydration, decreased oral intake in postoperative period leads to bacterial colonization in the oral cavity, resulting in retrograde migration of infection into the gland parenchyma.

Predisposing factors: Diabetes mellitus, medications (causing decreased salivary secretion), duct stricture.

Causative organisms: *Staphylococcus aureus* (most common), *Streptococcal* spp., *Hemophilus influenzae*

Clinical presentation: Patients present with acute pain and swelling of the affected gland along with fever and regional lymphadenopathy. Intraoral examination may reveal pus coming out from the parotid duct orifice.

Investigation: USG shows characteristic dilation of the acini.

Treatment: Treatment includes antimicrobial therapy against gram-positive and anaerobic organisms, administration of sialagogues, hydration, maintenance of oral hygiene. Incision and drainage is indicated if abscess develops.

Chronic Sialadenitis

Chronic sialadenitis most commonly affects the submandibular gland.

Pathophysiology: Salivary duct obstruction due to stones, strictures, tumor resulting in recurrent inflammation that leads to fibrosis of the gland parenchyma.

Clinical presentation: Patients present with enlarged gland with mild tenderness. The swelling may appear during eating. Bimanual examination reveals a firm, tender, enlarged gland.

Investigation: Workup primarily focused on identifying the underlying causes particularly stone or stricture.

Management: Treatment depends on the etiology. If no underlying etiology is detected, treatment is conservative (e.g., sialogogues, massaging of the gland, anti-inflammatory agents). Excision of the gland is indicated in refractory cases.

Autoimmune Sialadenitis

Seen in Sjögren syndrome

Sjögren syndrome is characterized by:

- Keratoconjunctivitis sicca
- Xerostomia
- Bilateral parotid swelling
- Rheumatoid arthritis.

Stafne Bone Cyst (Stafne's Bone Cavity)

- Asymptomatic, nonprogressive, unilateral, radiolucent defect near the angle of the mandible.
- The defect is either empty or contains salivary gland tissue, adipose tissue, muscles, blood vessels.

Sialolithiasis

Sialolithiasis is the most common cause of major salivary gland swelling. **About 80% of sialolithiasis occur in the submandibular gland**, 15% in the parotid gland, rest in the minor salivary gland.

Pathophysiology: The exact pathophysiology remains unknown. Several hypothesis have been proposed include: (i) Excretion of intracellular microcalculi into the duct as a nidus for further calcification and (ii) Migration of ailments, bacteria of the oral cavity into the duct as a nidus.

Clinical presentation: Classic presentation is acute pain and appearance of swelling beneath the jaw within a minute of starting the meal; both pain and swelling resolves after the meal but the pain resolves earlier **(Mealtime syndrome)**. This classic presentation is seen only when there is complete obstruction.

On examination, a congestive ostium of the submandibular duct may be found. In early periods of obstruction, the gland is not palpable in between meals. Later, a chronically infected gland becomes palpable with rubbery hard consistency.

Bimanual examination of the floor of the mouth has to be performed along the course of the submandibular duct to search for any thickening or induration of the duct.

Investigations:

- X-ray (classic occlusal view) detects most of the submandibular ductal stones (about 80% are radiopaque).
- Ultrasonography is an useful method for diagnosis but it is highly operator dependent.
- Computed tomography is useful imaging modality only in presence of large stone.
- Sialography is the old "gold standard" diagnostic modality that can provides a clear image of the ductal stone as well as ductal morphology.
- Newer diagnostic modalities are MR sialography and sialoendoscopy.

Treatment: Conservative management includes antibiotics, anti-inflammatory agents, gland massage after meal and administration of sialogogues. Definitive management includes extracorporeal lithotripsy, interventional sialoendoscopy and surgery.

Most of the sialolithiasis occur in the submandibular gland, because:

- Secretions contain mucus and more viscous
- Gland lies below the opening of its duct
- Secretion is more alkaline (predisposes to formation of calcium and phosphate salts)

Composition of Salivary Stone

Stones are composed of organic and iorganic substances.

Organic components: Cellular debris, bacteria, glycoproteins, mucopolysaccharides

Inorganic components: Calcium carbonates, calcium phosphates.

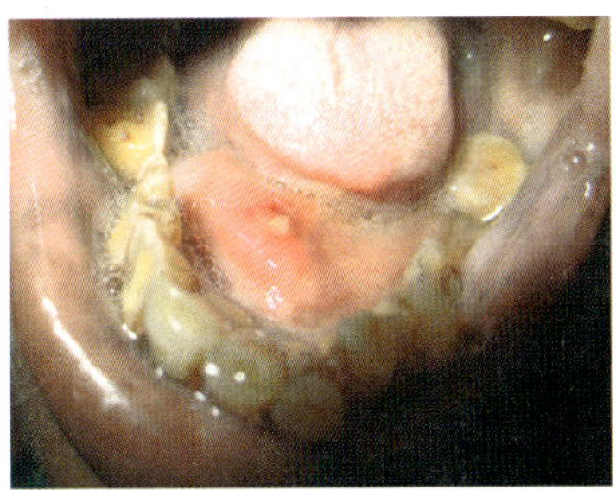

Stone in the submandibular duct (right)

Surgical Management of Submandibular Stone

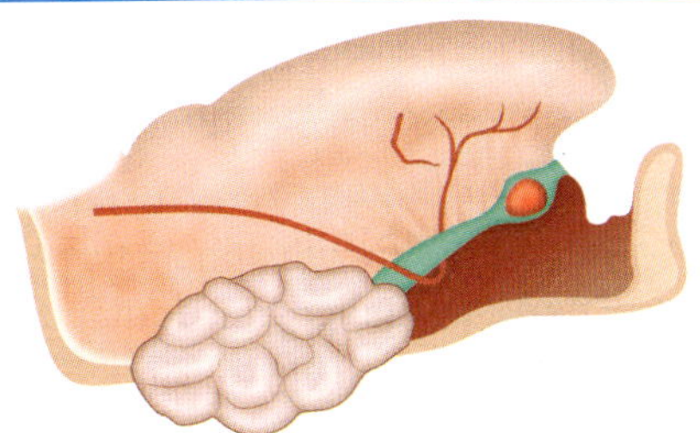

Stone in submandibular duct anterior to crossing point of lingual nerve and submandibular duct

↓

Removal of stone by incising the duct directly over the stone

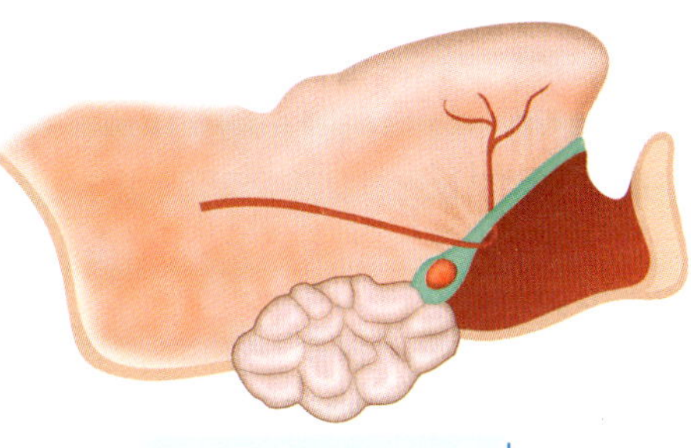

Stone lying distal to the crossing point or stone is very close to the gland

↓

Excision of submandibular gland

Mucocele (Mucus Retention Cyst)

- Mucus retention or extravasation cysts arise as a result of extravasation of salivary secretion due to damage of minor salivary gland or its ducts, most commonly following trauma
- It is a pseudocyst covered by fibrous capsule
- Most commonly present on the mucosal aspect of lower lip and in the posterior buccal mucosa
- Treatment is excision of the cyst along with underlying minor salivary glands.

Ranula

- Ranula is a large mucocele arising as a result of ruptured sublingual gland, rarely arises from submandibular gland
- Ranulas are classified as **simple and plunging ranula**
- Classically, **simple ranula presents** as large, tense, bluish, translucent, spherical swelling in the floor of the mouth.
- Occasionally, ranula extends through the mylohyoid muscle and enter the submental space, presenting as a fluctuant swelling in upper neck. This type of ranula is called **'plunging ranula'**.
- **Diagnosis** is based on classic clinical findings. **USG** is helpful if diagnosis is in doubt. **CT or MRI** is indicated in large plunging ranula to know the extent of the lesion.
- **Treatment** is excision of ranula along with the sublingual gland. Aspiration of cyst and marsupialization are not recommended due to high recurrence rate.

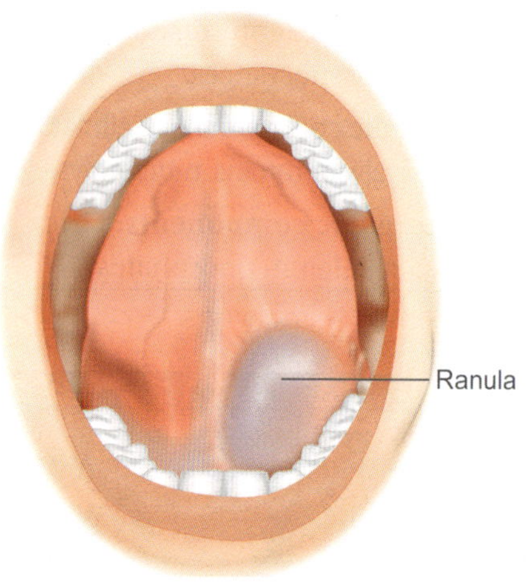

Simple Ranula

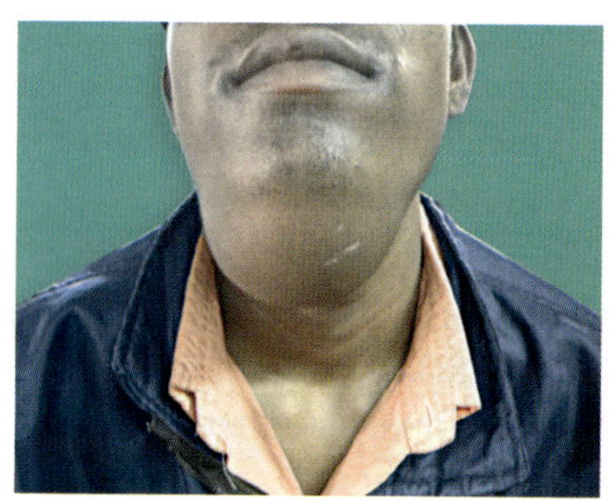

Plunging Ranula

Salivary Gland Tumors

- Tumors arise from both **major salivary glands** (parotid, submandibular and sublingual) as well as from **minor salivary glands.**
- **Majority of salivary gland tumors arise from parotid gland.**
- **Majority of parotid gland tumors** are benign (about 70–80%), **about 50% tumors of submandibular and sublingual glands** are benign, whereas **only 25% tumors arising from minor salivary glands** are benign.
- Most of the salivary gland tumors arise from ductal lining epithelium and underlying myoepithelial cells.

Clinical presentation: Parotid tumor usually present with slow growing, well-circumscribed painless swelling in the parotid region with rubbery hard consistency. Facial nerve palsy, skin invasion are suggestive of malignancy. Lymph node metastasis is uncommon in low grade salivary malignant tumor.

Submandibular and sublingual gland tumors present with slow-growing, well circumscribed, painless swelling in the neck or floor of the mouth.

Bimanual palpation is essential to evaluate the relationship of the tumor with floor of mouth, tongue and mandible.

Numbness in anterior two-thirds of the tongue suggests infiltration of the lingual nerve by malignant submandibular tumor. Level Ia, Ib, II, III groups of lymph nodes may be involved.

Minor salivary gland tumors present as painless mass in the oral cavity.

Investigations

- **CT and MRI**, both are useful imaging methods. They can define the extent of tumor, relationship of tumor to adjacent structures, status of cervical lymph nodes. MRI is more sensitive than CT.
- **FNAC** is useful to rule out malignancy. As facial nerve sacrifice may be necessary in malignant parotid tumors, preoperative counseling is indicated when a surgeon is planning for resection of malignant tumor.
- **Androgen receptor (AR) and HER2 status** should be assessed in malignant salivary tumor with distant metastases.
- **Open surgical biopsy is contraindicated to avoid microscopic spillage of tumor cells in surrounding tissues.**

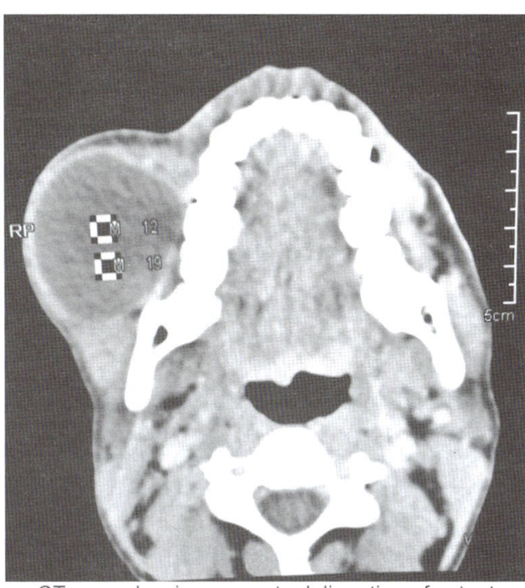

CT scan showing accurate delineation of extent and relationship of parotid tumor.

Benign Epithelial Tumors

- Pleomorphic adenoma
- Warthin tumor
- Oncocytoma
- Basal cell adenoma
- Clear cell adenoma

Low-grade Malignant Tumor

- Mucoepidermoid carcinoma
- Acinic cell carcinoma

Benign Nonepithelial Tumors

- Neural sheath tumor
- Hemangioma
- Lipoma
- Lymphangioma

High-grade Malignant Tumor

- Adenoid cystic carcinoma
- Adenocarcinoma
- Squamous cell carcinoma
- Undifferentiated carcinoma

Incidence of malignant salivary tumor:

- Parotid gland (about 20%)
- Submandibular gland (50%)
- Minor salivary glands (80%).

Mucoepidermoid carcinoma is the most common malignant tumor of parotid gland.

Adenoid cystic carcinoma is the most common malignant tumor of submandibular gland.

Pleomorphic Adenoma

- Pleomorphic adenoma is the **most common salivary gland tumor** as well as **most common benign salivary neoplasm**. It is **most commonly affects the parotid gland**, rarely develops in submandibular gland and minor salivary gland.
- Pleomorphic adenoma contains mesenchymal, epithelial and myxoid stromal components, that is why termed as **'pleomorphic' or benign mixed tumor**.
- It is a well demarcated **encapsulated lesion with incomplete capsule**. The tumor has **projections** that protrude beyond the capsule through the defects.
  [**This feature limits the scope of enucleation of the tumor and warrants excision of the involved lobe of the gland.**]
- This tumor develops at any age with equal male:female ratio.
- About two-third of parotid tumors and half of submandibular tumors are pleomorphic adenoma. Pleomorphic adenoma commonly affects the **superficial lobe of the parotid gland**.
- A slow growing, painless smooth mass with rubbery hard consistency, present in the typical site—**between angle of mandible and mastoid process** and usually causes eversion of the ear lobule. Tumor involving the deep lobe of the parotid gland presents as retrotonsillar or parapharyngeal mass.
- Rarely, this tumor may undergo malignant change (Carcinoma ex pleomorphic adenoma). This tumor is susceptible to **recurrence**.
- **Fine needle aspiration (FNA)** or core needle biopsy is required for tissue diagnosis. CT or MRI is particularly useful to define the extent of tumor, relationship of tumor to adjacent structures.
- Treatment is **superficial parotidectomy** if only superficial lobe of parotid is involved. **Total parotidectomy with preservation of facial nerve** is indicated if both lobes are involved.

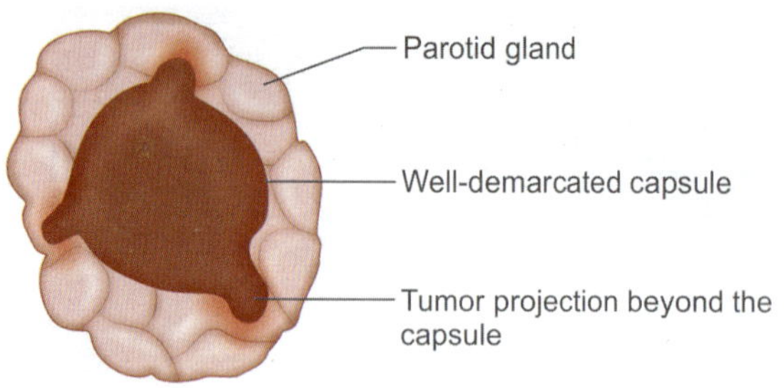

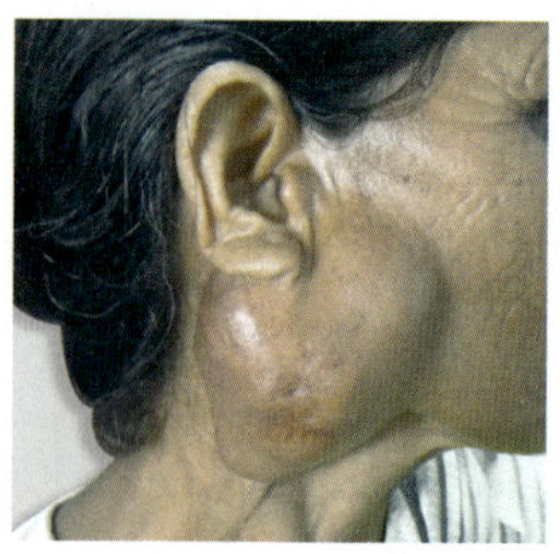
Recurrent parotid tumor.

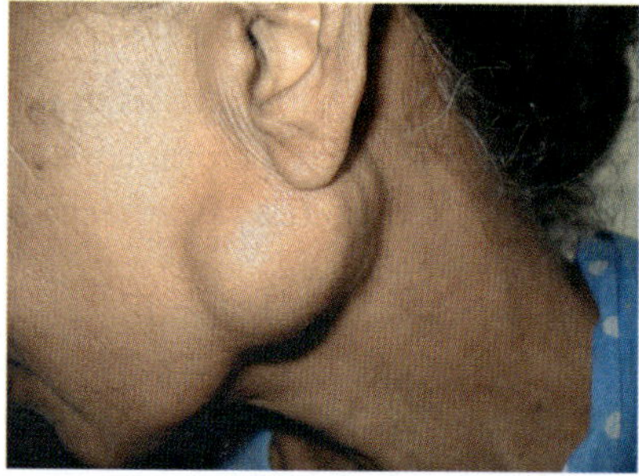
Left-sided parotid tumor (note the typical position).

Carcinoma ex Pleomorphic Adenoma

A high-grade salivary carcinoma arising due to malignant transformation of benign pleomorphic adenoma. Most commonly develops in parotid gland, rarely in submandibular gland.

Warthin's Tumor (Adenolymphoma)

- It is the **second most common benign tumor** of the salivary gland. It develops **only in the parotid gland**.
- A tumor of elderly population with a **male:female ratio 4:1**. Warthin tumor has **an association with history of smoking. Bilateral involvement** may found in 10–15% patients.
- This tumor contains two components:
  1. Epithelial element (originated from embryonic parotid ducts which have separated from main ductal system)
  2. Lymphoid element (originated from normal lymph tissues).
- Usually develops in the **lower part of the parotid gland**, level with the lower border of the mandible, **does not cause eversion of the ear lobule**, painless and soft in consistency.
- Malignant transformation is rare.

Mucoepidermoid Carcinoma

- It is the most common malignant salivary gland tumor.
- Adults (age 30–60 years) are more commonly affected, but it is also the most common malignant salivary tumor in pediatric population.
- Based on aggressiveness, this tumor exists in any form: Low grade and high grade. Low-grade mucoepidermoid carcinoma is composed of predominantly mucin secreting cells, whereas in high-grade tumors, epidermoid cells are more abundant.

Adenoid Cystic Carcinoma

- Second most common malignant salivary gland tumor
- This tumor has typical propensity for **perineural spread** and **local recurrence**
- **Distant metastasis** (most commonly in lungs) is more common than other malignant salivary tumors.

Androgen receptor (AR) and HER2 status should be assessed in malignant salivary tumor with distant metastases. Androgen receptor therapy (e.g., leuprolide, bicalutamide) is recommended for AR+ve tumors and trastuzumab is recommended for HER+ve tumors.

Parotid gland is a common site of metastases from skin cancer.

Nonepithelial Tumors

- In childhood, **hemangioma** and **lymphangioma** may develop in the salivary gland. Hemangioma usually regresses by the age of 2 years, but lymphangioma needs excision.
- **Neurofibroma** and **neurilemmomas** may develop in the adults.
- Most of the salivary gland **lymphomas** develop in the parotids. Treatment is total parotidectomy and adjuvant radiotherapy.

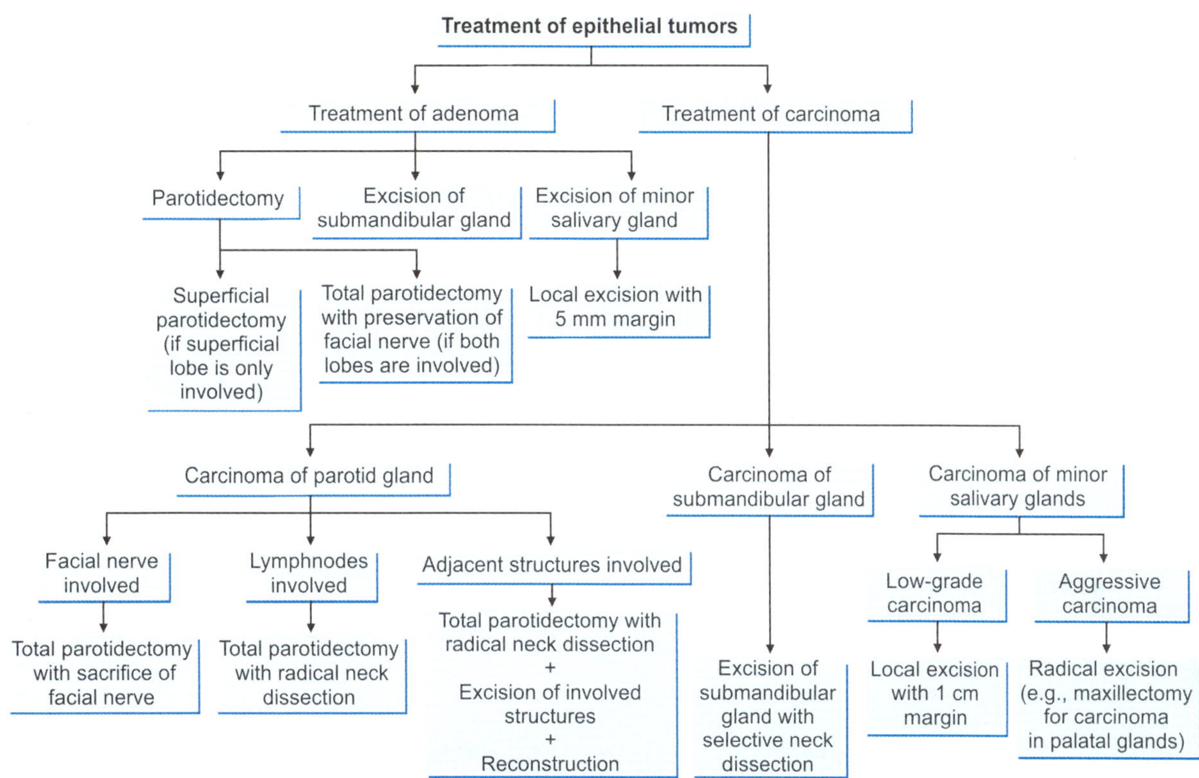

Surgical Procedures for Salivary Gland Pathology

Excision of Sublingual Gland

Indications: (i) Treatment of ranula and (ii) Neoplastic lesion of the sublingual gland.

Main operative steps:

- A linear incision is made in the floor of the mouth just lateral and parallel to the submandibular duct. The incision should not be extended beyond the 1st molar tooth to avoid injury to the lingual nerve.
- The submandibular duct, sublingual gland, and lingual nerve are identified.
- The sublingual gland is mobilized from the inner cortex of the mandible.

Complications: (i) Injury to the lingual nerve resulting numbness of the tongue and (ii) Injury to the submandibular duct.

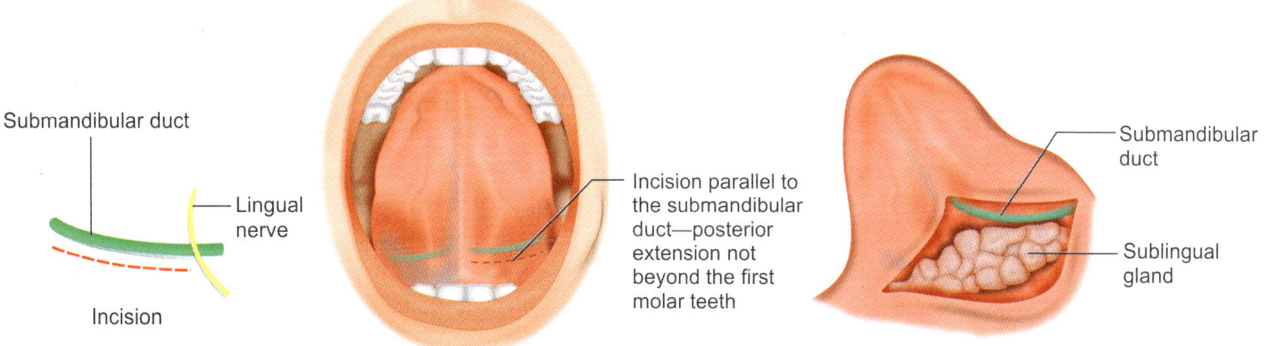

Injury to the submandibular duct and lingual nerve should be avoided.

Excision of Submandibular Gland

Indications
- Sialolithiasis
- Chronic sialadenitis
- Neoplastic lesion of the gland

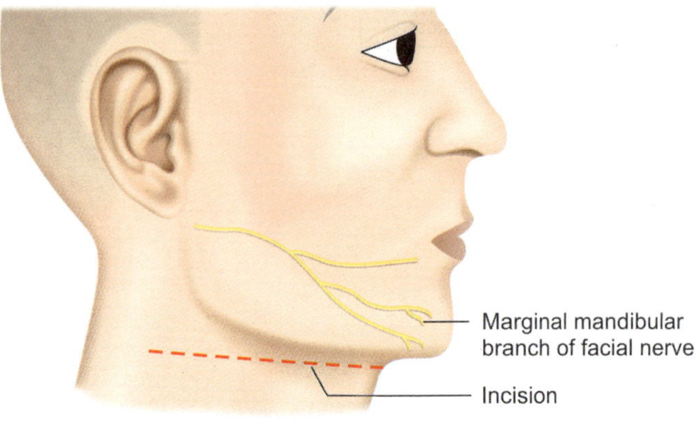

- A horizontal skin crease incision at least 3 cm below the ramus of the mandible (Risdon incision) to avoid injury to the mandibular branch of facial nerve.

Injury to marginal mandibular branch of facial nerve should be avoided.

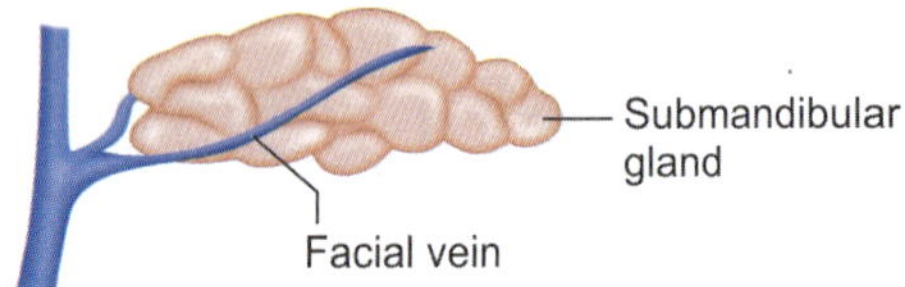

- Facial vein lies superficial to the gland and it is ligated and divided.
- Facial artery is dissected from the deeper surface of the gland and is ligated above and below.

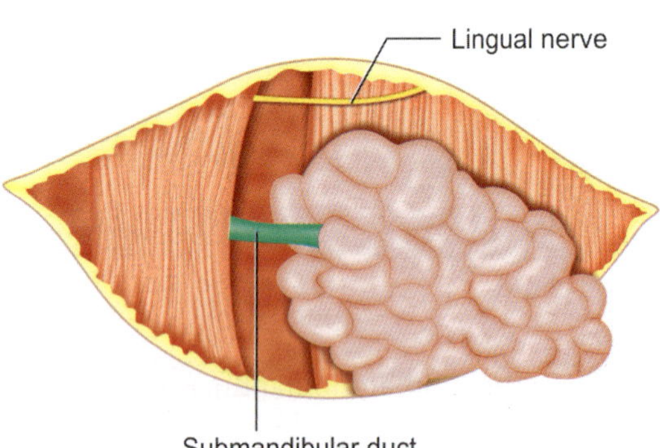

- The superficial part of the gland is dissected off mylohyoid.
- Mylohyoid is retracted anteriorly to expose the deeper part of the gland and its duct. Lingual nerve is now becomes visible.

Injury to lingual nerve should be avoided.

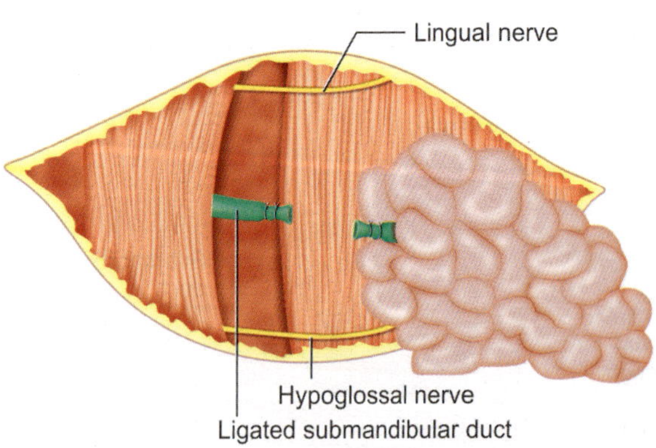

- Hypoglossal nerve is also visible at the lower part of the operative field, but in a deeper plane.
- Submandibular duct is ligated as anterior as possible.
- The only attachment of the gland, part of facial artery is again ligated at the lower border of the posterior pole of the gland, and is removed along with the gland.

Injury to hypoglossal nerve should be avoided.

Complications
- Injury to the marginal mandibular branch of facial nerve
- Injury to the lingual nerve
- Injury to the hypoglossal nerve.

Superficial Parotidectomy

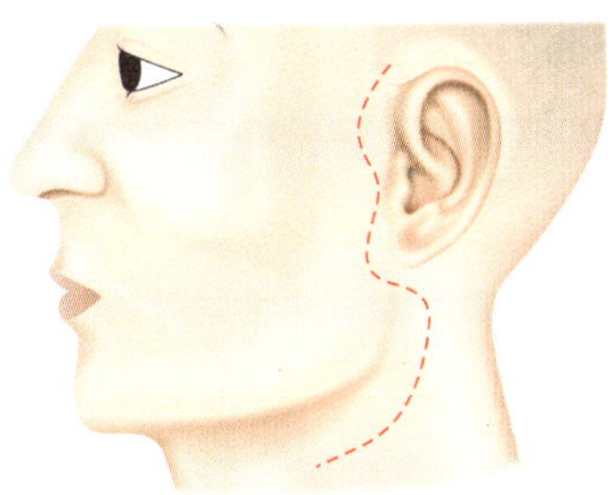

Indications
- Pleomorphic adenoma of parotid (involving superficial lobe only)
- Metastases to parotid lymph nodes from skin cancers

Incision
- **Modified Blair incision (Lazy S incision)**—Most commonly used incision for parotidectomy
- The cervicomastoidfacial incision was proposed by Blair in 1912
- Bailey proposed the modified incision (part of the incision parallel to the zygomatic arch is omitted) in 1941.

Other incisions for parotidectomy
- Modified facelift incision
- Periauricular incision

The principles of superficial parotidectomy is to:
- Identification of facial nerve before it enters the gland
- Following the nerve and it's branches, the gland is dissected superficial to the faciovenous plane.

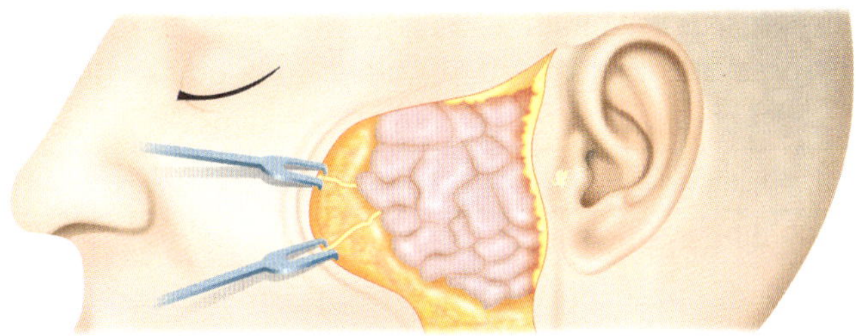

Anteriorly, skin and platysma flap is elevated to expose the parotid gland along with parotid fascia.

Injury to the branches of facial nerve emerging from the anterior border of the gland should be avoided during this step.

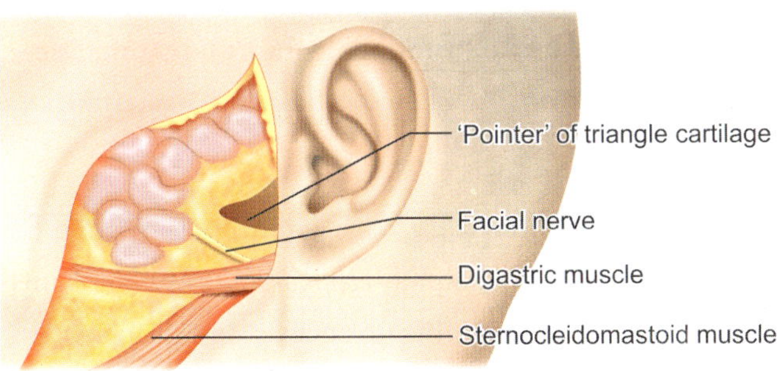

Identification of Facial Nerve

Method No. 1: A plane is made anterior to the external auditory meatus and dissection is done just superficial to styloid process and stylomastoid foramen. This plane is then opened in inferior direction by blunt dissection till facial nerve is visible.

Method No. 2: This method is particularly suitable when the tumor is large with posterior extension. Inferior pole of parotid is lifted off from sternocleidomastoid muscle through the cervical extension of the incision. Great auricular nerve is visible in this stage and needs sacrifice. Anterior border of sternocleidomastoid is retracted inferiorly, then posterior belly of digastric is identified. Digastric muscle is traced upwards to backwards upto its insertion to mastoid which lies immediately below the stylomastoid foramen.

The nerve can also be located 1 cm medial and inferior to the 'pointer' of tragal cartilage.

After leaving the stylomastoid foramen, the nerve becomes more superficial and divides into zygomaticofacial trunk and cervicofacial trunk.

Facial nerve divides into two main divisions, **temporofacial** and **cervicofacial** at the pes anserinus.

The temporofacial segment further divides into **temporal**, **zygomatic** and **buccal** branches; cervicofacial segment divides into **marginal mandibular** and **cervical** branches.

Dissection of Parotid

- The five branches of facial nerve are followed peripherally throughout the parotid. Between each branch of the nerve, the parotid tissue bridging between superficial and deep lobe must be divided carefully.
- Use of **unipolar diathermy is contraindicated during dissection**. Ligature or bipolar diathermy must be used for hemostasis.
- Following removal of superficial lobe, the nerve trunk and its branches can be seen.

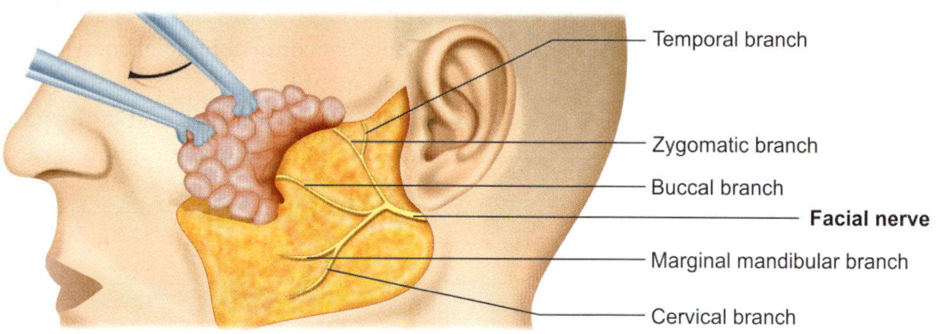

- **If deep lobe is involved**, total parotidectomy to be done by retracting the nerve with slings.
- **If nerve is injured or partially excised**, primary suturing or nerve grafting (using great auricular nerve or sural nerve) can be done using operating microscope if proper expertise is available.
- **During total parotidectomy for malignant tumor**, only branches that directly invaded must be sacrificed without disturbing others.

Facial nerve should be sacrificed during parotidectomy if:

- Preoperative facial nerve involvement with facial palsy
- Direct invasion of the tumor into the nerve.

Partial Superficial Parotidectomy

- Another surgical approach for pleomorphic adenoma of the parotid with relatively few postoperative complications.
- In this technique, main trunk of the facial nerve is identified followed by dissection of the nerve divisions adjacent to the tumor. Only the parotid tissue surrounding the tumor are excised.

Complications of Parotidectomy

Intraoperative

- Hemorrhage
- Transection of the facial nerve
- Rupture of the pseudocapsule of the tumor

Early Postoperative

- Facial nerve injury
- Hematoma
- Flap necrosis
- Parotid fistula
- Sialocele
- Hypoesthesia of the lobule

Late Postoperative

- Frey's syndrome
- Recurrence
- Hypertrophic scar or keloid

Facial Nerve Injury

Intraoperative transection of facial nerve is managed by: (i) Primary repair (if no tissue loss) and (ii) Nerve grafting with greater auricular nerve (if nerve length is inadequate). Most of postparotidectomy facial palsy are transient due to neuropraxia as a result of stretching during surgery. The injury may be in main trunk or the individual branches. Among the individual branches, marginal mandibular branch is most commonly injured. Most of the transient facial palsy resolves within 6 months.

Factors associated with increased risk of facial nerve injury: (i) Total parotidectomy; (ii) Larger tumor size; (iii) Malignant tumor; (iv) Revision surgery; and (v) Older age.

Clinical manifestations: (i) Facial contortion; (ii) Inability to close the eye completely; (iii) Corneal drying; and (iv) Difficulty in eating, drinking.

Management: (i) Measures to prevent exposure keratopathy (use of artificial tear during the day and application of ophthalmic ointment and eye taping at night, botulinum toxin injection, temporary or permanent tarsorrhaphy, external eyelid loading) and (ii) Facial exercise.

Frey Syndrome

- **Frey syndrome (Gustatory sweating)** following parotidectomy develops due to aberrant regeneration of sectioned parasympathetic secretomotor fibers of the auriculotemporal nerve to nearby denervated cutaneous facial sweat glands and blood vessels (normally innervated by cholinergic sympathetic fibers).
- **The syndrome is characterized by** flushing and sweating in the facial skin of parotid area during meal. During mastication, acetylcholine is released from parasympathetic nerve endings, induces sweating and flushing (before aberrant reinnervation, these was a sympathetic cholinergic response).
- **Diagnosis** is confirmed by Minor starch-iodine test.
- **Botulinum toxin injection is an effective treatment option.** Other treatment options are: (i) Temporoparietal fascia flap; (ii) Sternocleidomastoid muscle flap; and (iii) Superficial musculoaponeurotic system flap.

Parotid Fistula and Sialocele

- **Parotid fistula** develops when remaining parotid gland secretes saliva and that drains through the operative wound. **Sialocele** develops when this secretion collects beneath the skin flap of parotidectomy.
- **The secretion usually increases during chewing meals. If diagnosis is uncertain**, the fistula content is sent for amylase level.
- **Most of the fistula and sialoceles are managed by conservative management:** (i) Decreasing oral intake; (ii) Use of anticholinergics (to decrease salivary secretion); and (iii) Repeated needle aspiration and pressure dressing.
- **If these conservative managements fail, treatment options are:** (i) Botulinum injection; (ii) Tympanic neurectomy with or without chorda tympani section; (iii) Radiotherapy; and (iv) Completion of parotidectomy.

Case 1

History and Physical Examination

A 48-year-old male patient presented in the surgical OPD with a chief complaint of recurrent episodes of pain below the right jaw that was associated with chewing foods for last 2 months. Patient also complained of appearance of swelling in the same region for last one month. Both pain and swelling resolved after meal.

Clinical Examination

A firm, non-tender swelling was palpable in the right submandibular region. On intraoral examination, right submandibular duct opening was erythematous. On bimanual examination of the floor of the mouth, thickening along the course of the duct was revealed. Submandibular gland was rubbery hard in consistency on bimanual palpation.

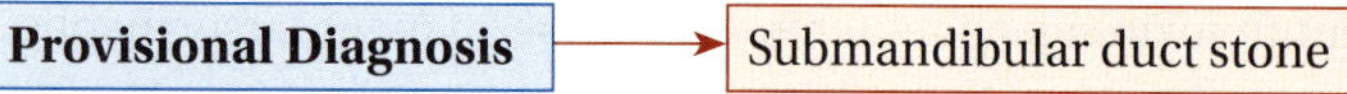

Investigations

Mandibular occlusal X-ray revealed single ovoid radiopacity from lateral incisor to the second premolar area. CT scan also revealed sialolithiasis in the submandibular region.

Discussion

History of recurrent episodes of pain and appearance of swelling in the submandibular region associated with taking meal was highly suggestive of submandibular duct stone. Clinical findings of erythematous duct opening along with thickened duct and palpable submandibular gland suggestive of ductal stone with chronic sialadenitis. X-ray and CT scan confirmed the diagnosis of right submandibular ductal stone. Submandibular gland excision was planned.

Management Algorithm

Preoperative work-up → Excision of submandibular gland

Case 2

History and Physical Examination

A 40-year-old female patient presented in the surgical OPD with complain of swelling around the right ear for last 6 years. The swelling was painless and gradually increasing in size. No other symptoms were present. Past medical and surgical histories were insignificant.

Clinical Examination

An ovoid, 4 cm × 3.5 cm, non-tender swelling with well-defined margin was seen on the right parotid region with slightly everted right ear lobule. The swelling was not fixed to the overlying skin or underlying structures. Intraoral examination was unremarkable. No clinical evidences of facial palsy.

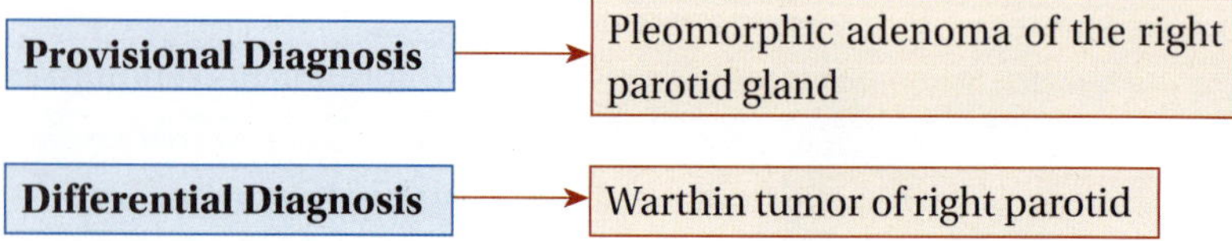

Investigations

FNAC was suggestive of pleomorphic adenoma. CT scan revealed a solid mass with heterogeneous enhancement. The tumor was not invading any adjacent structures.

Discussion

A non-tender, progressively increasing swelling in the parotid region without any clinical evidences of facial nerve involvement was highly suggestive of benign parotid tumor. Pleomorphic adenoma is the most common benign parotid tumor. FNAC confirmed the provisional diagnosis. CT scan excluded any local invasion of the tumor. Superficial parotidectomy was planned.

Management Algorithm

Preoperative work-up → Superficial parotidectomy

Chapter 23

Diseases of Skin and Adnexa

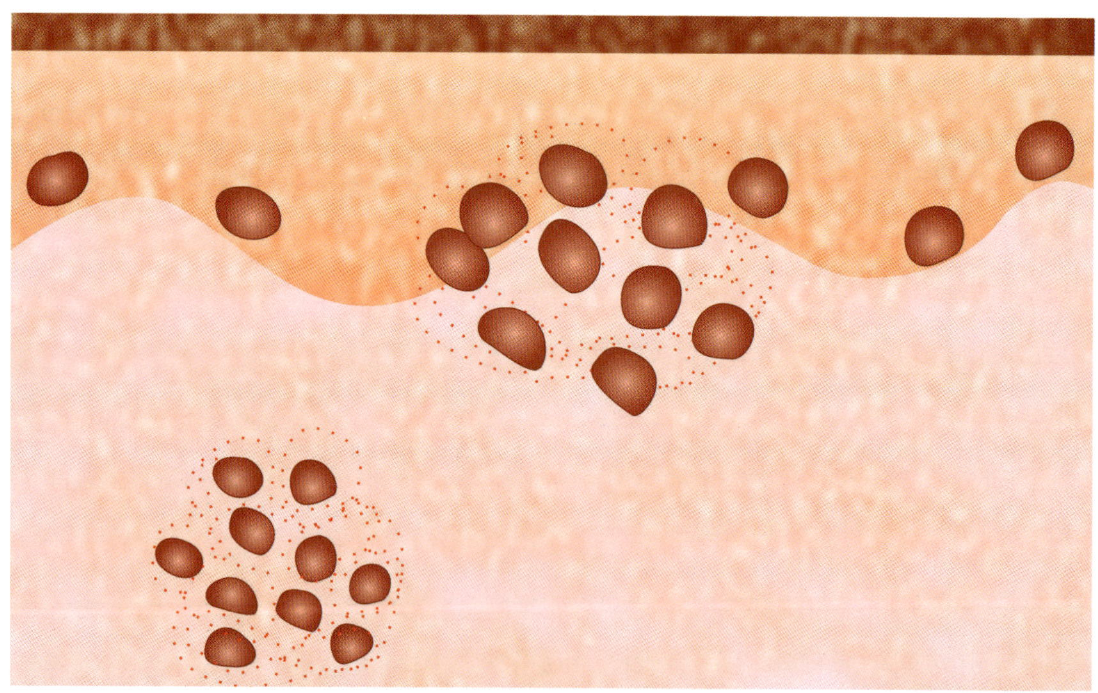

Important Topics

- Cystic Lesions of the Skin
- Common Vascular Anomalies
- Benign Tumors
- Skin Infections
- Benign Pigmented Lesions
- Premalignant Lesions
- Malignant Lesions

'If you cannot explain it to a six-year-old, you don't understand it yourself.'

Cystic Lesions of the Skin

Sebaceous Cyst (Epidermal Inclusion Cyst or Epidermal Cyst)

- Epidermal inclusion cyst (sebaceous cyst is a misnomer) is a **type of retention cyst** formed as a result of **obstruction of the pilosebaceous follicles**. The gland becomes distended by its own secretion. The cyst is lined by true, stratified-squamous epithelium.
- Develop in all ages.
- Can develop anywhere, but commonly occur in face, scalp, neck, and scrotum.
- **On clinical examination**, the cyst is smooth, soft or firm and sometimes a **pathognomonic keratin-plugged punctum** (attached to skin) is visible. Often, patient complains of foul smelling cheese-like material from the cyst. The rancid odor of the cyst content is most likely due to relative fat content and decomposition.
- **Complications** are infection, Cock's peculiar tumor and sebaceous horn.
- **Treatment** is excision of the cyst with complete cyst wall removal. [retained cyst wall may cause cyst recurrence.]
- Infected cyst (commonly found organisms are *Staphylococcus*, group A *Streptococcus*, *E. Coli*, pepto-*Streptococcus*, bacteroides) can be safely excised with antibiotic coverage and proper wound care.

Epidermal inclusion cyst may be associated with Gardner syndrome (multiple sebaceous cyst, osteoma, colonic polyposis, desmoid tumor) or Gorlin syndrome.

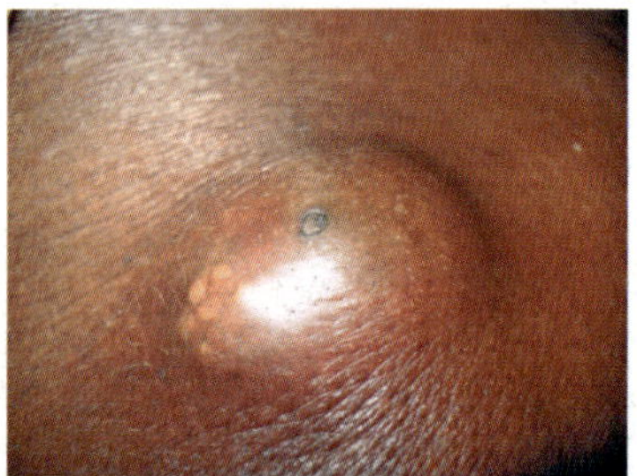

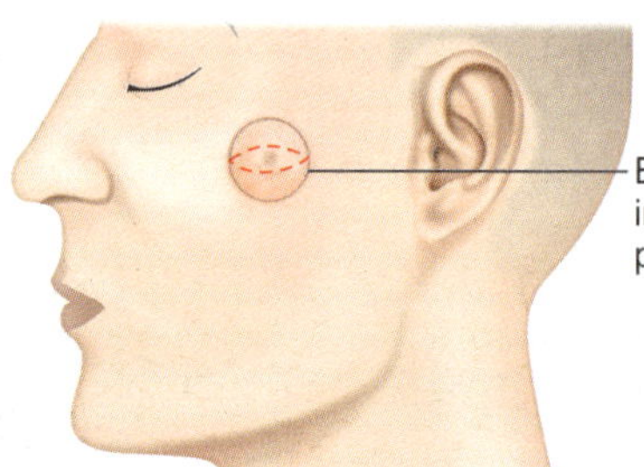

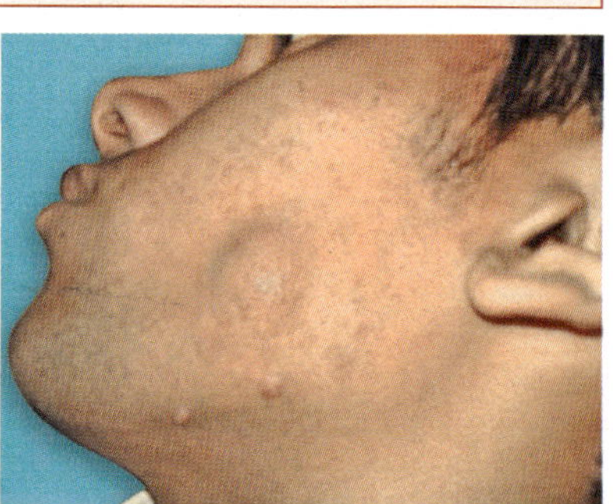

Epidermal cyst

Cock's Peculiar Tumor

- An infected, open, granulating sebaceous cyst.
- Granulation tissue arising from the lining of the cyst bursts through ruptured cyst and makes the lesion an angry looking lesion with an everted edge.
- **It looks like a squamous cell carcinoma.**

Dermoid Cyst

Congenital Dermoid Cyst (Sequestration Dermoid Cyst)

Congenital dermoid cyst arises from separated epidermal cells during fusion of the embryonic clefts and therefore found at the lines of fusion.

- External angular and root of the nose are two most common sites.
- Cyst contains thick opaque mixture of sebum, sweat, and desquamated epithelial cells.
- On clinical examination, it is soft, nontender, cystic swelling, not fixed to the skin but fixed to the underlying bone.
- Rarely, the cyst has a intracranial communication. So a skull X-ray or CT is essential to exclude this.
- Excision of the cyst is the treatment of choice.

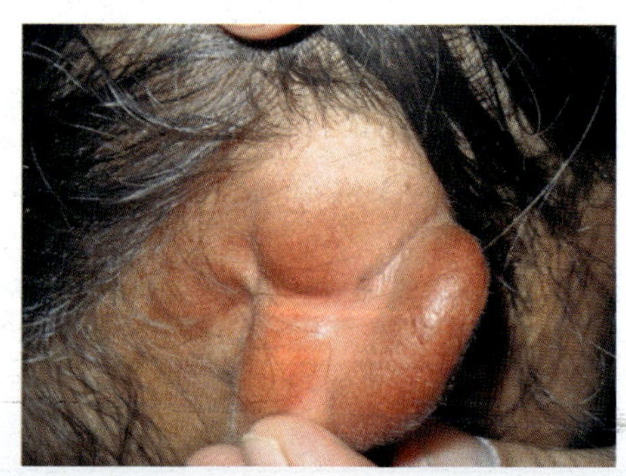

Postauricular sequestration dermoid cyst.

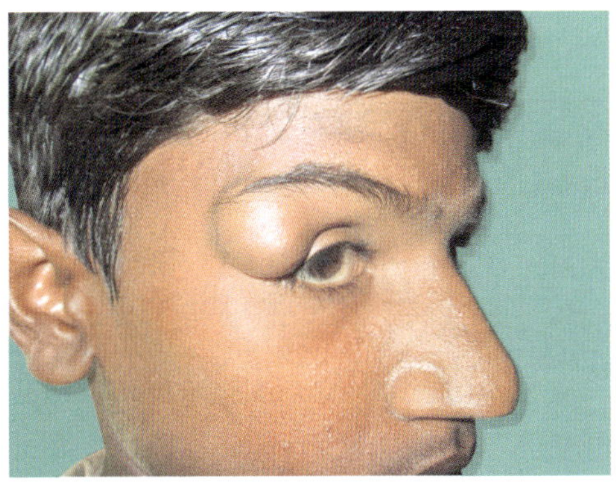

Congenital Dermoid Cyst in External Angular Region.

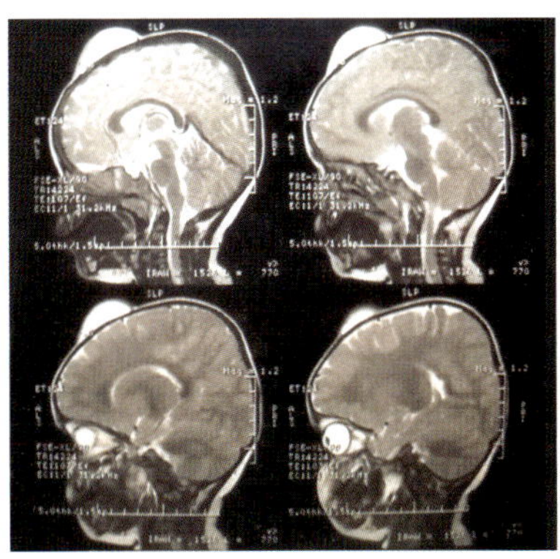

Skull CT is indicated to exclude intracranial communication.

Implantation Dermoid Cyst

- It is an acquired dermoid cyst, develops following an injury.
- Injury results in implantation of epithelial cells into the subcutaneous tissue.
- The cysts are often found in tailors, gardeners. In most of the cases, patient cannot remember the event of injury. Overlying skin is often scarred.
- Excision is the treatment of choice.

Ganglion

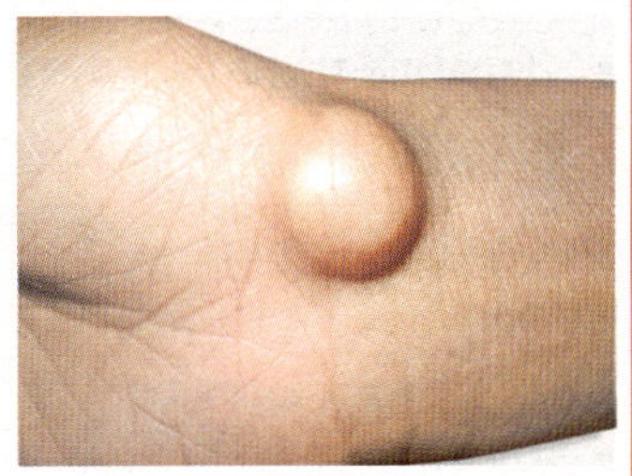

Volar ganglion cyst.

- A **unilocular, nonneoplastic, pseudocystic swelling** as a result of cystic, myxomatous degeneration of synovial tissue in relation to joints or tendons.
- **Most commonly present** in dorsum of the wrist, followed by volar wrist, flexor tendon sheath.
- **Clinically**, it is a nontender, smooth, firm swelling not fixed to the overlying skin. On compression, a ganglion may slip away between deeper structures, giving the false impression that the contents have reduced into the joint. **[A true ganglion is not connected with the joint.]** Mobility of ganglion is restricted when the underlying structures (joint capsule, tendon sheath) becomes tense.
- **Treatment** is excision or threading or intralesional sclerosant injection.
- **Definite therapy** is excision of the stalk of the ganglion and debridement of the synovial origin.

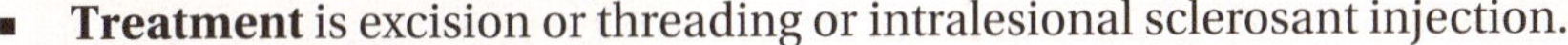

In Dorsal wrist ganglion, Excision of the stalk followed by debridement of dorsal wrist capsule over the scapholunate ligament. In volar wrist ganglion, Excision of the stalk followed by debridement of volar wrist capsule over the radioscaphocapitate ligament.

Care should be taken for protection of radial artery and superficial radial nerve during excision.

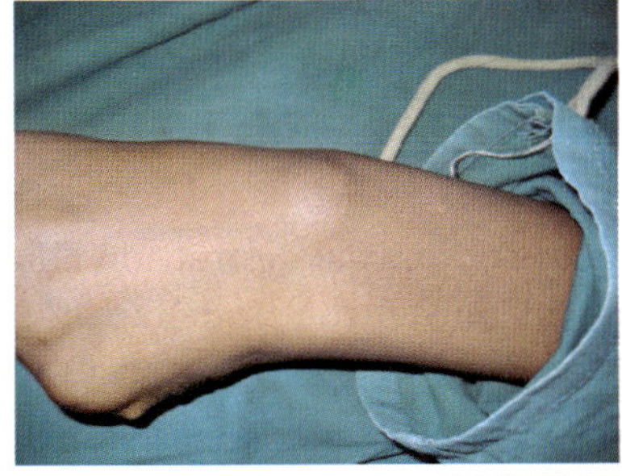

Ganglion in Dorsum of Wrist.

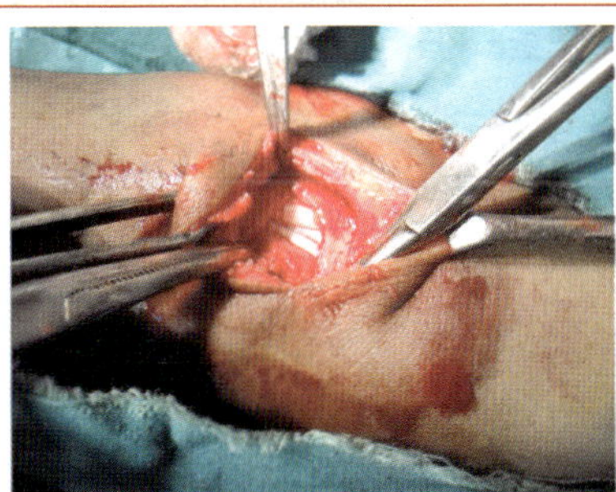

After Excision of Ganglion.

Common Vascular Anomalies

Strawberry Nevus

- Strawberry nevus or infantile hemangioma is the most common vascular tumor in infants and children.
- Small red mark is noted usually 1–3 weeks after birth, that rapidly increasing in size over a few weeks to take the shape of a strawberry.
- Raised, compressible, nonpulsatile lesion covered with smooth, pitted epithelium, commonly found in face, scalp and neck region.
- About 90% of the lesions regress spontaneously over time (within 5–9 years) with accepted cosmetic outcome.
- Treatment is conservative except in lesions causing difficulty in vision, feeding. Those lesions warrant early surgical intervention.

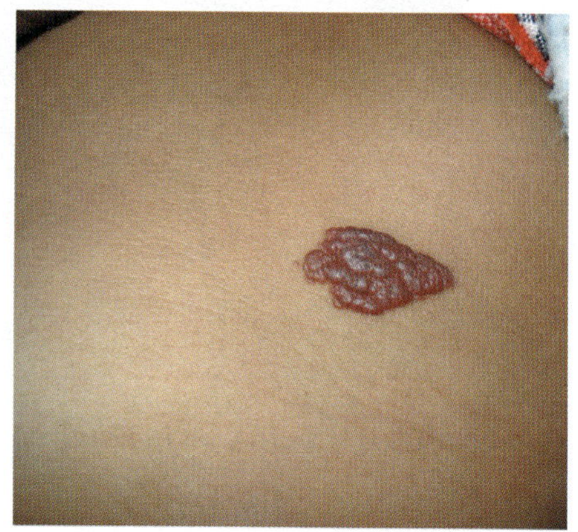

Port-wine Stain

- These are intradermal capillary malformation.
- **Histologically**, they are collections of ectatic capillaries lined by mature endothelium.
- **Commonly present** in face, shoulder, neck. Sometimes, they are confined to a single dermatome (along a trigeminal distribution in face).
- Occasionally, they present as a part of syndromes—**Sturge-Weber syndrome** (leptomeningeal angiomatosis, epilepsy, glaucoma); **Klippel-Trenaunay syndrome** (varicose vein, limb hypertrophy, port-wine stain).
- **Treatment** is pulsed dye laser therapy.

Venous Malformations

- Most common type of vascular anomalies.
- Venous malformations usually present as blue, soft, compressible lesion.
- Histologically, venous malformations are composed of thin-walled, dilated, sponge-like abnormal channels with surrounding smooth muscle.
- MRI is the most useful imaging modality.
- Treatment is sclerotherapy and surgery.

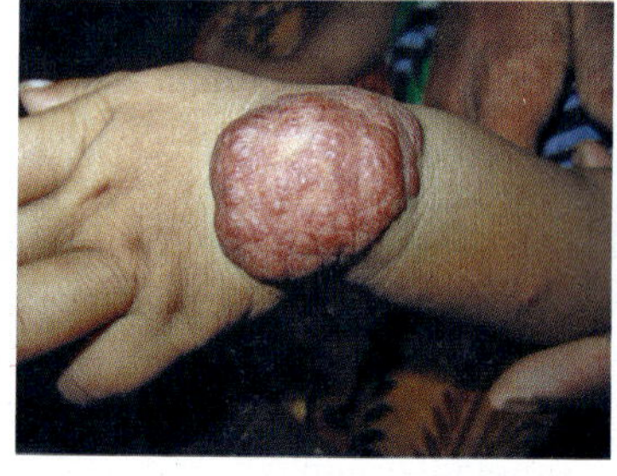

Lymphangioma

- Cluster of dilated lymph sacs in the skin and subcutaneous tissues, not connected with the main lymphatic system.
- Large, translucent lymph cysts mostly found in the neck—Known as '**Cystic hygroma**'.
- Lymphangioma is classified according to size—(1) Microcystic (<1 cm); (2) Macrocystic (>1 cm); and (3) Combined.
- Lymphangiomas are commonly located in cervicofacial region (70–80%), axilla, chest, mediastinum, buttock.
- Prenatal USG can detect macrocystic lymphangiomas at second or third trimester. USG can detect presence of macrocystic lymphangiomas, but MRI is the most useful imaging modality.
- **Treatment:** (1) Sclerotherapy and (2) Surgery.

Sclerotherapy: Sclerotherapy acts by obliterating lymphatic lumen by endothelial destruction followed by fibrosis. Commonly used sclerosants are sodium tetradecylsulfate, ethanol, bleomycin. Sclerotherapy is more effective in macrocystic lymphangiomas. Repeated sessions of sclerotherapy are required to achieve satisfying result.

Surgery: Staged excision is often necessary. During surgery, surgeon must keep in mind few principles. Attempts to minimize blood loss, focus on a defined anatomic region, thorough dissection as possible.

Pyogenic Granuloma

- It is an acquired, benign vascular tumor arises in skin or mucous membranes.
- At the phase of healing of ulcer or wound, sometimes capillary loops grow rapidly, thereby forming a protruding lesion consists of capillaries covered by epithelium. This mass becomes infected and forms a pyogenic granuloma.
- Typical natural history is usually present—History of minor injury followed by appearance of a nontender lump that rapidly grows and bleeds on minor touch.
- Treatment is excision.

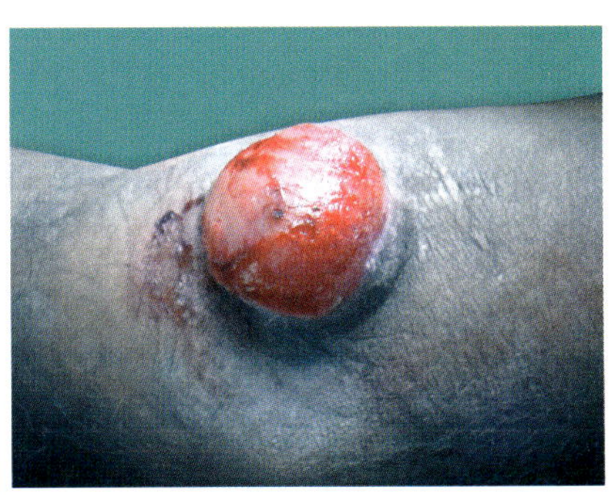

Glomus Tumor

- A tumor arises from glomus body [glomus body, an arteriovenous shunt in the skin that have a role in temperature regulation, are present throughout the skin with special preference in fingers and toes]
- Small, firm, bluish-gray, extremely tender nodules mostly found in subungual region. The clinical triad of: (1) Hypersensitivity to cold; (2) Paroxysmal pain; and (3) Pinpoint pain suggestive of glomus tumor.
- Three clinical tests can be performed for diagnosis:
  1. **Love's test:** Pressure is applied over the tumor by pin/paper clip ⇒ severe pain (positive result).
  2. **Hildreth's test:** Tourniquet is applied proximal to the tumor site ⇒ Love's test is performed ⇒ No pain (positive result).
  3. **Cold sensitivity test:** Increased pain with exposure to cold.

Arteriovenous Malformations

- AVMs are high-flow vascular malformations consist of disorganized arteries and veins that communicate.
- AVMs are manifested as warm, pink patch in the skin with underlying thrill or bruit.
- A clinical staging system exists: **Schobinger clinical staging system for AVMs**

Stage I (quiescence): Pink-bluish stain, warmth, and arteriovascular shunting by continuous Doppler scanning or 20 MHZ color Doppler scanning.

Stage II (expansion): Same as stage I plus enlargement, pulsations, thrill, bruit and tortuous/tense veins.

Stage III (destruction): Same as stage II plus either dystrophic skin changes, ulceration, bleeding, persistent pain, or tissue necrosis.

Stage IV (decompensation): Same as stage III plus cardiac failure.

- Doppler USG can detect the fast flow of AVM. CT, MR angiography can also detect the presence of AVMs.
- **Treatment** is angiographic embolization alone or in combination with surgical excision.

Treatment is indicated if symptoms (e.g., ischemic changes, pain, intermittent bleeding, ulceration) are present or endangering signs (e.g., recurrent ulceration, increased cardiac output, Schobinger stage III and IV) are present.

Benign Tumors

Papilloma

- Overgrowth of all layers of skin with a central core of connective tissue, blood vessels and lymphatics. With epithelial proliferation, it is thrown into folds and takes the shape of a papilloma. Along with epithelial proliferation, the connective tissue and blood vessels grow.
- It may present as **sessile** or **pedunculated** polypoidal lesion.
- Surgery is indicated if the lesion is cosmetically unacceptable or vulnerable to injury.

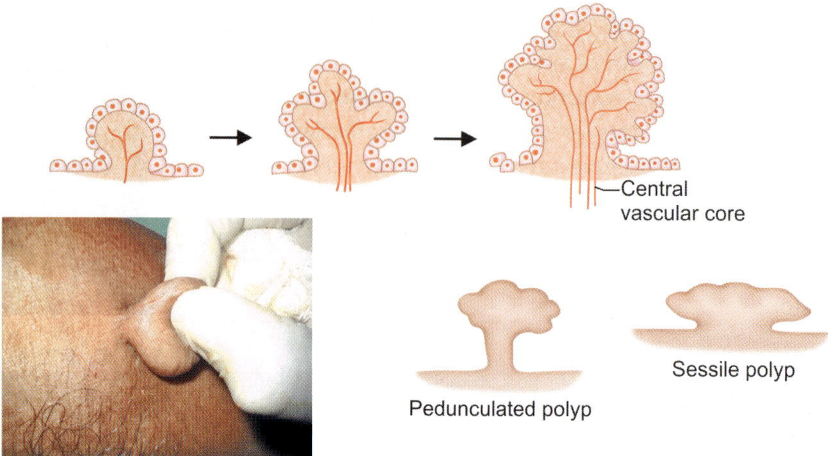

Lipoma

It is composed of adult type fat cells. Lipoma may present anywhere in the body, that is why it is also called **'universal tumor'**.

Different types:

1. **According to presence of edge:**
   - Encapsulated lipoma (has a definite edge)
   - Diffuse lipoma (no definite edge).
2. **According to number:**
   - Solitary.
   - Multiple lipomatosis (multiple lipomas of different sizes are present particularly in the trunk).
3. **According to presence of other tissues:**
   - Angiolipoma
   - Pleomorphic lipoma
   - Fibrolipoma
   - Neurolipoma
   - Naevolipoma
   - Myelolipoma.
4. **According to location:**
   - **Subcutaneous lipoma:**
     - Commonest type
     - Commonly found in the shoulder, back
   - Subfascial lipoma—Present deep to palmar and plantar fascia
   - Subsynovial lipoma—in the knee
   - Intra-articular lipoma.
   - Intermuscular lipoma—in thigh or shoulder
   - Retroperitoneal lipoma
   - Submucous lipoma—deep to mucous membrane of alimentary tract or respiratory tract

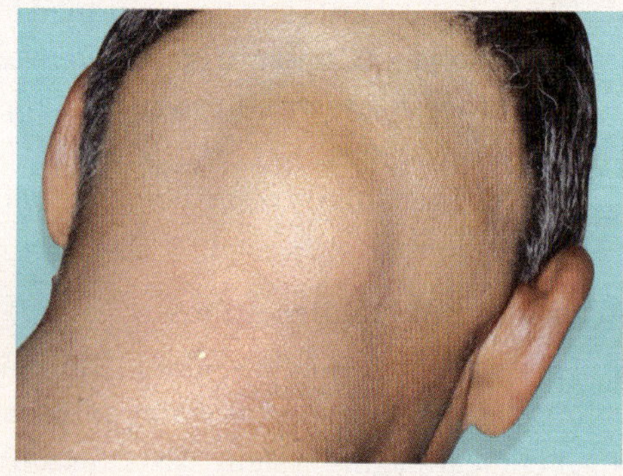

Lipoma in neck.

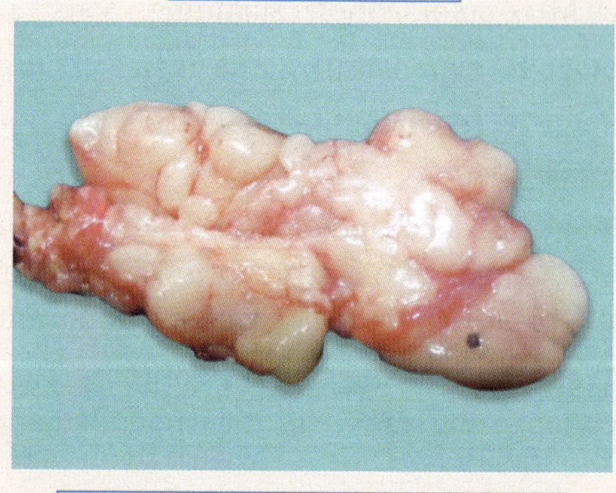

Operated specimen of lipoma.

Complications: (i) Myxomatous degeneration; (ii) Saponification; (iii) Calcification; and (iv) Sarcomatous change (rare)

On clinical examination, lipomas are usually spherical shaped, lobulated, slips away from examining finger (slip sign).

Investigation: Typical subcutaneous lipoma does not need preoperative imaging. Imaging (USG/CT/MRI) is indicated if lipoma >5 cm, irregular in shape or myofascial involvement. MRI is the most sensitive imaging modality.

Surgery is mostly indicated for cosmetic reasons. **Other indications of surgery are** nerve impingement, pain, functional limitation, increase in size, core needle biopsy showing atypical histology, involvement of deep fascia.

- **Lipoblastomas** are tumor composed of immature fat cells.
- **Hibernomas** are tumor composed of brown fat.

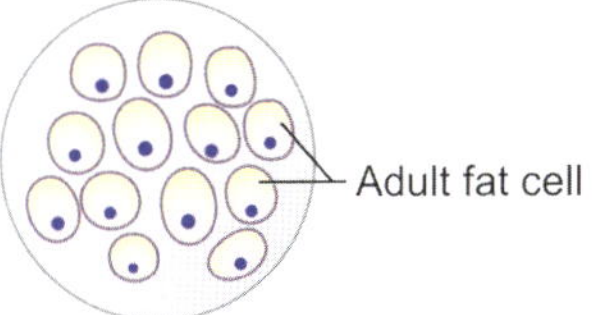
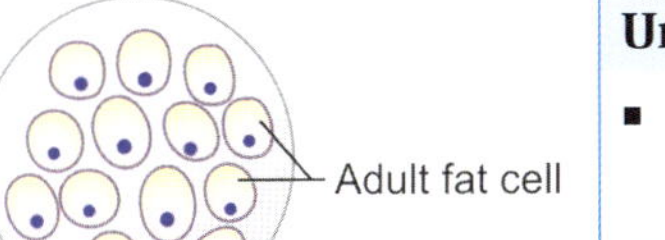

Uncommon Varieties of Lipoma

- **Adiposis dolorosa (Dercum's disease):** It is characterized by tender multiple lipomas in the trunk.
- **'Lipoma aborescens':** Pedunculated subcutaneous lipoma.

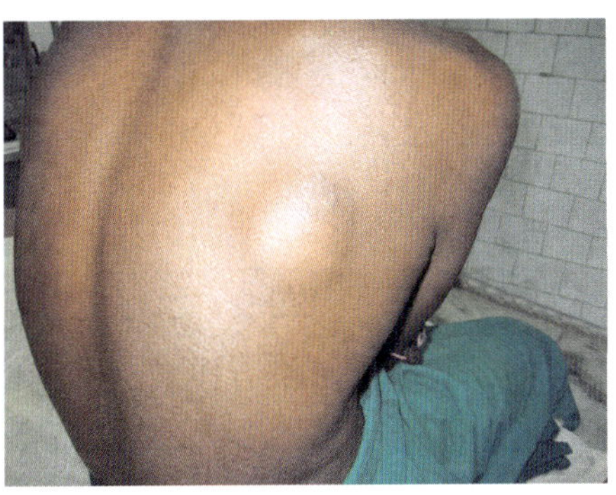

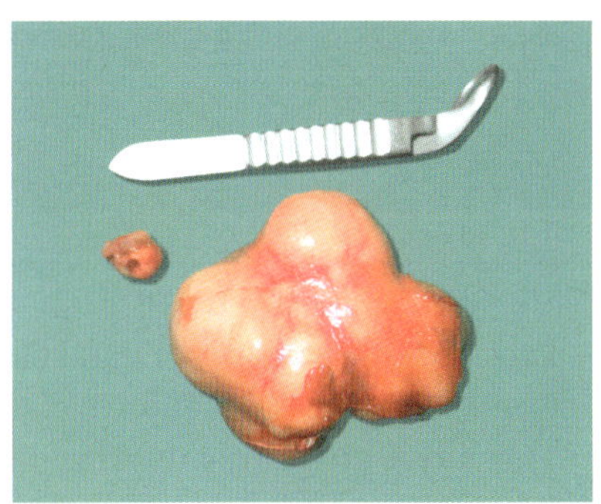

Syndromes Associated with Lipoma

- Adiposis dolorosa
- Benign symmetric lipomatosis (Madelung syndrome)
- Gardner syndrome
- Cowden syndrome
- MEN type 1
- Bannayan-Riley-Ruvalcava syndrome

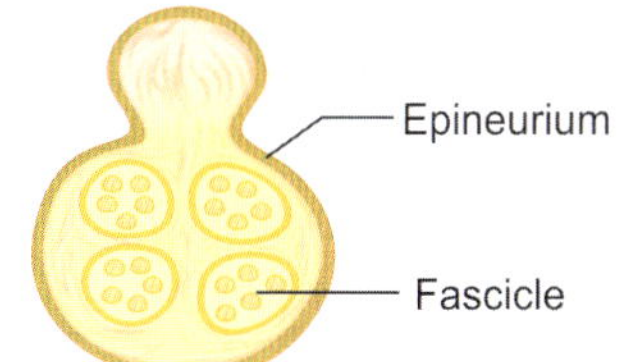

Neurofibroma

- Solitary benign tumor arising from connective tissue of a nerve sheath **(epineurium)**.
- Contains both neural (ectodermal) and fibrous (mesodermal) elements.
- **Present as** tender, subcutaneous, nodular swelling, most freely moves in right angle to the course of the nerve. Patient may present with tingling sensation in the distribution of the nerve from which it arises.
- **Treatment** is excision of the tumor.

Increased tendency for local recurrence.

Sarcomatous changes rarely develop in neurofibroma, particularly in multiple neurofibromatosis.

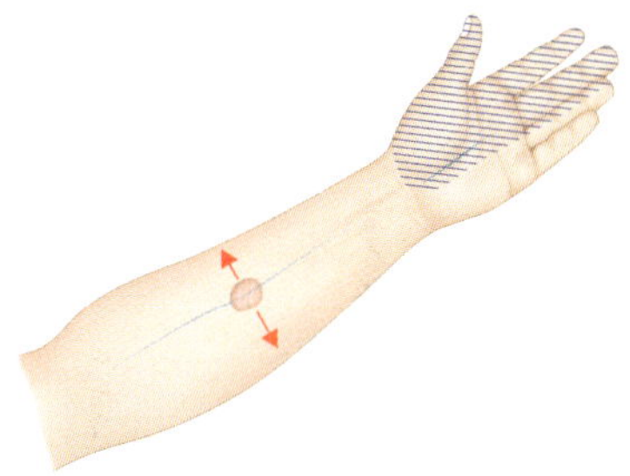

Multiple Neurofibromatosis

- This multiple, congenital, familial **(autosomal dominant inheritance)** neurofibromatosis is also called **von Recklinghausen's disease**.
- This is type 1 neurofibromatosis with mutation in **chromosome 17**.
- It arises from **endoneurium. Multiple neurofibromatosis is characterized by:** (i) Multiple cutaneous neurofibromas; (ii) Cutaneous hyperpigmented macules ('cafe' au 'lait spot); (iii) Pigmented nodules of the iris (lisch nodule); and (iv) Gliomas of the optic nerve.
- **Patients present** with nodules of varying sizes from a mili-meter sized to large varieties. Some of them in the skin, some are subcutaneous and few of them become pedunculated.
- Examination of the spinal nerve and hearing tests are essential to exclude major nerve involvement.
- Patient with *NF1* gene have a greater chance of malignant transformation of the tumors.
- Tumor with ulceration, large pedunculated and tumor with sarcomatous changes need excision.

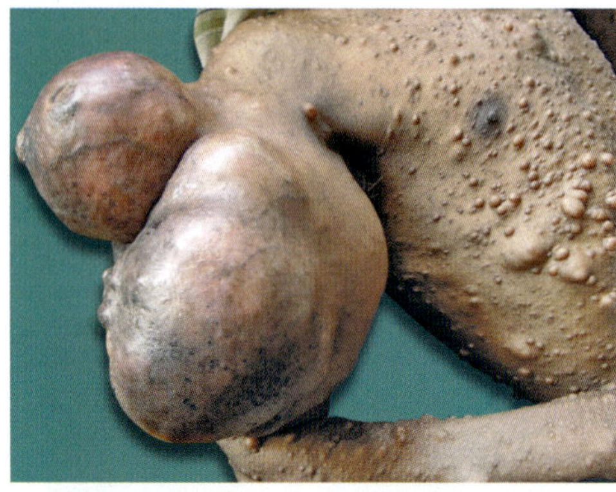

Multiple neurofibromatosis—some nodules having malignant transformation.

Plexiform Neurofibromatosis

- Excessive overgrowth of neural tissue in subcutaneous fat
- Commonly seen in relation to distribution of trigeminal nerve, sometimes seen in extremities.
- The nerves are heavily thickened due to myxomatous degeneration of endoneurium
- Presents as a folded, irregular mass hanging from the face with hyperpigmentation
- Very rarely, sarcomatous changes may develop.

Elephantiasis Neuromatosa

- Rare, congenital variety of plexiform neurofibromatosis
- Skin becomes coarse, dry and thickened, and resembles an elephant's skin.

Skin Infection

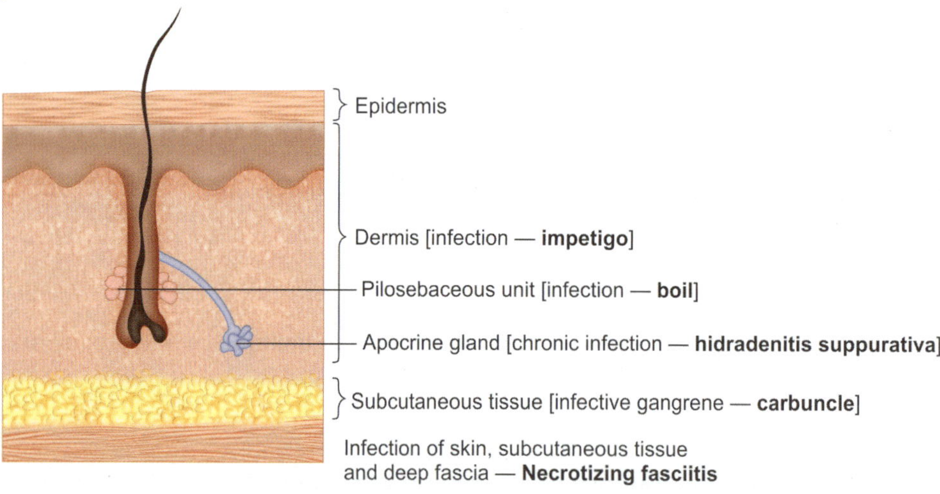

Furuncle (Boil)

- *Staphylococcal* infection of pilosebaceous unit with perifolliculitis. Infection proceeds to suppuration and then central necrosis.
- Commonly present in back and neck. Usually presents as tender, indurated swelling around a hair follicle with surrounding edema. Within a few days, the center softens, after that it bursts spontaneously.
- Commonly associated with generalized debility and diabetes mellitus.
- Incision is usually not necessary for drainage of pus. Local application of iodine aggravates spontaneous rupture.
- Removal of affected hair follicle also helps in drainage.
- Antibiotics coverage against *Staphylococcus* is indicated in blind boil (boil without suppuration).

Impetigo

- Intradermal bacterial infection caused by *Staphylococcus* and streptococci.
- Commonly involves the hand and face.
- Presents as vesiculopustular lesion and then ruptures and then formation of characteristic yellowish crust.
- Treatment is washing the lesion and removal of crust with chlorhexidine lotion.

Carbuncle

- Infective gangrene of the subcutaneous tissue with multiple openings in the skin.
- Usually caused by *Staphylococcus aureus*, sometimes streptococci and gram-negative bacilli are responsible.
- Commonly found in back, nape of the neck (vitality of the tissues are less in these region). Older diabetic patients are commonly affected.
- Antibiotics and local application of magnesium sulfate (helps to decrease the edema and softening the center of carbuncle) is necessary in initial stage.
- Surgical intervention is needed if the infection not responds to conservative management.

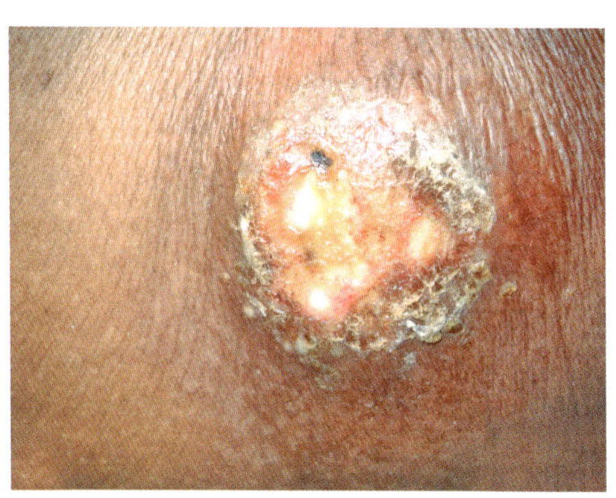

Carbuncle

Hidradenitis Suppurativa (Acne Inversa)

- Hidradenitis suppurativa is a **chronic, recurrent, inflammatory**, debilitating disease of the terminal hair follicle, affecting the **apocrine-gland bearing areas of the body**.
- More common in women in tropical countries. Most commonly found in **axilla**, but may also develop in groins, perianal regions (all apocrine gland bearing regions). **Perianal hidradenitis suppurativa** is more common in men.
- **Patients present** with multiple swellings in the axilla, which eventually discharges pus and then subsides spontaneously or after treatment. The swellings again appear after a few months.
- **Hurley staging system** is recommended for clinical grading of this disease. **Hurley stage I** for single or multiple abscesses with scarring; **Hurley stage II** for limited scarring and/or sinus tracts; **Hurley stage III** for extensive scarring and/or sinus tracts.
- **Commonly associated comorbid conditions** are diabetes mellitus, inflammatory bowel disease, inflammatory arthropathies, polycystic ovary syndrome, depression, anxiety.
- Cessation of smoking and weight reduction are effective **adjuvant therapy**.
- **Clindamycin 1% topical lotion** is the first-line therapy for HS management.
- Topical clindamycin (twice daily for 3 months) is particularly indicated for Hurley stage I and mild stage II.
- **Oral tetracyclines (e.g., doxycycline, minocycline)** are recommended for mild-to-moderate disease particularly if multiple anatomic sites are involved. The treatment is to be continued for 3 months, sometimes up to 4 months depending on the response. **Triple therapy** with moxifloxacin, metronidazole, and rifampin is recommended as second line treatment in moderate-to-severe disease.
- **Adalimumab, a fully-human monoclonal antibody targeting TNF-α**, is the only biologic approved for HS. This agent is particularly indicated for moderate-to-severe HS unresponsive to systemic antibiotics.
- **Procedural management includes:** (i) Photodynamic therapy; (ii) Intense Pulsed Light; (iii) Nd:YAG laser therapy; and (iv) Surgery.
- **Surgical management includes:** (i) Incision and drainage; (ii) Deroofing; and (iii) Wide local excision. Deroofing is indicated for recurrent nodules and sinus tracts. Wide local excision is indicated for severe disease refractory to systemic therapies.

Skin and Soft-tissue Infections (SSTIs)

Skin and soft-tissue infections are classified into three types (as per WSES guideline): (i) Surgical site infections (SSIs); (ii) Non-necrotizing SSTIs; and (iii) Necrotizing SSTIs.

Non-necrotizing soft-tissue infection includes erysipelas, impetigo, folliculitis, simple abscess and complex abscess. **Necrotizing soft-tissue infection** includes cellulitis, fasciitis, myositis, Fournier's gangrene.

Erysipelas is a fiery red, painful plaque with well-defined edges, caused by *Streptococcus pyogenes*. Treatment is antimicrobial therapy against gram-positive bacteria.

Impetigo is bacterial infection of the superficial layers of the epidermis., caused by β-hemolytic *Streptococci* spp. and *S. aureus*. Treatment is antimicrobial therapy.

Cellulitis is acute infection of the dermis and subcutaneous tissue. Treatment is antimicrobial therapy against gram-positive bacteria.

Simple abscess is characterized by: (i) Extension limited to superficial tissues and (ii) No multiloculated extension. Treatment is incision and drainage. **Complex abscess** is characterized by: (i) Extension into deeper tissues and (ii) Multiloculated extension. Treatment is early incision and drainage. Perioperative antimicrobial therapy is indicated if any signs of sepsis or significant cellulitis is present.

Necrotizing Soft Tissue Infection (NSTI)

It is a rapidly progressive, invasive, soft tissue infections with necrotizing component.

Pathophysiology of necrosis in NSTIs: (i) Endo or exotoxin mediated cellular injury; (ii) Thrombosis of blood vessels; and (iii) Inflammatory edema within closed tissue compartment causing impaired tissue perfusion.

Diagnosis: (i) Clinical findings; (ii) Plain X-ray (if gas is in the soft tissues, it is characteristic); (iii) MRI (imaging modality of choice for necrotizing fasciitis); (iv) Finger test; and (v) LRINEC scoring (score ≥8 suggests 75% chance of NSTIs).

Finger test: A 2-cm incision is made under LA deep-to-deep fascia. Minimal resistance to finger dissection, absence of any bleeding, presence of necrotic tissue, presence of murky and grayish ("dishwater") fluid are all suggestive of NSTIs.

Management: (i) Fluid resuscitation; (ii) Management of sepsis; (iii) Empirical broad-spectrum antibiotic therapy (coverage against gram-positive, gram-negative and anaerobic organisms); and (iv) Aggressive surgical debridement.

Fournier's Gangrene

Fournier's gangrene is a **type of necrotizing soft-tissue infection involving the genital area and or perineum.** This infection may extend through the fascial planes into the abdominal wall, thigh, perirectal, and gluteal region.

Clinical manifestations include erythema, patchy areas of gangrene, foul smell, tenderness, wound discharge.

Diagnosis is based on clinical findings. US, CT, and MRI are particularly helpful to confirm the diagnosis and to determine the extent of soft-tissue involvement. **FGSI (Fournier's Gangrene Severity Index)** more than 9 indicated a 75% likelihood of mortality.

Management is early and aggressive surgical debridement along with antimicrobial therapy. Often multiple debridements are necessary. To protect the perineal wound from fecal contamination, diverting colostomy may be indicated. Fecal diversion tube is an effective alternative method of diversion.

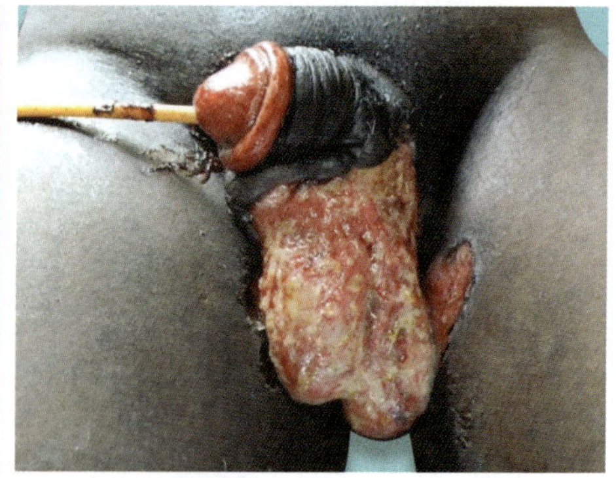

Fournier's gangrene.

Benign Pigmented Lesion

Normally, melanocytes are present in the basal layer of the epidermis.

Normal skin

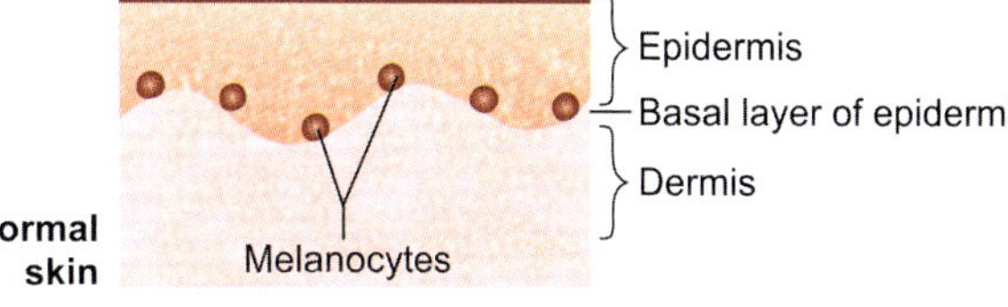

Nevi are benign pigmented lesions of the skin due to increased number of melanocytes. **According to microscopic appearance, nevi are classified into:**

Lentigo

- Increased number of melanocytes within the basal layer of epidermis.
- Usually found in face and hand of elderly person.

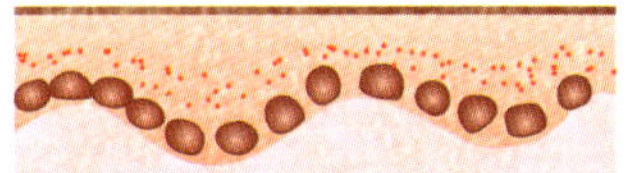

Junctional Nevus

- Develops due to increased number of melanocytes at dermo-epidermal junction. Usually found during or before puberty, as a smooth, flat pigmented lesion.
- **Majority of malignant melanoma arise from junctional nevus.**

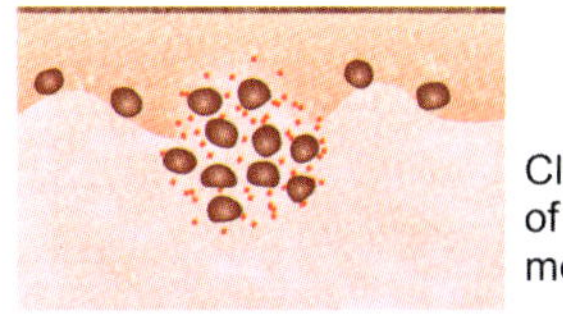

Dermal nevus

- Excess number of melanocytes cluster within the dermis.
- Presents as pigmented, elevated fleshy lesion in adults.

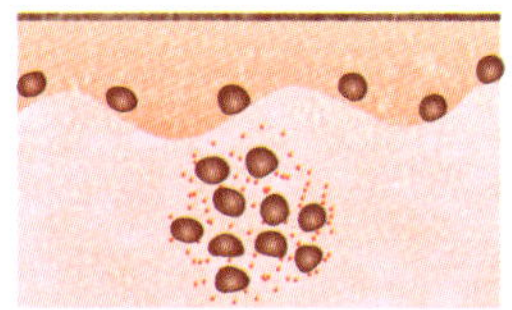

Compound nevus

- Excess melanocytes both at the dermo-epidermal junction and within the dermis.
- Presents as dermal nevus or junctional nevus.

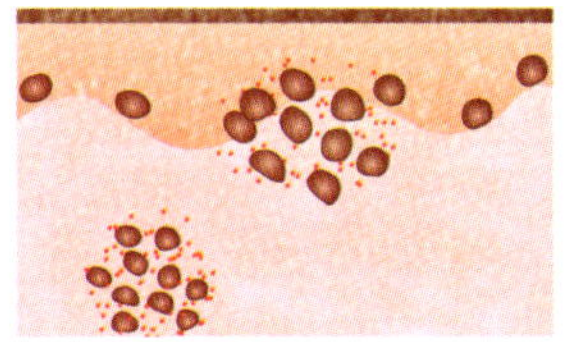

Blue nevus

- Excess melanocytes in the deeper layer of dermis. Most commonly found in face, dorsum of hand and feet.
- As the clusters of melanocytes present deep in the dermis, the lesion appears bluish rather than brown.

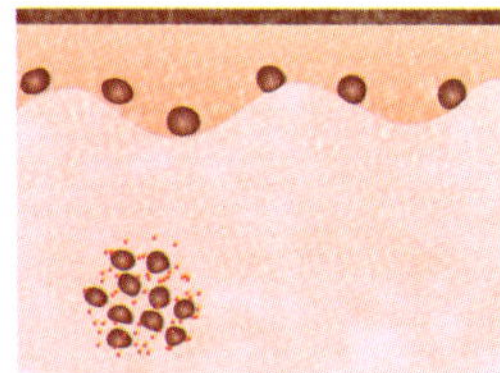

Different Types (According to Clinical Presentation)

a. **Hairy mole:**
   - Flat, slightly raised lesion with warty epidermal covering
   - Hairs grow from its surface
   - Microscopically, intradermal nevi.

b. **Nonhairy mole:**
   - Epithelium is smooth and not elevated
   - Microscopically, junctional or compound nevi.

c. **Blue nevus:**
   - Overlying skin is smooth and shiny.
   - More often seen in children.
   - Commonly found in face, dorsum of hands and feet, over the sacrum (mongolian blue spot).

d. **Hutchinson's lentigo:**
   - Large area of hyperpigmentation.
   - Seen in the face and neck of older people.
   - Surface is smooth, but may be raised (areas of junctional activity) as well as pale areas (areas of regression). **[Increased chance of malignant transformation]**

Treatment

Most of the nevus are benign and do not require treatment.

Conditions where excision is indicated:

- Patient wants for aesthetic reasons.
- Recently discovered lesion in an adult.
- Lesions undergone change in color (more darker), change in surface (loss of skin crease), increase in size, shape and thickness.
- Lesion starts itching (early symptom).
- Lesion starts bleeding (a late symptom).
- Lesion in sole of foot or palm of the hand.

Premalignant Lesions

Solar Keratosis (Actinic Keratosis, Senile Keratosis)

- Areas of epidermal dysplasia and hyperkeratosis in sunexposed areas of skin in elderly fair skinned males
- Ultraviolet B-induced P53 mutation have been observed in these lesions
- Commonly seen in back of fingers and hands, face, rim of ears
- Presents as raised erythematous plaque of skin with rough surface
- **Three possible behavior patterns:** (i) Spontaneous regression; (ii) Persistence; and (iii) Progression to carcinoma
- These lesions are potentially malignant (squamous/basal cell carcinoma)

Prevention:

- Use of hat
- Use of sunprotective clothings, sunscreen.

Treatment:

- Cryotherapy with CO_2 or liquid nitrogen (in solitary lesion)
- Topical 5-FU cream application (in multiple lesion)
- Thermocautery + curettage
- Topical imiquimod
- Photodynamic therapy
- Laser resurfacing
- Chemical peel with trichloroacetic acid.

Solar keratosis not responding to treatment or presents with bleeding, rapid growth or pain—Think of SCC and should be confirmed by biopsy.

Bowen's Disease

- It is an intraepidermal squamous cell carcinoma in situ.
- Clinically presents as flat, pink papular patches with well-defined margins, covered with crusts.
- Exposure to arsenic is sometimes associated as an etiological factor.
- Local cytotoxic therapy, e.g., 5-FU, cryotherapy, cauterization is useful but increased chance of recurrence.
- Surgical excision is the best treatment option.

Erythroplasia of Queyrat

- It is the Bowen's disease of glans penis.
- Most commonly found in uncircumcised males.

Xeroderma Pigmentosum

- Autosomal recessive disorder where sunexposed skin is mostly affected.
- Patients are in increased risk of developing squamous cell carcinoma, basal cell carcinoma and malignant melanoma.

Malignant Lesions

Basal Cell Carcinoma (Rodent Ulcer)

Second most common skin cancer.

Locally invasive malignancy of skin arising from basal layer of the epidermis.

Risk Factors Associated with BCC

- UV-A and UV-B radiation (persons with fair skin, red or blond hair, and light eye color are at increased risk of UV radiation induced damage)
- Ionizing radiation
- Albinism
- Xeroderma pigmentosum
- Radiation therapy (particularly at a young age)

Genetics associated with BCC

- The sonic hedgehog signaling pathway
- Mutations in PTCH1, p53 gene.

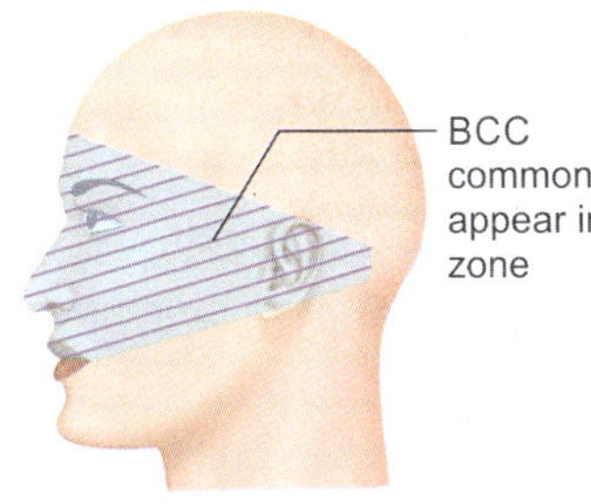

Anatomic Location

- Most common location is face, especially a zone above a line from lobe of the ear to corner of mouth.
- BCC can develop any skin sites exposed to UV radiation and radiation therapy.
- BCC develops in the "**H-zone**" are at increased risk of recurrence.

"H zone": "Mask areas" of face [central face, eyelids, eyebrows, periorbital, nose, lips (cutaneous and vermilion), chin, mandible, preauricular and postauricular skin/sulci, temple, and ear], genitalia, hands and feet.

Low-risk Histologic Subtypes

- Superficial
- Nodular
- Keratotic
- Infundibulocystic
- Fibroepithelial BCC

Pathology

- Characteristic feature is proliferation of basaloid cells resembling basal layer of epidermis.
- Masses of basaloid cells with single, outer layer of cells with palisaded appearance in dermis.

High-risk Histologic Subtypes

- Basosquamous
- Infiltrative
- Sclerosing/morpheaform
- Micronodular
- BCC with carcinosarcomatous differentiation.

Basosquamous basal cell carcinoma behaves more like a squamous cell carcinoma. So this type of carcinoma should be treated aggressively.

Clinical Presentation

- **Clinically** starts as nodular lesion (covered by fine vessels which give it a pink hue), that soon become ulcerated centrally. The resulting ulcer has a rolled pearly edge.
- In advanced stage, the tumor erodes bone, muscle, cartilage. BCC grows slowly, BCC does not metastasize.

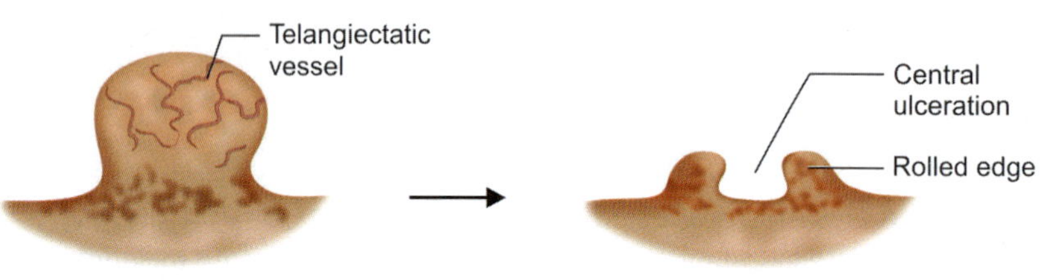

Types of BCC According to Clinical Appearance

- Nodular (most common)
- Cystic
- Pigmented (difficult to distinguish clinically from nodular melanoma)
- Morpheiform
- Infiltrated
- Superficial
- Fibroepithelioma of Pinkus (difficult to distinguish clinically from amelanostic melanoma)

Workup includes:

(i) Complete skin examination; (ii) Skin biopsy (must include deep reticular dermis); and (iii) Imaging (if bone involvement, perineural invasion or soft tissue involvement)—CT or MRI.

Management

Surgery

In low-risk BCC: Surgical excision (with 4-mm clinical margin) followed by postoperative pathologic evaluation of margins.

In high-risk BCC: Mohs micrographic surgery **(MMS)** is the preferred surgical option. Excision with complete circumferential peripheral and deep-margin assessment **(CCPDMA)** using intraoperative frozen section assessment is an alternative option to MMS.

Adjuvant Radiation Therapy

Indications: (i) Any BCC showing evidence of substantial perineural involvement (i.e., Involvement of more than just a few small sensory nerve branches or large nerve involvement) and (ii) Margins are positive after MMS or CCPDMA.

Contraindications: (i) In genetic diseases predisposing to skin cancer (e.g., basal cell nevus syndrome, xeroderma pigmentosum) and (ii) Connective tissue disorders (e.g., lupus, scleroderma).

Superficial Therapy

Superficial therapies are indicated when surgery or radiation is contraindicated or not feasible.

Superficial therapies include: (i) Topical therapies with 5-FU or imiquimod; (ii) Photodynamic therapy; and (iii) Cryotherapy

Targeted Therapy

Vismodegib and Sonidegib, hedgehog pathway inhibitors are recommended for locally advanced BCC that has recurred following surgery or radiotherapy.

Vismodegib may be used for prophylaxis in **nevoid BCC syndromes**.

Moh's Micrographic Surgery (MMS)

Serial horizontal excision

⇓

Each piece of tissue is undergone frozen section biopsy [entire margin of resection is examined]

⇓

Resection process to be continued until the margin is free.

This technique is particularly useful for BCC in eyelids and nose where tissue loss is undesirable, in recurrent lesions and in lesion with indistinct borders (morpheaform).

Least sacrifice of uninvolved tissue.

The procedure is lengthy (takes upto several days).

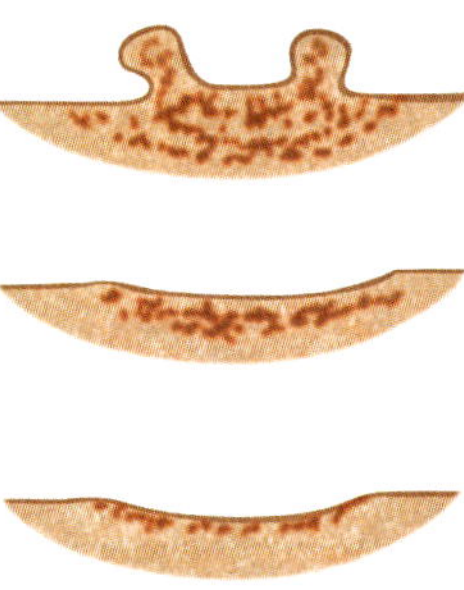

	Low-risk	High-risk
Location/size	Area L <20 mm; Area M <10 mm	Area L ≥20 mm; Area M ≥10 mm; Area H
Borders	Well defined	Poorly defined
Immunosuppression	(–)	(+)
Site of prior irradiation	(–)	(+)
Pathological subtype	Nodular, superficial	Aggressive growth pattern
Perineural involvement	(–)	(+)

Area M: Cheeks, forehead, scalp, neck, and pretibia.

Area L: Trunk and extremities (excluding hands, nail units, pretibia, ankles, and feet).

Squamous Cell Carcinoma

Anatomic Location

- Most commonly found in exposed areas—Head region (about 75%), face, pinna, back of hands
- Mucocutaneous junctions—Lip, anal canal, glans penis.

SCC in external ear have increased tendency to recur and regional lymph node metastasis.

- **Chimney-sweeper's cancer**—Cancer of scrotal skin due to repeated exposure to soot.
- **Kangari cancer**—SCC of skin of inner side of thigh and lower abdomen in natives of Kashmir
- **Marjolin's ulcer**—SCC in old scar, most commonly old burn scar. This ulcer may also develop in osteomyelitis, venous stasis ulcer, radiation dermitis.

Kangari is an earthenware pot containing glowing charcoal—people keep this pot close to abdomen to keep warm.

- Cutaneous squamous cell carcinoma (cSCC) arises from the **keratinocytes in epidermis**.
- Squamous cell carcinoma and basal cell carcinoma are collectively termed as **nonmelanoma skin cancers** or **keratinocyte carcinomas**.
- Commonly found in men than women.

Risk Factors Associated with cSCC

- Prolonged exposure to sunlight (Amount of exposure is proportional to risk, persons with fair complexion, blonde hair are more susceptible than individual with dark complexion)
- Indoor tanning
- Solar keratoses
- Bowen's disease
- Xeroderma pigmentosa (1,000-fold increased risk)
- Oculocutaneous albinism
- Immunosuppression (Four-fold increased risk)
  - Risk is related to degree of and duration of immunosuppression.
  - Patient of organ transplantation (on immunosuppressive drugs, e.g., azathioprine, cyclosporine, prednisolone)
  - Patient with immunosuppressive diseases (e.g., HIV and HPV infection, autoimmune diseases, lymphoma, leukemia)
- Exposure to certain chemicals (e.g., organic hydrocarbons)
- Exposure to arsenic
- Old burn scar (higher incidence of recurrence and metastases)
- Long standing venous ulcer
- Chronic osteomyelitis (higher incidence of recurrence and metastases)
- Tobacco use

Pathology

Microscopically, well differentiated SCC have a characteristic appearance—**Whorled arrangement** of malignant squamous cells, in which the center of it contains **laminated keratin material**.

SCC stains positive for cylokeratin 1 and 10.

Histological Grading of SCC

- Well or moderately differentiated
- Poorly differentiated.

Normal epithelium

SCC

Ulcerated growth

Everted edge

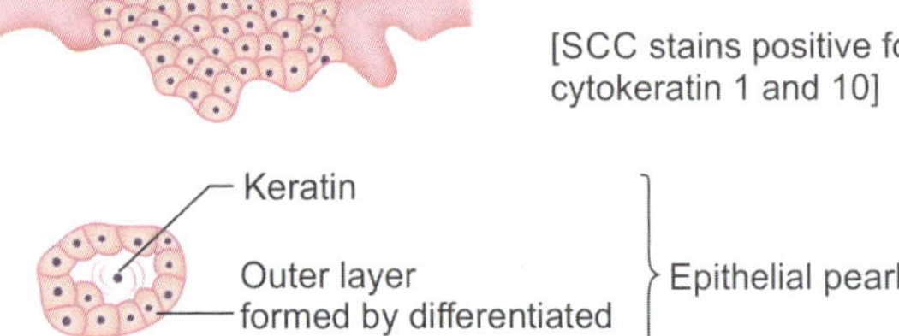

Clinical Presentation

- Clinically presents as slightly raised hyperkeratotic macule or papule. Gradually the surface breaks down and an **ulcerated growth with everted edge** with indurated base develops.
- Regional lymph nodes may become involved, either due to metastasis or from infection.

Patients with Increased Risk of Multiple SCC

- Patients with immunocompromised state (solid organ transplant recipients, HIV, drug induced immunosuppression)
- Patients with albinism or xeroderma pigmentosa

Workup

- Full skin examination (to rule out other precancerous or cancerous lesions in other sun-exposed sites)
- MRI with contrast or contrast CT (if bone or soft tissue involvement, perineural, lymphatic or vascular invasion is suspected)
- Biopsy of the lesion (preferably incisional biopsy)
- FNA or core biopsy of palpable or image detected regional lymph nodes.

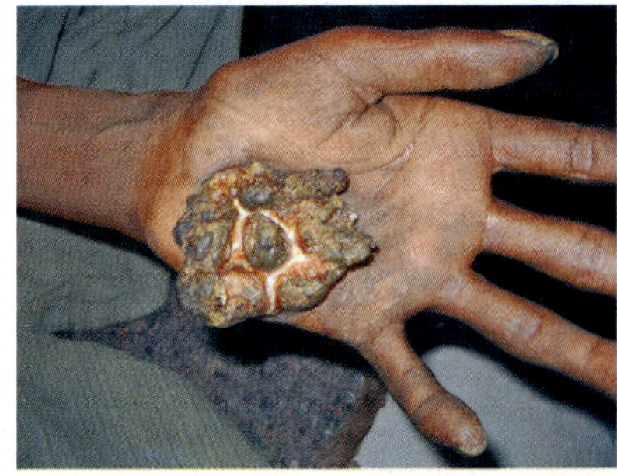

Treatment

Treatment Options

- Curettage and electrodesiccation
- Standard surgical excision
- Mohs Micrographic Surgery **(MMS)**
- Excision with Complete Circumferential Peripheral and Deep Margin Assessment **(CCPDMA)**
- Radiation therapy (as primary therapy)
- Superficial therapies (Topical 5-FU, topical imiquimod, photodynamic therapy, cryotherapy).

SCC in situ: Superficial therapies are indicated for patients with SCC in situ.

Low-risk SCC: Treatment options are: (i) Curettage and electrodesiccation (in areas with hair growth, e.g., scalp, pubic and axillary area, beard area; (ii) Standard surgical excision with 4–6 mm margin; and (iii) Radiation therapy for non-surgical patients.

High-risk SCC: Treatment options are: (i) Standard surgical excision with wider margin than low-risk lesions; (ii) Mohs Micrographic Surgery; (iii) CCPDMA; and (iv) Radiation therapy for nonsurgical patients.

MMS or CCPDMA may be considered as primary therapy or as second-line therapy if negative margin cannot be achieved after standard surgical excision.

Adjuvant radiation therapy is indicated if extensive perineural involvement or tissue margins are positive after surgical excision.

Management of regional lymph node involvement: Parotidectomy and/or neck dissection with or without adjuvant radiation therapy for SCC in face. For lesion in other areas, regional lymph node dissection for clinically palpable lymph nodes or nodes detected on imaging.

Indications for Mohs Micrographic Surgery for Nonmelanoma Skin Cancer

- High-risk anatomic locations (eyelids, nose, ears, lips, genitalia, fingers)
- Tumors >0.6 cm on face or >2.0 cm on the body and extremities
- Recurrent tumors
- Tumors occurring in sites of previous radiation therapy or in chronic scars
- Tumors with indistinct clinical margins or incompletely excised margins (positive margin after surgical resection)
- Tumors with aggressive patterns (micronodular, infiltrative and morpheaform BCC, basosquamous carcinoma, and poorly differentiated or deeply invasive squamous cell carcinomas).
- Tumors in immunosuppressed patients.

Verrucous Carcinoma

- A special variety of SCC which is well-differentiated, invade locally and rarely metastasize
- Commonly found in palms and soles
- Superficial part of the tumor resembles verruca (hyperkeratosis, parakeratosis, acanthosis, papillomatosis)
- Treatment is surgical excision.

Cutaneous Melanoma

- **Melanoma** is a malignant neoplasm arising from **melanocytes**.
- **Cutaneous melanoma** arises from malignant transformation of melanocytes at the dermoepidermal junction.
- **More than 98% of melanomas are cutaneous melanomas.**
- **Melanocytes are also found** in mucous membranes, meninges, upper esophagus and eyes (sites where precursor melanocytes migrate from neural crest during embryonic development).

Classification of Melanoma

- Cutaneous melanoma
- Noncutaneous melanoma

Noncutaneous melanoma develop on: (i) Mucosal membrane; (ii) Uveal tract of the eye; and (iii) Lepto-meninges.

Mucosal melanomas commonly develop in headneck sinuses, oral cavity, anorectum, vulva and vagina, but may develop in any mucosal membranes lining the GI and urogenital tract.

Cutaneous Melanoma

- Arise from epidermal melanocytes
- The median age at diagnosis is lower than mucosal melanoma
- Often, patients diagnosed at early stage
- Definite risk factors (e.g., exposure to sunlight etc.) are present
- BRAF and NRAS mutations are commonly associated
- Not associated with KIT mutation
- Role of SLN mapping is established.

Mucosal Melanoma

- Arise from melanocytes in epithelial lining of the respiratory, gastrointestinal and genitourinary tracts
- The median age at diagnosis is higher
- Often, patients have advanced disease at the time of initial diagnosis
- No definite risk factors are present
- BRAF and NRAS mutations are rare in mucosal melanomas
- Associated with activating mutations and/or amplifications in KIT
- Role of SLN mapping is not established.

Risk Factors

(i) Male; (ii) Age >60 years; (iii) Atypical mole or dysplastic nevus pattern; (iv) Fitzpatrick skin type I; (v) History of actinic keratosis or nonmelanoma skin cancer; (vi) Xeroderma pigmentosum; (vii) Family history of multiple cutaneous melanoma; (viii) Chronic sun exposure; (ix) Immunosuppression related to solid organ transplantation, HIV infection; (x) Use of tanning bed; and (xi) Genetic predisposition.

Pathophysiology

Progression from normal melanocytes to metastatic melanoma is a stepwise process induced by multiple genetic mutations and involves several histologic intermediates.

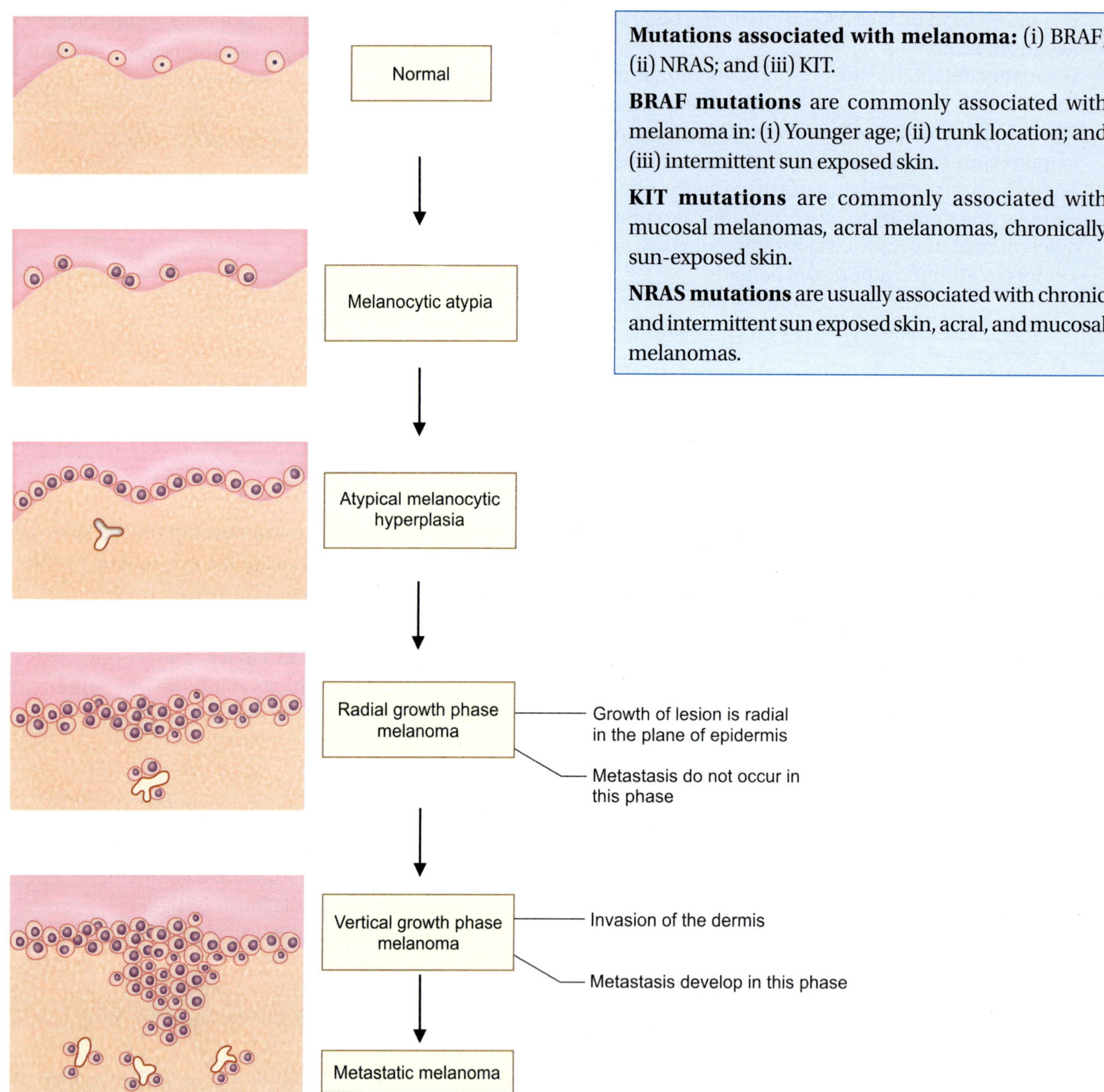

Mutations associated with melanoma: (i) BRAF; (ii) NRAS; and (iii) KIT.

BRAF mutations are commonly associated with melanoma in: (i) Younger age; (ii) trunk location; and (iii) intermittent sun exposed skin.

KIT mutations are commonly associated with mucosal melanomas, acral melanomas, chronically sun-exposed skin.

NRAS mutations are usually associated with chronic and intermittent sun exposed skin, acral, and mucosal melanomas.

Cells in the vertical growth phase are different from **cells in radial growth phase** in respect of morphology, cell surface antigens, behavior in cell culture.

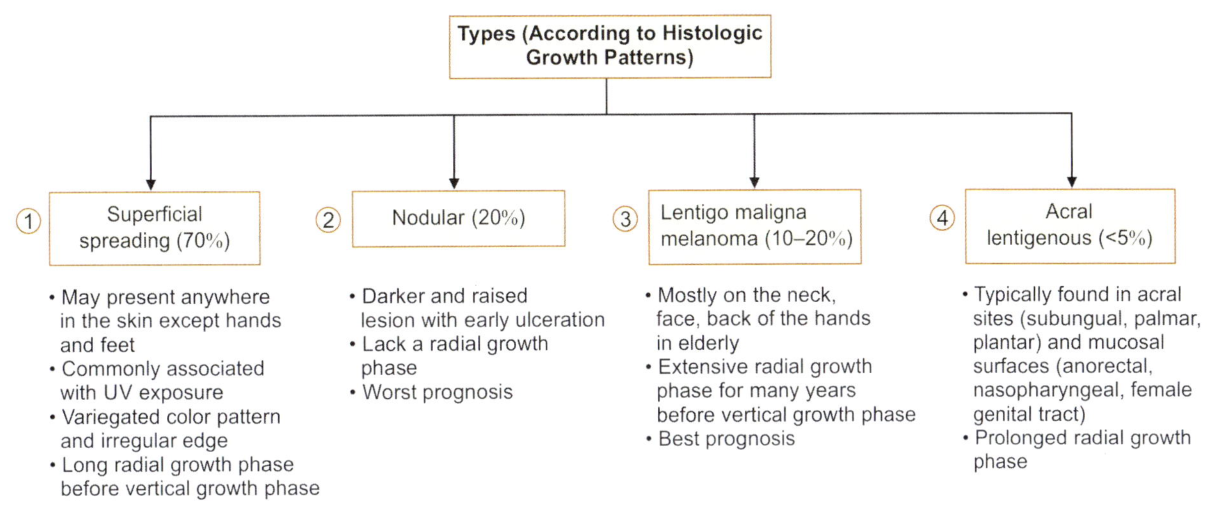

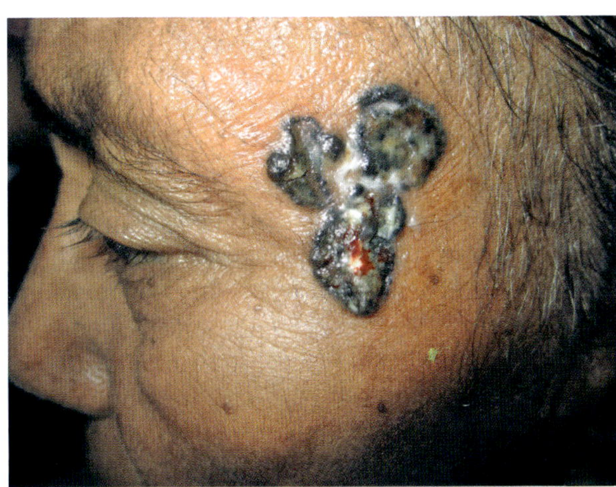

- Etiology of acral lentiginous melanoma (ALM) is most likely independent of UV exposure.
- ALM is more common in African, Asian and Hispanic population than in fair skinned population.
- Subungual lesions present as blue-black discoloration of the posterior nail fold.
- Additional presence of discoloration in proximal or lateral nail folds **(Hutchinson's sign)** is diagnostic of subungual melanoma.

Any pigmented subungual lesion should be biopsied.

Spread of Tumor

Lymphatic spread: Tumor may spread to regional lymph node by embolism. Lymphatic permeation causes local satellite lesion.

Hematogenous spread: Lungs, liver, brain, spinal cord, adrenals are common sites of metastasis.

Unusual sites of metastasis—Small intestine, heart, breast.

In-transit metastases or satellite lesions are subcutaneous or cutaneous lymphatic deposits of tumor cells in between the primary tumor site and the draining lymph nodal basin.

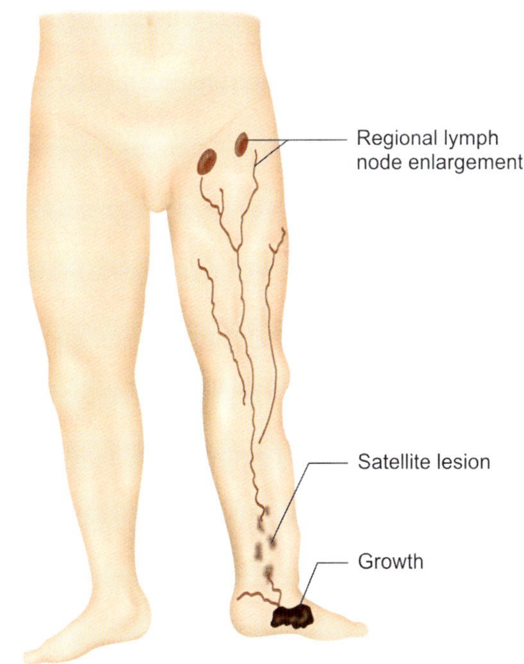

Diagnosis

- **Malignant melanoma can be differentiated from benign pigmented lesions** by examining the features: **A**symmetry, **B**order irregularity, **C**olor change, **D**iameter >6 mm, **E**levation (**ABCDE**).
- **Clinical examination** is to be done to assess the site of primary lesion, any satellite lesion, all major lymph nodal basins, thorough evaluation of regional lymph node basins along with complete skin examination.
- Suspicious pigmented lesion should undergo an **excisional biopsy** (elliptical/punch/saucerization) with 1–3 mm negative margins.
- Where excisional biopsy is not appropriate, **full-thickness incisional or punch biopsy** (from the thickest part of the lesion) is indicated.
- **Shave biopsy** is not preferred because it compromises complete assessment of Breslow thickness.

Excisional biopsy is not appropriate in:

- Large lesions
- Palmar surface of the hand
- Sole of the foot
- Distal digit
- Face
- Subungual lesions

Sentinel Lymph Node Biopsy

Indications

- Clinical stage IB, T1b or T1a lesions with Breslow depth <0.8 mm and with other adverse features (e.g., mitotic index ≥ 2/mm^2, lymphovascular invasion, or combination of these factors
- Clinical stage IB (T2a) or II (>1 mm thick, any feature, N0)
- Isolated in-transit metastases or local recurrence of a primary melanoma without clinically or radiologically evident regional nodal or distant metastases.

All patients with positive sentinel lymph node biopsy warrant completion lymph node dissection (CLND). If sentinel lymph node biopsy is negative, regional lymph node dissection is not indicated. Patient with clinically positive lymph nodes without distant metastases should undergo CLND of involved nodal basin.

Prognostic Factors

Age of the patient: Melanoma-associated mortality increases with age.

Gender: Prognosis is better in women

Location of tumor:

- Prognosis is better in melanoma on extremities in comparison to melanoma in trunk, head-neck
- Melanoma on acral sites have also poorer prognosis
- Significant poor prognosis in mucosal melanoma.

Ulceration: Ulceration of the lesion is a negative prognostic indicator.

Histologic growth pattern: Lentigo maligna melanoma have a better prognosis and acral lentiginous melanoma have a worse prognosis independent of Breslow thickness.

Metastasis:

- **Lymph node metastasis:** Regional lymph node involvement is a poor prognostic sign. The number of positive lymph nodes is related with survival rates.
- Distant metastasis is also a grave prognostic sign.

Depth of invasion: Breslow tumor thickness

Mitotic rate

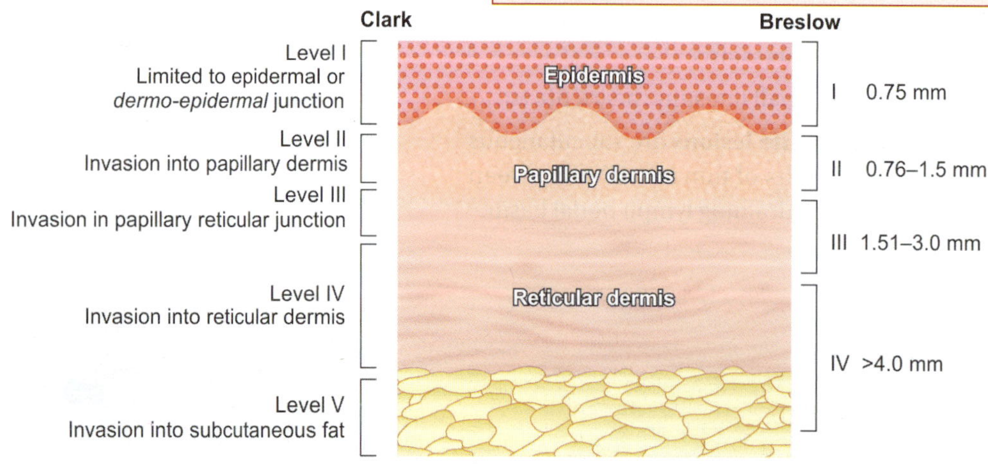

Treatment

Excision of primary lesion:

Wide excision is the treatment of choice for all types of melanomas. The defect is closed by either primary closure or by skin graft or local flap.

Lymph node dissection:

Complete lymph node dissection (CLND) is indicated in patients with clinically positive nodes. All patients with positive sentinel lymph node biopsy warrant completion lymph node dissection.

Pelvic dissection is indicated for clinically positive inguino-femoral nodes and for iliac and/or obturator node involvement detected by pelvic CT.

In lesion on the face, anterior scalp and ear, superficial parotidectomy to remove parotid nodes and appropriate neck dissection of the draining nodal basins are indicated.

Adjuvant radiation therapy is indicated in: (i) Desmoplastic neurotropic melanoma (a locally aggressive variant) and (ii) Clinically positive lymph nodes with features suggestive of increased risk of nodal basin prolapse.

Adjuvant systemic therapy is indicated in stage III disease (regional disease).

FDA-approved systemic therapy are: (i) Immune checkpoint inhibitors (Ipilimumab, Nivdumab, Pembrolizumab) and (ii) BRAF/MEK combinations (Dabrafenib/trametinib).

Surgical Margin for Wide Excision

Tumor thickness	*Margin*
In situ	0.5–1.0 cm
≤1 mm	1 cm
1.01–2.0 mm	1–2 cm
≥2 mm	2 cm

Treatment of In-transit Metastases

Complete surgical excision with histologically negative margin (most preferred)

Unresectable stage III in-transit disease-intralesional T-VEC (Talimogene Laherparevec) is recommended. Other options are intralesional IL-2, BCG, IFN.

Low-volume cutaneous metastases—topical imiquimod.

Multiple in-transit metastases confined to an extremity—Isolated limb perfusion (ILP) or Isolated limb infusion (ILI).

Isolated Limb Perfusion (ILP) and Isolated Limb Infusion (ILI)

These regional therapies are indicated for regionally recurrent melanomas not suitable for local or topical therapies. In these techniques, high doses of cytotoxic chemotherapeutic agents are administered to the diseased extremity under hyperthermic conditions (40°C) while avoiding systemic toxicities.

Melphalan is the most commonly used chemotherapeutic agent. Often, actinomycin D is used along with melphalan.

ILI is simpler, less invasive and safer in comparison to ILP.

Other Malignancies of the Skin

Kaposi Sarcoma

- Kaposi sarcoma is a HHV-8-related angiosarcoma affecting the skin and viscera
- Clinically presents as rubbery red or brown papules in the extremities
- Four form of Kaposi's sarcoma:
  1. **Classic:** Locally aggressive, slowly progressive, commonly involve the lower extremities, visceral involvement is rare, more common in males, other malignancies are commonly associated
  2. **Endemic:** Occurs in children and younger adults of equatorial Africa, more aggressive than classic form, predilection to spread to lymph nodes, more common in males.
  3. **Epidemic (AIDS-associated):** Occurs exclusively in male homosexuals, not in IV drug abusers and hemophiliacs, disease become more aggressive if immunosuppression is more advanced.
  4. **Iatrogenic or transplant-associated:** Usually develops 2–8 months after initiation of immunosuppressive therapy, more common in males.

- Treatment is surgical excision. Other treatment options are: (i) Radiotherapy; (ii) Cryosurgery; and (iii) Laser ablation.

Angiosarcoma

- Highly aggressive malignant tumor of endothelial cells
- Clinically presents as 'bruise' like lesion that spontaneously bleeds or enlarges, in elderly males
- **Four forms of angiosarcoma:**
  1. As of scalp and face
  2. As associated with lymphedema
  3. Radiation-induced AS
  4. Epithelioid AS.
- Radical excision is the treatment of choice
- Prognosis is poor.

Lymphangiosarcoma

Lymphangiosarcoma is a rare malignancy arises in the setting of **chronic lymphedema**. It may arise in areas of chronic lymphedema of the arm following mastectomy **(Stewart–Treves syndrome)**.

Prognosis is very poor. Early amputation offers the best chance of long-term survival. Chemotherapy and radiotherapy are used for palliation.

Skin Metastases

Common primary sites in male: Lung, large intestine, melanoma, oral cavity, kidney, breast.

Common primary sites in female: Breast, ovary, oral cavity, melanoma, lung, large intestine.

Cutaneous metastases may present as papules, plaques, nodules, tumors, ulcers.

Sister Mary Joseph nodule, a specific variety of cutaneous metastasis, presents as indurated umbilical nodule.

Case 1

History and Physical Examination

A 10-year-old boy presented with a swelling in the face near the outer part of right eye for last 6 years. The swelling was like a peanut in the beginning, gradually increasing in size and now attained the size of a marble. No history of pain in the swelling. No history of trauma.

Clinical Examination

A 2 cm × 2 cm cystic, non-tender, non-pulsatile swelling with well-defined margin was present at the upper part of lateral canthus of right eye. The swelling was not fixed to the overlying skin but some fixity to the underlying structures.

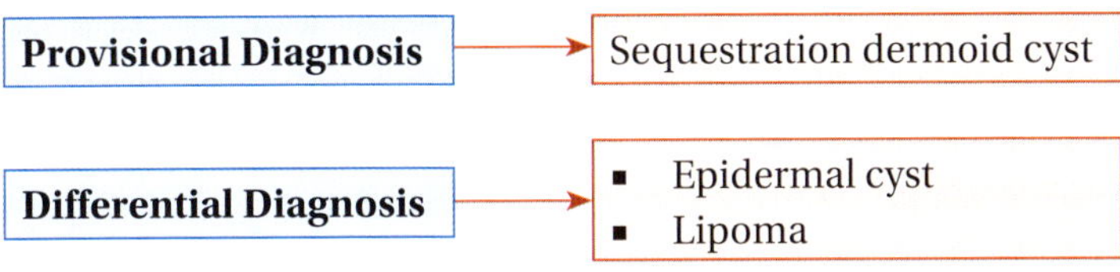

Provisional Diagnosis → Sequestration dermoid cyst

Differential Diagnosis →
- Epidermal cyst
- Lipoma

Investigations

FNAC suggestive of dermoid cyst. CT scan excluded any intracranial communication of the cyst.

Discussion

A non-tender cystic swelling over the lines of fusion and almost fixed to the underlying bone was highly suggestive of sequestration dermoid cyst. CT scan was done to exclude any intracranial communication.

Management Algorithm

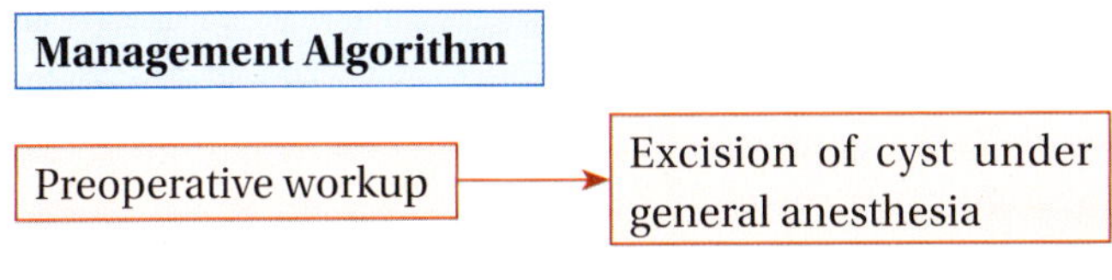

Preoperative workup → Excision of cyst under general anesthesia

Case 2

History and Physical Examination

A 50-year-old female patient presented in the surgical OPD with complain of ulceration of the previous burn scar in her right leg for last 4 months. The hypertrophic scar in her leg following burn injury developed about 10 years back. About 4 months back, she noticed mild erythematous changes over the scar followed by breaching of the skin and development of this ulcer. Patient was treated by local physician but no improvement. No history of diabetes mellitus or hypertension.

Clinical Examination

An irregular shaped ulcer with everted edge was seen over the burn scar in the posterior aspect of right leg. Base was indurated and bleeds on touch. Multiple inguinal group of lymph nodes were palpable on the right side.

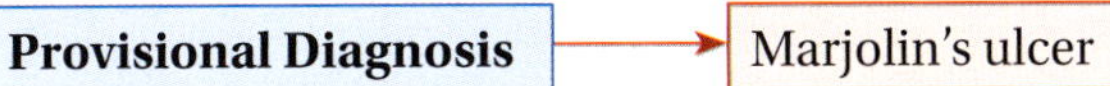

Provisional Diagnosis → Marjolin's ulcer

Investigations

Incisional biopsy revealed squamous cell carcinoma. FNAC from inguinal lymph nodes revealed metastatic squamous cell carcinoma.

Discussion

Formation of an ulcerated lesion with an everted margin in an old burn scar was highly suggestive of Marjolin's ulcer. Incisional biopsy confirmed the diagnosis. Wide local excision along with inguinal lymph node dissection was planned.

Management Algorithm

Preoperative work-up → Wide local excision of the ulcerated lesion with 1 cm margin along with right inguinal lymph node dissection.

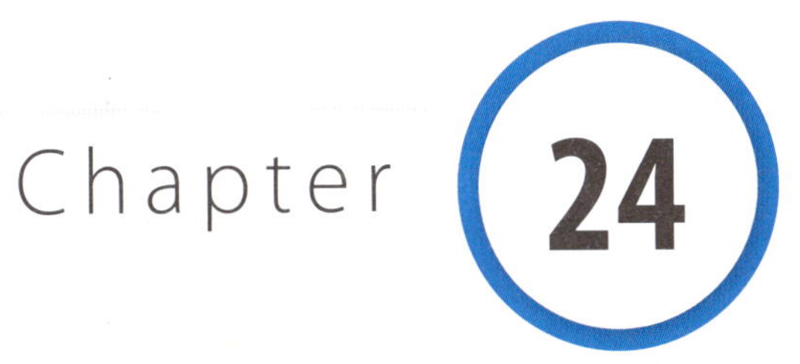

Chapter 24

Ulcer, Sinus, and Fistula

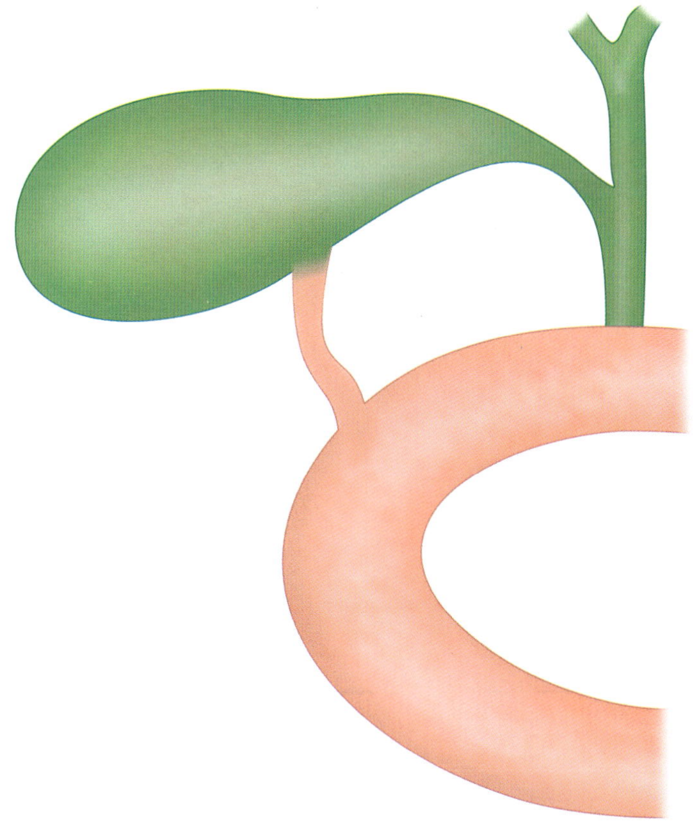

Important Topics

- Types of Ulcer
- Sinus
- Fistula

'Learn from yesterday, live for today, hope for tomorrow. The important thing is to not stop questioning.'

Ulcer

An ulcer is a discontinuity of an epithelial surface.

Ulcer has some features that must be examined in clinical examination:

- **Edge:** It is the junction between healthy and diseased tissue. It takes characteristic form according to underlying disease.
- **Floor:** Floor is that which is seen by a clinician.
  Floor may be covered by—
  - Granulation tissue—In healing ulcer
  - Dead tissues (slough)—In active ulcer
  - Malignant tissue—In malignant ulcer.
- **Base:** Base is that which can be palpated.
  - Marked induration of the base—In squamous cell carcinoma.
  - Base is attached to deeper structures—Varicose ulcer (attached to tibia).
- **Discharge:** Serous, serosanguinous, purulent, offensive. Discharge should be sent for culture-sensitivity.

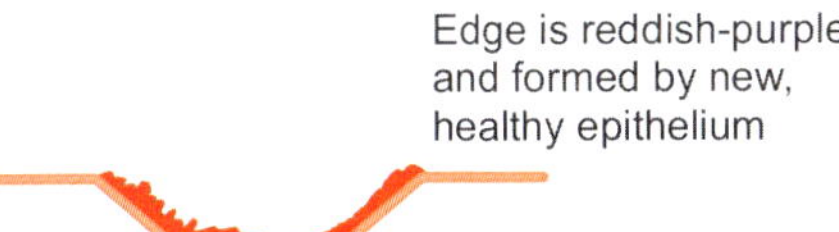

Sloping edge: The edge gently slopes from normal epithelium to base of the ulcer.
For example, all healing ulcers

Surrounding tissue is less affected

Punched-out edge: The edge drops down at right angles to the skin surface.
For example, deep trophic ulcer, gummatous ulcer

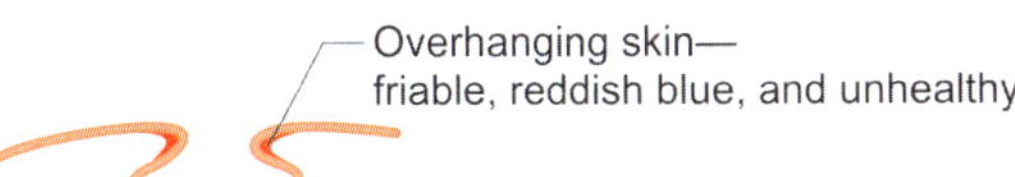

Undermined edge: The disease destroys the subcutaneous tissue faster than the overlying skin.
For example, tuberculous ulcer

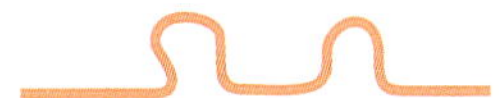

Rolled edge: Lesion becomes necrotic at its center but grows rapidly at its periphery.
For example, basal cell carcinoma

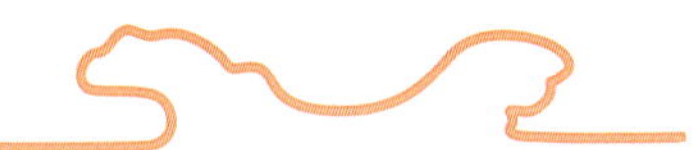

Everted edge: When ulcer caused by fast growing disease, the edge of the ulcer heaps up due to excessive growth.
For example, squamous cell carcinoma, ulcerated adenocarcinoma

Types of Ulcer

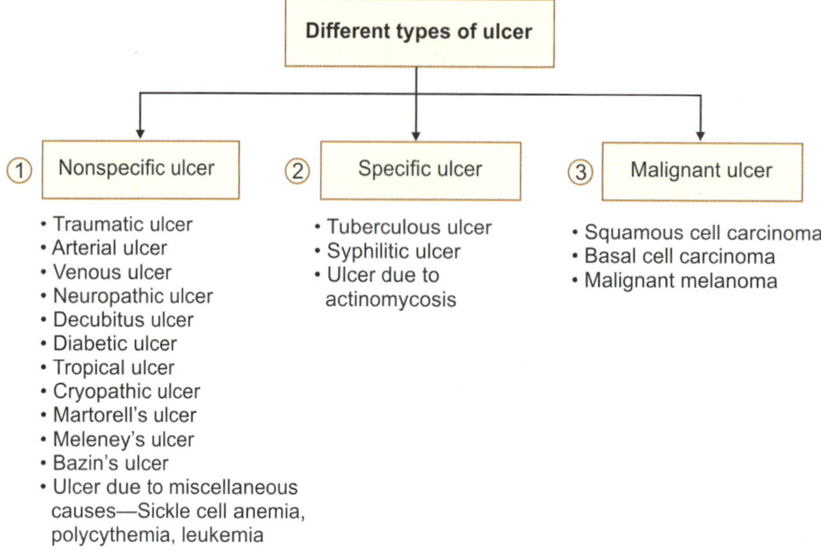

Traumatic Ulcer

- The ulcer may present in the body but more commonly found where skin is closely applied to the bony prominences, e.g., shin, medial and lateral malleoli, back of heel.
- They are painful, circular-shaped ulcers.

Arterial Ulcer (Ischemic Ulcer)

- An ulcer that develops due to inadequate blood supply.
- Arterial ulcer develops due to: (i) **Large artery occlusion** (e.g., atherosclerosis) and (ii) **Small artery occlusion** (e.g., Buerger's disease, Diabetes, Raynaud's disease, Embolism, Pressure necrosis)
- These ulcers are commonly developed **in the tip of the toes and fingers and over the pressure areas.**
- Floor is often infected, the blood supply is not adequate enough to form healthy granulation tissue.
- Clinically presents as **painful, deep ulcer in the distal part of the extremities** associated with symptoms of PAD (intermittent claudication, rest pain, exacerbation of pain at night) and signs of peripheral ischemia (dryness of skin, hair loss, blackish discoloration, gangrene).
- **Treatment:** Care of the ulcer + revascularization. Unless revascularization is successful, the healing of ulcer is not satisfactory.

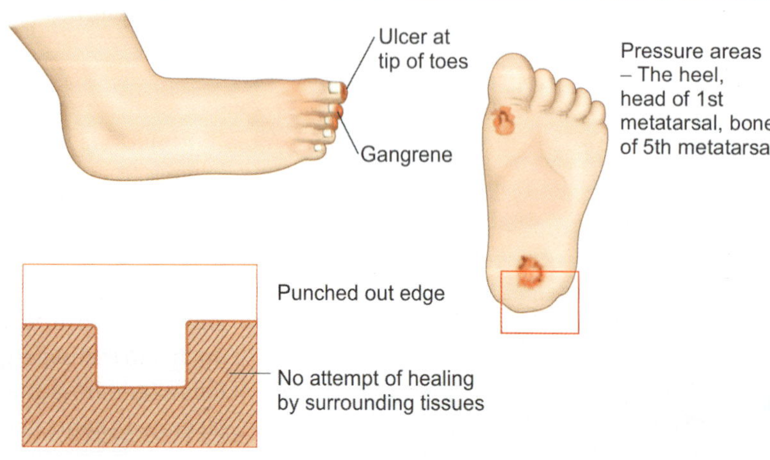

Venous Ulcer

- Commonly found around the **'gaiter' area of the lower leg** (lower third) and on the medial side of the leg. The ulcers particularly develop at the sites of incompetent perforators—Most common over Cockett's perforator (above the medial malleolus). The typical location of ulcer, characteristic skin changes and history of venous incompetence—Suggestive of venous ulcer.
- **Treatment**—Care of the ulcer + compression therapy.

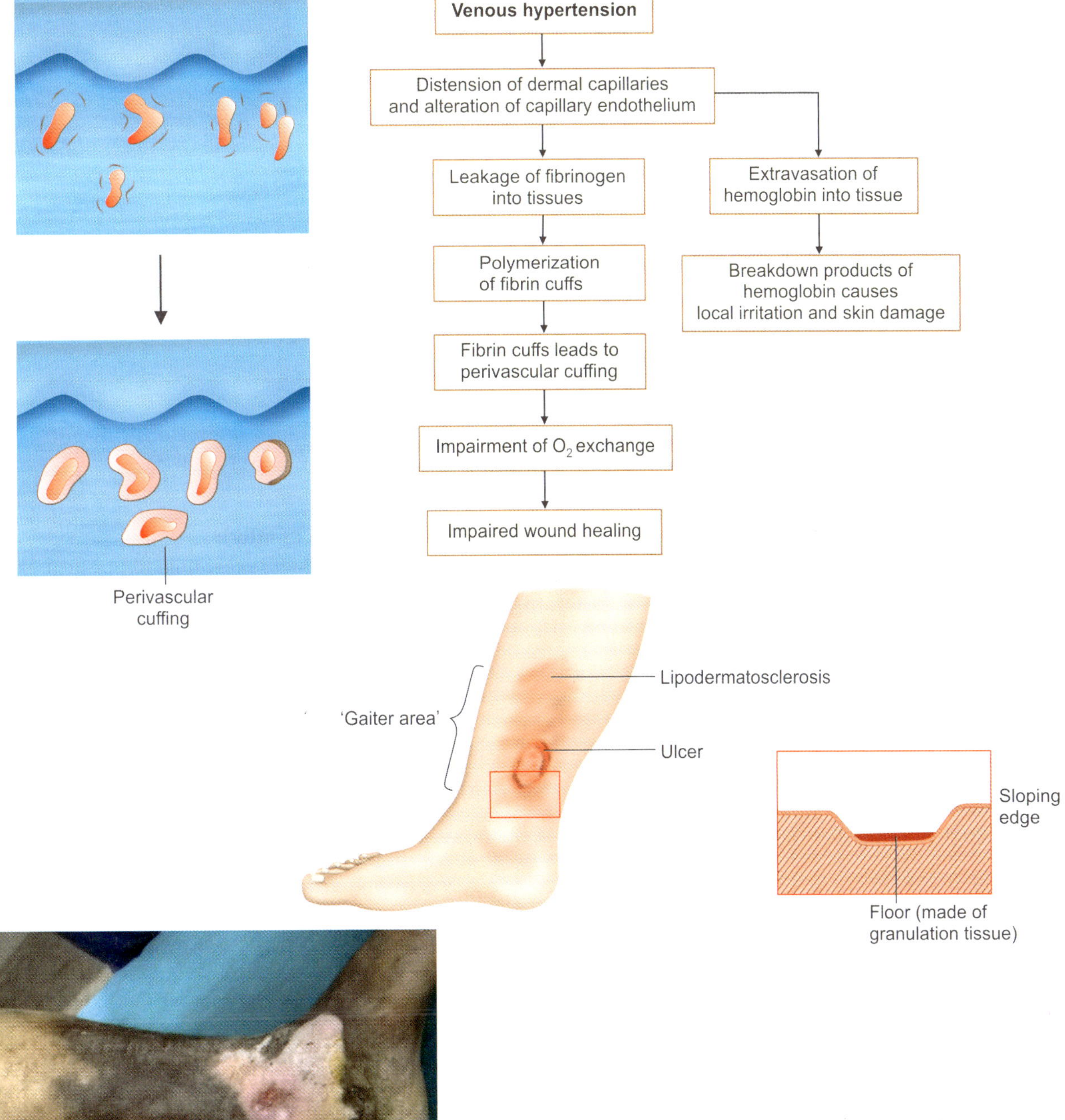

Neuropathic Ulcer

- The ulcer develops due to repeated injury or pressure in an area unable to appreciate pain.
- These ulcers develop due to (i) **Peripheral nerve lesion** (e.g., diabetes, leprosy, alcoholic neuropathy, peripheral nerve injury) and (ii) **Spinal cord lesion** (e.g., Spinal bifida, Syringomyelia, Tabes dorsalis, Paraplegia).
- The ulcers are seen on the **heel, base of 5th metatarsal, head of 1st metarsal** in ambulatory patients; on the **buttock and on the back of the heel** in nonambulatory patients.
- **Characteristic features of this ulcer:**
  - Painless ulcer
  - Loss of sensation in the surrounding tissues
  - Normal vascularity in the surrounding tissues.
- **Clinically,** neuropathic ulcers must be differentiated from ischemic ulcer by neurological examination.
- **Treatment:** Care of the ulcer + use of appliances to reduce pressure + treatment of the cause.

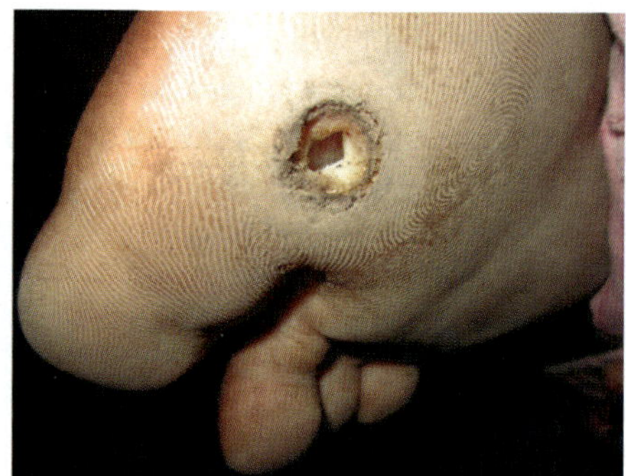

Diabetic Foot Ulcer (DFU)

Definition of Diabetic Foot

Infection, ulceration, or destruction of tissues of the foot of a person with currently or previously diagnosed diabetes mellitus, usually accompanied by neuropathy and/or PAD in the lower extremity (IWGDF).

Etiology

- **Neuropathic (sensory neuropathy, motor neuropathy, autonomic neuropathy):**
  - In sensory neuropathy, loss of protective sensation (LOPS) makes patient susceptible to physical, thermal, or chemical trauma.
  - In motor neuropathy, there is development of foot deformities (hammer toes, claw foot) may result in abnormal pressure over bony prominences.
  - Autonomic neuropathy is associated with dry skin, resulting in formation of fissures, cracks, callus.
- **Ischemic:**
  - Diabetic patients are commonly associated with peripheral arterial disease.
  - Diabetic microangiopathy is also responsible for ulcer formation.
- **Neuroischemic:**
  - Both neuropathic and ischemic causes are responsible for ulcer development.

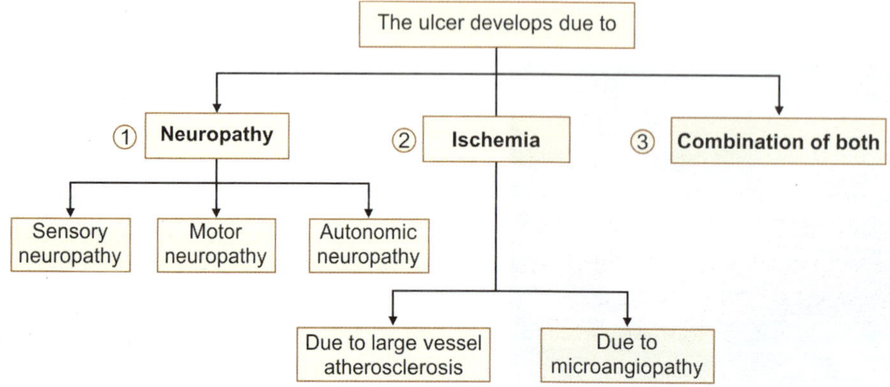

Features of Diabetic Foot Ulcers According to Etiology [Adapted from Wound International Guideline]

Feature	Neuropathic	Ischemic	Neuroischemic
Sensation	Sensory loss	Painful	Degree of sensory loss
Callus/necrosis	Callus present and often thick	Necrosis common	Minimal callus, prone to necrosis
Wound bed	Pink and granulating, surrounded by callus	Pale and sloughy with poor granulation	Poor granulation
Foot temperature and pulses	Warm with bounding pulses	Cool with absent pulses	Cool with absent pulses
Typical location	Weight-bearing areas of foot	Tips of toes, nail edges and between the toes	Margins of the foot and toes
Prevalence	35%	15%	50%

Risk Factors for Developing Foot Ulcer or Amputation

Low risk: No risk factors except callus

Moderate risk:
- Deformity of foot
- Neuropathy
- Non-critical limb ischemia

High risk:
- Previous ulcer formation
- Previous amputation
- Presence of both neuropathy and non-critical limb ischemia
- Presence of both neuropathy and callus and/or foot deformity

Assessment

Assessment of DFU includes: (i) Physical examination of the ulcer; (ii) Tests for loss of sensation; (iii) Assessment of vascular status; (iv) Identifying infection; and (v) Assessment of foot deformities.

Physical examination of ulcer:
- Neuropathic/ischemic/neuroischemic
- Site, size, depth, edge of the ulcer
- Color of the wound bed
- Any malodor, pain
- Any necrosis or gangrene
- Presence of any signs of infection
- Presence of exudates
- Any exposed bone.

Tests for loss of sensation:
- Tests used for peripheral neuropathy are: (i) 10 g (Semmes-Weinstein) monofilament; (ii) Standard 128 Hz tuning fork; and (iii) Biothesiometer.
- The 10 g monofilament is applied at various sites along the plantar aspect of the foot (over first metatarsal, third metatarsal, fifth metatarsal, etc.) for about 2 seconds. A positive result is the inability to feel the monofilament when it is pressed against the foot with enough force to bend it.

Assessment for vascular status:

- Evaluation is done by—Doppler arterial waveforms in combination with ankle systolic pressure and ankle brachial index (ABI) or toe systolic pressure and toe brachial index (TBI).
- Peripheral artery disease is less likely present if—ABI 0.9–1.3, toe brachial index ≥0.75 and triphasic pedal Doppler waveforms.

Identifying infection:

- About half of the DFUs become infected and about 20% of infected DFUs will undergo amputation.
- Risk factors associated with likelihood of infection: (i) DFU present for >30 days; (ii) Recurrent DFUs; (iii) PAD in the affected limb; (iv) Loss of protective sensation; and (v) Presence of renal insufficiency.
- Clinical symptoms and signs along with culture is needed for identifying infection. Sometimes, classic signs of infection are absent and 'secondary signs' of infection (e.g. friable granulation tissue, wound undermining, malodor, presence of wound exudates) may present.

Assessment of foot deformities:

- Assessment is done to identify foot deformities causing high plantar pressure areas, development of Charcot-foot.
- Foot deformities with high risk of ulcer development are: (i) High-arch foot; (ii) Clawed lesser toes; (iii) Hallux valgus; (iv) Hallux rigidus; and (v) Fatty pad depletion.

Meggitt-Wagner Wound Classification

- Assessment of **ulcer depth** along with presence of **gangrene and loss of perfusion**
- **Six grades (0–5)**
- Does not allow for identification of PAD or infection.

The University of Texas Wound Classification

- Assesses **ulcer depth, presence of infection** and presence of **signs of lower extremity ischemia** using a matrix of **four grades with four stages**
- Helpful for predicting the outcome of DFU.

Management

- Optimal control of diabetes
- Management of hypertension, hyperlipidemia
- Avoidance of smoking
- Treatment of PAD, if present
- **Local wound care:** (i) Debridement-sharp debridement (most effective)/larval/autolytic/ultrasonic/hydrosurgical; (ii) Control of inflammation and infection- for superficial (mild) infections, systemic antibiotics and for deep (moderate or severe) infections, broad spectrum antibiotics, change after culture and sensitivity report; (iii) Wound bed preparation; and (iv) Dressing of the wound.
- **Pressure offloading:** The gold standard offloading device is Total contact cast (TCC). Other offloading devices are: Removable cast walkers, Scotchcast boots, Healing sandals, Crutches, Walkers.

Prevention of Foot Ulcer

- Identifying the at-risk foot
- Regularly inspecting and examining the at-risk foot
- Educating the patient, family, and healthcare professionals
- Ensuring routine wearing of appropriate footwear
- Treating risk factors for ulceration.

Patient (with At-risk for Foot Ulceration) Education on Foot Care [Adapted from IWGDF Guideline]

- Avoid walking barefoot, in socks without footwear, or in thin-soled slippers, whether at home or outside.
- Do not wear shoes that are too tight, have rough edges or uneven seams
- Visually inspect and manually feel inside all shoes before you put them on
- Wear socks/stockings without seams (or with the seams inside out); do not wear tight or knee high socks and change socks daily.
- Wash feet daily (with water temperature always below 37°C), and dry them carefully, especially between the toes.
- Do not use any kind of heater or hot-water bottle to warm feet.
- Do not use chemical agents or plasters to remove corns and calluses.
- Use emollients to lubricate dry skin, but not between the toes.
- Cut toenails straight across.
- Have your feet examined regularly by a healthcare professional.

Pressure Ulcer

Definition: A pressure ulcer is localized injury to the skin and/or underlying tissue usually over a bony prominence, as a result of pressure, or pressure in combination with shear. [NPUAP/EPUAP/PPPIA 2014]

Alternative terms: Decubitus ulcer, bed sore, pressure sore.

Factors responsible for pressure ulcer development:

Extrinsic factors:

- Pressure on skin and underlying soft tissues
- Friction and shear
- Microclimate (increased tissue temperature and skin moisture)

Intrinsic factors:

- Immobility
- Reduced sensation
- Extremes of age
- Acute illness
- Presence of edema

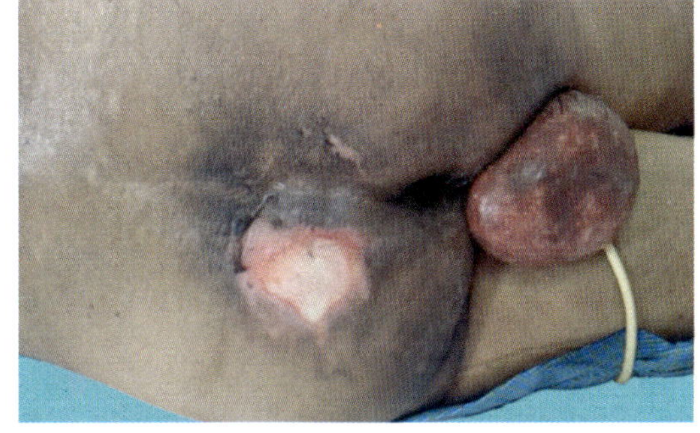

Decubitus ulcer (Pressure ulcer).

Sites at Risk

- **In adults:** Sacrum and heel are common sites. Other sites are- ischium, ankle, hip, elbow.
- **In children and neonates:** Skin over the occiput.
- **Vulnerable pressure points can be remembered by the acronym "BESTSHOT"** [Adapted from SSKIN bundle]: **B**: Buttocks (ischial tuberosities); **E**: Elbows/Ears; **S**: Sacrum (bottom); **T**: Trochanters (hips); **S**: Spine/shoulders; **H**: Heels; **O**: Occipital area (back of the head); **T**: Toes.

Prevention

SSKIN bundle outlines five critical areas of ulcer prevention: **S**: Skin assessment; **S**: Surface; **K**: Keep moving; **I**: Incontinence; **N**: Nutrition.

Skin assessment:

- Redness/erythema- nonblanching when finger pressure applied
- Pain, soreness
- Warmer or cooler area over bony prominence
- Boggy feeling
- Hardened area
- Discoloration- dark red, purple, black
- Broken skin/ulcer
- If any such changes develop, close monitoring is essential.
- In darkly pigmented skin, assessment includes: (i) Skin temperature; (ii) Edema; and (iii) Change in tissue consistency in relation to surrounding tissues.

Surface:

- For individuals at risk of pressure ulcer—High specification reactive foam mattress.
- For individuals sitting in a chair whose mobility is reduced—Pressure redistributing seat cushion.
- For category/stage I and II pressure ulcer—High specification reactive foam mattress or nonpowered pressure redistribution support surface.
- For category/stage III, IV and unstageable pressure ulcers—A support surface that provides enhanced pressure redistribution, shear reduction, and microclimate control.

Keep moving (Repositioning and early mobilization):

- Unless contraindicated, repositioning should be considered in all patients at risk of, or with existing pressure ulcers.
- Repositioning frequency should be determined with consideration of multiple factors: (i) Type of support surface; (ii) Level of activity and mobility; (iii) General medical condition; and (iv) Skin condition.
- Lift-don't drag-the individual while repositioning.
- Use different positions, e.g. 30° tilted side-lying position, right side, back, left side, prone position if patient can tolerate or his/her medical condition permits.

Incontinence: Incontinence-associated dermatitis (IAD), a variety of moisture-associated skin damage may act as an initiating factor in development of pressure ulcer.

Nutrition: Following recommendations for patients at risk of malnutrition are: (i) 30–35 Kcal/kg body wt for adult; (ii) 1.25–1.5 g protein/kg body wt; and (iii) Diet with good source of vitamins and minerals.

NPUAP (National Pressure Ulcer Advisory Panel) Classification	EPUAP (European Pressure Ulcer Advisory Panel) Classification
Stage I • Non-blanchable erythema of intact skin usually over a bony prominence • Darkly pigmented skin may not have visible blanching; its color may differ from the surrounding area • The area may be painful, firm, soft, warmer, or cooler compared to surrounding tissue	**Grade 1** • Non-blanchable erythema of intact skin • Discoloration of the skin, warmth, edema, induration or hardness may also be used as indicators, particularly in individuals with darker skin
Stage II • Partial thickness loss of dermis presenting as a shallow open ulcer with a red pink wound bed • Presents as a shiny or dry shallow ulcer without slough or bruising • May also present as an intact or open/ruptured serum-filled blister	**Grade 2** • Partial thickness skin loss involving epidermis, dermis or both • The ulcer is superficial and presents as an abrasion or blister **Grade 3** • Full thickness skin loss involving damage or necrosis of subcutaneous tissue that may extend down to but not through umderlying fascia
Stage III • Full thickness skin loss • Subcutaneous fat may be visible, but not bone, muscle or tendon	**Grade 4** • Extensive destruction, tissue necrosis or damage to muscle, bone or supporting structures, with or without full thickness skin loss
Stage IV • Full thickness skin loss with exposed bone, tendon or muscle	
Unstageable Full thickness tissue loss in which the base of the ulcer is covered with slough and/or eschar	
Deep tissue injury Purple or maroon localized area of discoloured intact skin or blood-filled blister due to damage of underlying soft tissue from pressure and/or shear. The effect may be preceded by tissue that is painful, firm, mushy, boggy, and warmer or cooler than adjacent tissue. Evolution may be rapid exposing additional layers of tissue even with optimal treatment	

Medical Device-related Pressure Ulcer (MDRPU)

Type of device: (i) Nasogastric tube; (ii) Tracheostomy tube; (iii) Ventilation mask; (iv) Oxygen saturation probe; (v) Cervical collar; (vi) Immobilization splint; (vii) Fixation tapes; (viii) Catheter (arterial, hemodialysis catheter, ECMO catheter); (ix) Nasal cannula; and (x) Intermittent pneumatic compression device.

Preventive measures: (i) Correct positioning and care of the equipment/device; (ii) Repeated assessment of the skin underneath the device; (iii) Use of thin hydrocolloids, film dressings or barrier products underneath the device; and (iv) Use of pressure reducing dermal gel pads.

Tuberculous ulcer:

- Usually develops following spontaneous rupture of cold abscess in neck, chest wall, groin.
- Ulcer is often multiple, oval-shaped with irregular crescentic border and undermined edge. The ulcer is tender with caseating material in the floor.
- **Slight induration is the characteristic feature.** Regional lymph nodes are often enlarged.

Bazin's ulcer:

- This ulcer is associated with 'Erythrocyanosis frigida'.
- E. Frigida is a disease exclusively occurs in young women with thick ankles (due to increased subcutaneous fat), characterized by diminished arterial supply to the ankle skin as a result of absence or small perforators arising from posterior tibial and peroneal arteries.
- Clinically presents as blue, tender, cold ankle in cold weather and hot, swollen, tender ankle in hot weather. Superficial, tender nodules around the ankle develops, which breakdown to form small, multiple ulcers.
- Sympathectomy is necessary, particularly if patient lives in a cold climate. Tuberculosis is responsible in many of these patients. ATD is effective in that patients.

Actinomycotic ulcer:

- Caused by gram-positive mycelia (***Actinomyces israelii***).
- Multiple ulcers develops which discharge granules ('sulfur granules')
- Commonly found in—Facio cervical region **(most common)**
- Thorax
- Liver
- Presence of 'sulfur granules' in the discharge is almost diagnostic. On microscopy, the granules consist of gram-positive mycelia.

Basic Principles of Ulcer Dressing

Primary aim of ulcer dressing:

- To remove the dead, necrotic tissues
- To hasten the granulation process
- To accelerate the healing.

During dressing, followings must be kept in mind:

- Excess exudate to be removed
- All dead and necrotic tissues should be excised
- Dressing must be permeable to oxygen, CO_2, moisture and impermeable to microorganisms
- Dressing must be such that there will be minimal trauma during dressing change.

Sinus

A blind track lined by granulation tissue from an epithelial surface into surrounding tissues.

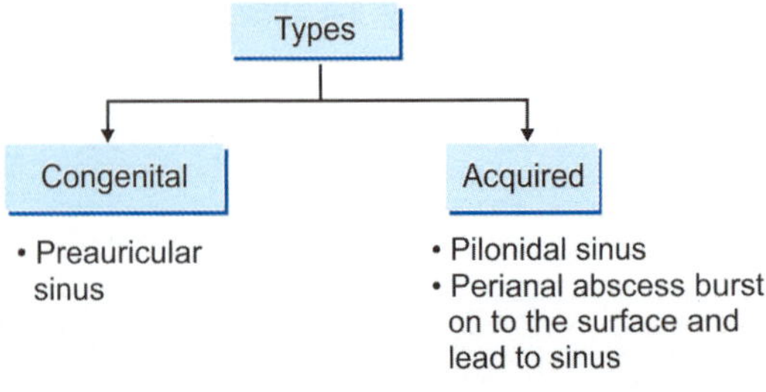

Fistula

- A communicating track lined by granulation tissue between two epithelial surfaces.
- Communication may develop between hollow viscus and skin **(external fistula)** and between two hollow viscus **(internal fistula)**.

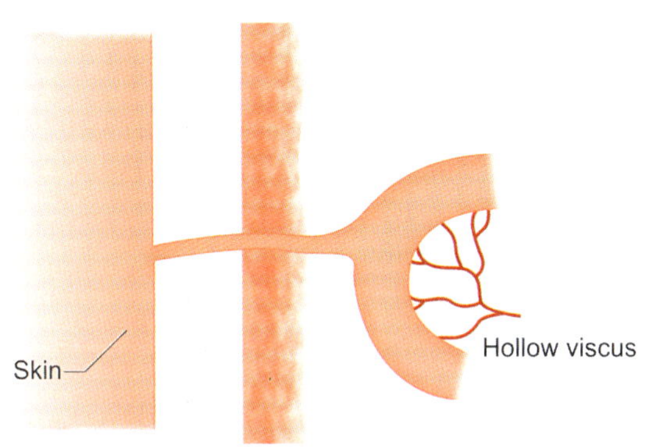

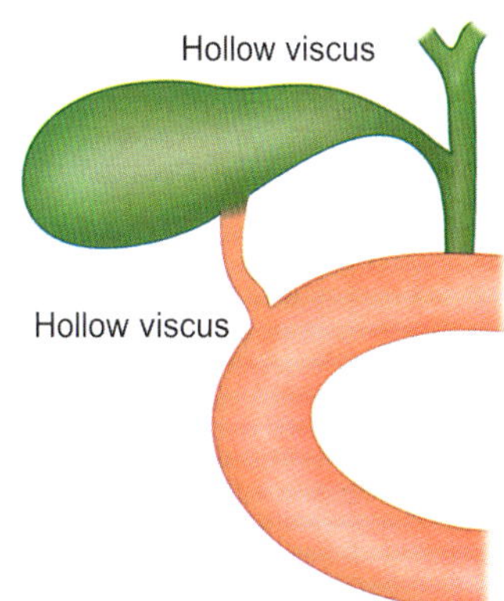

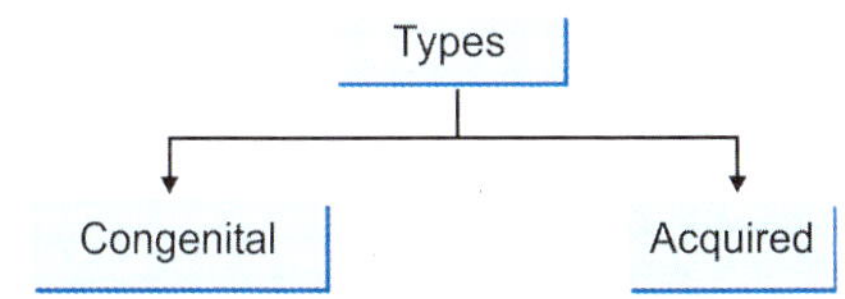

- Congenital
  - Branchial fistula
  - Tracheoesophageal fistula
  - Arteriovenous fistula
- Acquired
  - Thyroglossal fistula
  - A-V fistula (following trauma/for renal dialysis)
  - Fistula-in-ano
  - Cholecystoenteric fistula
  - Enterocutaneous fistula

Causes of Persistence of Sinus or Fistula

- Presence of foreign body or necrotic tissue (e.g., suture material, sequestrum, tuft of hair)
- Presence of distal obstruction
- Chronic infection (e.g., tuberculosis, actinomycosis)
- History of radiotherapy
- Nondependent drainage
- Malignancy.

Case 1

History and Physical Examination

A 38-year-old male patient attended surgical OPD with a chief complain of multiple ulcers in the right neck for last 1 month. About 4 months back, patient noticed multiple swelling over the neck for which he consulted with local physician. Patient was advised antibiotics and biopsy from the swelling. Patient did not follow the advice of biopsy. In the last month, these swelling gradually increasing in size and spontaneously ruptured. No history of swelling in axilla or groin. Patient had no history of evening rise of temperature, loss of appetite. Patient's father was treated for pulmonary tuberculosis about 8 years back.

Clinical Examination

Multiple, oval-shaped tender ulcers in the both anterior and posterior triangles of the right neck with irregular crescentic border and undermined edges. Multiple fluctuant tender lymph nodes were palpable in the left neck. Lymph nodes were not palpable in axilla or groin. No hepatomegaly or splenomegaly.

Provisional Diagnosis

→ Tubercular ulcer in neck

Investigations

- Hb: 10.6 gm%, ESR: 100 mm/hr
- Incisional biopsy from ulcer margin suggestive of tuberculous lesion
- Chest X-ray revealed no significant abnormality.

Discussion

- History of multiple swelling in neck followed by spontaneous rupture was highly suggestive of rupture of cold abscess.
- Incisional biopsy confirmed the diagnosis of tuberculous ulcer.

Management Algorithm

Antitubercular therapy for 6 months

Case 2

History and Physical Examination

A 52-year-old male patient presented in the surgical OPD with a chief complain of nonhealing ulcer in his right foot for last 3 months. About 4 months back, patient sustained trauma in his right foot resulting in lacerated wound. Even after multiple course of antibiotic therapy and dressing, the wound did not healed completely. Patient also complained of impaired sensation in his both foot for last 1 year. No history suggestive of intermittent claudication or rest pain. History of diabetes for last 10 years for which he was taking oral antidiabetics. No history of smoking. No history of hypertension.

Clinical Examination

An ulcer over the dorsum of right foot measuring about 4 cm × 3 cm, slough in base with minimal granulation tissue. Surrounding skin was shiny and mild erythematous changes. No deformities of foot was present. Arteria dorsalis pedis pulsation was absent, but other peripheral pulses were present.

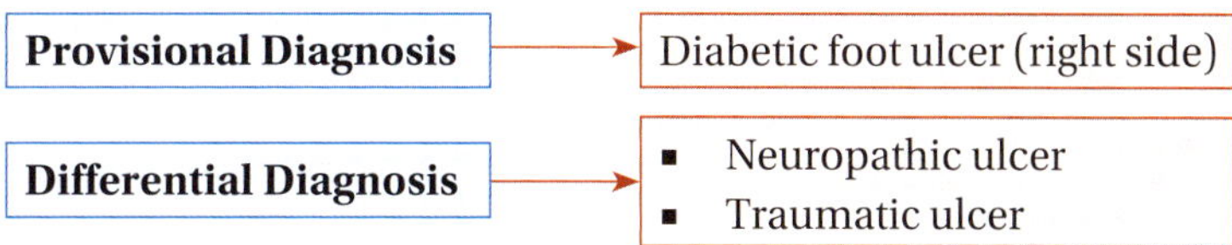

Investigations

Hb: 10.5 gm%, Total WBC: 14,000/cumm, Blood sugar (F): 170 mg/dL, Blood sugar (PP): 290 mg/dL, HbA1c: 8.0, Serum creatinine: 1.2 mg/dL, Lipid profile within normal limit.

Doppler USG of arterial system of both lower limbs revealed mild atherosclerotic changes without any luminal narrowing.

Discussion

A diabetic patient presented with a non-healing ulcer in his foot without any features of peripheral vascular disease (no history of intermittent claudication or rest pain, absence of any pre-gangrenous or gangrenous changes in foot) was highly suggestive of diabetic foot ulcer. Laboratory investigations were also suggestive of uncontrolled diabetes. Doppler USG excluded any peripheral occlusive arterial disease.

Management Algorithm

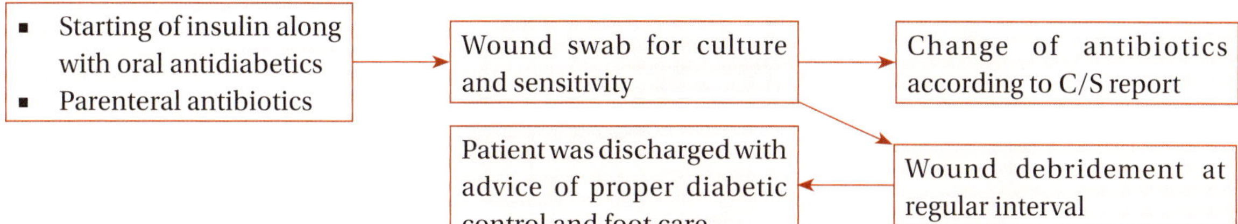

Chapter 25

Urology

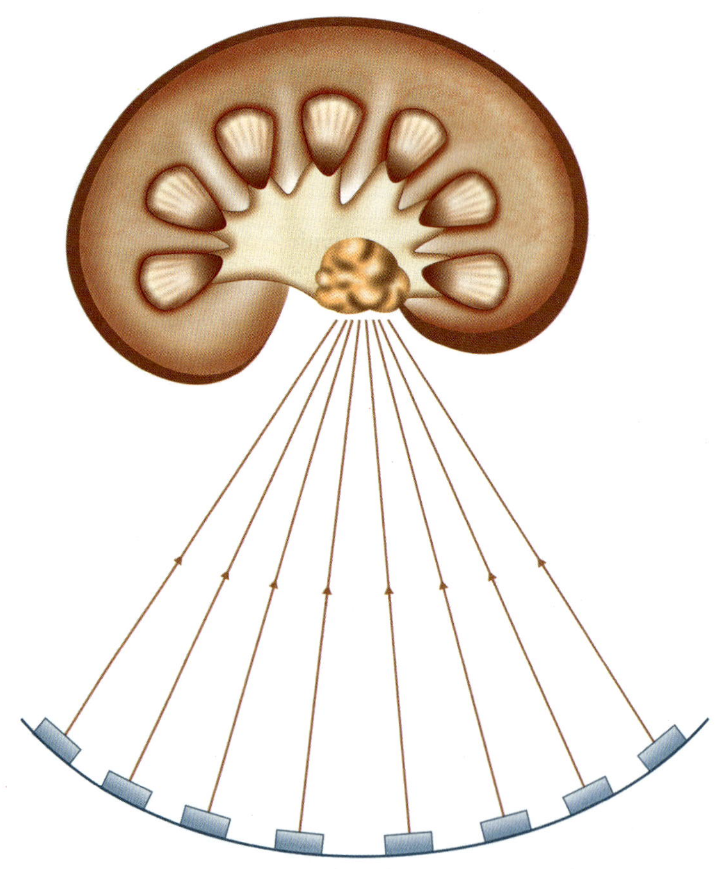

Important Topics

- Urinary Symptoms
- Congenital Malformations of Kidney and Ureter
- Hydronephrosis
- Renal Stone
- Infections of Kidney
- Kidney Tumors
- Ureteral Calculi
- Urothelial Tumors of Renal Pelvis and Ureter
- Bladder Calculi
- Schistosomiasis of the Urinary Bladder
- Bladder Tumor
- Benign Prostatic Hyperplasia
- Prostatitis
- Prostate Carcinoma
- Urethral Stricture
- Hypospadias
- Priapism
- Peyronie's Disease
- Carcinoma of Penis
- Testicular Cancer

'The person who never made a mistake never tried anything new.'

Urinary Symptoms

Hematuria

Presence of blood in the urine is called hematuria. Hematuria is either gross or microscopic.

Gross hematuria is commonly associated with significant pathology in comparison to **microscopic hematuria**.

Hematuria associated with pain is commonly due to obstruction by clots or due to inflammation.
Malignancies of kidney and bladder usually present with **painless hematuria**.

Patients with gross painless hematuria have a urinary tract malignancy until proved otherwise.
Clot indicates significant degree of hematuria. Amorphous clot indicates bladder or prostatic urethral origin whereas vermiform clot indicates upper urinary tract origin.

Hematuria should be differentiated from pseudohematuria.

Microscopic Hematuria

Presence of three or more RBCs per high-powered field on microscopic examination of one properly-collected non-contaminated urinalysis.

Causes: (i) Urinary tract infection; (ii) Urinary calculi; (iii) Benign prostatic hypertrophy; (iv) Nephropathy; (v) Nephritis; (vi) Vigorous exercise; and (vii) Menstruation

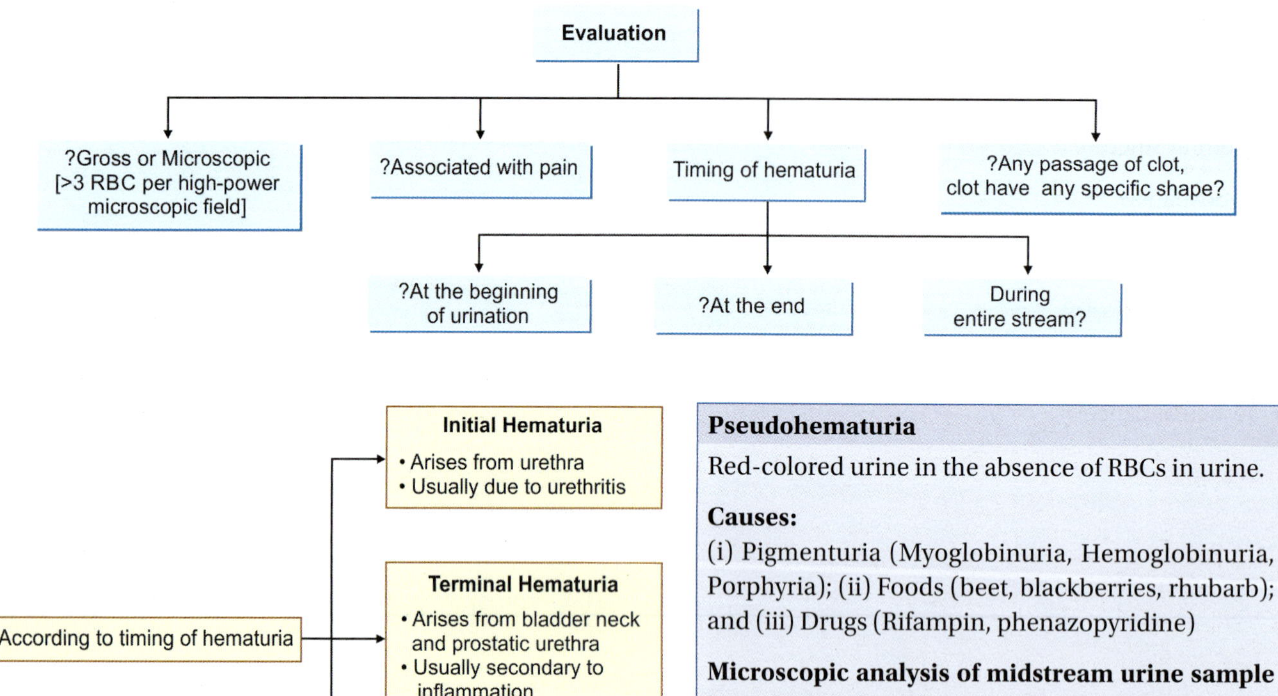

Pseudohematuria

Red-colored urine in the absence of RBCs in urine.

Causes:

(i) Pigmenturia (Myoglobinuria, Hemoglobinuria, Porphyria); (ii) Foods (beet, blackberries, rhubarb); and (iii) Drugs (Rifampin, phenazopyridine)

Microscopic analysis of midstream urine sample is necessary for differentiation between hematuria and pseudohematuria. The urine dipstick is sufficient because it may give false-positive result.

Causes of Hematuria

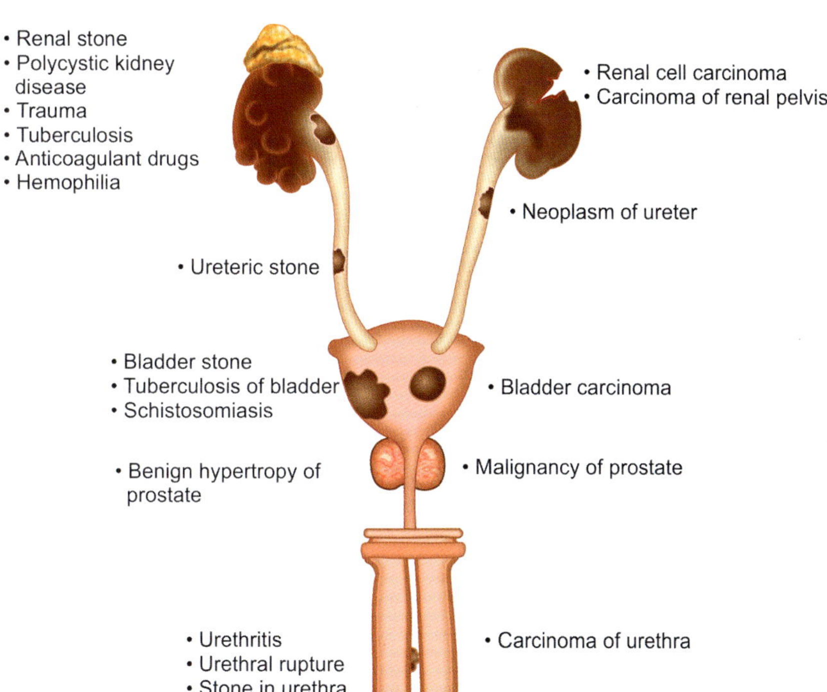

Pain

Renal Pain

- Caused by acute distension of renal capsule due to obstruction or inflammation.
- Pain due to inflammation is steady; pain due to obstruction is colicky.
- Renal pain may be associated with GI symptoms due to:
  - Reflex stimulation of celiac ganglion
  - Proximity of organs of GI system.

Site of pain- Ipsilateral renal angle (junction of lateral border of erector spinae and 12th rib)

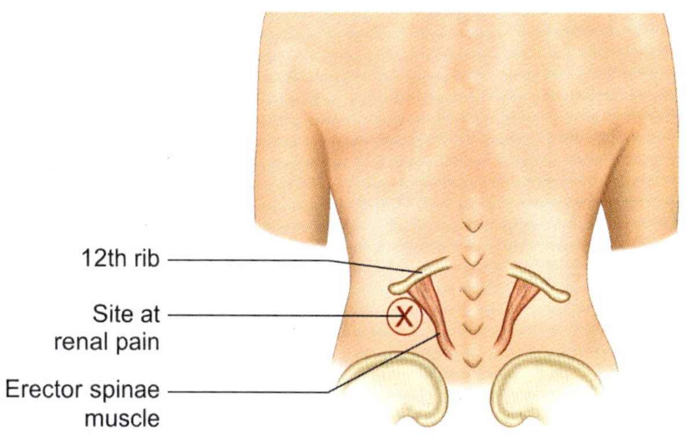

Ureteral Pain

- Acute colicky pain in the loin that usually radiates to the ipsilateral groin and genitalia. The patient rolls around in agony. Pain-free periods persist between each attack.
- Site of radiation of pain is determined by site of obstruction. **In obstruction of right midureter**, pain is referred to right iliac fossa (simulate appendicitis) and in **obstruction of left midureter**, pain is referred to left iliac fossa (simulate diverticulitis). In midureter obstruction, pain may also referred to scrotum and labium. **In obstruction of lower ureter**, patient may experience pain that radiates along the urethra to the tip of penis, along with frequency, urgency.
- Pain is due to hyperperistalsis of the ureter to relieve the obstruction.

Radiation of ureteral pain

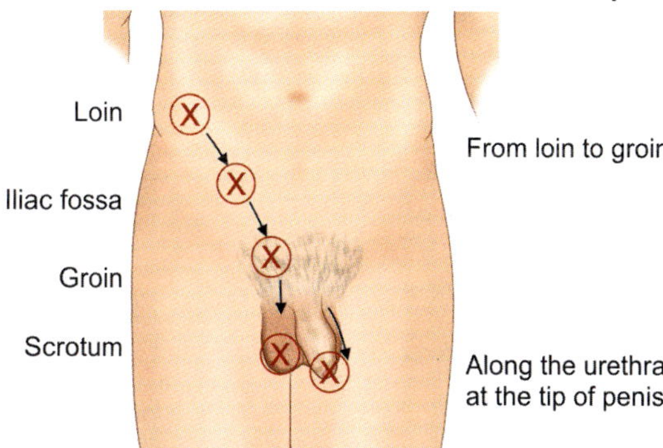

Bladder Pain

- Usually caused by overdistension of urinary bladder or by inflammation of urinary bladder.
- Pain is felt in the suprapubic region and is most severe when the bladder is full.
- Sometimes, in cystitis, patient may complain sharp, stabbing suprapubic pain at the end of micturition-called 'Strangury' (due to final contraction of the inflammed detrusor muscle).

Prostatic Pain

- Usually caused by distension of prostatic capsule as a result of inflammation.
- Patient experiences a penetrating ache in perineum or rectum that is poorly localized and usually associated with dysuria and frequency.

Urethral Pain

Scalding or burning sensation in penis or vulva during voiding due to inflammation of bladder or urethra.

Irritative Symptoms

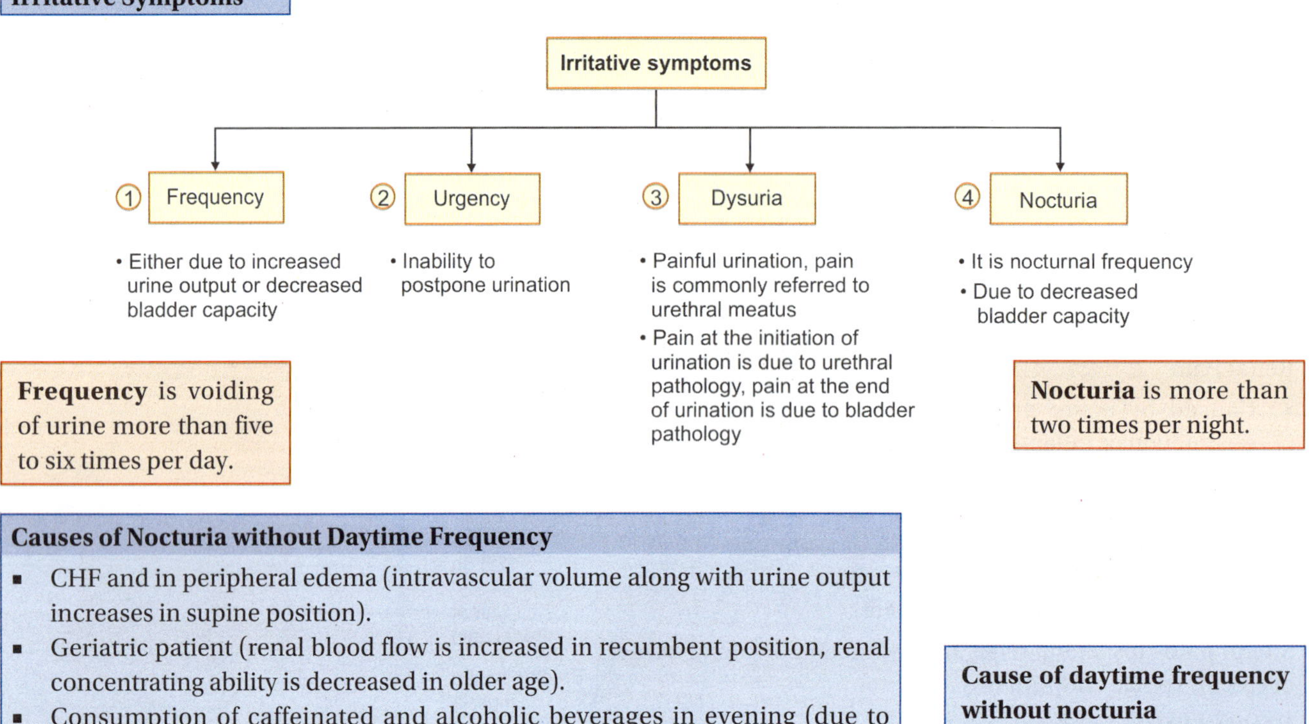

Frequency is voiding of urine more than five to six times per day.

Nocturia is more than two times per night.

Causes of Nocturia without Daytime Frequency

- CHF and in peripheral edema (intravascular volume along with urine output increases in supine position).
- Geriatric patient (renal blood flow is increased in recumbent position, renal concentrating ability is decreased in older age).
- Consumption of caffeinated and alcoholic beverages in evening (due to diuretic effect).

Cause of daytime frequency without nocturia

- Anxiety

Obstructive Symptoms

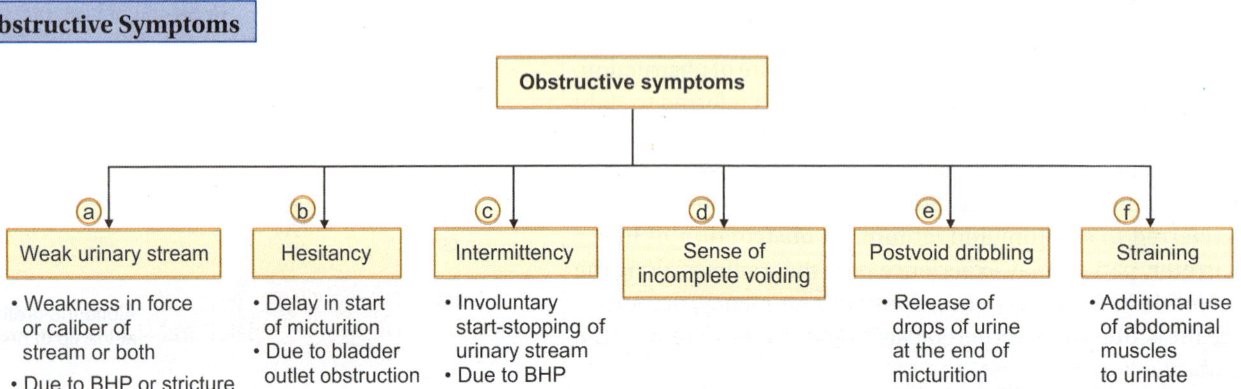

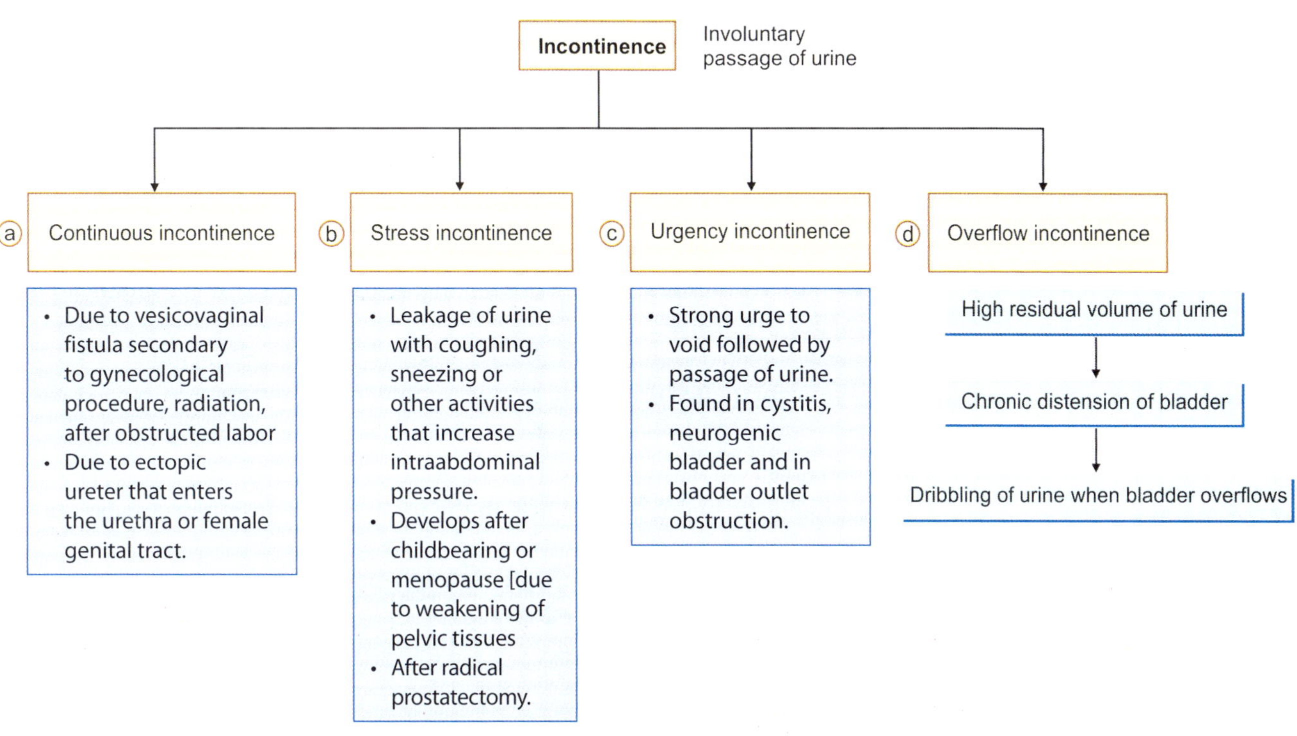

Enuresis

- Urinary incontinence during sleep
- Children older than 6 years with enuresis warrants thorough urologic evaluation.

Congenital Malformations of Kidney and Ureter

Bilateral Renal Agenesis

- Children who are born alive cannot survive beyond 48 hours due to associated pulmonary hypoplasia.
- Presence of oligohydramnios and Potter facies (prominent fold and skin crease beneath eyes, blunt nose, depression between lower lip and chin, low set ears) are pathognomonic.

Unilateral Renal Agenesis

- Occurs once in 1100 births.
- Most commonly associated with cardiovascular anomalies. Sometimes the GI system and musculoskeletal systems are affected.
- Unilateral agenesis (commonly left side) with contralateral normal kidney can lead to normal life. Genital anomalies are commonly associated with this congenital anomaly.
- Contact sports or strenuous physical exertion must be avoided.

Supernumerary Kidney

- Very rare anomaly (about 100 cases have been reported).
- Supernumerary kidney has its own collecting system, blood supply and distinct capsule.
- The kidney is located either separately or loosely attached to the main kidney of the ipsilateral side, commonly caudal to the dominant kidney.

Duplication of Ureter

- In most of the cases, the ureters join in the lower third of their course.
- Sometimes, the ureters open independently into the bladder. The ureter from the upper pelvis opens distal and medial to the ureter from lower pelvis.
- Infection, stone formation and PUJ obstruction are more common in duplication of renal pelvis or ureter.
- In male, the aberrant opening may be above the external urethral sphincter, at the apex of bladder trigone, in the posterior urethra **(most common site of termination of ectopic ureter)**, in seminal vesicle or ejaculatory duct.
- In female, ectopic opening may be below the urethral sphincter or into the vagina **(urethra and vestibule are the most common site of termination of ectopic ureter)**.
- If atrophic or nonfunctioning chronically infected segment of kidney is present—Partial nephrectomy
- Incontinence due to ectopic ureter—Implantation of ureter into bladder or into the fellow ureter.

Horseshoe Kidney

- Most common of all renal fusion anomalies.
- Most medial subdivisions of the mesonephric bud meet and fuse in the midline. The fusion occurs before the rotation on their long axis.
- The kidneys usually fused at their lower poles. The inferior mesenteric artery prevents ascent by obstructing the isthmus. As kidneys fail to rotate, the calyces are pointed posteriorly.
- The ureter may insert high on the pelvis and a characteristic angulation while crossing over and anterior to isthmus. Ureter enters the bladder normally.
- The blood supply is variable. Sometimes duplicate and triplicate renal arteries supply the kidneys.
- Isthmus is supplied by main renal artery or artery originating from aorta and sometimes branches arising from inferior mesenteric artery or common iliac artery.
- Associated anomalies present—Genitourinary, skeletal, cardiovascular and CNS defects.
- Patient may presents with vague abdominal pain radiated to lumbar area. Sometimes, patient may present with midline abdominal mass.
- Many of the patients present with ureteropelvic junction obstruction. As a result, increased incidence of infection and calculus formation in these patients.
- Classic radiologic features (in Urogram)—Lower pole calyces on both sides are directed towards midline, ureters have vase-like curves.
- Division of isthmus is not indicated for relief of pain.

Anomalies of Renal Vasculature

- Accessory vessel—Two or more arterial branches supplying the same renal segment.
- Aberrant vessel—Kidney supplied by vessels originate from other than aorta or main renal artery.
- Multiple vessels—Any kidney supplied by more than one vessel.

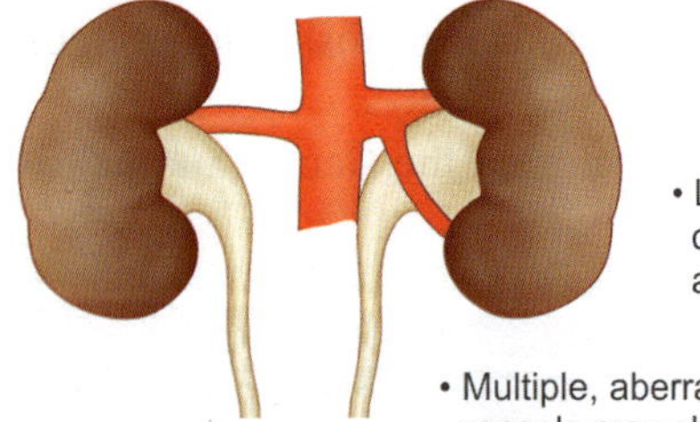

- Lower renal segment is commonly supplied by an accessory vessel
- Multiple, aberrant, accessory vessels may obstruct major calyx or PUJ, leads to hydronephrosis

Horseshoe Kidney

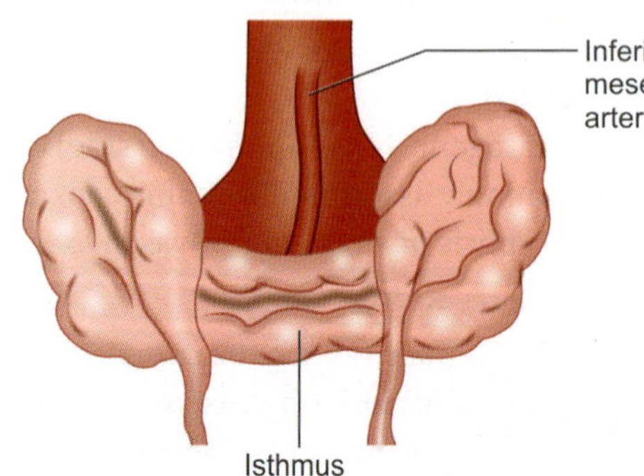

Autosomal Dominant (Adult) Polycystic Kidney Disease (ADPKD)

Pattern of inheritance is **autosomal dominant with mutation in *PKD* gene.** Three PKD genes are identified:

1. *PKD1* gene (in 85% cases)—Located in chromosome 16
2. *PKD2* gene (5–10% cases)—Located in chromosome 4
3. *PKD3* gene—About 5% cases.

Symptoms and signs usually manifest between 30 to 50 years.
Associated anomalies: (i) Multiple cysts in liver, pancreas, spleen, lungs (appears later than renal cysts); (ii) Aneurysm of the circle of Willis; (iii) Colonic diverticula; (iv) Aortic aneurysm; and (v) Mitral valve prolapse.

Clinical manifestations: (i) Dull aching pain in the lumbar region; (ii) Irregular abdominal mass; (iii) Hematuria; (iv) Infection; (v) Hypertension; (vi) Subarachnoid hemorrhage (due to rupture of berry aneurysm); and (vii) End-stage renal failure.

Diagnosis:

- For diagnosis, positive family history is important but not essential. Bilateral renal cysts associated with 3 or more hepatic cyst, presence of berry aneurysm or solitary cyst in pancreas or spleen are sufficient enough for establish the diagnosis.
- Ultrasonography and CT abdomen reveals multiple cysts in both kidneys and sometimes cysts in liver, pancreas.
- On intravenous urography—Bilateral renal enlargement, calyceal distortion (like spiders' legs), Swiss cheese appearance in nephrogram phase.
- MRI is helpful when patient is in compromised renal function.

Treatment: According to symptoms. No definite surgical procedure is helpful.

[50% of the children of patient will be affected. The children should be screened by ultrasonography.]

Characteristic Features of Kidneys and Cysts

- Kidneys are bilaterally enlarged and lobulated appearance due to underlying cyst.
- Cysts are of varying sizes, from few mm to 4–5 cm in diameter.
- Cysts do not communicate with the pelvis of the kidney.
- Cysts derived from entire nephron (Only 1% of nephrons changed into cysts).

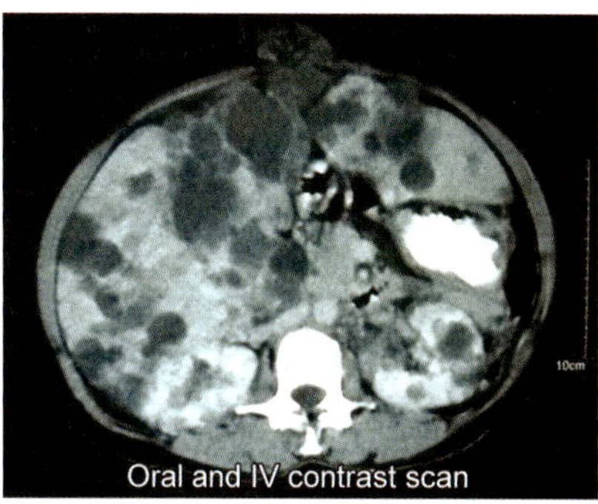

CT scan showing multiple cysts in liver, spleen, and kidneys.

Autosomal Recessive (Infantile) Polycystic Kidney Disease

A rare disease—1 of every 40,000 live births.
Pattern of inheritance is autosomal recessive.

Mutations of a single gene *PKHD1*, located on chromosome 6 is responsible.
Age of presentation may be—Perinatal, Neonatal, Infantile, Juvenile.

Clinical manifestations depend on when the disease presents. Earlier the disease presents, more severe the disease. Newborn presents with huge, normal reniform-shaped, nonbosselated, hard flank mass and sometimes history of difficult delivery due to the mass. Also, history of oligohydramnios may be present. If disease appears later in childhood, patient may present with renal failure and hypertension.

All affected individuals have **associated congenital hepatic fibrosis, which may lead to portal hypertension and splenomegaly.**

Cysts are formed from dilatation of collecting tubules.
Diagnosis: The disease may be suspected during prenatal USG screening. Newborn presenting with ARPKD can be diagnosed by USG. In delayed films of IVU, functioning kidneys with characteristic radial streaking (sunburst pattern) may be present.

Treatment: Patients to be treated for hypertension, renal and hepatic failure. Hemodialysis and renal transplantation may be considered in some of these patients.

Simple Cyst of the Kidney

- A common incidental finding in USG of abdomen.
- Rarely seen in infants and children.
- If cyst causes pain or pressure effects, laparoscopic unroofing either transperitoneally or retroperitoneally, is the treatment.

A simple cyst must be differentiated from a cystic neoplasm or early stage of ADPKD.

Postcaval Ureter (Retrocaval Ureter)

- The right ureter deviates medially behind the IVC, winding about and crossing in front of it form a medial to lateral direction, then follows the normal course to drain in the bladder.
- Most of the patients are present in the 3rd or 4th decades. Patient may present with pain in the flank or hydronephrosis.
- MRI is superior to demonstrating the course of IVC and ureter in comparison to CT and retrograde pyelography.
- Treatment is excision of retrocaval segment of ureter followed by ureteral relocation.

Ureterocele

- A cystic dilatation of the intramural part of ureter, associated with stenotic ureteral opening.
- Found mostly in females (4 :1).
- Large ureterocele can obstruct the bladder neck or contralateral ureteral orifice resulting in hydroureter and hydronephrosis.
- The **'adder head' found in IUV** is typical. Voiding cystourethrography can delineate the size and location of ureterocele and also can detect the presence or absence of vesicoureteral reflux.
- Treatment is indicated for symptomatic ureterocele (bilateral hydronephrosis).

Endoscopic incision (transverse incision) through the full thickness of ureterocele using cutting diathermy is the preferred surgical approach.

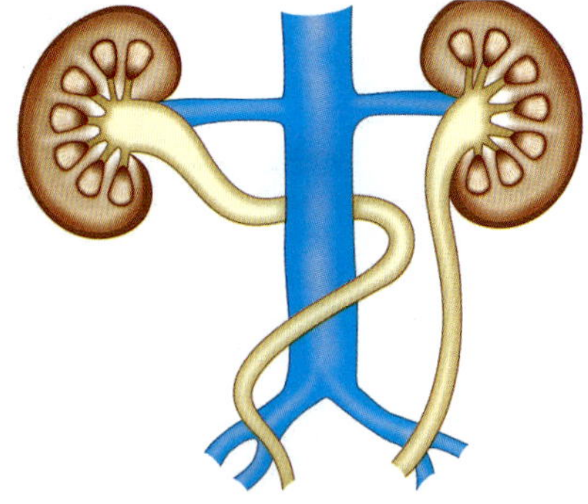

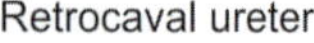
Retrocaval ureter

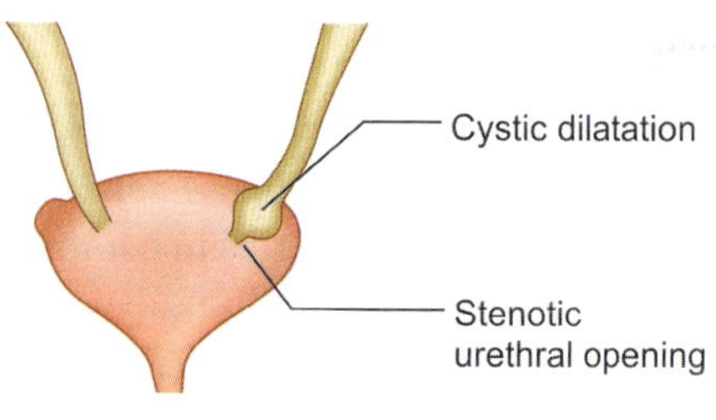

Ureterocele

Hydronephrosis

Aseptic dilatation of the calyces and pelvis of the kidney due to partial or complete obstruction to the outflow of urine.

Causes of Hydronephrosis

Unilateral Hydronephrosis

- Tumor infiltrating the ureter, e.g., carcinoma cervix, rectum, colon prostate
- Retrocaval ureter
- Congenital PUJ stenosis
- Calculus in renal pelvis or ureter
- Ureterocele
- Neoplasm of ureter
- Neoplasm of bladder involving ureteric orifice

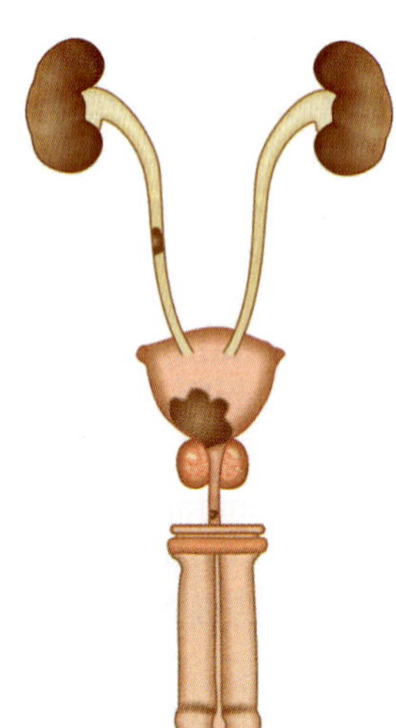

Bilateral Hydronephrosis

- Carcinoma bladder
- Bladder neck contracture.
- Prostatic enlargement (benign or malignant)
- Urethral stricture.
- Posterior urethral valve
- Retroperitoneal fibrosis

Causes of Hydronephrosis

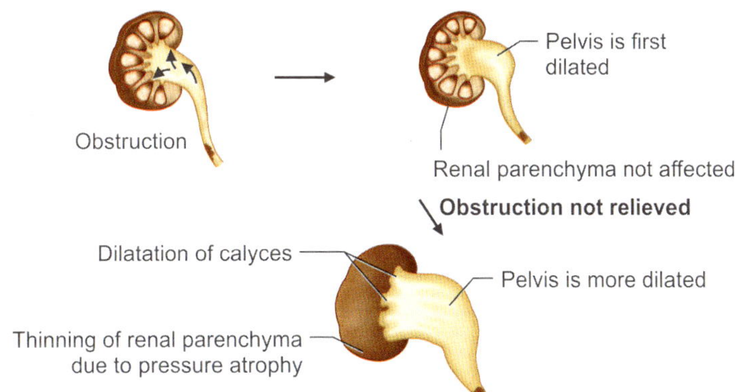

Clinical Features

- Insidious onset of dull, persistent aching pain in the loin is the commonest symptom
- Sensation of dragging heaviness
- Pain or heaviness may be exacerbated by taking excess water or alcohol
- Intermittent hydronephrosis—After attack of pain, swelling appears in loin, few hours later, after passage of large amount of urine, the pain relieved and swelling disappears, also called **'Dietl's crisis'**.

Diagnosis

USG imaging:

- Initial screening test for detection of hydronephrosis
- Can also detect hydronephrosis in utero.

Intravenous urography—Pelvis appears dilated, and calyces lose their cupping and become clubbed.

DTPA (diethylenetriaminepentaacetic acid) Renography—^{99m}Tc labelled DTPA is injected intravenously. If there is distal obstruction, the marker is trapped in renal pelvis and will not be washed out even after diuresis.

Treatment

Indications for surgical intervention: (i) Recurrent episodes of pain; (ii) Progressive hydronephrosis; (iii) Pyonephrosis; and (iv) Evidence of parenchymal damage.

Surgical options: Management of hydronephrosis with definite management of cause of hydronephrosis.

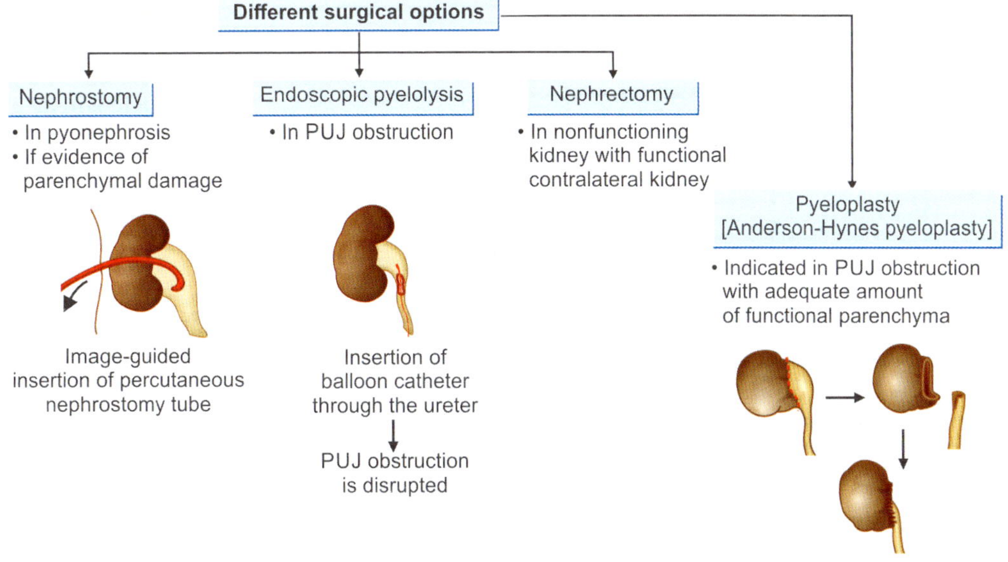

Renal Stone

Stone diseases is one of the common urologic diseases worldwide. Commonly affects adult men than adult women.

Pathophysiology

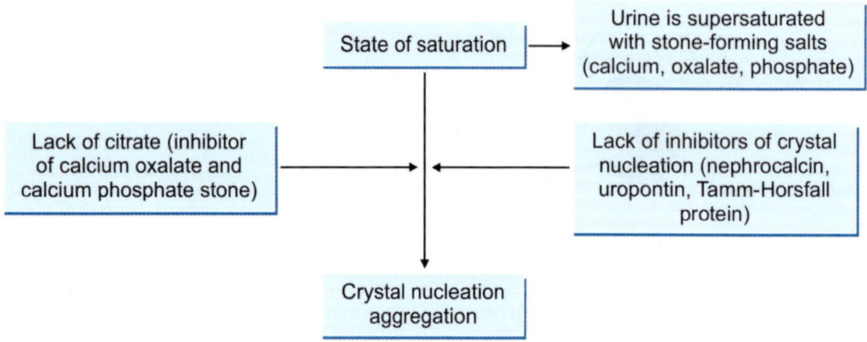

Randall's Plaque

- A plaque of calcium deposited in the interstitial tissue of the renal papilla.
- Randall's plaque acts as a nidus for stone formation.

Risk Factors

- Hypercalcuria
- Hyperoxaluria
- Hyperuricosuria
- Low urine pH (<5.5)
- Dehydration
- Urinary tract infection (particularly caused by urease-producing bacteria)
- Type I renal tubular acidosis

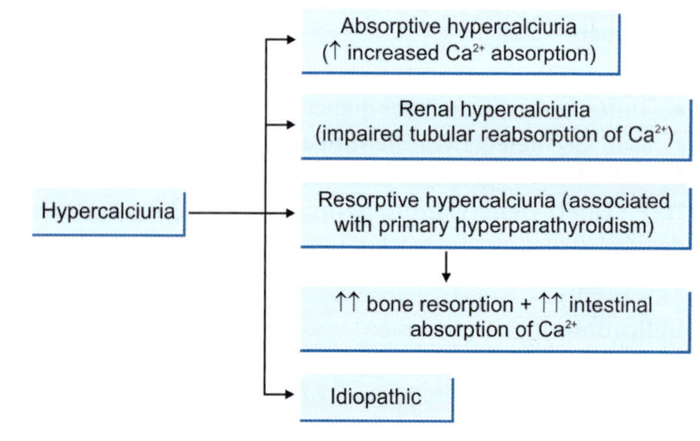

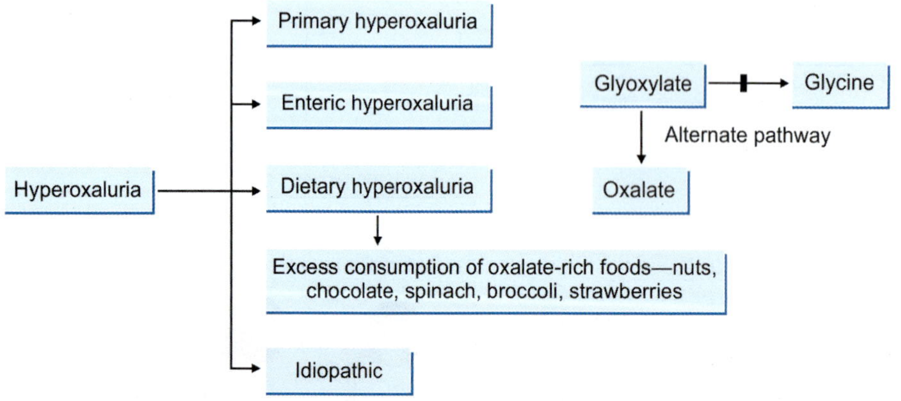

Diseases Associated with Hyperuricosuria

- Gout
- Myeloproliferative disorders
- Multiple myeloma

Urease-producing Bacteria

- *Proteus spp.*
- *Ureaplasma urealyticum*
- *Corynebacterium urealyticum*
- *Klebsiella spp*
- *Pseudomonas*

Diseases Associated with Stone Formation

- Primary hyperparathyroidism
- Nephrocalcinosis
- Polycystic kidney disease
- Malabsorptive syndrome
- Crohn's disease
- Jejuno-ileal bypass, intestinal resection
- Bariatric surgery
- Neurogenic bladder

Anatomical Abnormalities Associated with Stone Formation

- Ureteropelvic junction obstruction
- Horseshoe kidney
- Ureteral stricture
- Ureterocele
- Calyceal diverticulum
- Medullary sponge kidney

Genetic Disorders Associated with Stone Formation

- Cystinuria (type A, B, and AB)
- Primary hyperoxaluria
- Xanthinuria
- Renal tubular acidosis type I
- Cystic fibrosis

Drugs Associated with Stone Formation

- Allopurinol
- Indinavir
- Acetazolamide
- Quinolones
- Ascorbic acid
- Furosemide

Types of Renal Calculi

Calcium Oxalate Stone

- Calcium oxalate stone is the most common type of renal stone.
- Most of the calcium oxalate stones (calcium oxalate monohydrate and calcium oxalate dihydrate) are formed due to idiopathic hypercalciuria without hypercalcemia. In few patients, stones are formed due to absorptive or renal hypercalciuria.
- Oxalate stones are usually small, hard, irregular in shape and surface covered with sharp projections. These projections tend to cause bleeding due to repeated trauma. Surface is dark brown colored due to pigments of altered blood.
- These stones are radiopaque.

Calcium Phosphate Stone

- Calcium phosphate stones are most commonly appear as hydroxyapatite crystal form in kidney stones.
- These stones more commonly found in women and presents at a younger age.
- These stones are radiopaque.

Brushite Stone

- Brushite is considered as precursor phase of hydroxyapatite. Brushite stone is the rare subtype of calcium phosphate stone.
- It is the hardest urinary stone and resistant to shock wave lithotripsy.
- This stone disease is associated with high risk of recurrence despite aggressive surgical and medical interventions.
- These stones are radiopaque.

- **Calcium is the most common component of urinary calculi.**
- **Randall plaques** act as a potential precursor in calcium-containing stone formation.

Diseases Associated with Calcium Phosphate Stone Formation

- Hyperparathyroidism
- Renal tubular acidosis
- Urinary tract infection

Uric Acid Stone

- **Uric acid stone formation is associated with** hyperuricemia and hyperuricosuria in gout, myeloproliferative disorders (e.g., leukemia), patient on chemotherapy, use of uricosuric drugs (e.g., salicylates and probenecid).
- **Three determinant factors of uric acid stone formation are:** (i) Acidic urinary pH; (ii) Low urine volume; and (iii) Hyperuricosuria. In acidic urinary pH, the solubility of uric acid decreases, resulting in precipitation of uric acid crystals.
- These stones are hard, smooth, yellow to reddish brown in color and often multiple. On cut section, they have multifaceted appearance.
- **Pure uric acid stones are radiolucent**. In IVU, they appear as filling defect.

Infection Stone

- Infection stones are either **struvite stones** or **calcium carbonate apatite stones. Struvite stones are composed of magnesium ammonium phosphate.**
- Infection of the urinary tract with **urea-splitting organisms** is a prerequisite for formation of infection stones. Urease splits urea into ammonia and carbon dioxide. Ammonia reacts with water to become ammonium and hydroxide ions. In this alkaline environment, precipitation of components of struvite stone develops.
- Stones are dirty white and smooth.
- Sometimes, large solitary stone takes the shape of renal pelvis and major calyces—**'Staghorn calculus'.** Staghorn calculus may present as mixed stones—composed of calcium carbonate apatite and struvite.
- **They are radiopaque stones**.

- **Low urine pH (<5.5)** is the most common factor associated with **uric acid stone formation.**
- **Infection stone form in alkaline urine.**

A Swedish Geologist discovered **magnesium-ammonium phosphate** and named it **'struvite'** after his mentor, **Naturalist hCG Von Struve**.

Factors Predisposing to Struvite Stone Formation

- Foreign body
- Indwelling urinary catheter
- Urethral stricture
- Neurogenic bladder
- Bladder diverticulum
- Cystocele

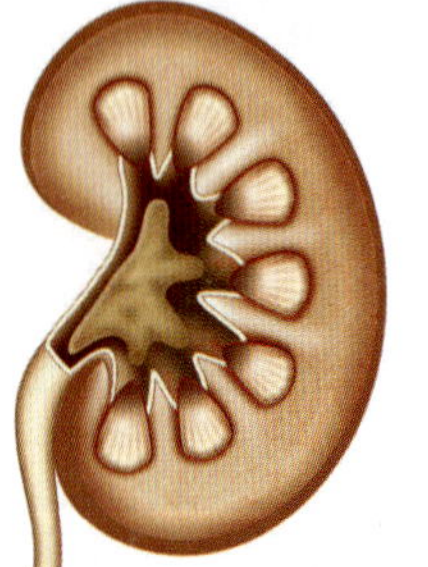

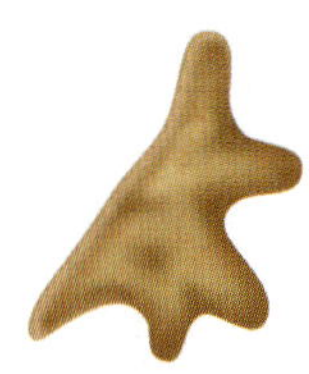

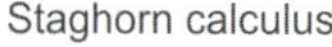

Staghorn calculus

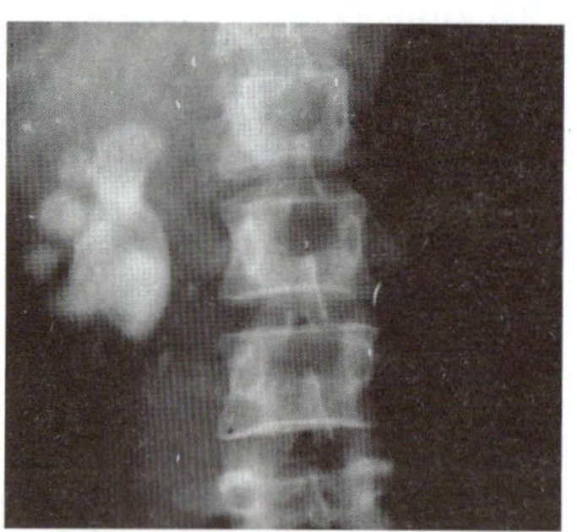

Straight X-ray of KUB showing staghorn calculus in right kidney.

Staghorn Calculus

- Struvite calculi often involve the renal pelvis and extend into at least two calyces, resulting in **characteristic shape of antlers of a stag** (adult male deer).
- Staghorn stones may be **'partial'** (involves at least two calyces) or **'complete'** (at least 80% of the renal collecting system is involved).

Cystine Stone

- Cystine stones are uncommon urinary stones. This stone develops **due to cystinuria** as a result of congenital defect in transport of cystine and other amino acids
- They are small, rounded, smooth, waxy, yellowish, multiple and very hard
- **Cystine stones are associated with presentation at younger age group, more risk of recurrence**.
- They are **lightly radiopaque** because of its sulfur content.

Xanthine Stone

- Xanthine stone is a rare type of urinary stone
- Develops as a result of **hereditary xanthinuria**
- They are **radiolucent stones**.

Classification of Urinary Stones According to X-ray Characteristics

Radiopaque

Calcium oxalate dihydrate Calcium oxalate monohydrate Calcium phosphate

Poor Radiopacity

- Magnesium ammonium phosphate
- Apatite
- Cystine

Radiolucent

- Uric acid
- Ammonium urate
- Xanthine
- Drug-stone

Clinical Presentation

- Pain is the most common symptom in patients with renal calculi.
- Most of the patients experience a fixed renal pain at the renal angle.
- Microscopic hematuria is commonly associated with renal stone, gross hematuria is not so common.
- Staghorn calculi becomes asymptomatic for a long period of time.

Complications of Renal Stone

- Hydronephrosis
- Pyonephrosis
- Renal parenchymal damage

Diagnosis

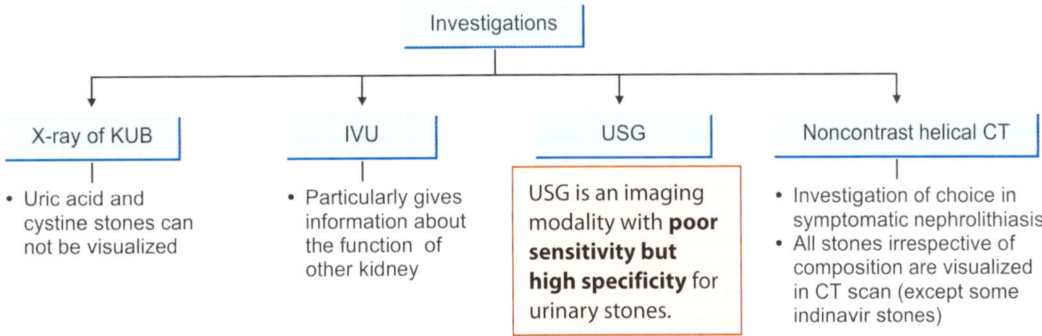

Role of MRI

MRI is indicated in pregnant patients with acute flank pain when USG is nondiagnostic.

Non-contrast CT scan is the imaging modality of choice for diagnosing acute flank pain.

- **Advantages:** (i) High sensitivity and specificity; (ii) Can detect uric acid and xanthine stones (radiolucent on plain X-ray); (iii) Can determine stone density; (iv) Can provide detailed anatomic details of the kidneys; and (v) Can determine skin-to-stone distance.
- **Limitations:** (i) More expensive imaging modality; (ii) Exposure to ionizing radiation; and (iii) Cannot detect indinavir stone and pure matrix stone.

Workup After Diagnosis

- **Thorough history** (chronic diarrhea, gout, diabetes mellitus, history of bariatric surgery or bowel resection, family history of urinary stones, amount of fluid consumption and certain type of foods)
- **Blood biochemistry:** Serum electrolytes (sodium, potassium, chloride, bicarbonate), serum creatinine, calcium, uric acid
- **Urinalysis:** Urinary pH, urine culture, crystalluria
- **Stone analysis**
- **Metabolic evaluation** (for specific group of patients)

Indications of Metabolic Evaluation

- Family history of urinary stone disease
- Cystine, uric acid and struvite stone disease
- Recurrent stone formers
- Patients with anatomic abnormalities of the urinary tract
- Pediatric patients with urinary stone
- High-risk stone formers (renal tubular acidosis, primary hyperparathyroidism, gout, diabetes mellitus, chronic diarrhea).

Appearance of Crystals in Urine

Calcium oxalate stone: Tetrahedral "envelopes"

Struvite calculi: Rectangular, "coffin-lid" crystal

Cystine stone: Hexagonal crystal

Uric acid stone: Amorphous fiber

Management

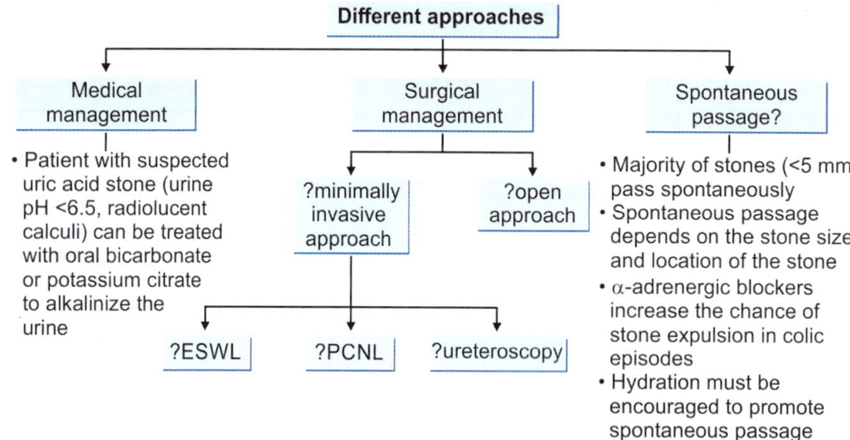

Medical Management

- **Fluid intake:** Increased fluid intake (at least 3 liters/day to achieve urine output of at least 2.5 liters/day
- Avoidance of increased consumption of sugar-sweetened beverages, animal protein
- Consumption of DASH diet
- Intake of citrus juices (lemonade and orange juice)
- Medical expulsion therapy—with alpha antagonist (most commonly used agent is tamsulosin).

DASH (Dietary Approaches to Stop Hypertension) Diet

Diet rich in fruits and vegetables, moderate in low-fat dairy products, low in animal protein.

Surgical Management

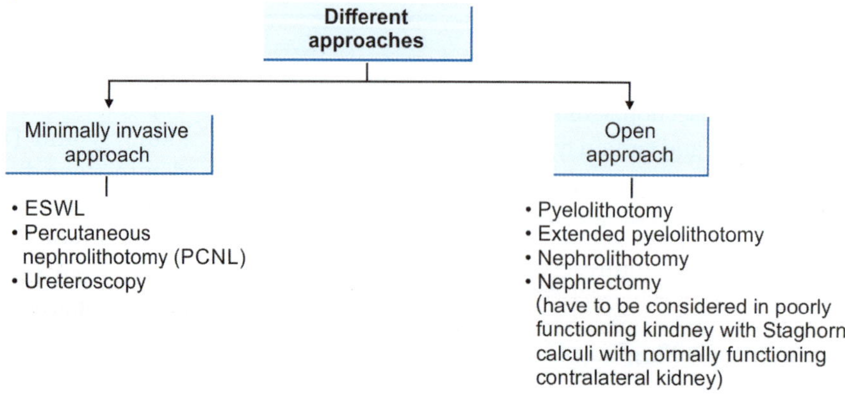

Following Factors to be Considered for Choosing the Most Appropriate Treatment

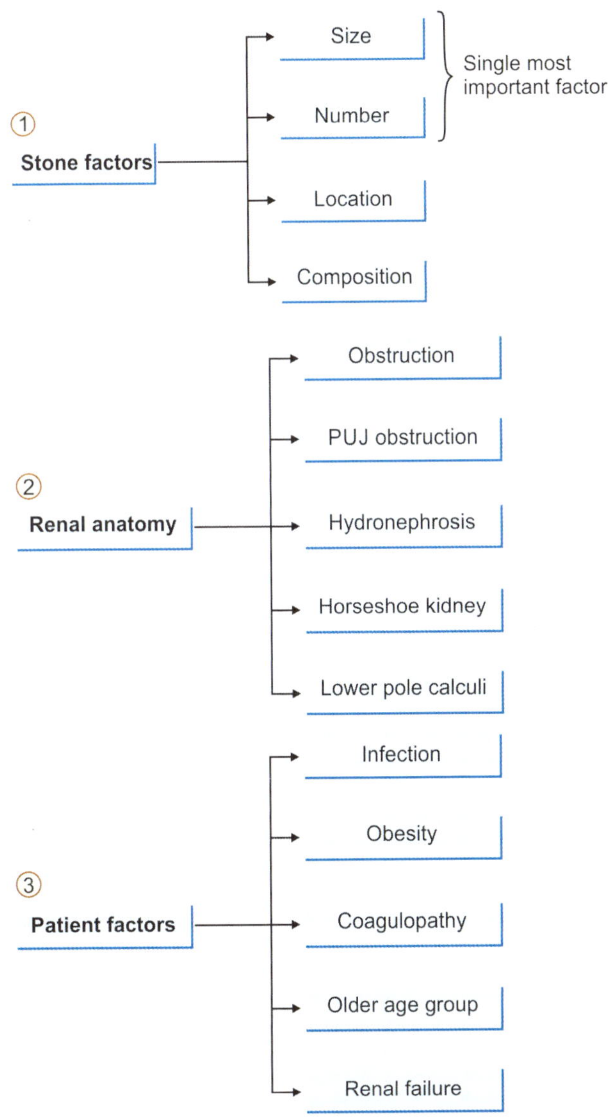

Non-Staghorn Calculi

- **>20 mm**—First choice: PNL
  Second choice: Retrograde renal surgery/SWL
- **10-20 mm—Upper and middle pole:** SWL/PNL/Ureterorenoscopy
  Lower pole: SWL or PNL or URS
- **<10 mm**—First choice: SWL or RIRS
  Second choice: PNL.

Staghorn Calculi

- PNL followed by SWL or PNL followed by repeat PNL.
- SWL should be considered in a background of sterile urine and absence of distal obstruction.
- Stone-free rate for SWL to lower pole calculi is lower (60%) in comparison to PNL (90%).

Extracorporeal Shock Wave Lithotripsy (ESWL)

- Shock waves are generated by a source (shock wave generator) external to the patient's body. Shock wave is propagated into the body focusing on the stone. Shock waves harmlessly propagate through the body tissues.
- Stone is positioned in the focal point of shock waves
- Shock waves is focused by using USG or fluoroscopy or USG + Fluoroscopy.

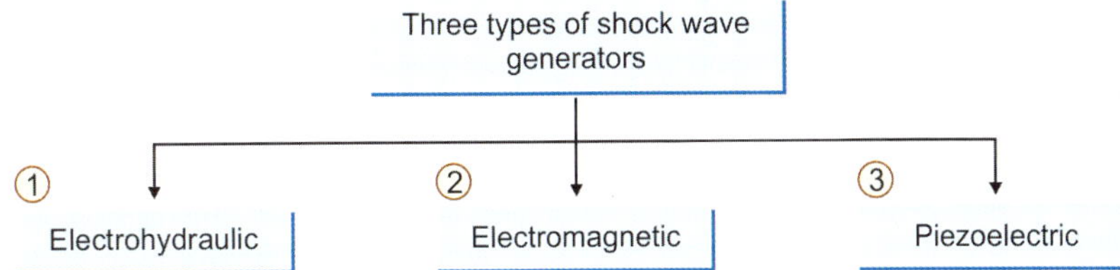

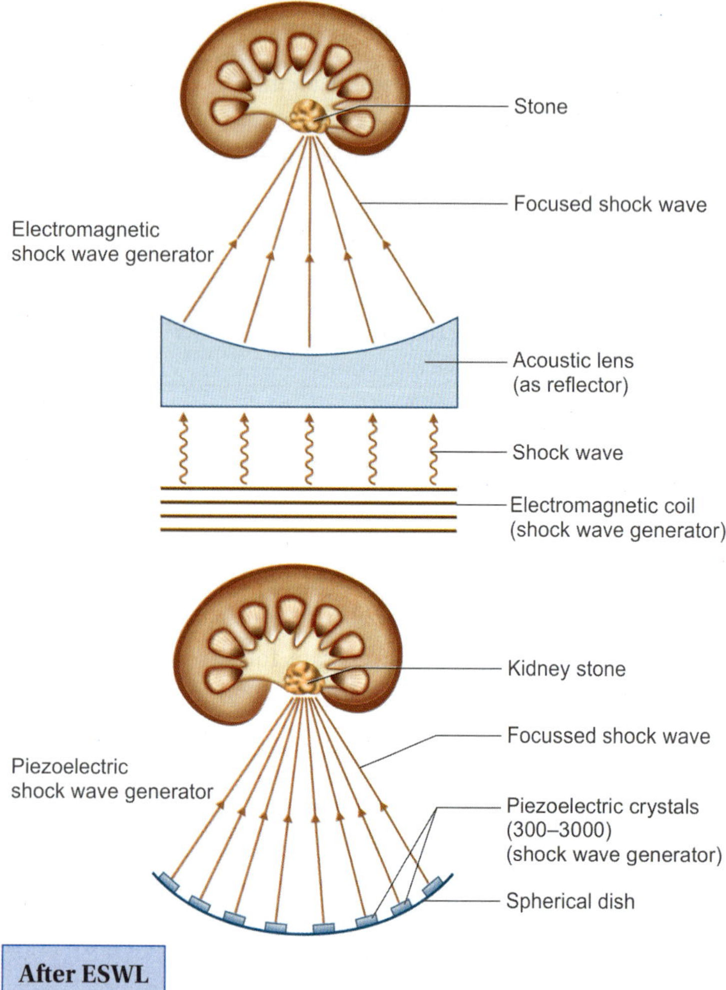

After ESWL

ESWL

Ureteric colic (to be treated with NSAID and antispasmodic)

Impacted stone—Stent is placed to passage the fragments

Residual fragment

Release of organisms causing infection

'Steinstrasse' (accumulation of stone fragment in the ureter causing obstruction)

Shock Waves Break Stones by Different Mechanisms

- Spall fracture—At the sites of impedance mismatch (stone-fluid interface, crystalline-matrix interface)
- Circumferential compression
- Shear stress
- Cavitation
- Dynamic fracture

Fragmentation depends on:

- Consistency of stone
- Size of stone
- Site of stone
- Obesity

Most oxalate and phosphate stones are well-fragmented after ESWL.

Unfavorable Factors for SWL Success

- **Shock-wave-resistant stones** (e.g., calcium oxalate monohydrate, brushite, cystine)
- Steep infundibular-pelvic angle
- Long calyx
- Narrow infundibulum (<5 mm)
- Long skin-to-stone distance (>10 cm)

Contraindications of SWL

- Pregnancy
- Bleeding diatheses
- Uncontrolled UTI
- Morbid obesity
- Severe skeletal malformation
- Anatomical obstruction distal to the stone

Complications of SWL

- Steinstrasse
- Regrowth of residual stone fragments
- Renal colic
- Perirenal hematoma
- Hematoma in liver, spleen
- Bacteriuria
- Sepsis

Percutaneous Nephrolithotomy

Contraindications of Percutaneous Nephrolithotomy (PNL)

(i) Anticoagulant therapy; (ii) Untreated UTI; (iii) Pregnancy; and (iv) Potential malignant kidney tumor.

Calculi

Balloon catheter

1. PNL is initiated by **placement of 7 Fr occlusion balloon catheter:**
   - To prevent migration of fragments into the ureter
   - To instill contrast during the procedure.

2. Selection of point of puncture and selection of calyx: **A posterior calyx is the preferred site of entry.**

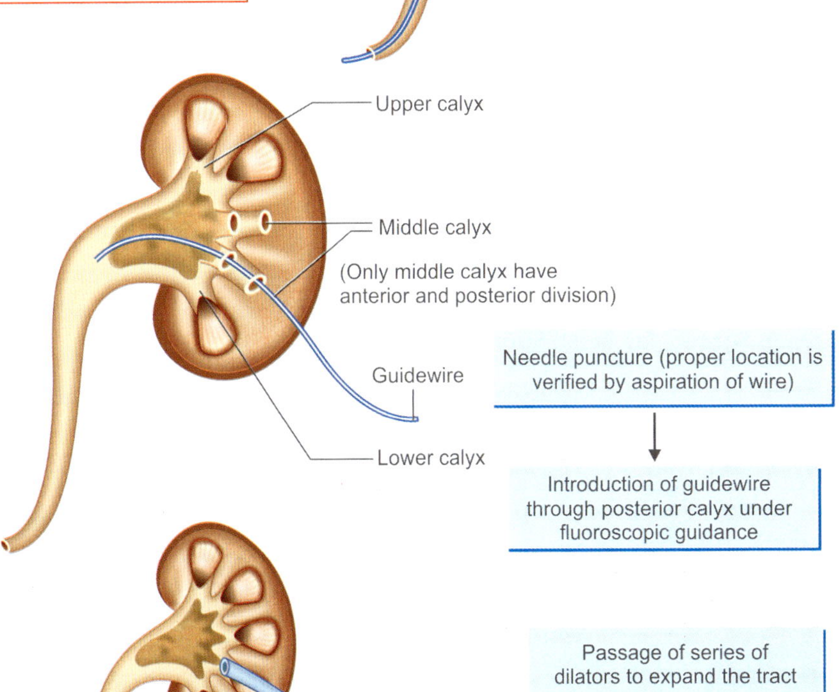

Needle puncture (proper location is verified by aspiration of wire)

↓

Introduction of guidewire through posterior calyx under fluoroscopic guidance

3. **Introduction of nephroscope**

Passage of series of dilators to expand the tract

↓

Introduction of nephroscope

Stone ≤1 cm

Nephroscope

Grasper

4. **Removal of stone**
   - Stones upto 1 cm can be grasped with graspers or stone baskets
   - Stones >1 cm require fragmentation by intracorporeal lithotripters.

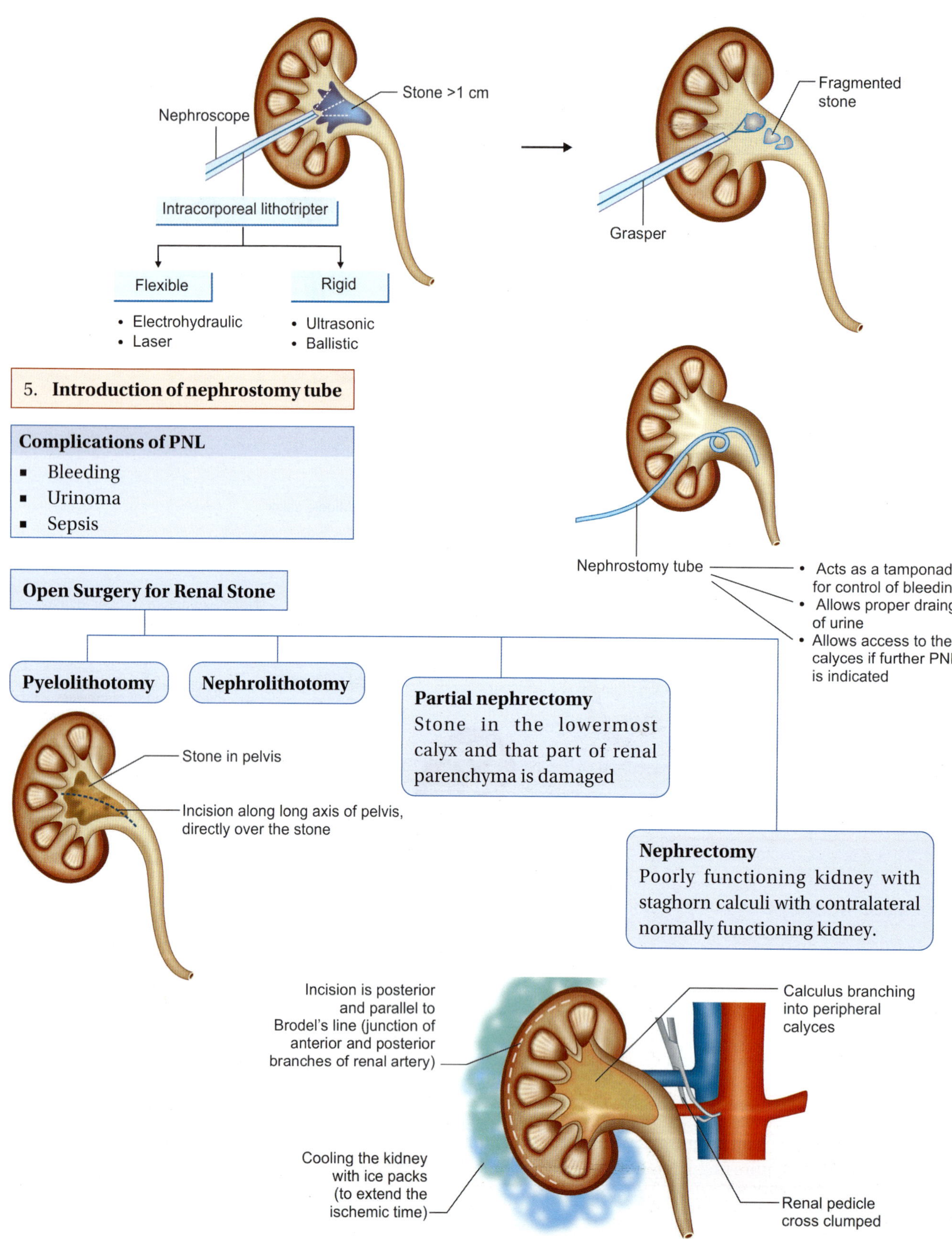
Nephroscope
Stone >1 cm
Intracorporeal lithotripter
Flexible
Rigid
• Electrohydraulic
• Laser
• Ultrasonic
• Ballistic
Fragmented stone
Grasper
5. Introduction of nephrostomy tube
Complications of PNL
▪ Bleeding
▪ Urinoma
▪ Sepsis
Nephrostomy tube
• Acts as a tamponade for control of bleeding
• Allows proper drainge of urine
• Allows access to the calyces if further PNL is indicated
Open Surgery for Renal Stone
Pyelolithotomy
Nephrolithotomy
Partial nephrectomy
Stone in the lowermost calyx and that part of renal parenchyma is damaged
Nephrectomy
Poorly functioning kidney with staghorn calculi with contralateral normally functioning kidney.
Stone in pelvis
Incision along long axis of pelvis, directly over the stone
Incision is posterior and parallel to Brodel's line (junction of anterior and posterior branches of renal artery)
Cooling the kidney with ice packs (to extend the ischemic time)
Calculus branching into peripheral calyces
Renal pedicle cross clumped

Prevention of Recurrence of Urinary Stone

- Increased fluid intake (at least 3 liters/day to achieve urine output of at least 2.5 liters/day
- Avoidance of increased consumption of sugar-sweetened beverages, animal protein, oxalate-rich foods (e.g., spinach, beet, chocolate and nuts),
- Excess consumption of vitamin C supplements (should not be more than 2 g/day)
- Consumption of DASH diet
- Intake of citrus juices (lemonade and orange juice)

Infections of Kidney

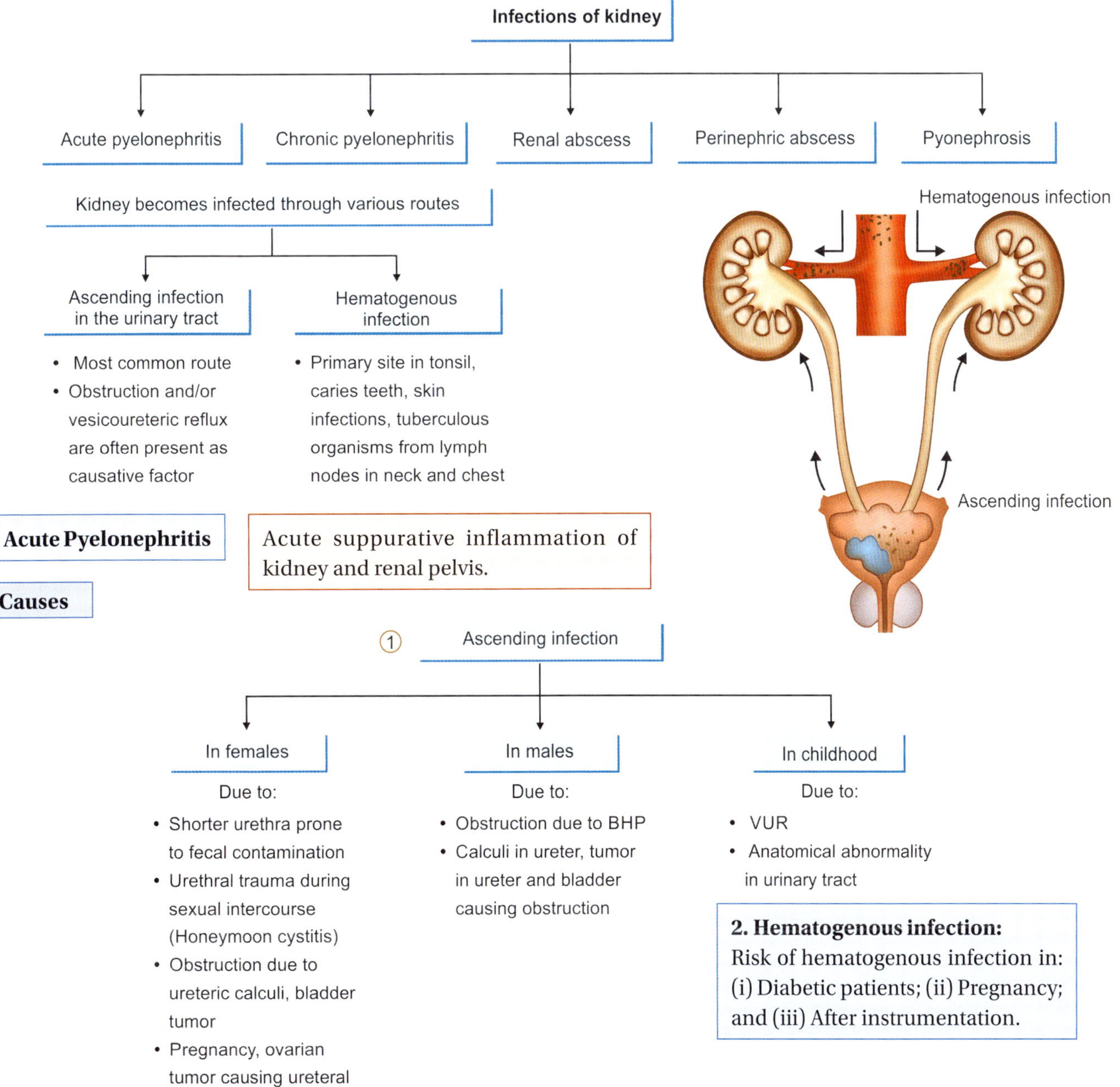

Acute Pyelonephritis

Acute suppurative inflammation of kidney and renal pelvis.

Causes

2. Hematogenous infection:
Risk of hematogenous infection in: (i) Diabetic patients; (ii) Pregnancy; and (iii) After instrumentation.

Pathology

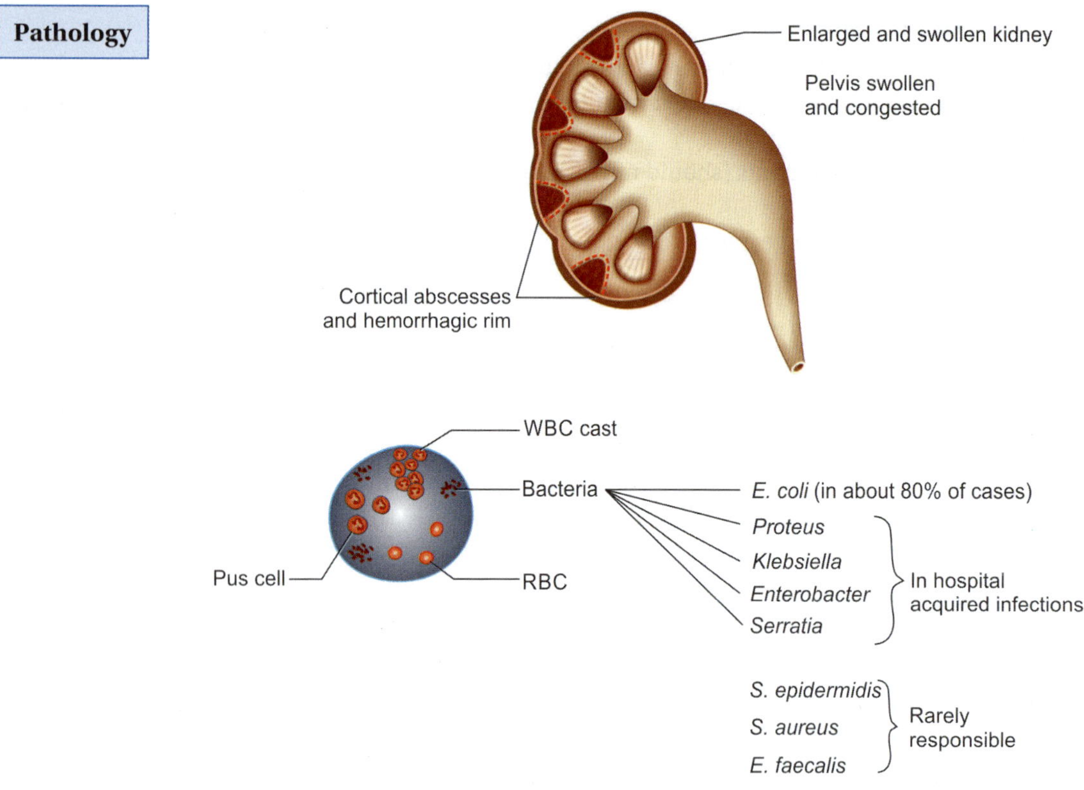

Clinical Presentation

- Patient presents with abrupt onset of fever, chill, pain and tenderness in renal angle.
- Dysuria, increased frequency and urgency are often present.

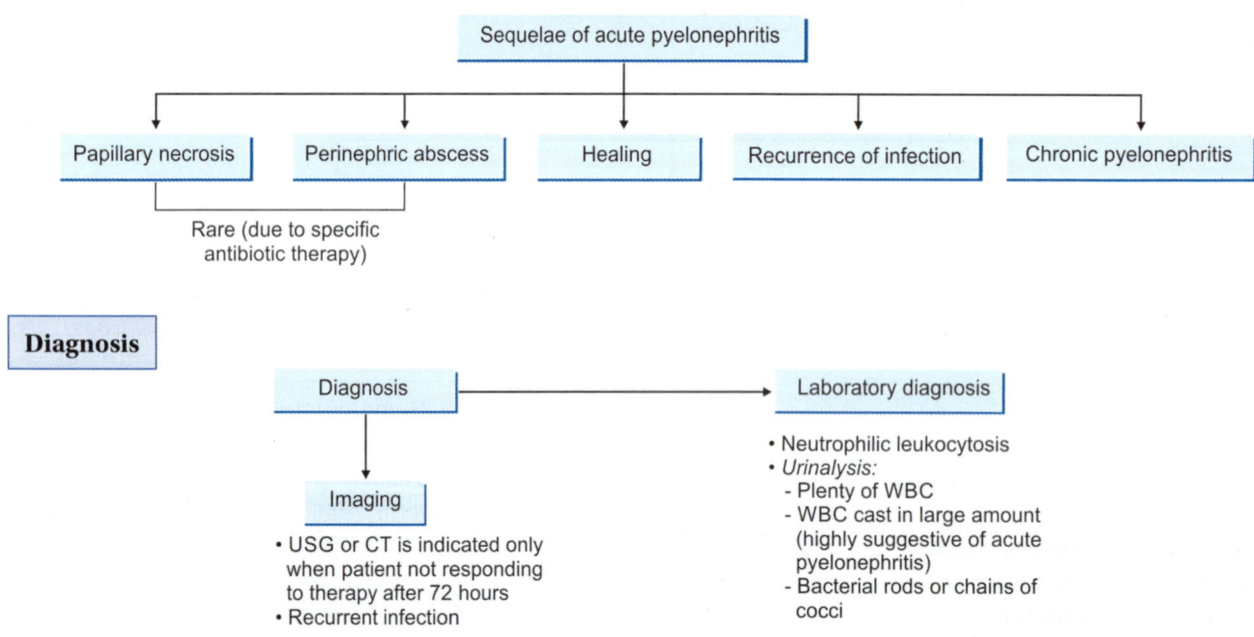

Diagnosis

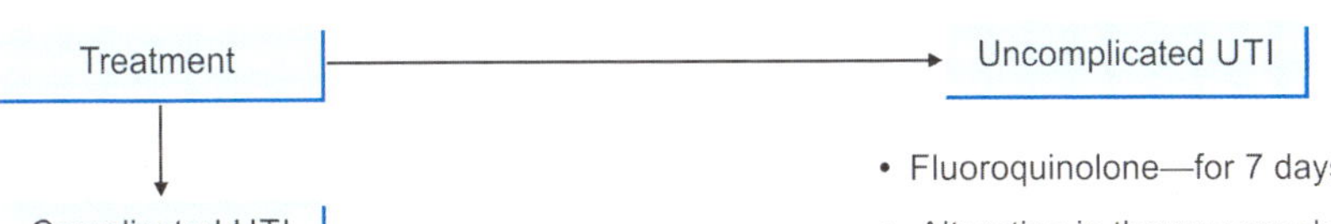

Complicated UTI

- Bed rest
- IV fluid
- Antipyretics
- Emperical antibiotic therapy—Parenteral fluoroquinolone/ aminoglycoside with or without ampicillin. Extended-spectrum cephalosporin ± aminoglycoside — 7 days
- Antibiotic may be changed after getting C/S report

Uncomplicated UTI

- Fluoroquinolone—for 7 days
- Alteration in therapy may be needed after C/S report

> - **If fever persists more than 72 hours,** radiologic investigation (USG/CT) have to be done to rule out obstructive uropathy, anatomic abnormalities or perirenal infections.
> - **Repeat urine culture on** 5–7th day, on 10–14th day and 4–6th week.

Chronic Pyelonephritis

A chronic tubulointerstitial disease resulting from repeated attacks of inflammation and healing.

Types

Chronic obstructive pyelonephritis

Obstruction at different levels of urinary tract results in recurrent episodes of infection followed by fibrosis and scarring of cortex.

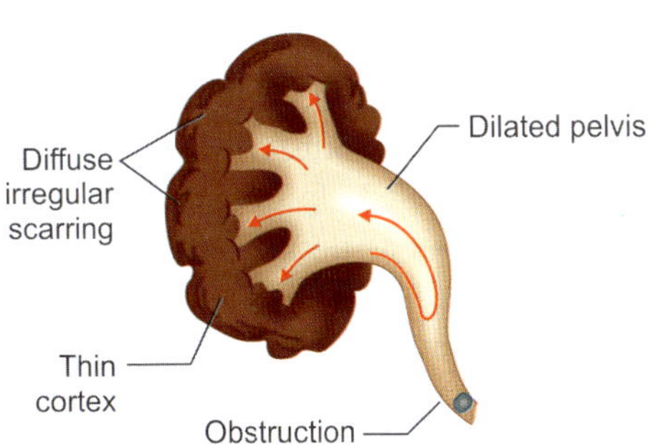

Reflux-associated pyelonephritis

- Major cause of pyelonephritis
- Reflux may be unilateral or bilateral

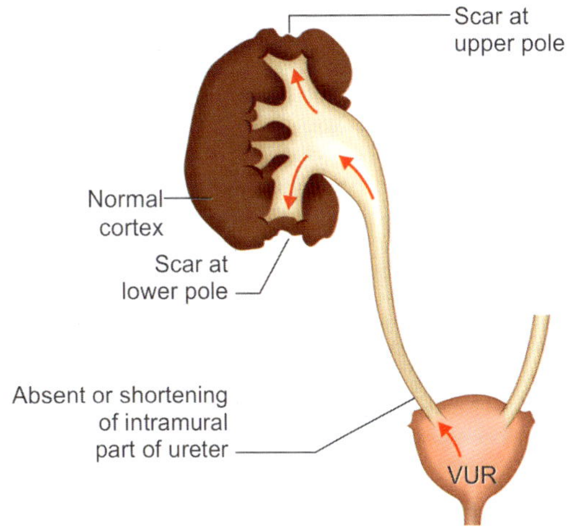

Characteristic Features of Chronic Pyelonephritis

- One or both kidneys may affected. Either kidney is diffusely or scatteredly involved.
- Grossly, the kidney is small, contracted with irregular scarring. Scarring involves the pelvis and calyces leads to blunting of calyces.
- Chronic interstitial inflammation is present.
- Tubules show varying degrees of atrophy and dilatation. Glomeruli are usually unaffected except in advanced stage.

Clinical Features

- Usually, no symptoms are present until chronic renal failure develops.
- If it is a sequele of recurrent attacks of acute pyelonephritis, then symptoms like fever, loin pain and dysuria may be present.
- Hypertension is present in about 40% of patient and may be of malignant type.

Diagnosis

- Urine culture commonly reveals the presence of *E. coli, Proteus, and Pseudomonas.* Urine culture may be negative.
- Casts are usually absent. Plenty of WBCs are found in microscopical examination of urine.
- IVU findings are almost diagnostic. The usual findings are: (i) Asymmetrical kidney outline and (ii) Blunting or dilatation of one or more calyces and cortical scars at the corresponding site.

Treatment

- Treatment of bacterial infection (emperical, then according to C/S report)
- Prevention of future infections
- Treatment of causative factors (stone/VUR)
- Nephrectomy/partial nephrectomy
- Renal transplantation (in patient with end stage renal failure)

Perinephric Abscess

Causes

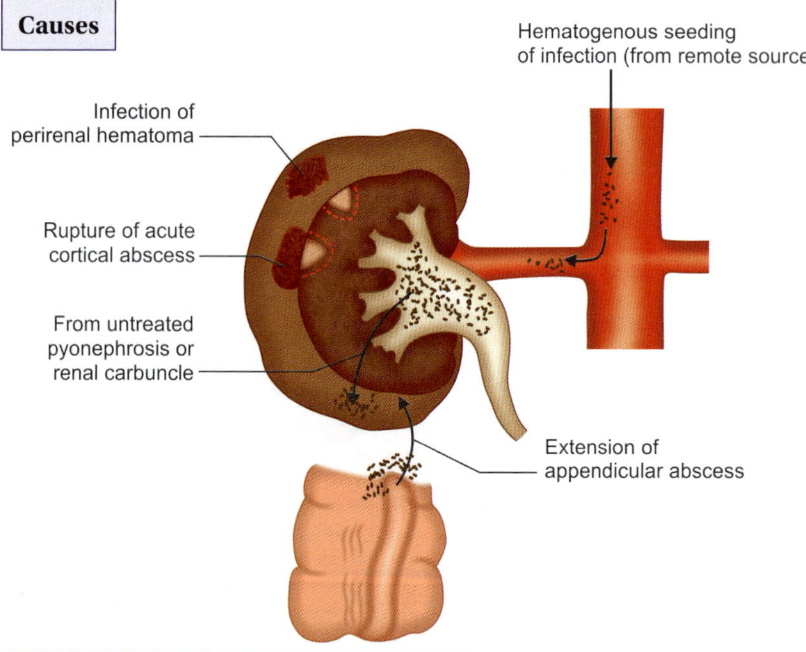

Diagnosis

Laboratory investigation:
Leukocytosis

Urine examination:

- Pyuria
- **Culture of urine:** *E. coli, Proteus, S. aureus* are found in most of the cases.

Plain X-ray of KUB:

- Absence of psoas shadow
- Reactionary scoliosis—Concavity of vertebral column toward the abscess
- Elevated and immobile diaphragm on the affected side.

CT is specifically helpful to identify the abscess as well as detailed information about the spread of infection.

CT is also helpful for planning surgical drainage.

Clinical Presentation

- High swinging pyrexia
- Abdominal or flank mass
- Tenderness in loin

Treatment

Treatment includes: (i) Antimicrobial therapy; (ii) Drainage of abscess; and (iii) Treatment of the cause. Image-guided (USG or CT) drainage is indicated for small abscess. For larger abscess, open drainage (through lumbar incision) is a better option.

Pyonephrosis

Pyonephrosis is infected hydronephrosis along with suppurative destruction of renal parenchyma.

- **Clinical presentation:** Patient looks toxic, high rise of temperature with chill, flank pain, tenderness in loin, swelling in loin
- History of urinary tract calculi, UTI may be present.
- **Diagnosis:** USG reveals dilated pelvicalyceal system; CT is nonspecific; IVU shows a poorly functioning or nonfunctioning hydronephrotic kidney.
- **Treatment includes:** (i) Antimicrobial therapy and (ii) Urgent drainage of pus through percutaneous nephrostomy followed by treatment of cause of obstruction and source of infection. Nephrectomy is indicated for pyonephrosis of nonfunctioning kidney if contralateral kidney is normally functioning.

Renal Abscess or Carbuncle

Collection of purulent material confined to renal parenchyma.

- **Risk factors:** (i) Diabetes mellitus; (ii) IV drug abuse; and (iii) Immunosuppression
- **Etiopathogenesis:** Renal abscess may develop via following routes: (i) Hematogenous spread; (ii) Ascending infection (associated with obstruction or stasis); and (iii) Vesicoureteral reflux
- **Clinical presentation:** Fever with chill, flank pain, tender swelling in loin are the usual symptoms and signs.
- **Diagnosis:** Laboratory investigations reveal marked leukocytosis, positive blood and urine culture. USG and CT both are useful imaging modalities to differentiate renal abscess from other inflammatory renal diseases. CT is the investigation of choice.
- **Treatment:** Parenteral antibiotic therapy is adequate if abscess size less than 3 cm. Drainage of abscess (image-guided or open) is indicated if disease is not responding to antibiotic therapy or abscess is more 3 cm or patient is immunocompromised.

Tuberculosis of Kidney

Etiopathogenesis

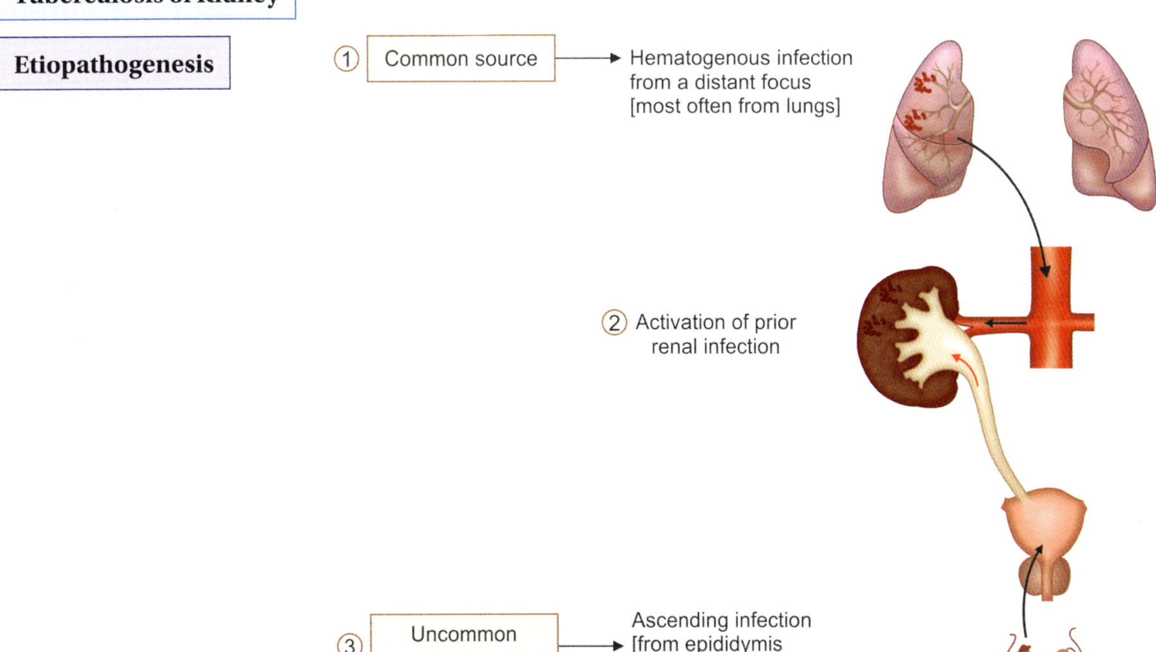

Development of Tubercular Ulcer

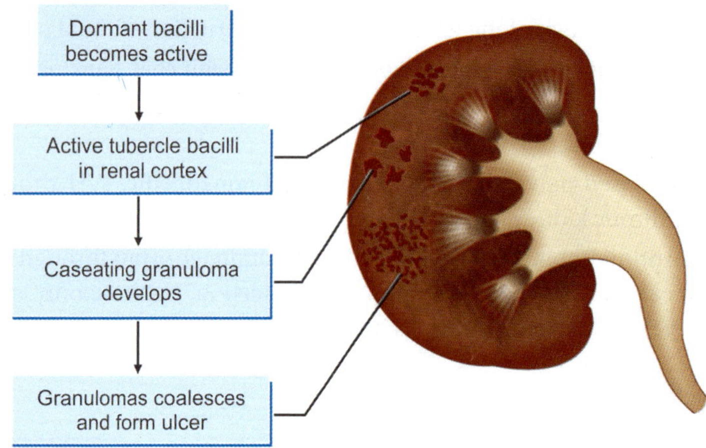

Types of Tubercular Lesion

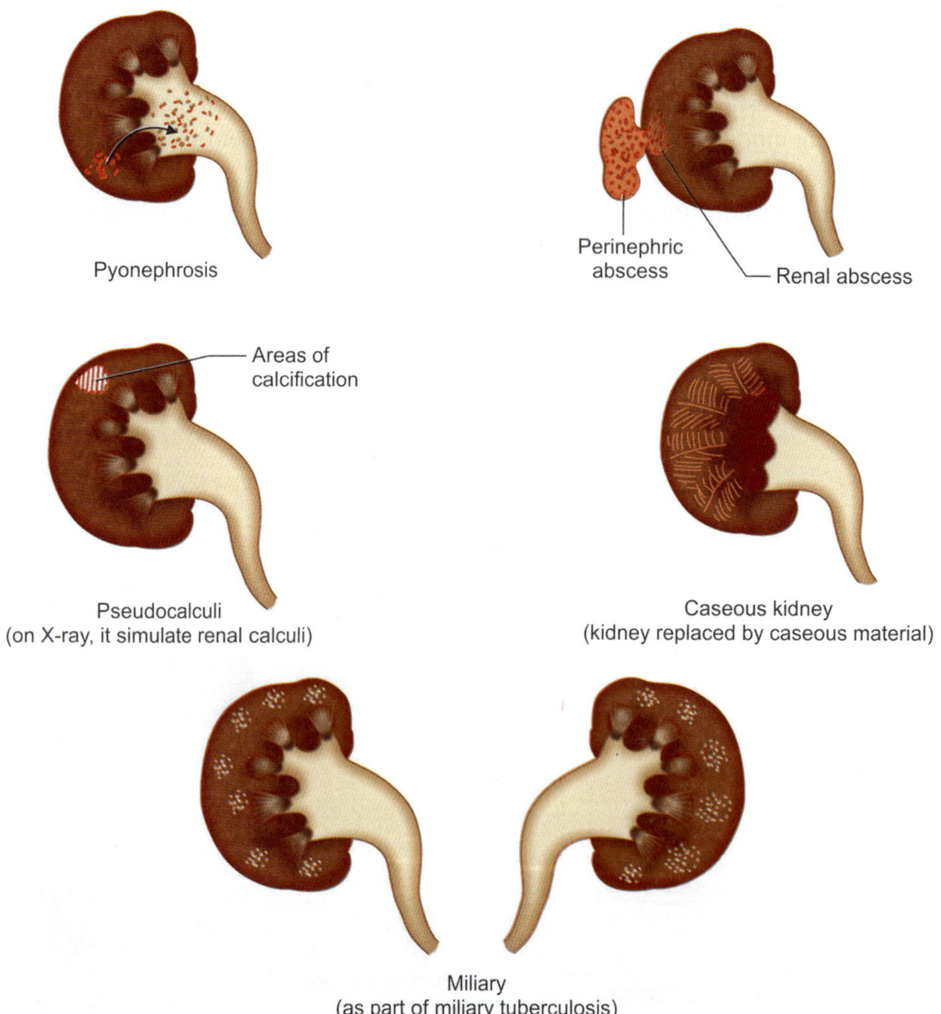

Clinical Presentation

- Usually common in 20–40 years of age. Genitourinary TB is very uncommon in children.
- More common in men (2:1)
- Right kidney is more affected.
- Increased frequency of micturition—**Often the earliest symptom**
  - Hematuria
  - Dull aching pain in loin
  - Constitutional symptom—Weight loss, evening rise of temperature

Genitourinary TB should be suspected if patient presenting with vague, persistent urinary symptoms without any obvious cause.

Diagnosis

- **Urine examination:** Sterile pyuria is the classic finding on routine urinalysis and culture. Z–N staining rarely shows the presence of acid-fast bacilli. Urine culture on Lowenstein- Jensen medium takes 6–8 weeks as the bacteria is slow growing. 3–5 consecutive early morning samples of urine should be cultured (because the organism is intermittently excreted). PCR technique can be used to detect mycobacterial DNA in urine.
- **Imaging:** Plain X-ray, IVU and CT are imaging modalities to detect tuberculous lesions in kidney. Calcification in kidneys is a common radiological finding in plain X-ray. IVU findings include distortion of calyx, calyceal and parenchymal destruction. CT is the imaging modality of choice. CT with 3D reconstruction is helpful to identify calyceal abnormalities, hydronephrosis, hydroureter. Chest X-ray is indicated to exclude any active lung lesion.

Treatment

- Prognosis is good if patient completes the course of ATD (6–9) months
- Surgical intervention—Aim is to preserve the organ and reconstruction rather than excision. Surgery should be done at least after 4–6 weeks of chemotherapy. Nephrectomy or partial nephrectomy may be indicated.

Kidney Tumors

Benign Tumor

- Adenoma
- Oncocytoma
- Transitional cell papilloma
- Mesoblastic nephroma
- Angiomyolipoma

Malignant Tumor

- Renal cell carcinoma
- Transitional cell carcinoma
- Wilms' tumor

Metastatic Tumor

- Most common malignant tumor of kidney.
- Usually, hematogenous route of spread.
- Lung, breast, GI tumors, malignant melanoma are the common primary sites.

Oncocytoma

- A benign epithelial tumor arising from collecting ducts.
- Ultrastructurally, these tumors are packed with numerous large mitochondrias.
- Most of the oncocytomas cannot be differentiated from RCC by clinical or radiological means. That is why, most urologists treat this tumor aggressively (thermal ablation, partial nephrectomy, radical nephrectomy).

Angiomyolipoma

Angiomyolipoma is a benign mesenchymal tumor. **This tumor is a member of the perivascular epithelioid cells tumor group (PEComas)**. This tumor is four times more common in females. Most of the tumors occur as sporadic entities. In about 20–30% of cases, this tumor is associated with **tuberous sclerosis**.

Angiomyolipomas are composed of variable amounts of irregular and aneurysmatic blood vessels, smooth muscle and mature adipocytes. Typically, AMLs are benign, but **epithelioid variant is potentially malignant**.

Clinical presentation: Most of the AMLs are asymtomatic. Sporadic AMLs are usually single, small, with a slow and consistent growth rate, rarely progress to cause significant morbidity.

AMLs associated with Tuberous sclerosis are multiple, bilateral, large, rapidly progressive, with more risk of significant morbidity. Tuberous sclerosis-associated AMLs are usually present at a younger age group with equal gender distribution.

A significant complication is retroperitoneal bleeding or bleeding into the urinary collecting system.

Diagnosis: On CT scan, presence of fat within a renal lesion is diagnostic of AML and excludes RCC.

Positivity to HMB-45, a monoclonal antibody, is characteristic of AML.

Treatment: Treatment options include- (i) Active surveillance; (ii) Selective arterial embolization; (iii) Nephron-sparing surgery; (iv) Complete nephrectomy; (v) Radiofrequency ablation; and (vi) mTOR inhibitor.

Small (<4 cm), asymptomatic AML can be observed expectantly with active surveillance.

Solitary, large, symptomatic (e.g., life-threatening hemorrhage) AML can be managed by nephron-sparing surgery; some patients require complete nephrectomy.

In tuberous sclerosis patients, bilateral AML, patients with pre-existing renal insufficiency: A nephron-sparing surgery or selective embolization should be considered. The volume of tumor can be reduced by mTOR inhibitor, everolimus.

Renal Cell Carcinoma

- Most lethal of all the urologic malignancies
- Common in elderly patients—in 6th and 7th decades
- Male-female ratio 3:2
- Most of the RCCs are sporadic.
- These tumors are derived from tubular epithelium. So, they are located predominantly in the cortex.
- Usually arises from poles of the kidney, usually from the upper pole.
- Most sporadic RCCs are unilateral and unifocal.

Hereditary Kidney Cancer Syndromes

- VHL syndrome
- Hereditary papillary RCC
- Birt-Hogg-Dube syndrome
- Tuberous sclerosis
- Non-polyposis colorectal cancer syndrome
- Hyperparathyroidism—jaw tumor syndrome

Risk Factors

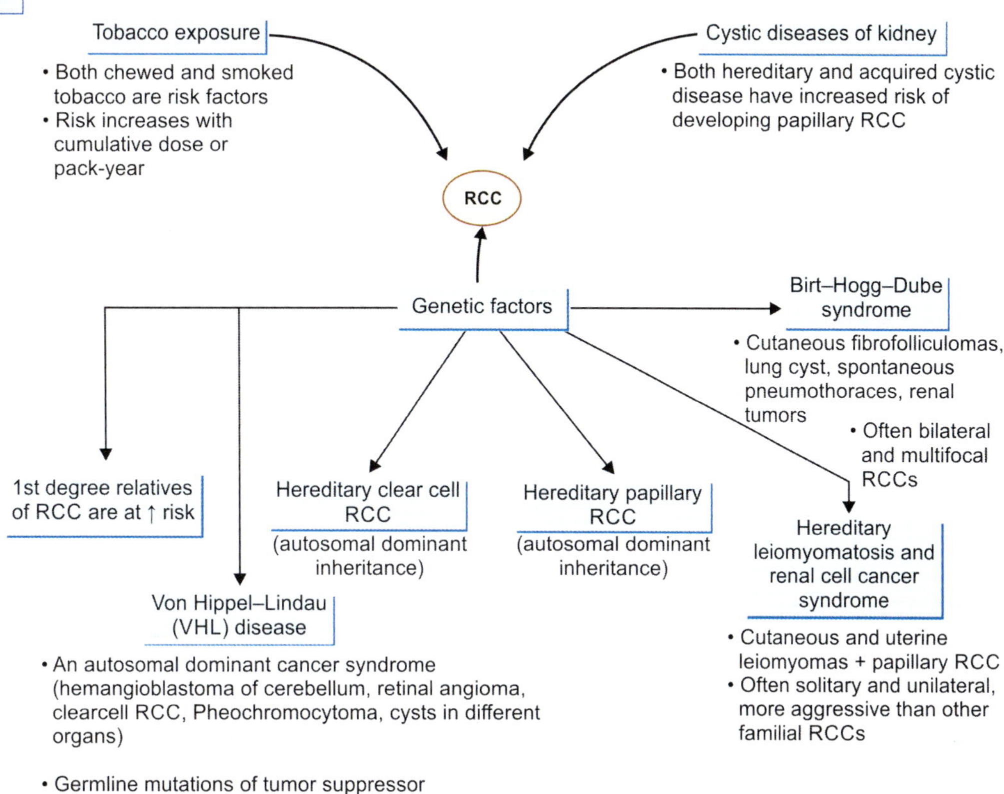

Pathology

- Most RCCs are round to avoid in shape, golden yellow in color, usually varies in size from 5–8 cm, circumscribed by a pseudocapsule (composed of compressed parenchyma and fibrous tissue).
- The cut section shows areas of necrosis, hemorrhage and cystic changes.

[RCC with cystic degeneration is associated with better prognosis than solid RCC.]

The three most common histologic RCC types are: (i) Clear cell RCC; (ii) Papillary RCC; and (iii) Chromophobe RCC.

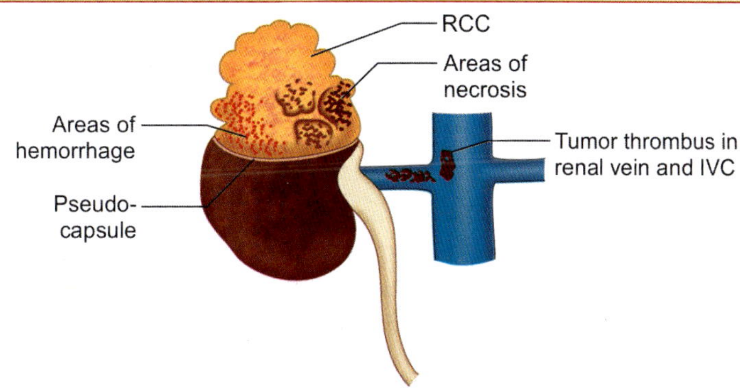

Clear Cell Renal Cell Cancer (ccRCC)	Papillary Renal Cell Cancer (pRCC)	Chromophobe Renal Cell Cancer (chRCC)
▪ Most common histologic type ▪ Well-circumscribed tumor and capsule is usually absent ▪ Cut surface is golden-yellow with hemorrhage and necrosis ▪ The cells contain lipid, glycogen which are removed during processing of tissues, thus appears as cells with clear cytoplasm (clear cell) ▪ Worse prognosis compared to pRCC and chRCC.	▪ Second most common histologic type ▪ pRCC is well circumscribed with pseudocapsule, yellow or brown in color ▪ The tumor cells arranged in papillary pattern over fibrovascular stalks. ▪ They tend to be bilateral and multiple ▪ Better prognosis than ccRCC.	▪ chRCC is homogenous, well-demarcated mass without capsule ▪ Arise from intercalated cells of collecting ducts. Stains more darkly than clear cell type. Perinuclear halo and presence of numerous microvesicles are distinctive features ▪ Better prognosis.

Spread of Tumor

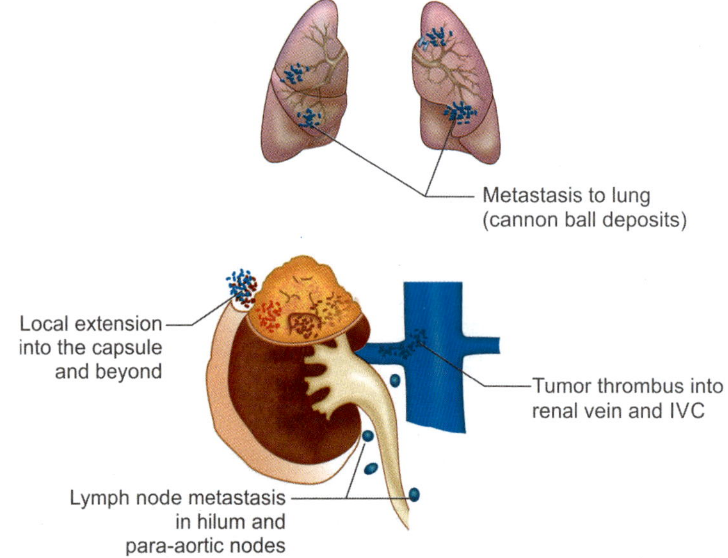

Clinical Presentation

- Most of the patients with RCC are asymptomatic. **The classic traid** of flank pain, gross hematuria, and palpable abdominal mass is rare, found in advanced disease only.
- **Other symptoms due to advanced disease:** Weight loss, Varicocele (left), fever, bilateral lower extremity edema, night sweat.
- **Symptoms due to metastatic disease:** Bone pain, persistent cough.
- **Paraneoplastic syndrome:** Hypercalcemia, hypertension, polycythemia, nonmetastatic hepatic dysfunction (Stauffer's syndrome).

Diagnosis

- **Contrast enhanced multi-phasic CT:** Highly sensitive and specific for detection and characterization of primary tumor, tumor invasion, tumor thrombus and metastasis
- **MRI:** Higher sensitivity and specificity for small renal masses and tumor thrombus compared to CT
- **Contrast enhanced ultrasound (CEUS):** A useful imaging modality for characterization of renal mass.
- **For metastatic workup:** CT abdomen and CT chest are indicated for staging. Routine bone scan is not indicated.
- **Tumor biopsy** is not necessary if surgery is planned based on imaging findings. Tumor biopsy is indicated if ablative therapy or systemic therapy is planned.

Treatment

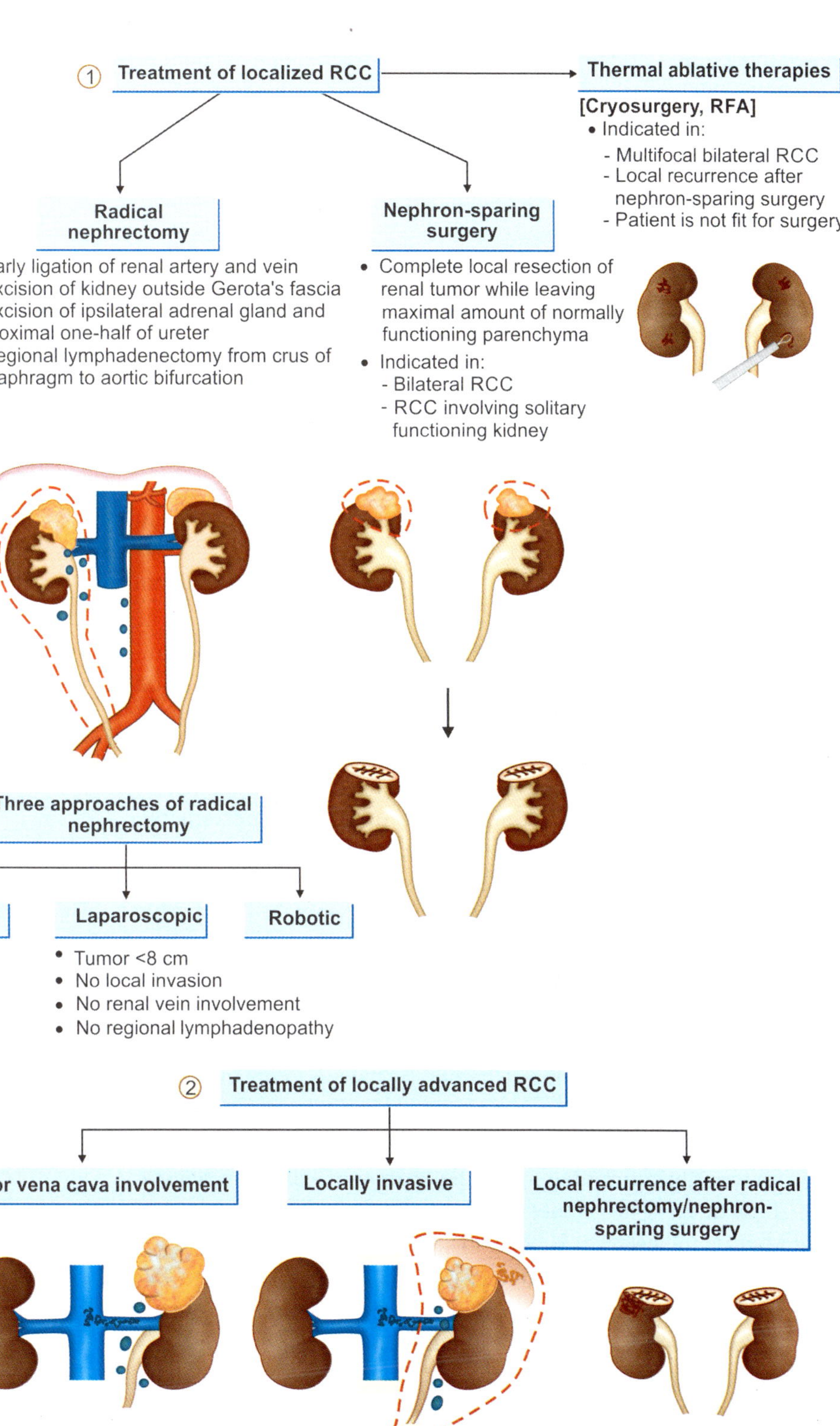
① Treatment of localized RCC
Thermal ablative therapies
[Cryosurgery, RFA]
• Indicated in:
- Multifocal bilateral RCC
- Local recurrence after nephron-sparing surgery
- Patient is not fit for surgery
Radical nephrectomy
• Early ligation of renal artery and vein
• Excision of kidney outside Gerota's fascia
• Excision of ipsilateral adrenal gland and proximal one-half of ureter
• Regional lymphadenectomy from crus of diaphragm to aortic bifurcation
Nephron-sparing surgery
• Complete local resection of renal tumor while leaving maximal amount of normally functioning parenchyma
• Indicated in:
- Bilateral RCC
- RCC involving solitary functioning kidney
Three approaches of radical nephrectomy
Open
Laparoscopic
Robotic
• Tumor <8 cm
• No local invasion
• No renal vein involvement
• No regional lymphadenopathy
② Treatment of locally advanced RCC
Inferior vena cava involvement
Locally invasive
Local recurrence after radical nephrectomy/nephron-sparing surgery
Radical nephrectomy + Removal of thrombus from IVC after getting vascular control
Radical nephrectomy + en bloc resection of involved organs (bowel, spleen, etc.)
Thermal ablative therapy

Treatment of Metastatic RCC

- **Palliative nephrectomy** followed by systemic treatment. Palliative nephrectomy is particularly indicated if a patient presenting with hematuria or symptoms related to a primary tumor.
- **Pazopanib and sunitinib** are recommended as first-line treatment in relapsed or medically unresectable clear cell stage IV RCC with good-risk features. **Nivolumab and ipilimumab** in combination is recommended as first-line treatment for relapsed, medically unresectable, clear cell, stage IV RCC with intermediate and poor risk features.

Wilms' Tumor

This is an embryonal tumor that originated from remnants of immature kidney. Most common primary malignant renal tumor of childhood. Most commonly seen in children between 1–5 years.

Genetics: More than 90% of Wilms' tumors arise from somatic mutations. Very few tumors arise as result of germline mutations. These tumors have an inherited predisposition.

Pathology: Grossly, the tumor is large, spheroidal, compresses the adjacent normal renal parenchyma to form a pseudocapsule.

Microscopically, it is composed of primitive epithelial and mesenchymal elements (e.g., muscle, cartilage, bone and fibrous tissue).

Wilms' tumor histologically classified into: (i) Favorable histology (predominant epithelial differentiation); (ii) Anaplastic (resistant to chemotherapy); and (iii) Nephrogenic rests (precursor of WT).

Clinical features: Palpable abdominal lump is the most common clinical presentation. The lump may be large comparing to the size of the patient. Other clinical presentations are abdominal pain, fever, hematuria, hypertension. Uncommon presentations include varicocele, hernia, enlarged testicle, congestive heart failure, acute abdomen, tumor rupture, shock.

During clinical examination, signs of syndromes associated with this tumor must be searched—aniridia, macroglossia, genitourinary anomalies, hemihypertrophy.

Diagnosis:

Ultrasonography should be the initial imaging modality. It is helpful to evaluate whether the mass originated from kidney or whether the mass is cystic or solid.

Abdominal CT or MRI is indicated to differentiate renal tumors from extrarenal tumors and benign renal conditions (e.g., angiomyolipoma, dysplastic kidney, hydronephrosis, metanephric tumors, polycystic kidney disease, multicystic kidney disease). These imaging modalities are also helpful to evaluate extension of the tumor and whether metastatasis is present.

Chest CT should be done to exclude pulmonary metastases (most common site of distant metastases). Biopsy is not necessary if surgery is planned based on imaging findings. **Biopsy (image-guided core needle biopsy or open biopsy)** is indicated if neoadjuvant therapy is planned.

Treatment: Radical nephroureterectomy is the treatment of choice for resectable, unilateral tumors. **Nephron-sparing surgery** is reserved for bilateral disease, those with predisposing conditions and at risk of renal failure.

Neoadjuvant therapy is indicated in unresectable unilateral tumor, bilateral tumor, those with predisposing conditions.

Syndromes Associated with Wilms' Tumor

- Beckwith-Wiedemann syndrome (omphalocele, nephromegaly, hepatomegaly, macroglossia and hemihypertrophy)
- Denys-Drash syndrome (male pseudohermaphroditism, renal mesangial sclerosis, nephroblastoma)
- WAGR syndrome (Wilms' tumor, aniridia, genital anomalies and mental retardation).

Germline Mutations Associated with Wilms' Tumor

- WT1 mutation (11p13)-associated with WAGR syndrome, Denys-Drash syndrome, Frasier syndrome; associated with bilateral tumor
- WT2 mutation (11p15)-associated with Beckwith-Wiedemann syndrome.

Intraabdominal Malignancies Presenting as Flank Mass

- Neuroblastoma
- Hepatoblastoma
- Extrarenal Wilms' tumor
- Burkitt lymphoma
- Ewing sarcoma Rhabdomyosarcoma

Ureteral Calculi

Ureteral calculi almost always originated in kidney.

Clinical features:

Ureteric colic: Character and radiation of pain- Acute colicky pain in the loin that usually radiates to the ipsilateral groin and genitalia. The patient rolls around in agony. Pain-free periods persist between each attack. Site of radiation of pain is determined by site of obstruction. **In obstruction of right midureter**, pain is referred to right iliac fossa (simulate appendicitis) and **in obstruction of left midureter**, pain is referred to left iliac fossa (simulate diverticulitis). In midureter obstruction, pain may also referred to scrotum and labium. **In obstruction of lower ureter**, patient may experience pain that radiates along the urethra to the tip of penis, along with frequency, urgency. Pain is mediated by prostaglandins in response to obstruction. Prostaglandin increases the ureteral peristalsis and sensitize nociceptors to stimuli such as bradykinin.

Hematuria: Microscopic hematuria is commonly associated with attacks of ureteric colic.

[If macroscopic hematuria is present, think of other causes of colicky pain (e.g., clot) rather than stone.]

On clinical examination, tenderness may be present over the course of ureter according to the site of impaction of stone.

[Right-sided ureteric colic and appendicitis are almost similar in clinical presentation].

Usually, the pain in ureteric colic is more but patient is less ill.

Diagnosis: Same as renal stone.

Treatment: Goal of treatment is complete stone clearance with minimal morbidity.

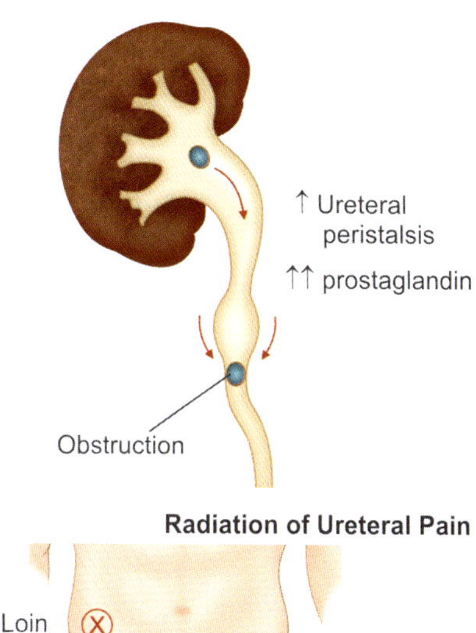

Radiation of Ureteral Pain

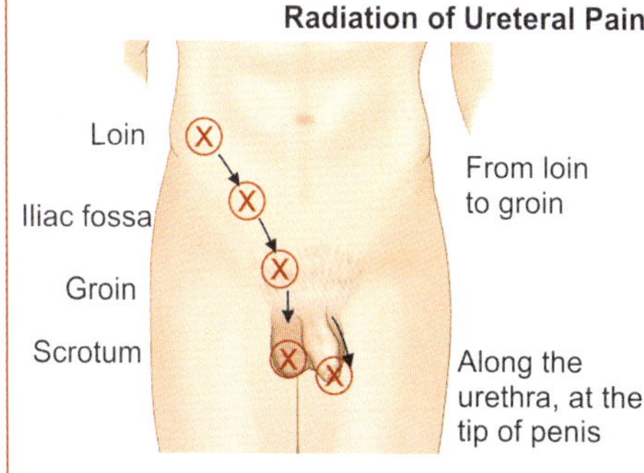

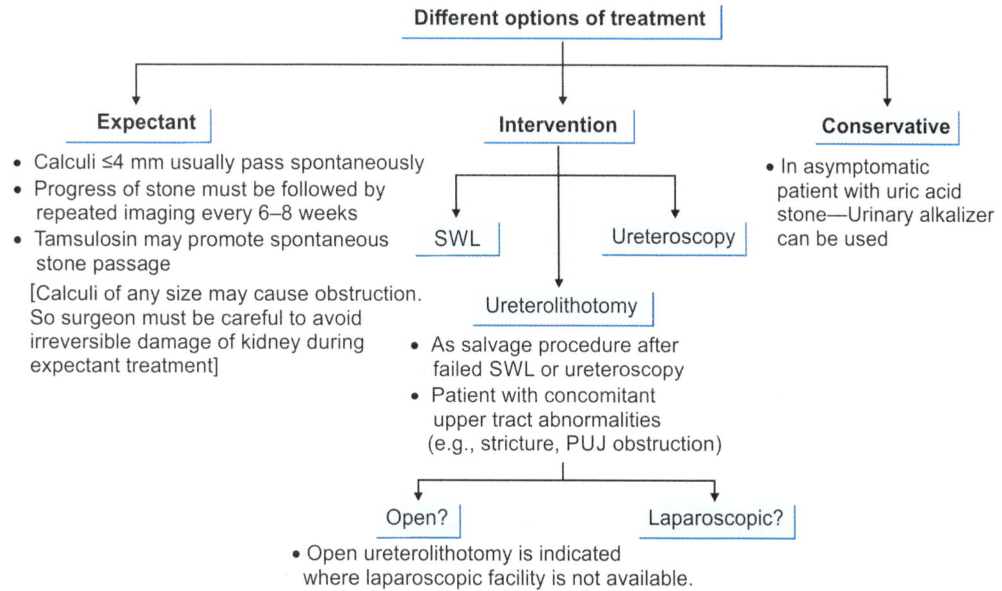

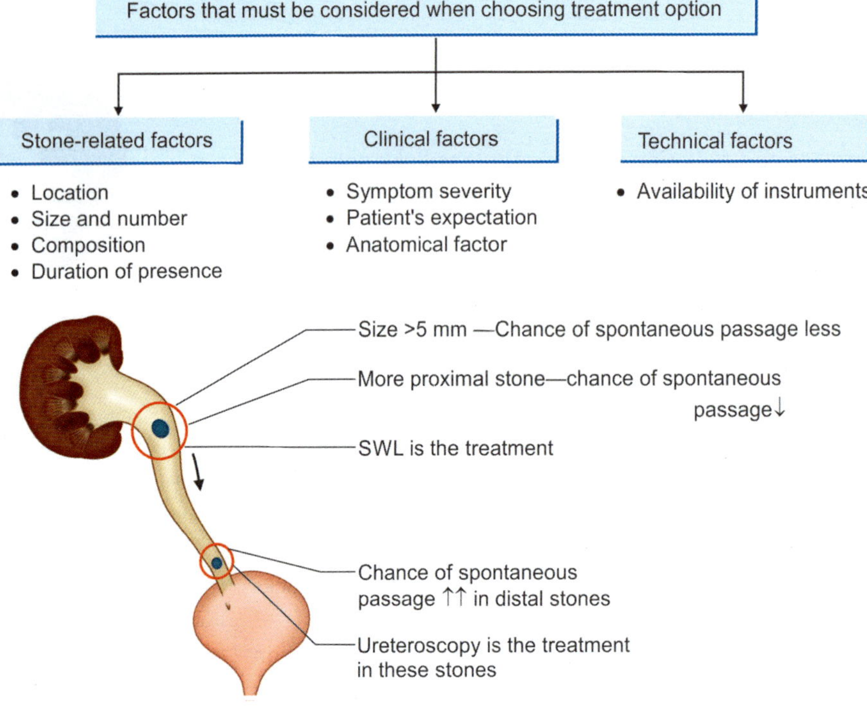

Proximal Ureteral Stone
>10 mm First choice—URS; second choice—SWL
<10 mm SWL or URS
Distal Ureteral Stone
>10 mm First choice—URS; second choice—SWL
<10 mm URS or SWL

Ureteroscopy is more effective for larger stones.

- **Calcium oxalate dihydrate stone (fragile)**—SWL is a better option.
- **Cystine and brushite stone**—Ureteroscopy ± intracorporeal lithotripsy.
- **Pyelonephritis or pyonephrosis due to obstruction needs urgent drainage of the tract (by ureteral catheter/ percutaneous nephrolithotomy)**—Definite treatment after infection resolves.
- Ureteral stone obstructing a solitary kidney warrants active intervention.

Urothelial Tumors of Renal Pelvis and Ureter

- Urothelial carcinomas can be located in the upper (pyelocaliceal cavities and ureter) and lower (bladder and urethra) urinary tract.
- Upper tract urothelial carcinomas are uncommon in comparison to lower tract urothelial carcinoma.
- **Transitional cell carcinoma (TCC)** is the most common type of urothelial cancer (Renal pelvis, ureter, bladder and proximal urethra are lined by transitional epithelium). Other uncommon histological types are squamous cell carcinoma, sarcomatoid carcinoma, lymphoepithelioma.
- Men are commonly affected.

Genetic Events Associated with Urothelial Cancer

- Mutations in *MMR* genes
- Mutations in *p53* gene
- Abnormalities in chromosome 9

Risk Factors

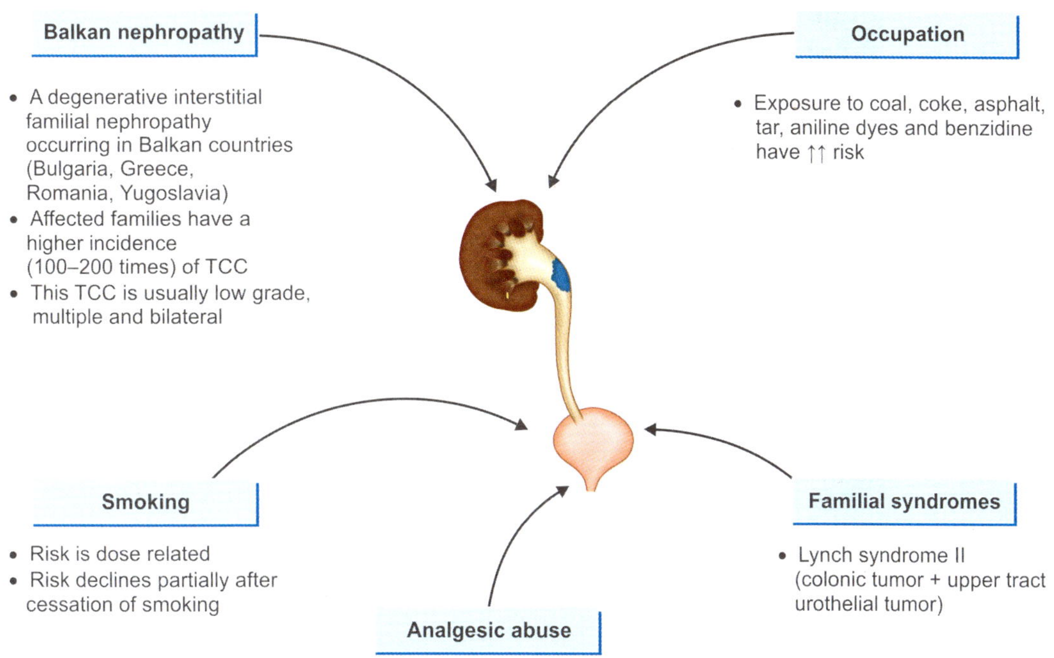

Clinical Presentation

- Hematuria (gross or microscopic) is the most common symptom. Flank pain may be present in 20–40% of patients.
- Abdominal mass, weight loss, anorexia, fatique, bone pain are usually associated with advanced disease.

Diagnosis

CT urography is the most accurate imaging modality for upper tract urothelial cancers.
MR urography is indicated only when CT urography is contraindicated.
Urinary cytology should be done as a diagnostic work-up.
Cystoscopy is mandatory in all patients of upper tract tumors to rule out coexisting bladder tumor.
Flexible ureteroscopy is particularly indicated if diagnosis is uncertain after imaging, kidney-sparing treatment is considered or in patients with a solitary kidney.

Treatment

Treatment options are: (i) Endoscopic treatment; (ii) Segmental ureterectomy; and (iii) Radical nephroureterectomy.
Endoscopic treatment is indicated in patient with solitary kidney, bilateral upper tract tumor or patient with contralateral nonfunctioning kidney. This approach is also indicated in low-stage, low-grade lesions.
Segmental ureterectomy is indicated for low-grade tumors.
Radical nephroureterectomy is the standard surgical approach for high-risk upper tract urothelial carcinoma, regardless of tumor location.

Endoscopic Management

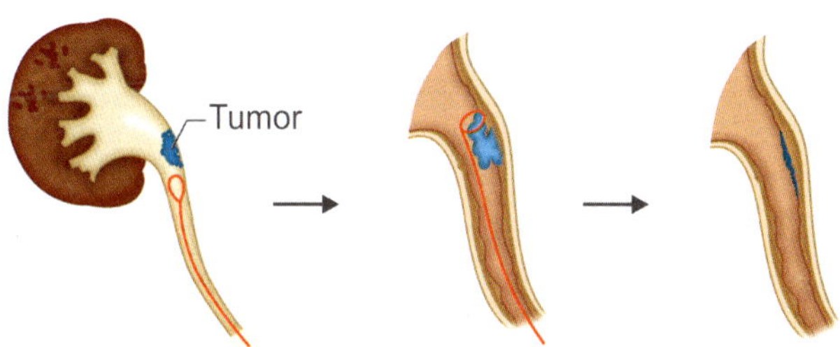

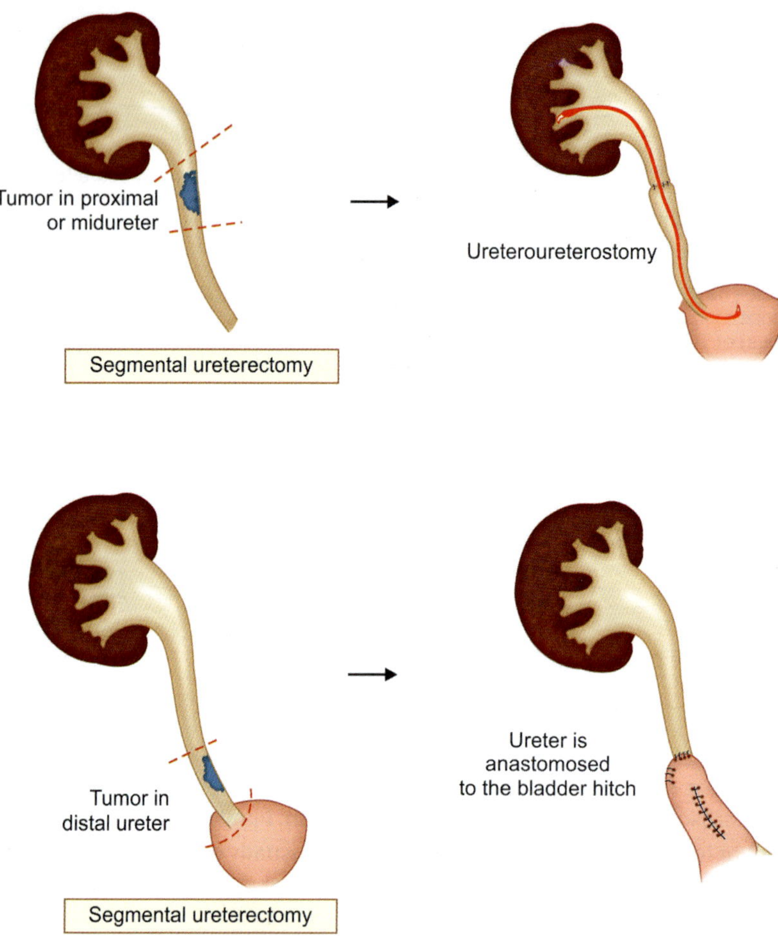

Radical Nephroureterectomy

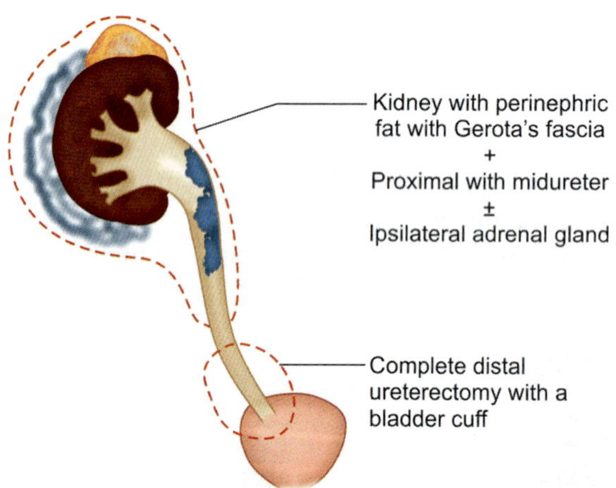

Patent Urachus

- Patent urachus develops due to failure of urachal canal to obliterate.
- **Clinically presents as** continuous or intermittent discharging umbilicus. This pathology may present as edematous umbilicus with delayed healing of cord stump.
- **Diagnosis** is done by retrograde fistulogram or voiding cystourethrogram.
- **Treatment** is complete excision of patent urachus including a bladder cuff.

Ectopia Vesicae (Exstrophy of the Bladder)

Exstrophy of the bladder is one of the components of exstrophy–epispadias complex of genitourinary malformations. In classic bladder exstrophy, the defects are in the bladder, abdominal wall, pelvic skeletal structure, pelvic floor, anorectum and genitourinary tract.

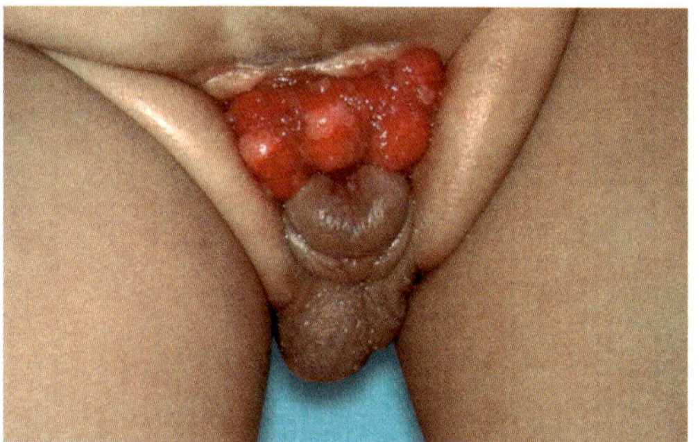

Ectopia vesicae.

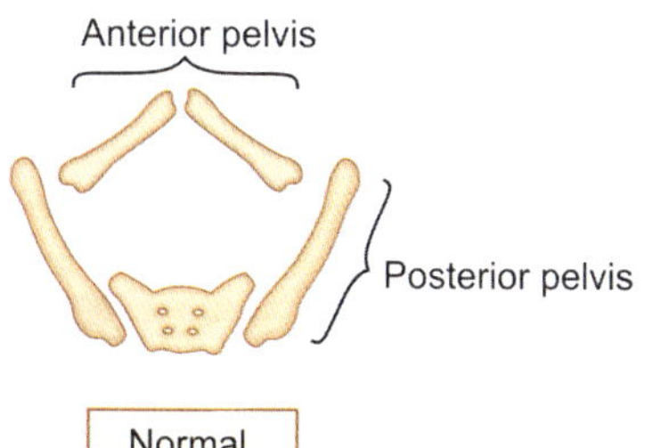

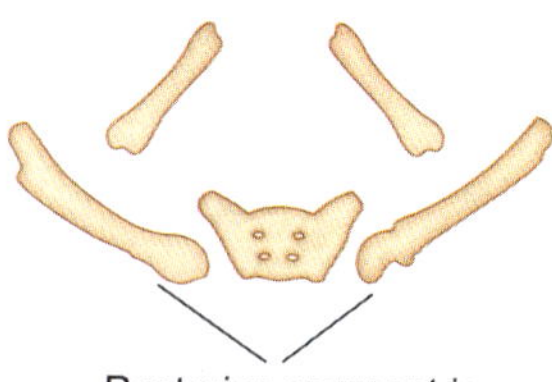

Skeletal Defects

- Anterior segment of the pelvis is externally rotated and shortened
- Posterior segment is externally rotated
- No change in length.

Pelvic Floor Defects

- Levator ani group is more posteriorly placed
- Puborectal sling becomes flattened than its normal conical shape.

Anorectal Defects

- Perineum is short and broad
- Anus is present directly behind the urogenital diaphragm.

Genital Defects

In male: Epispadias, prominent dorsal chordee, wide separation of crural attachments, deficiency of anterior corporal tissue, shorter penis.

In female: Bifid clitoris, shorter vagina, stenotic and anteriorly placed vaginal orifice.

Abdominal Wall Defects

- Triangular defect in the abdominal wall occupied by exstrophy bladder and posterior urethra.
- At the upper end of the fascial defect, umbilicus is present.
- Umbilical hernia is usually present.
- Indirect inguinal hernia (unilateral/bilateral) is usually associated.

Urinary Defects

- Horseshoe kidney, hypoplastic kidney or pelvic kidney may present
- Ureters are abnormally terminated resulting in VUR in all patients.

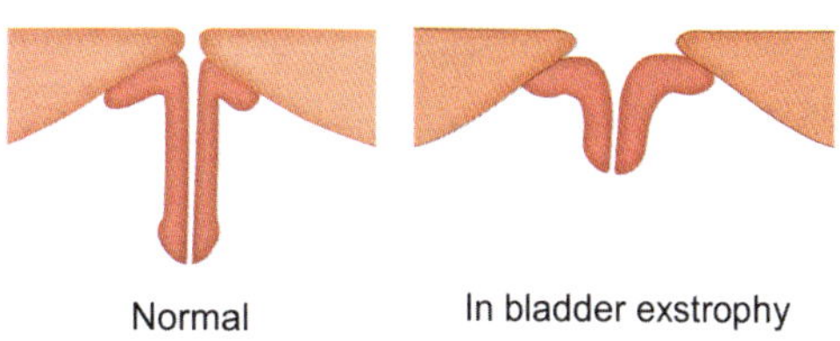

Diagnosis

- In conventional USG imaging, prenatal diagnosis is difficult
- 3D USG and fetal MRI is helpful in prenatal diagnosis.

Treatment

- Management is based on **staged surgical approach**.
- **In the newborn period**, surgical procedures include bladder closure, abdominal wall closure, urethral closure on to the penis, bilateral innominate and vertical iliac osteotomy.
- **On 6 months to 1 year of age**, epispadias repair is planned followed by bladder neck reconstruction **at the age of 4–5 years**.

Bladder Calculi

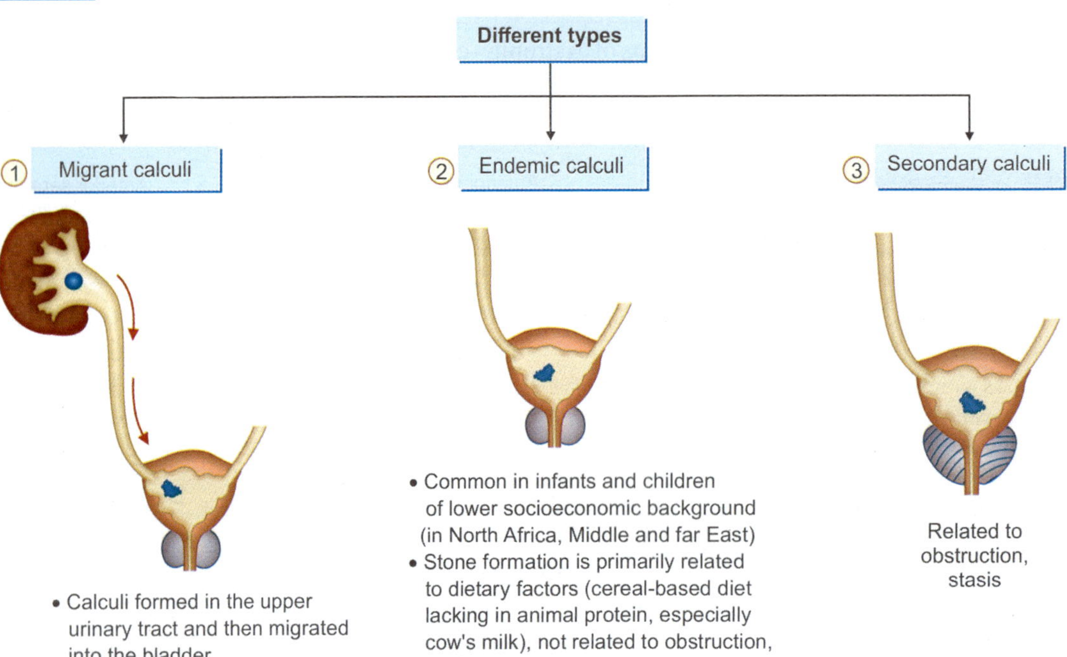

Secondary Calculi

Related to bladder outlet obstruction:

- Main cause of bladder calculi
- Mostly related to BHP
- Stones are composed of uric acid, calcium oxalate or triple phosphate.

Related to infection:

- Urease producing bacteria's are responsible
- Usually triple phosphate and carbonate apatite calculi are found.

Related to catheterization:

- Patients with urethra or suprapubic catheter have increased (9-fold) risk of stone formation.

Calculi related to foreign body:

- Calculi may develop following self-induced (e.g., hairpin, pen) foreign body or iatrogenic FB (e.g., balloon catheter, ureteral stent).

Calculi related to bladder augmentation and urinary diversion.

- Incidence is **higher in males**
- The age distribution is **bimodal** (peak at 3 years in childhood and 60 years in adulthood)
- **Bladder outlet obstruction is the most common predisposing factor in adults.**

Clinical Features

Most of the bladder calculi are asymptomatic.

Symptomatic presentation:

Pain: Usually located in the suprapubic region, exacerbated after exercise and sudden movement, usually felt at the end of micturition. Detrusor overactivity is seen in most of the patients and particularly common in patients with larger stones (>4 cm). Pain may be referred to the tip of penis, scrotum, labia majora or perineum.

Frequency: More common during daytime.

Hematuria: Terminal hematuria is due to abrasion of bladder trigone by the stone.

Interruption of urinary stream

Symptoms of UTI.

In pediatric patients, clinical presentations include pulling of the penis, difficulty in micturition, urinary retention, enuresis, rectal prolapse.

Diagnosis

X-ray of KUB: Most of the bladder calculi are radiopaque.

USG: US of the bladder has low sensitivity but high specificity for detecting bladder stones

CT: A useful imaging modality for detecting bladder stones

Cystoscopy: Most accurate method of detecting bladder calculi.

X-ray KUB showing bladder calculi.

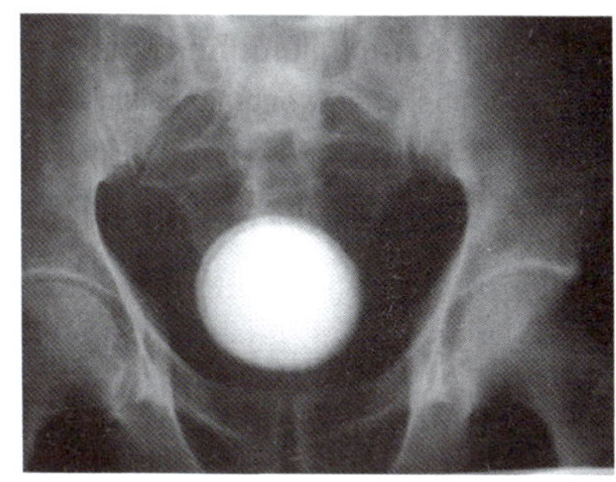

Management

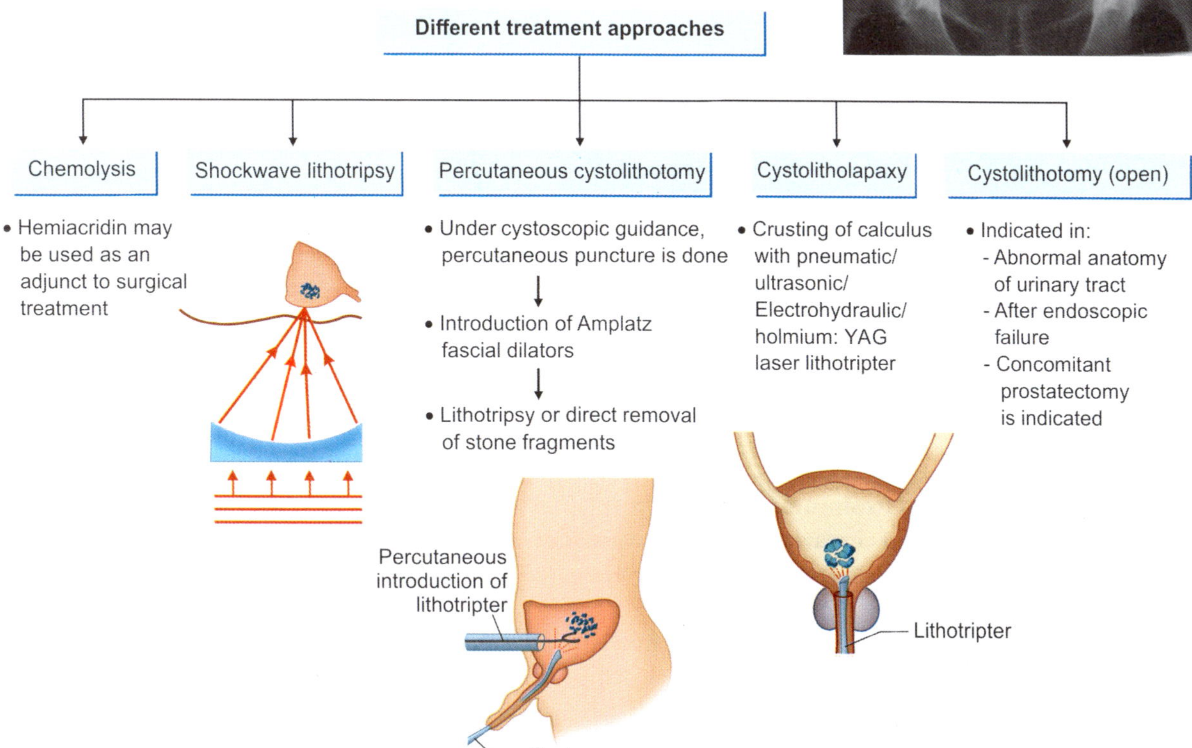

- In both adult and pediatric patients, **transurethral cystolithotripsy** is the preferred treatment option.
- **Percutaneous cystolithotripsy** is another option if transurethral approach is not feasible or risk of urethral stricture is high.
- **In adult patients with BOO and bladder stone**, both pathologies can be treated simultaneously without any significant risk of increased morbidity.

Schistosomiasis of the Urinary Bladder

- Schistosomiasis is a disease caused by Schistosomes, a digenetic trematode.
- *S. haematobium* pairs (adult male and female) reside in the prevesical venous plexus—**Urinary schistosomiasis**.
- *S. mansoni* and *S. japonicum* reside in the mesenteric veins—**GI and hepatic schistosomiasis**.
- Urinary schistosomiasis is endemic in parts of Africa and Middle East.

Mode of Infestation

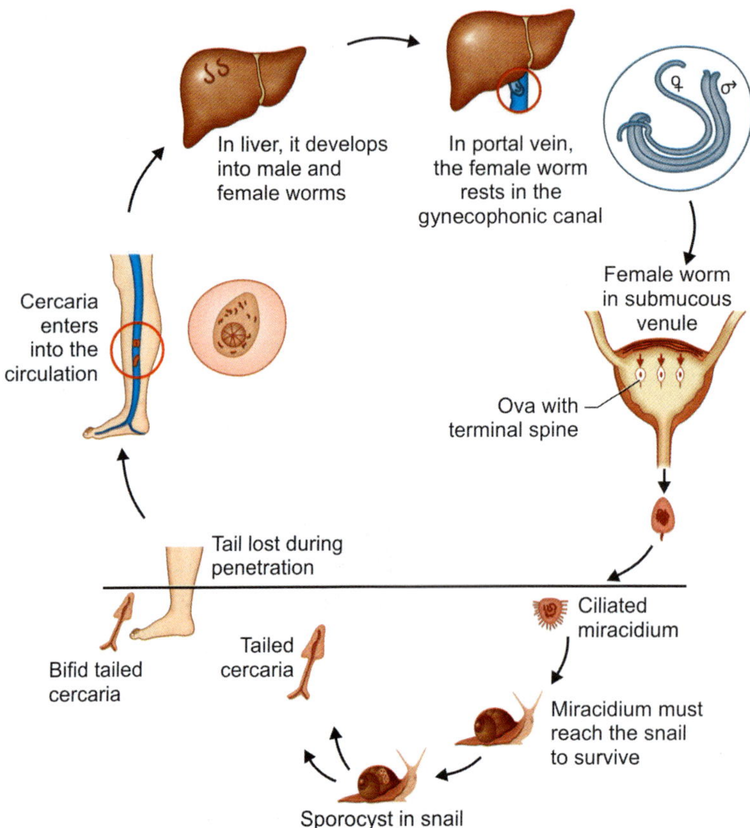

Man is the definitive host and freshwater snail (Bulinus truncatus) is the intermediate host.

Free-swimming bifid-tailed cercaria is the **infective stage**. Cercaria penetrate the unbroken skin while bathing in infected water. It lost its tail during penetration. Cercaria enters into the circulation and reaches to the liver where it develops into male and female worms.

In liver, it attains sexual maturity and leaves the liver and enters the portal vein. **In portal vein**, the male worm bends to take the shape of a gutter (the gynecophonic canal), into which the female worm rests, and then the pair proceed to the inferior mesenteric vein. **Through the portosystemic anastomotic channel**, the pair ultimately reaches the vesical **venous plexus**. After reaching the vesical venous plexus, the female worm moves forward and enters into the submucous venule and then lay ovas in a chain (each ovum has a terminal spine). This ova penetrate the wall of venules and reaches the **urinary bladder**.

An infected person excretes hundreds of ova through urine. If the ova reaches fresh water, the envelope bursts and **ciliated miracidium** emerges. To survive, the miracidium must reach the intermediate host (snails of Bulinus species), where they develop into sporocyst, daughter sporocysts and then cercariae. These cercariae emerge into the water from snail's surface. The cercariae, if fail to penetrate human skin within a few hours, they die.

Clinical Features

- Men are commonly affected.
- Urticaria may develop at the site of penetration by cercaria **(Swimmer's itch)**
- Classic presentation is painless recurrent hematuria with terminal dysuria.
- Polypoidal lesion in bladder may develop. Bladder ulcer usually develops in the posterior bladder wall (**"sandy batches"** is dried up bladder mucosa with patches of granular floor) and clinically presents as dysuria, intense pelvic and suprapubic pain. Most of these patients present with gross hematuria and pyuria. **'Schistosomal contracted bladder'** syndrome presents as chronic suprapubic and pelvic pain, frequency, urgency and incontinence.

Diagnosis

Microscopic examination of urine:

Terminally spined eggs in urinary sediment is the gold standard diagnostic tool for active *S. haematobium* infection (egg excretion peaks between 9 AM–3 PM). The egg usually appears between 8 and 12 weeks after initial infection (when oviposition begins).

Serological tests:

- FAST-ELISA followed by Western blot analysis- highly sensitive and specific but cannot distinguish between active and chronic infection.
- PCR- highly sensitive and specific for diagnosis of urogenital schistosomiasis from vaginal lavage sample or urine sample.
- Detection of CAA and CCA (circulating anodic antigen and circulating cathodic antigen) by ELISA- specific for active infection, also useful for determining infection severity.

Biopsy: Rectal snip biopsy and bladder biopsy may be considered for detection of eggs if eggs are not found in urine or stool, but clinical features and serological tests are suggestive of schistosomiasis infection.

Imaging:

- **Plain X-ray:** A calcified bladder which looks like a fetal head in pelvis is diagnostic of chronic urinary schistosomiasis.
- USG may reveal focal thickening of urinary bladder, polypoidal lesion, as well as hydroureter or hydronephrosis.
- IVU may reveal striations in the ureter and renal pelvis (earliest change in IVU), hydroureter, hydronephrosis, bladder or ureteral filling defects.
- CT can detect calcified lesions in the urinary tract and changes due to obstructive uropathy.

Treatment

Medical:

- Praziquantel is the drug of choice (active in all stages of diseases)
- 2 oral dose—each dose 20 mg/kg 6–8 hours apart for 1 day.

Surgical:

Indications: (i) Intractable bladder hemorrhage; (ii) 'Contracted bladder'; (iii) Bladder cancer secondary to schistosomiasis; and (iv) Residual ureteral stenosis after chemotherapy.

Katayama Fever

- Acute schistosomiasis is also known as Katayama fever. It occurs most commonly with ***S. japonicum*** infections and less commonly with *S. mansoni* and *S. haematobium* infections.
- Patients present with fever, dry cough, fatigue, headache, urticaria, eosinophilia.

Schistosoma-associated Bladder Cancer

- ***Schistosoma haematobium*** infection is associated with development of bladder cancer. The histological type of bladder cancer associated with schistosomiasis is **squamous cell carcinoma.**
- This cancer tends to develop at **younger age** with **more advanced local stage** but **lower incidence of nodal and metastatic disease.**

Bladder Tumor

Types of Bladder Tumor

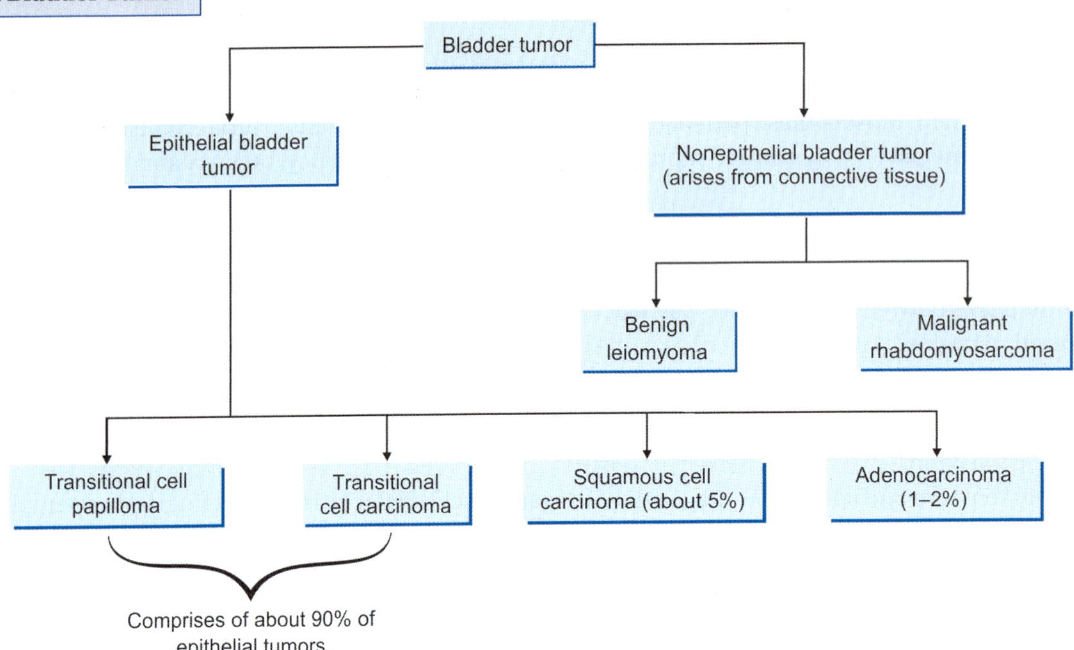

Transitional Cell Papilloma

- Rare bladder tumor.
- Usually solitary, small (0.2–1 cm), frond like structure having a delicate fibrovascular core covered by multi-layered (≤7), well-differentiated transitional epithelium.
- Looks like a red sea-anemone.
- Noninvasive
- Almost never recurs after endoscopic resection.

Bladder Cancer

- Bladder cancer is the fourth most prevalent cancer in both sexes worldwide. It is the most common cancer of the lower urinary tract.
- More common in men (3 times). Incidence increases with age [Younger patients have more favorable prognosis as they present with well-differentiated tumors]

Risk Factors

Genetic factors:

- RAS (oncogene) mutation
- Absence or abnormal expression of tumor suppressor genes (*TP53*, and retinoblastoma gene)
- Overexpression of ERBB1 and ERBB2 oncogenes.

Occupational factors:

- Workers with exposure to β-naphthylamine, aniline dyes, dyes used in rubber, textile industries.
- Cigarette smoking.
- Higher incidence (4-fold) of bladder carcinoma.
- Risk related with number of cigarets smoked, duration of smoking, degree of inhalation of smoke.

Other bladder lesions:

- Chronic cystitis in presence of catheter or calculi is associated with increased risk of SCC of urinary bladder.
- Cystitis caused by *S. haematobium* is associated with increased risk of SCC.
- Ectopia vesicae, diverticulum, urinary diversion in defunctionalized bladder are associated with increased risk.

Cyclophosphamide—9-fold increased risk of bladder carcinoma.

Pelvic irradiation—Radiation for carcinoma cervix or ovary is associated with increased risk.

Arsenic—Ingestion of high arsenic contaminated water is associated with increased risk.

Analgesic abuse—Large amount of phenacetin containing analgesic use is associated with TCC of bladder.

Renal transplant recipients.

Pathology

Urothelial (Transitional cell) carcinoma is the most common histologic type. The histologic variants of urothelial carcinoma are- (i) Micropapillary variant; (ii) Sarcomatoid variant; (iii) Plasmacytoid variant; and (iv) Nested variant. Micropapillary and nested variant carry a poor prognosis. Other histologic types are squamous cell carcinoma, adenocarcinoma, small cell carcinoma.

Squamous cell carcinomas (SCCs) are usually sessile and associated with muscle invasion. **Nonbilharzial SCCs** are caused by urinary calculi, indwelling catheter, chronic UTI and bladder diverticula. **Bilharzial SCCs** are usually exophytic, fungating lesions (caused by *S. haematobium*) and present early (10–20 years earlier than TCC). Prognosis not good.

Adenocarcinomas arise in exstrophic bladder, urachal remnants and in intestinal urinary conduits and augmentations.

Small cell carcinoma is a poorly differentiated neuroendocrine neoplasm, primarily occur in lung but may develop in prostate and urinary bladder.

Secondary metastasis in bladder: Primary sites are rectum, stomach, breast and prostate.

Different Patterns of Tumor Growth

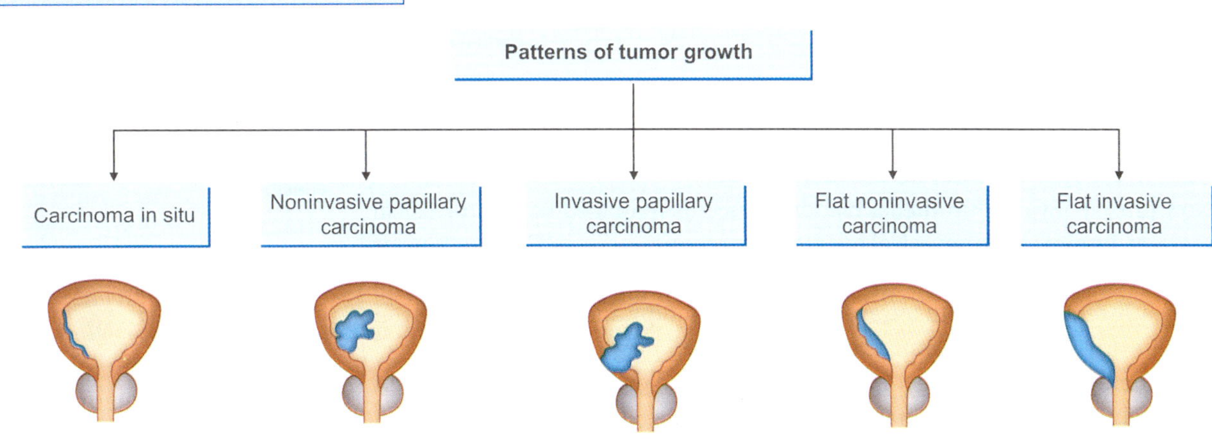

Clinical Presentation

Most common presentation is **painless gross hematuria**. Hematuria is typically intermittent. Symptom complex of frequency, urgency and dysuria are present, particularly in patients with carcinoma in situ (CIS). Flank pain due to obstructive uropathy, lower extremity edema and pelvic mass may be present in advanced disease.

[An elderly patient with painless gross hematuria—bladder carcinoma should be suspected unless proved otherwise.]

Diagnosis

- **Cystoscopy:** The gold-standard test for diagnosis of bladder cancer is cystoscopy and biopsy. **White light cystoscopy (WLC)** is the current standard in the evaluation and staging of bladder cancer. WLC has high sensitivity for papillary lesions, but low sensitivity for non-papillary and flat lesions, small or multifocal lesions. **Blue light cystoscopy (BLC) or narrow band imaging in conjunction with WLC**, increases the sensitivity for detecting different types (papillary, non-papillary, flat, multifocal, etc.). Location, number and nature of tumor can be assessed by cystoscopy. Local invasion such as involvement of ureteral orifices or prostatic urethra also can be assessed.
- **Conventional microscopic cytology of urinary sediment or bladder washings:** This test is more sensitive for high-grade tumors or CIS. The chance of false-positivity and false-negativity is high. Flow cytometry is not much valuable.

Staging

- Treatment decision is based on whether tumor is muscle invasive or not.
- Primary TUR of the tumor (TURBT) is done to assess the depth of tumor invasion and also to remove all visible tumors. After TURBT, persistence of a palpable mass suggests locally advanced disease.
- Then, assessment of local extension and distant metastasis is done by—

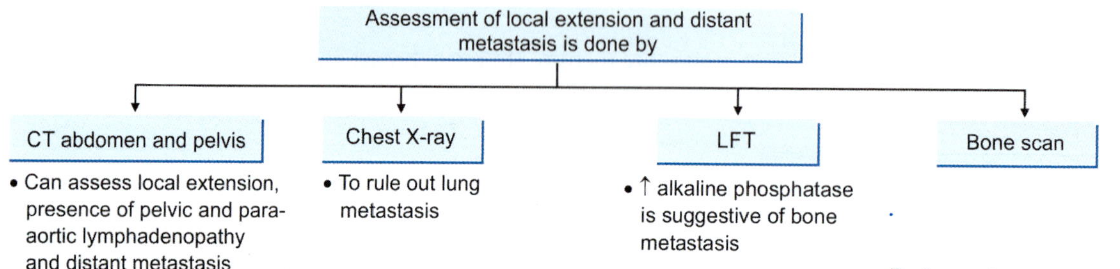

Treatment

Non-muscle invasive urothelial bladder cancer:

- Non-muscle invasive urothelial bladder cancer is managed with intravesical therapy. Immediate intravesical instillation of chemotherapy (Gemcitabine or Mitomycin C) within 6 hours of TURBT, can prevent tumor cell implantation and early recurrence. Both intravesical chemotherapy and BCG may be given as adjuvant therapy in nonmuscle invasive cancer.
- BCG therapy is given once a week for 6 weeks, followed by a rest period of 4–6 weeks, with a full re-evaluation at 3 months. Side effects of BCG instillation are flu like symptoms, dysuria.

Muscle-invasive urothelial blader cancer:

The gold standard treatment is radical cystectomy with neoadjuvant cisplatin-based chemotherapy.

Endoscopic management

TURBT under regional or general anesthesia

↓

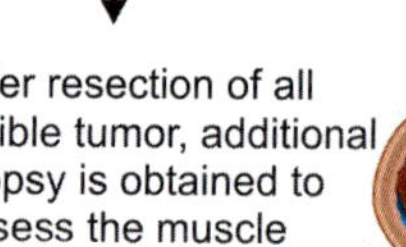

↓

Mitomycin C (single dose) is administered intravesically through the 3-way catheter within 6 hours of TURBT

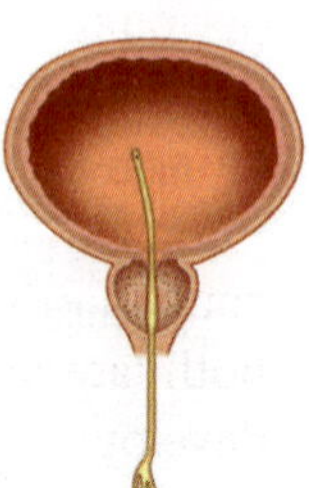

Radical cystectomy is the primary treatment for both **squamous cell carcinoma and adenocarcinoma**. No definite supportive evidence regarding the advantage of chemotherapy in neoadjuvant or adjuvant settings.
Platinum-based chemotherapy is the primary treatment for **small cell carcinoma** of urinary bladder.

Benign Prostatic Hyperplasia

Characterized by **both glandular and stromal hyperplasia** resulting in enlargement of the gland.

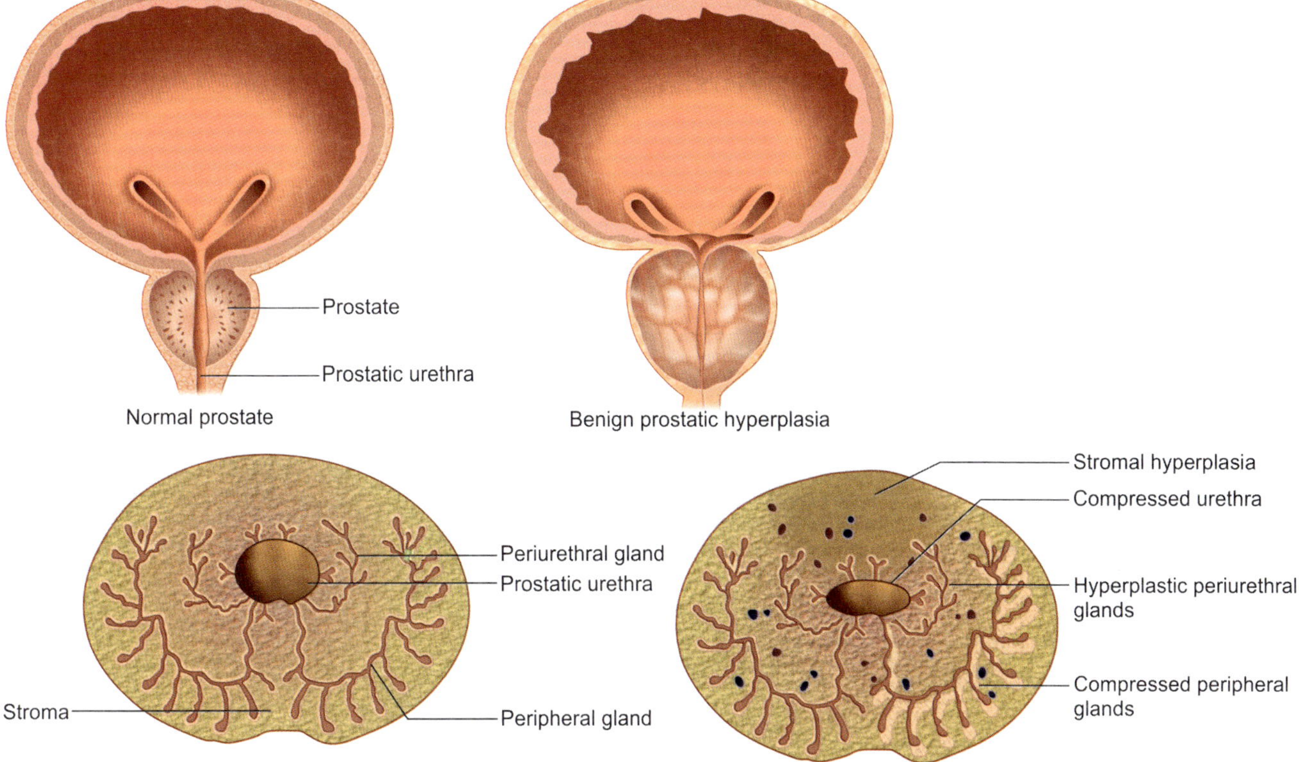

Prostate is divided into several biologically distinct regions:
Peripheral, central, transitional and periurethral zone.
Hyperplasia initially develops in the **periurethral transition zone** of the prostate, resulting in nodular enlargement.
Glandular and stromal component of peripheral zone are compressed and take the appearance of typical **'lateral lobe' enlargement.**
If hyperplasia primarily affects the central zone, **'middle lobe' develops.** Sometimes both lateral and middle lobe enlargement develops.

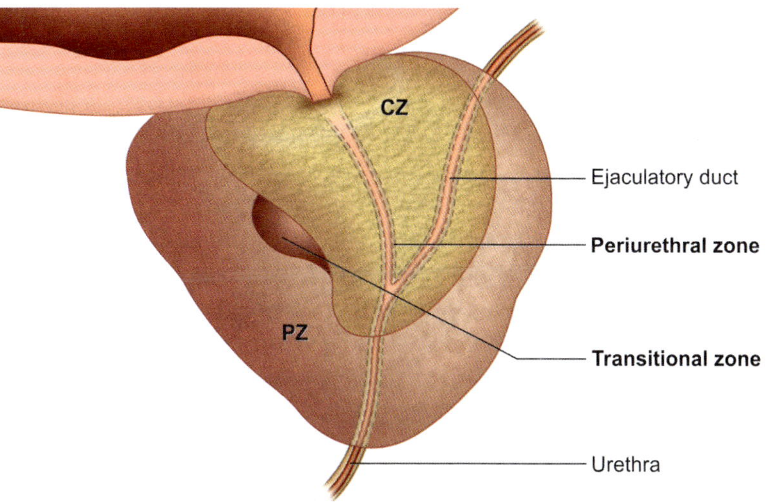

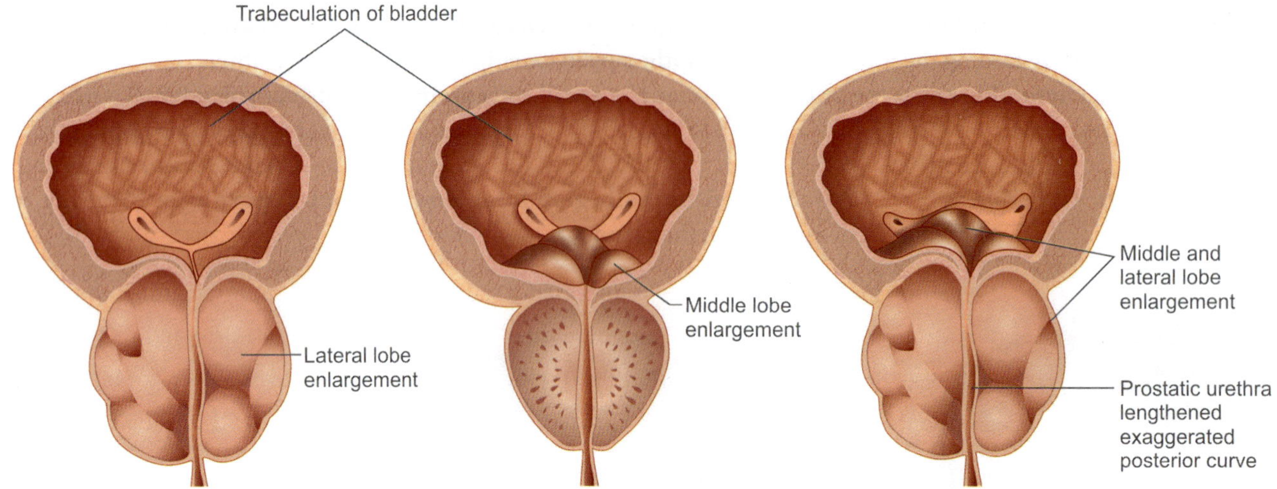

Pathophysiology

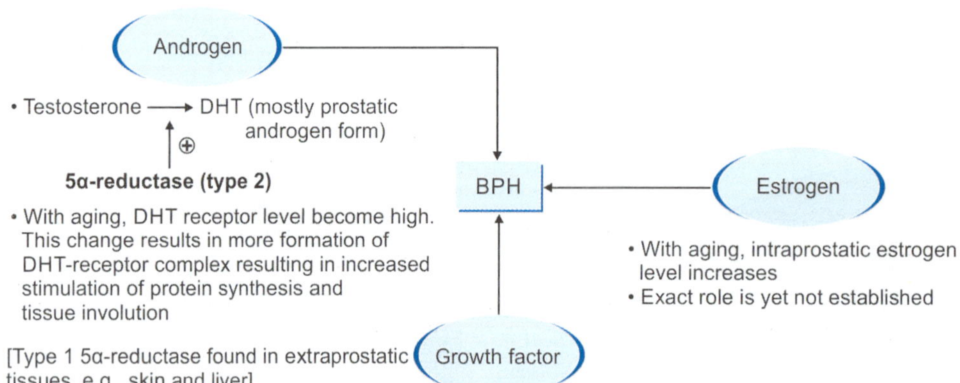

Clinical Presentation

- Lower urinary tract symptoms (LUTS)
- Recurrent urinary tract infection
- Hematuria
- Acute retention of urine

Causes of LUTS in Male

- Benign prostatic hyperplasia
- Detrusor underactivity and overactivity
- Neurogenic bladder dysfunction
- Bladder tumor
- Urinary tract infection
- Urethral stricture
- Distal ureteric stone
- Foreign body

Lower Urinary Tract Symptoms (LUTS)

Obstructive symptoms:

- Sensation of incomplete emptying
- Intermittency
- Urinary straining
- Weak urinary stream

Irritative symptoms:

- Frequency
- Urgency
- Dysuria

Initial Evaluation

History:

- History of hematuria, UTI, retention of urine
- History of lower urinary tract surgery (to exclude the possibility of urethral stricture or bladder neck contracture)
- History of medical illness (e.g., diabetes, Parkinson's disease and CVA)
- History of medication (e.g., anticholinergics, α-adrenergics).

Clinical Examination:

Examination of nervous system—To exclude tabes dorsalis, Parkinson's disease, cervical spondylosis (these diseases may present as prostatic obstruction). Elicitation of perianal sensation and anal tone is helpful to detect Cauda equina lesion.

Examination of lower abdomen and external genitalia—

- To detect palpable bladder
- To exclude meatal stenosis, palpable urethral mass.

Digital rectal examination (DRE)—

- To assess the size, consistency and nodularity of prostate. **In BPH, the posterior surface of prostate is convex, smooth. Rectal mucosa can be moved over the prostate**.

Symptom Assessment:

Symptom severity is assessed by **IPSS (International Prostate Symptom Score)** or **AUA symptom index (AUA-SI)**. According to scoring, symptoms are classified as **mild (0–7), moderate (8–19)** and **severe (20–35)**. IPSS is used to grade symptom severity, to choose the optimal treatment, assess the response to therapy and assess disease progression in the follow-up period.

Urinalysis: To exclude UTI and microscopic hematuria.

Urine cytology should be done in patients with severe irritable symptoms and dysuria.

Prostate-specific Antigen (PSA):

- Prostate carcinoma may coexist with BPH. So measurement of PSA in patients with greater life expectancy should be done to detect early prostate carcinoma.
- PSA velocity, free versus complexed PSA ratio, PSA density are more specific than serum PSA.

Additional Evaluation

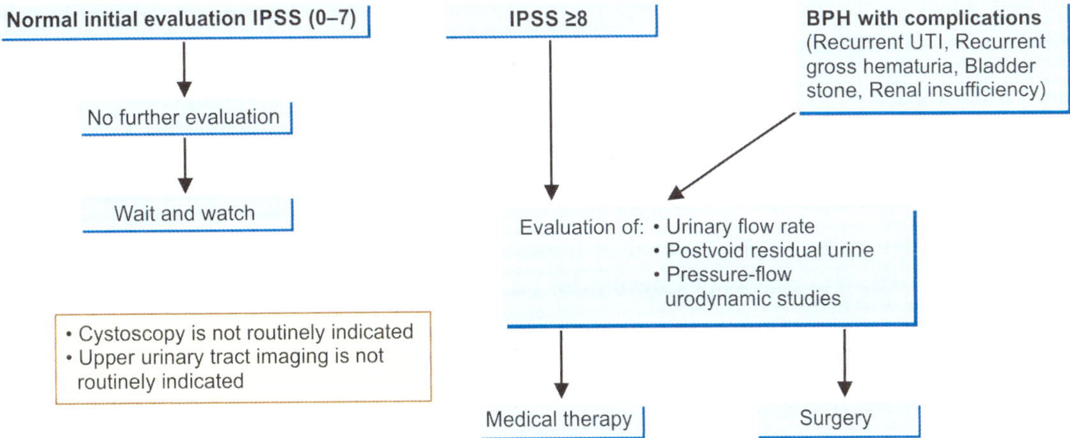

- **The IPSS is an 8-item questionnaire**, consisting of seven symptom questions and one QOL question.
- **AUA-SI is a seven-question questionnaire** with a response scheme from 0 to 5 for each question for a total score ranging from 0 to 35.

- **Uroflowmetry:** A noninvasive urodynamic test to record the urinary flow rate throughout the act of micturition.
- **Postvoid residual urine (PVR):** Urine remains in the bladder immediately after completion of micturition. PVR measurement is done by noninvasive method (ultrasound) or invasive method (catheterization).
- **Pressure-flow urodynamic studies:** If an invasive treatment is planned and flow rate and PVR are not suggestive of BOO.

Management

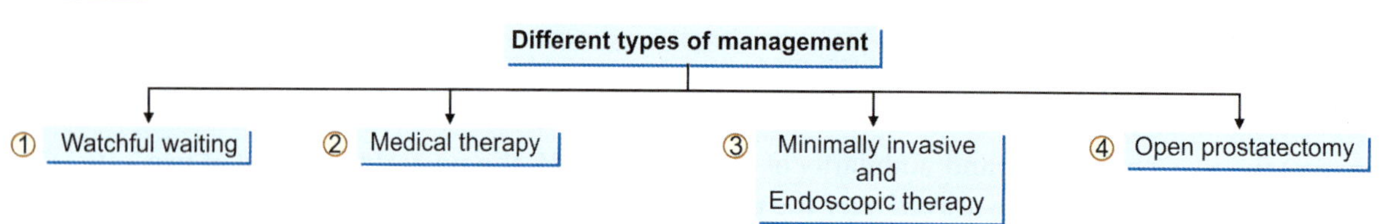

Watchful Waiting

Watchful waiting is the preferred management option in patients with mild symptoms of LUTS secondary to BPH (AUA-SI score <8) and with moderate-to-severe symptoms (AUA-SI score ≥8) without complications of LUTS and bladder outlet obstruction (e.g., renal insufficiency, recurrent UTI, refractory urinary retention). Carcinoma of the prostate must be excluded before adopting this treatment policy.

Symptoms can be managed by: (i) Decreasing total fluid intake before bedtime; (ii) Avoid over intake of alcohol and caffeine; and (iii) Maintenance of time-voiding schedule.

Medical Therapy

Medical therapy is the treatment of choice except absolute indications for surgery. Medical therapies are: (i) **Alpha-blockers** (alfuzosin, doxazosin, terazosin, tamsulosin, silodosin); (ii) **5α –reductase inhibitors** (finasteride, dutasteride); (iii) **Anticholinergic agents**; and (iv) **Combination therapy** (alpha-blocker and 5-alpha reductase inhibitor, alpha-blocker and anticholinergics).

Alpha-adrenergic blockers are effective for bothersome, moderate-to-severe LUTS secondary to BPH (AUA-SI score ≥8) without complications of LUTS and BOO.

Tamsulosin is a third-generation alpha-blocker with greater specificity for α-1A adrenoreceptor compared to α-1B adrenoreceptor. The dose is 0.4 mg daily. Adverse effects are: (i) dizziness; (ii) headache; (iii) decreased libido; and (iv) erectile dysfunction. Alpha-blockers, particularly tamsulosin, should be avoided if patient is waiting for cataract surgery. Intraoperative floppy iris syndrome may develop, resulting in posterior capsule rupture with vitreous loss.

Finasteride is less effective than alpha-blocker in improving LUTS and not appropriate for LUTS not due to prostatic enlargement. Adverse effects of finasteride- (i) decreased libido; (ii) ejaculatory dysfunction; and (iii) erectile dysfunction.

TURP (Transurethral Resection of Prostate)

- Gold standard surgical management of BHP
- Indicated in moderate to severe symptom severity and that interfere with quality of life.

Absolute indications: (i) Acute retention; (ii) Recurrent UTI; (iii) Recurrent hematuria; and (iv) Renal insufficiency.

[Not indicated if associated bladder diverticula or large bladder stone is present.]

- **Commonly used irrigation fluid** is 1.5% glycine (nonhemolytic, hypotonic)

Standard technique is described by Nesbit (1943)—Nesbit technique is divided into 3 stages.

- Resection starts at the bladder neck at 12'o clock position.
- Verumontanum is the distal-most point of resection.
- Strips of prostatic tissue are resected from the bladder neck to verumontanum using diathermy.
- Irrigation with glycine is applied whenever necessary.
- At the end of the resection, 3-way self-retaining catheter is introduced into the bladder. After completion of TURP procedure, the color of irrigation fluid should be light pink.

Complications: (i) TUR syndrome; (ii) Hemorrhage; and (iii) Bladder neck contracture.

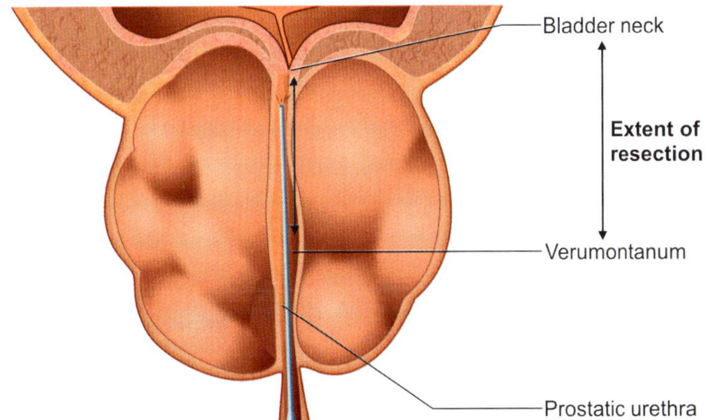

TUR Syndrome

- An immediate postoperative complication due to excess systemic absorption of glycine leads to dilutional hyponatremia.
- Risk is increased if gland >45 gm, resection time >90 minutes, Irrigant fluid >70 cmH_2O.
- Syndrome is manifested as mental confusion nausea, vomiting, hypertension, bradycardia and visual disturbance.
- Treatment includes—Diuretic (furosemide)

+Decreasing the fluid overload

In severe cases, 200 mL of 3% saline (very slow infusion).

Bipolar resectoscope uses 0.9% NaCl solution as irrigant fluid, so risk of TUR syndrome is nil.

Hemorrhage

- Arterial bleeding must be controlled with electrocoagulation.
- Venous bleeding can be controlled by placing the catheter on traction for few minutes and over inflating the balloon of the catheter.

Transurethral Radiofrequency Needle Ablation (TUNA)

The lumen of the prostatic urethra is visualized with an endoscope and two radiofrequency needles are inserted into the adenoma under guidance of endoscopic viewing. Each needle simultaneously delivers radiofrequency energy, resulting in necrosis of adenomatous tissues.

Advantages: (i) Low perioperative complications including bleeding; (ii) Minimal incidence of sexual dysfunction; and (iii) Significant improvement of urinary flow rate.

Disadvantages: High retreatment rate.

Transurethral microwave thermotherapy:
Delivery of the microwave energy by a microwave antennae mounted on a urethral catheter resulting in formation of heat energy, lead to delayed coagulation necrosis, apoptosis and denervation of alpha-receptors.
Advantages: (i) Can be performed as an OPD procedure and (ii) No sexual dysfunction.

Transurethral Holmium Laser Ablation of the Prostate (HoLAP):
The holmium: YAG laser is used transurethrally using a 550 micron side-firing laser fiber in a noncontact mode, delivering laser energy at a wavelength of 2120 nm.

Transurethral Holmium Laser Enucleation of the Prostate (HoLEP):
This technique enucleates the adenoma from the surgical capsule, from apex to base.

Holmium Laser Resection of the Prostate (HoLRP):
The adenoma is resected using a holmium laser fiber and specially adapted resectoscope.

Photoselective vaporization of the prostate:
This technique uses laser energy of 532 nm wave length (green visible spectrum) using a 600 micron side-firing fiber in a noncontact mode.

Transurethral incision of the prostate (TUIP):
This procedure is effective in smaller prostate size (<30 mL).
Advantages: (i) Symptomatic improvement similar to TURP and (ii) Minimal risk of ejaculatory dysfunction.

Open Prostatectomy

Indications of Open Prostatetectomy

- Prostate volume more than 80–100 mL
- Associated bladder diverticula
- Associated large bladder stone

Risk of hemorrhage, transfusion requirement and hospital stay are more in comparison to TURP.

Approaches for Open Prostatectomy

- Retropubic prostatectomy (Millin)
- Transvesical prostatectomy (Frayer's)

Complications

- Hemorrhage
- Perforation of bladder or prostatic capsule
- Incontinence
- Urethral stricture
- Bladder neck stricture
- Retrograde ejaculation

Retropubic Prostatectomy

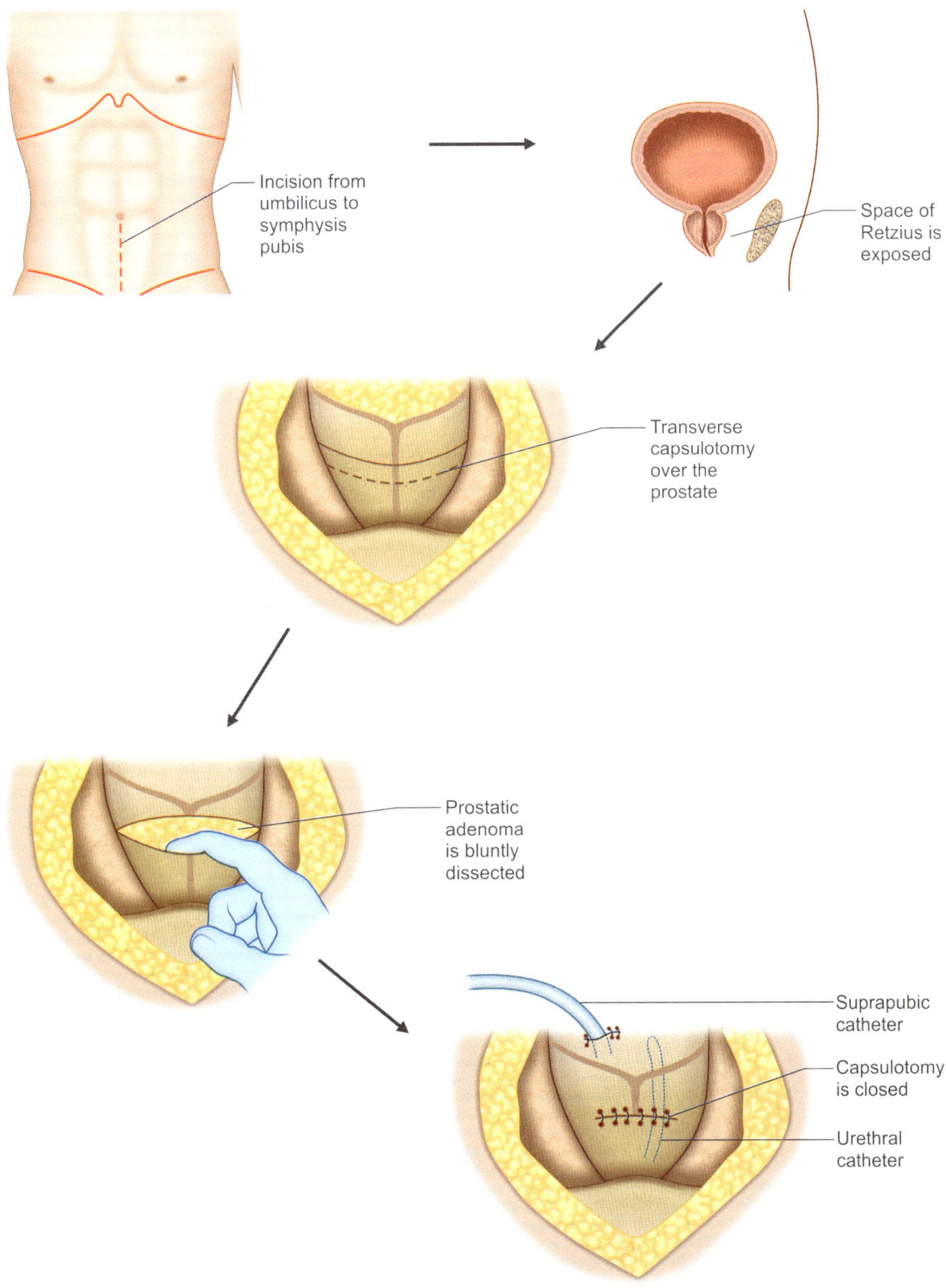

Transvesical Prostatectomy

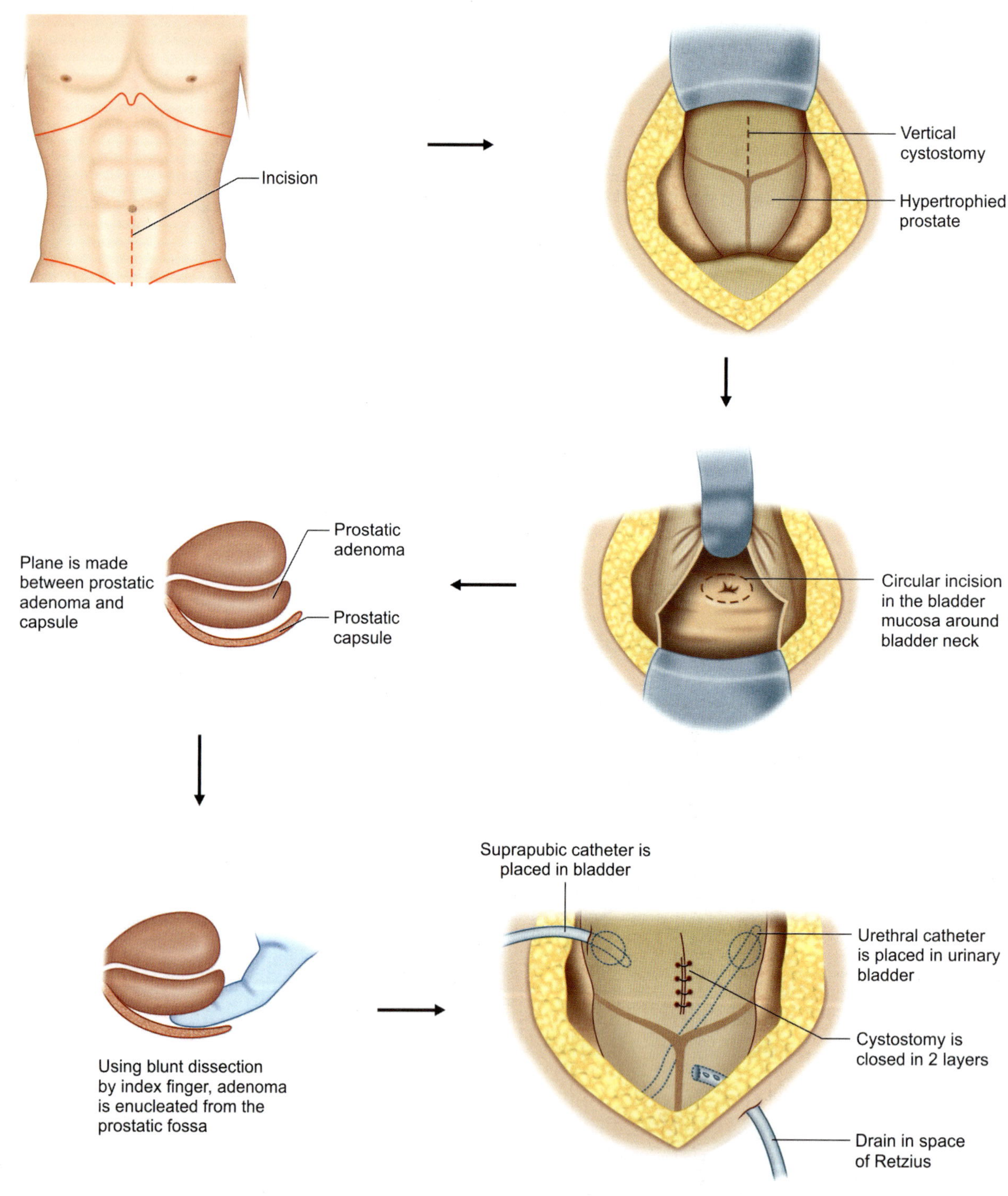

Prostatitis

Types of Prostatitis

Traditional Classification

- Acute bacterial prostatitis
- Chronic bacterial prostatitis
- Nonbacterial prostatitis
- Prostatodynia

NIH Classification

Category I
Category II
Category III A (inflammatory CPPS)
Category III B (noninflammatory CPPS)
Category IV (asymptomatic inflammatory prostatitis)

CPPS (Chronic pelvic pain syndrome)

Clinical Presentation

Category I: Acute onset of perineal or suprapubic pain associated with irritative and obstructive urinary symptoms along with systemic symptoms (e.g., fever, malaise, nausea, vomiting).

Category II: History of recurrent UTI

Category III A and B: Pain in the perineum, suprapubic area and penis, pain during or after ejaculation.

Category IV:

- Asymptomatic
- Evidence of prostatitis detected during workup for other prostatic pathologies.

Assessment of Symptoms

Objective assessment of symptoms:

By NIH—CPSI (The National Institutes of Health-Chronic Prostatitis Symptom Index)

This symptom index covers 3 domains:

1. Pain (location, frequency, severity)
2. Urinary symptoms (irritative and obstructive symptoms)
3. Quality of impact

Diagnosis

- In acute prostatitis, on DRE, prostate gland presents as a hot, boggy and exquisitely tender swelling. (DRE is better avoided due to sphincter spasm)
- **4-glass test (Meares Stamey test)**—A four-glass collection technique to differentiate between urethral, bladder and prostate infections.
- **Urine culture**—*E. coli, Klebsiella, Proteus, Pseudomonas* are the most common uropathogens found in prostate specimens.

Gram-positive enterococci are the next common organisms.

Cytology

Treatment

Antibiotics: Fluoroquinolones are effective in chronic prostatitis caused by *Enterobacteriaceae*, but not against *P. aeruginosa* or enterococci.

α-adrenergic blockers: May improve outflow obstruction and thereby intraprostatic ductal reflux is diminished.

Prostate Carcinoma

- Carcinoma of prostate is the most common malignant tumor in men of 65 years or more and the second most common cancer in men worldwide.
- It is predominantly a disease of older males.
- Prostate carcinoma is unique among solid tumors—it exists in two forms: (1) Histologic (Latent) form and (2) Clinically evident form.

Risk Factors

Genetic factors: Various susceptibility genes have been identified. Among them, HPC1 is the best characterized. Others are *SR-A/MSR* and *MIC-1* gene.

Chronic inflammation: There is a significant association of prostate carcinoma with history of sexually transmitted disease.

Androgen: A variable lifetime exposure of prostate to androgens have important role in carcinogenesis. No dose response relationship is yet established.

Estrogen: Estrogen increases risk by initiating inflammation and producing mutagenic metabolites.

Vitamin D: Vitamin D deficiency is associated with increased risk of prostate carcinoma.

Dietary factors: Diects rich in fat particularly polyunsaturated fat are associated with increased risk.

Obesity: Higher BMI is associated with increased risk.

Pathology

- Adenocarcinoma is the most common histologic type.
- The tumor may show variable degrees of differentiation and based on that; a grading system was devised—Gleason system.

Gleason Score

A grading system of prostate cancer based on patterns of tumor cells in prostate biopsy specimens. The score of most predominant pattern and the second predominant pattern are added. Score 6 is low-grade, score 7 is intermediate grade and score of 8–10 is high-grade cancer.

A new prostate cancer grading system is developed by International Society of Urological Pathology (ISUP) consensus conference. The new system assigns grade groups from 1 to 5.

Grade Group 1 [Gleason score ≤6]; **Grade Group 2** [Gleason score 7 (3 + 4)]; **Grade Group 3** [Gleason score 7 (4 + 3)]; **Grade Group 4** [Gleason score 8]; **Grade Group 5** [Gleason score 9–10].

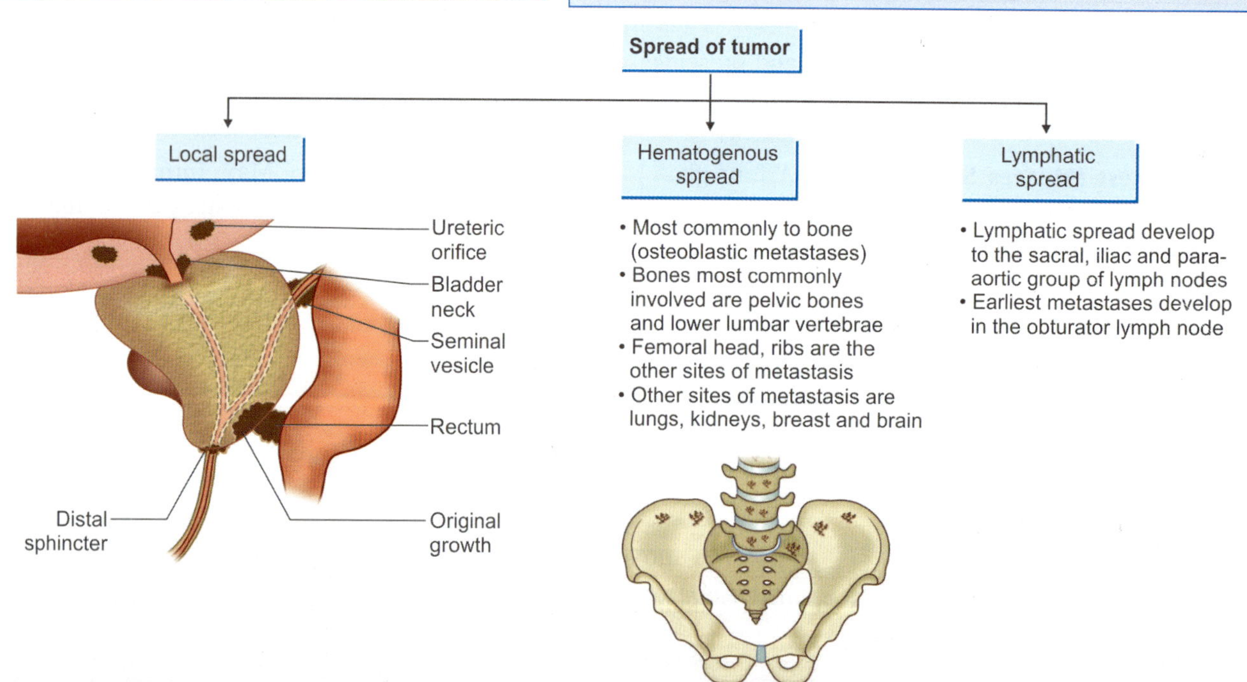

Presence of osteoblastic metastases in older male—prostate carcinoma with bony metastases should be keep in mind.

Clinical Presentation

- In early stage, patient become asymptomatic.
- Incidentally, it is detected during histologic examination of prostatic tissue excised for BPH.
- Clinically, it may be detected as hard nodular prostate with obliteration of median sulcus during routine DRE.
- In locally advanced stage, patient may present with symptoms of LUTS, hematuria, or local discomfort.
- In the stage of metastases, patient may present with bone pain.

Investigations

- For diagnosis, serum PSA and TRUS-guided prostate biopsy is indicated.
- Men with PSA >4 ng/mL should undergo a TRUS-guided prostate biopsy.
- **PSA velocity** (rate of change of PSA values with time), **PSA density** (ratio of serum PSA value and volume of prostate gland) and **free versus bound forms of PSA** are the most useful tests when PSA is in between 4–10 ng/mL (Gray zone).
- Pelvic and abdominal CT or MRI is indicated as staging work-up.
- Bone scan is the standard imaging modality for detecting bony metastases. Bone scan is not necessary if PSA <10 ng/mL. Bone scan is indicated if PSA >20 ng/mL or patient presents with bone pain.

Prostate Specific Antigen (PSA)

- A proteolytic enzyme produced by normal and neoplastic prostate epithelium.
- PSA is secreted in high concentration (mg/mL) in seminal fluid and maintains the seminal secretions in a liquid phase.
- Serum PSA is elevated when normal prostatic architecture is disrupted, and PSA is diffused from prostatic tissue to circulation.
- Serum PSA is elevated in other prostate pathologies (e.g., BPH, prostatitis), after prostatic massage, prostate biopsy, after TURP.

TRUS-guided Prostate Biopsy

- TRUS is not helpful to detect early prostate carcinoma.
- TRUS is helpful to locate the suspicious lesions targeted for biopsy.
- A 18-gauge core biopsy device is attached to the ultrasound probe and biopsy is taken (sextant biopsy).

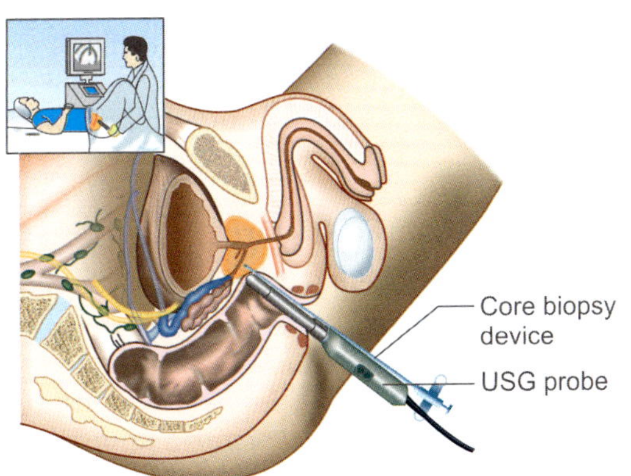

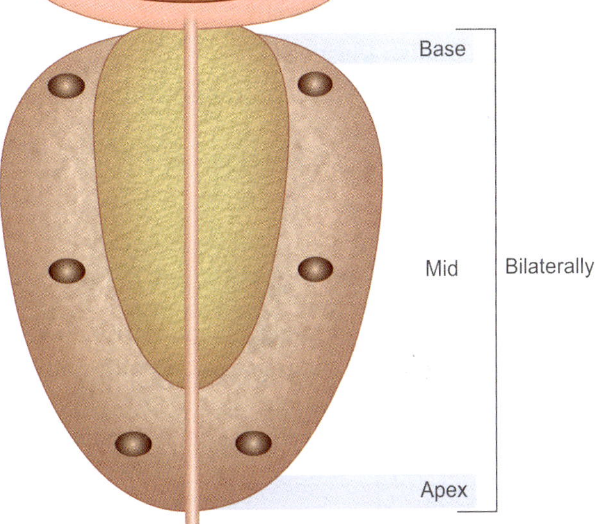

Treatment of Localized Disease

- **Active surveillance**—is particularly indicated for men with life expectancy <10 years and low-grade tumor. Patient should be evaluated with DRE and serum PSA monitoring quarterly and prostatic biopsy annually.
- **Radical prostatectomy or Radiotherapy (EBRT)** is indicated for men with life expectancy >10 years and without any comorbid illness.
- No long-term data are available regarding oncological outcomes of **Cryosurgical ablation of prostate (CSAP) and High-intensity focused ultrasound (HIFU)** compared with radical prostatectomy and EBRT.

Treatment of Locally Advanced Disease

- **Radical prostatectomy:** Most of the patients are not benefited by this treatment modality. Adjuvant radiotherapy Improves local control after radical prostatectomy
- **EBRT with brachytherapy boost**
- **Androgen ablation**

Treatment of Metastatic Disease

Androgen ablation

Radical Prostatectomy

Radical prostatectomy includes complete removal of prostate along with seminal vesicles along with modified pelvic lymph node dissection.

Approaches of radical prostatectomy:

- Open
- Laparoscopic
- Robot assisted (RARP)

Methods of Androgen Ablation

By ablating the source: Bilateral subcapsular orchiectomy

Antiandrogens: Cyproterone acetate, Flutamide, Bicalutamide

LHRH agonist: Leuprolide, goserelin

LHRH antagonist: Degarelix

For castration-resistant patients: Abiraterone acetate, enzalutamide.

Complications of Radical Prostatectomy

Early complications:

- Hemorrhage
- Nerve injury (obturator nerve)
- Ureter injury
- Rectal injury
- Urinary fistula

Late complications:

- Erectile dysfunction
- Urinary incontinence
- Urethral stricture

In radical prostatectomy, **blood loss can be reduced by:** (i) Laparoscopic or robotic assisted surgery and (ii) Careful control of dorsal vein complex and periprostatic vessels in open approach.

Urinary incontinence can reduced by: (i) Preservation of urethral length beyond the apex of the prostate; (ii) Avoiding damage to distal sphincter mechanism; and (iii) Preserving bladder neck.

Urethral Stricture

Classically, **urethral stricture** means scarring involving the **anterior urethra** and sometimes along with spongy erectile tissue of corpus spongiosum.
Narrowing of **posterior urethra** is better termed as **'stenosis'.**

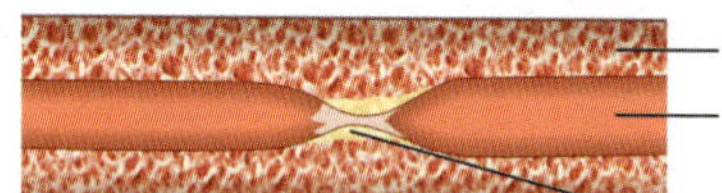

The posterior urethra includes prostatic urethra and membranous urethra. **The anterior urethra** includes the bulbar urethra, penile urethra and fossa navicularis.

The anterior urethra is completely surrounded by corpus spongiosum. Posterior urethra lacks corpus spongiosum.

Etiologies of Urethral Stricture

(i) Trauma; (ii) Iatrogenic (prolonged urethral catheterization, transurethral resection, hypospadias surgery); and (iii) Idiopathic.

Sites of Urethral Stricture

- Bulbar urethra is the most common site of urethral stricture.
- Bulbar urethra and posterior urethra are common sites of traumatic stricture or stenoses.
- Hypospadias and lichen sclerosus-related strictures commonly develop in penile urethra. Lichen sclerosus-related strictures are usually longer and associated with increased risk of urethral cancer.

Clinical Presentation

- Decreased urinary stream
- Incomplete bladder emptying
- Urinary spraying
- Recurrent UTI
- Decreased force of ejaculation.

In well-developed stricture, the stricture can be palpated along the line of urethra.

Evaluation

- Location, length, depth and density of the stricture must be determined to make appropriate line of management.
- **Initial assessment** includes uroflowmetry and USG.
- **Diagnosis is confirmed by:** (i) Retrograde urethrography (with or without voiding cystourethrography) and (ii) Urethroscopy.

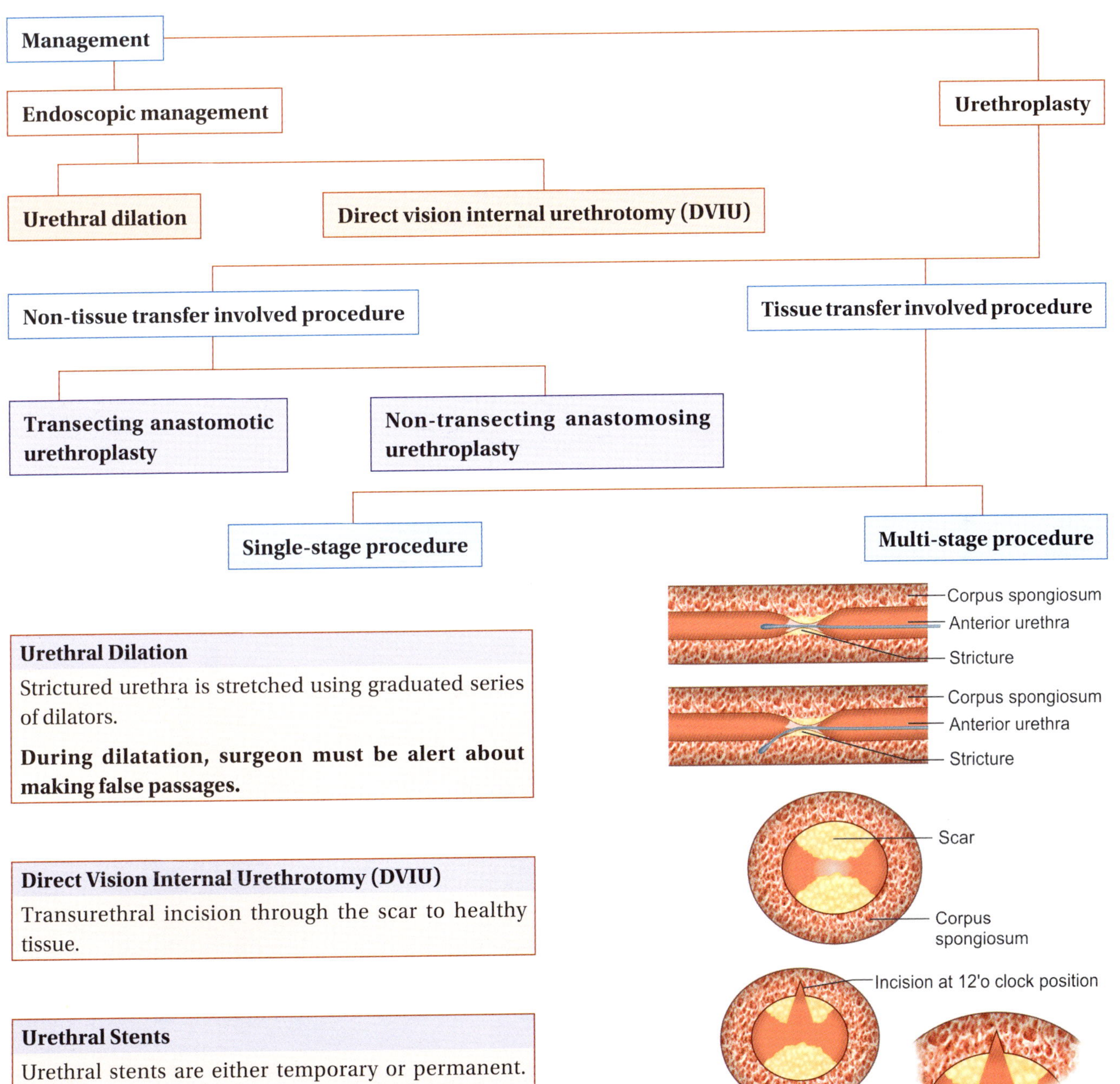

Urethral Dilation

Strictured urethra is stretched using graduated series of dilators.

During dilatation, surgeon must be alert about making false passages.

Direct Vision Internal Urethrotomy (DVIU)

Transurethral incision through the scar to healthy tissue.

Urethral Stents

Urethral stents are either temporary or permanent. Stents prevent the process of epithelialisation.

Transecting Anastomotic Urethroplasty

Transection and removal of strictured segment of urethra and corresponding spongiofibrosis, followed by anastomosis of urethra.

Non-transecting Anastomotic Urethroplasty

Placement of longitudinal incision over the strictured segment and closed in a Heineke-Mikulicz fashion.

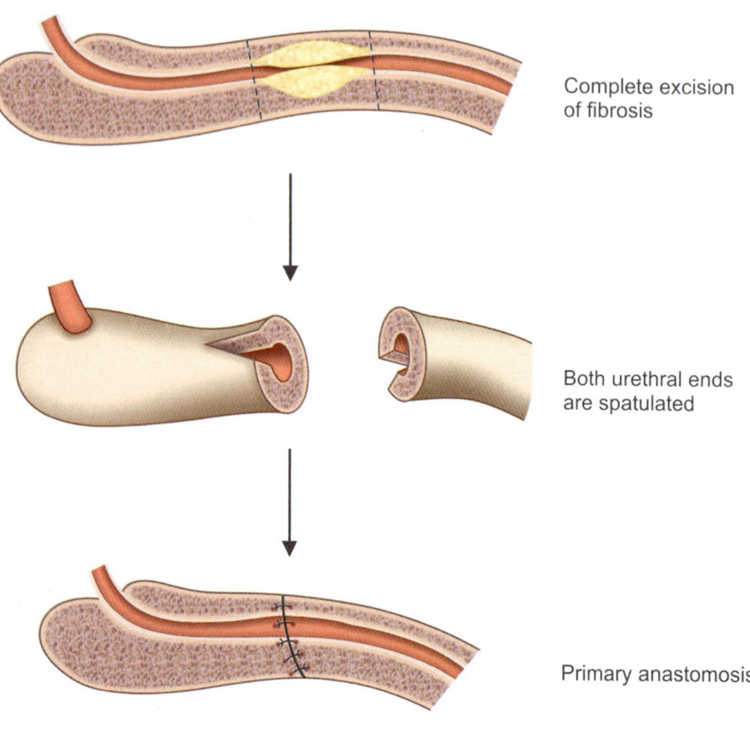

Complications of Urethroplasty

- Urethral leak
- Urinoma
- Urethrocutaneous fistula
- Erectile dysfunction
- Ejaculatory dysfunction.

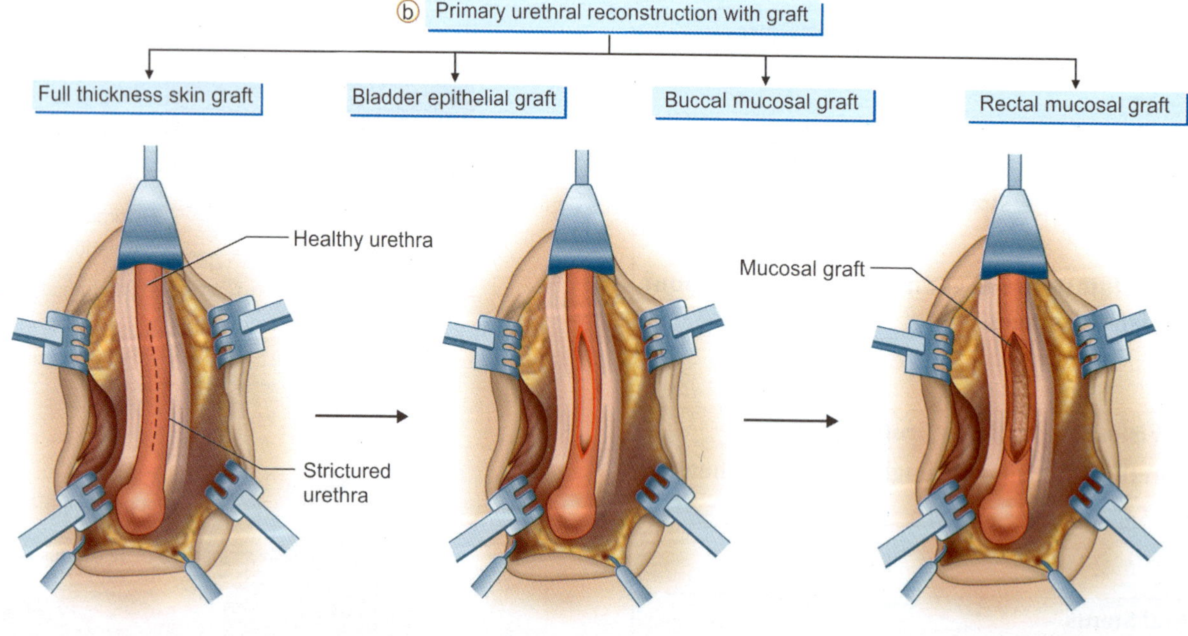

Hypospadias

A congenital abnormality in which urethral meatus open on the ventral aspect of the penis, scrotum or perineum.
The classic triad of hypospadias are: (i) Dorsally hooded foreskin; (ii) Proximal urethral meatus; and (iii) Ventral penile curvature.
Development: Due to incomplete fusion of urethral plate during development of penis.
Risk factor: Risk is increased by history of maternal intake of estrogen or progesterone during pregnancy.
Associated anomalies include: Cryptorchidism, inguinal hernia
Classification: based on location of the urethral meatus

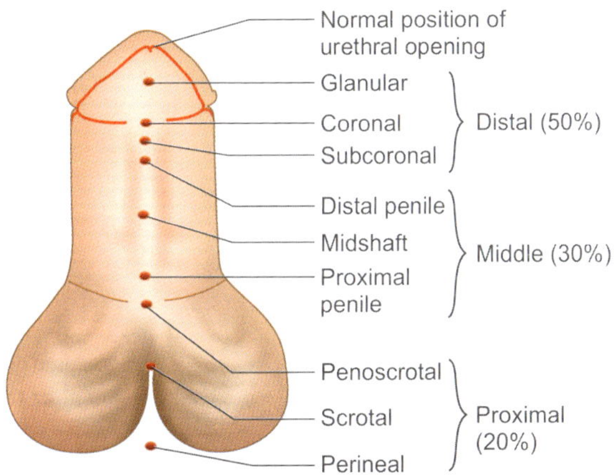

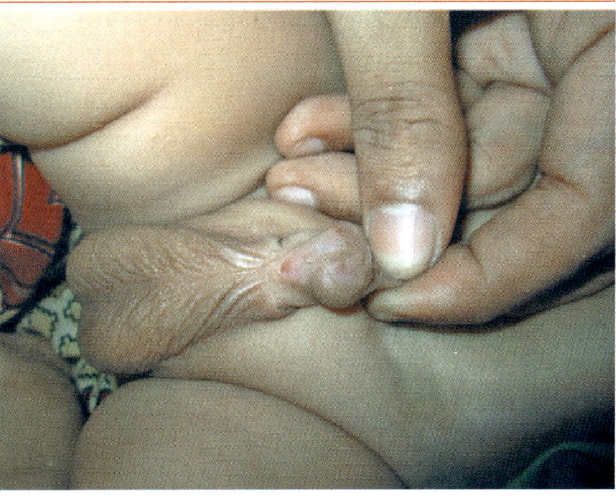

Middle hypospadias with a proximal penile meatus.

Penoscrotal or perineal hypospadias may represent intersex state. Hypospadias along with cryptorchidism also may represent intersex disorder. So **chromosomal study must be done in these conditions.**

Management

The ideal age of surgery is between 6–12 months of age. [Newborn with hypospadias should not be circumcised.]
Principles of hypospadias repair:
- Correction of penile curvature
- Urethroplasty

Correction of penile curvature is done by 2 steps: (i) Assessment of penile curvature by inducing erection and (ii) Correction of curvature

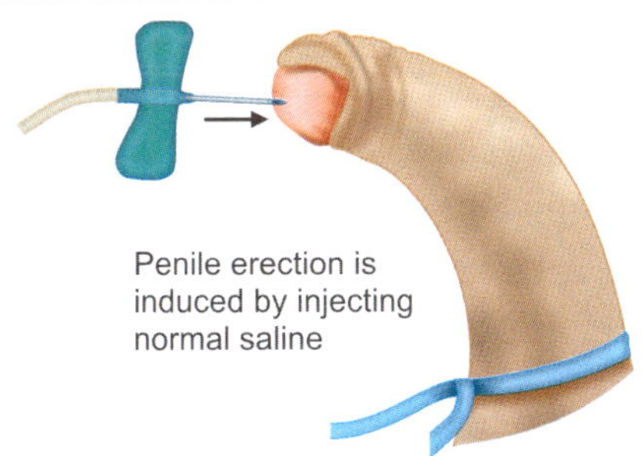

Syndromes Associated with Hypospadias
- WAGR syndrome
- Beckwith-Wiedemann syndrome
- Denys-Drash syndrome

GMS (Glans Meatus and Penile Shaft) Score
- This score is used to stratify severity of hypospadias at the time of procedure.
- This scoring system includes a 1–4 scale for each component:

G-Glans size/urethral plate quality
M- Meatal location
S- Degree of shaft curvature.

Inducing erection by injecting **normal saline into** corpora cavernosa or by injecting **prostaglandin E1** into corpora cavernosa

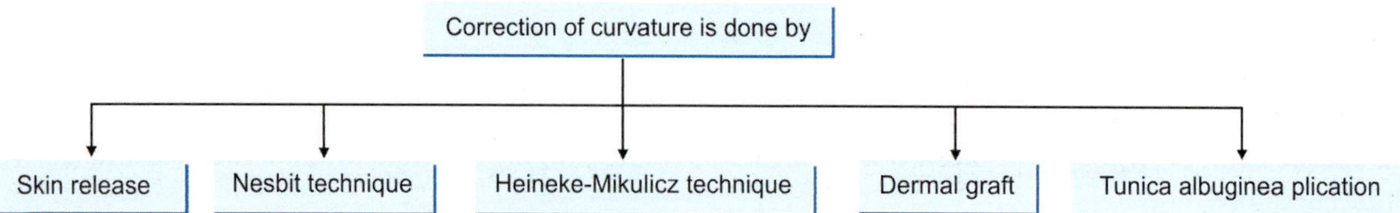

Urethroplasty

For distal hypospadias:

Meatoplasty and glanuloplasty (MAGPI)—All glanular and some coronal hypospadias are repaired by this technique.

Tubularization technique—is a Snodgrass modification of Thiersch-Duplay technique.

Critical steps are:

- A 'relaxing' incision of the urethral plate distal to the hypospadias opening.
- Tubularization of the relaxed urethral plate.

For middle and proximal hypospadias:

- Onlay island flap
- Transverse preputial island flap (TPIF).

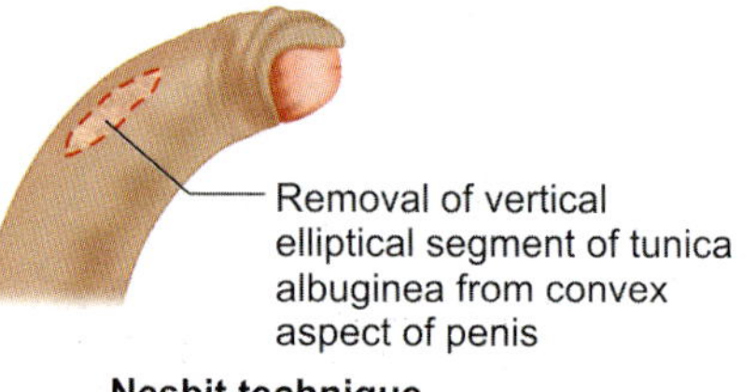

Nesbit technique

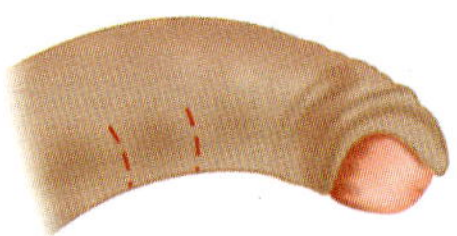

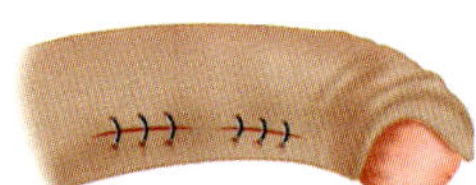

Heineke-Mikulicz technique

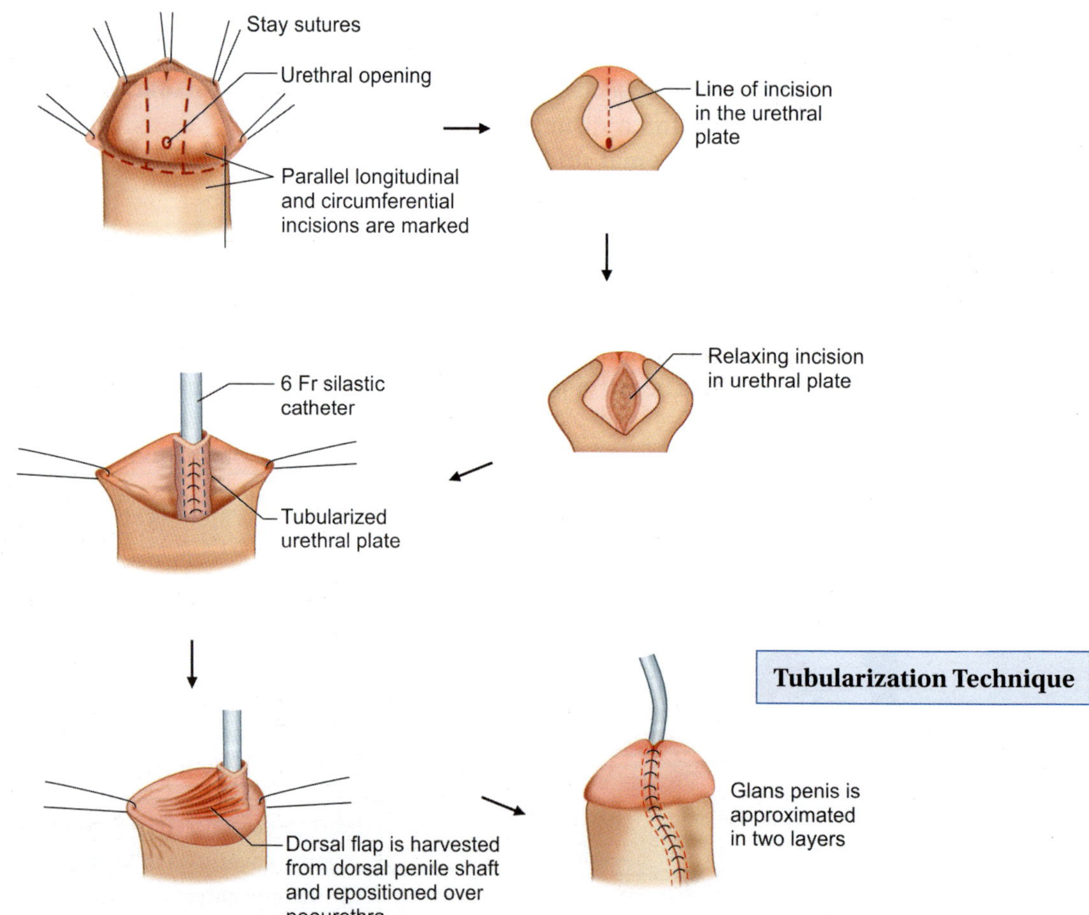

Tubularization Technique

Priapism

- Priapism is persistent penile erection of more than four hours duration, unrelated to sexual stimulation.
- **Subtypes:** (i) Ischemic (veno-occlusive, low flow); (ii) Nonischemic (arterial, high flow); and (iii) Stuttering (intermittent).

Ischemic Priapism

The most common type of priapism. **This type of priapism is a surgical emergency.**
It is characterized by: (i) Minimal or no cavernous blood flow; (ii) Abnormal cavernous blood gases (hypoxic, hypercarbic, and acidotic); and (iii) Corpora cavernosa rigid and tender.

Causes of ischemic priapism:

- **Hematological disorders:** Sickle disease, leukemia, multiple myeloma
- **Neurologic disorders:** Spinal cord injury, cauda equina syndrome
- **Metabolic disorders:** Amyloidosis, gout
- **Medications:** Papaverine, phentolamine, alprostadil, hydralazine, trazodone, fluoxetin, sertraline, alcohol, marijuana, cocaine.

Nonischemic Priapism

This type is characterized by: (i) Unregulated cavernous inflow; (ii) Cavernous blood gases are not hypoxic, or acidotic; and (iii) Penis is neither fully rigid nor painful.

- This type of priapism is commonly caused by **blunt perineal or penile trauma.**
- **This priapism does not require emergent treatment.**

Stuttering Priapism

This type of priapism is characterized by: (i) Recurrent form of ischemic priapism and (ii) Repeated painful erections with intervening period of detumescence.

- Patient with **sickle cell disease** may develop stuttering priapism.

History of priapism includes: (i) Duration of erection; (ii) Erection is painful or not; (iii) Previous history of priapism and its treatment; (iv) History of perineal trauma; (v) History of sickle cell disease; and (vi) Medication history.

Diagnosis

- Low-flow priapism can be differentiated from high-flow priapism by corporal blood gas analysis.
- **Blood aspirated from corpora cavernosa** in ischemic priapism is dark (hypoxic blood), blood from corpora cavernosa in nonischemic priapism is bright red (oxygenated blood).
- **Blood gas analysis and color duplex USG** are the most reliable diagnostic modalities to differentiate between ischemic and nonischemic priapism.

Management of Ischemic Priapism

Initially **therapeutic aspiration** (with or without irrigation). If priapism persists following aspiration, **intracavernous injection** of sympathomimetic drug should be considered. Repeated injection may be tried before planning for any surgical intervention. **Phenylephrine is the most preferred sympathomimetic drug** because of its minimal cardiovascular side effects. **Other sympathomimetic drugs that may be used for intracavernosal injection are-** epinephrine, norepinephrine, phenylephrine, ephedrine, metaraminol. **Phenylephrine or other sympathomimetics are less effective if priapism persisting for more than 72 hours.** In this condition, surgical shunting is often indicated.

Phenylephrine is to be diluted with normal saline to a concentration of 100–150 μg/mL, 1 mL of diluted phenylephrine is injected every 3–5 minutes for about 1 hour. Adverse effects are- acute hypertension, reflex bradycardia, arrhythmia.

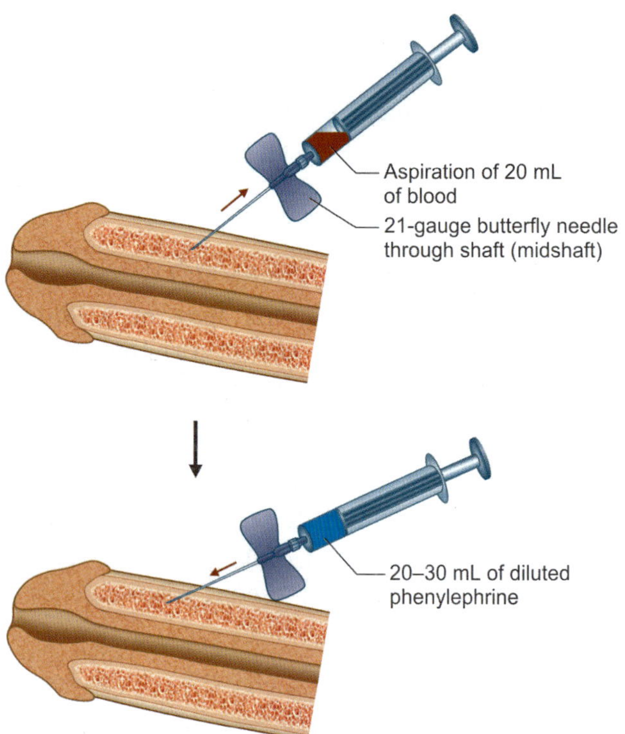

Proximal Shunts
Quackel shunt (Cavernospongious shunt)
Grayhack shunt (Cavernosaphenous shunt
Distal Shunts

- **Al-Gharab** (excising a piece of tunica albuginea at the tip of the corpora cavernosa)
- **Winter** (insertion of large biopsy needle percutaneously through the glans)
- **Ebbehoj** (insertion of a scalpel percutaneously through the glans)
- **Disadvantages of proximal shunting:** (i) Technically demanding; (ii) Urethral fistula; (iii) Purulent cavernositis; and (iv) Pulmonary embolism (following Grayhack shunt).

- **If intracorporeal injection fails, shunt is necessary**. Two types of shunts are effective for ischemic priapism- **Proximal shunt** and **Distal shunt**.
- **A distal shunt is preferred over proximal shunt**. If distal shunt fails, then proximal shunting is indicated. Among the distal shunt, Al-Gharab shunt is the most effective.

Management of nonischemic priapism:

- Observation
- Nonpermanent selective arterial embolization (using autologous clot or absorbable gels)
- Permanent selective arterial embolization (using coils, polyvinyl alcohol particles, acrylic glue)
- Color duplex US-guided selective ligation of the fistula through transcorporeal approach- last treatment option.

Management of stuttering priapism:

Prevention of future episodes and management of each episode (as in ischemic priapism).

Management of priapism due to Sickle cell disease:

- Can be managed conservatively with hydration, alkalinization with bicarbonate and oxygenation
- Chance of recurrent priapism is high, so transfusion or exchange transfusion should be considered.

Peyronie's Disease

- An acquired penile abnormality characterized by fibrosis of the tunica albuginea.
- **Pathophysiology:** Penile buckling in the erect or semi-erect state during sexual activity most likely causes microvascular trauma to the penile shaft.
- This type of repetitive trauma initiates a cascade of events that includes extravascular protein deposition, fibrin trapping, changes in elastin content of tunica albuginea, that ultimately results in scarring of tunica.

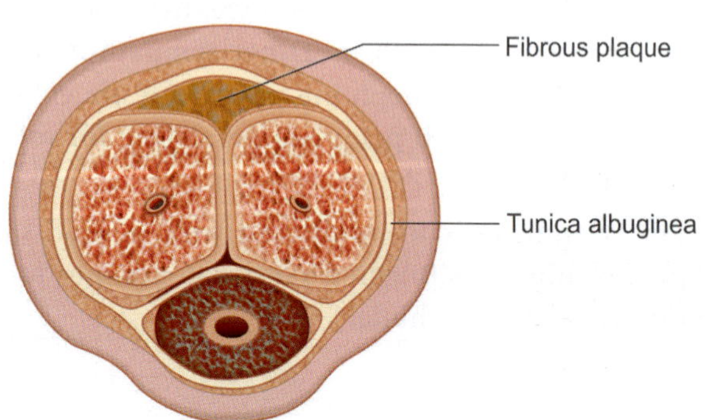

Clinical Presentation

Most common presentation- Recent onset penile curvature along with penile pain. No plaque is palpable in the non-erect state.
Other presentations are penile curvature with penile pain along with palpable plaque in the non-erect state or erectile dysfunction only.

Plaque most commonly palpable on the dorsal aspect of the midshaft of penis.

Diagnosis

History taking- to assess penile deformity, penile pain (related to erection or not), interference with intercourse, erectile dysfunction.

Physical examination includes location of plaque (if any), presence of deformity, area of tenderness, length of penis, any associated anomalies (e.g., hypospadias)

Intracavernosal injection (ICI) test with or without duplex Doppler US- ICI test can assess deformity, plaques and pain in erect state. Duplex Doppler is helpful to assess the size and density of the plaques as well as to differentiate calcified from non-calcified plaques.

Treatment

- Role of vitamin E, tamoxifen, procarbazine, omega-3 fatty acids, vitamin E with L-carnitine are doubtful.
- **Intralesional collagenase clostridium histolyticum along with modeling by the clinician and by the patient**—for stable disease with penile curvature more than 30° and less than 90° and intact erectile function
- **Intralesional interferon** α**-2b**
- **Surgical management** is indicated if erectile dysfunction develops or curvature interferes with sexual intercourse.

Plication and corporoplasty, Incision and grafting have excellent results.

Significant erectile dysfunction in Peyronie's disease warrants **penile prosthesis**.

Carcinoma of Penis

Commonly presents in the sixth decode of life, but may develop in earlier age.

Risk Factors

Phimosis—Definitive role of smegma in carcinogenesis is still lacking. Neonatal circumcision is protective for invasive penile carcinoma, not so much protective for CIS. Circumcision at puberty or at adult life do not have any protective role.

HPV infection—particularly HPV-16 and 18

Exposure to tobacco products—cigarette smoking, chewing tobacco, snuff—all are associated with increased risk.

Psoriasis patients undergoing PUVA treatment
Balanitis xerotica obliterans.

Pathology

Macroscopically, penile carcinomas are either **exophytic** or **ulcerative**.
More than 95% of carcinomas are squamous cell carcinoma. Other histological types are melanoma, mesenchymal tumor, lymphoma. Malignant lesion rarely involve corporal bodies because **Buck's fascia** acts as a natural barrier.
Distant metastases to lungs, liver, bone and brain are uncommon.

Premalignant Penile Lesions

- Erythroplasia of Queyrat
- Bowen's disease
- Giant condylomata (Buschke-Lowenstein)
- Paget's disease
- Intra-epithelial neoplasia grade III

Penile intraepithelial neoplasia (PIN or PEIN) is a premalignant condition includes clinical entities of-

Bowenoid papulosis (does not progress to invasive disease)

Erythroplasia of Queyrat (involves the glans penis and prepuce)

Bowen's disease (involves the penile shaft).

Clinical Presentation

- Patient may present with small papular, warty growth or in advanced cases, an exophytic lesion.(Phimosis may obscure the tumor.)
- Patient may present with inguinal lymphadenopathy or ulceration in the inguinal region.
- Urethral involvement is very rare.
- On clinical examination, location, fixity, involvement of corporal bodies must be assessed. **Bilateral palpation of inguinal area** must be done to assess lymphadenopathy (number of nodes in each inguinal region, unilateral or bilateral localization, size of the nodes, fixity to the adjacent structures and/or overlying skin).

SCC Variants with Excellent Prognosis

- Verrucous
- Papillary
- Warty
- Pseudohyperplastic
- Carcinoma cuniculatum

These tumors are locally invasive, rarely metastasise.

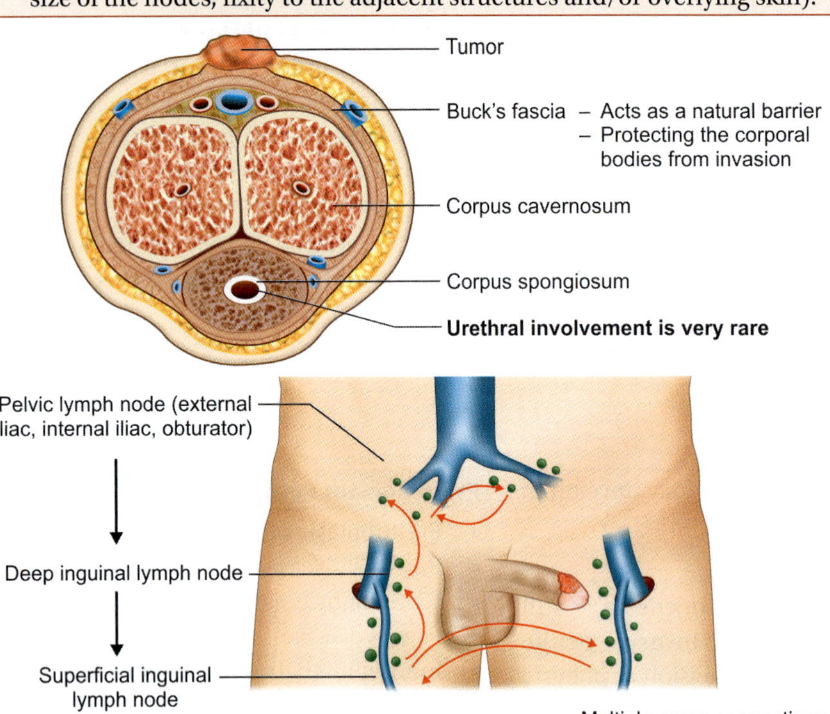

Intermediate-risk SCC Variants

- Common SCC
- Mixed forms
- Pleomorphic form of warty carcinomas

High- risk SCC Variants

Basaloid

Sarcomatoid Adenosquamous

These tumors are associated with early metastasis and high. mortality rate.

Investigations

- The diagnosis of penile carcinoma is confirmed by biopsy. Assessment of depth of invasion, presence of vascular invasion and for histologic grading, biopsy is essential. A dorsal slit is often necessary for adequate exposure for biopsy.
- High-grade lesions suspected of involving corporal bodies, and if partial penectomy is being considered—**Contrast-enhanced MRI** with an artificially induced erection is helpful to give additional informations.
- **For assessment of inguinal lymph nodes, clinical assessment is sufficient enough. Pelvic CT scan** is indicated to assess the pelvic lymph nodes.

CT scan of chest, abdomen and pelvis are recommended for patients with inguinal lymph node metastases.

Treatment

Treatment of the primary tumor: Treatment depends on stage, location and size of the tumor as well as patient preference.

Different treatment options are available: (I) **Organ-sparing approaches** [(i) Topical therapy; (ii) Laser therapy; (iii) Glansectomy; (iv) Moh's micrographic surgery; (v) Glans resurfacing; (vi) Radiotherapy]; (II) **Partial penectomy**; and (III) **Total penectomy**. Organ-sparing approach is particularly indicated in Tis, Ta, T1 lesions.

Topical therapy: 5-fluorouracil (5-FU) as first-line therapy and Imiquimod as second-line therapy. Topical 5% 5-FU cream twice daily for 2–6 weeks. Imiquimod 5% cream at night 3 times per week for 4–16 weeks.
Laser therapy: Four types of lasers can be used- (i) CO_2 laser; (ii) Nd:YAG laser; (iii) Argon laser; and (iv) Potassium titanyl phosphate (KTP) laser. Nd:YAG and CO_2 lasers are most commonly used.
Glansectomy may be considered in tumors on glans or prepuce (clinical stage Ta, Tis, T1).
Radical circumcision may be indicated if tumor is confined to the prepuce.
Glans resurfacing may be offered as primary treatment modality in superficial non-invasive disease confined to glans penis. This surgical approach includes complete abrasion of the glandular epithelium followed by coverage with split-thickness skin grafting.
Mohs surgery is particularly indicated in small superficial lesion on proximal shaft to avoid amputation of penis.
Radiotherapy (EBRT or brachytherapy) can be used if a young patient with small superficial lesion in distal penis who is willing to preserve his organ or patient is unfit for surgery.
Partial penectomy can be offered for invasive distal penile lesion if after surgery, remaining penile stump will allow the patient to void in standing position and to perform sexual intercourse.
Total penectomy is reserved for invasive tumor involving the midshaft and base of penis.

Partial Penectomy

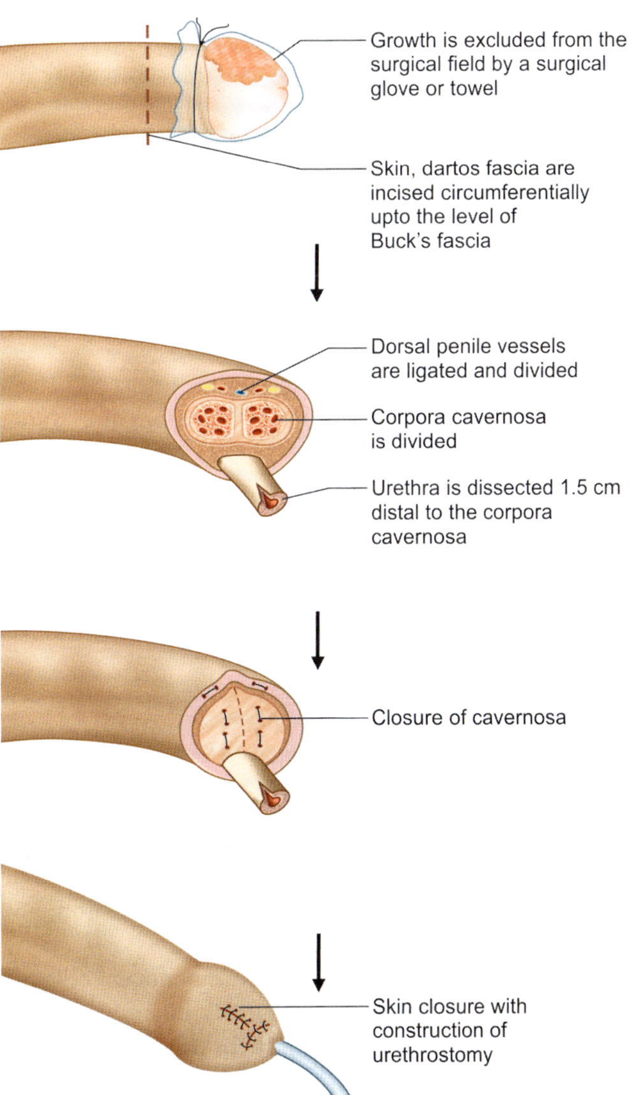

Total Penectomy

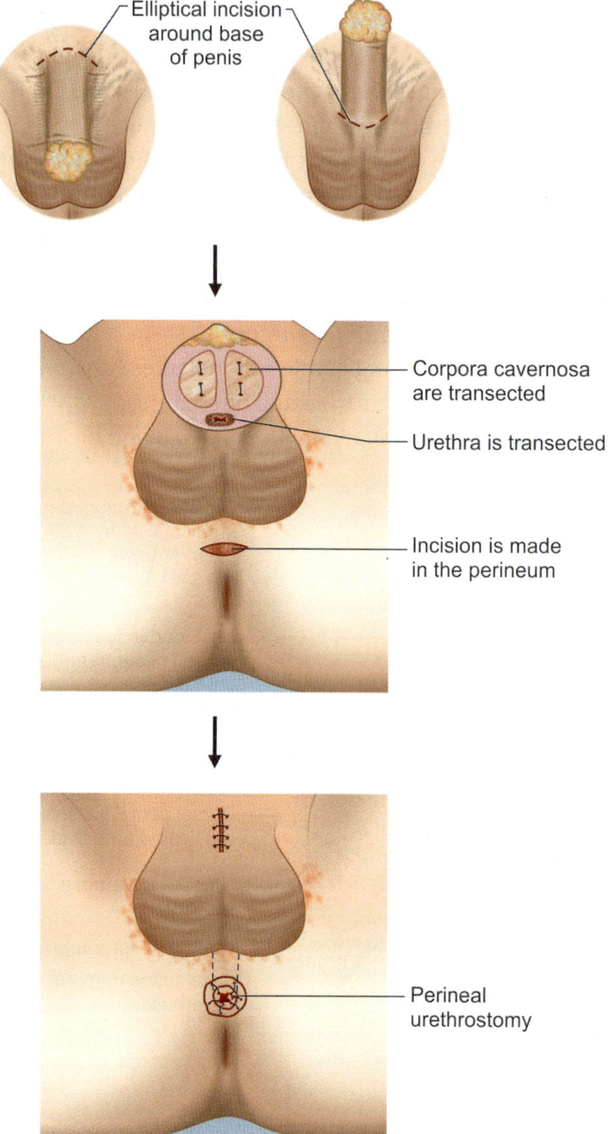

Management of Regional Lymph Nodes
Presence and extent of lymph node metastases is the most important prognostic indicator in invasive penile SCC.
Clinically N0
▪ **Tis, Ta, T1 tumor with grade 1 or 2**- Active surveillance ▪ Standard or modified inguinal lymph node dissection (ILND) or Dynamic sentinel node biopsy (DSNB) is indicated if **high-risk features (≥pT1G3 or ≥T2 any grade, lymphovascular invasion, >50% poorly differentiated)** for nodal metastases are found in primary tumor. ▪ Following DSNB, if positive lymph nodes are found, ILND is recommended. Unilateral Pelvic lymph node dissection **(PLND)** is indicated if ≥2 positive lymph nodes are found in ILND. Bilateral PLND is indicated if ≥4 positive lymph nodes are found in ILND. **Superficial inguinal dissection with intraoperative fozen section biopsy** is another option for staging. ILND is recommended if positive lymph nodes are found in frozen section biopsy.

Clinically N1

- **Unilateral mobile, <4 cm node:** High-risk features (high grade, lymphovascular invasion, poor differentiation in more than half of the tumor cells) are absent—percutaneous lymph node biopsy followed by bilateral ILND if biopsy is positive. Excision biopsy of the lymph node if biopsy is negative; High-risk features present- Standard or modified bilateral inguinal lymph node dissection. Unilateral Pelvic lymph node dissection (PLND) is indicated if ≥2 positive lymph nodes are found in ILND. Bilateral PLND is indicated if ≥4 positive lymph nodes are found in ILND.
- **Unilateral mobile, ≥4 cm node:** Percutaneous lymph node biopsy followed by bilateral ILND if biopsy is positive. Excision biopsy of the lymph node if biopsy is negative. Neo-adjuvant cisplatin based chemotherapy may be administered before ILND. Unilateral Pelvic lymph node dissection (PLND) is indicated if ≥2 positive lymph nodes are found in ILND. Bilateral PLND is indicated if ≥4 positive lymph nodes are found in ILND. Adjuvant chemoradiotherapy may be considered if pelvic lymph nodes are positive.
- **Unilateral fixed or bilateral inguinal nodes:** Percutaneous lymph node biopsy followed by neoadjuvant chemotherapy if biopsy is positive. ILND and PLND should be performed after neoadjuvant therapy. Bilateral PLND is indicated if ≥4 positive inguinal lymph nodes are found.
- **Enlarged pelvic lymph nodes detected on imaging:** Image-guided percutaneous lymph node biopsy from the pelvic nodes. If positive, resectability should be assessed. Neoadjuvant chemotherapy followed by bilateral superficial and deep ILND and unilateral/bilateral PLND should be considered for resectable disease. Chemoradiotherapy is indicated for unresectable disease.

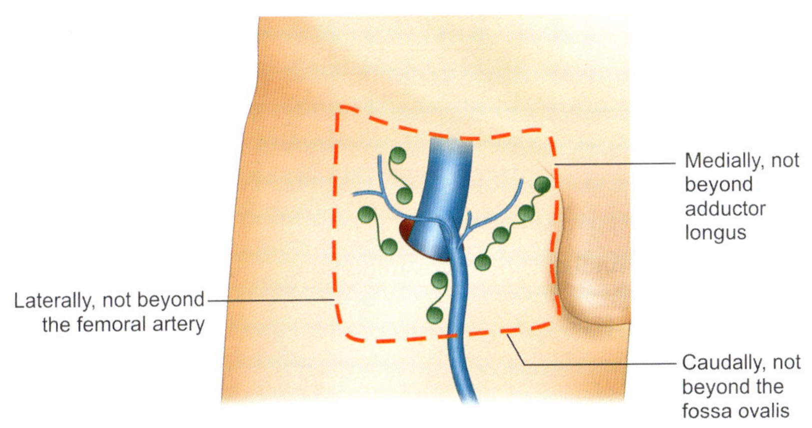

Modified inguinal lymphadenectomy

[Saphenous vein is preserved]

[Bilateral inguinal lymphadenectomy is indicated as due to high chance of bilateral drainage]

The boundaries of the standard, full-template inguinal lymph node dissection (i.e., Daseler's quadrilateral area) are:

Superiorly, the inguinal ligament; **inferiorly,** the fossa ovalis; **laterally,** the medial border of Sartorius muscle; and **medially,** the lateral edge of adductor longus.

Pelvic lymphadenectomy includes external iliac, internal iliac and obturator lymph nodes

Testicular Cancer

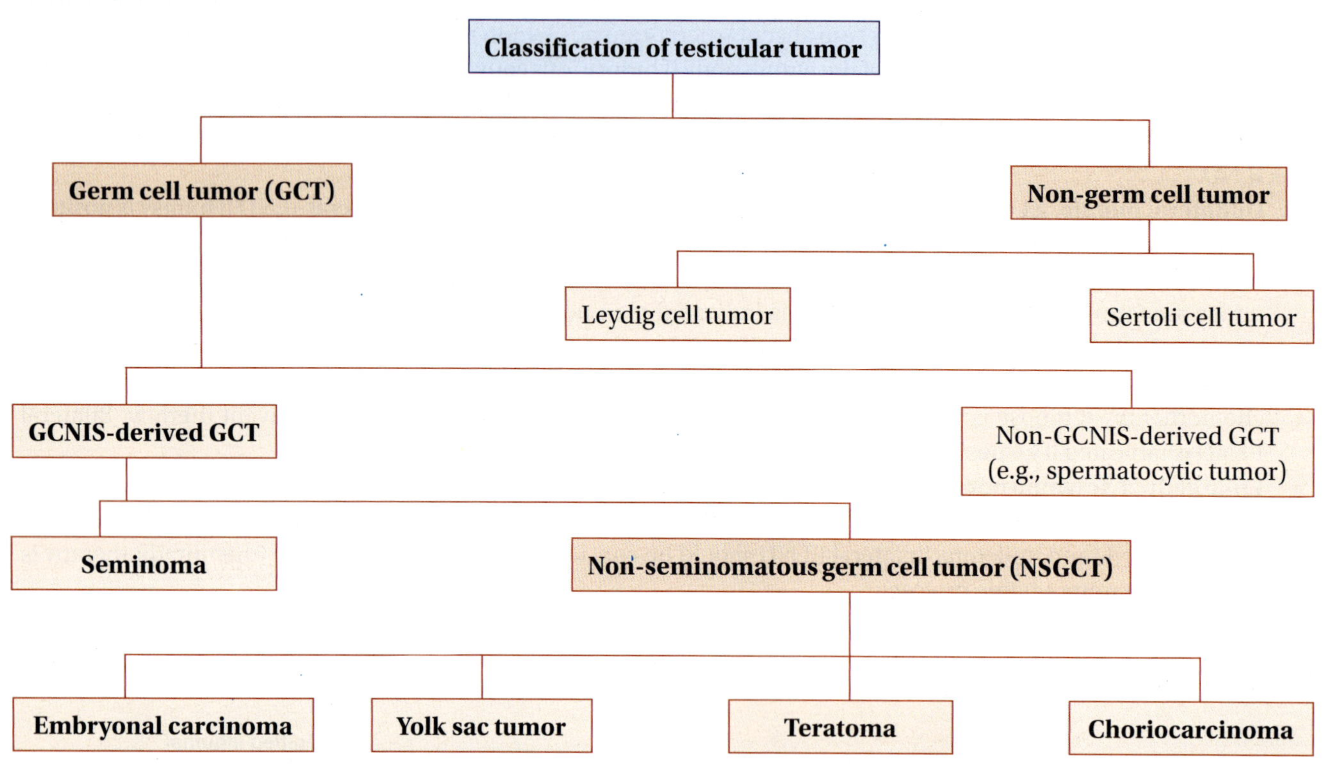

Germ Cell Tumor Neoplasia in situ (GCNIS)

- GCNIS is considered as a precursor of all postpubertal testicular GCTs except spermatocytic tumor.
- GCNIS composed of undifferentiated germ cells confined within the seminiferous tubules.

Seminoma

- Seminoma is the **most common type of GCT**.
- Seminoma arises from GCNIS and has the ability to transform into NSGCT elements.
- Seminomas are less aggressive than nonseminomatous GCTs. **Prognosis is better among all GCTs.**
- If germ cell tumors have both seminoma and non-seminomatous element, the management of the tumor will be as per nonseminomatous GCTs.
- Highly **radiosensitive**.

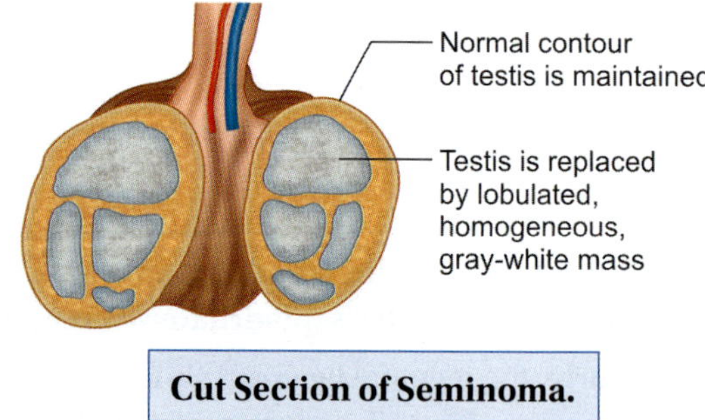

Cut Section of Seminoma.

Teratoma

- Teratoma composed of two or more germ cell layers-Ectoderm, mesoderm, and endoderm.

Different types of teratoma are: (i) Mature teratoma; (ii) Immature teratoma; and (iii) Teratoma with malignant transformation (teratoma with somatic-type malignancy)

"Teratoma with malignant transformation" type may transform into somatic malignancy such as rhabdomyosarcoma, adenocarcinoma

- Teratoma is histologically benign
- The genetic unstabilty makes teratoma a tumor with unpredictable biological behavior.
- Teratoma usually develops in younger age
- Teratoma is chemoresistant.

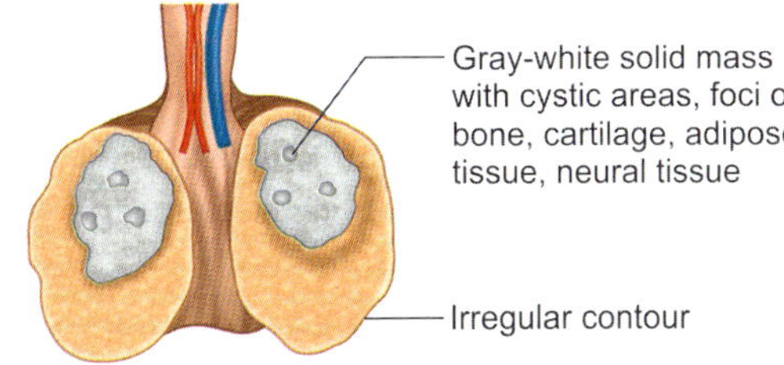

Cut Section of Teratoma.

- **Leydig cell tumor:** Secretes androgen, thereby causes sexual precocity.
- **Sertoli cell tumor:** Secretes estrogen, thereby causes gynecomastia and loss of libido.

Embryonal carcinoma (EC) is the most undifferentiated type NSGCT. EC can differentiate to other types of NSGCT. This tumor is highly aggressive and carries increased risk of mestastases.

Choriocarcinoma is also a highly aggressive NSGCT, usually diagnosed at advanced stage. This tumor is associated with highly elevated serum HCG, increased risk of distant metastases (lungs, liver, brain) and spontaneous hemorrhage in primary tumor site as well as in metastatic sites.

Yolk sac tumor is an uncommon type of post pubertal testicular GCT, more commonly associated with pediatric and mediastinal GCTs. Characteristic histological findings are eosinophilic hyaline globules and Schiller-Duval bodies. This tumor almost always produces AFP.

Extragonadal Germ Cell Tumor

Extragonadal GCTs are most commonly located in **retroperitoneum** and **mediastinum**. **Retroperitoneal GCTs** are biologically similar to testicular GCTs.

Mediastinal seminomas are similar to testicular seminomas in respect to prognosis. **Mediastinal NSGCTs** are associated with yolk-sac tumor components, poor prognosis and less sensitivity to chemotherapy.

Clinical Presentation

The pathognomonic presentation is painless testicular mass. Vague scrotal discomfort may be present.

Presentation due to metastases: Palpable abdominal mass, abdominal pain, swelling of lower extremities may be found in bulky retroperitoneal metastases. Patient may present with cough, respiratory distress due to pulmonary metastases.

Uncommon presentation: Gynecomastia, diminished fertility.

On clinical examination, testis is enlarged and firm. Testicular sensation is lost. Lax secondary hydrocele may present.

A solid mass in testis detected by clinical examination or imaging should be considered as a malignant tumor unless proved otherwise.

Diagnosis

Measurement of serum tumor markers (AFP, hCG, LDH) and **scrotal ultrasound with Doppler** should be done prior to any treatment in patients with suspected testicular neoplasm.

If serum tumor markers are within normal range and sonographic findings are equivocal- Repeat imaging with USG should be done after 6-8 weeks or MRI with enhancement.

Testicular microlithiasis without any solid mass lesion in USG—no further evaluation is indicated.

Patients with suspected testicular neoplasm and a normal contralateral testis should undergo radical inguinal orchiectomy (testis and spermatic cord en bloc).

Serum Tumor Markers

Serum tumor markers should be measured **at diagnosis, after orchiectomy** (for staging and risk stratification), **before chemotherapy** (for IGCCCG risk stratification), **after chemotherapy** (to monitor response) and during surveillance (to detect any relapse).

AFP (Alpha-fetoprotein): Nonseminomatous GCTs (embryonal carcinoma, yolk sac tumor) produce AFP. Choriocarcinomas and pure seminomas do not secrete AFP. So, AFP is a indicator of presence of nonseminomatous component in GCT.

hCG (Human chorionic gonadotropin): Most of the choriocarcinomas, about 50% of embryonal carcinoma and few percentage of seminomas secrete hCG. Beta-subunit of hCG is measured for diagnosis and further workup of testicular carcinoma.

LDH (Lactate dehydrogenase): LDH is a less specific tumor marker for testicular cancer than AFP and beta-hCG. A direct relationship is present between tumor burden and LDH level. It is a useful prognostic marker of GCT at diagnosis. Among the five isoenzymes, LDH-1 is most commonly elevated in GCT.

Other Causes of Elevated AFP

- Hepatocellular carcinoma
- Gastric carcinoma
- Pancreatic cancer
- Cancer of the biliary tract
- Alcoholic liver disease

Other Causes of Elevated hCG

- Cancers of liver, biliary tract, pancreas
- Cancer of kidney and bladder
- Lymphoma
- Pituitary tumor (alpha-subunit is elevated)
- Hypogonadism
- Marijuana use

Radical Inguinal Orchiectomy

Patients with suspected testicular neoplasm and a normal contralateral testis should undergo radical inguinal orchiectomy (includes early control of the spermatic cord, complete removal of the testis, epidymis and spermatic cord to the level of deep inguinal ring). Radical orchiectomy makes the histologic diagnosis and provides T staging, presence of GCNIS as well as information about lymphatic and vascular invasion.

Transcrotal orchiectomy is contraindicated because this approach is associated with increased risk of local recurrence and inguinal and pelvic lymph node metastases.

Testis-sparing surgery (partial orchiectomy) is an alternative approach to radical orchiectomy in selected patients.

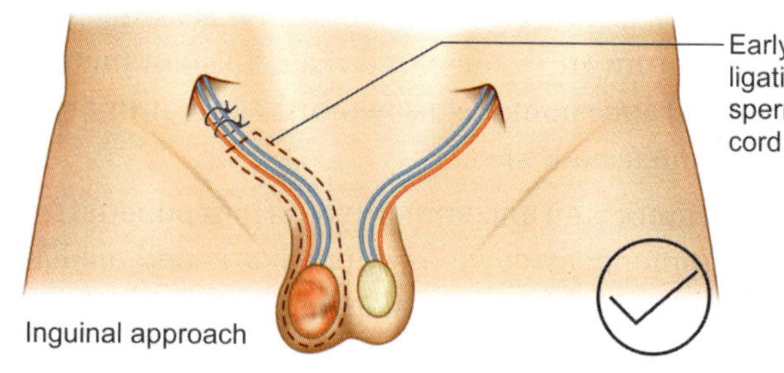

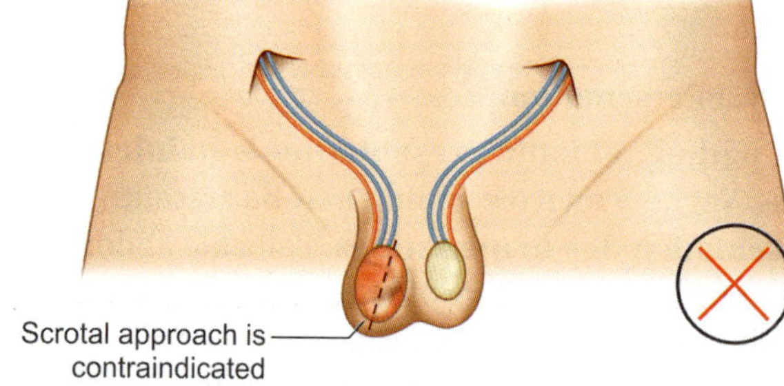

- **Sperm banking** may be considered before orchiectomy in patients with atrophic contralateral testis or history of infertility.
- **Placement of testicular prosthesis** during orchiectomy may be considered if patient wishes.

Testis-sparing Surgery

Indications are: (i) Tumor of less than 2 cm in a solitary testis and (ii) Synchronous bilateral tumors with tumor size less than 2 cm.

- Multiple biopsies of the adjacent testicular parenchyma should be obtained.

Patients considering testis-sparing surgery should be counselled regarding: (i) Increased risk of local recurrence; (ii) Role of adjuvant radiotherapy; and (iii) Radiotherapy related testicular atrophy and impaired sperm and testosterone production.

Staging

Clinical staging depends on histopathological diagnosis, pathological stage of the primary tumor, post-orchiectomy tumor markers and status of metastases.

To assess metastases, CT scan of abdomen with pelvis with IV contrast or MRI (if CT is contraindicated) and chest X-ray are indicated. Imaging should be done within 4 weeks prior to initiation of chemotherapy

CT chest is indicated if: (i) Post-orchiectomy elevated serum tumor markers; (ii) Evidence of metastases on CT abdomen and pelvis; and (iii) Abnormal or equivocal findings on chest X-ray.

FDG-PET is not indicated in staging workup.

All patients should be assigned a **TNM category** that also incorporates serum marker levels (S0-3).

IGCCCG (The International Germ Cell Cancer Consensus Group) risk group should be determined in advanced GCT for evaluation of prognosis and selection of chemotherapy regime.

Retroperitoneum is the initial site of metastases via lymphatic spread in most of the GCTs.

In right testicular tumor, primary site of metastases is inter-aortocaval lymph nodes inferior to the renal vessels, followed by paracaval and para-aortic nodes.

In left testicular tumor, primary site of metastases is para-aortic lymph nodes followed by inter-aortocaval lymph nodes.

Hematogenous spread is the most common route of metastases in choriocarcinoma.

The International Germ Cell Cancer Consensus Group (IGCCCG) Classification for Advanced GCT

Nonseminoma

- **Good risk**

Testicular or retroperitoneal primary tumor
And
No pulmonary visceral metastases
And
Post-orchiectomy markers all of:
AFP <1,000 ng/mL
hCG <5000 iu/L
LDH <1.5X upper limit of normal

- **Intermediate risk**

Testicular or retroperitoneal primary tumor
And
No nonpulmonary visceral mestastses
And
Post-orchiectomy markers-any of:
AFP 1,000–10,000 ng/mL
hCG 5,000–50,000 iu/L
LDH 1.5–10 X upper limit of normal

- **Poor risk**

Mediastinal primary tumor
Or
Nonpulmonary visceral metastases
Or
Post-orchiectomy markers-any of:
AFP>10,000 ng/mL
hCG>50,000 iu/L
LDH>10 X upper limit of normal

Seminoma

- **Good risk**

Any primary site
And
No nonpulmonary visceral metastases
And
Normal AFP
Any hCG
Any LDH

- **Intermediate risk**

Any primary site
And
Nonpulmonary visceral metastases
And
Normal AFP
Any hCG
Any LDH

- **Poor risk**

No patients classified as poor prognosis

Treatment
GCNIS: Radical orchiectomy or cisplatin-based chemotherapy followed by low-dose radiotherapy.
Seminoma
Stage I: Surveillance is the most preferred management option. One or two cycles of carboplatin-based chemotherapy or radiotherapy are the less preferred approach.
Stage IIA and IIB: Radiotherapy or chemotherapy (3 cycles of BEP or 4 cycles of EP) [BEP—bleomycin, etoposide, cisplatin; EP—etoposide, cisplatin].
Stage IIC and III: 3 cycles of BEP or 4 cycles of EP for good-risk disease and 4 cycles of BEP or 4 cycles of VIP (etoposide, mesna, ifosfamide, cisplatin) for intermediate risk disease.
Nonseminomatous GCT
Stage I: Surveillance is the recommended management option. Nerve-sparing retroperitoneal lymph node dissection (RPLND) or Chemotherapy (1 cycle of BEP) are alternative treatment options.
Stage IS: Induction chemotherapy (3 cycles of BEP or 4 cycles of EP)
Stage IIA: Nerve-sparing RPLND or Chemotherapy with 3 cycles of BEP or 4 cycles of EP
Stage IIB: 3 cycles of BEP or 4 cycles of EP or nerve-sparing RPLND (in selected patients).
Advanced Nonseminomatous GCT
IGCCCG Good-risk group [IS, IIA (S1), IIB (S1), IIC, IIIA]: 3 cycles of BEP or 4 cycles of EP **Intermediate-risk (Stage IIIB):** 4 cycles of BEP or 4 cycles of VIP **Poor-risk (stage IIIC) nonseminoma:** 4 cycles of BEP

Retroperitoneal Lymph Node Dissection (RPNLD)

RPNLD may be either full bilateral template dissection or modified template dissection.

- **A full bilateral template dissection** is indicated for retroperitoneal metastases detected in CT imaging or intraoperative assessment.

  It includes removal of the para-aortic, retro-aortic, pre-aortic, left common iliac, interoartocaval, pre-caval, para-caval, retro-caval, and right common iliac lymph nodes in addition to the ipsilateral gondal vessels.
- **Modified template dissection** may be considered in patients with clinically negative retroperitoneal lymph node.
- **For right-sided tumors, the modified template must include** the right common iliac, para-caval, pre-caval, retro-caval, interaortocaval, pre-aortic, and retro-aortic lymph nodes in addition to the right gonadal vessels.
- **For left-sided tumors, the modified template must include** the left common iliac, para-aortic, pre-aortic, and retro-aortic lymph nodes.

  Modified template dissection is associated with decreased risk of ejaculatory dysfunction.
- **Nerve-sparing RPNLD should not be performed compromising the quality of lymph node dissection.**

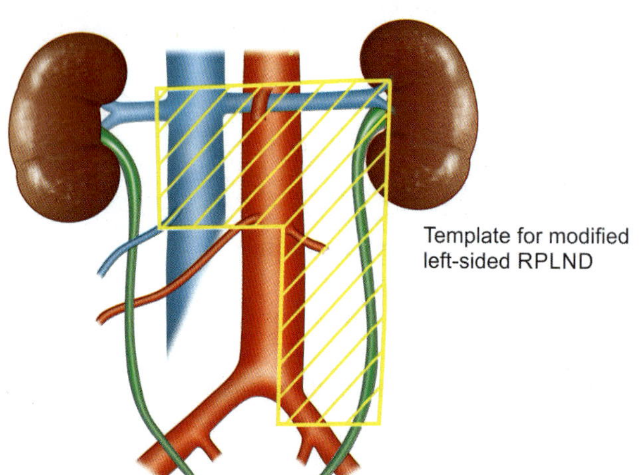

Complications of RPNLD

- Ejaculatory dysfunction
- Chylous ascites
- Symptomatic lymphocele
- Ureteral injury
- Paralytic ileus

Case 1

History and Physical Examination

A 25-year-old female patient presented in the surgical emergency with acute onset pain in the right loin radiating to the groin. As per description of the patient, she rolled around in agony during the attack of pain. Patient experienced similar types of pain for 3–4 times in the last 2 weeks. The pain is sometimes associated with nausea. No history of dysuria, increased frequency of micturition, hematuria.

Physical Examination

Pulse: 100/min, Surface temperature: Normal

Mild tenderness in the right loin

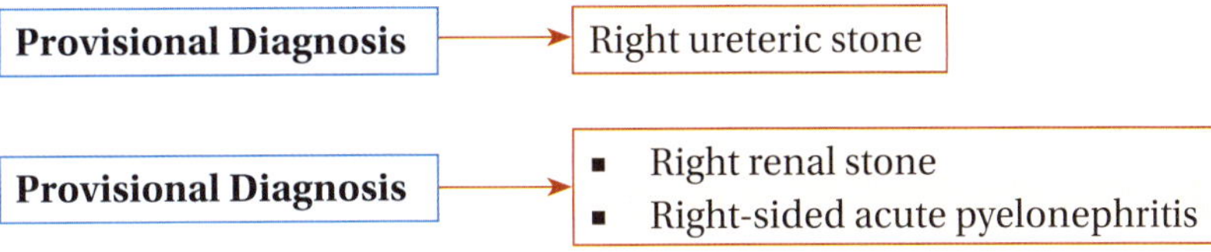

Investigations

- X-ray KUB revealed no significant findings as it was almost obscured by gas shadow.
- Non-contrast CT KUB suggestive of stone measuring 7 mm in the right upper ureter with mild hydronephrosis.
- Urine for RE and ME revealed no significant abnormalities.

Discussion

The history of acute onset pain in the loin radiating to the groin is highly suggestive of ureteric stone. Non-contrast CT KUB confirmed the diagnosis. As 7 mm stone in upper ureter with hydronephrotic changes, chances of spontaneous passage was less. Though Shock Wave Lithotripsy (SWL) is the preferred option in this patient, laparoscopic ureterolithotomy was planned as facility of SWL was not available.

Management Algorithm

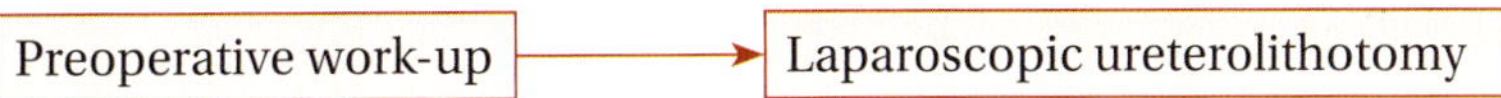

Case 2

History and Physical Examination

A 49-year-old male patient presented in the surgical OPD with an ulcerated lesion over the penis for last 4 months. Patient noticed a nodular lesion about 5 months back that became ulcerated. The ulcer was painful. He also noticed swelling in his right groin for last 3 months. History of smoking for last 20 years. No history of diabetes or hypertension.

Physical Examination

A tender ulcer-proliferative lesion over the glans penis also encroaching the proximal shaft. Multiple inguinal lymph nodes were palpable, size less than 3 cm, not fixed to the overlying skin or underlying structures in the right side.

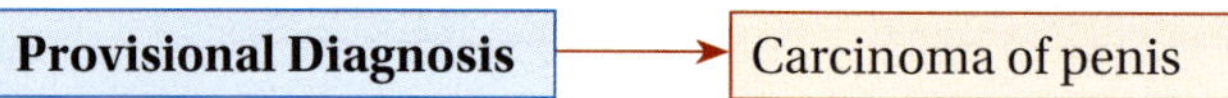

Investigations

- Incisional biopsy from the lesion revealed squamous cell carcinoma. FNAC from the inguinal lymph nodes revealed metastatic lymph nodes.
- CT abdomen and chest revealed no distant metastases.

Discussion

A middle-aged patient presented with ulcero-proliferative growth in penis along with inguinal lympadenopathy highly suggestive of carcinoma penis. Histopathology report confirmed the diagnosis and cytology of inguinal lymph nodes revealed presence of inguinal lymph node metastases. CT abdomen and chest excluded any distant metastases. Based on the location of tumor, partial penectomy followed by bilateral inguinal lymph node dissection was planned.

Management Algorithm

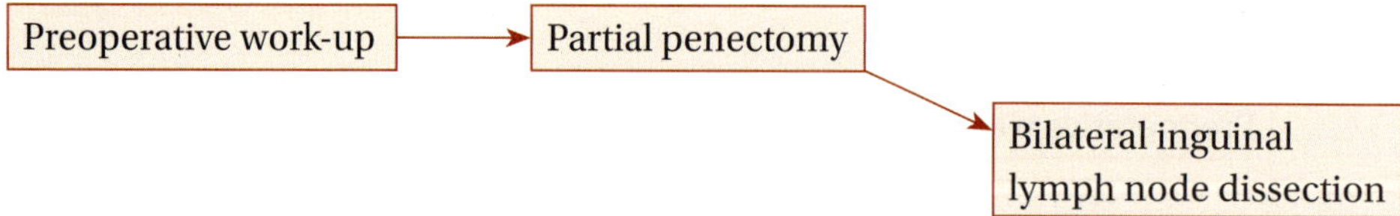

Chapter 26

Minimally Invasive Surgery

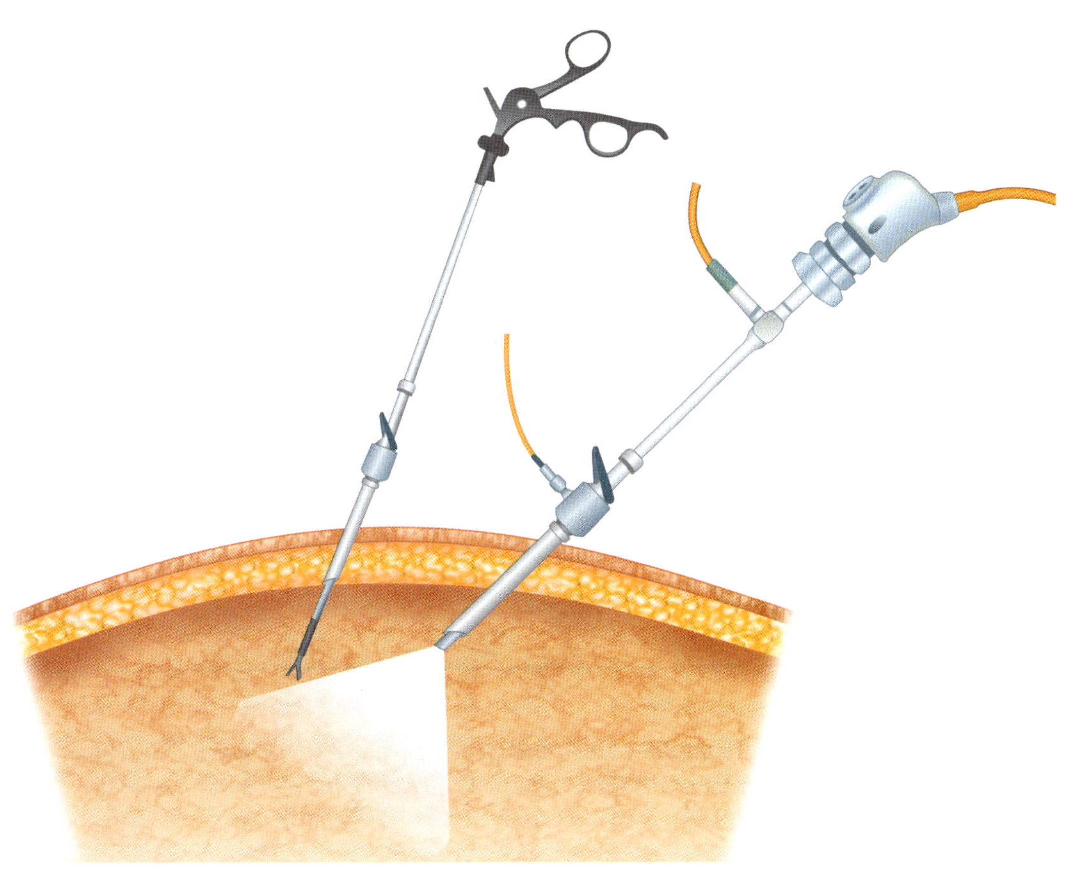

Important Topics

- Different Minimal Access Techniques
- Physiology of Pneumoperitoneum
- Laparoscopic Access
- Principles of Port Placement
- Instrumentation
- Sterilization of Laparoscopic Instruments
- Energy Sources in Minimally Invasive Surgery
- Complications of Laparoscopy
- NOTES and SILS
- Robotic Surgery

'The mind likes a strange idea as little as the body likes a strange protein and resists it with a similar energy. It would not perhaps, be too fanciful to say that a new idea is the most quickly acting antigen known to science.'

Wilfrid Batten Lewis Trotter (1872–1939)
British Surgeon and Sociologist

Different Minimal Access Techniques

Laparoscopy

Access to the inflated peritoneal cavity (pneumoperitoneum) through port (cannula).

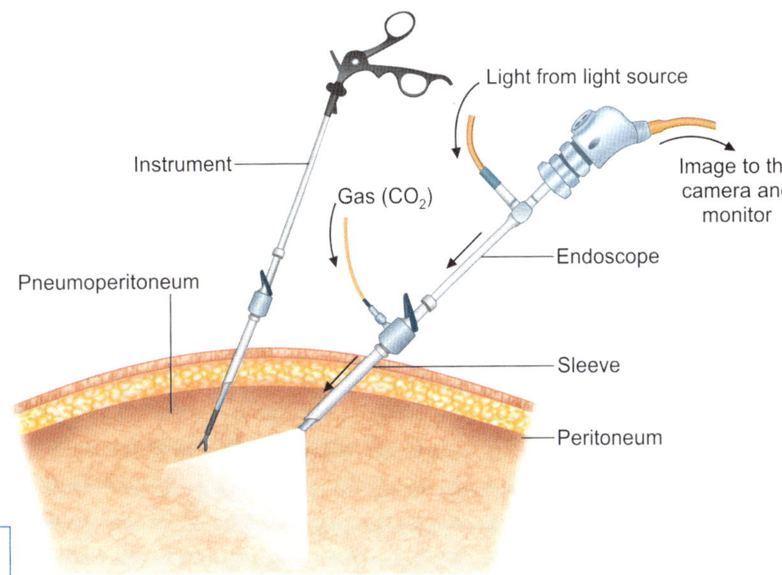

Extracavitary Minimally Invasive Surgery

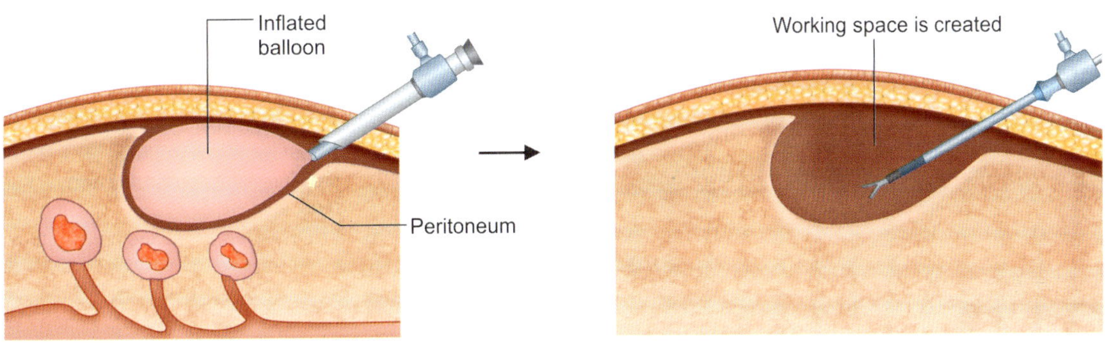

Different extracavitary body planes, e.g., retroperitoneal space, space of Retzius, extraperitoneal space, subfascial space of leg are accessed after creating working space by balloon inflation. *Examples:* TEP repair of inguinal hernia, laparoscopic nephrectomy, and subfascial perforator ligation.

Endoluminal Endoscopy

Rigid or flexible endoscopes are introduced into the urinary tract (cystoscopy), gastrointestinal tract (upper and lower GI endoscopy), respiratory tract (bronchoscopy).

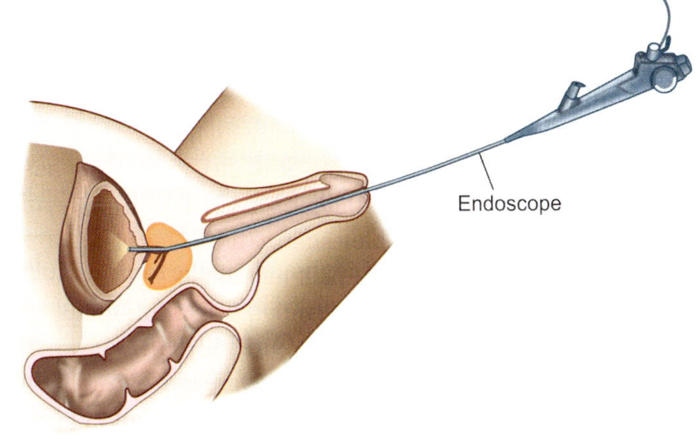

Thoracoscopy

Thoracic cavity is accessed through a rigid endoscope.

Physiology of Pneumoperitoneum

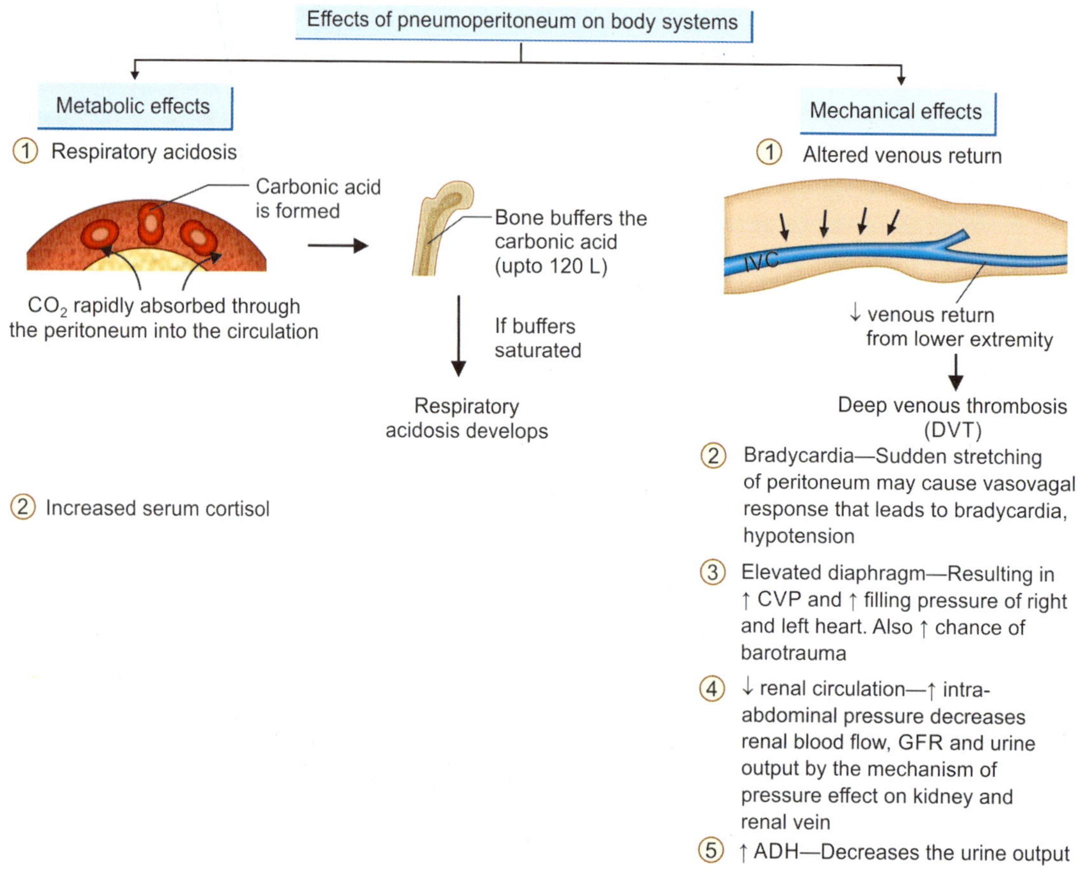

Laparoscopic Access

Methods of access to the abdominal cavity for creating pneumoperitoneum:

(i) Closed technique (by Veress needle); (ii) Direct trocar insertion (DTI); (iii) Open technique (Hasson's technique or Fielding technique); and (iv) Optical trocar technique

Access Locations

Umbilical point:

- Most common location where Veress needle is inserted.
- Easy access because it is the thinnest part of the abdominal wall.
- Significant blood vessels are not present.
- In umbilical point, 3 possible sites of incision: (i) Superior crease; (ii) Inferior crease; and (iii) Transumbilical.
- Contraindications are previous midline incision, portal hypertension, presence of urachal cyst or umbilical hernia.

Palmer's point:

- 2 cm below the left subcostal margin in the midclavicular line.
- This access should be considered in patients with previous laparotomy, in obese and extremely thin patients, very thin women with android pelvis and prominent sacral promontory.
- Gastric decompression is mandatory before access in this location.
- Access in this point should be avoided in patients with gastric or splenic surgery, hepatosplenomegaly, portal hypertension.

Lee-Huang point:
- Midway between xiphoid process and umbilicus
- This access point can overcome adhesions caused by previous low-midline incision.
- Provides central vision rather than lateral vision.
- Contraindications are previous midline vertical incision, hepatosplenomegaly.

Closed Technique (By Veress Needle)

Before closed entry, following measures should be taken: (i) Insertion of nasogastric tube and urinary catheter (a distended urinary bladder or stomach increases the chance of iatrogenic injuries); (ii) Patient should be in horizontal position; and (iii) Checking of the Veress needle for spring action, opening of its tip and unrestricted CO_2 flow.

Skin incision: The ideal site of skin incision is the deepest point of the umbilical pit. This is the thinnest point of the abdominal wall (at this point, skin, subcutaneous tissue, fascia and parietal peritoneum fuse).

Access locations: (i) Umbilical point (most common); (ii) Palmer's point; and (iii) Lee-Huang point. Umbilicus is the preferred site of access because: (i) Thinnest point of the abdominal wall; (ii) Better cosmesis; and (iii) Better ergonomics (because of its central position in abdomen).

Trajectory and insertion angle of the Veress needle: If access location is the umbilical point, the trajectory of the Veress needle should be towards the foot end. The insertion angle should vary between 45° in non-obese patient and 90° in morbidly obese patients.

Elevation of the abdominal wall: The Veress needle is introduced after lifting the abdominal wall with towel clip or firm hand grip. Surgeon can feel two clicks as the needle penetrate the fascia and the peritoneum. Lateral movements of the needle should be avoided (to avoid enlargement of any vessel or visceral injury).

Verification of correct placement of Veress needle: Different tests for verification of correct placement are: (i) Aspiration test; (ii) Saline hanging-drop test; and (iii) Quadro-manometric test.

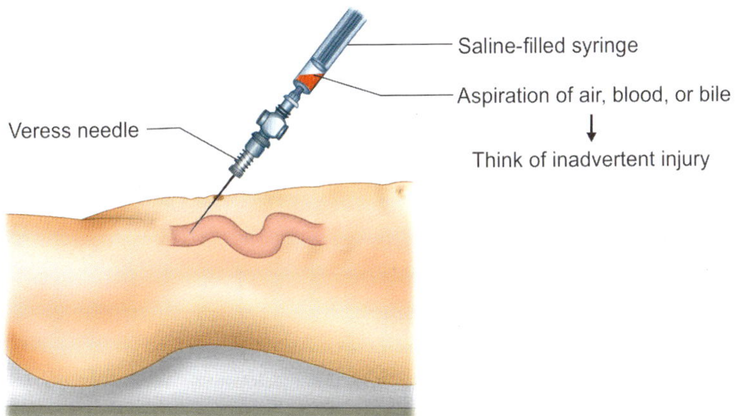

Aspiration Test

Saline is injected through the Veress needle. The irrigated fluid cannot be aspirated if needle is in peritoneal cavity. If needle is in pre-peritoneal space or muscle layer, some amount of fluid is aspirated back. If more fluid is coming, either bladder injury or ascites should be suspected. If bile or fecal matter is aspirated, bowel injury should be suspected.

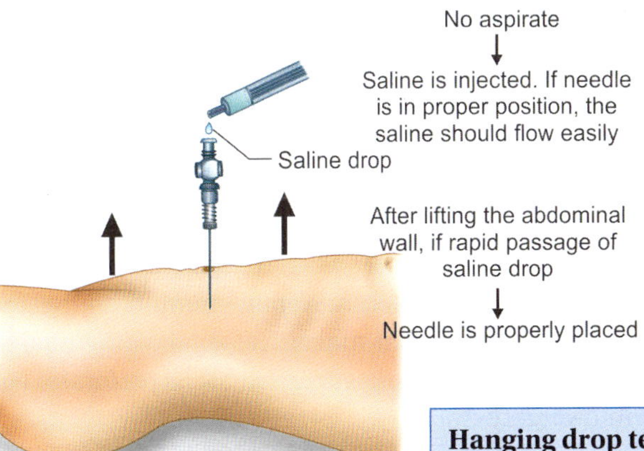

Hanging drop test

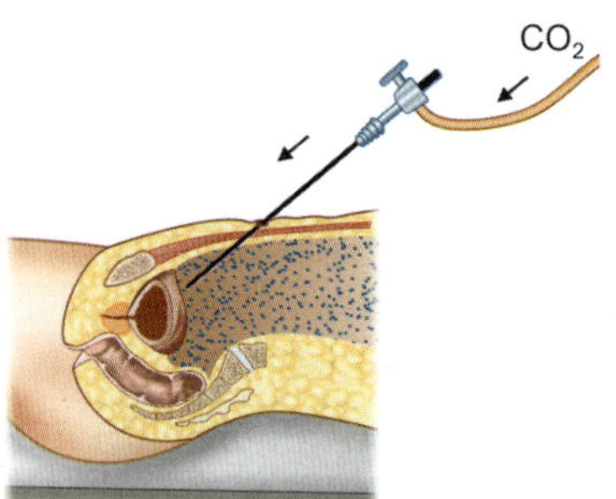

After confirming the correct placement of Veress needle, insufflation tubing is attached to the needle for creating pneumoperitoneum.

Important Indicators of Insufflator

i. **Preset insufflation pressure:** Preset pressure should be 12 mm Hg. It should not be more than 18 mm Hg.
ii. **Actual intra-abdominal pressure:** The pressure sensed by the insufflator.
iii. **Flow rate:** Initial flow rate should be adjusted to 1 liter/minute.
iv. **Total gas used:** About 1.5 liter of gas is needed to achieve intra-abdominal pressure of 12 mm Hg.

Open Technique (Hasson's Technique)

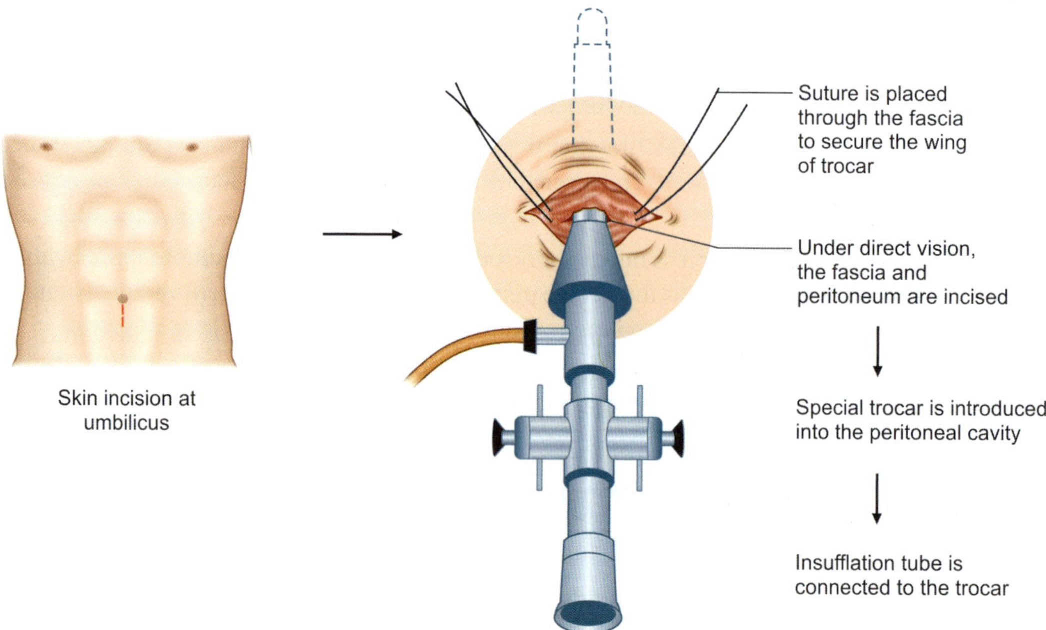

Advantages of Open Technique

- No chance of extraperitoneal insufflation
- Less risk of vascular or intestinal injuries
- Retrieval of surgical specimen is easier through the larger umbilicus incision.

Extraperitoneal and Subcutaneous Access

Access to retroperitoneum: Nephrectomy, ureterolithotomy, adrenalectomy
Access to preperitoneal space: TEP repair of inguinal hernia
Access to subcutaneous space: Subfascial perforator ligation, minimally invasive thyroid surgery

Hand-assisted Laparoscopic Access

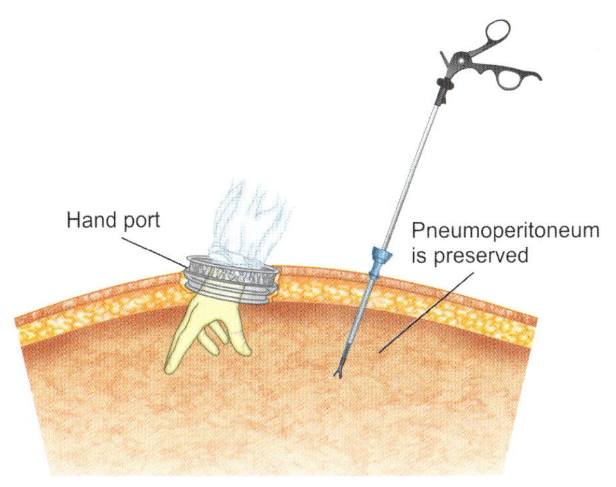

- A sleeve appliance is used to maintain pneumoperitoneum while the Surgeon's hand can be inserted.
- Particularly indicated in advanced colon surgery.
- **Advantages:** (i) Maintenance of tactile sensation and (ii) Advantages of digital dissection and digital pressure in intraoperative bleeding.

Principles of Port Placement

Baseball Diamond Concept of Port Positioning

1. The laparoscopy instruments should be work like type 1 lever.
2. Half of the instruments should be inside and half should be outside.
3. The **manipulation angle** should be 60° (±15°) and **azimuth angle** should be 30° on either side.

Manipulation angle	Azimuth angle	Elevation angle
Angle between the two instruments (active and assisting)	Angle between the instrument and the optical axis of the endoscope	Angle between the instrument and the horizontal plane
Ideally it should be 60° ±15°	Ideally it should be 30°	Should be 60°

Instrumentation

Imaging System

The imaging chain in laparoscopy requires seven pieces of equipment: (i) Telescope (visual channel with fiber-optic light channel); (ii) Light source; (iii) Fiber-optic light cable; (iv) Camera head; (v) Video signal processor; (vi) Video cable; and (vii) Monitor, known as the 'Magnificent Seven'.

Telescope

Standard telescope is a metal shaft containing series of **quartz-rod lenses (Hopkins rod lens system)** and **optical fibers**.

Length of telescope: 24 cm; Diameter of telescope: (i) 10 mm (most commonly used); (ii) 5 mm (for use through 5 mm ports); and (iii) 1.5 mm (for pediatric laparoscopy).

Angle of laparoscope: (i) Flat-end (0°)—provides straight view and (ii) Angled-end (30° and 45°)—provides oblique view as well as wider field of view.

Total field of view: The 0° telescope provides field of view of 76° and the 30° telescope provides field of view of 152°.

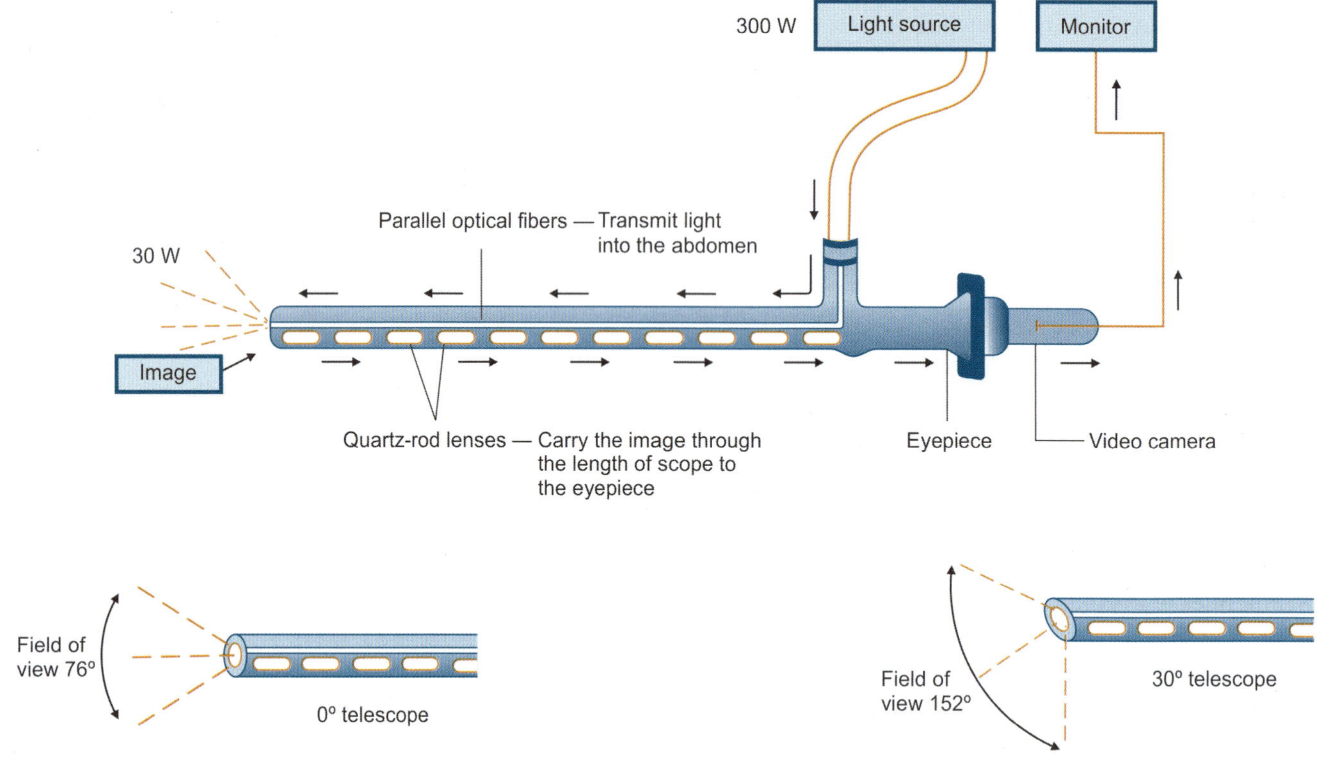

Video Camera

Video camera is attached to the eyepiece of the telescope. For proper color representation, three-chip camera is required. Three charge-coupling device (CCD) is used for each red, green, and blue (RGB) color. In minimally invasive procedures, illumination is the 1st priority, followed by resolution and then color.

Light Source

Three types of light sources are available: (i) Halogen light source (150 watt); (ii) Xenon light source (300 watt); and (iii) Metal halide light source (250 watt)

Video Monitor

Video monitor is used to display the images. High-definition monitors have a resolution of up to eight times more than a standard NTSC/PAL monitors.

Hand Instruments

Hand instruments are longer and narrower than instruments used in open surgery. Standard hand instruments are 36 cm long and 5 mm in diameter. Shorter and narrower instruments are used in pediatric laparoscopy and longer instruments are used in bariatric surgery.

Ports

Ports are of different varieties: (i) Resusable or disposable; (ii) Blunt-ended or sharp-ended; and (iii) 5 mm or 10 mm. All ports have attachments for insufflation and valves to prevent gas leak.

Insufflator

Insufflator supplies the CO_2 and maintains the pneumoperitoneum. It maintains the gas flow according to preset pressure values.

Dimension of Laparoscopic Instruments

Instrument	Dimension
Telescope	**Diameter:** 1.5–15 mm (common is 5 mm and 10 mm) **Length:** 24–33 cm **Angle of view:** 0° to 120° (0° and 30° are common)
Insufflator	**Insufflation pressure:** 0–30 mm Hg **Total gas flow volume:** 0–9.9 liters/mm
Veress needle	**Length:** 80 mm, 100 mm, 120 mm
Port (cannula)	**Diameter:** 3–30 mm (common is 5 mm and 10 mm)
Hand instruments	**Length:** 18–45 cm (for adult, 36 cm)
Clips	**Length:** 7 mm, 9 mm, 11 mm

Types of clips: (i) Titanium clips and (ii) Hem-o-lok clip (nonabsorbable polymer clip with lock-engagement feature as well as teeth within the jaws).

Size of titanium clips	Cartridge color	Pcs/cartridge
Small	Blue	6
Medium	White	6
Med-large	Green	6
Large	Yellow	6

Cleaning and Sterilization of Laparoscopic Instruments

1. **Cleaning of endoscope:**
    - All three optical surfaces (distal optic, fiber optic surface and eyepiece/proximal optic surface) must be cleaned.
    - Cleaning should be done with warm water and recommended pH-neutral cleaning and disinfecting solution. The endoscope should be rinsed thoroughly to remove the cleaning solution.
    - Each optical surface should be checked with reflective light for foreign particles and scratches.
    - Ultrasonic cleaners should not be used (it will damage the optical system).
2. **Sterilization of endoscope:**
    - By chemical sterilization. During the sterilization process, there should not be any contact between the endoscope and any other metal parts.
    - Endoscope cannot be autoclaved unless it is "AUTOCLAVABLE".
3. **Cleaning of hand instruments:**
    - Cleaning removes most of the bioburden (debris, blood, tissues), which interfere with the action of disinfectants.
    - Soft nylon brush is used to remove exterior dirt and debris. Instruments that are equipped with LUER-LOCK connection, should be opened and force flushed with water under pressure.
    - During cleaning, any damaged, worn, corroded area in the instrument should be noted.
    - In ultrasonic cleaners, all jointed instruments should be placed in an open position.

4. **Sterilization of hand instruments:**
   - By steam sterilization or chemical sterilization
   - During steam sterilization, instrument jaws and rachets must be in open position. Cutting edges and tips of instruments must be protected with soft cloth.

Different Methods of Chemical Sterilization

1. **Ethylene oxide (ETO) sterilization:**
   - It is a low-temperature (37–63°) sterilization process.
   - Effectiveness of sterilization depends on: (i) Gas concentration (450–1200 mg/L); (ii) Temperature (37–63°); (iii) Relative humidity (40–80%); and (iv) Exposure time (1–6 hours).
   - Available ETO gas mixtures are: (i) 8.5% ETO + 91.5% CO_2 and (ii) ETO + hydrofluorocarbon.
   - This method of sterilization is used to sterilize critical items and some semicritical items that are moisture and heat sensitive and cannot be sterilized by steam sterilization.
2. **Activated 2% aqueous glutaraldehyde solution (Cidex):**
   - A high-level disinfectant for semi-critical, heat-sensitive medical devices.
   - Provides sterilization in 10 hours at 25°C in especially designed tray (Cidex tray).
   - Once activated, the solution must be discarded after 21 days.
3. **0.55% Orthophthalaldehyde (Cidex OPA):**
   - A quick and high-level disinfectant for semicritical, heat-sensitive medical devices.
   - No activation or mixing is required.
   - Provides sterilization in an automatic endoscope reprocessor in 5 minutes at 25°C or in 12 minutes at 20°C manually.
   - The solution must be discarded after 14 days.
4. **Formaldehyde:**
   - Sterilization of heat-sensitive instruments by formaldehyde in especially designed cabinet.
   - Eight to ten formalin tablets (paraformaldehyde 96%) wrapped with moist gauge are placed in the chamber.
   - Tablets have to be changed after 1 week.

Energy Sources in Minimally Invasive Surgery

Radiofrequency Electrosurgery

Radiofrequency electrosurgery is the most popular energy source in minimally invasive surgery. RF electrosurgery delivers an alternating current of 300–500 KHz. This causes tissue heating that results in coagulation (60°C), dessication (100°C), and carbonization (>200°C). The radiofrequency can be delivered by monopolar or bipolar electrodes.

Components of a monopolar electrosurgical circuit: (i) Electrosurgical generator; (ii) Active electrode; (iii) Patient; and (iv) Return electrode.

Components of a bipolar electrosurgical circuit: (i) Electrosurgical generator and (ii) Bipolar electrode.

Electrosurgical tissue effects are: (i) Cutting; (ii) Fulguration (noncontact coagulation); and (iii) Dessication (contact coagulation).

Fulguration (Spray coagulation) is a type of non-contact coagulation effect by using high voltage, low frequency waveform. The active electrode is held away from the tissue (3–4 mm). Significant tissue charring and small vessel (<1 mm) hemostasis can be achieved. With repeated application, temperature increase beyond 100°C. Lateral thermal spread is more than the deeper tissue spread.

Desiccation is a contact type of coagulation in which active electrode is in direct contact with the tissues. It causes greater lateral thermal spread as well as deeper tissue necrosis.

Electrosurgical tissue effects depend on following factors: (i) Current density; (ii) Time duration of activation of active electrode; (iii) Electrode size; (iv) Tissue conductivity; (v) Current waveforms; and (vi) Manipulation of the electrode (contact with tissues or noncontact).

Unipolar Electrosurgery

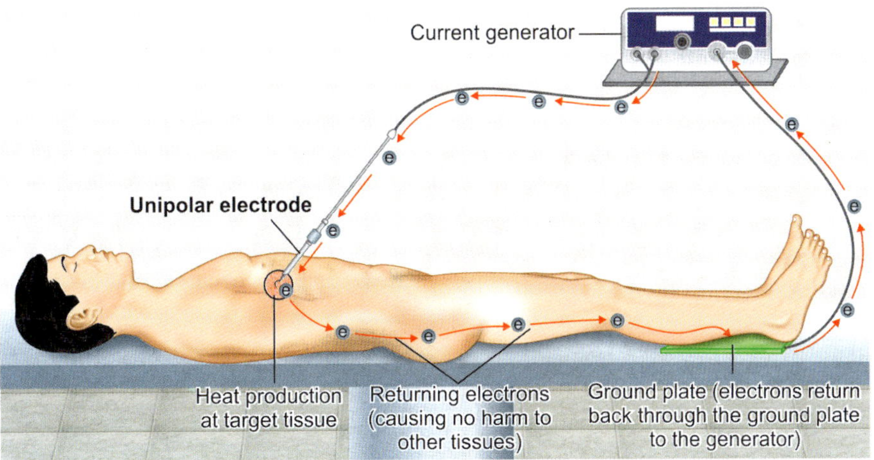

Proper Positioning of Return Electrode (Ground Plate)

- Site should be as close to operative site.
- Site should be well-vascularized muscle mass.
- Any bony prominences or irregular body contour site must be avoided.
- Area of vascular insufficiency should be avoided.

Bipolar Electrosurgery

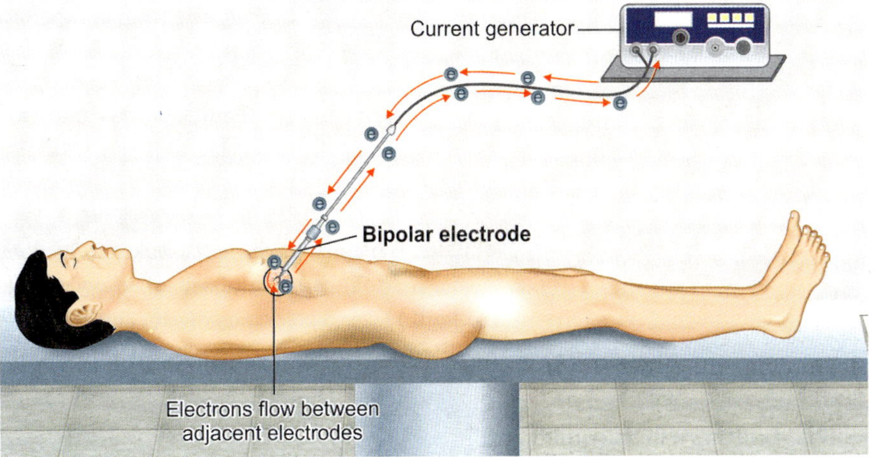

Electrosurgery	Electrocautery
Uses alternating current	Uses direct current
Flow of radiofrequency electric current (in the range of 300–500 KHz) generates heat in the tissues	Heated wire directly transfers the heat in the tissues
Patient is included in the circuit.	Patient is not in the circuit.

Unipolar Electrosurgery	Bipolar Electrosurgery
Patient is included in the circuit	Patient is out of the circuit
Can be used for both cutting and coagulation	Not suitable for tissue cutting
Can seal only smaller vessels (<2 mm)	Can seal vessels upto 5 mm
Chance of burn injury in return electrode site	No chance of such burn
More lateral thermal spread	Lateral thermal spread is less
Interfere with pacemaker function	Not interfering with pacemaker function

Waveforms of Electrosurgical Unit

Cutting waveform Continuous (100% duty cycle), unmodulated, undamped	**Low voltage, continuous waveform** is applied through the monopolar active electrode near the tissue, create a spark gap, through which current arcs to the tissue. ⇩ Rapid production of heat with rise in temperature (>100°C) ⇩ Rapid tissue vaporization ⇩ Cutting Depth of tissue necrosis is minimal, smoke production is minimal, energy loss is more.
Coagulation waveform Interrupted (6% duty cycle), modulated, damped	**High voltage, low frequency waveform** is applied by direct contact to the tissues ⇩ Temperature reaches between 70–80°C ⇩ Formation of coagulum ⇩ Coagulation Tissue damage is more, more smoke production
Blended waveform • Combination of both cutting and coagulation waveform – Blend 1 (80% cut, 20% coagulation) – Blend 2 (60% cut, 40% coagulation) – Blend 3 (50% cut, 50% coagulation)	**Blend 1** produces maximum heat, **Blend 3** produces minimum heat. **Blend 1** is used predominantly for **cutting,** Blend 2 for predominantly cutting with hemostasis, whereas **Blend 3** is used predominantly for **hemostasis**.

Complications of Electrosurgery

- **Electrothermal injury of organs adjacent to target organ**—due to unintended activation of active electrode or lateral thermal spread.
- **Insulation failure**—due to break in insulation of the instrument caused by repetitive use, repeated sterilization, high intensity of current flowing through the wire (most common site of insulation failure is distal third of laparoscopic hand instruments).
- **Residual heat**—in tip of the energy devices
- **Direct coupling**—when active electrode is touched by another metal instrument or scope.
- **Capacitive coupling**—when electrical current is established in the metal instrument running parallel to the active electrode, but not in direct contact. Metal instrument (metal cannula) can discharge the charge into the body but hybrid instruments (metal with plastic) cannot discharge as plastic act as a insulator.
- **Antenna coupling**—during use of monopolar energy use, radiofrequency energy from a insulated wire/cable is transmitted into nearby conductors (cables, instruments).
- Burn in return electrode site (in monopolar electrosurgery)
- Interaction with electronic devices (e.g., cardiac monitor, pacemaker)
- Operating room fire

Safety Precautions for Electrosurgery

- The ESU should not be used in the presence of inflammable agents (i.e., alcohol and/or tincture-based agents) [AORN Recommendation 2003]
- "The active electrode(s) should be placed in a clean, dry, well-insulated safety holster when not in use". [AORN Recommendation 2003]
- Insulation of the instrument should be checked carefully before surgery.
- Use lowest possible power setting.
- Use a low voltage waveform (cutting mode).
- Use short intermittent activation rather than prolonged activation.
- Do not activate in open circuit.
- Bipolar electrosurgery should be used when appropriate.
- Hybrid cannula system (metal with plastic) should not be used.
- Active and dispersive electrode cords should be separated from other nearby cables/wires to prevent antenna coupling.
- Use of monopolar energy should be avoided in single incision laparoscopic surgery to prevent antenna coupling.
- Newer technology, i.e., tissue response generator (to reduce capacitive coupling), active electrode monitoring system (to reduce risk of insulation failure and capacitive coupling), return electrode monitoring system (to reduce risk of burn in return electrode site) should be used, if available.
- Red rubber catheter or other plastic materials should not be used as a sheath on active electrodes (these materials may ignite with high-power settings).
- Cords should not be wrapped around metal instruments (current leakage, if happens, may conducted via metal instruments).

Return Electrode Monitoring System

A technology to protect burn in return electrode site. REM™-equipped generators actively monitor the level of impedance at the patient-return electrode pad interface. If the system detects a high level of impedance at patient-pad interface, the electrosurgical generator is deactivated.

Advanced Bipolar Devices

ENSEAL®

- An bipolar electrosurgical technology that combines pressure and energy to create a permanent seal.
- Can seal **vessels upto 7 mm in diameter** and tissue bundles.
- Can adjust dose energy in a tissue bundle according to impedance characteristics.
- Minimal thermal spread.

LigaSure™

- An bipolar electrosurgical technology that combines pressure and energy to create a permanent seal
- Can seal **vessels upto 7 mm in diameter** and tissue bundles
- Delivers pulsed energy with continuous feedback control
- Automatically cuts off energy supply when sealing effect is achieved
- Minimal thermal spread.

THUNDERBEAT®

- An energy device that can **deliver both advanced bipolar energy and ultrasonic energy**.
- The 'seal' mode delivers advanced bipolar energy whereas its 'seal and cut' mode delivers both type of energy.
- Can seal **vessels upto 7 mm**.
- Faster precise tissue dissection.

Harmonic Scalpel

- An ultrasonic energy device for cutting and coagulation.
- The piezoelectric transducers in the instrument **convert electrical energy into mechanical vibrations (55,000 cycles/second)**.
- The cutting mechanisms are: (i) Cavitational cutting and fragmentation (due to large pressure changes, cellular water vaporizes) and (ii) Protein denaturation (by breaking down the hydrogen bonds in tissues caused by vibrations).
- Can seal vessels upto 2–3 mm. Newer generation devices can seal **vessels upto 7 mm (Harmonic ACE® + 7 shears)**.
- Advantages are: (i) Less risk of thermal injury; (ii) No smoke production; and (iii) Less chance of charring and dessication of tissues.

FUSE (Fundamental Use of Surgical Energy): An educational program (by the SAGES) on energy-based surgical devices. The curriculum contains ten sections: (i) Fundamentals of electrosurgery; (ii) Mechanism and prevention of adverse events with electrosurgery; (iii) Monopolar devices; (iv) Bipolar devices; (v) Radiofrequency for soft-tissue ablation; (vi) Endoscopic devices; (vii) Ultrasonic energy devices; (viii) Microwave energy systems; (ix) Energy-based systems in pediatric surgery; and (x) Integration of energy systems with other devices.

Advantages of Minimally Invasive Surgery

- Smaller incisions
- Cosmetically better
- Minimal tissue trauma
- Earlier return to activity
- Reduced hospital stay
- Less risk of HIV, hepatitis B and C exposure
- Video recording of operative procedures

Disadvantages of Minimally Invasive Surgery

- Difficulty in depth perception due to 2D representation of the operative field
- Hand-eye coordination is required
- Tactile feedback is absent
- Technical expertise and infrastructure facility is required.

Absolute Contraindications of Minimally Invasive Surgery

- Generalized peritonitis
- Acute intestinal obstruction
- Refractory coagulopathy

Relative Contraindications of Minimally Invasive Surgery

- Pregnancy
- Cirrhosis of liver
- History of multiple abdominal operations

Complications of Laparoscopy

Related to pneumoperitoneum	Related to portinsertion	Related to procedure	Delayed complications
CO_2 embolus	Injury to vessels, viscera	Electrosurgery-related thermal injury	Port-site infection (e.g., atypical mycobacterial infection)
Respiratory acidosis	Hemorrhage	Inadvertent organ injury (e.g., CBD ligation)	Port-site hernia (commonly in umbilical port)
Cardiorespiratory compromise		Hemorrhage	

NOTES (Natural Orifice Transluminal Endoscopic Surgery)

NOTES is a type of hybrid endoscopic/surgical procedure that involves access within the abdominal cavity through a natural orifice (mouth, vagina, urethra, rectum).

Transvaginal and transgastric approaches are common in NOTES.

Examples of NOTES procedure are: Transgastric cholecystectomy, transvaginal appendectomy, transanal TME.

Advantages of NOTES are better cosmetic outcome, reduced postoperative pain, reduced risk of wound-related complications (e.g., wound infection, incisional hernia).

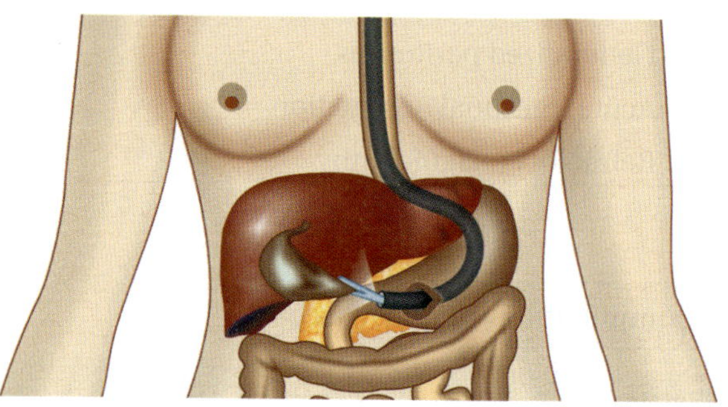

SILS (Single Incision Laparoscopic Surgery)

- SILS involves use of single port device with multiple port sites. Umbilicus is the most common site for port insertion.
- **Advantages of SILS** are better cosmetic outcome (virtually 'scarless'), reduced risk of wound related complications.
- **Technical challenges in SILS** procedure are loss of triangulation, restricted range of movements of instruments, difficulty in maintaining pneumoperitoneum.

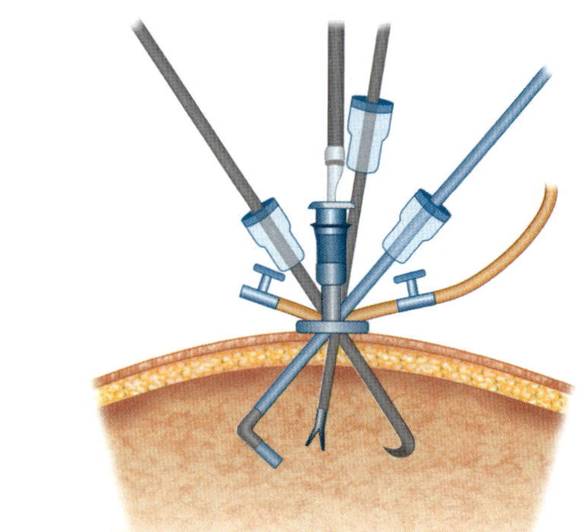

Robotic Surgery

The da Vinci® surgical system is the surgical robotic system that is used worldwide. In this system, surgery is performed by a surgeon with the help of robotic arms. This system consists of the control console, the vision system cart, and the patient (robotic) cart.

Control console: The surgeon sits at the control console and moves the "masters" or controls for the surgical instruments after viewing the 3-D image of the operative field. These movements of the surgeon are exactly translated to the robotic arms, but with more degree of freedom, more preciseness and without any tremor or fatigue.

The vision system cart: The vision system cart includes 3-D high-resolution endoscope, camera (3-chip) with camera control unit, light source and other equipment related to endoscopic camera. This system provides 3D stereoscopic vision to the surgeon.

The patient (robotic) cart: This cart provides 4 robotic arms—one for the camera and other for the instruments.

Advantages: (i) High definition 3-D stereoscopic vision. Surgeon can achieve depth perception and image detailing; (ii) More degrees of freedom of movement of instruments—enables to perform complex maneuvers in difficult anatomic areas (e.g., pelvis); (iii) Better hand-eye coordination due to visual and spatial alignment; and (iv) Motion scaling—it scales down-coarse movements of the surgeon to precise and finer movements made by the robotic arm and the tip of the instruments.

Disadvantages: (i) Higher cost; (ii) Needs adequate setup; and (iii) Needs proper training.

Uses: (i) Nissen fundoplication; (ii) Heller myotomy; (iii) Liver resection; (iv) Single-incision robotic cholecystectomy; (v) Robotic radical prostatectomy (RRP); and (vi) Robotic radical cystectomy (RRC)

Control Console

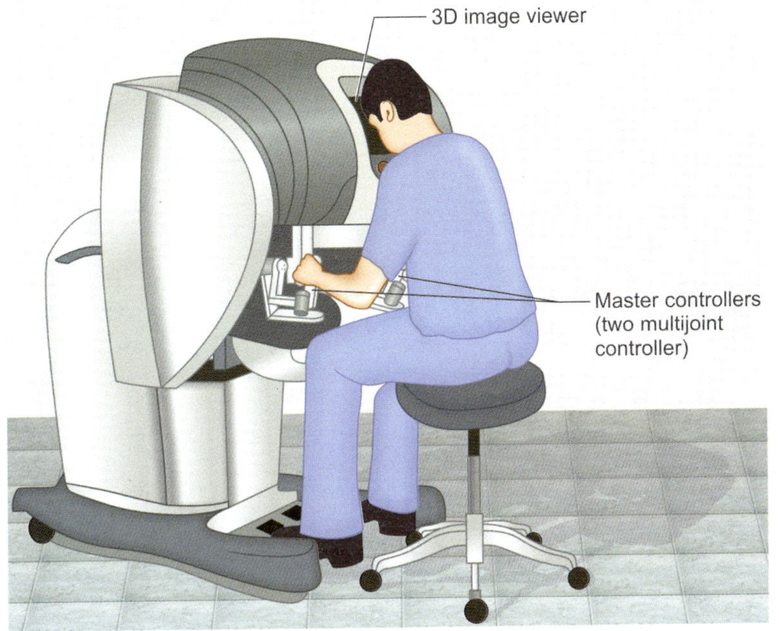

3-D High Resolution Endoscope

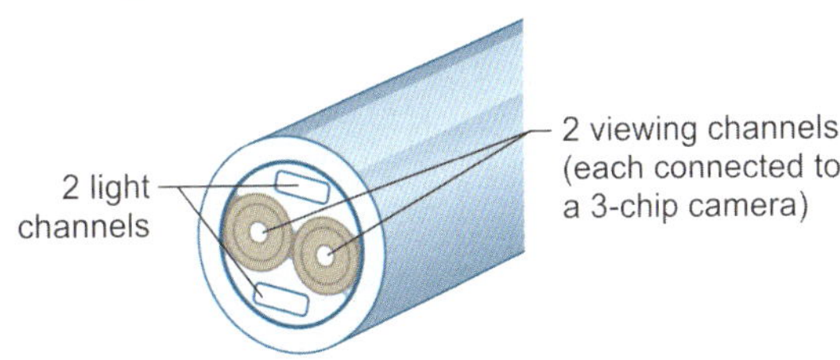

The Patient (Robotic) Cart

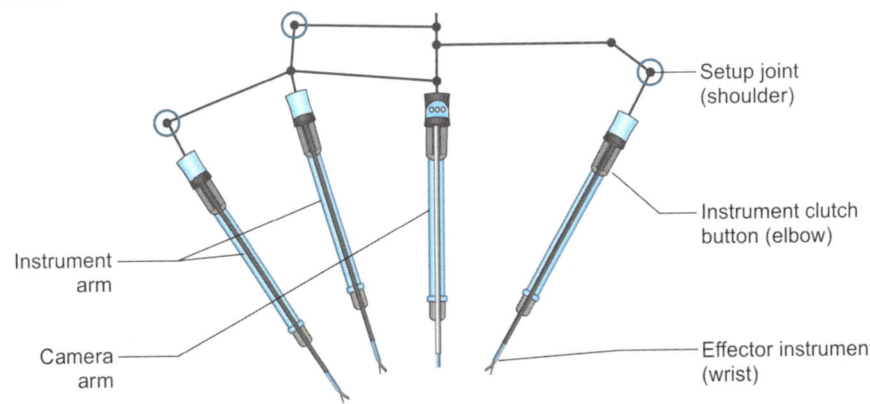

Each robotic arm has three joints:

1. Setup joint
2. Instrument clutch button
3. Effector instrument

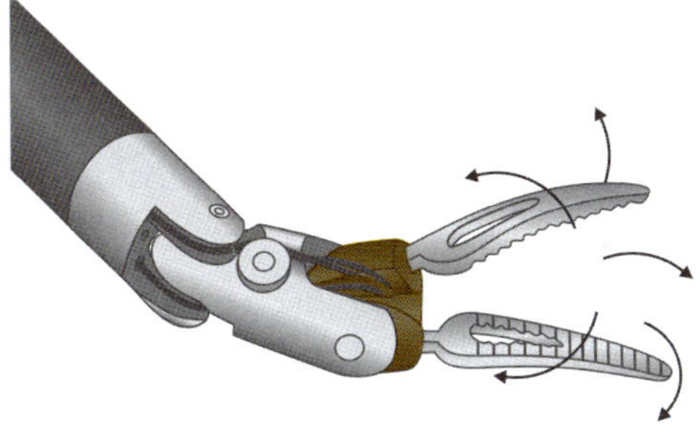

Each instrument has a wrist: The wrist provides six degrees of freedom at the tip and the seventh degree of freedom is by the instrument itself.

Chapter 27

Nerve Injury

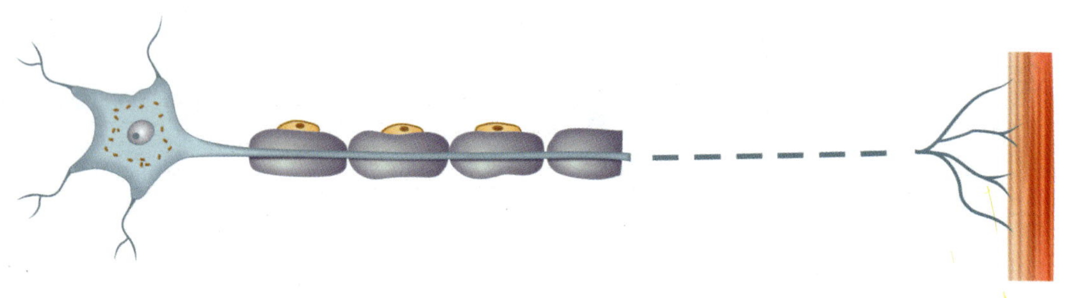

Important Topics

- Anatomy of Nerve
- Classification of Nerve Injuries
- Principles of Nerve Repair
- Injuries of Important Nerves

'Look at the sky. We are not alone. The whole universe is friendly to us and conspires only to give the best to those who dream and work.'

Anatomy of Nerve

- A **peripheral nerve trunk** is made up of many nerve fibers. Each **nerve fiber** consists of an axon which is surrounded by myelin sheath formed by Schwann cells.
- **Axon** is the process of a nerve cell (neuron). Each **neuron** consists of a cell body, dendrites and one axon.
- Group of nerve fibers form **fascicles**. Each fascicle is surrounded by a layer of connective tissue, the **perineurium**. Many such fascicles are surrounded by connective tissue sheath, called the **epineurium**. Fascicles surrounded by the epineurium form the nerve fiber.

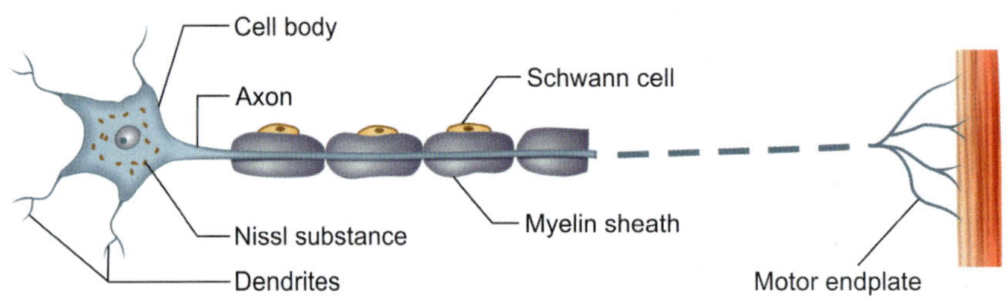

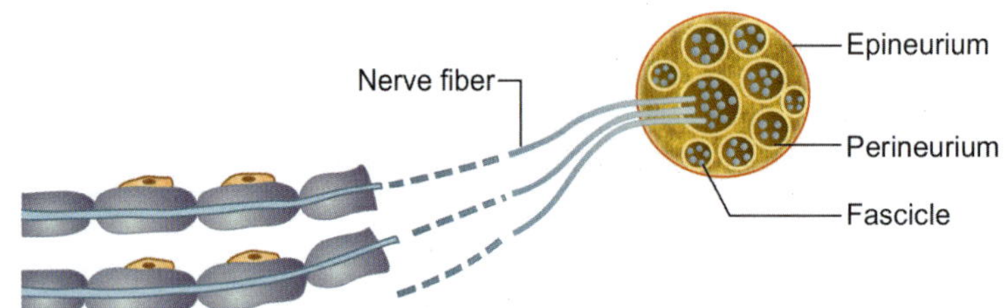

Classification of Nerve Injuries

Seddon's Classification

Neuropraxia: Local block of conduction of nerve fibers due to localized demyelination of axon
Axonotmesis: Disruption of axons and myelin sheath but perineurium and epineurium is intact

Neurotmesis: The nerve is completely severed.

Sunderland's Classification

1st degree: Neuropraxia

2nd degree: Axonotmesis

3rd degree: Disruption of axon and endoneurial tube, intact perineurium and epineurium

4th degree: Only epineurium is intact

5th degree: Epineurium is also disrupted.

[Schwann cell basement membrane along with endoneurial collagen fiber form the **endoneurial tube**]

Neuropraxia

Local block of conduction of nerve fibers due to localized demyelination of axon. Caused by compression of the nerve, mild stretching, etc. Recovery occurs spontaneously (takes days to weeks). In neuropraxia, paralysis of specific muscle groups but sensory and autonomic function is preserved.

Axonotmesis

Disruption of axons and myelin sheath but perineurium and epineurium is intact. Wallerian degeneration occurs distal to the site of injury, so distal conduction is lost. This type of nerve injury is caused by severe stretch injury of the nerve. Recovery occurs by spontaneous regeneration (1–2 mm/day). Restoration of motor and sensory function is almost normal. In axonotmesis, complete paralysis of specific muscle groups, sensory function, and autonomic function (e.g., sweating) is also lost.

Neurotmesis

The nerve is completely severed. This injury is caused by cut injury (after trauma or iatrogenic), severe traction injury. No recovery is possible unless surgical repair is undertaken. Recovery is not so perfect, in aspect of both motor and sensory function.

Neuropraxia

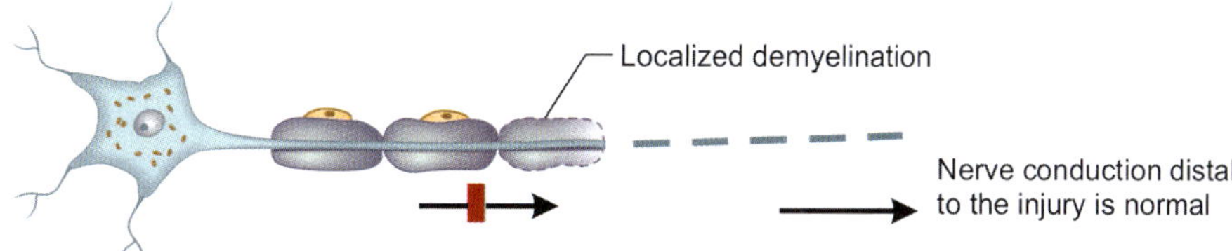

Axonotmesis

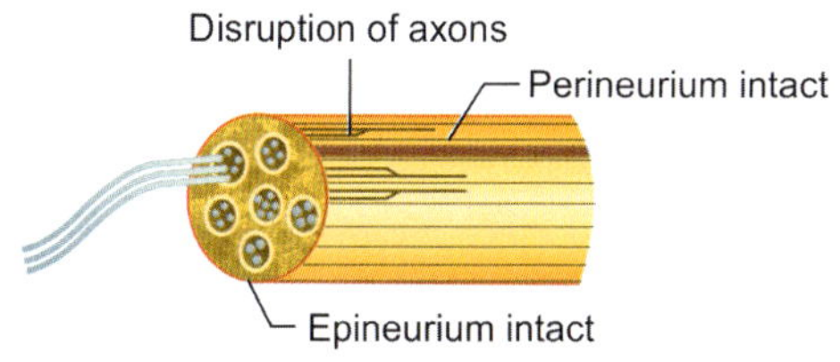

Neurotmesis

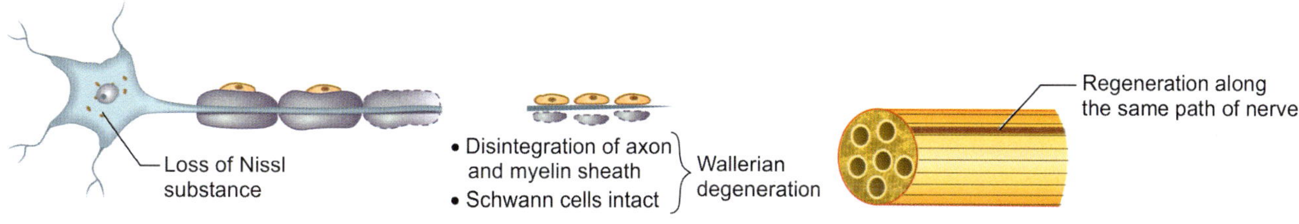

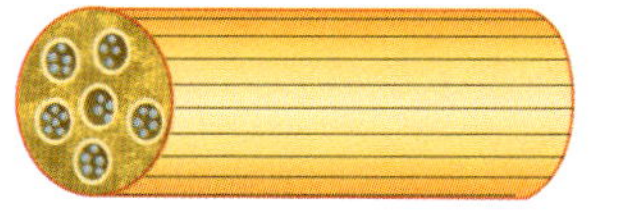

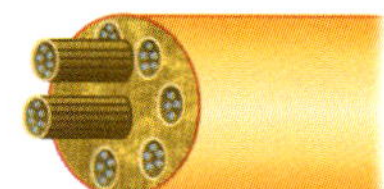

Management of Nerve Injury in Closed Wound

A loss of nerve function in a closed injury is usually due to stretch or compression. The type of injury is usually neuropraxia or axonotmesis. These types of injuries recover spontaneously, but if it is axonotmesis, recovery is usually delayed for few weeks. If any doubt about neurotmesis type of injury, the wound should be explored, as early repair carries better prognosis.

Management of Nerve Injury in Open Wound

After control of hemorrhage, the surgical exploration should be continued for search of injured nerve, if any clinical evidence of nerve injury is present. Routine exploration without any evidence of neurological deficit should be done in flexor compartment of forearm (in this region, nerves are vulnerable to damage).

Principles of Nerve Repair

Timing of Repair

- Primary repair is indicated if: (i) Wound is clean and incised; (ii) Surgeon has proper expertise; and (iii) Proper instruments (e.g., loupes, operating microscopes) available.
- Secondary repair is preferable if: (i) Wound is highly contaminated and (ii) Proper expertise and instruments are not available.

Type of Repair

- Nerve suturing is indicated if there is clean division of the nerve and after mobilization, suturing is technically possible.
- Nerve grafting is indicated if length of nerve is lost and after mobilization, suturing is technically not possible.

Choice of suture material:
Fine (8/0 or fine), nonabsorbable (e.g., prolene or nylon) suture is preferable for median nerve, 6/0 for sciatic nerve and 10/0 for digital nerve.

Basic Steps of Primary Repair

- Minimal trimming of nerve ends.
- Correct orientation of the nerve ends to minimize crossover during recovery (pattern of nerve fascicles and surface blood vessels act as guide for proper alignment).
- Sutures are placed in the epineurium (epineurial repair). No need of interfascicular repair.
- Sufficient suturing to provide epineurial cover.
- Excessive suturing must be avoided.

Basic Steps of Secondary Repair

- During wound exploration, if primary repair is technically not feasible, secondary repair to be planned.
- The severed ends should be fixed to surrounding tissue to prevent further retraction.
- During secondary repair, first to identify the nerve before dissecting the scar tissue.
- The neuroma of both ends must be excised until nerve bundles sprout from the cut surface.
- Orientation and suturing techniques are same as primary suturing.

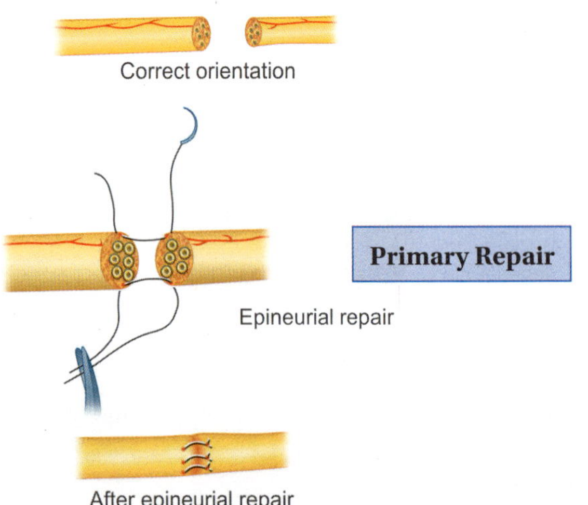

Primary Repair

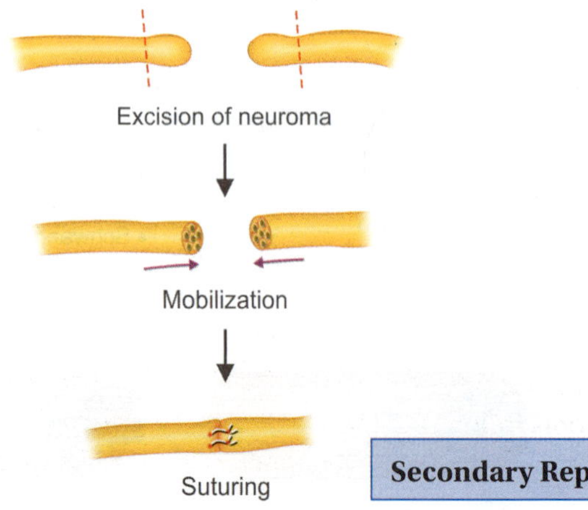

Secondary Repair

Nerve Grafting

- When direct nerve suturing is technically not feasible (defect >3 cm), nerve grafting (cable grafting) is indicated.
- The nerves that can be used as graft are sural nerve, saphenous nerve, medial cutaneous nerve of forearm (these are nerves of long length carries sensation of small areas).

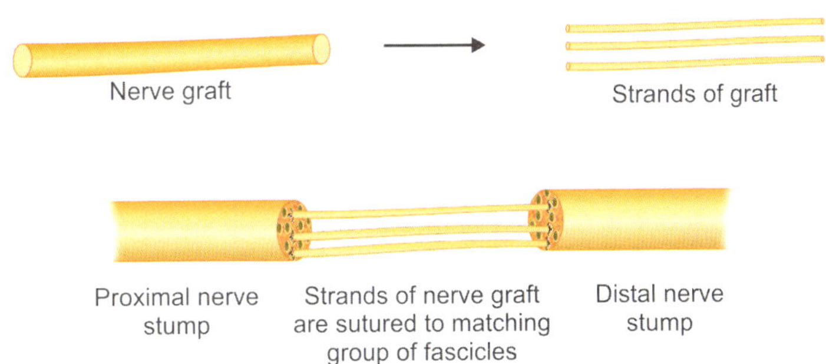

Postoperative Management

- Immobilization for 3 weeks to protect the suture line from undue tension
- Regular physiotherapy to prevent contracture and muscle atrophy
- Tinel's sign is regularly elicited to monitor axon regeneration.

Injuries of Important Nerves

Facial Nerve

Neuropraxia after superficial parotidectomy is not uncommon. Recovery within a few days is the rule. **Intraoperative transection of facial nerve is managed by:** (i) Primary repair (if no tissue loss) and (ii) Nerve grafting with greater auricular nerve (if nerve length is inadequate). Most of post-parotidectomy facial palsy are transient due to neuropraxia as a result of stretching during surgery. The injury may be in main trunk or the individual branches. Among the individual branches, marginal mandibular branch is most commonly injured. Most of the transient facial palsy resolves within 6 months.

Recurrent Laryngeal Nerve

Chance of recurrent laryngeal nerve injury is more in thyroid surgery (particularly in total thyroidectomy or re-do thyroid surgery). Neuropraxia due to dissection recovers spontaneously. In unilateral axonotmesis or neurotmesis, force of voice is reduced. In bilateral injury, both vocal cords is shifted medially. Thereby, tracheostomy is indicated to maintain the airway.

Management includes: (i) Voice therapy; (ii) Vocal cord injection technique (injection of autologous fat, minced autologous fascia lata); (iii) Open vocal cord medialization (Medialization thyroplasty); (iv) Tension-free primary anastomosis of the nerve; (v) Nerve transfer (ansa cervicalis-to-RLN anastomosis) with epineural microsuturing; and (vi) Arytenoid cartilage resection.

Brachial Plexus

Caused by: (i) Traction injuries (in motorcycle accidents); (ii) Penetrating injuries in axilla; and (iii) Iatrogenic (during axillary lymph node dissection).

In traction injury, any grade of injury like neuropraxia, axonotmesis, neurotmesis, preganglionic injury (avulsion of the roots from the spinal cord) may occur. According to degree of injury, the neurological deficit varies from paralysis and sensory loss of whole upper limb to only a specific group of muscles.

Median Nerve

- Usually injured at elbow (fracture distal humerus or dislocation of elbow joint) or at wrist (laceration or fracture distal radius).
- Paralysis of pronators and flexor muscles of wrist and fingers (except flexor carpi ulnaris and medial part of flexor digitorum profundus). Thenar muscles are also paralyzed. Sensory loss over the palmar aspect of thumb, index, middle finger, and radial half of ring finger.
- ***Ape-hand deformity*** (median claw hand deformity) may be seen due to loss of ability to abduct and oppose the thumb due to paralysis of the thenar muscles.
- ***Pointing finger*** (inability to flex the index finger) sign is seen in high median nerve palsy.

Radial Nerve

- Commonly injured in the radial groove in fracture of humeral shaft. Recovery after repair is satisfactory.
- ***Saturday night palsy*** is neuropraxia or axonotmesis of radial nerve due to pressure over the nerve, as arm is placed over the sharp back of a chair in deep sleep.
- Paralysis of brachioradialis, extensor digitorum and extensors of wrist and sensory loss over the dorsum of the thumb and first webspace develops after this nerve injury.

Ulnar Nerve

- Commonly injured following lacerations in forearm. Paralysis of small muscles of hand (except thenar muscles and lateral two lumbricals). Sensory loss over the medial one and half of the ring finger.
- ***Claw hand deformity*** (hyperextension at the metacarpophalangeal joints and flexion at the proximal and distal interphalangeal joints of the 4th and 5th fingers) may develop following ulnar nerve injury due to paralysis of the lumbricals.

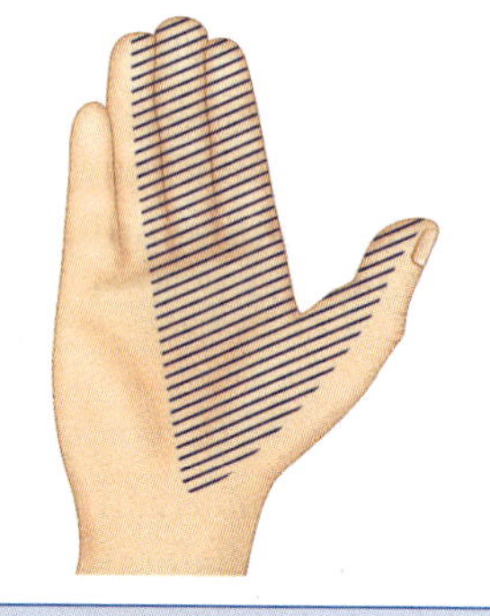

Areas of Sensory Loss in Median Nerve Injury

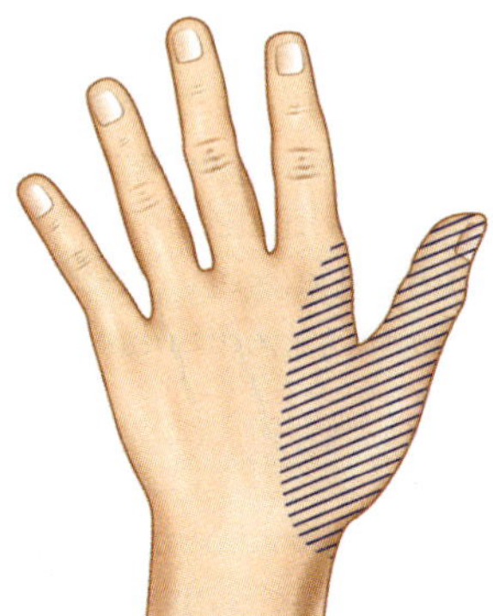

Areas of Sensory Loss in Radial Nerve Injury

Case 1

History and Physical Examination

A 40-old-year male patient presented in the surgical emergency with complains of inability to extend the right wrist and decreased sensation of the right thumb from the morning. Patient had history of falling asleep after alcohol intoxication last night. No history of any weakness, tingling or numbness in the same limb in the recent past. No history of trauma.

Clinical Examination

Inability to extend the right wrist joint and inability to extend the fingers at the metacarpophalangeal joint. Sensory loss over the dorsum of right thumb and first webspace.

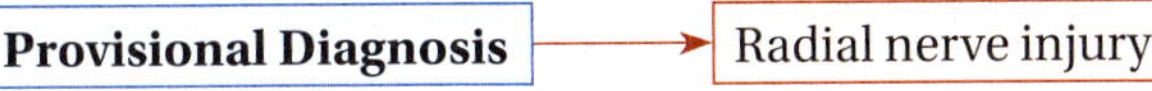

Investigations

The classic history and clinical findings suggestive of radial nerve palsy **(Saturday night palsy)**. No need of any investigations for confirmation of diagnosis.

Discussion

The classic history of falling asleep after alcohol intoxication and weakness and sensory loss in the right hand suggestive of 'Saturday night palsy'. This diagnosis is primarily clinical, so investigations are usually not indicated. Treatment is primarily physical rehabilitation.

Management Algorithm

- NSAIDs
- Systemic corticosteroids
- Wrist splint for maintaining wrist in extension

→ Dynamic splint

Surgery of Hand

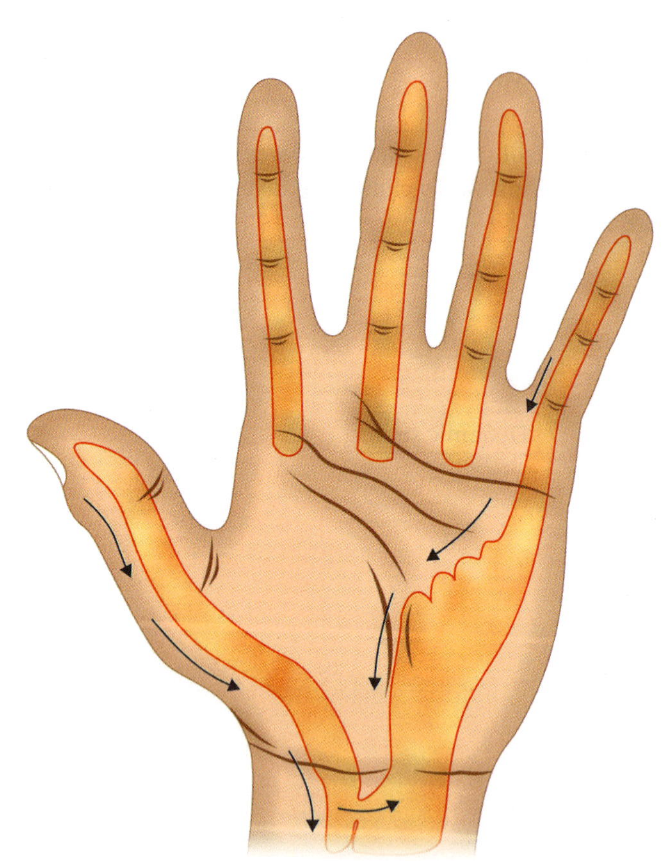

Important Topics

- Hand Infections
- Hand Injuries

'However many holy words you read, however many you speak, what good will they do you if you do not act on upon them?'

Surgery of Hand

Anesthesia in Hand Surgery

- General anesthesia
- Digital nerve block (without adrenalin)
- Brachial plexus block

Tourniquet

To make a bloodless operative field for better visualization of structures.

Different types

- **Finger tourniquet** by sterile gloves 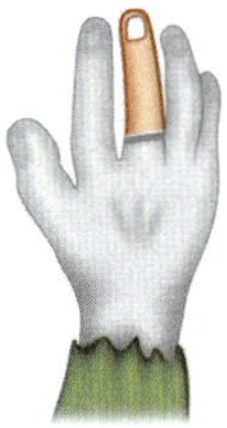
- **Pneumatic tourniquet** 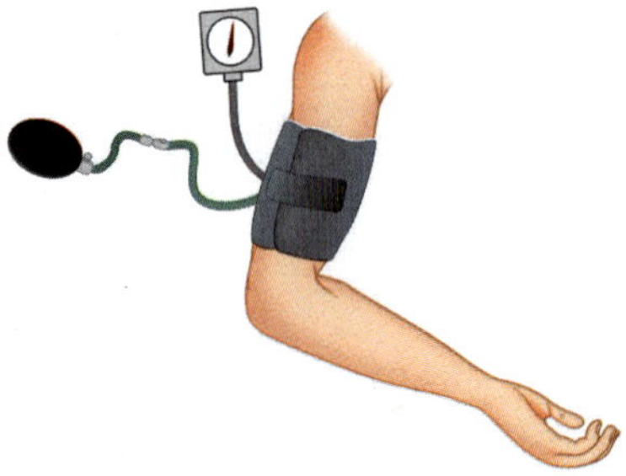
  - Pressure is 75 mm Hg over the systolic blood pressure.
  - Tourniquet time should not be more than 2 hours.
- **Esmarch bandage** 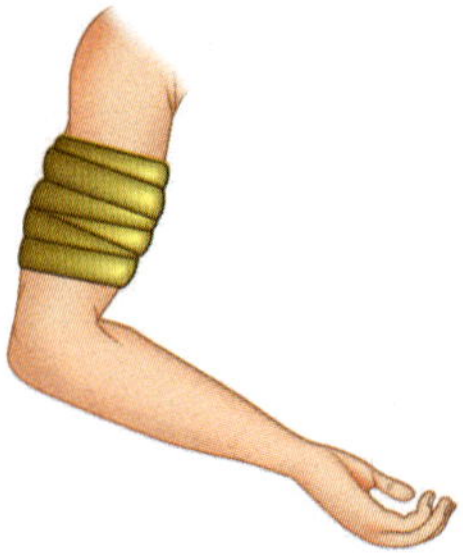
  - Should be avoided in presence of tumor or infection to avoid systemic spread.

Incisions

- Shorter incision in palmar aspect is better placed through flexion crease.
- If longer exposure is needed, a 'mid-lateral incision' is preferable.
- To prevent scar contracture formation, the incision should not cross the skin creases at right angle.
- Incision should not cross the wrist at right angles.

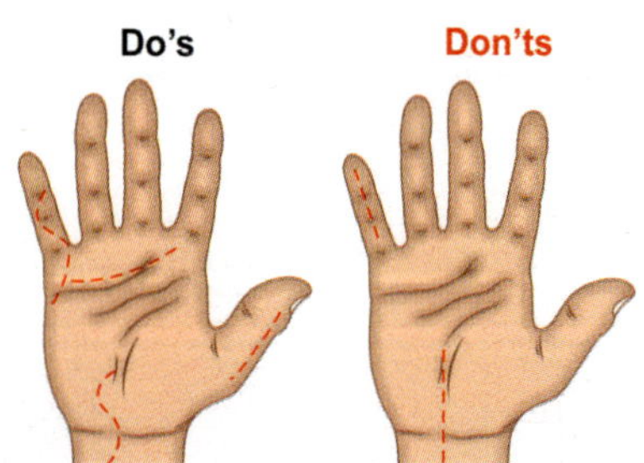

Position of Immobilization

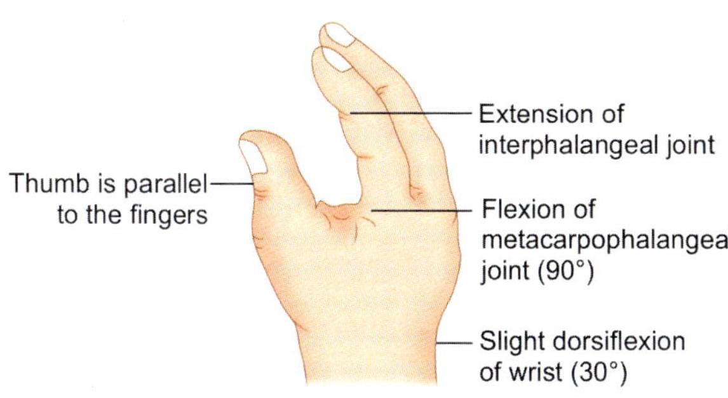

The position of immobilization is maintained by **boxing glove dressing along with plaster back slab**.

Measures to Prevent Swelling and Stiffness

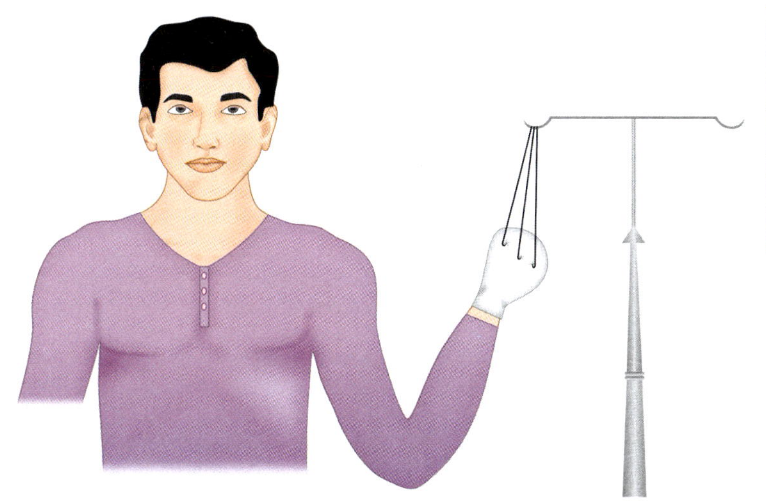

- **Elevation:** Hand must be elevated in a high sling.
- **Immobilization**
- **Early joint movement:** Movement of the joints should be restored as early as possible.

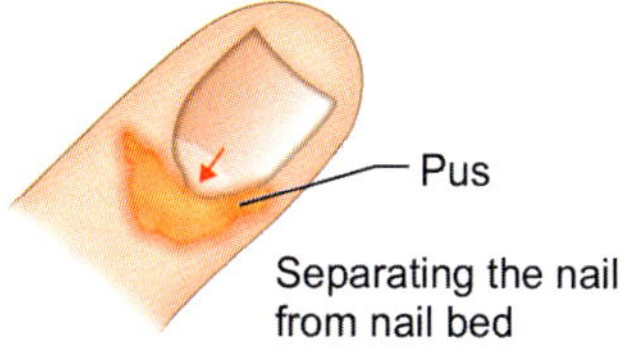

Hand Infections

Acute Paronychia

- Acute infection of the nail fold.
- Mild infection can be treated by antibiotics. If any pus collection, it must be drained by either separating the nail from nail bed or by partial excision of proximal part of nail.

Chronic Paronychia

- A chronic fungal infection of the nail fold
- Treatment—keep the hands dry and application of antifungal ointment.

Pulp Space Infection

- Infection of the terminal pulp space does not spread proximally into the other pulp spaces due to fibrous septa, but it causes a rapid rise of pressure with sloughing of skin and osteomyelitis of terminal phalanx.
- Incision is made over the maximum point of tenderness.

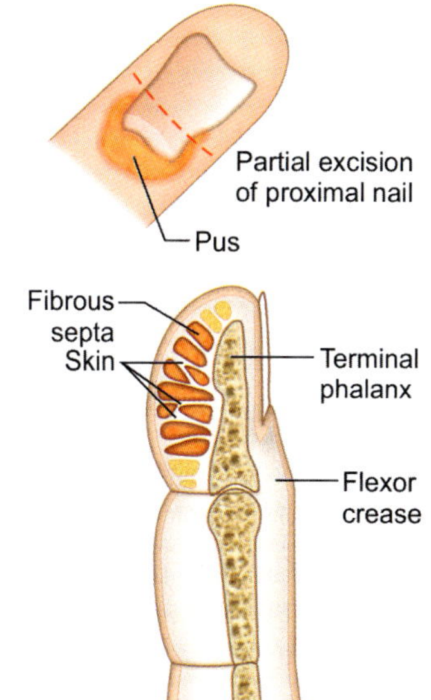

Webspace Infection

- The webspaces are connected with the dorsum of the hand and proximal pulp spaces of the fingers.
- **Natatory ligament** is a fascial support in webspace and acts as a partial barrier between volar and dorsal webspace.
- At the stage of cellulitis, antibiotic therapy is sufficient. If abscess develops, it must be drained. The abscess should be drained through the most direct route. Incision should be in such position that digital nerves and vessels will least likely injured.

Flexor Tendon Sheath Infection

- The synovial sheath of the flexor tendons, those of index, middle and ring finger end proximally at the level of metacarpophalangeal joints. The synovial sheath of thumb is continuous with the **radial bursa** and synovial sheath of little finger is continuous with **ulnar bursa**.
- **Infection in the tendon sheath of index, middle and ring finger** cannot spread to the palm or forearm.
- **Infection in the tendon sheaths of thumb and little finger** can spread to the palm and forearm.
- Patient complains of throbbing pain and swelling of the fingers. Passive movements cause severe pain. **Infection of synovial sheath of thumb or radial bursa** causes swelling of thumb and thenar eminence and makes the thumb slightly flexed.
- **Infection of the ulnar bursa** causes swelling of the whole hand, sometimes involvement of the wrist.
- Surgical exploration of the affected tendon sheath or infected bursa is absolutely necessary if the infection has not subsided after 48 hours of antibiotic management.

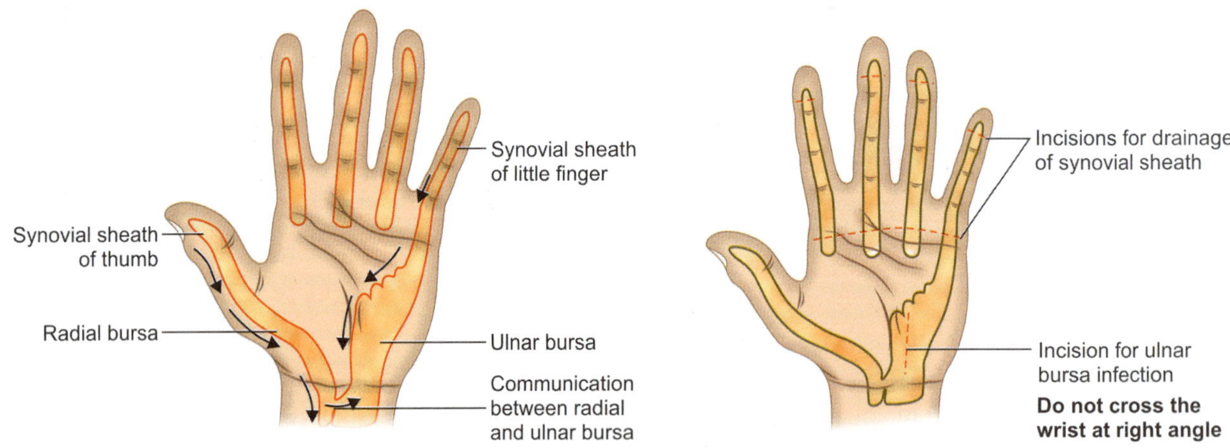

Palmar Space Infection

- The deep fascial spaces consist of **hypothenar, midpalmar, and thenar spaces**.
- These spaces are prone to infection by penetrating trauma or from spreading from a neighboring compartment.
- The characteristic presentation is loss of normal concavity of the palm along with swelling of the dorsum of the hand. Passive movements of the fingers cause extreme pain.
- Drainage of the pus is done through appropriate **lumbrical canal**.

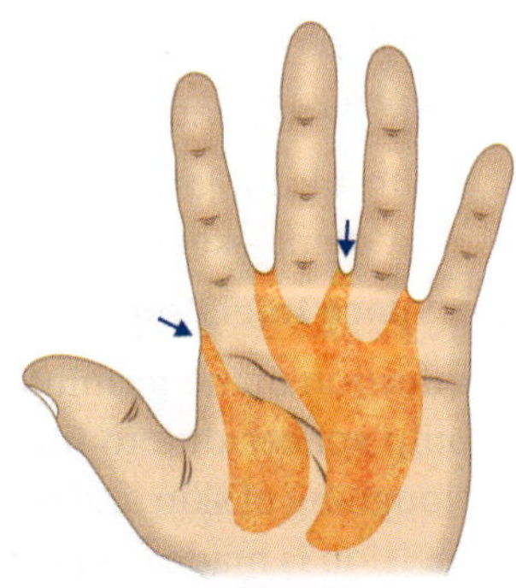

Injuries in Hand

Nerve Injury

Median Nerve Injury

- Wasting of thenar eminence
- Inability to abduction and opposition of thumb
- Absence of flexion of terminal interphalangeal joint of index finger

Ulnar Nerve Injury

- Wasting of hypothenar eminence
- Inability to flexion of little and ring fingers
- Inability to adduct and abduct the fingers

Radial Nerve Injury

- Inability to extend the wrist
- Inability to extend the MCP joint of digits and interphalangeal joint of thumb

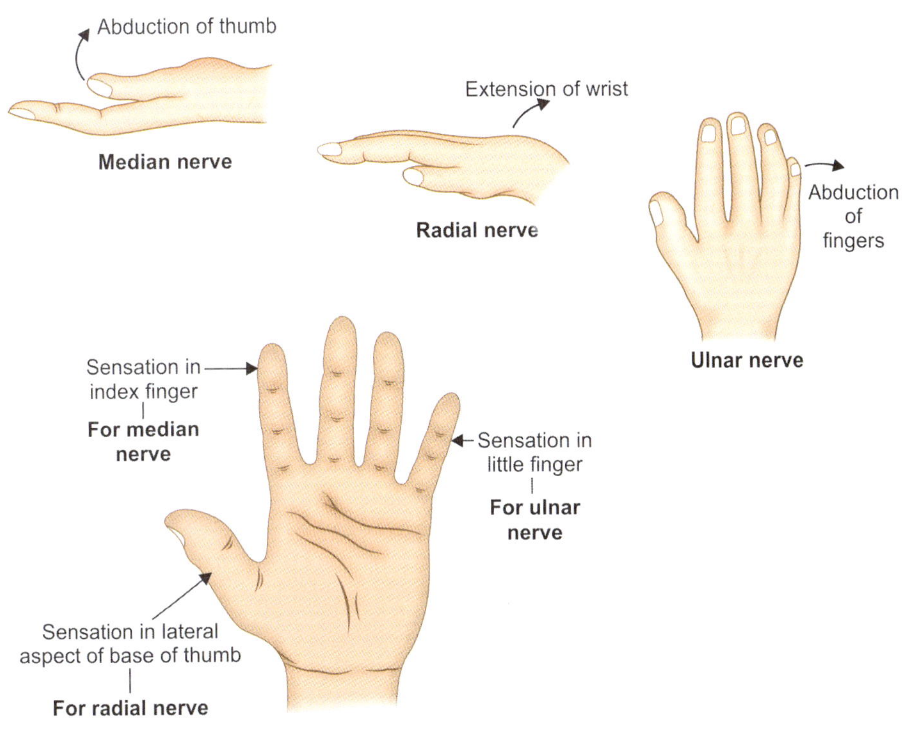

Tendon Injury

Injury of Extensor Tendons

- Repair is done by classic tendon suturing technique (with nonabsorbable, monofilament suture—Polypropylene).
- Recovery is satisfactory.

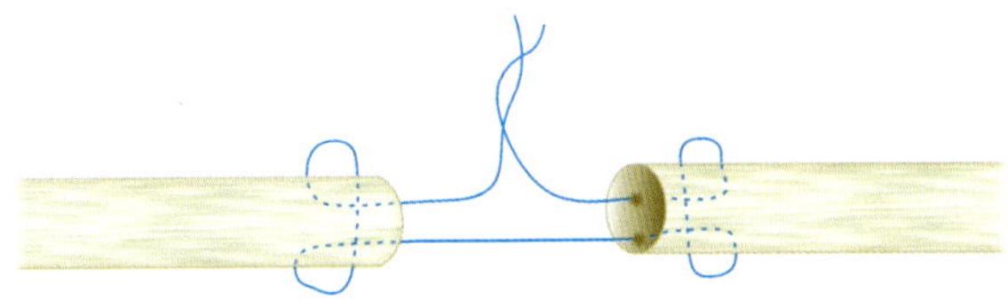

Injury of Flexor Tendons

- **Injury in zone 2 and 4:** Primary repair should not be attempted. Repair should be done by a tendon graft of palmaris longus or plantaris.
- **Injury in zone 1, 3, and 5:** Primary repair is satisfactory.

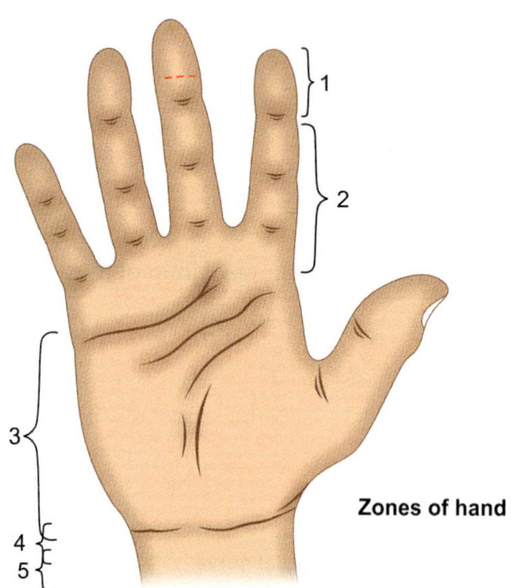

Vascular Injury

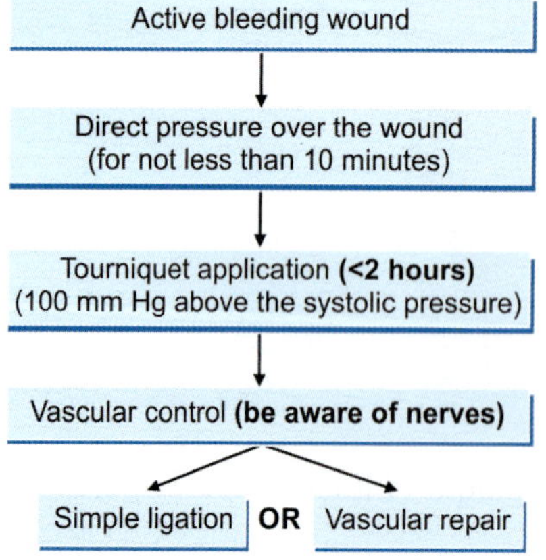

Case 1

History and Physical Examination

A 43-year-old male patient presented in the surgical OPD with complain of pain and swelling in his right hand for last 3 days. Patient had a history of thorn prick about 1 week back. Patient was suffering from diabetes mellitus for last 3 years for which he was taking oral hypoglycemics.

Clinical Examination

Swelling of the right hand with loss of concavity of the palmar surface. Pain on passive movements of the fingers.

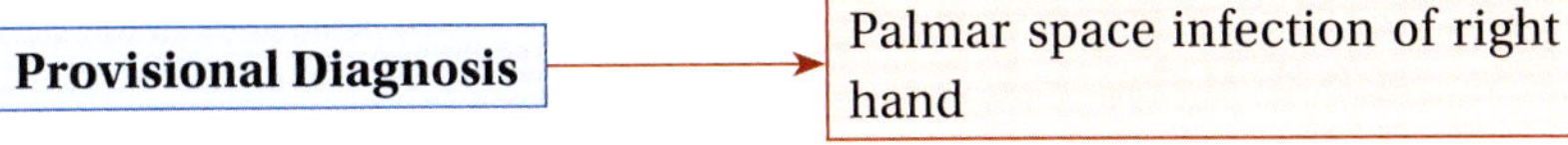

Investigations

Palmar space infection is primarily a clinical diagnosis. No investigations were indicated to confirm the diagnosis. USG may be indicated for better localization of pus collection.

Management Algorithm

Drainage of pus through appropriate lumbrical canal under wrist block.

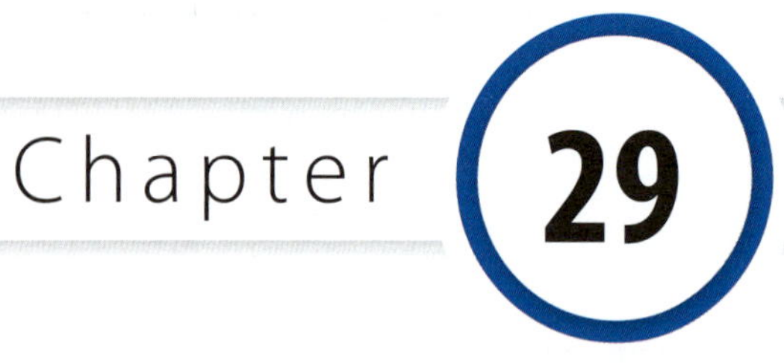

Neck Swelling

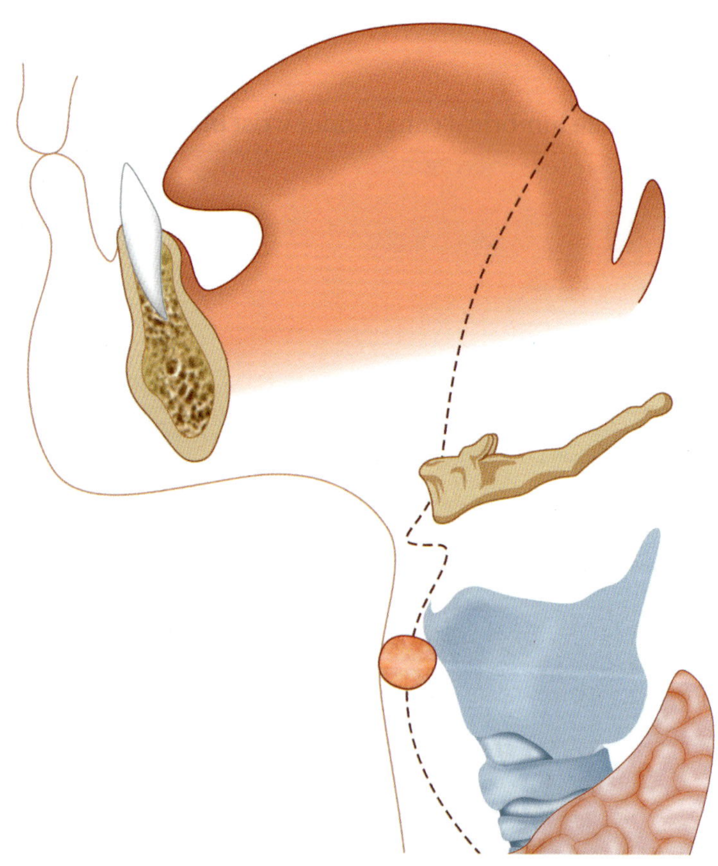

Important Topics

- Lymphatic Levels of Neck
- Types of Neck Swelling
- Lymphadenopathy
- Tubercular Lymphadenitis
- Cervical Lymph Node Metastases
- Neck Dissection
- Branchial Cleft Cyst
- Branchial Fistula
- Carotid Body Tumor
- Cystic Hygroma
- Sternomastoid Tumor
- Thyroglossal Cyst

'Technology is just a tool. In terms of getting the kids working together and motivating them, the teacher is the most important.'

Triangles of neck

- Anterior triangle
- Posterior triangle

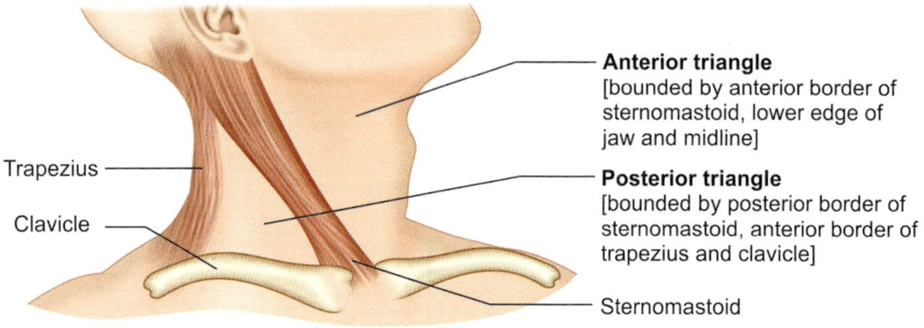

Trapezius

Clavicle

Anterior triangle
[bounded by anterior border of sternomastoid, lower edge of jaw and midline]

Posterior triangle
[bounded by posterior border of sternomastoid, anterior border of trapezius and clavicle]

Sternomastoid

Facial layers of neck

- Superficial cervical fascia
- Deep cervical fascia
  - External layer of deep cervical fascia → Invests the strap muscles, sternomastoid, and trapezius
  - Middle layer of deep cervical fascia → Invests the trachea, esophagus, and thyroid gland
  - Deep layer of deep cervical fascia (prevertebral fascia) → Encloses the vertebral column and deep muscles of neck

Lymphatic Levels of Neck

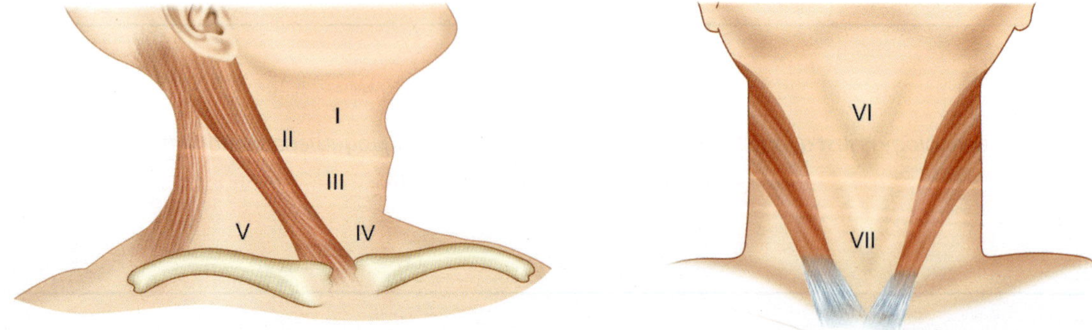

Submental (Sublevel IA)

- Lymph nodes within the triangular boundary of the anterior belly of the digastric muscles and the hyoid bone.
- Metastases from floor of the mouth, anterior tongue, anterior mandibular alveolar ridge, lower lip.

Submandibular (Sublevel IB)

- Lymph nodes within the boundaries of the anterior belly of the digastrics muscle, the stylohyoid muscle, and the body of the mandible.
- Metastases from oral cavity, anterior nasal cavity, soft tissue structures of the midface, submandibular gland.

Upper Jugular (includes Sublevels IIA and IIB)

- Lymph nodes located around the upper third of the internal jugular vein and adjacent spinal accessory nerve extending from the level of the skull base (above) to the level of the inferior border of the hyoid bone (below). The anterior (medial) boundary is the stylohyoid muscle, and the posterior boundary is the posterior border of the sternocleidomastoid muscle.
- **Sublevel IIA** nodes are located anterior (medial) to the vertical plane defined by the spinal accessory nerve.
- **Sublevel IIB** nodes are located posterior (lateral) to the vertical plane defined by the spinal accessory nerve.
- Metastases from oral cavity, nasal cavity, nasopharynx, oropharynx, hypopharynx, larynx, and parotid gland.

Middle Jugular (Level III)

- Lymph nodes located around the middle third of the internal jugular vein extending from the inferior border of the hyoid bone (above) to the inferior border of the cricoid cartilage (below). The anterior (medial) boundary is the lateral border of the sternohyoid muscle, and the posterior (lateral) boundary is the posterior border of the sternocleidomastoid muscle.
- Metastases from oral cavity, nasopharynx, oropharynx, hypopharynx, and larynx.

Lower Jugular (Level IV)

- Lymph nodes located around the lower third of the internal jugular vein extending from the inferior border of the cricoid cartilage (above) to the clavicle (below). The anterior (medial) boundary is the lateral border of the sternohyoid muscle, and the posterior (lateral) boundary is the posterior border of the sternocleidomastoid muscle.
- Metastases from hypopharynx, thyroid, cervical esophagus, and larynx.

Posterior Triangle Group (includes Sublevels VA and VB)

- This group is composed predominantly of the lymph nodes located along the lower half of the spinal accessory nerve and the transverse cervical artery. The supraclavicular nodes are also included in the posterior triangle group. The superior boundary is the apex formed by convergence of the sternocleidomastoid and trapezius muscles, the inferior boundary is the clavicle, the anterior (medial) boundary is the posterior border of the sternocleidomastoid muscle. And the posterior (lateral) boundary is the anterior border of the trapezius muscle.
- Sublevel VA is separated from sublevel VB by a horizontal plane marking the inferior border of the anterior cricoid arch.
- Metastases from nasopharynx, oropharynx, cutaneous structures of the posterior scalp and neck.

Anterior Compartment Group (Level VI)

- Lymph nodes in this compartment include the pretracheal and paratracheal nodes, precricoid (Delphian) node, and the perithyroidal nodes including the lymph nodes along the recurrent laryngeal nerves. The superior boundary is the hyoid bone, the inferior boundary is the suprasternal notch, and the lateral boundaries are the common carotid arteries.
- Metastases from thyroid gland, glottis and subglottic larynx, apex of the piriform sinus, and cervical esophagus.

Neck Swelling

Congenital Neck Swelling

- Cystic hygroma
- Branchial cyst
- Thyroglossal cyst
- Vascular malformation
- Dermoid cyst
- Torticollis

Neck Swellings due to Infective Etiology

- Tuberculous lymphadenitis
- Sialadenitis
- Mononucleosis
- Cat scratch disease
- Odontogenic

Neoplastic Neck Swelling

- Metastatic neck node
- Primary salivary neoplasm
- Lymphoproliferative disorder
- Soft tissue sarcoma

Midline Neck Swelling

- Thyroid swelling
- Thyroglossal cyst
- Ranula
- Dermoid cyst (sublingual)
- Ludwig's angina
- Enlarged submental lymph node
- Subhyoid bursitis

Cystic Neck Swelling

- Thyroglossal cyst
- Branchial cleft cyst
- Lymphangioma (cystic hygroma)
- Dermoid cyst
- Laryngocele
- Ranula

Features Highly Suggestive of Malignant Neck Mass

- Mass present for more than 2 weeks or of uncertain duration
- Neck mass size >1.5 cm
- Firm consistency
- Reduced mobility or fixed neck mass
- Ulceration of overlying skin

Lymphadenopathy

Enlargement of the cervical lymph node is the most common cause of neck swelling.

Causes:

- **Infection:** Tuberculosis, tonsillitis, infective focus in oral and nasal cavity, larynx, pharynx, ear, face, toxoplasmosis.
- **Metastatic deposit:** Carcinoma in head-neck region (nasopharynx, tonsil, piriform fossa, supraglottic larynx), carcinoma in chest and abdomen.
- **Primary neoplasms of lymphatic system:** Hodgkin's lymphoma and non-Hodgkin's lymphoma.
- **Sarcoidosis**

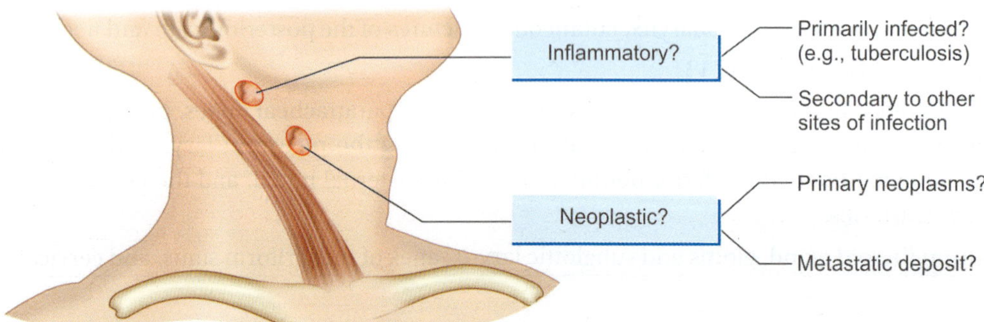

Nonspecific Lymphadenitis

- Due to infective focus in oral and nasal cavity, larynx, pharynx, and face
- Enlarged lymph nodes are tender. Systemic symptoms such as fever, malaise are usually present.
- Treatment is antibiotic therapy. If abscess develops, then incision and drainage is indicated along with antibiotics.

Tuberculous Lymphadenitis

- Common cause of cervical lymphadenopathy in developing countries
- Both human and bovine strain may be responsible.
- Tubercular bacilli can enter the body through the tonsil, from where it enters the cervical lymph nodes.
- In most of the cases, disease is limited to clinically affected cervical lymph nodes. Associated pulmonary and renal tuberculosis is rare. If any suspicion, then it have to be investigated.
- Common in children and young adults but can occur at any ages.
- The upper deep cervical lymph nodes are most commonly affected.
- In the early stage, the nodes are appeared firm and discrete. If no treatment is instituted, caseation increases, infection spreads beyond the capsule of nodes. The nodes now become coalesce and appear as matted. Abscess develops in the center of the matted glands.
- Initially, the pus is confined by the deep cervical fascia, but later it bursts through it and reach the subcutaneous tissue. Now it has two compartments, one on either side of the deep fascia connected by a track. This is now called **'collar stud abscess'**. The superficial abscess gradually enlarges, the skin overlying the abscess becomes eroded and then the discharging sinus develops.
- Treatment is **antitubercular chemotherapy**.

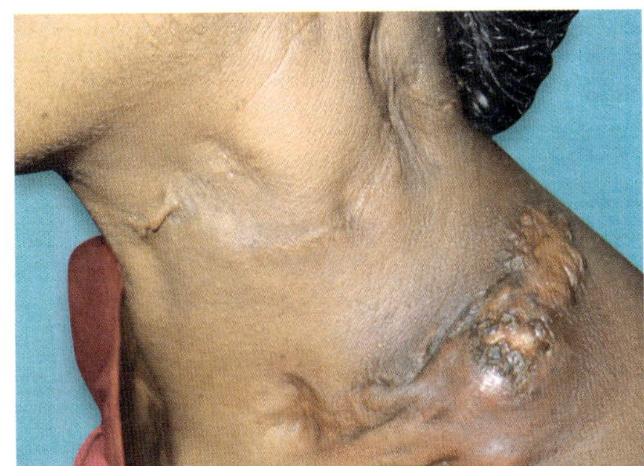

Tubercular lymphadenitis.

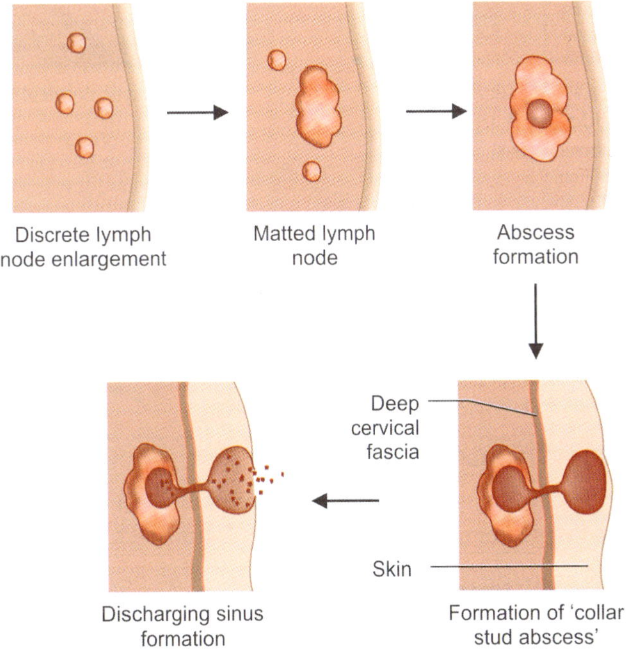

The Jones and Campbell Stages of Tuberculous Lymphadenitis

Stage 1: Enlarged, firm, mobile, discrete nodes showing non-specific reactive hyperplasia

Stage 2: Large rubbery nodes fixed to the surrounding tissue owing to periadenitis

Stage 3: Central softening due to abscess formation

Stage 4: Collar stud abscess formation

Stage 5: Sinus tract formation

Cervical Lymph Node Metastases

- The most common cause of cervical lymphadenopathy in adults.
- The primary one is most commonly present in the buccal cavity (tongue, lip, buccal mucosa) and larynx.
- **Other sites that have to be searched for:** (i) Skin of scalp, ear, and external auditory meatus; (ii) Nose, nasopharynx and maxillary antrum; (iii) Thyroid; (iv) Upper limb and both sides of chest wall; (v) Lungs; (vi) Breast; (vii) Stomach, pancreas, ovaries; and (viii) Testis
- Presents as painless lump in neck. They are hard, irregular, and tethered to the surrounding structures.
- Enlarged left supraclavicular lymph node is called **Virchow's node**. The presence of Virchow's node is called **Troisier's sign**.
- **Work-up:** Complete head and neck examination, thorough examination of the skin, palpation of the oropharynx, mirror and fiberoptic examination of the nasopharynx, oropharynx, hypopharynx and larynx, and FNA (preferably USG-guided) of the cervical lymph node. Based on the FNA report, further work-up includes CECT of head and neck (from base of the skull to thoracic inlet), CECT of chest and abdomen, high-risk HPV and EBV testing for squamous cell carcinoma or undifferentiated type, thyroglobulin and calcitonin and PAX8 for adenocarcinoma and anaplastic type. If primary site cannot be found in CECT, FDG PET/CT is indicated.
- **Treatment:** Treatment of the primary disease along with radiotherapy/neck dissection for the lymph node, if indicated.

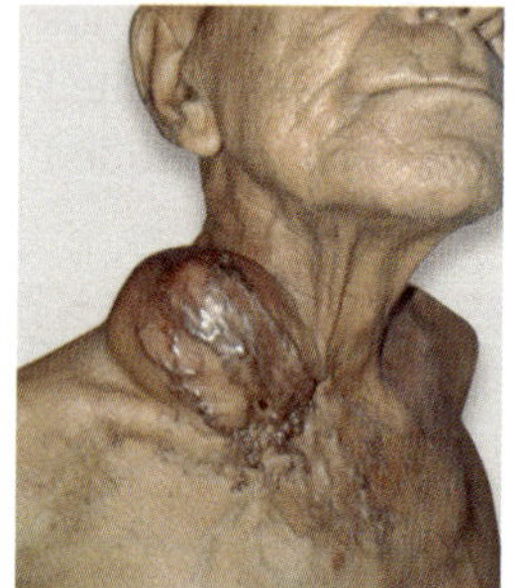

Metastatic cervical lymph node (note the venous prominences).

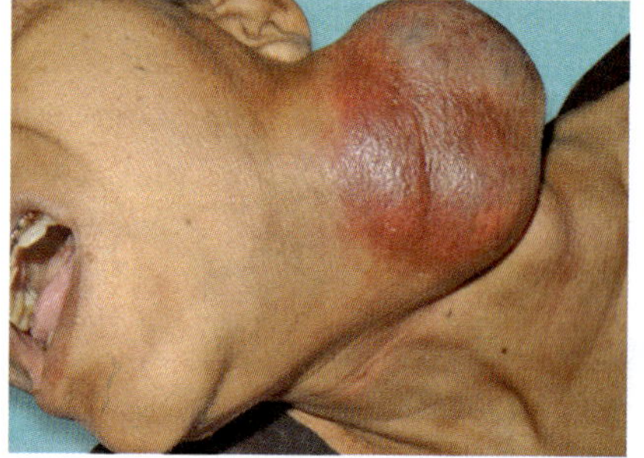

Metastatic cervical lymph node.

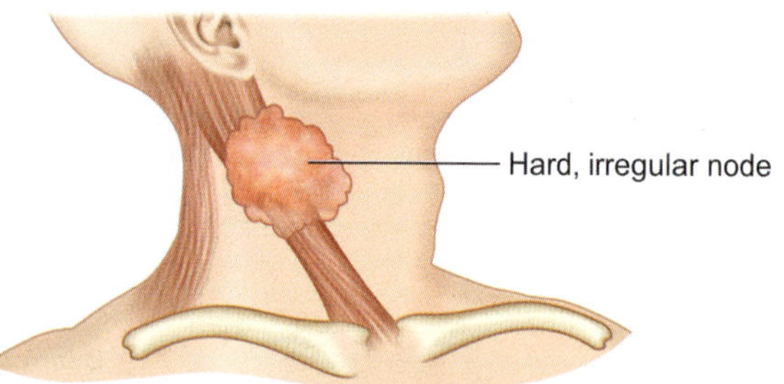

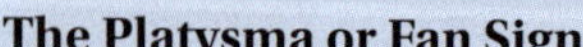

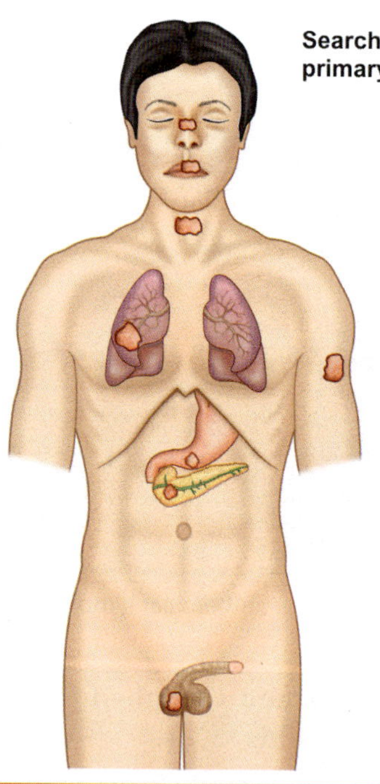

The Platysma or Fan Sign

The platysmal fibers become prominent like a Japanese fan when stretched due to involvement of platysma by metastatic neck nodes.

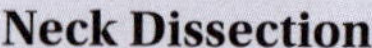

Neck Dissection

Classification of neck dissection proposed by the American Head and Neck Society and the American Academy of Otolaryngology—Head and Neck Surgery.

Radical neck dissection:

- Removal of all ipsilateral cervical lymph node groups extending from the inferior border of the mandible to the clavicle, from the lateral border of the sternohyoid muscle, hyoid bone, and contralateral anterior belly of the digastric muscle medially, to the anterior border of the trapezius muscle.

- Included all lymph nodes from Level I to V.
- Spinal accessory nerve, internal jugular vein, and sternocleidomastoid muscle are also removed.
- Does not remove suboccipital nodes, periparotid nodes (except intraparotid nodes located in the posterior aspect of the submandibular triangle), buccinators nodes, retropharyngeal nodes, and anterior compartment nodes.

Modified radical neck dissection (MRND):

- Removal of all lymph nodes routinely removed by radical neck dissection with preservation of one or more nonlymphatic structures (i.e., The spinal accessory nerve (SAN), internal jugular vein, and sternocleidomastoid muscle).
- The structure(s) preserved should be specifically named, e.g., MRND with preservation of SAN.

Selective neck dissection:

- Preservation of one or more of the lymph node groups that are routinely removed in the radical neck dissection.
- The lymph node groups removed are based on the primary site of disease. *Example:* For oral cavity cancer, selective neck dissection level I-III; for medullary thyroid cancer- selective neck dissection level VI.

Extended neck dissection:

- Removal of one or more additional lymph node groups or nonlymphatic structures, or both, not encompassed by the radical neck dissection.
- Examples of additional lymph node groups are parapharyngeal, superior mediastinal, perifacial (buccinator), and paratracheal lymph nodes.
- Examples of additional nonlymphatic structures are carotid artery, hypoglossal nerve, vagus nerve, and paraspinal muscles.

As per NCCN panel, Neck dissection is classified into: (i) Comprehensive neck dissection (removes all lymph node groups in classic radical neck dissection irrespective of preservation of any structures) and (ii) Selective neck dissection (same as previous classification).

Incisions for Neck Dissection

- Reverse Hockey-stick incision
- Hockey-stick incision
- Modified Schobinger incision
- Macfee double horizontal incision
- Wide apron flap
- Apron flap with lateral extensions

Complications of Neck Dissection

Early complications: (i) Hemorrhage; (ii) Airway obstruction; (iii) Nerve injury (spinal accessory nerve, hypoglossal nerve, vagus nerve, lingual nerve, phrenic nerve); (iv) Pneumothorax; and (v) Increased intracranial pressure.

Intermediate complications: (i) Chylous fistula and (ii) Deep vein thrombosis

Late complications: (i) Lymphoedema; (ii) Hypertrophic scar; and (iii) Recurrence

Primary Neoplasm of the Lymph Node

- Malignant lymphoma (Hodgkin's lymphoma and Non-Hodgkin's lymphoma) are most common primary tumor of lymphoid tissue.
- Painless lymphadenopathy, particularly in the posterior triangle along with systemic symptoms (e.g., fever, malaise, weight loss, pallor). Other groups of lymph nodes (e.g., inguinal, axillary) are commonly enlarged.
- Lymph nodes are smooth, discrete, and rubbery in consistency.
- Chemotherapy is the treatment of choice.

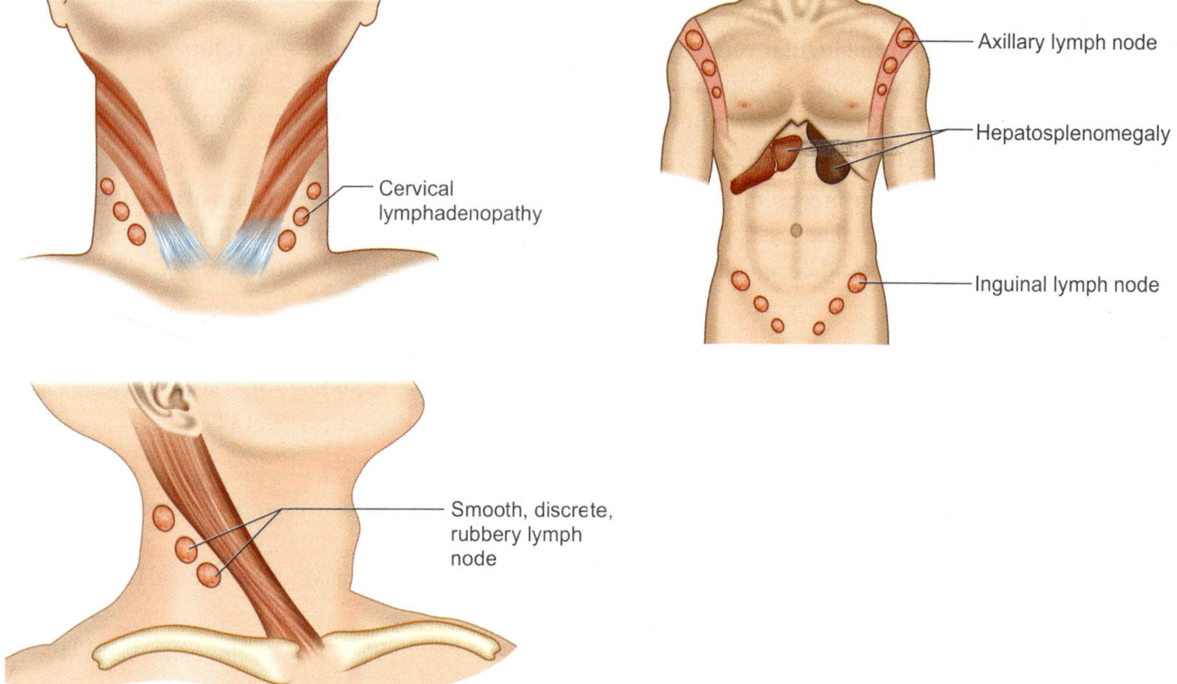

Branchial Cleft Cyst

- The word **'branchial'** came from the Greek word **'bragchia' meaning 'gills'**.
- Branchial or cervical lymphoepithelial cysts originate **due to failed obliteration of branchial clefts.**
- It is lined by squamous epithelium and contains turbid, thick white fluid full of fat globules and cholesterol crystals secreted by sebaceous glands of epithelial lining.
- **Classified as** first, second, third and fourth branchial cleft cyst. **Second branchial cleft cyst is the most common type of branchial cyst.**
- **Bailey classification of second branchial cleft cyst:** *Type I:* Deep to platysma, anterior to sternocleidomastoid; *Type II (most common type):* Abutting internal carotid artery and adherent to internal jugular vein; *Type III:* Extending between internal and external carotid arteries; *Type IV:* Abutting pharyngeal wall and potentially extending superiorly to skull base.
- **Second branchial cyst commonly presents as** nontender, soft, smooth, fluctuant, mobile swelling deep to the anterior border of sternocleidomastoid (at the junction of upper one-third and lower two-thirds), but may present in the palatine tonsil or between internal and external carotid arteries.
- **USG** is the first-line imaging modality. **CECT and MRI** are useful for assessment of relationship of the cyst with adjacent structures.
- **Differential diagnosis** includes cystic hygroma, lymphadenopathy, lipoma, carotid body tumor, and hemangioma.
- **Treatment of choice** is surgical resection.
- Incision over the cyst along the skin crease. Incision should be atleast 2 cm below the angle of jaw to avoid the injury of marginal mandibular branch of facial nerve. **The anterior (superficial) part of the cyst** can be easily enucleated. **If deep extension is present**, then it must be excised with careful dissection. The deeper part of the cyst extends backwards and upwards in between the internal and enternal carotid artery to the region of tonsillar fossa. **The hypoglossal and spinal accessory nerves are encountered during dissection of deeper extension.**
- **Complications of surgical resection** includes recurrence, persistent fistula, injury to the cranial nerves (e.g., glossopharyngeal, vagus, hypoglossal, spinal accessory nerve).

Branchial Fistula

- It is due to **persistence of second branchial cleft**.
- **The external opening** is near the lower third of sternomastoid at its anterior border, **the internal opening** in the tonsillar fossa. If the upper end of the fistula obliterates, then it is called **branchial sinus**.
- The tract is lined by ciliated columnar epithelium.
- **Course of the fistula tract:** External opening is in mid or lower third of neck in the line of anterior border of sternocleidomastoid, then passes proximally deep to platysma along the carotid sheath and then turns medially and **passes between internal and external carotid arteries** and then courses behind the posterior belly of digastrics and stylohyoid muscles and then end in the tonsillar fossa.
- **Patient presents** with small dimple in the lower part of the neck that discharges mucous or mucopurulent discharge with recurrent interval.
- **CT fistulogram** delineates the fistula tract path and reveals its relationship with important structures along its course.
- **Treatment of choice** is excision of the fistula tract. Standard surgical approach is **transcervical stepladder approach. One elliptical incision** around the external opening and a **higher transverse incision** for better delineation of fistula tract. The higher incision should be bigger because the fistula tract courses deeper proximally with close proximity to important neurovascular structures.
- **Other surgical approach** is combined transcervical and oral approach. In this approach, chance of recurrence is lower in comparison to transcervical approach.

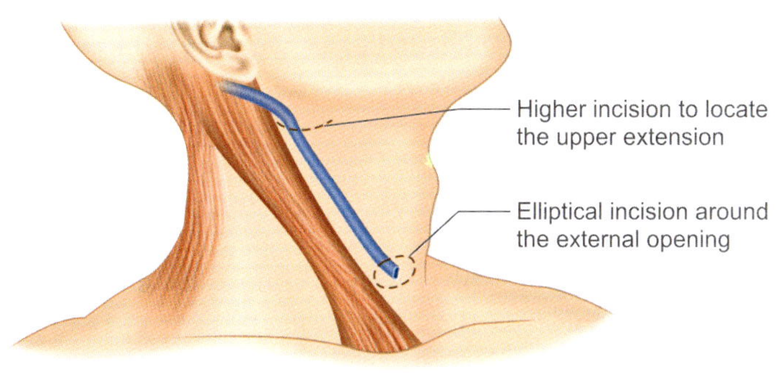

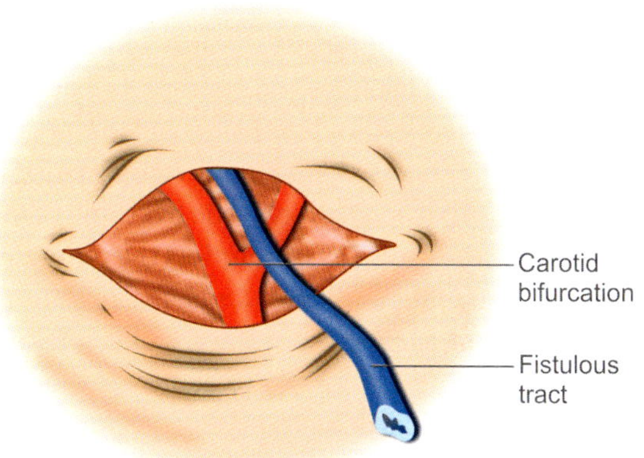

Carotid Body Tumor

- Rare neoplasm originates from **neural crest cells (extra-adrenal paragangliomas)**. Most of carotid body tumors are parasympathetic paragangliomas.
- A painless neck mass **beneath the anterior edge of the sternocleidomastoid muscle** just lateral to the tip of the hyoid bone.
- This tumor is mobile in the lateral plane but restricted mobility in the cephalocaudal direction **(Fontaine sign)**.
- **Functional tumors (catecholamine producing)** may present with palpitation, episodic headache, fluctuating hypertension. If tumor is increasing in size, then patient may present with odynophagia, dysphagia, hoarseness of voice (cranial nerve X involvement), tongue weakness and atrophy (cranial nerve XII involvement), and Horner syndrome (involvement of sympathetic chain).
- **Shamblin classification** is based on size of the tumor and degree of arterial invasion (Type I, II and III). **Modified Shamblin classification** (by Luna-Ortiz et al.) classified this tumor into Type I, II, IIIa and IIIb. **Type I** is small tumors and minimally attached to carotid vessels; **Type II** tumors are larger and more adherent to the adventitia but still removable without reconstruction; **Type IIIa** tumors are larger and densely adherent to the artery, and **Type IIIb** tumors are any size of tumor with densely adherent and surrounding the carotid arteries.

- **CT angiography (CTA)** and **MR angiography (MRA)** are diagnostic.
- **Resection of the tumor** is the treatment. Type I tumor can be easily dissected from the artery. For Type II tumor resection, subadventitial dissection is required. Arterial excision and reconstruction is indicated for type IIIa and type IIIb tumors.

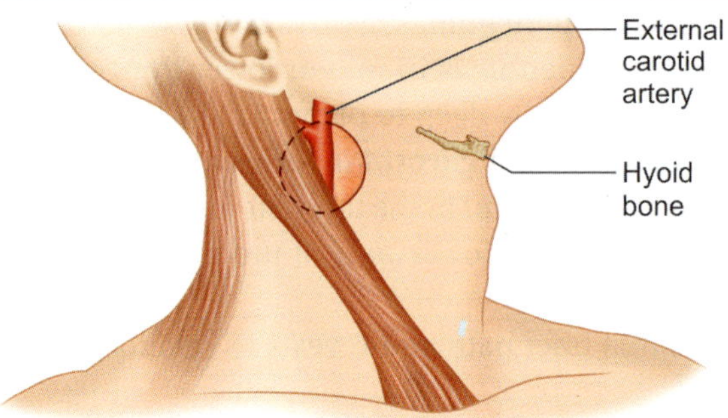

Cystic Hygroma

- Cystic hygroma is a **cystic variety of lymphangioma** (other types of lymphangiomas are capillary and cavernous).
- **Congenital anomalies** that may be associated with cystic hygroma—Down's syndrome, Turner's syndrome, Trisomy 18, Trisomy 13, Noonan syndrome.
- **Common locations** are cervico facial regions (particularly posterior triangle of neck), axilla, mediastinum, groin.
- **Commonly present as** soft, non-tender, partially compressible, brilliantly translucent swelling.
- **USG reveals** multicystic lesions with internal septations and no blood flow in Doppler study. **CT scan** and **MRI** are particularly useful when surgical excision is planned because these imaging modalities can reveal exact extent of the lesion and its relationship with adjacent structures.
- **Complications that may develop are** secondary infection, spontaneous hemorrhage in the cyst, respiratory distress (particularly in cystic hygroma of neck and oral cavity).
- **Treatments options include:** (i) Complete surgical excision and (ii) Sclerotherapy. Recent approaches include radiofrequency ablation and Laser excision.
- **Complete surgical excision is a difficult job due to:** (i) Infiltrative nature of the lesion; (ii) Thin wall of endothelium; and (iii) Close proximity to neurovascular structures (particularly if lesion is present in neck). Aggressive blunt and electrosurgical dissections should be avoided because of excessive lymphatic leakage that may result in infection.
- **Complications of surgical excision:** (i) Wound infection; (ii) Hemorrhage; (iii) Lymphatic leakage; and (iv) Recurrence.
- **Other treatment options are** Sclerotherapy with bleomycin or OK-432 (lyophilized incubation mixture of group A *Streptococcus pyogenes* of human origin). **Bleomycin** acts by initiating nonspecific inflammatory process resulting in fibrosis. **OK-432** acts by inducing cytokine synthesis, resulting in increased endothelial permeability and thereby increased lymph flow within the cystic spaces of this lesion.

Sternomastoid Tumor (Fibromatosis colli)

- **A benign, self-limiting disease of neonates with unknown etiology.** Breech presentation, primiparous birth are commonly associated with this lesion.
- **The lesion commonly presents** as firm, nontender mass involving the mid or lower part of sternocleidomastoid muscle.
- Mother notice a lump in neck with slight torticollis. If muscle damage is more and causes fibrosis, the tilting of head to one side will become prominent as the child grows.
- **USG** is the imaging modality of choice. **Differential diagnosis** includes cervical lymphadenopathy, branchial cyst, hemangioma, rhabdomyoscarcoma.
- **Most of the lesions resolve spontaneously** without sequelae. Progressive torticollis or facial asymmetry are indications for surgery.

Thyroglossal Cyst

- Most common congenital anomaly of the neck. The cyst represents the persistence of a part of **thyroglossal duct**, which begins at the foramen cecum and ends at the thyroid isthmus.
- The cyst can present anywhere between base of tongue and isthmus of thyroid. The two sites are common—**subhyoid and suprahyoid at the midline**.
- The swelling moves with deglutition as well as with protrusion of tongue.
- **USG** is the initial imaging modality of choice.
- Thyroglossal cyst may be the only thyroid tissue present in the body. So, before excision, **thyroid scan** should be done.
- Treatment is excision of cyst along with whole thyroglossal tract including the body of hyoid bone. This is called **Sistrunk's operation**.

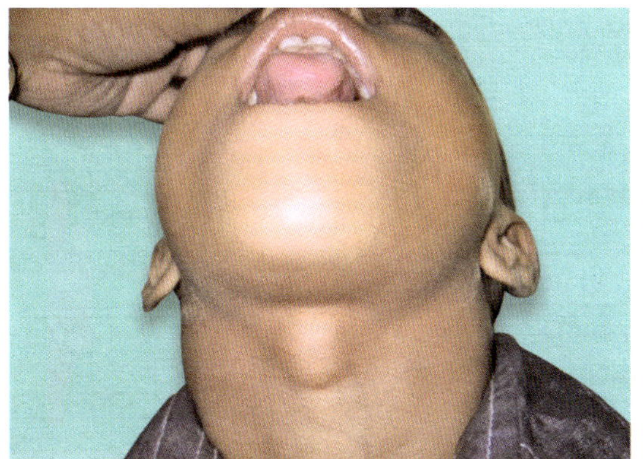

Thyroglossal cyst—moves with protrusion of the tongue.

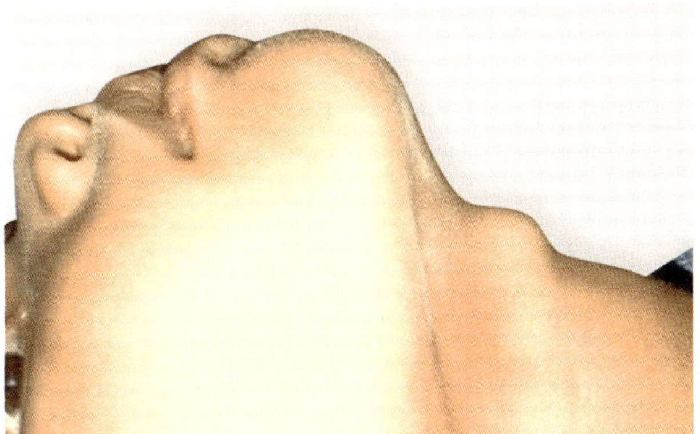

Thyroglossal cyst.

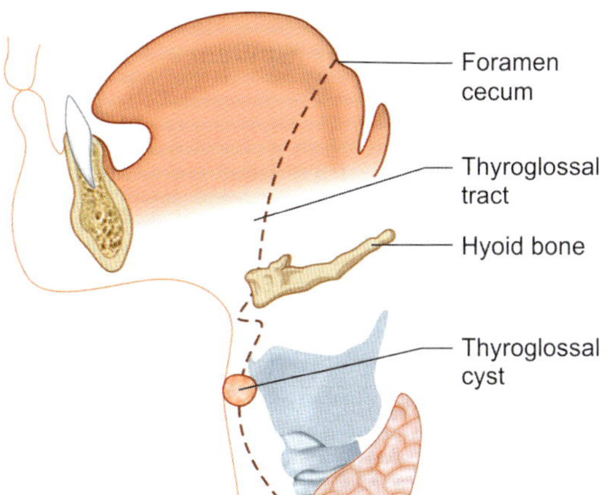

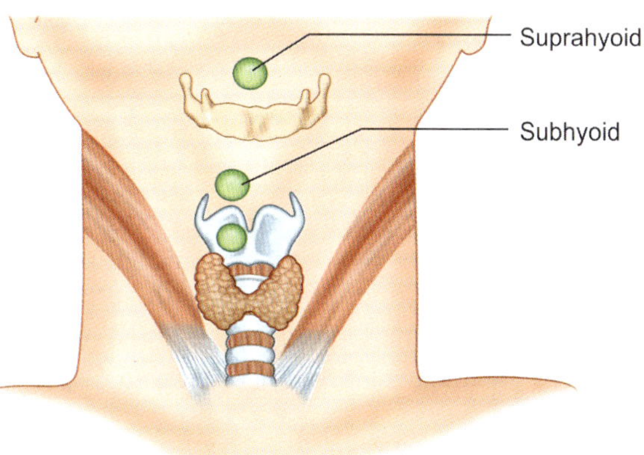

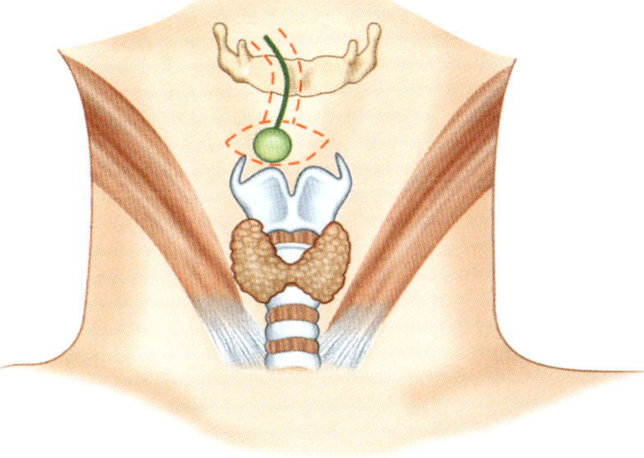

Case 1

History and Physical Examination

A 34-year-old male patient presented with multiple neck swellings for last 3 months. These swellings gradually increasing in size and became soft in consistency. He consulted with local physician and on antibiotic therapy for about 2 weeks. The swelling not subsided after antibiotic therapy. No history of swellings in other parts of the body. No history of loss of appetite, weight loss, evening rise of temperature. No past history or family history of pulmonary tuberculosis. No history of diabetes or hypertension.

Clinical Examination

Multiple matted lymph nodes were palpable in level II and III, predominantly on the right neck. The consistency was soft. Two to three discrete lymph nodes also palpable, firm in consistency, at level III. No lymph nodes were palpable in axilla or groin.

Liver and spleen not palpable. No palpable abdominal lump.

Chest examination revealed no abnormalities.

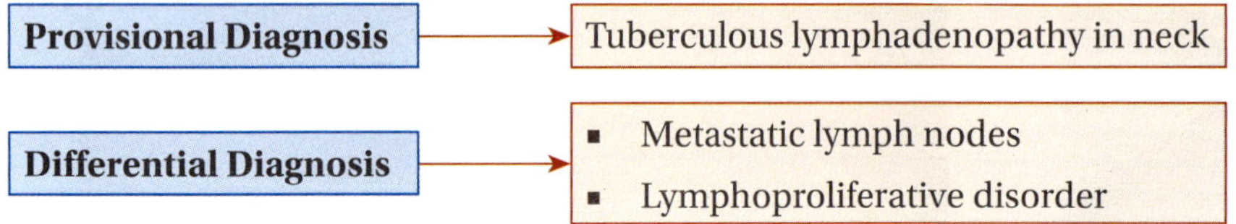

Investigations

FNA of cervical lymph nodes suggestive of tubercular lymphadenitis. Chest X-ray and sputum for AFB revealed no abnormalities. Laboratory parameters were within normal limit.

Discussion

A young-aged patient presented with multiple lymph node swellings in neck for last 3 months and clinical examination findings revealed matted lymph nodes with soft consistency highly suggestive of tubercular lymphadenopathy. In most patients with tubercular lymphadenitis, constitutional symptoms of tuberculosis are usually not present. FNA confirmed the diagnosis and Chest X-ray and sputum test excluded associated pulmonary tuberculosis.

Management Algorithm

Antitubercular therapy

Case 2

History and Physical Examination

A 13-year-old boy presented in the surgical OPD with complain of mucopurulent discharge from an opening in the right neck. The discharge appeared on regular interval. Patient had no history of any swelling in other part of neck. No history of any surgical interventions in neck. No other history suggestive of any congenital abnormalities.

Clinical Examination

A dimple was visible in the lower third of right neck in the line of anterior border of sternocleidomastoid. No active discharge was present. No inflammatory changes were present around the opening. Neck nodes were not palpable.

Provisional Diagnosis

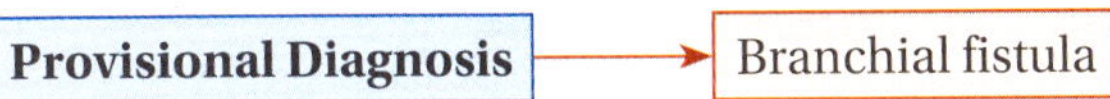

Investigations

CT fistulogram revealed a contrast-delineated fistula tract traversing anterior to the right sternocleidomastoid muscle, then in between the external and internal carotid arteries and finally ended in the right tonsillar fossa.

Discussion

The classic clinical presentation was suggestive of branchial sinus or fistula. CT fistulogram confirmed it as branchial fistula as well as delineated the entire tract that was helpful for surgery.

Management Algorithm

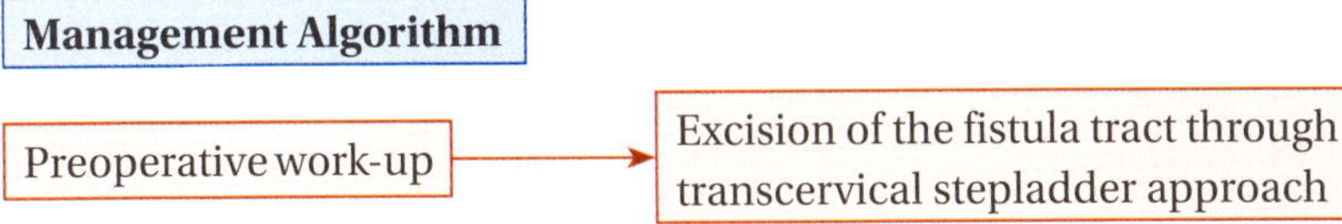

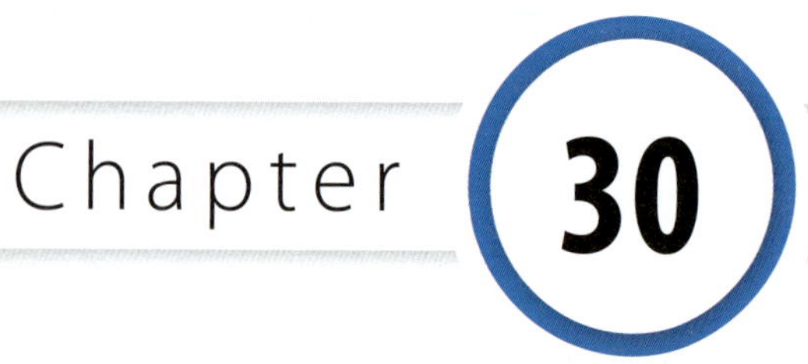

Cleft Lip and Palate

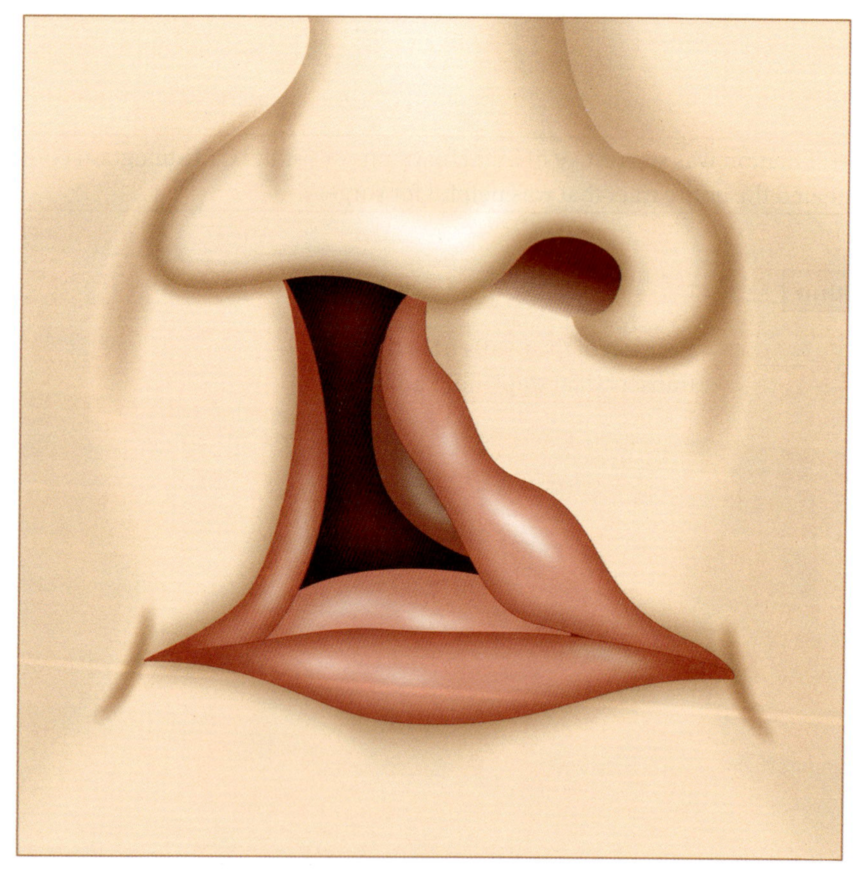

Important Topics

- Cleft Lip and its Management
- Cleft Palate and its Management

'When books are opened, we discover that we have wings.'

Cleft Lip

- Congenital defects in head and neck is one of the common pathologies encountered by Pediatric and Plastic Surgeons. Among head-neck defects, cleft lip and palate is the most common problem encountered.

Development

- During embryogenesis, the five facial elements (one frontonasal, two lateral maxillary and two mandibular segments) merge to form the face and jaw.
- **The frontonasal process** forms the nose, the nasal septum, the nostrils, the philtrum of the upper lip and the premaxilla. **The maxillary processes** form the cheek, the upper lip (except the philtrum), the upper jaw and palate. **The mandibular processes** form the lower jaw and lower lip.
- **In classic theory, failure of fusion of the maxillary process and frontonasal process causes the cleft.**

Incidence

- Racial difference is noted in prevalence
- Cleft lip and palate—45%
- Isolated cleft lip—15%
- Isolated cleft palate—40%
- Cleft lip and other malformations is about 14%
- In cleft lip, the deformity in left side is about 60%

Etiology

Multifactorial

- Hereditary factors
  - If one sibling has cleft lip or palate, the probability of next child being affected is 4%.
  - When both a parent and child are affected, the likelihood of the next child having a cleft lip or palate is 17%.
- Environmental factors
  - Parental age
  - Maternal drug intake (e.g., phenytoin, steroid, diazepam)
- Genetic factors
  - Cleft lip and palate may be associated with some syndromes, e.g., Down syndrome, Apert and Treacher-Collins syndrome

Classification of Cleft Lip

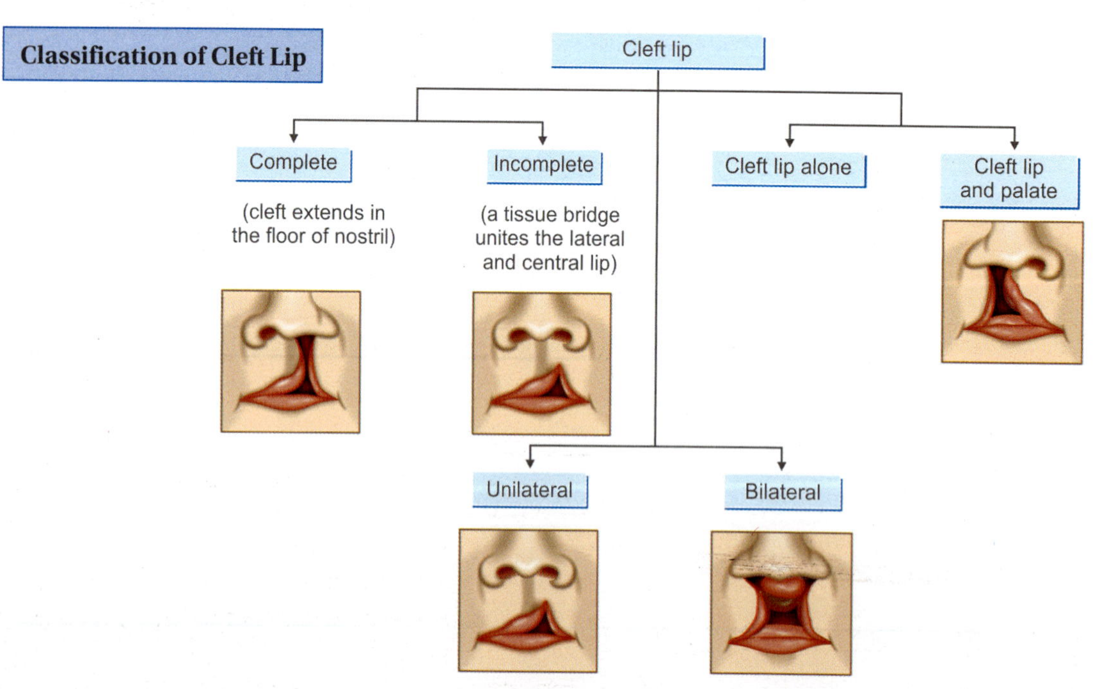

Defects in Cleft Lip (Unilateral)
- Ill-defined philtral ridge on the cleft side
- Columella shorter on cleft side
- Lateral inferior and posterior displacement of the alar cartilage
- Vermilion thining
- Nasal floor defect
- Hypoplastic muscles and abnormal muscle insertions

Defects in Cleft Lip (Bilateral)
- Premaxilla is outwardly rotated and projected.
- Prolabium is devoid of muscle.
- Short columella

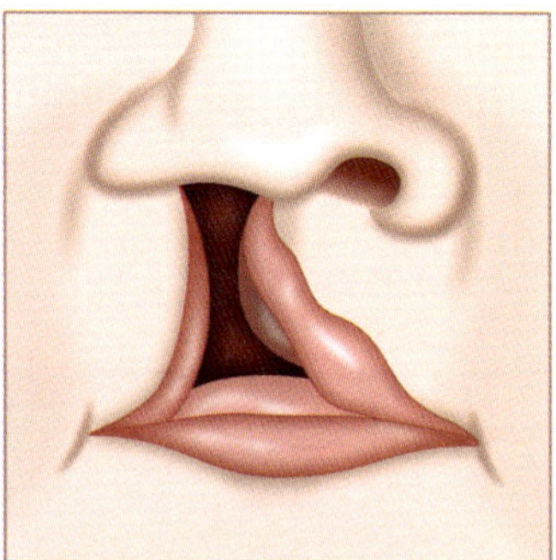

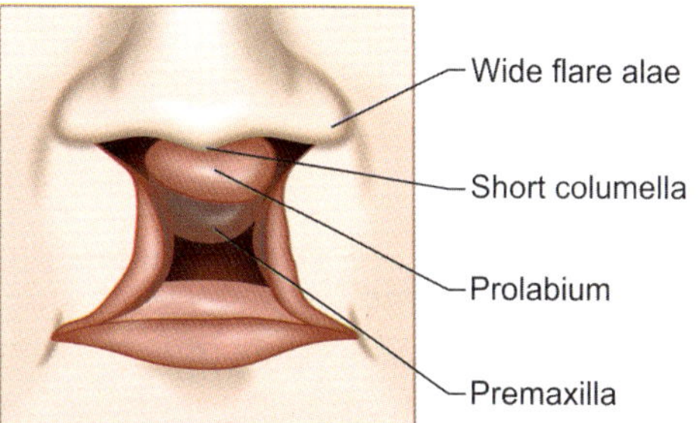

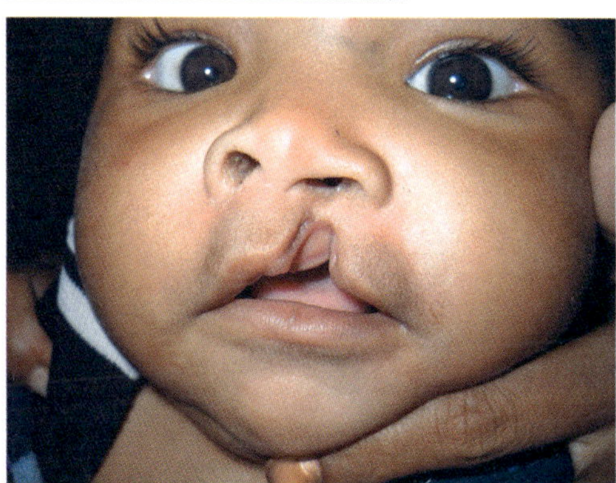

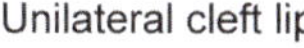
Unilateral cleft lip

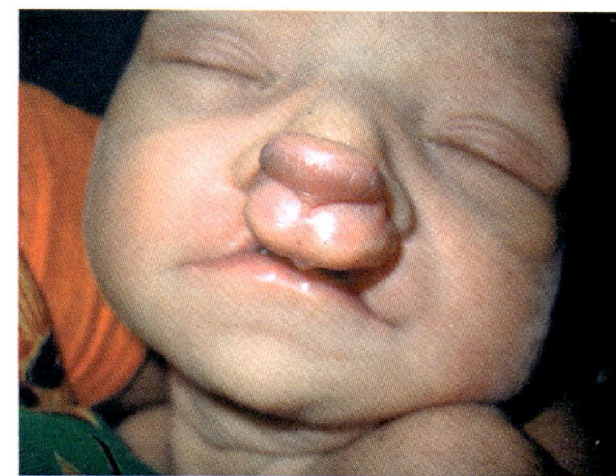

Bilateral cleft lip

Treatment
- A **multidisciplinary team** consists of plastic surgeon, pediatric dentist, otorhinolaryngologist, speech therapist, pediatrician, and psychologist is necessary for highest level of care.
- **Timing of repair:** Usually follow the 'rule of tens.'
    - 10 weeks of age
    - 10 lbs body weight
    - Hb% 10 mg/dL
- **Presurgical procedure:** Presurgical orthodontics such as nasoalveolar segment alignment
- **Goal of repair:** To make the appearance of lip, nose and face normal and also to make the development of speech, dentition and facial growth almost normal
- **Principles of cleft lip repair:**
    - Layered repair of skin, muscles and mucous membrane to restore symmetric shape and function
    - To level cupid's bow and reconstruct the central philtrum of the lip
    - Primary closure of the alveolar cleft (gingivoperiosteoplasty) at the time of primary lip repair
    - Primary nasoplasty at the time of lip repair.
- **The Millard rotation:** Advancement flap technique is widely used for unilateral cleft lip repair.
- **Delaire technique** is another option.
- **Mulliken technique** is commonly used for bilateral cleft lip repair.

Cleft Palate

Due to failure of fusion of the **two palatal processes**.

Classification

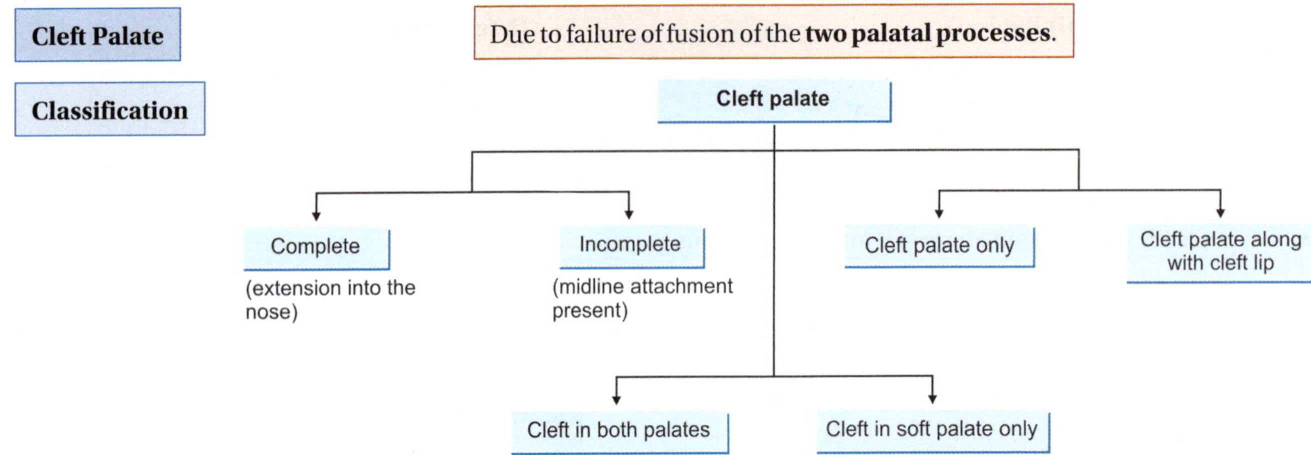

Problems due to Cleft Palate

- Ineffective suckling and feeding (due to failure of creating negative intraoral pressure because of nasal and oral cavity continuity)
- Speech difficulties (due to velopharyngeal incompetence)
- Improper facial growth
- Recurrent otitis media

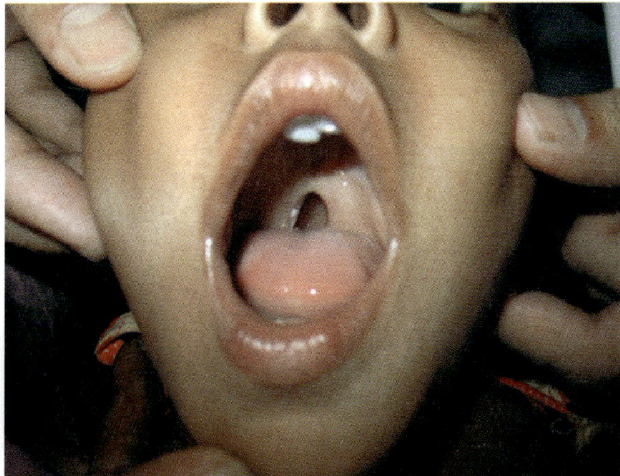

Cleft palate.

Timing of repair: Before speech development (6–18 months of age)
Goal of surgical repair: To separate the oral and nasal cavities and formation of tight velopharyngeal valve.
Different techniques of repair:

- **Furlow palatoplasty:** Double opposing z-plasty of soft palate.
- **Von Langenbeck repair:** Bipedicled hard palate mucoperiosteal flap repair.
- **Wardill-Veau-Kilner repair:** Unipedicled hard palate mucoperiosteal flap repair.

Secondary management:
Hearing difficulty: Child with cleft lip and palate are at increased risk of sensorineural deafness and conductive deafness (due to secretory otitis media). All children with cleft lip and palate should undergo assessment for deafness by auditory brainstem responses (ABR) and tympanometry before 1 year of age. Sensorineural deafness are treated with hearing aid and treatment of conductive deafness is controversial.
Speech difficulty: Speech assessment should be started from 1½ years of age and at regular interval.
Assessment is done by: (i) Videofluoroscopy; (ii) Aerophonoscopy; and (iii) Nasoendoscopy.
Difficulties are managed by: (i) Speech therapy; (ii) Veloplasty; and (iii) Pharyngoplasty.
Dental abnormalities:

- Child with cleft lip and palate should undergo regular dental examination.
- Delayed eruption, variation in number and ill health teeth may present.
- Preventive measures, e.g., fluoride supplements, maintenance of dental hygiene is essential for disease-free dentition.

Orthodontic management: By alveolar bone graft/maxillary osteotomy.

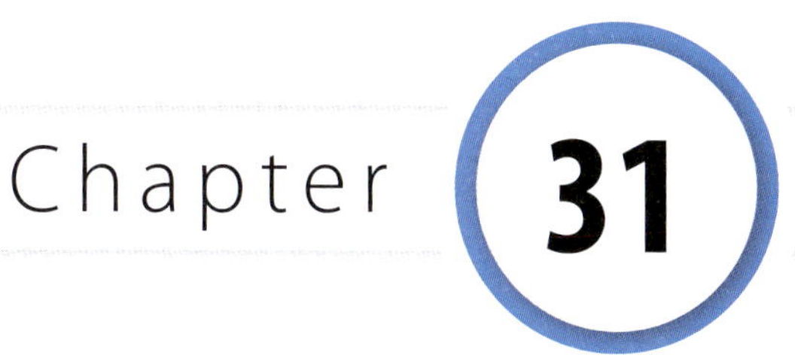

Anesthesia

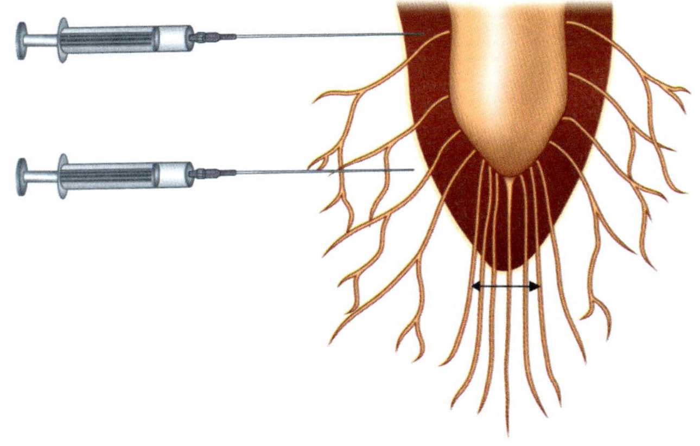

Important Topics

- Local Anesthesia
- Spinal Anesthesia
- Epidural Anesthesia and Analgesia
- General Anesthesia
- ERAS Pathway

'I keep six honest serving men; they taught me all I know.
Their names are what, why, when, how, where, and who.'

Types of Anesthesia

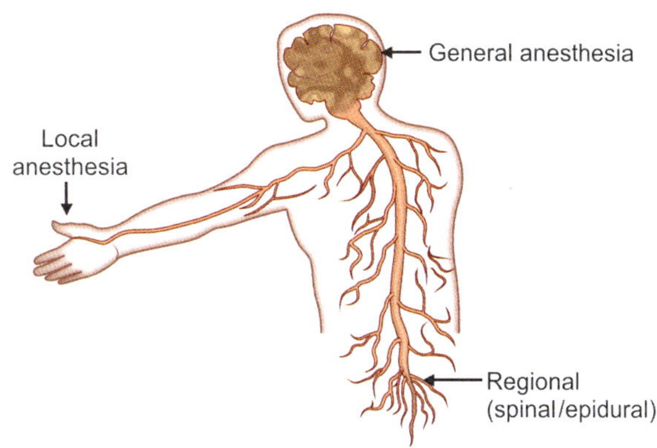

Local Anesthesia

Local anesthesia reversibly block impulse conductions along nerve axons by blocking voltage-gated sodium channels (small-diameter unmyelinated fibers, such as type C pain fibers are most sensitive whereas heavily myelinated, thicker fibers are least).

According to chemical structure, local anesthetics are of two types: (i) Amides (Lidocaine, bupivacaine, prilocaine, ropivacaine) and (ii) Esters (Cocaine, procaine, benzocaine). Amides are metabolized in the liver. Esters are hydrolyzed in the blood by pseudocholinesterase.

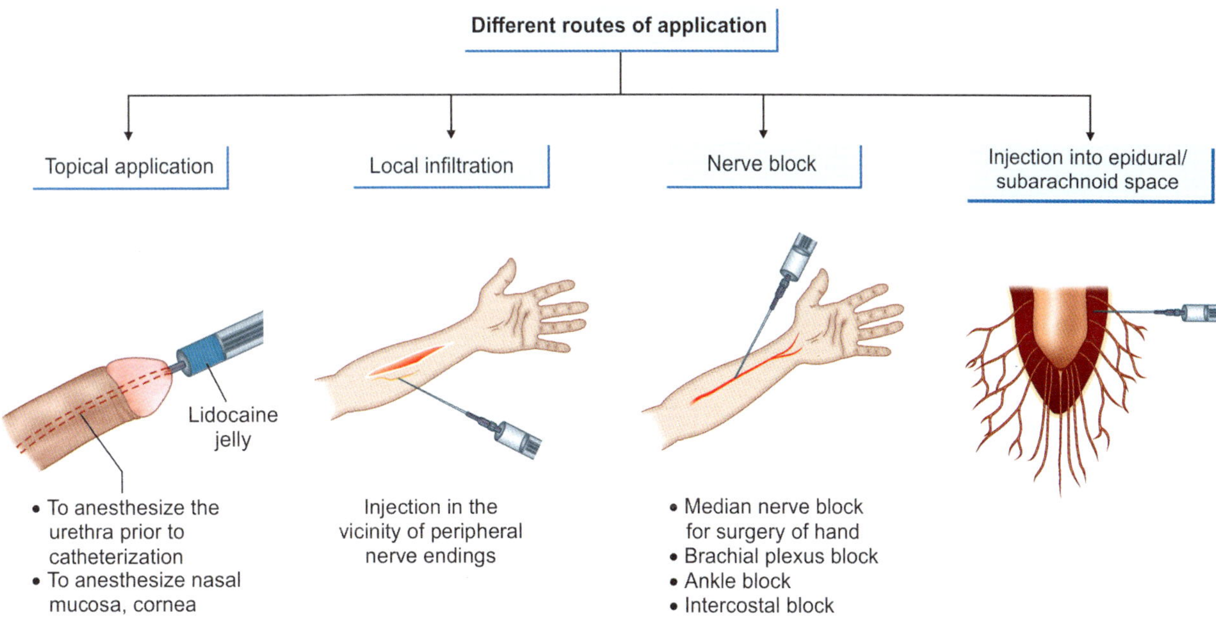

Topical Local Anesthetics

- **EMLA® (2.5% lidocaine, 2.5% prilocaine)**
- LET® (4% lidocaine, 1:2000 epinephrine, 0.5% tetracaine)
- LMX® 4/5 (4% or 5% liposomal lidocaine)
- Topicaine® (4% lidocaine)
- Pliaglis® (7% lidocaine, 7% tetracaine)
- Betacaine® Plus (15% lidocaine, 5% prilocaine)

Among topical local anesthetics, most commonly used is EMLA cream. EMLA cream is an eutectic mixture of lidocaine 2.5% and prilocaine 2.5%. It delivers maximal benefit after being in place for 30 to 60 minutes with an occlusive dressing.

- Lidocaine (pH 6.6) is less acidic than lidocaine with epinephrine (pH 4.6).
- Lidocaine 1% is less acidic than lidocaine 2%.
- Lidocaine is less acidic than bupivacaine.
- The lower the pH level of the anesthetic, the more intense the infiltration pain.

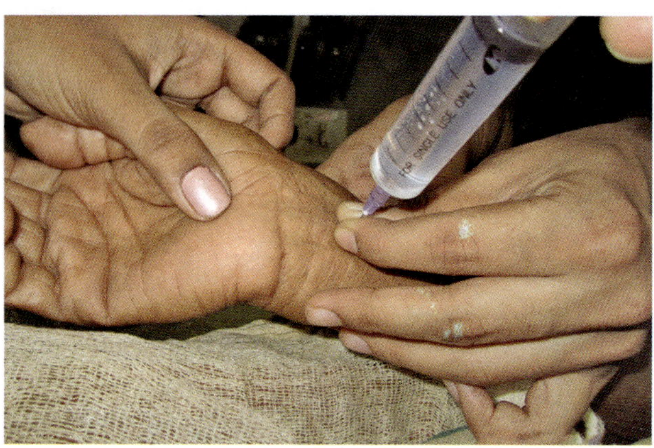

Nerve Block

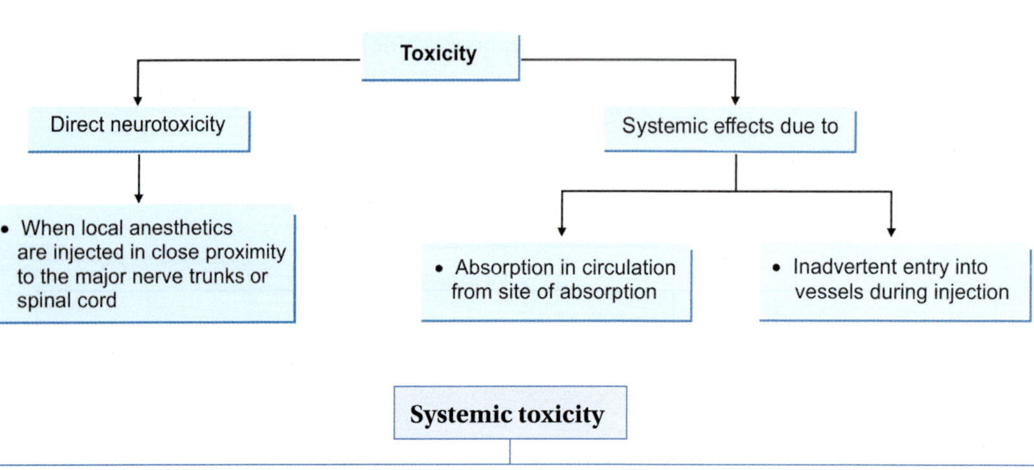

Systemic toxicity

CNS manifestations

- Sleepiness
- Circumoral and tongue numbness
- Metallic taste
- Tinnitus
- Visual disturbances
- Slurred speech
- Seizures

CVS manifestations

- Hypotension
- ↑P–R interval
- Bradycardia
- Cardiac arrest

[Bupivacaine is more cardiotoxic than other local anesthetics.]

Inadvertent IV injection of bupivacaine results in profound hypotension, VT, VF, complete A–V block that is refractory to treatment.

Measures to Minimize the Toxicity of Local Anesthetics

- Using the lowest concentration of local anesthetic.
- Using enough LA to achieve maximum anesthetic effect.
- Modify the dose of LA or epinephrine in patients at risk for toxicity.
- Using epinephrine to slow the absorption of LA into circulation and to prolong anesthetic effect.
- Avoiding direct injection into blood vessels.

Treatment of Local Anesthetic Systemic Toxicity (LAST) [Adapted from ASRA (American Society of Regional anesthesia and Pain Medicine) Checklist]

- Stop injecting local anesthetic
- Ventilate with 100% oxygen
- Seizure control with benzodiazepines
- Treatment of hypotension and bradycardia; CPR if patient is pulseless
- **Lipid emulsion therapy:**
  - **Patient's body weight >70 kg:** Bolus 100 mL lipid emulsion 20% rapidly over 2–3 minutes followed by lipid emulsion infusion 200–250 mL over 15–20 minutes.
  - **Body weight <70 kg:** Bolus 1.5 mL/kg lipid emulsion 20% rapidly over 2–3 minutes followed by lipid emulsion infusion 0.25 mL/kg/min
  - If patient remains unstable, rebolus once or twice at same dose and double infusion rate.
- **Monitoring:** 4–6 hours after a cardiovascular event, atleast 2 hours after a limited CNS event.

Epinephrine as an Additive

- Reduces local bleeding
- Absorption of local anesthetic from injection site is delayed, so the anesthetic will work for a longer period
- Systemic absorption is delayed, so chance of toxicity will be less.

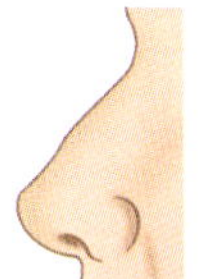
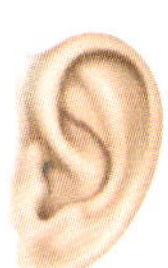
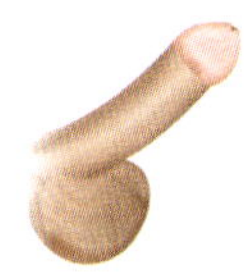
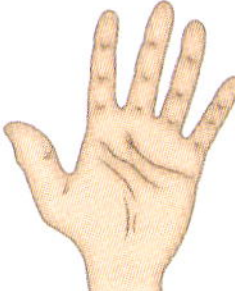
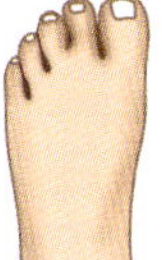

Only lidocaine
No adrenaline

Epinephrine containing anesthetics should not be injected in body parts which are supplied by end arteries.

Spinal Anesthesia

- Spinal anesthesia is a type of **neuroaxial anesthesia.** Other neuroaxial anesthesia techniques are epidural and caudal anesthesia.
- Local anesthetic is injected in the **intrathecal space (subarachnoid space)** resulting in sensory, motor and sympathetic blockade below the level of blockade.
- Site of injection is usually **below L1 or L2** (needle is passed between two lumbar spinous processes).
- **Lidocaine and bupivacaine** are the commonly used anesthetic agents.
- Spinal anesthesia is commonly indicated for surgical procedures in the lower abdomen, pelvis, perineum, lower extremity.

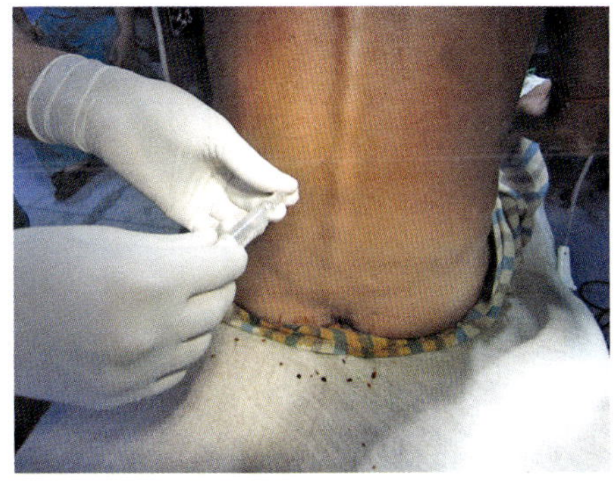

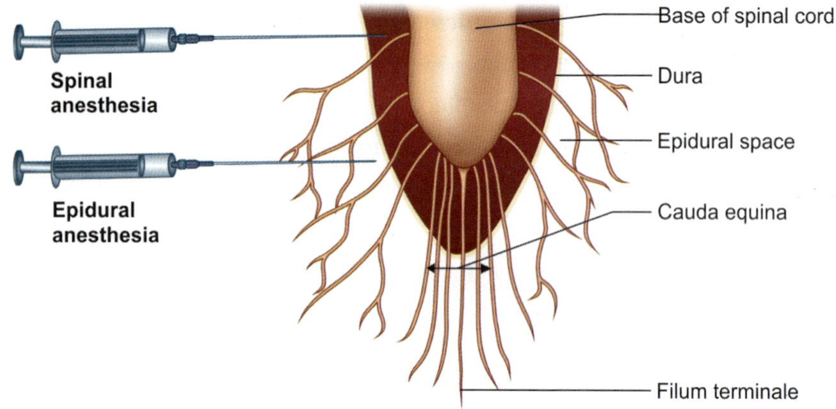

Anesthetics Used in Spinal Anesthesia

Local anesthetics	Onset of action	Duration of action (Plain)	Duration of action (with epinephrine)
Bupivacaine 0.75%	5–8 min	90–110 min	100–150 min
Lidocaine 5%	3–5 min	60–70 min	75–100 min
Tetracaine 0.5%	3–5 min	70–90 min	120–180 min
Ropivacaine 0.75%	3–5 min	140–200 min	

Absolute contraindications	Relative contraindications
Patient refusal	Preexisting neurological disease (particularly that wax and wane, e.g., Multiple sclerosis)
Increased intracranial pressure	Coagulopathy
Infection at the site of injection	Uncorrected hypovolemia
	Fixed cardiac output states (e.g., severe mitral and aortic stenosis, hypertrophic obstructive cardiomyopathy)

Minor complications	Major complications
Nausea and vomiting	Total spinal anesthesia
Mild hypotension	Direct needle trauma to spinal nerves or spinal cord
Itching	Meningitis
Postdural puncture headache	Arachnoiditis
Shivering	Spinal hematoma
Postoperative urinary retention	Cauda equina syndrome
Low-frequency hearing loss	Cardiovascular collapse

Epidural Anesthesia and Analgesia

Epidural anesthesia is another neuroaxial technique of anesthesia where local anesthetic is administered in epidural space. It is also an effective modality for perioperative pain management.

Indications of epidural anesthesia: Thoracic surgery, spine surgery, major intra-abdominal surgery.

Indications of epidural analgesia: Perioperative pain management, labor analgesia.

Benefits: (i) Reduce the risk of postoperative pulmonary complications (e.g., atelectasis, pneumonia); (ii) Decrease the incidence of postoperative pulmonary embolism and DVT; (iii) Early return of bowel function; (iv) Decreased stress response; and (v) Shortens length of hospital stay.

Absolute contraindications: (i) Increased intracranial pressure; (ii) Infection at the injection site; and (iii) Patient refusal

Relative contraindications: (i) Anatomic deformities of spine; (ii) Coagulopathy; (iii) Significant aortic stenosis; and (iv) Pulmonary hypertension

Complications: (i) Hypotension; (ii) Bradycardia; (iii) Inadvertent penetration of the dural space; (iv) Epidural hematoma; (v) Epidural abscess; (vi) Transient neurological syndrome; (vii) Paraplegia—rare (due to epidural hematoma); and (viii) Opiod-induced respiratory depression (following epidural analgesia).

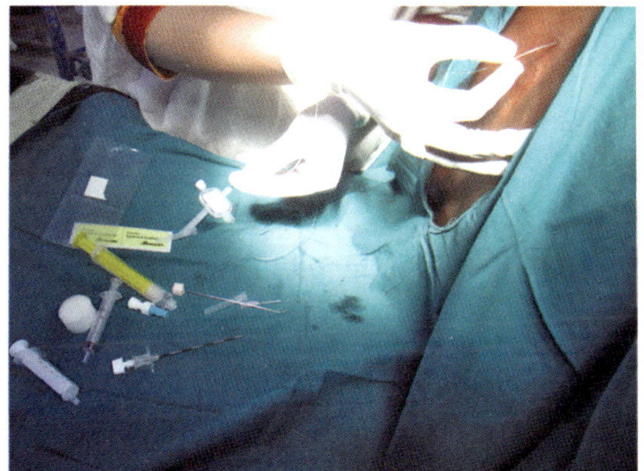

Introduction of Epidural Catheter

General Anesthesia

Effects of General Anesthesia

- Unconsciousness and Amnesia
- Analgesia
- Muscle Relaxation

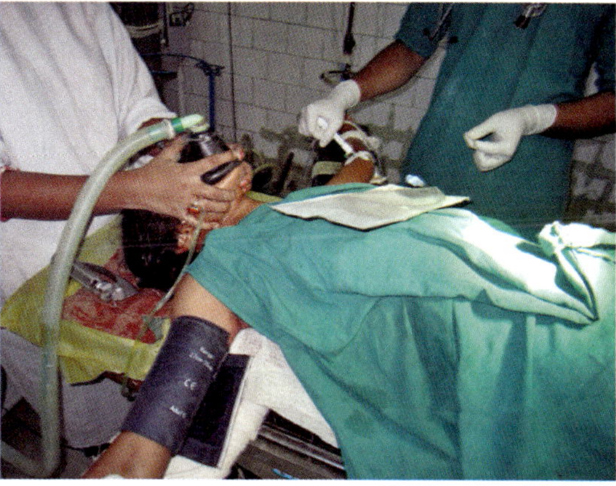

General anesthesia is achieved by both **intravenous** and **inhalational** agents.

IV Agents (causing Unconsciousness and Amnesia)

- **Barbiturates:** Thiopental is a barbiturate that is commonly used. They act on GABA receptor, resulting in inhibition of excitatory synaptic transmission. Barbiturates are anticonvulsants and reduces cerebral metabolism. In higher doses, it is myocardial depressant.
- **Propofol:** It acts on GABA receptor resulting in inhibition of synaptic transmission. It has bronchodilator property. It may cause hypotension. It is the anesthetic of choice for ambulatory surgery.
- **Etomidate:** It acts on GABA receptor.
- **Ketamine:** It acts on NMDA receptor. It is a dissociative anesthetic, producing analgesia also. Patient may present with delirium and hallucinations while regaining consciousness. It increases heart rate and BP. It can maintain BP in hypovolemic patients by sympathetic stimulation. It is myocardial depressant.

IV Agents (causing Amnesia and Reduction of Anxiety)

Benzodiazepines: It acts on GABA receptor. This agents cause peripheral vasodilation and hypotension. They are also good anticonvulsants. When it is combined with opioid analgesics, it may cause respiratory depression. Commonly used benzodiazepines are diazepam, lorazepam, midazolam.

IV Agents (causing Analgesia)

- **Opiod analgesics:** Acts on μ-receptor in brain and spinal cord. Commonly used opiod analgesics are: morphine, codein, fentanyl (Synthetic opiod).
- **Nonopiod analgesics:** Ketamine and Ketorolac. Ketorolac acts by inhibiting both COX-1 and COX-2.

IV Agents (causing Neuromuscular Block)

- Acts on postsynaptic receptors in the neuromuscular junction to antogonize the effects acetylcholine.
- Two types of neuromuscular blockers: (i) Nondepolarizing agents (Vecuronium, Pancuronium, Atracurium) and (ii) Depolarizing agents (Succinylcholine).
- **Succinylcholine:** Rapid acting (<60 seconds) depolarizing neuromuscular blocker also with rapid offset (5–8 minutes) property. This agent is rapidly hydrolyzed by plasma cholinesterase. It causes hyperkalemia. Patient with severe burn or trauma may develop arrhythmia or cardiac arrest. It can increase intraocular, intracranial, and intragastric pressures. Malignant hyperthermia is a rare but fatal complication.
- **Vecuronium:** Intermediate duration (<1 hour), nondepolarizing neuromuscular blocker. It is metabolized by both kidneys and liver.
- **Pancuronium:** Longest-acting (>1 hour) nondepolarizing blocker. It is excreted by kidneys in unchanged form.
- **Atracurium:** Intermediate-acting (<1 hour) nondepolarizing blocker. It is metabolized in plasma by a unique method—Hofmann elimination.

Reversal of neuromuscular blockade:

Neostigmine, pyridostigmine inhibit the acetylcholinesterase, thereby increased circulatory level of acetylcholine. So, more acetylcholine is available for competition for postsynaptic receptors.

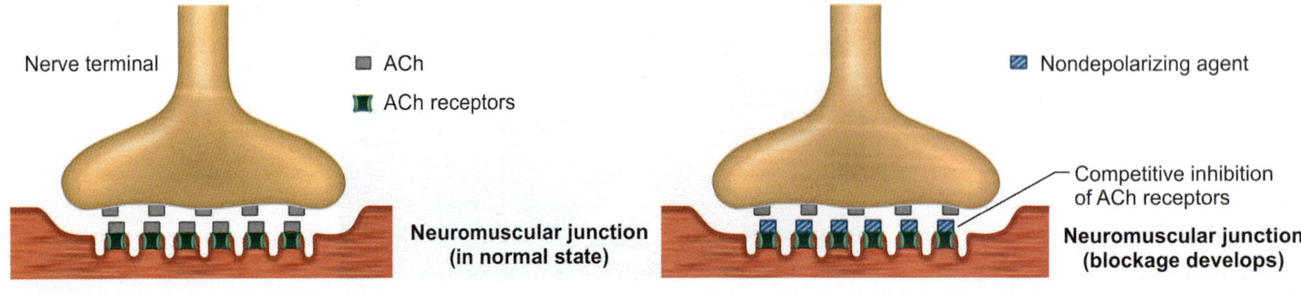

Inhalational Agents

Inhalational agents produce three aspects of GA—unconsciousness, analgesia, and muscle relaxation. These agents act on GABAA receptor-chloride channel, resulting in inhibition of synaptic transmission.

Inhalational agents are: Nitrous oxide, Halothane, Sevoflurane, Desflurane, Isoflurane.

To provide adequate anesthesia, the anesthetic agent requires transfer from the alveolar air to the blood and from the blood to the brain.

Minimum alveolar concentration (MAC) is the measure of potency of an inhalational anesthetic. Higher the MAC, less potent the agent is.

Nitrous oxide (MAC 105%): A weak anesthetic agent with most rapid onset and offset. When combined with other inhalational agents, it reduces the required dose and side effects of other inhalational agents. It readily diffuses into any closed gas space, thereby increases the presence of the space. It should not be administered in intestinal obstruction or pneumothorax.

Halothane (MAC 0.75%): Halothane has rapid onset of action. It is a preferable induction agent in pediatric patients due to less irritating effect on airway and a preferable agent for asthmatics due to its bronchial smooth muscle relaxing properties. Halothane use is associated with increased chance of ventricular arrhythmia. It increases intracranial pressure. So, it should be used cautiously in patients with brain lesions.

Isoflurane (MAC 1.15%): Characteristic properties are: (i) Less cardiovascular depression and (ii) Low rate of metabolism.

Sevoflurane (MAC 1.17%): Pleasant smell, therefore ideal for mask induction. Sevoflurane has less tissue and blood solubility, therefore rapid induction and recovery.

Desflurane (MAC 6%): Desflurane has rapid induction and recovery. This agent causes increase in cerebral blood flow. So, it is better avoided in patients with intracranial lesion. It is not used as an induction agent because it causes upper airway irritation (cough, bronchospasm).

Preoperative Evaluation

History taking:

- Detailed medical history also includes any history of exposure to anesthesia.
- History of atopy (atopy to food, medications, etc.)
- History of medication (e.g., anticoagulants, antihypertensives, antidiabetics)

Physical examination: Examination of CNS, CVS and respiratory system

Investigations:

- Specific investigations
- Routine investigations

Risk Assessment

ASA physical status scale is to assess the risk of an individual during anesthesia and surgery.

Scale: P1 to P6

P1: Normal healthy patient

P2: Patient with mild systemic disease

P3: Patient with severe systemic disease

P4: Patient with severe systemic disease that is a constant threat to life

P5: Moribund patient who is not expected to survive without the operation

P6: A declared braindead paitent whose organs are being removed for donor purposes.

Assessment of Patient with Comorbid Illness

Ischemic heart disease: Assessment of severity and functional limitations induced by the disease.

Pulmonary disease: Assessment is essential for thoracic and upper abdominal surgical procedures.

Renal disease: Patient with chronic renal disease needs vigorous attention to intraoperative fluid management and control of ventilation. Doses of anesthetic agents, particularly opioids and neuromuscular blockers must be reduced.

Hepatobiliary disease: Selection of a proper inhalational anesthetic is crucial. Halothane has the greatest potential and desflurane has the least potential for hepatotoxicity. Selection of neuromuscular blocker (e.g., vecuronium, pancuronium) is better avoided in impaired hepatic function.

Metabolic disease: The three metabolic diseases, diabetes mellitus, hypothyroidism and obesity are mostly associated with increased risk.

CNS disease: Propofol decreases cerebral blood flow, intracranial pressure. Etomidate also decreases cerebral blood flow and ICP. It has also excitatory effect on the brain.

Assessment of the Airway:

- Assessment of the airway is important to identify the chance of difficulty during conventional endotracheal intubation.
- Mallampati classification is based on how much posterior pharynx is visualized after maximal mouth opening and tongue protrusion in sitting position.

Mallampati Classification

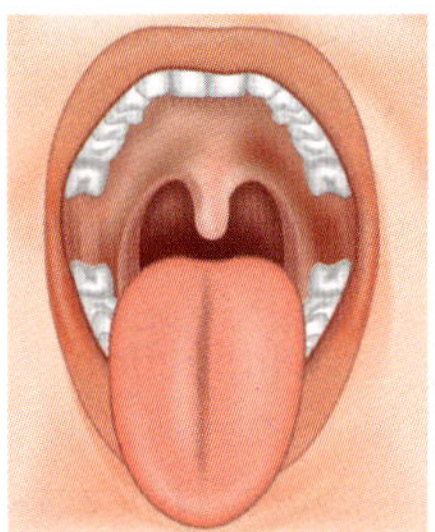

Class 1
(soft palate, fauces, uvula, pillars)

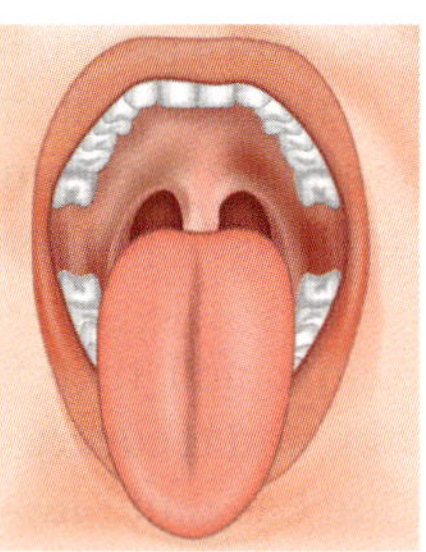

Class 2
(soft palate, fauces, part of uvula)

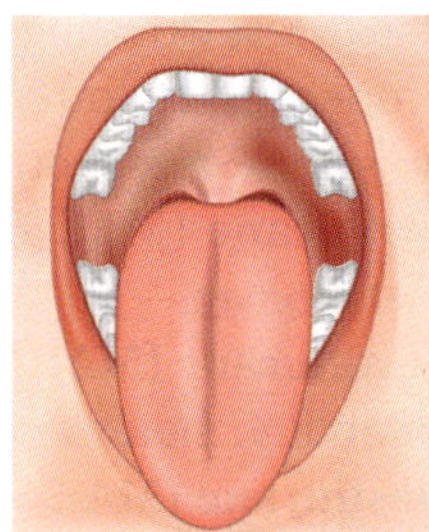

Class 3
(soft palate, base of uvula)

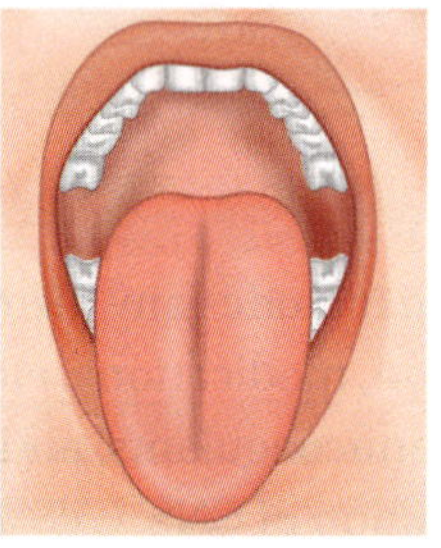

Class 4
(hard palate only)

Intraoperative Management

1. **Induction of anesthesia:**
   - Most vital phase of anesthesia, as most of the catastrophes occur during this phase.
   - During induction, patient becomes unconscious and apneic, myocardial function is being depressed.

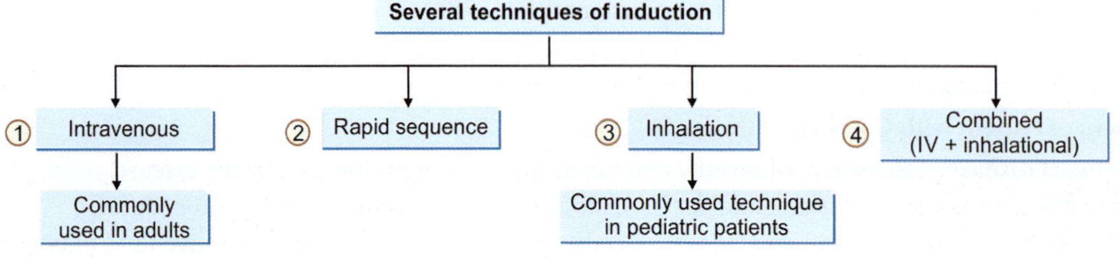

2.

Management of airway

- **Mask ventilation**
  Used in peripheral procedures that do not required neuromuscular blockade [Contraindicated in patient with risk of aspiration]
- **Endotracheal intubation**
  - It secures the airway and can control the ventilation
  - It can be performed usually with the aid of laryngoscope, but sometimes performed with the aid of fiberoptic bronchoscope
- **Laryngeal mask airway (LMA)**
  - It is inserted blindly into the pharynx
  - It makes a seal around the laryngeal inlet and permit positive pressure ventilation

3. **Neuromuscular blockade:**
   - It optimizes ventilatory support.
   - It relaxes the muscles, thereby provides satisfactory working conditions.
   - Done by nondepolarizing neuromuscular blockers
4. **Maintenance of anesthesia:**
   - With the help of both inhalational as well as intravenous agents
5. **Fluid therapy** is to replace the perioperative fluid losses.
6. **Recovery from anesthesia:**
   - The goal of smooth recovery is to achieve a smooth and rapid return to consciousness, stable hemodynamics, return of protective airway reflexes, and continued analgesia.
7. **Postanesthesia care unit (PACU):**
   - All patients awakening from anesthesia are to be observed in PACU, to detect immediate postoperative nausea and vomiting, hypotension requiring pharmacologic support, abnormal bleeding, dysrhythmia. Once patient become oriented, hemodynamically stable and without signs of anesthetic or surgical complications, patient can be shifted to the ward.

Indications of general anesthesia: (i) Surgery that requires deep relaxation for a longer period; (ii) Surgeries where regional or local anesthesia is not sufficient; (iii) Failure of regional anesthesia; and (iv) Uncooperative patient.

Relative contraindications of general anesthesia: (i) Medical conditions are not optimized prior to elective surgery; (ii) Patient with a difficult airway; and (iii) Patient with significant comorbidities (e.g., severe aortic stenosis, congestive heart failure etc.)

Complications of general anesthesia: (i) Postoperative nausea and vomiting; (ii) Laryngospasm; (iii) Hypothermia; (iv) Malignant hyperthermia; and (v) Nerve injury.

Recommendations for Preoperative Fasting before Procedures Requiring General Anesthesia, Regional Anesthesia, or Procedural Sedation and Analgesia [Adapted from ASA Guidelines]

Type of food	Preoperative minimum fasting period
Clear liquids (e.g., water, fruit juice without pulp, carbonated beverages, clear tea, black coffee)	2 hours
Breast milk	4 hours
Infant formula	6 hours
Light meal and nonhuman milk	6 hours
Fried food, fatty foods, meat	8 hours or more

ERAS (Enhanced Recovery after Surgery) Pathway

A new concept in surgical and anesthetic discipline to improve the quality of perioperative care. This pathway includes multiple elements to reduce surgical stress, maintaining postoperative physiological function, enhance mobilization after surgery, resulting in reduced morbidity, faster recovery, and shorter length of stay in hospital.

Elements of ERAS: (i) Preoperative; (ii) Intraoperative; and (iii) Postoperative.

ERAS elements:

1. **Preoperative counseling:** Preoperative counseling about the surgical and anesthetic procedures may reduce the fear and anxiety and may enhance postoperative recovery.
2. **Preoperative optimization:** Four weeks of abstinence from smoking and alcohol consumption reduces the postoperative morbidity. Pharmacological support and individual counseling should be offered to every patient who smokes and to alcohol abusers undergoing elective surgery. Optimization of medical conditions, e.g., cardiovascular diseases, anemia, diabetes, etc. should follow international recommendations.
3. **Preoperative fasting and carbohydrate loading:** Clear fluids should be allowed upto 2 hours and solids should be allowed upto 6 hours before induction of anesthesia. Preoperative treatment with oral carbohydrate should be routinely administered except in patients with documented delayed gastric emptying or slow gastrointestinal motility.
4. **Preoperative bowel preparation:** Mechanical bowel preparation should not be used in colonic surgery, pelvic surgery, in pancreaticoduodenectomy.
5. **Preanesthetic medication:** Patient should not receive short-or long-acting sedative or anxiolytic medications because it may delay discharge.
6. **Prophylaxis against thromboembolism:** Patient who have had major cancer surgery in abdomen or pelvis should use compression stockings or intermittent pneumatic compression and receive pharmacological prophylaxis with LMWH. Extended prophylaxis should be continued for 28 days in patients with colorectal cancer or with increased risk of VTE.
7. **Antimicrobial prophylaxis and skin preparation:** Routine prophylaxis with intravenous antibiotics should be given 30–60 min before skin incision. Repeat dose may be necessary during intraoperative period depending on the half life of the antibiotic and duration of surgery. Chlorhexidine-alcohol should be used for skin preparation.
8. **Prevention and treatment of postoperative nausea and vomiting (PONV):** A multimodal approach to PONV prophylaxis should be adopted in all patients with 2 or more risk factors for PONV. If PONV is present, treatment should be given using multimodal approach.
9. **Standard anesthetic protocol:** A standard anesthetic protocol allowing rapid awakening should be given. The anesthesist should control fluid therapy, analgesia, and hemodynamic changes to reduce metabolic stress response. In open surgery, mid-thoracic epidural blocks using local anesthetics and low dose opiods are indicated. In laparoscopic surgery, spinal analgesia or morphine PCA is an alternative to epidural anesthesia.
10. **Surgical techniques:** Laparoscopic surgery for gastrointestinal surgery is recommended when expertise is available.
11. **Preventing intraoperative hypothermia:** Intraoperative hypothermia should be avoided using active warming devices and warm intravenous fluids.
12. **Perioperative fluid management:** Patients should receive perioperative fluids in such a manner to attain a near-zero fluid balance and to avoid fluid excess and organ hypoperfusion. Postoperatively, intravenous fluid should be discontinued as soon as practicable and oral intake is encouraged.

13. **Perioperative glycemic control:** Glucose level should be kept as close to normal as possible without compromising safety. ERAS protocols that affect insulin action/resistance without risk of hypoglycemia, should be implemented.
14. **Nasogastric intubation:** Routine use of nasogastric tube in postoperative period should be avoided.
15. **Use of drain:** Routine use of intraperitoneal drain is discouraged after colorectal surgery and pancreatic surgery.
16. **Urinary catheter:** Early removal of routine urinary catheter (1st or 2nd postoperative day) is recommended.
17. **Postoperative pain management:** Opiod-sparing analgesic strategies, including regional analgesia techniques should be implemented.
18. **Prevention of postoperative ileus:** Multimodal preventing strategies (e.g. laparoscopic surgery, mid-thoracic epidural analgesia, avoidance of fluid overload and nasogatric tube) should be adopted to facilitate recovery of gastrointestinal function.
19. **Early mobilization:** Patient should be actively mobilized from the morning of first postoperative day and encouraged to meet daily targets for mobilization.

Chapter 32

Instrument

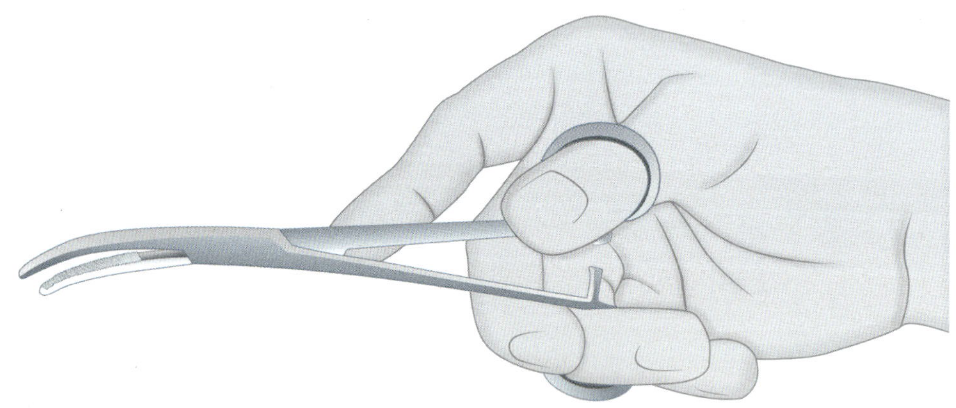

Important Topics

- Instruments Used for Antiseptic Dressing
- Instruments Used for Giving Incision
- Instruments Used for Hemostasis
- Instruments Used for Holding Tissues
- Instruments Used for Suturing
- Scissors
- Urinary Catheter
- Suture Material
- Miscellaneous Instruments
- Intravenous Cannula

'Medicine rests upon four pillars—philosophy, astronomy, alchemy, and ethics ...., the fourth shows the physician those virtues which must stay with him up until his death, and it should support and complete the three other pillars.'

Paracelsus (C. 1493–1541)
Swiss Doctor and Chemist

Basic Anatomy of a Surgical Instrument

Blades—a pair of blades

Joint: (i) Box joint—slot in each shaft, fits with each other and (ii) Pivot joint—two shafts are joined by a screw at one point

Shaft—a pair of shafts

Catch or rachet

Finger bow—two finger bows

Instruments Used for Antiseptic Dressing and Draping

Rampley's Swab Holding Forceps

Blades are oval, fenestrated, and serrations on the inner aspect.

Uses:

- Antiseptic dressing prior to any surgical procedure [antiseptic most commonly used is povidone-iodine (both antibacterial and antifungal)]. Antiseptic dressing is essential to remove the transient and resident bacterial flora of skin.
- During blunt dissection of Calot's triangle in open cholecystectomy
- During retroperitoneal dissection—to strip off the peritoneum
- For removal of laminated membrane and daughter cyst of hydatid cyst
- May be used as a substitute of Moynihan cholecystectomy forceps.

Sterilization: Autoclaving

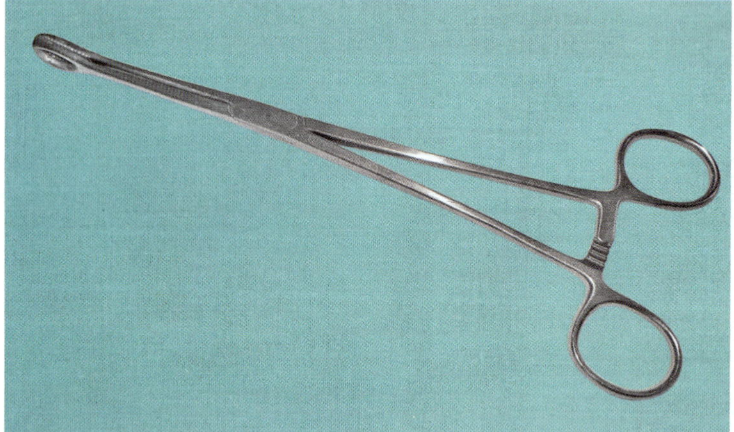

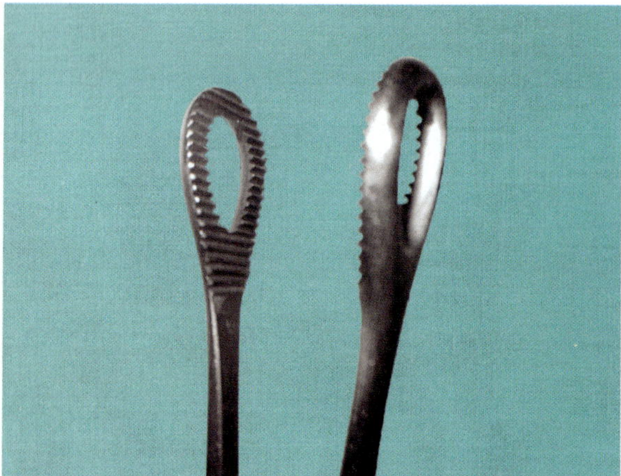

Instruments Used for Fixation

Towel Clip

- Towel clips are of two types: (i) Doyen's cross action type and (ii) Corner clip

Uses:

- For fixing the draping sheets
- For fixing the diathermy cables, suction tubes, and other cables
- May be used as a tongue-holding forceps.

Sterilization: Autoclaving

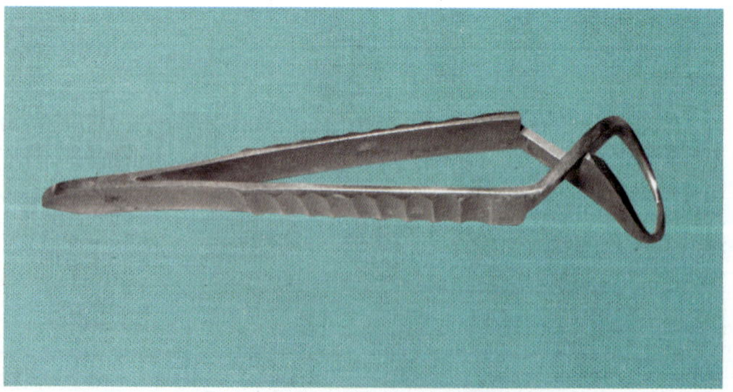

Doyen's cross action type towel clip

Instruments Used for Giving Incision

Bard Parker (BP) Handle

It has a slot on one end for attachment of the surgical blade.

Various sizes are available: No. 3, No. 4, No. 5 and No. 7. Handle No. 3 and 4 are commonly used.

Handle No. 3 is compatible with Blade no. 10, 11, 12, 15

Handle No. 4 is compatible with Blade No. 20, 21, 22, 23, 26

Handle No. 7 is compatible with Blade No. 10, 11, 12, 15

Sterilization: Autoclaving

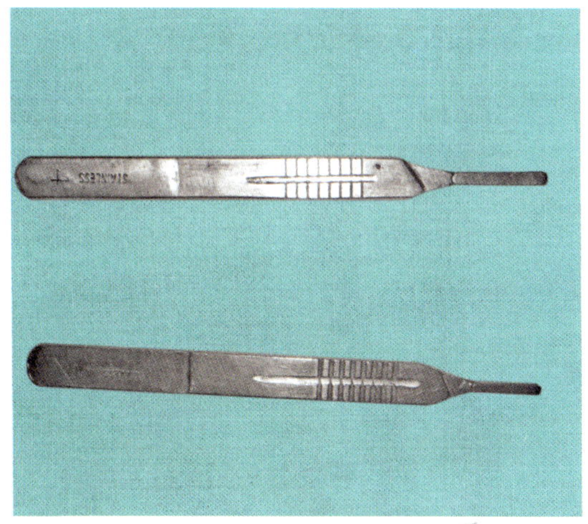

Surgical Blades (Scalpel Blades)

- Scalpel (Bard Parker handle with surgical blade) is the most common instrument used for giving incision.
- Blades are of varying sizes and slots, for attachment with the BP handles of different sizes.

Uses:

- To make skin incisions in all operations
- To make skin flaps in mastectomy, thyroidectomy, neck dissection
- For incision and drainage of abscess (by blade number 11—also called 'stab knife')

Blade No. 10: Blade with a sharp-edged curved belly, used for making skin incisions.

Blade No. 11: Blade with a straight and an angled edge with a pointed end, used for making stab incisions.

Blade No. 12: Crescent-shaped blade with sharp inner side, used for suture removal, cleft palate surgeries.

Blade No. 15: Blade with a sharp-edged curved belly like No. 10 but smaller cutting edge, used for making precise, small incision.

Blade No. 20: Blade with a sharp-edged curved belly similar to No. 10 but larger, used for making skin incisions.

Blade No. 21: Blade with a sharp-edged curved belly larger than No. 20, used for making skin incisions.

Blade No. 22: Blade with a small-cutting edge, similar to No. 10 but larger than No. 21.

Blade No. 23: Leaf-shaped blade with a curved cutting edge, used for making long incisions.

Blade No. 26: Blade with a straight cutting edge and opposite side is blunt with a downward angle.

Methods of holding scalpel: (i) Pen-holding grip and (ii) Finger-tip grip.

Methods of safe handling of scalpel: (i) Always pass the scalpel to the surgical members in a kidney tray and (ii) Always fit and remove the surgical blade with the hemostatic forceps, not with the hand.

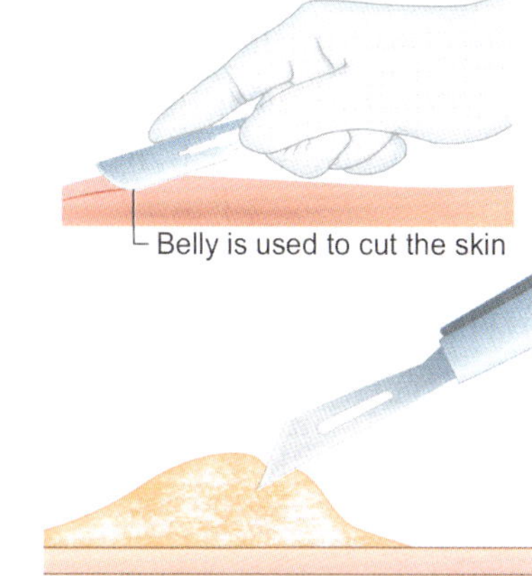

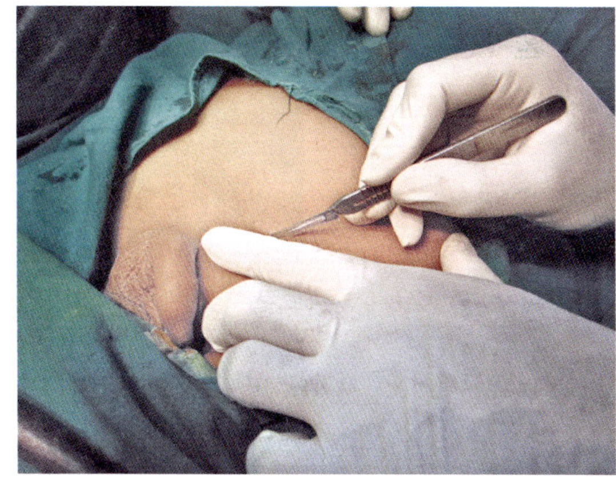

Pen-holding grip.

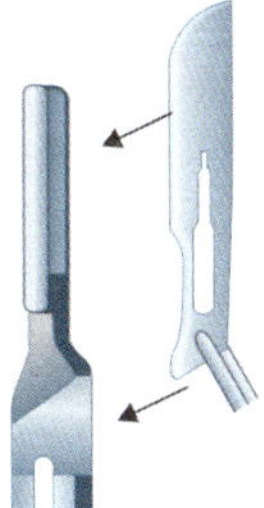

Fit and remove the blade with the hemostatic forceps, not with the hand

Instruments Used for Hemostasis

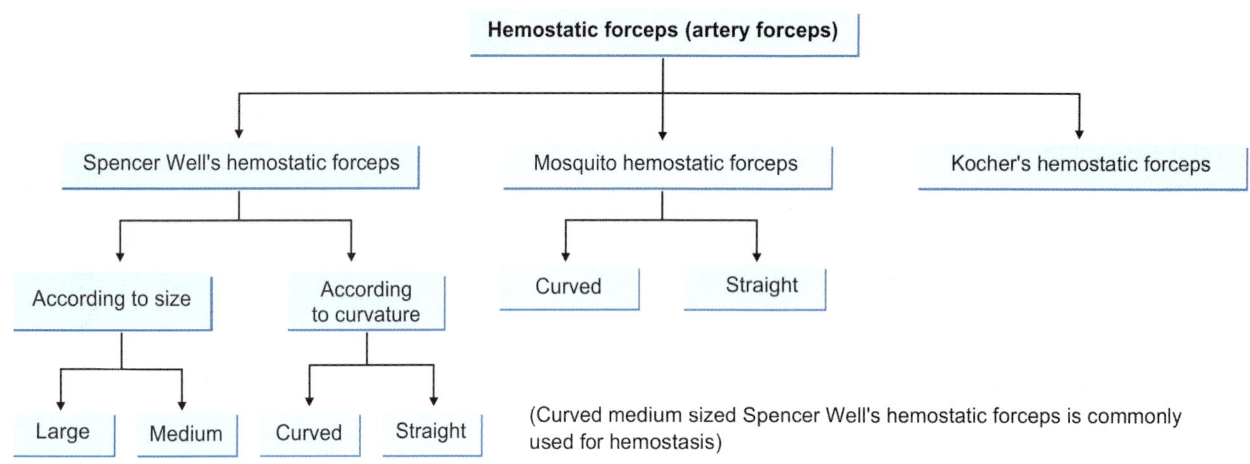

(Curved medium sized Spencer Well's hemostatic forceps is commonly used for hemostasis)

Spencer Well's Hemostatic Forceps

Uses:

- Used to hold the bleeding points
- Used to hold the vessel and ligate it
- To hold the cut margins of rectus sheath, aponeurosis, and peritoneum
- For blunt dissection during excision of lipoma, sebaceous cyst
- May be used in drainage of abscess as an alternative to sinus forceps
- To hold the end of a ligature during anastomosis, sheath, or skin closure.

Sterilization: Autoclaving

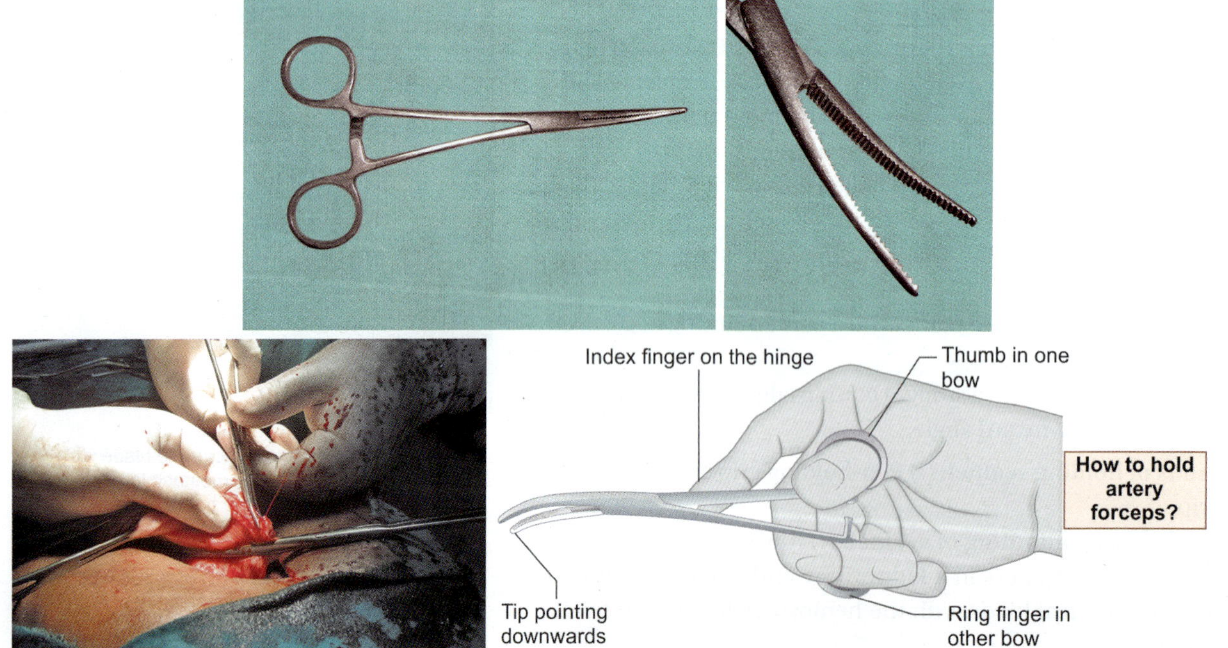

Mosquito Hemostatic Forceps

- Lighter and smaller than Spencer Well's hemostatic forceps
- *2 varieties:* Straight and curved

Uses:

- In appendicectomy (Mesoappendix is punctured by mosquito forceps for tying the appendicular artery)
- In circumcision
- In cleft lip operation
- For holding delicate vessels

Sterilization: Autoclaving

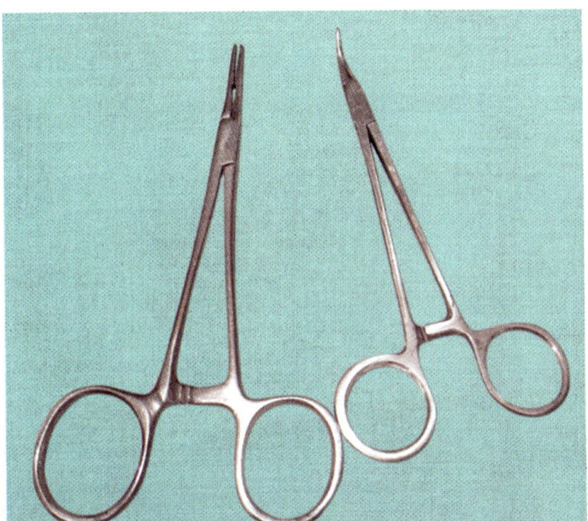

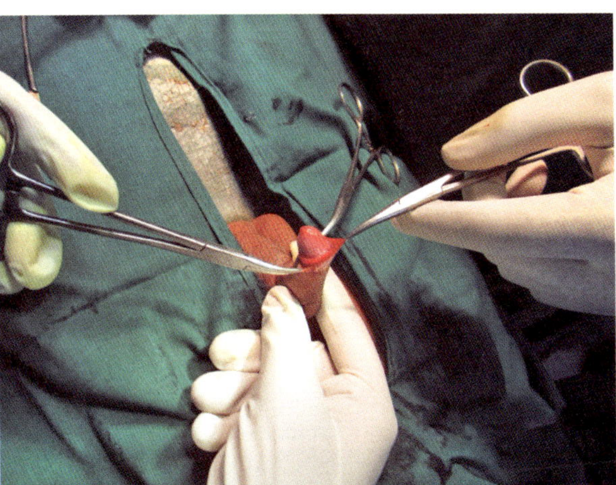

Kocher's Hemostatic Forceps

Uses:

- To hold the bleeding vessels in palm, sole, and scalp (vessels tend to retract)
- To crush the base of appendix
- In subtotal thyroidectomy

Sterilization: Autoclaving

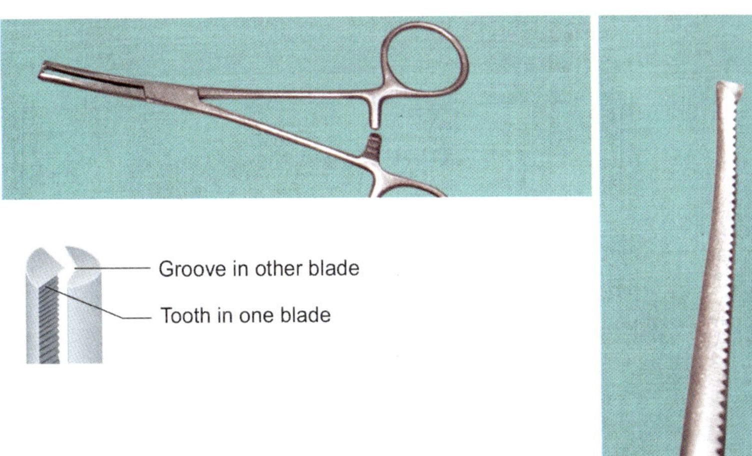

Instruments Used for Holding Tissues

Allis Tissue Forceps

Uses:

- During mastectomy or thyroidectomy, to raise the skin flaps.
- During midline incision, the skin margins are retracted by it when linea alba is incised.
- During closing the midline incision, the linea alba is held by this instrument.
- During excision of lipoma, sebaceous cyst, the skin margins are held by it.
- During creation of stoma, the skin is grasped by it.

Sterilization: Autoclaving

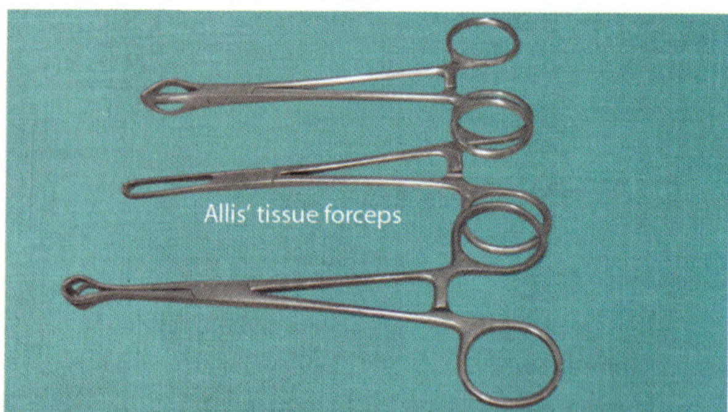

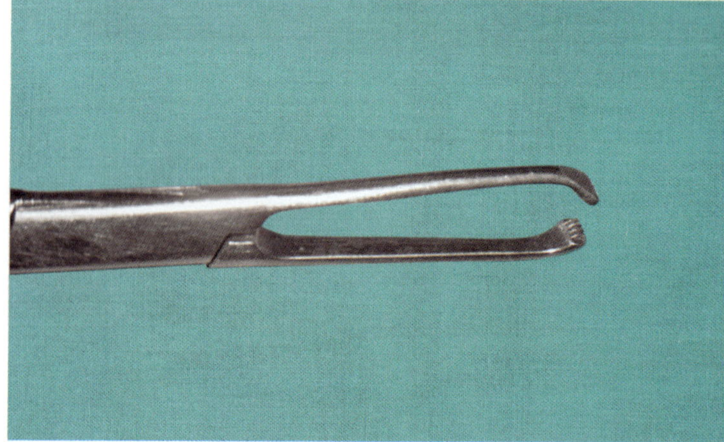

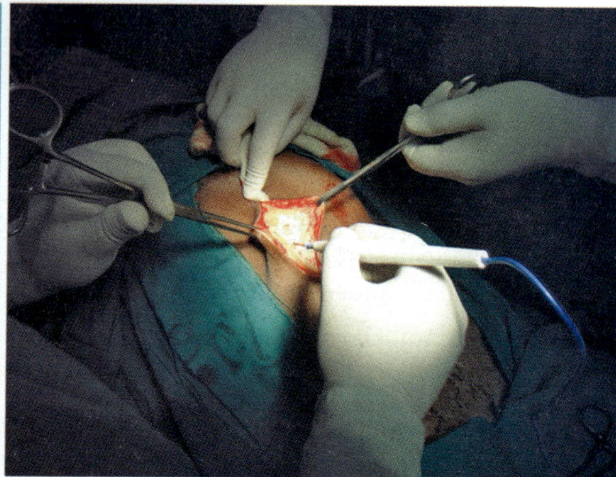

Babcock Tissue Forceps

No teeth in blades, so minimal trauma to the tissues. Fenestration in the blade allows tissues to be accommodated.

Uses:

- In appendectomy
- During resection anastomosis
- During gastrectomy
- During open prostatectomy or suprapubic cystostomy

Sterilization: Autoclaving

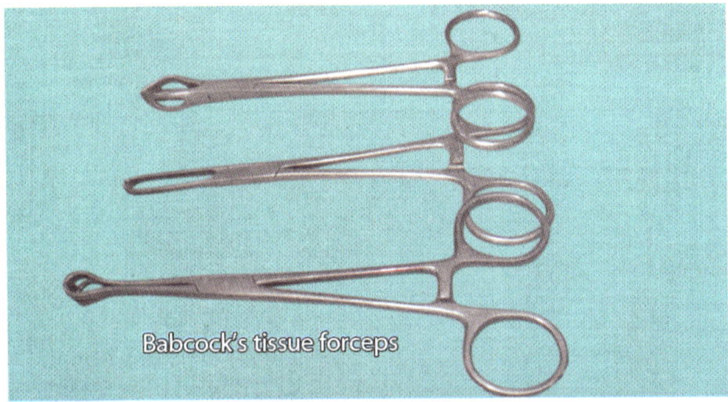

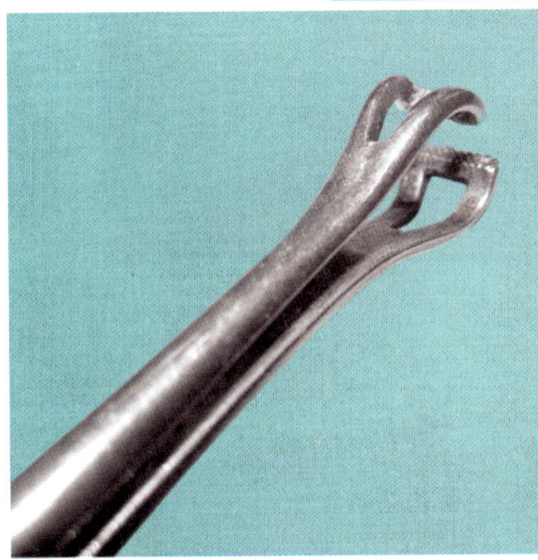

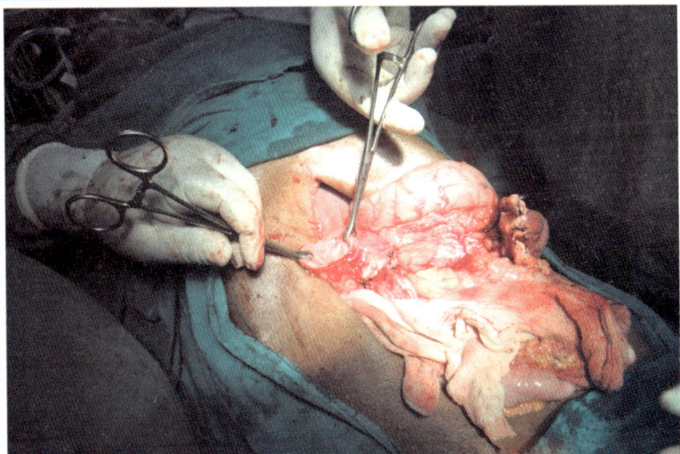

Lanes Tissue Forceps

At the tip of the blade, tooth in one blade and groove in the other blade.

Uses:

- As an alternative to towel clip
- During mastectomy, to hold the breast tissue when dissecting it from the pectoral muscle.

Sterilization—Autoclaving.

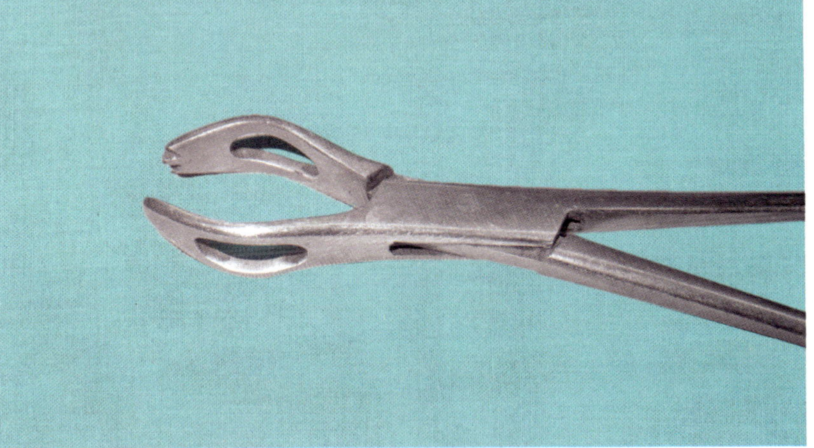

Dissecting Forceps

Dissecting forceps are of two types: (i) Plain and (ii) Toothed.

Uses of plain dissecting forceps:

- During hernia repair, to dissect the sac from cord structures as well as during ligation of the sac
- During resection anastomosis or in gastrojejunostomy, to hold the gut margins during suturing
- During choledocholithotomy, to hold the cut margins of common bile duct for closure.

Uses of plain dissecting forceps:

- To hold the skin margins during skin closure
- Suturing of aponeurosis in appendectomy
- During closure of midline incision, to hold the linea alba

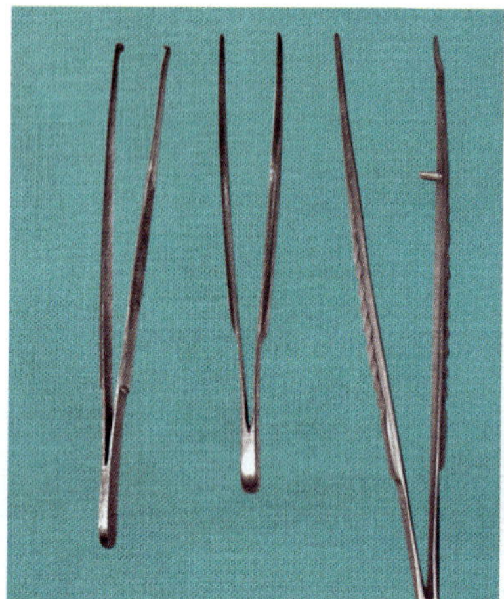

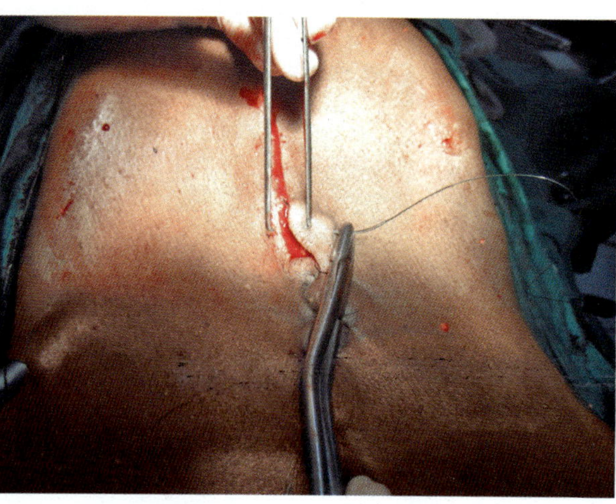

Instruments Used for Suturing

Needle Holder

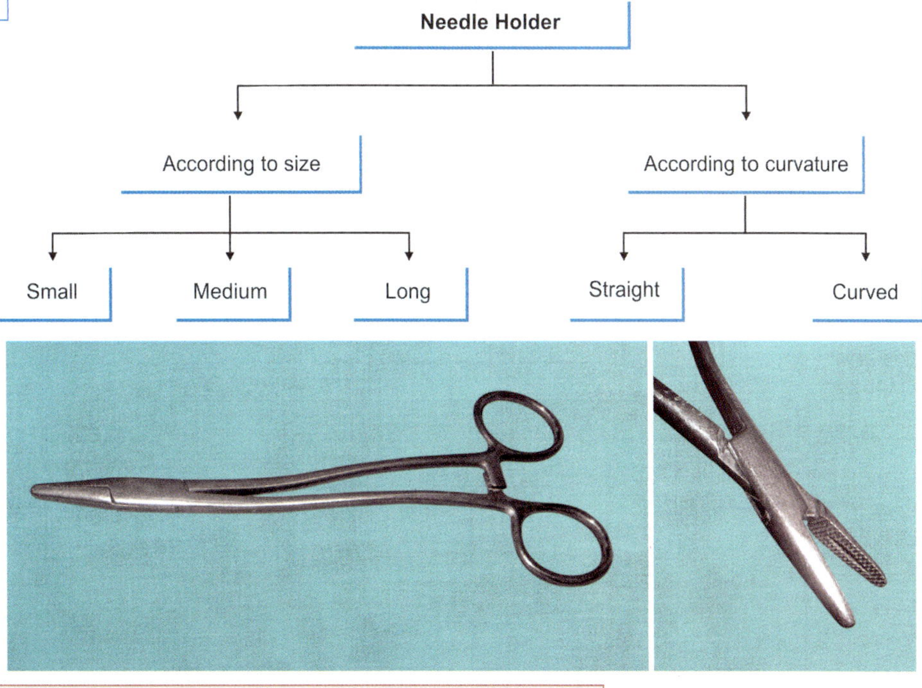

How to Hold Needle by Needle Holder?

Needle should be grasped by the tip of the needle holder at the junction of 2/3rd and 1/3rd of the needle.

Movements of the Hand during Suturing

Hand should be fully pronated at the start of suturing, then progressive supination and then full supination.

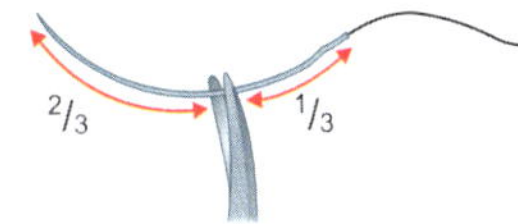

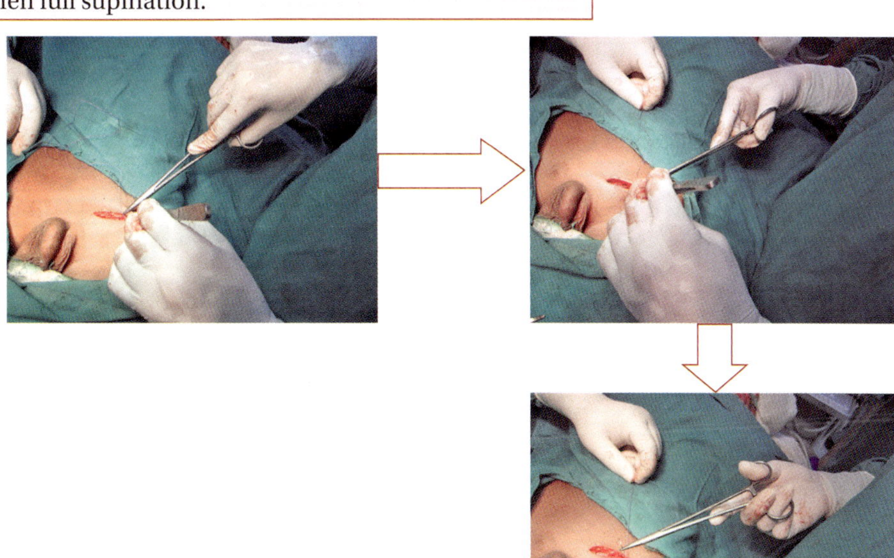

Surgical Needle

Properties of an Ideal Surgical Needle

- Made of high-quality stainless steel
- As slim as possible without compromising strength
- Sharp enough to penetrate tissue with minimum resistance
- Rigid enough to resist bending
- Ductile enough to resist breaking
- Stable in the grasp of needle holder

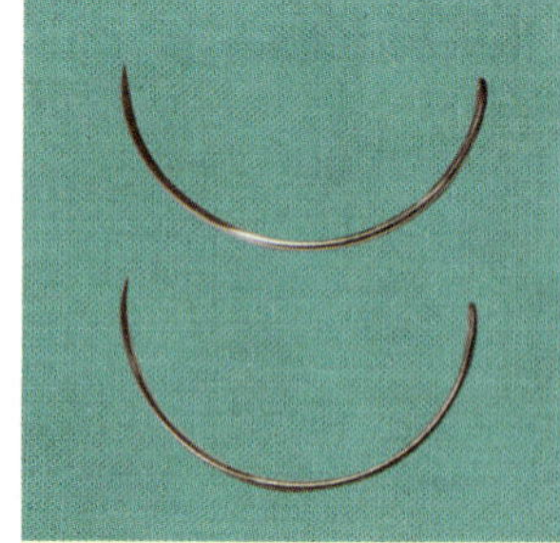

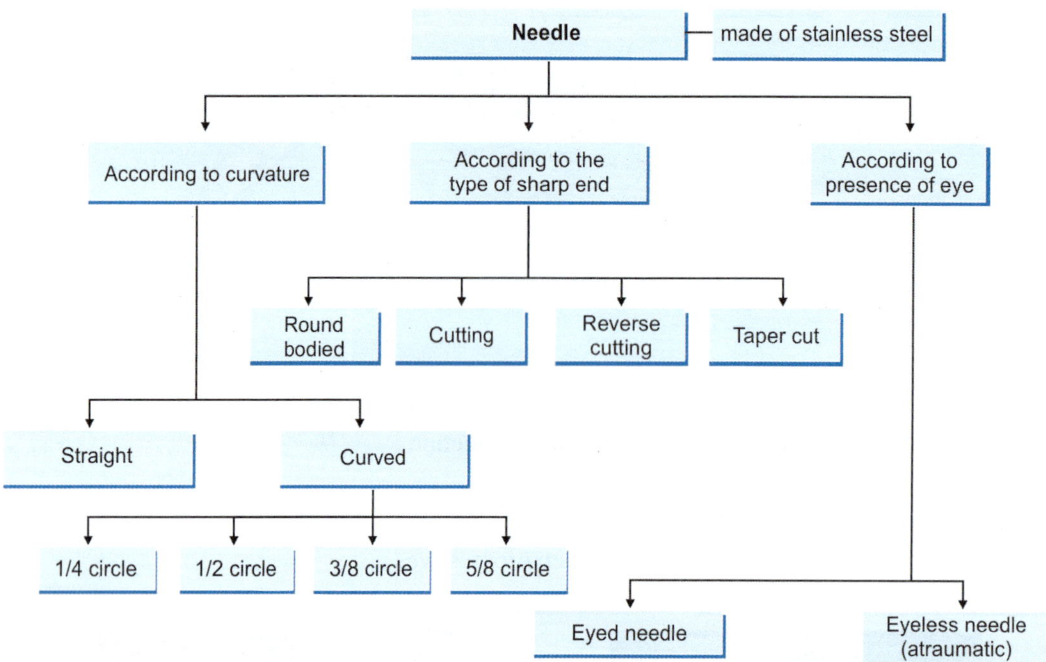

- **Parts of a needle:** (1) Eye; (2) Body; and (3) Point (extends from the tip to the maximum cross-sectional area of the body)
- **Needle performance is determined by:** (1) Sharpness; (2) Strength; (3) Surface finish; (4) Temper; (5) Rigidity; (6) Malleability; and (7) Ductility
- **Sterilization of eyed needle:** Lysol
- **Sterilization of eyeless needle:** Packed after sterilization (Gamma radiation)

Round Bodied Needle

Use: For suturing delicate tissues like intestines, vessels

Cutting Needle

Use: For suturing tough structures, e.g., skin

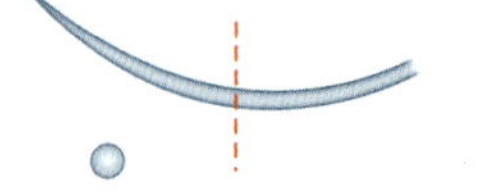

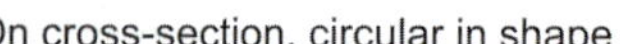

On cross-section, circular in shape

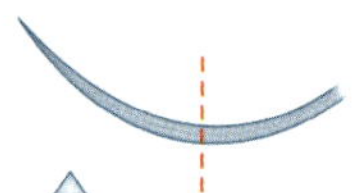

On cross-section, a triangle with apex on the concavity of the needle

Reverse Cutting Needle

Use: During closure of midline in mass closure technique

Taper Cut Needle

Use: Particularly used in vascular surgery

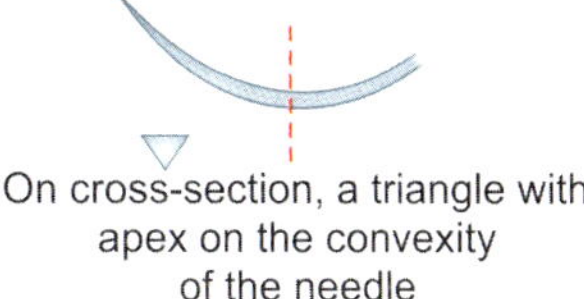

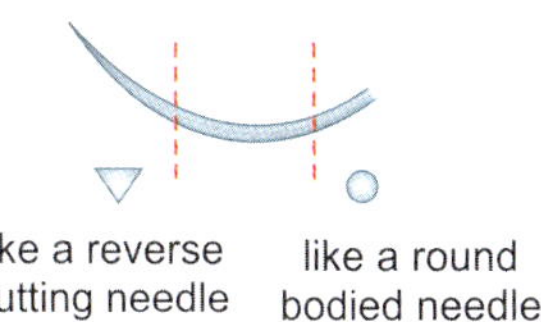

Eyed and Swaged (Atraumatic) Needle

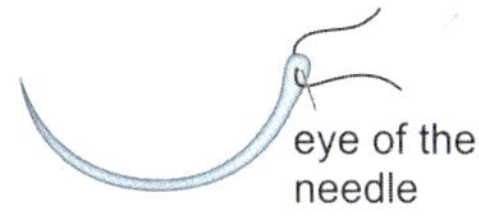

- Causes more trauma to the tissues as two layers of suture material pass through the tissues
- **Use:** Skin suturing

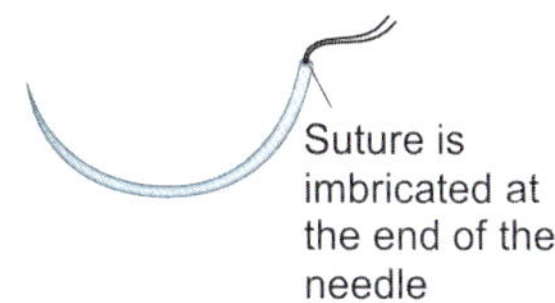

- Causes least trauma to the tissues
- **Use:** Suturing delicate tissues

Needle with Different Curvature

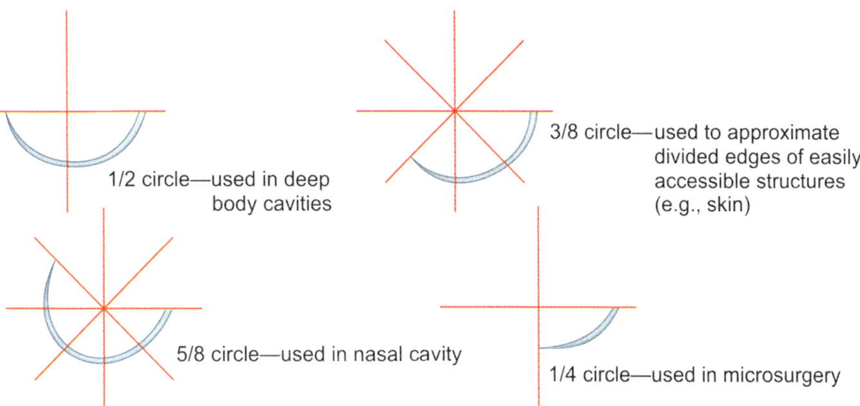

Retractor

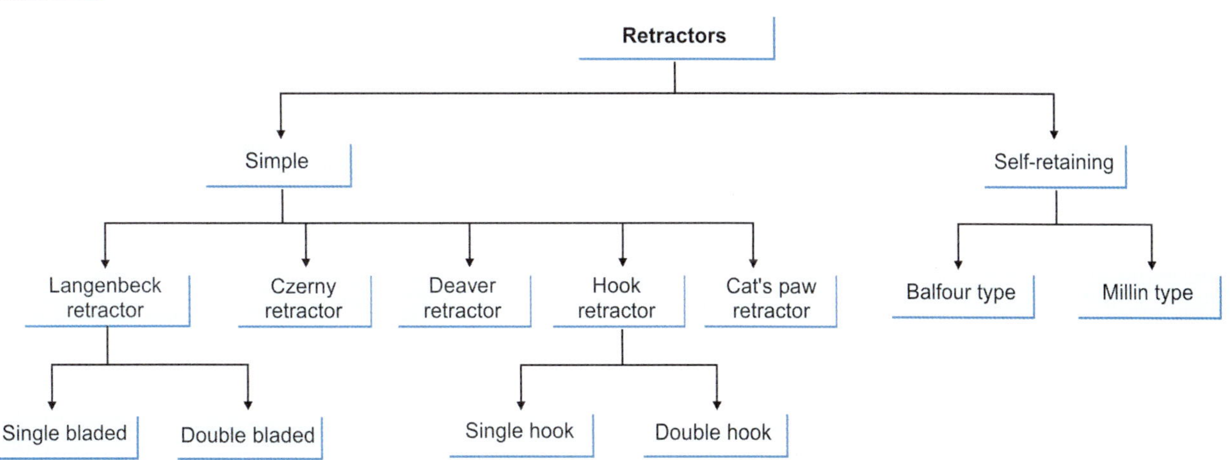

Uses of Langenbeck Retractor

- During appendicectomy, the abdominal wall is retracted to visualize the cecum.
- During modified radical mastectomy, pectoralis major and minor is retracted for proper axillary dissection.
- During hernia repair, retraction is required for repair of the posterior wall of inguinal canal.
- During neck dissection, retraction of sternocleidomastoid is required for adequate exposure.

Uses of Czerny Retractor

Same as Langenbeck retractor

Uses of Deaver Retractor

- During open cholecystectomy, to retract the right lobe of liver.
- During right hemicolectomy, to retract the abdominal wall laterally, during mobilization of colon.
- During APR or anterior resection, to retract the urinary bladder or pelvis during pelvic dissection.

Uses of Hook Retractor

- To retract the skin flap during excision of sebaceous cyst, lipoma.
- To retract the skin and isthmus of thyroid during tracheostomy.

Uses of Self-retaining Retractor

- During truncal vagotomy and gastrectomy
- During hepatic resection
- During APR and anterior resection of rectum.

Sterilization of retractors: Autoclaving

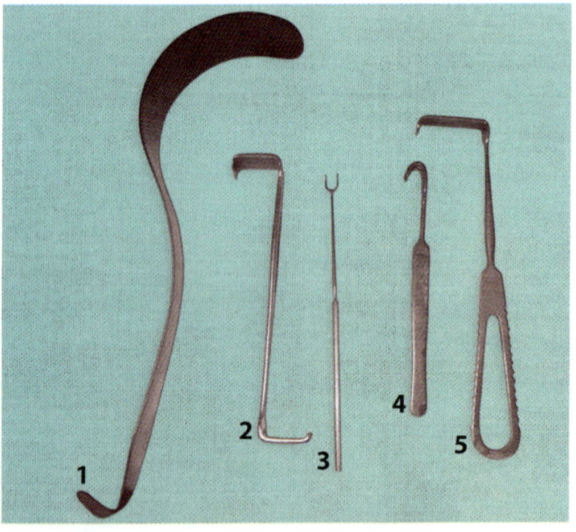

1. Deaver retractor; 2. Czerny retractor; 3 and 4. Double hook retractor; 5. Langenbeck retractor.

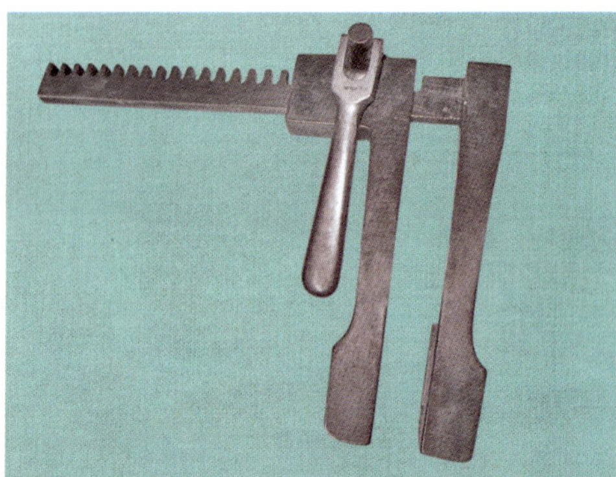

Self-retaining retractor.

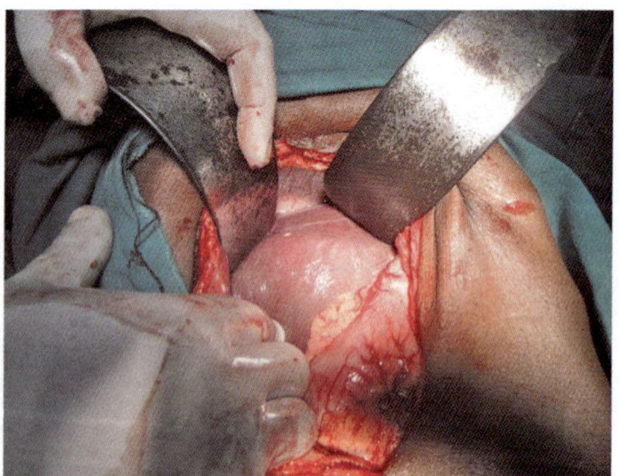

Use of Deavor retractor.

Scissors

Uses of Mayo's Scissors

- To cut external oblique aponeurosis, rectus sheath
- To cut sutures

Uses of Mcindoe Scissors

- To raise the skin flap during thyroidectomy and mastectomy
- To cut the cystic duct and artery during cholecystectomy, to cut the splenic artery and vein during splenectomy

Use of Metzenbaum Scissors

Same as Mcindoe scissors

Sterilization: Lysol

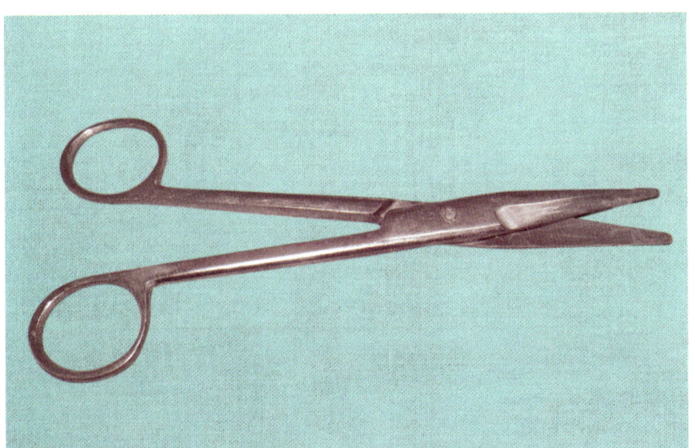
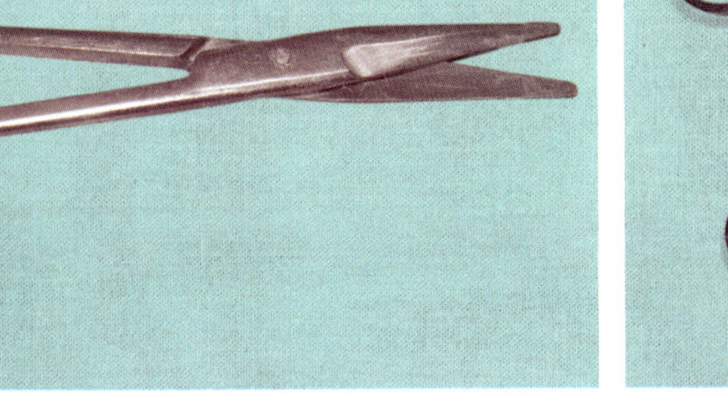
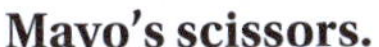

Mayo's scissors.

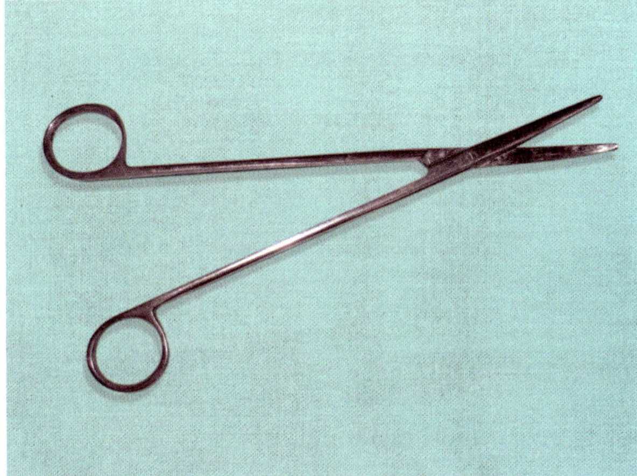

Metzenbaum scissors.

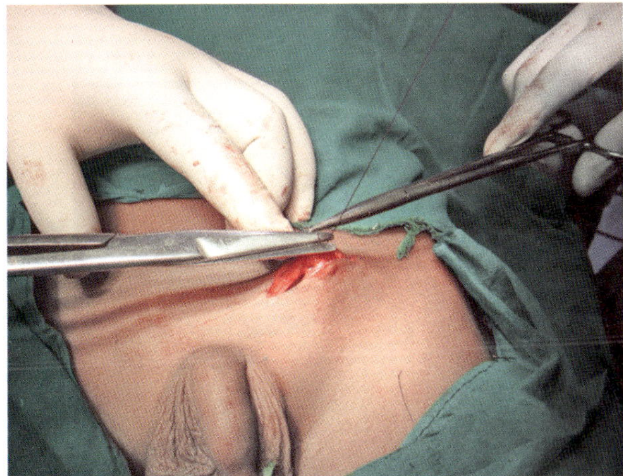

Use of Mayo's scissors.

Moynihan Cholecystectomy Forceps

Use: During open cholecystectomy, for traction of gallbladder

Sterilization: Autoclaving

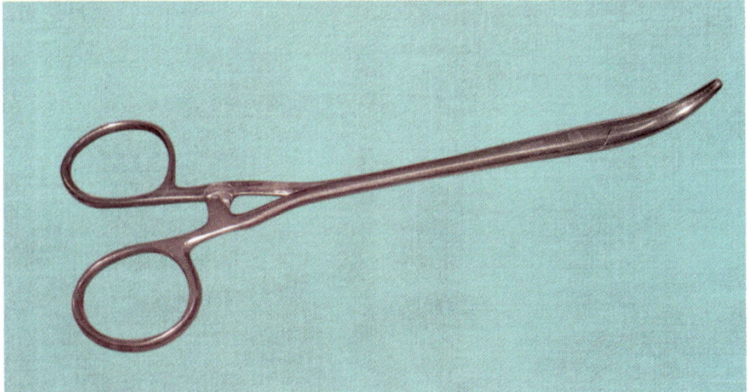

Desjardin's Choledocholithotomy Forceps

Uses:

- During choledocholithotomy, to remove the stones from the common bile duct.
- During laparoscopic cholecystectomy, while extracting the gallbladder through the umbilical or epigastric port, the stones are removed from the gallbladder for easy delivery of the gallbladder specimen from port site.

Sterilization: Autoclaving

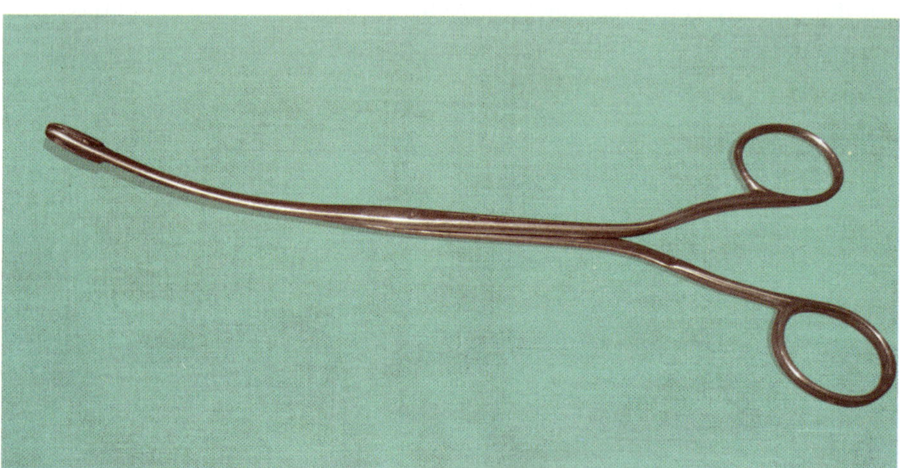

Right-angled Forceps

Uses:

- During truncal vagotomy, to dissect the anterior and posterior vagal trunk.
- During open cholecystectomy, to dissect the cystic duct and artery.
- During thyroidectomy, to dissect the middle thyroid vein, superior thyroid pedicle, and inferior thyroid pedicle.
- During gastrectomy, to dissect the vascular pedicles.

Sterilization: Autoclaving

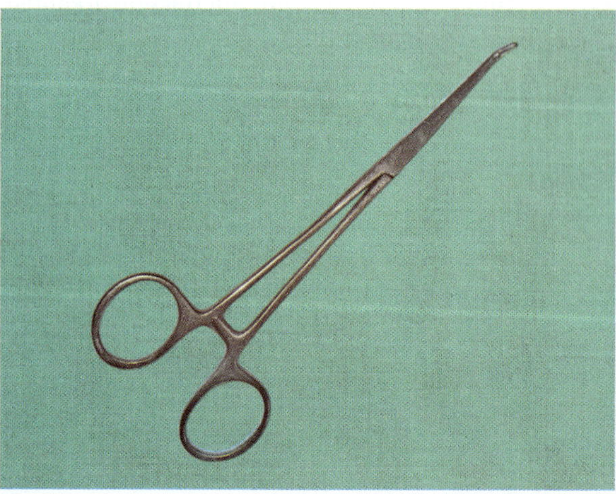

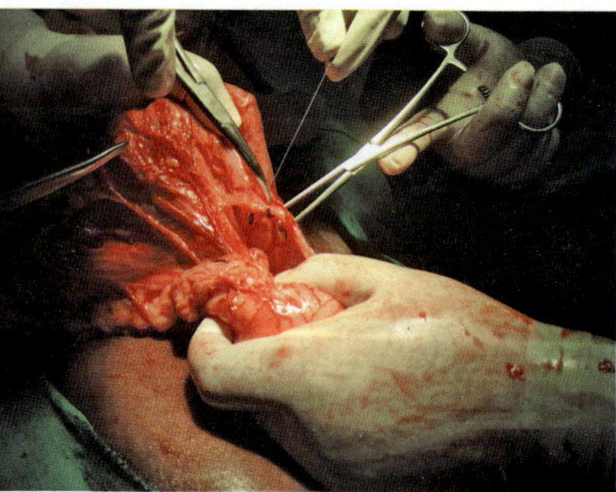

T-tube

Made up of PVC/Latex/Silastic

Uses: During open choledocholithotomy, to place it as a stent as well as drainage.

Sterilization: Supplied in pack (Sterilized pack)

Urinary Catheter

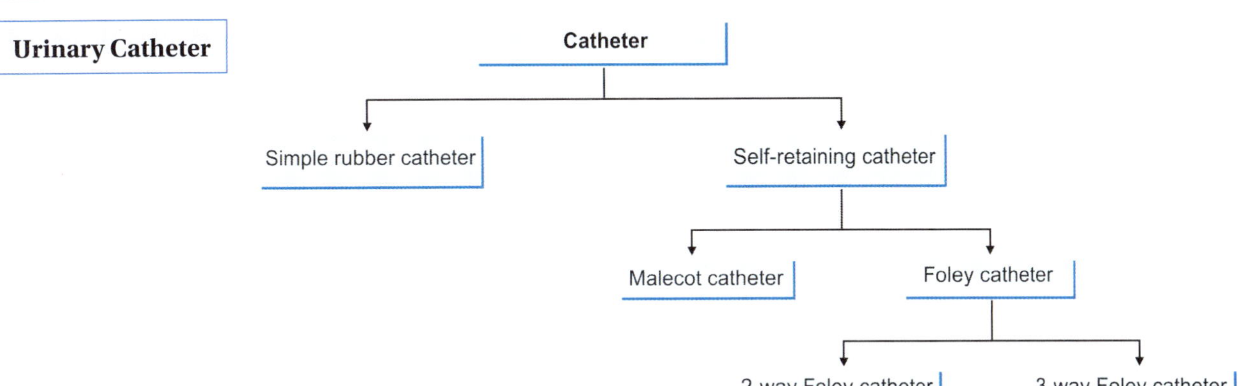

Simple Rubber Catheter

Made of India rubber

Variety of sizes: No. 8, 10, etc.

The diameter of catheter (in mm) = No. of catheter/2 + 1

Diameter of No. 10 catheter = 10/2+1= 6 mm

Uses:

- To differentiate between anuria and retention of urine
- In acute retention of urine (particularly in females)
- For performing cystography
- May be used as a substitute of umbilical tape to sling the esophagus during truncal vagotomy.
- Used to flush the bile duct during open choledocholithotomy.

Sterilization: Autoclaving

Foley Self-retaining Catheter

- Foley catheter are of two types: (i) 2-way catheter and (ii) 3-way catheter
- Size of catheter (circumference)—in French (Fr)
- Diameter of catheter (in mm) = French scale/3
- Diameter of a 16-Fr catheter =16/3 = 5.33 mm
- Balloon capacity varies according to size of catheter.

In 2-way catheter, one is for drainage of urine, and another is for inflation of balloon. In 3-way catheter, the third one is for irrigation.

Uses of 2-way Catheter

- In retention of urine, for relief the retention
- In postoperative patient, for proper monitoring of urine output
- In suprapubic cystostomy
- In feeding jejunostomy, as feeding tube

Uses of 3-way Catheter

- For bladder irrigation in patient with hematuria
- After open prostatectomy

Sterilization: By gamma irradiation

Dimensions of Urethra

	Length	Caliber
• Male urethra	18–20 cm	• Meatus—24 Fr • Bladder neck—28 Fr • Prostatic urethra—32 Fr
• Female urethra	4 cm	• 22 Fr

Contraindications of urethral catheterization:
Absolute contraindications: Suspected or confirmed urethral injury, history of bladder neck repair.
Relative contraindications: Urethral stricture, history of recent urethral surgery, and history of artificial urinary sphincter.

Precautions to be taken during male urethral catheterization: (i) Catheter should be inserted completely before inflation of balloon; (ii) Balloon should not be inflated until flow of urine through the catheter is seen; (iii) Foreskin must be replaced over the glans, if it is retracted; and (iv) If child has physiologic phimosis, then forceful retraction should be avoided, gentle retraction is to be done to locate the meatus.

Technical tips for male urethral catheterization: (i) Distal glans is pinched after injecting lubricant or anesthetic jelly to prevent the reflux of jelly; (ii) During insertion of catheter, penis is pulled straight and taut; (iii) Slow, steady pressure is to be maintained to overcome mild resistance by sphincters or prostate; and (iv) Catheter may be irrigated with saline or sterile water, if flow of urine is not seen after complete insertion of catheter (lubricant or anesthetic jelly may obstruct the catheter).

Complications of urethral catheterization: (i) Urinary tract infection; (ii) Urethral injury; (iii) Urethral stricture; (iv) Balloon malfunction; (v) Catheter knotting; and (vi) Bladder cancer.

Metallic Bougie

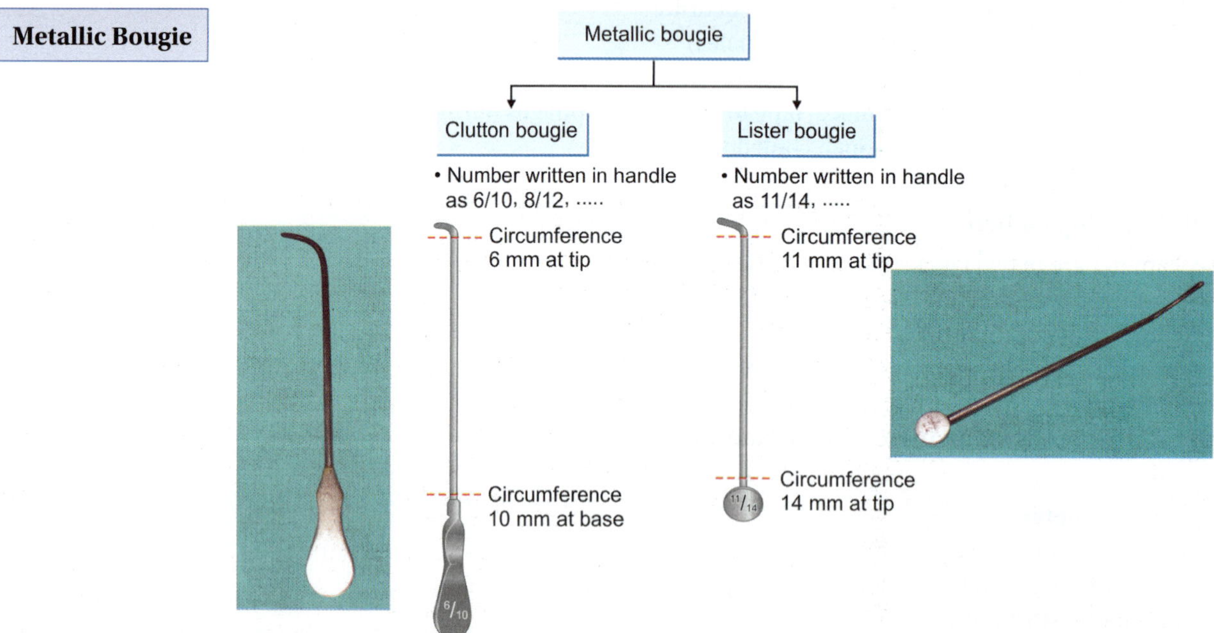

Uses:
- For dilatation in urethral stricture
- For dilatation prior to cystoscopy

Sterilization: Autoclaving

Rectal Speculum (Proctoscope)

Two parts: Speculum and obturator

Uses:

- Diagnosis of anorectal pathologies (e.g., hemorrhoids, carcinoma rectum, internal opening of fistula-in ano)
- For sclerosant injection in hemorrhoids (in 2nd degree)
- To take biopsy from rectal and anal canal growth

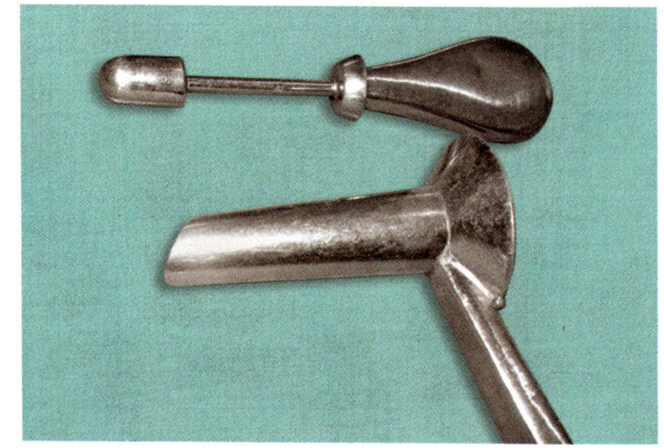

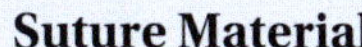

Suture Material

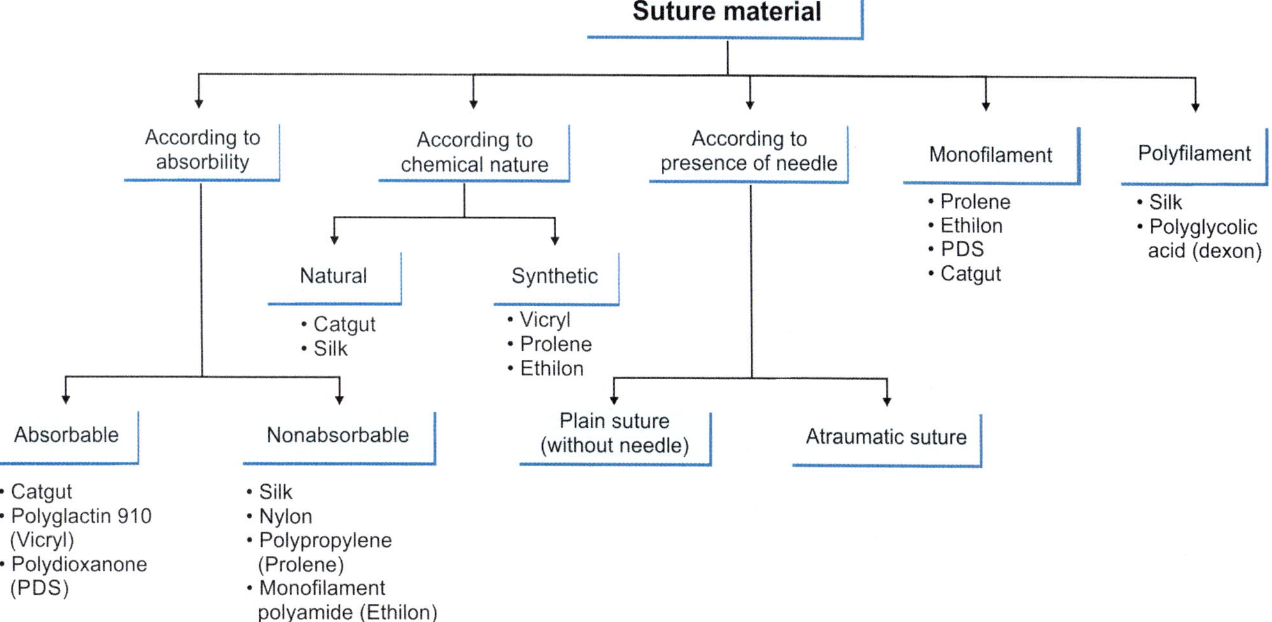

Properties of Suture Materials

- **Tensile strength:** Measured force (in pounds) that a suture can withstand before it breaks. Tensile strength of the suture never exceed the tensile strength of the tissue.
- **Tissue absorption:** Absorbable or nonabsorbable
- **Coefficient of friction:** How easily a suture passes through tissues?
- **Knot security:** A quality of a suture that allows it to be tied securely with minimum number of throws per knot.
- **Elasticity:** Ability of the suture material to return to its original length after stretching
- **Plasticity:** Capacity of a suture to be permanently molded or altered.
- **Memory:** Capacity of a suture to assume a stable linear configuration after removal from packaging and after stretching.
- **Handling:** Depends on elasticity, plasticity, and memory of suture materials.
- Tissue reactivity
- Cross-sectional diameter
- **Origin:** Natural/synthetic
- **Physical configuration:** Monofilament/multifilament
- **Capillarity:** The physical property of transporting liquids along the suture strands.
- Fluid absorption
- Ease of removal
- Color

Properties of an Ideal Suture Material

- High uniform tensile strength
- High tensile strength retention, holding the wound securely throughout the critical healing period, followed by rapid absorption
- Consistent uniform diameter
- Pliable for ease of handling and knot security
- Sterile
- Nonallergenic
- Noncarcinogenic

Principles of Suture Selection

- Tissues that usually heal slowly (skin, fascia, tendons) must be closed with nonabsorbable sutures.
- Tissues that heal rapidly (e.g., stomach, colon, bladder) must be closed with absorbable sutures.
- Where good cosmetic outcome is expected, smallest, inert, monofilament sutures (e.g., nylon, polypropylene) should be used.
- In urinary bladder and biliary tracts, rapidly absorbed sutures should be used.
- Use the finest size suture commensurate with the natural strength of the tissue.

Absorbable sutures	Raw materials
Surgical gut (plain, chromic, fast absorbing)	Submucosa of sheep intestine or serosa of beef intestine
Polyglactin 910(Vicryl, Vicryl rapid, coated Vicryl plus)	Copolymer of glycolide and L-lactide (polyglactin 370) and calcium stearate, if coated
Polyglycolic acid	Homopolymer of glycolide
Poliglecaprone 25 (Monocryl)	Copolymer of glycolide and epsilon-caprolactone
Polyglyconate	Copolymer of glycolide and trimethylene carbonate
Polydioxanone (PDS II)	Polyester of poly (p-dioxanone)

Non-absorbable sutures	Raw materials
Nylon (Ethilon)	Polyamide polymer
Polypropylene (Prolene)	Polymer of propylene
Surgical silk	Raw silk spun by silkworm
Polyester fiber (uncoated, coated)	Polymer of polyethylene
Stainless steel wire	Especially formulated iron-chromium-nickel-molybdenum alloy

Surgical Gut

- They are natural, absorbable, and monofilament sutures.
- Classified as plain, chromic, and fast-absorbing plain gut.
- Consists of processed strands of highly purified collagen prepared from the submucosal layers of the small intestine of sheep or the serosal layer of the small intestine of cattle.
- The plain gut is untreated, strength retention is 7 days and absorption occurs in 10–14 days by proteolysis.
- The chromic gut is tanned with chromic salts to increase the strength retention capacity, strength retention is 7 days with absorption in 21 days.
- Fast-absorbing plain gut is heat-treated to accelerate absorption property. These sutures have less tensile strength than plain gut. They are used primarily for epidermal suturing where sutures are required for only 5–7 days.

Polyglactic 910 (Vicryl)

- Synthetic, absorbable, braided suture made of polyglactin 910 coated with a copolymer of L-lactide and glycolide (Polyglactin 370) and calcium stearate.
- Retains 65% of its tensile strength at 2 weeks and 40% at 3 weeks.
- Complete absorption occurs between 60 and 90 days by hydrolysis.
- Less inflammatory response compared to surgical gut
- Available in clear undyed and violet-dyed form
- **Uses:** (i) For closure of right or left subcostal incision (with 1-0 Vicryl); (ii) Biliary-enteric anastomosis; and (iii) Small and large gut anastomosis.

Coated Polyglactic 910 (Vicryl Rapide)

- Synthetic, absorbable, braided suture made of polyglactin 910 and coated with polyglactin 370 and calcium stearate.
- Hydrolyzed in a buffer solution accelerates absorption property and maintain the mechanical properties.
- Retains 50% of tensile strength at 5 days. At 2 weeks, the tensile strength is 0%.
- Absorption occurs between 7 and 14 days by hydrolysis.

Coated Vicryl Plus

Synthetic, absorbable, braided suture made of polyglactin 910 and coated with polyglactin 370 and calcium stearate and Triclosan (an antimicrobial agent).

Polyglycolic Suture (Dexon II)

- Synthetic, coated, braided, absorbable, and suture made of polyglycolic acid polycaprolate.
- The lubricant coating (consists of calcium stearate and polycaprolactone) decreases the coefficient of friction.
- Retains 89% of its tensile strength at 7 days, 63% at 14 days, and 17% at 21 days.
- Absorption occurs within 90 days by hydrolysis.

Poliglecaprone (Monocryl)

- Synthetic, absorbable, monofilament suture made of a copolymer of glycolide and e-capralactone.
- Superior pliability for easy handling and knot tying
- Available in dyed and undyed form
- Dyed Monocryl retains 30–40% of its tensile strength at 2 weeks, undyed Monocryl retains 25% at 2 weeks and 0% at 3 weeks.
- Absorption occurs within 90–120 days by hydrolysis.

Polydioxanone (PDS)

- Synthetic, absorbable, monofilament suture made of polyester of poly (p-dioxanone).
- Available in a looped configuration for abdominal fascial closure.
- A low reactivity suture that maintains its integrity in presence of bacterial infection.
- Retains 70% of its tensile strength at 2 weeks, 50% at 4 weeks, and 25% at 6 weeks.
- Absorption is minimal until 90 days and absorption complete in 180–210 days by hydrolysis.
- **Uses:** (i) Same as polyglactin suture and (ii) Closure of midline incision.

Nylon (Ethilon)

- Synthetic, nonabsorbable, and monofilament suture made of polyamide polymer fiber.
- These sutures have high tensile strength and extremely low tissue reactivity.
- Good handling property as well as significant memory (need extra throws for knot security)
- Tensile strength is high upto 2 weeks with gradual loss of 15–20% per year by hydrolysis.
- **Use:** Closure of skin incision

Polypropylene (Prolene)

- Synthetic, nonabsorbable, and monofilament suture made of catalytic polymerization of propylene.
- These sutures have low tissue reactivity, high tensile strength, significant memory, high plasticity, and extremely smooth surface.
- These sutures are easy to remove and therefore ideal for running, subcuticular suture.
- Not degraded by tissue enzymes.
- **Uses:** (i) For closure of midline incision; (ii) For repair of tendon and nerves; (iii) Repair of vascular injuries; (iv) In herniorrhaphy; and (v) For fixing the prolene mesh during hernioplasty

Surgical Silk

- Natural, nonabsorbable, and braided suture made of raw silk spun by silkworm.
- This suture is braided for easy handling and dyed for better visibility.
- This suture has good knot security, high tissue reactivity, prone to infection.
- It loses most of its tensile strength in about 1 year and usually cannot be detected in tissue after 2 years.
- Available in various forms: (i) Silk in sterile pack (Sutupak); (ii) Silk in reel (unsterilized form); and (iii) Silk mounted on a atraumatic needle (mersilk).
- **Uses:** (i) To ligate the cystic duct and artery during open cholecystectomy; (ii) To ligate the appendicular artery during open appendectomy; (iii) To ligate the vessels during resection anastomosis; and (iv) Mersilk is used for suturing seromuscular layer in gut anastomosis.

Polyester Fiber Suture

- Synthetic, nonabsorbable, uncoated, braided suture made of polymer of polyethylene.
- This suture has minimal tissue reaction, high coefficient of friction.
- Tensile strength is high upto 2 weeks.

Stainless Steel Wire

- Synthetic, nonabsorbable, and monofilament or twisted multifilament suture made of especially formulated iron-chromium-nickel-molybdenum alloy.
- These sutures made of minimal tissue reaction, high tensile strength, and good knot security.
- Disadvantages are difficulty in handling, fragmentation, barbing, kinking, potential buckling, wire fracture, wire fatigue, and injury during handling.

Different Suturing Techniques

- Simple interrupted suture
- Vertical mattress suture
- Horizontal mattress suture
- Subcuticular continuous suture
- Buried suture
- Purse-string suture
- Figure-of-eight or far-near-far pulley suture
- Retention suture
- Running continuous suture
- Horizontal continuous suture
- Half-buried horizontal mattress or 3-corner suture
- Continuous locking suture

To Appose Skin and other Tissues
- Subcuticular
- Vertical mattress
- Horizontal mattress

To Invert Tissues
- Lembert
- Connell
- Purse-string

To Evert Tissues
Horizontal mattress

Techniques of Skin Closure (Other than Suturing)

Staples

Nonabsorbable staples:
- Made of stainless steel
- High tensile strength and low tissue reactivity
- Excellent wound edge eversion without strangulation of tissue
- Minimal cross-hatch scarring
- Faster closure than suturing
- Lower incidence of wound infection in presence of contaminated wounds
- Staples can be removed by especially designed extractors or by a hemostat.

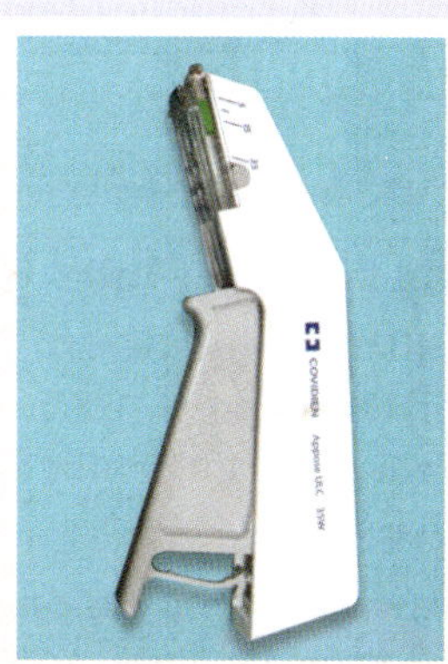

Skin stapler.

Absorbable staples:
- Made of absorbable copolymer of predominantly polylactide and lesser component of polyglycolide.
- MRI compatible
- Eliminates the pain and discomfort of metal skin staples.
- Eliminates potential "railroad track" scars.

Topical Tissue Adhesives
- The topical skin adhesive is 2-octyl cyanoacrylate (Dermabond).
- A sterile, liquid topical adhesive designed to hold closed, easily approximated skin edges, punctures in minimally invasive surgery.
- This chemical utilizes the skin moisture to form a strong, flexible, three-dimensional bond.
- This should not be applied to tissues within wounds.
- Should not be used in—mucosal surfaces, across mucocutaneous junctions (e.g., lip, oral cavity), contaminated wounds, deep wounds, wounds under tension, wound in area with dense hair (e.g., scalp).
- The adhesive film usually remain in place for 5–10 days and naturally falls off the skin.

Adhesive Tapes

- Steri-strips are an effective alternative to sutures or staples where there is minimal tension to the wound.
- Also be used to complement suture or staple closures.
- Linear wounds with minimal tension can be easily approximated by tapes alone.
- Wound edge approximation is less precise with tape alone.
- Chance of dislodgement and dehiscence are more common than sutures or staples.

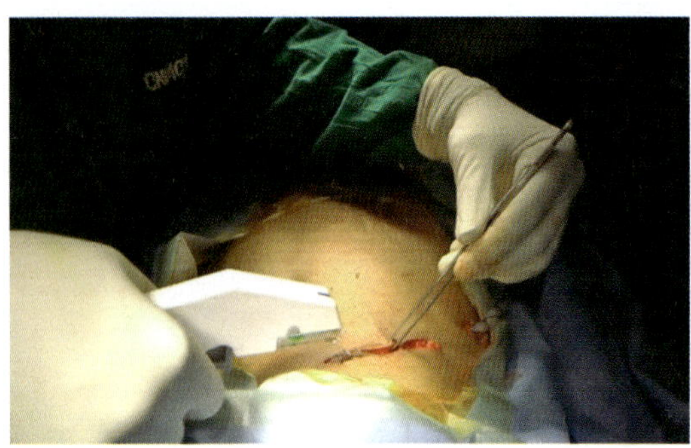

Technique of skin closure by skin stapler.

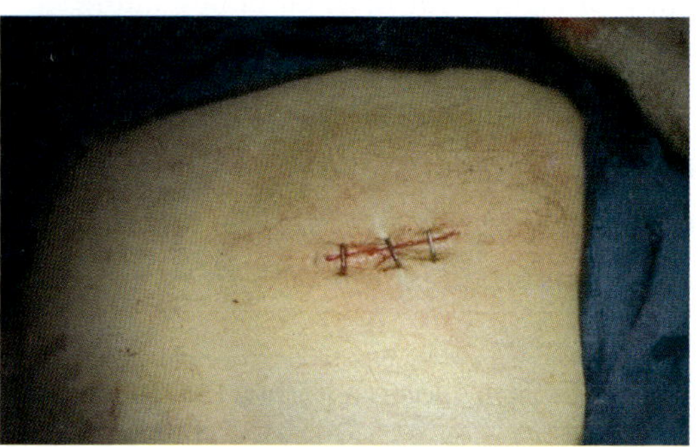

Skin closure by staples.

Tracheostomy Tube

Different varieties: (i) Metallic tracheostomy tube and (ii) Cuffed portex tracheostomy tube

Two parts: Inner tube and outer tube

Uses:

Emergency indications:

- Acute laryngeal edema
- Airway obstruction following RTA
- Ludwig's angina causing laryngeal obstruction
- Foreign body in larynx
- Cut-throat injury
- Bilateral recurrent laryngeal nerve palsy

Elective indications:

- Following laryngectomy
- Following respiratory paralysis in GB syndrome, bulbar palsy.

Ryle's Tube

- One meter long plastic tube with lead shots (radiopaque) near the rounded tip of the tube.
- A number of side holes near the tip of the tube

The body of the tube has four black circular markings:

First mark: 40 cm from the tip—when tube is inserted upto this mark, the tip of the tube lies at G-E junction.

Second mark: 50 cm from the tip—when tube is inserted upto this mark, the tip of the tube lies at body of the stomach.

Third mark: 60 cm from the tip—when tube is inserted upto this mark, the tip of the tube lies at the pylorus of the stomach.

Fourth mark: 70 cm from the tip-when tube is inserted upto this mark, the tip of the tube lies at the duodenum.

Uses:

- For nasogastric suction
- For feeding through the tube

IV Cannula

Consists of plastic cannula and metal needle.

Uses:

- For intravenous fluid infusion
- For blood transfusion

Fluid flow rate depends on: (i) Type and viscosity of the fluid; (ii) Size of the cannula; (iii) Fluid temperature; and (iv) Height of the fluid container

Different sizes of cannula—color codes according to the size:

Color	Gauze	Length	Flow rate	Uses
Orange	14 G	45 mm	240 mL/min	Massive traumatic hemorrhage, rapid blood transfusion
Gray	16 G	45 mm	180 mL/min	Traumatic hemorrhage, rapid blood transfusion, rapid fluid replacement
Green	18 G	32 mm	90 mL/min	Routine fluid replacement in adult during surgery, fluid replacement in burn, blood transfusion
Pink	20 G	32 mm	60 mL/min	Routine fluid replacement, blood transfusion
Blue	22 G	25 mm	36 mL/min	Infusion in neonate, pediatric and older patients
Yellow	24 G	19 mm	20 mL/min	Infusion and blood transfusion in neonates, pediatric and older adult patients
Purple	26 G	19 mm	13 mL/min	Infusion in neonates and pediatric patients

Chapter 33

Do's and Dont's in Surgery

'A good surgeon doesn't just concentrate on technical ability, but also on the appropriateness of what you're doing.'

—Dr Benjamin Carson

DO'S IN SURGERY

1.	A surgeon should convert a untidy wound to a tidy one by saline irrigation, and thorough debridement of all devitalized tissues.
2.	Any trauma patients should be examined as per advanced trauma life support (ATLS) protocol.
3.	Surgeon should recognize normal landmarks (e.g., lip vermilion, eyelid, nostril free margin, hair lines) during repair (to avoid any misaligned scar).
4.	Surgeon should take responsibility regarding placement of passive diathermy electrode pad (to avoid electrosurgical burn) and positioning of patient in operating table (to avoid pressure-induced nerve injury).
5.	All port sites above 5 mm in diameter should be repaired (to reduce the risk of port-site hernia).
6.	Surgeon should ensure before anastomosis that the bowel edges are pink and bleeding.
7.	Surgeon must ensure that the anastomosis is under no tension.
8.	After anastomosis, the mesenteric defect should be closed (to avoid risk of internal hernia).
9.	During removal of suction drain, suction should be taken off prior to removal of the drain.
10.	During removal of chest drain, patient should be asked to breath in and hold his/her breath (to avoid sucking of air into pleural cavity).
11.	Surgeon should keep all conducting surfaces of the instruments within the visual field when applying electrosurgical current during laparoscopic surgery.
12.	In open surgery of abdomen in children, surgeon should choose supraumbilical transverse incision rather than vertical midline one.
13.	To detect free air in chest X-ray to diagnose hollow viscus perforation, surgeon should search free air under the right hemidiaphragm, not under the left hemidiaphragm (to avoid misinterpretation of gastric air bubble).
14.	Before planning for a major intra-abdominal or intrathoracic surgery, surgeon should identify the patients who have high perioperative risk of major adverse cardiovascular events including myocardial infarction.
15.	Surgeon should take opinion of a cardiologist before surgical intervention if: (i) Patient have poor left ventricular function or cardiomegaly; (ii) Ischemic changes in electrocardiogram (ECG); (iii) Arrhythmia in ECG; and (iv) Clinically patient is symptomatic and murmur is present.
16.	If patient having pacemaker, bipolar diathermy should be used. If monopolar diathermy have to be used, the cardioversion overpace modes must be turned off and converted to 'VOO' mode.
17.	Surgeon should put the diabetic patient first on the operating list.
18.	Surgeon should consider nutritional support if any patient has sustained 5 days of inadequate intake or possibility to have inadequate intake for the same duration or more.
19.	In tube feeding, tube should be flushed with water at least twice daily.
20.	In tube feeding, if aspirate amount exceeds 200 mL in any 2-hour, feeding should be temporarily stopped or rate of feeding have to be reduced.
21.	Surgeon should access central venous route for total parenteral nutrition (TPN), if feeding have to be continued for more than 2 weeks.
22.	For central venous route, surgeon should choose the most suitable position for feeding, the infraclavicular subclavian route.
23.	If liver enzymes are persistently abnormal during TPN, it should be temporarily discontinued.
24.	Surgeon should identify at risk patients for deep vein thrombosis (DVT) and implement DVT prophylaxis measures.
25.	Surgeon should encourage early mobilization of postoperative patients (to decrease the risk of DVT, atelectasis, pressure sores, fecal impaction).
26.	In discharge certificate, surgeon should mention final diagnosis, preoperative findings, any perioperative complications, medications to be taken at home, possible complications, collection of histopathology report (if indicated) and time of follow-up.
27.	Surgeon should initiate enteral nutrition as soon as feasible after elective surgery.
28.	Surgeon should achieve 'Critical view of safety' before dividing the cystic duct and artery during laparoscopic cholecystectomy.
29.	Before clipping of the cystic duct and artery, surgeon should visualize the posterior jaw of the clip applicator just before application of clips.

Contd...

Contd...

30. Cystic artery is dissected upto its termination at the gallbladder wall before ligation to avoid ligating aberrant or anterior right hepatic artery.
31. Surgeon should aware of the common anatomical variations of the cystic duct, artery, relationship of cystic duct with extrahepatic biliary tree during laparoscopic or open cholecystectomy.
32. During open common bile duct (CBD) exploration, the choledochotomy incision should be placed in the lowest part of the supraduodenal CBD.
33. During open CBD exploration, aspirated bile from CBD and biliary stent (if present) should be sent for culture.
34. During placement of T-tube in CBD, surgeon should take care that proximal limb is not entering in one of the hepatic ducts or the distal limb not entering into the duodenum.
35. Surgeon should consider diagnosis of autoimmune pancreatitis and assess serum IgG4 level, if malignancy is not confirmed after repeat biopsies in borderline resectable pancreatic carcinoma.
36. In locally advanced pancreatic carcinoma presenting with gastric outlet obstruction, life expectancy more than 3–6 months, good performance status, surgeon should consider open or laparoscopic gastrojejunostomy as palliative option instead of endoscopic stenting.
37. Cervical spine immobilization should be done by hard cervical collar in all blunt trauma patients until spine injury is excluded.
38. ECG should consider in all patients with electrical injury.
39. During laparoscopic cholecystectomy, if clip does not fit across the entire width of the cystic duct, surgeon should reconsider before transection of the duct.
40. Surgeon can safely perform laparoscopy in any trimester of pregnancy without an increased risk to the mother or fetus.
41. In laparoscopy in pregnancy, surgeon should choose the initial access to the abdomen via subcostal approach (to avoid gravid uterus).
42. During laparoscopy in pregnant patients, intraoperative CO_2 monitoring by capnography should be used.
43. Coagulopathy and thrombocytopenia should be corrected before planning laparoscopic cholecystectomy in Child's A or B cirrhosis patients.
44. During laparoscopic cholecystectomy in cirrhotic patients, dilated pericholecystic vein, abdominal wall veins or recanalized umbilical veins should be handled with extreme care.
45. If preoperative biliary drainage is indicated in malignant extrahepatic biliary obstruction, surgeon should consider decompression via endoscopic retrograde cholangiopancreatography (ERCP) approach rather than percutaneous or surgical approach.
46. A registry of patients with biliary stents (particularly for benign biliary diseases) should be maintained to recall them for stent removal or exchange in due time.
47. Plastic biliary stent placed due to incomplete clearance of CBD stone should be removed or replaced within 3–6 months.
48. During open exploration of amebic liver abscess, surgeon should be careful because vascular and biliary structures may traverse the abscess cavity and may mistakenly taken as septa in abscess (injury of these structures may lead to hemorrhage, bile leak).
49. If intercostal tube drainage is indicated due to pulmonary complications of amebic liver abscess, the tube should be placed on right lateral side of the chest near the axilla (right hemidiaphragm is significantly elevated and may injured if tube is placed at lower level).
50. Surgeon should exclude cysto-biliary communication before PAIR technique.
51. Surgeon should ensure periinterventional chemotherapy with albendazole 4 days before PAIR and at least 1 month thereafter.
52. Before surgical intervention of hydatid cyst of liver, a recent CT scan of abdomen and chest should be done to exclude occult pelvic, retroperitoneal or pulmonary hydatid cyst.
53. If hydatid cyst of liver is close to hilum or cysto-biliary communication is suspected, MRCP should be done before any intervention.
54. During surgery of hydatid cyst of liver or other abdominal organs, any hydatid fluid spillage should be avoided.
55. During surgery of hydatid cyst of liver, before injecting the scolicidal agent into the cyst cavity, surgeon must sure that the cyst fluid is not bile stained.
56. Surgeon should ensure perioperative prophylaxis with albendazole 1 week before the intervention and 3–8 weeks after intervention.

Contd...

Contd...

57.	24-hour pH test should be done prior to antireflux surgery.
58.	In patients with gastroesophageal reflux disease (GERD), if adequate symptom control on proton pump inhibitor (PPI) therapy, it should be continued instead of antireflux surgery.
59.	Diagnostic workup (to exclude esophageal pathologies) should be done after extraction of impacted food bolus in esophagus.
60.	Surgeon should keep in mind during gastrointestinal (GI) surgery that the submucosal layer has the greatest suture-holding capacity.
61.	After completion of the laparoscopic procedure, all trocars should be removed under direct vision and trocar sites should be inspected for bleeding.
62.	Grossly contaminated wounds should be allowed to heal by secondary intention.
63.	Surgeon should examine the small bowel for Meckel diverticulum if abdomen is opened with a diagnosis of acute appendicitis but appendix is normal appearing.
64.	An incidentally discovered Meckel diverticulum should be removed unless absolute contraindication (e.g., Crohn disease).
65.	Norepinephrine (instead of dopamine) should be used as first-line vasopressor agent to correct hypotension in septic shock (dopamine is more arrhythmogenic than norepinephrine).
66.	The curvature radius of the light cable in laparoscopic surgery should not be less than 15 cm in radius during handling (to avoid breakage of the optical fibers).
67.	For focus adjustment of laparoscopic camera, the laparoscope should be placed approximately 5 cm away from the target.
68.	Before the use of Veress needle, surgeon should check its patency and spring action.
69.	All port sites should be closed in laparoscopic cholecystectomy in cirrhotic patients.
70.	Before access in laparoscopy, urinary bladder should be emptied.
71.	During laparoscopic surgery, surgeon should use the cutting current (lowest voltage) for both cutting and coagulation (high voltage current compromise insulation integrity more).
72.	Surgeon should test for insulation defects in hand instruments before starting the laparoscopic surgery.
73.	Surgeon should use brief intermittent activation of low voltage waveform ("cutting" mode) rather than prolonged activation during laparoscopic surgery.
74.	Surgeon should close the fascial defect in port site (10 mm or more) under direct vision, incorporate all layers of the abdominal wall.
75.	During laparoscopic hernia surgery, surgeon must be alert during dissection and fixation on Cooper's ligament (if "Corona mortis" is present, it may cause significant hemorrhage).
76.	Surgeon should be vigilant during adhesiolysis in laparoscopic ventral hernia repair to recognize any type of bowel injury.
77.	Infected ePTFE mesh must always be explanted (if infected, it is difficult to manage because the micropores allow bacteria to pass and form biofilm).
78.	While fitting or removing the scalpel blade in BP handle, surgeon should always hold the blade by forceps.
79.	During surgery, always pass the sharp instruments in kidney dishes (to avoid injuries by instruments).
80.	Periareolar incision should be made just outside the areola in darker-skinned patients and immediately inside the areola in lighter-skinned patients (because of the lighter shade of scar tissue).
81.	Surgeon should rule out MEN1 syndrome by measuring serum calcium level before surgery for gastrinoma.
82.	A knot should have at least 3 throws with 3-mm long ends.
83.	When elliptic skin incision is made, the long axis should be four times greater in length than the smaller axis.
84.	During albendazole chemotherapy for hydatid cyst, leucocyte count should be measured at 2 weeks interval during the first 3 months (leucopenia may develop in early phases of chemotherapy).
85.	Before giving incision for emergency appendectomy, surgeon must palpate the right iliac fossa to rule out any appendicular lump (sometimes lump cannot be palpated due to guarding during clinical examination).
86.	In traumatic brain injury patients, during examination of the pupillary light reflex, Surgeon should wait for several seconds before assessing light reflex in contralateral eye (pupil may be temporarily constricted due to consensual pupillary response).
87.	During insufflation in laparoscopic surgery, Surgeon must observe for hypercarbia, hypotension, or arrhythmia and if anyone develop, immediate desufflation should be initiated.

Contd...

Contd...

88. Surgeon should call for help of an experienced colleague if during laparoscopic or open cholecystectomy, any bile duct injury happens.
89. In laparoscopic cholecystectomy, Surgeon should always dissect cephalad to Rouvier's sulcus.
90. Pneumothorax must be excluded in trauma patients before initiating positive pressure ventilation because simple pneumothorax can be converted into tension pneumothorax.
91. IV potassium supplementation should be administered in normal saline, not in dextrose solution.
92. Urgent endoscopic intervention should be considered in patients with esophageal obstruction who cannot swallow the saliva (to reduce the risk of aspiration, a potentially life-threatening condition).
93. Preoperative ureteric stent insertion should be considered in reoperative pelvic surgery to avoid the risk of ureter injury.
94. A reoperative pelvic surgery should be delayed for at least 6 months.
95. In reoperative pelvic surgery, initial entry into the peritoneal cavity should be in the upper abdomen.
96. In reoperative pelvic surgery, surgeon must be cautious during the opening of abdomen at the level of symphysis pubis, because at this level, urinary bladder may be adherent with the undersurface of the abdominal wall.
97. Prophylactic antibiotic should be administered within 1 hour before surgical incision. Re-administration should be considered if the duration of operative procedure exceeds the recommended redosing schedule.
98. Preoperative hair removal should be done by clipping, not by shaving.
99. Skin antisepsis with the antiseptic solutions (e.g., chlorhexidine, povidone-iodine, isopropyl alcohol, chlorhexidine-alcohol combination) should be done before surgery to reduce the risk of surgical site infection (SSI).
100. Timely decision of establishing an airway should be taken in elderly patients with trauma because of significant loss of protective airway reflexes in older age group.
101. A reef knot must be kept 'square' by pulling the ligatures in appropriate directions.
102. In skin suturing, stitches should be tied in such a way that skin edges are brought together without constriction and knots are positioned laterally away from the incision.
103. Skin sutures should be removed at around 5 days in face, around 2 weeks in back and below the knee and at least 7 days in other parts of the body.
104. For continuous subcuticular suturing, monofilament synthetic suture should be preferred because of minimal tissue reaction and easy removal.
105. Underlying brain injury or pulmonary contusion should be strongly suspected in pediatric patients with skull or rib fracture.
106. Intraosseous infusion should be considered after two failed attempts of peripheral IV access in pediatric trauma patients with hypovolemic shock.
107. The fluid resuscitation in burn patients should be titrated based on a urine output target of 0.5 mL/kg/h in adults and 1 mL/kg/h in children below 30 kg.
108. In burn patients with inhalation injury and electrical burn injury, additional fluid should be considered during fluid resuscitation.
109. In infants and children (≤30 kg) with burn injury, sugar-containing solution (5% dextrose in Lactated Ringers) in maintenance rate should be considered along with resuscitation fluid (in young children, hepatic glycogen stores are depleted after 12–14 hours of fasting).
110. Glucose-containing fluids and hyponatremia should be avoided in brain injury patients.
111. A surgeon should consider a trauma patient is in hemorrhagic shock if patient's extremities are cool and tachycardia is present.
112. Surgeon should ensure a healthy, pink, flat granulating surface of the recipient area by scraping away the exuberant, soft granulation tissues before skin grafting.
113. Dressing of the recipient skin grafting site should be left undisturbed for 5–8 days unless evidence of infection are present.
114. Incision in the superomedial quadrant of the breast should be avoided, if possible, to decrease the risk of development of hypertrophic scar.
115. The amount of IV fluid administration and the dose of medications should be always based on the weight in pediatric patients.
116. A chest X-ray should be done after central venous catheterization to confirm the proper location of the catheter tip and to exclude pneumothorax.

Contd...

Contd...

117.	Irrigation fluids should be warmed to body temperature in abdominal surgery in pediatric patients.
118.	The orientation of the scalpel or diathermy blade should be perpendicular to the skin surface to facilitate proper reapproximation of the wound margin during wound closure.
119.	Additional periods of preoperative fasting should be considered in patients with impaired gastric emptying (i.e., diabetes mellitus, hiatal hernia).
120.	Evaluation of normal thyroid tissue in neck should be evaluated by imaging (e.g., thyroid scintigraphy or USG) before considering excision of thyroglossal cyst and lingual thyroid.
121.	The superior thyroid artery and vein should be individually ligated during thyroidectomy to avoid injury to the external branch of superior laryngeal nerve (EB-SLN).
122.	Surgeon should use the belly of the scalpel blade, not the tip for giving incisions.
123.	Sharp instruments should always keep and pass in kidney dishes.
124.	Surgeon should use scissors to cut in the transverse plane from the dominant side to the nondominant side. If surgeon needs to cut from nondominant side to the dominant side, scissors should be used in the nondominant hand or swing the scissors round in the dominant hand.
125.	Skin should be grasped by the toothed forceps, not by the instruments that crush the skin, because crushing is more damaging for skin than puncture.
126.	Blunt-tipped forceps should be preferred over fine-tipped forceps for tissue holding because the exerted pressure per unit area is more in between the tips of the fine-tipped forceps.
127.	Needles should be handled with needle-holders or forceps, not by the hands.
128.	Surgeon should closely examine any old scars particularly burn scars on routine physical examination to detect any changes suggestive of malignant degeneration (Marjolin ulcer).
129.	Surgeon should choose the size of the suture material depending on the size of the structures.
130.	Cervical spine injury must be excluded before endotracheal intubation in trauma patients.
131.	Surgeon should dissect near a ductal structure along the expected line of the duct, rather than at right angles to it, to prevent any transection of the duct.
132.	During dissection of a ductal structure, Surgeon should be careful to preserve its blood and nerve supply.
133.	Mesenteric defect should be closed (with interrupted sutures) to avoid internal herniation of intestines.
134.	Surgeon should handle blood vessels as minimal as possible because any type of trauma increases the risk of thrombus formation.
135.	During dissection of CBD, Surgeon must aware of the anomaly that right hepatic artery may pass in front of the bile duct.
136.	In portal hypertension patients, during mobilization of the sides of the liver, the ligamentous attachments should be ligated before division because venous collateral may develop in these ligaments.
137.	Hepatic duct should be dissected together with the surrounding Glissonian sheath during any biliary reconstruction. Any attempt to dissect the duct from the hilar plate increases the risk of disruption of its blood supply.
138.	During cholecystectomy, dissection of the gallbladder from the cystic plate should be in a correct plane. Any deep dissection into the cystic plate may cause major bleeding and bile leak.
139.	During cholecystectomy, anterior and posterior branches of the cystic artery should be separately ligated, if present.
140.	Gallbladder perforation or gangrenous cholecystitis should be suspected if features of peritonitis are present in acute cholecystitis patients.
141.	Internal defibrillators should be turned off during surgery.
142.	Noncardiac elective surgeries should be delayed for at least 6 weeks after coronary angioplasty or bare metal stenting.
143.	Smoking cessation should be encouraged preferably 4–6 weeks prior to surgery.
144.	Aminoglycosides and NSAIDs should be avoided in patients at high risk for postoperative acute renal failure.
145.	Blood glucose should be less than 180 mg/dL during perioperative period in diabetic patients. Insulin therapy should be initiated if blood glucose become more than 180 mg/dL.
146.	Subcutaneous insulin pump should be inactivated in the morning of surgery.

Contd...

Contd...

147. Catheter should be removed on postoperative day 1 or 2 to prevent catheter-associated urinary tract infection (CAUTI).
148. Tranexamic acid should be considered in adults undergoing surgery with expected blood loss of more than 500 mL.
149. Intraoperative cell salvage with tranexamic acid should be considered for patients who are expected very high volume of blood loss (e.g., in cardiac surgery, complex vascular surgery).
150. The blood sample collection from the patient for grouping and Rh typing, the sample labeling and filling of the request form for blood units should be a continuous, uninterrupted event involving one patient and one healthcare worker at a time.
151. All blood components should be transfused through a blood transfusion set (170–200 μm integral mesh filter).
152. Blood transfusion should be completed within 4 hours of leaving the storage area.
153. Blood transfusion set should be changed every 12 hours (to reduce the risk of bacterial infection).
154. Intravenous fluids and blood products should be warmed to 37°C before infusion in patients undergoing elective or emergency surgery.
155. Elective surgery should be delayed if HbA1c is more than 7%.
156. Metformin should be stopped on the day of contrast-enhanced imaging and for the next 48 hours (to decrease the risk of lactic acidosis).
157. The probable sites of nerve injury should be padded during positioning of the patient in operating theater (OT) table before the surgery.
158. FNA should be considered to detect cancer in a neck mass. Open biopsy is associated with increased risk of tumor seeding and local and regional tumor recurrence.
159. Workup for malignancy should be initiated in adults if the neck mass does not resolve with two weeks of antibiotic therapy.
160. Imaging should be considered prior to fine needle aspiration (FNA) for clinically suspected vascular lesion.
161. To repair a transverse defect in an artery, suturing should be from the outside in on the upstream side, and from the inside out on the downstream side (to avoid the risk of 'dissection').
162. USG-guided FNA should be considered for evaluation of neck mass if the previous FNA showed an indeterminate cytology. (USG-guided FNA facilitates acquisition of sample from solid component of the lesion rather than cystic or necrotic component).
163. FNA should be considered as first-line tissue sampling method in all cystic neck masses in adults.
164. During thyroid surgery, Surgeon should aware that branching of recurrent laryngeal nerve ('anterior' and 'posterior' branch) may present and anterior branch should be preserved.
165. Non-recurrent recurrent laryngeal nerve (RLN) should be searched during thyroidectomy if retro-esophageal subclavian artery is detected during preoperative CT evaluation of neck.
166. A second look after 24 hours should be considered for a wound with suspected tissue viability.
167. Surgeon must be careful during the control of hemorrhage from the inferior laryngeal artery (a posterior branch of inferior thyroid artery) near the ligament of Berry to avoid thermal or mechanical injury to the recurrent laryngeal nerve.
168. Surgeon should be cautious during excision of thyroid tissue near the ligament of Berry to avoid injury to the recurrent laryngeal nerve.
169. A chest X-ray should be done after insertion of chest drain.
170. Chest drain insertion should be done through the 'triangle of safety' except: (i) breast tissue covers the area; (ii) a better position for drainage is determined after ultrasonography (USG).
171. It should be ensured during chest drain insertion that the most distal tube hole is within the pleural space.
172. Before injecting the local anesthetic, syringe piston should be withdrawn each time to ensure that the needle is not in a blood vessel.
173. During ring block of the finger, the local anesthetic should be injected on the web space, not around the base of the finger.
174. Slight eversion, rather than inversion of the skin edges should be considered during skin approximation.
175. Peripheral venous catheters should be removed if signs of phlebitis (increased local temperature, tenderness, erythema or palpable venous cord) are present.
176. In adults, a lower extremity peripheral vascular catheter should be replaced by an upper extremity catheter as soon as possible.

Contd...

Contd...

177.	Sterile gloves should be worn during insertion of central venous catheter and arterial catheter.
178.	Triphasic CT scan should be advised if hepatocellular carcinoma (HCC) or hypervascular liver metastases are suspected.
179.	Routine CT evaluation of the liver should be done using portal venous phase imaging.
180.	Aponeurotic fibers should be separated parallel to the fibers, whenever possible (because the muscle tone pulls the fibers along their length and closes the gap).
181.	Adequate fluid resuscitation should be done prior to exploratory laparotomy in patients with acute intestinal obstruction.
182.	For fluid resuscitation in hypovolemic shock, the IV access should be through short, wide-bore cannula. Central venous catheter should be better avoided.
183.	Dissection should be started away from the diseased area, if the disease process distorted the plane of dissection.
184.	Debridement of the wound (following RTA, firework explosion) should be done with scrubbing brush and copious irrigation of normal saline to remove all dirt to prevent development of dirt tattooing.
185.	During wound debridement, devitalize tissues should be excised until bleeding starts.
186.	Bedridden patients should be turned at least every 2 hours to minimize the risk of development of pressure sores.
187.	Prophylactic antibiotic should be administered to cover the 'decisive period' (a 4-hour interval before bacterial growth becomes established after incision) to prevent surgical site infection.
188.	Mycobacterial or Actinomyces infection should be suspected if chronic abscess is present, particularly if associated with sinus or fistula.
189.	Abscess cavity should be left open after incision and drainage.
190.	Every surgeon should know their immune status to hepatitis B and be vaccinated, if indicated. Antibody titer should be measured one month after completion of immunization schedule.
191.	Surgeon should seek expert medical advice and measurement of antibody titer if he/she is exposed to an hepatitis C infection risk (this infection is potentially curable with ribavirin and interferon-alpha therapy).
192.	The HBV and HCV infection status of the patient and surgeon should be confidential.
193.	Double gloves should be worn during any invasive procedures where chance of exposure to body fluids is high or extended duration of procedure is expected.
194.	During surgery, surgeon should routinely check their gloves for perforation. If the outer glove is perforated, it is better to change both layers.
195.	Preoperative skin shaving should be done immediately before surgery to minimize the risk of SSI.
196.	Clippers should be used for preoperative skin shaving, if available (lowest risk of SSI).
197.	Perioperative hypothermia, dead space and hematoma should be avoided during surgery to minimize the risk of SSI.
198.	All practicable measures should be taken to minimize the number of OT personnels and in-out movement in the operation theater to decrease the risk of SSI.
199.	The dose of prophylactic antibiotic should be repeated 4 hourly if surgery is continuing for more than 4 hours or unexpected contamination happens.
200.	Sutures or clips should be removed to drain the pus if clinical evidence of suppuration is present in the operative wound. Pus should be sent for culture and sensitivity before starting empirical antibiotic therapy.
201.	Topical application of antiseptic agents in the operative wound should be avoided because it impair wound healing.
202.	If intestinal perforation due to roundworm is found in exploratory laparotomy, it is better to deliver the perforation site as ileostomy instead of closure of perforation or anastomosis (increased risk of anastomotic failure due to worm activity).
203.	Extra care should be taken in obese, elderly and emaciated patients during positioning in the OT table to avoid nerve injuries (nerves at risk are brachial plexus, ulnar nerve, common peroneal nerve).
204.	Skin incision should be made in the exposed area of the body bearing in mind the cosmetic result but without compromising exposure for the operative procedure.
205.	'Dog ears' at the corner of skin incisions must be excised for a satisfactory cosmetic outcome.
206.	Peritoneum should be excised very carefully during emergency abdominal surgery to avoid bowel injury (dilated bowel loops may present just underneath the peritoneum).

Contd...

Contd...

207. During resection of the malignant tumor, Surgeon must anticipate increased vascularity, involvement of vital structures by tumor infiltration, displacement of important structures.
208. Trainee surgeons should revise the surgical anatomy and basic steps of the procedure before assisting the operation.
209. During laparoscopic surgery, all secondary trocars should be inserted and removed under direct vision.
210. During suturing of the incision, the needle should be inserted and exit at right angles to the incision.
211. Drain should be removed whenever the requirement has been met.
212. Every surgeon should know the basic principles and practice of diathermy, its complications and how to avoid such complications.
213. Any laparoscopic procedures should be converted to an open procedure, if indicated.
214. Before any laparoscopic procedure, informed consent related to conversion to open procedure should be taken from the patient.
215. Optical port entry should be considered, if possible, for creating pneumoperitoneum in laparoscopic procedures in morbidly obese patients.
216. If stone spillage occurs during laparoscopic cholecystectomy, every attempt should be made to extract the stones from the peritoneal cavity.
217. In laparoscopic surgery, all conducting surfaces of the hand instruments should be within the visual field while applying the electrosurgical current.
218. Suctioning should be avoided in closed proximity to placed clips.
219. Nasogastric tube should be removed just after the completion of laparoscopic surgery, if it is placed during surgery for a distended stomach.
220. In children, abdominal wounds should be closed with absorbable suture (layered closure or mass closure).
221. Nonoperative management (NOM) should be strongly considered for isolated blunt liver or splenic injury in pediatric patients.
222. The scrotum should be urgently explored if testicular torsion cannot be excluded in patient with acute scrotum.
223. Patients should be allowed to refuse treatments that may save their lives.
224. The informed consent for surgery should be ideally taken by the surgeon who will carryout the surgical procedure.
225. Beside the informed consent, Surgeon should make a note in patient's clinical records about the communication with the patient regarding the proposed treatments and their risks.
226. All near miss and adverse events in surgery should be reported.
227. Portable X-ray should be avoided whenever possible (uses more radiation to achieve the same image quality).
228. Injudicious repeat imaging using radiation should be avoided.
229. Diabetic patients should be put first in the endoscopy list.
230. Surgeon and endoscopist must be alert to the symptoms suggestive of perforation (e.g., neck or chest pain, abdominal pain, dysphagia, surgical emphysema) after endoscopy, particularly therapeutic endoscopy.
231. Rectal administration of diclofenac or indomethacin should be considered immediately before or after ERCP in all patients without contraindication to reduce the risk of post-ERCP pancreatitis.
232. Tissue samples for routine histology should be placed in a fixative, i.e. formalin (10% formaldehyde) to preserve morphology.
233. Tissue samples for frozen section biopsy should be sent without any fixative.
234. Request form for histology should be sent to the pathological laboratory with relevant clinical details, provisional diagnosis, cytological findings (if any), biopsy site, name of the operative procedure (if any), details of neoadjuvant therapy (if any such).
235. During preoperative assessment, women of child-bearing age should be asked about her LMP, and if any doubt, pregnancy should be excluded by laboratory test or pregnancy kit.
236. During preoperative assessment, a cardiologist's opinion should be taken if ischemic changes or arrhythmia is seen in ECG or echocardiography reveals poor left ventricular function.
237. During preoperative management of patient with hypertension, if a new antihypertensive agent is introduced, a period of at least 2 weeks should be allowed for stabilization of blood pressure.

Contd...

Contd...

238.	Temporary or permanent pacemaker placement should be considered if symptomatic heart block or asymptomatic second or third-degree heart block is detected during preoperative assessment.
239.	H_2 blocker or proton pump inhibitors should be considered along with preoperative fasting to avoid the risk of acid aspiration syndrome in patients with high risk of aspiration (e.g., obesity, pregnancy, diabetes, hiatus hernia).
240.	Estrogen-containing oral contraceptive pills (OCPs) and hormone replacement therapy should be stopped 4 weeks before elective surgery.
241.	Combined-oral contraceptive pill (OCP) should be stopped 4 weeks before major surgery with a expected prolonged period of immobility.
242.	Chest physiotherapy and incentive spirometry should be considered during postoperative period to decrease the risk of postoperative respiratory complications.
243.	Resuscitation facility and oxygen should be available during any surgical procedures using local anesthesia (life-threatening adverse reactions may develop).
244.	The abdominal drain should be placed in the most dependent part of the peritoneal cavity where body fluid collection likely to accumulate.
245.	Hands should be checked for cuts, and abrasions before scrubbing. Waterproof adhesive dressing should be applied if any such injuries.
246.	Blood clots and accumulated blood should be removed from the peritoneal cavity (blood is a good culture medium for bacterias).
247.	A clean and clean-contaminated wound of more than 6 hours old should be managed by delayed primary closure (immediate cleaning and debridement of the wound followed by closure after 48 hours).
248.	The shifting of postoperative patient from the recovery room to the ward should be considered only when patient is awake, breathing spontaneously and comfortably, can lift head on command, pulse and BP are stable.
249.	If a postoperative patient is restless in the recovery room, following reasons should be suspected—hypoxia, hemorrhage, hypotension, hypothermia, inadequate analgesia.
250.	All jeweleries should be removed from fingers and hands before hand washing for surgery.
251.	Hands should be cleaned with soap and water after removing gloves.
252.	Surgical cricothyroidotomy should be considered in any patient with airway obstruction where intubation has been attempted twice and failed and/or the patient cannot be ventilated.
253.	In the discharge note of a surgical patient, following things should be mentioned—diagnosis on admission and final diagnosis, details of operation (if any), summary of patient's course in hospital, instructions for medications, other relevant investigations and follow up, advice for consultation to other discipline (if indicated).
254.	Instruments and sponge counting should be done just before beginning of a surgical procedure, before closure of a cavity (e.g., closure of peritoneum), at skin closure.
255.	Sponges used for surgical procedures should be X-ray detectable.
256.	When sponges are used for packing in damage control surgeries (e.g., perihepatic packing for liver injury), the number and type of sponges should be documented on the intraoperative record and confirmed by the surgeon. When the sponges will be removed, the number and types should be verified from the intraoperative record and should be recorded in the patient's record.
257.	Members of the surgical team should account for breakage and/or separation of parts of sharps or other instruments in open as well as minimally invasive surgery. It must be verified during counting that all broken or separated parts are present or accounted.
258.	The first scrub of the day should be longer (minimum 5 minutes) than any subsequent scrubs (minimum 3 minutes).
259.	During incision and drainage of abscess, if there is any doubt about the etiology, a part of abscess wall should be sent for histopathology.
260.	Before the initial access for pneumoperitoneum, it must be ensured that the urinary bladder is empty.
261.	Surgeon should keep in mind that the patient may be allergic to iodine (used for antiseptic skin preparation before surgery), latex (may present in gloves).
262.	Opioid analgesics beyond the minimum doses needed to achieve adequate perioperative analgesia should be avoided in older patients (more than 65 years).
263.	Nutritional support should be considered in any patients with inadequate or no oral intake of food for 5 days or more.

Contd...

Contd...

264. Tube-feeding (e.g., Ryle's tube, nasojejunal tube, jejunostomy tube, gastrostomy tube) should be temporarily discontinued if aspirate volume is more than 200 mL in any 2-hour period.
265. All tubes for tube-feeding should be flushed with water at least twice daily to avoid tube blockage.
266. If long-term requirement of parenteral nutrition is anticipated, central venous line should be considered. Peripheral venous access is appropriate only for short-term parenteral nutrition (less than 2 weeks).
267. Before commencement of TPN via central venous access, a chest X-ray should be done to confirm that the catheter tip lies in the distal superior vena cava (SVC) and to exclude pneumothorax.
268. Before starting the operative procedure, surgeon should check the availability of special instruments (if any needed) appliances (e.g., mesh, implant), functioning of machines (e.g., diathermy).
269. Before the administration of anesthesia, surgeon makes sure that the correct patient is on the operating table and he/she is planning to do the surgical procedure on the correct side.
270. Rough handling of tissues should be avoided (increased risk of delayed wound healing and wound infection).
271. Drain should be monitored on regular interval in the first 24 hours after surgery (postoperative bleeding is most common in this period).
272. Infective focus (e.g., chest infection, UTI, SSI) should always be searched in patients with postoperative pyrexia.
273. Drain should be removed once there is no drainage or drain amount become less than 30 mL in 24 hours.
274. Mechanism of injury should be strongly considered during assessment of trauma patients.
275. During assessment of penetrating injuries in torso, it should be kept in mind that the abdominal organs may be present at a higher level than anticipated, particularly during expiration.
276. During exploration of high-velocity projectile injuries, surgeon should explore and debride the apparent wound along with adequate margin of surrounding tissues (high-velocity projectiles cause both permanent and temporary cavitation, temporary cavitation is not evident during surgical exploration).
277. Trauma patients should be completely exposed during primary survey to search for some specific external injury marks (e.g., seatbelt marks) that indicate obvious specific internal injuries.
278. Whole body CT (WBCT) should be considered judiciously in trauma patients (risk of exposure to high radiation dose).
279. Tranexamic acid should be administered within 3 hours of injury to all trauma patients (blunt and penetrating) suspected to have significant hemorrhage.
280. Pelvic binder should be applied (at the level of the greater trochanter) in all trauma patients with hypovolemic shock suspected to have major pelvic disruption.
281. In a patient with multiple operative scar marks in different quadrants, open technique should be used for initial access for pneumoperitoneum.
282. A laparoscopic surgeon should be well-oriented about the principles of instruments used for laparoscopic surgery.
283. Trocar and cannula should be held in a proper grip during entry into the peritoneal cavity (head of the trocar on the thenar eminence, middle finger over the gas inlet and index finger towards the tip).
284. Cleaning of the hand instruments after laparoscopic surgery should be done carefully to avoid any breach of insulation. If any breach is noticed, the instrument should be replaced by a new one.
285. Laparoscopic instruments should be dismantled (if technically feasible) before cleaning and sterilization.
286. During focusing of the camera, the distance between the tip of the telescope and the gauze piece should be between 6 to 8 cm.
287. During introduction of Veress needle in obese patients, the patient should be in supine position and the direction of needle entry should be perpendicular to the abdominal wall.
288. Removal of the last port should be done after introducing any blunt hand instrument or telescope through this port to avoid inadvertent entrapment of omentum or intestine inside the port wound.
289. Blood and other body fluids of all patients should be considered as potentially infectious unless proved otherwise.
290. The patient's stay in the hospital before an elective surgery should be as minimum as possible. Most of the preoperative investigations should be completed on an outpatient basis.

Contd...

Contd...

291.	The side to be operated should be clearly marked. It should be rechecked from the clinical notes and from the patient before surgery.
292.	The clinical notes, laboratory reports, imaging must accompany the patient to operating theater.
293.	Surgeon must communicate with the anesthesiologist during the surgical procedure if any unexpected findings are identified or unexpected event is occurred that might change the operative procedure.
294.	Surgeon should keep in mind that smaller amount of blood loss may be life threatening in children.
295.	Meticulous hemostasis at all stages of surgical procedures must be practiced to minimize the requirement for blood transfusion.
296.	Suture removal must be considered as early as 3 days if suture marks are unacceptable in that area (e.g., face). The wound should be reinforced with skin tapes after suture removal.
297.	Dressing of the debrided wound should be changed whenever it becomes soaked with blood or serosanguinous fluid.
298.	During surgical debridement of the lacerated wound, lacerated small vessels should be ligated whether they are bleeding or not.
299.	In emergency, repair of nerves and flexor tendons of fingers should be avoided. The ends of nerves and tendons should be loosely apposed by suturing to prevent retraction.
300.	Proper anatomical alignment should be seriously considered during repair of lip, ear, and nose injuries.
301.	During diagnostic workup of mastitis, inflammatory carcinoma of breast should be keep in mind as differential diagnosis. If any suspicion, biopsy should be sent to rule out inflammatory carcinoma.
302.	If clinical diagnosis is lymphoma, lymph node biopsy rather than FNA should be considered.
303.	Digital rectal examination in children should be done by the little finger rather than index finger.
304.	Repeated clinical examination should be done in acute abdomen with equivocal abdominal findings. Even opinion of an experienced colleague should be taken, if feasible.
305.	Surgeon should keep in mind that clinical presentation of peritonitis may not be so obvious in very young, elderly and immunosuppressed patients.
306.	For urinalysis, the sample should be a midstream urine sample (to avoid contamination of the urine specimen by skin and urethral organisms).
307.	In pregnant women with groin swelling, round ligament varicosities should be excluded before reaching the diagnosis of groin hernia.
308.	Intraosseous puncture should be considered in children with shock if venous access is failed or technically not feasible.
309.	Cuffed endotracheal tube should be avoided for tracheal intubation in children less than 10-year-old (to minimize the risk of subglottic swelling and ulceration).
310.	In pregnant trauma patients, resuscitation should be performed in lateral position (to prevent aortocaval compression).
311.	Anticholinergics agents, corticosteroids, sedative hypnotics should be avoided in elderly postoperative patients (to minimize the risk of postoperative delirium).
312.	Patients with type 1 diabetes mellitus should be more closely monitored for blood glucose level in the perioperative period than patients with type 2 diabetes mellitus (type 1 DM patients are more at risk of hypoglycemia and ketoacidosis).
313.	Flexor tendon injuries should be repaired as an elective procedure in the operating theater but the time interval between injury and repair should be as minimal as possible.
314.	The nerve injuries should be repaired as an elective procedure in the operating theater but the time interval between nerve injury and repair should be as minimal as possible (early repair increases the chance of primary repair).
315.	If replantation for amputated digit is planned, the amputated digit should be wrapped in moistened gauze and then placed in a sealed plastic bag and that plastic bag is placed in ice water bath.
316.	High-pressure injection injuries in the digits should be explored within 6 hours of injury (these are digit-threatening injuries).
317.	If any clinical suspicion of compartment syndrome, early fasciotomy should be performed (not to wait for the florid presentations with established muscle necrosis).
318.	To prevent painful neuroma in amputation stump, the nerve stump should be resected as far proximally in the wound as possible.

Contd...

Contd...

319. Diffuse axonal injury (DAI) should be suspected in high-velocity RTA patients if cognitive and neurological impairment seems disproportionate to the CT findings.
320. Early intubation and ventilation should be considered for airway control in severe brain injury patients.
321. Imaging of the whole spine should be done if spinal fracture is detected in cervical spine X-rays.
322. In multinodular goiter, the fine needle aspiration cytology (FNAC) should be performed under USG guidance (USG can detect the nodules with features of concern).
323. Routine patient observations should be done at least hourly for the first 6 hours following thyroid surgery for early recognition of potential airway compromise secondary to hematoma (hemorrhage and subsequent hematoma most commonly develop within first 6 hours).
324. A post-thyroidectomy patient should be in a bed near to the nursing station (direct visibility by the nursing staff allows early recognition of alarming features of airway compromise).
325. Emergency box containing instruments for opening the neck wound should be kept at the bedside of post-thyroidectomy patients.
326. If signs of airway compromise due to suspected hematoma develop following thyroidectomy, 'SCOOP' approach (Skin exposure; Cut sutures; Open skin; Open muscles; Pack wound) should be taken at bedside.
327. Tracheal intubation should be considered if no resolution of airway compromise after hematoma evacuation in post-thyroidectomy patients.
328. Synacthen test should be considered to assess adrenal function prior to stopping supplemental cortisol after unilateral adrenalectomy.
329. Patient must be counseled about the inability to breastfeeding and altered nipple sensation before Hadfield operation (cone excision of the major ducts).
330. Any patient with lumpy breast (without any discrete lump) should be clinically reviewed at a different point in the menstrual cycle.
331. Recurrence should be excluded if post-mastectomy patient presents with painful lymphoedema of the arm (neoplastic infiltration of the brachial plexus and lymphatics cause pain and lymphoedema).
332. The emergency tracheostomy in small children and thick necked adults should be done by a more experienced medical personnel (anatomical landmarks are difficult to locate).
333. In emergency tracheostomy, hemostasis of the operative field should be secured only after the establishment of the airway.
334. The pressure within the tracheostomy tube cuff should be low enough (high cuff pressure increases the risk of subglottic stenosis).
335. Humidification and suction of tracheostomy should be considered at regular interval to keep the airway free from secretions.
336. Cricothyroidotomy should be converted to a tracheostomy as soon as possible.
337. Lung cancer should be considered as the etiology of left vocal cord palsy until proved otherwise.
338. Other associated injuries (e.g., head injury, spinal injury, chest or abdominal injuries etc.) should be excluded in burn injury patients, particularly following explosion or escape attempt from fires.
339. Continuous cooling of burn wounds with cool tap water (soaks, compress, lavage) for the first 10 minutes should be considered in pre-hospital settings.
340. Early elective intubation should be considered in patients with suspected airway burn injury.
341. Inhalational injury should be suspected if burn injury occurs in a closed space.
342. Adequate amount of blood should be available for transfusion before considering escharotomy of the burn wound.
343. Burn injury with indeterminate depth should be reassessed after 48 hours.
344. Topical application of silver sulphadiazine (1%) should be avoided in pregnant and nursing mothers and infants of less than 2 months of age (increased risk of development of kernicterus).
345. The skin excision should be kept to a minimum during debridement of traumatic wound.
346. The exposed blood vessels and joint surfaces should be covered with adjoining muscles during emergency management of traumatic wound not ideal for primary closure.

Contd...

Contd...

347.	During debridement of facial injuries, the skin and soft tissue excision should be kept to a minimum to maintain maximum functional and cosmetic outcome.
348.	Any positive result on Fecal Occult Blood Test (FOBT) should be followed up with colonoscopy.
349.	Lactating mothers should be advised for nursing or breast pumping just prior to mammography (sensitivity is increased due to decrease in density of breast parenchyma).
350.	Surgeon should provide splenectomy wallet card (mentioning his/her name, blood group, indication of splenectomy, date of splenectomy, immunization status) to the patient along with discharge certificate.
351.	Patients with blunt splenic injury who are treated with conservative management should be advised to avoid contact sports for at least 3 months.
352.	Patients with temporary or permanent stoma should be well informed about the stoma complications and stoma care.
353.	Counseling of the patients must be well advance prior to mastectomy, orchidectomy, stoma formation.
354.	Patient should be advised to stop smoking at least 4 weeks before hernia surgery.
355.	Site of tru-cut biopsy or incisional biopsy should be planned in such a way so that if wide local excision is to be planned subsequently, then the biopsy site can be encompassed without a larger surgical defect.
356.	Surgeon should know optimal surgical margin of that cancer while resecting that tumor (optimal surgical margin of breast carcinoma and malignant melanoma are not same).
357.	Excision biopsy should be done with a curative intent (adequate tissue surrounding the tumor to ensure negative surgical margin).
358.	Marking of the margins of the excisional biopsy specimen with sutures or clips should be done (to know whether all margins are free from tumor or any margin is involved by microscopic disease).
359.	Antimicrobial regimen of sepsis patient should be reassessed daily for appropriate de-escalation of antimicrobial therapy from broad-spectrum therapy to directed antimicrobial agent therapy.
360.	Nonemergent, nonobstetric surgery in the pregnant patients should be planned in the second trimester of pregnancy (increased risk of spontaneous abortion in the 1st trimester and risk of preterm labor in 3rd trimester).
361.	The foreskin should be returned back to its normal anatomical position after catheterization if Foley catheter is placed in an uncircumcised patient to avoid paraphimosis.
362.	Isolated right-sided varicoceles should be evaluated with further imaging workup to rule out retroperitoneal SOL or aberration of venous anatomy.
363.	Cord lipoma, if found during hernia repair should be resected or reduced into the preperitoneal space to avoid any future confusion with a recurrent hernia.
364.	Occult incarcerated femoral hernia should be in the differential diagnosis of any patient presenting with acute small intestinal obstruction, particularly if there is no history of abdominal surgery.
365.	Peripherally inserted central catheters (PICCs) should be considered as venous access of choice in patients who require long-term administration of IV medications (antibiotics, antifungals, chemotherapeutic agents) in outpatient setting.
366.	Internal jugular central venous cannulation should be performed under ultrasound guidance, if available.
367.	During removal of subclavian, internal jugular catheter or PICCs, patient should be placed in Trendelenburg position and manual pressure over the insertion site for a minimum of 5 minutes should be applied.
368.	Subcutaneous knots of polypropylene sutures must be buried to avoid the complications of localized tenderness or sinus formation.
369.	During the closure of skin by staples, the coaptation of the dermal margins must be accurate avoiding inversion or eversion.
370.	Surgeon must look that the surfaces of the two organs are in apposition throughout the intended anastomosis and no extraneous tissue lies in between the stapling ring during the firing of staples for GI anastomosis.
371.	It is better to achieve the proximal and distal control of a major blood vessel by a vascular sling during dissection adjacent to the vessel so that vascular clamps can be readily applied if any hemorrhage occurred.
372.	During vascular control by clips, it should be applied in such a way that it must encompass the vessel totally and it is placed at right angles to the long axis of the vessel.

Contd...

Contd...

373.	The vessel should be divided at some distance from the ligature or clip so that splayed-out cuff is adequate because it prevents the slippage of ligature or clip.
374.	During vascular control of a tributary, flush control should be achieved so that parent vessel is not constricted or blind outpouch is left. In both these situations, there is an increased risk of thrombosis of the parent vessel.
375.	Surgeon should use the cutting mode of electrosurgery when doing wedge biopsy.
376.	During wedge biopsy, the wedge should be handled gently with minimal grasping to minimize crushing damage of tissue architecture.
377.	Vascular lesions should be biopsied with extreme care and if possible, excised intact.
378.	Lymph nodes should be biopsied intact if possible. If technically not possible, the wedge biopsy should be done in such a way that the biopsy specimen contains a capsule and the surrounding stroma.
379.	The lymph node specimen should send to the pathology department as early as possible because special immuno-histochemical staining and electron microscopy may be required.
380.	The frozen section facility should be used by the surgeon if only the biopsy findings will influence the nature of the surgical procedure carried out at that time.
381.	Life-threatening injuries should be suspected in all road traffic accident victims with rollover or ejection until proven otherwise.
382.	Pregnancy tests should be done in all trauma patients with childbearing age.
383.	Personal protective equipment should be donned by all the members of trauma team on arrival of trauma patients in designated trauma centers.
384.	ICU admission should be strongly considered in elderly patients with thoracic trauma because of increased risk of complications and mortality.
385.	Repeated assessment should be considered in all trauma patients with suspected intra-abdominal injury because concomitant CNS, chest, and musculoskeletal injuries may obscure signs and symptoms of abdominal injury.
386.	High level of clinical suspicion and judicious use of adjunctive imaging should be strongly considered in patients with suspected injury to the retroperitoneal part of the hollow viscus because often these patients present with non-specific symptoms.
387.	Laparotomy should be strongly considered in trauma patients with seatbelt sign and free fluid in FAST.
388.	All penetrating wounds should be marked with radiopaque clips before the X-ray or CT scan so that trajectory of the bullet or knife and associated injuries can be assessed.
389.	Patients with hard signs of vascular injury should be immediately transferred to the operating room.
390.	During the repair of scalp wound, the local anesthesia must be injected in the connective tissue layer (nerves are located in this layer) and the aponeurosis must be closed (to prevent stretching of the scar).
391.	Surgeon must look for a second perforation nearby while doing laparotomy for peptic ulcer perforation because simultaneous perforation of two ulcers may develop, particularly in patients with Zollinger-Ellison syndrome.
392.	The nerve should be divided proximally to the level of bone resection during amputation to prevent development of stump neuroma.
393.	Surgeons should take every possible measure against pulmonary complications in emergency surgery patients because these patients are at increased risk of these complications.
394.	Patients should be encouraged to share their feelings with relatives and medical staff to cope the 'postoperative blues'.
395.	In any acutely confused patient, surgeon should exclude hypoxia, metabolic abnormalities, severe sepsis, intracranial injury, or acute lack of sleep.
396.	Pulse oximeter readings must be interpreted with extreme caution in patients with hypovolemic shock or in patients with carboxyhemoglobin.
397.	In trauma patients, surgeon must take adequate measures for pain relief as part of initial trauma care because physiological responses to pain may alter the outcome of the patient (e.g., by increasing intracranial pressure).

Contd...

Contd...

398.	Penetrating missile wounds should be explored throughout the whole length of the wound to reveal damage to the underlying structures.
399.	Before attempting to remove a foreign body, surgeon must consider whether or not there is real indication for immediate exploration. The surgeon should also be prepared to abandon the procedure after a certain period of time, if no foreign body is found.
400.	Surgeon should be more vigilant to identify multiple traumas in patients with history of trauma because polytrauma patients have higher rates of deaths, ICU admission, higher number of surgeries and complications.
401.	It is always better to describe each component of the GCS scale separately rather than a total score.
402.	Prior to initiating DEC therapy for lymphatic filariasis, onchocerciasis should be excluded in all patients with constant exposure history because of the possibility of severe exacerbations of skin and eye involvement (Mazzotti reaction).
403.	In breast core biopsy, the skin entry site should be optimized for both cosmesis and accurate targeting. The lateral, inferior, and periareolar skin entry sites are preferable.
404.	During core biopsy of the breast lesions, during firing, the needle should be kept as near as possible parallel to the chest wall to minimize the risk of pneumothorax.
405.	Chemotherapy should be avoided during the first trimester of pregnancy due to higher risk of teratogenicity and intrauterine fetal death.
406.	Colposcopic examination by a gynecologist should be recommended in patients with HIV(PWH) diagnosed with anal cancer to search for the presence of vulvar, vaginal, or cervical disease.
407.	Interruption of antiretroviral therapy (ART) should be avoided during cancer treatment because it increase the risk of opportunistic infection and death.
408.	All patients with anal cancer should be tested for HIV if already not done.
409.	Surgeon must consider a wider lateral perianal margin in APR for anal cancer than APR for rectal cancer.
410.	Flap reconstruction (e.g., rectus abdominis myocutaneous flap) for closure of the perineal wound should be considered for patients with anal cancer undergoing an APR because of increased risk of poor perineal wound healing due to prior radiation therapy.
411.	Skin biopsy for any lesion suspicious of skin cancer should include deep reticular dermis because infiltrative histology may be present at the deeper margin of the tumor.
412.	Full skin examination should be considered in any patients with basal cell carcinoma because precancers or cancers may locate in any sun-exposed skin sites.
413.	Biliary protocol imaging (preferable CT) should be planned before stenting in patients with cholangiocarcinoma because stenting related reactive changes may compromise the ability to delineate complete extent of biliary tract involvement.
414.	HER2 testing should be done in all new primary or newly metastatic breast cancers.
415.	Repeat or consultative HER2 testing should be considered if a grade 1 of any histologic type, pure mucinous, pure tubular, or pure cribriform breast carcinoma becomes HER2 positive.
416.	Repeat testing or consultative review should be considered if invasive ductal carcinoma, classic type lobular carcinoma, pure tubular, mucinous, or cribriform carcinomas, encapsulated or solid papillary carcinomas are ER-negative.
417.	Repeat testing or consultative review should be considered if metaplastic carcinomas of all subtypes, adenoid cystic carcinoma or other salivary gland-like carcinomas of the breast, secretory carcinoma, and carcinomas with apocrine differentiation are ER-positive.
418.	Surgeon must advise his/her patient not to conceive during radiation therapy, chemotherapy, endocrine therapy, or during or within 6 months of completing trastuzumab or pertuzumab.
419.	Breastfeeding should be discouraged during chemotherapy, endocrine therapy, or during or within 6 months of completing trastuzumab or pertuzumab.
420.	Hormone-based birth control methods should be discouraged regardless of hormone receptor status of breast cancer.
421.	Patients with risk factors (e.g., smoking, WHO Class 2 and 3 Obesity) should be counseled about the increased risk for complications following breast reconstruction (e.g., flap necrosis, total flap failure, implant failure) including donor site complications (e.g., abdominal wall hernia, abdominal wall bulging).

Contd...

Contd...

422. Patient should be encouraged to stop smoking before breast reconstruction.
423. Ultrasound should be considered as first-line imaging modality in pregnant and lactating patients with palpable breast lesions.
424. Pregnant and lactating patients should be counseled about the risk of milk fistula and increased risk of bleeding before any biopsy procedure of palpable breast lesions.
425. Breastfeeding or pumping should be encouraged in lactating patients before mammography to optimize the sensitivity of mammography.
426. Transthoracic echocardiography (TTE) resting should be considered as first-line imaging modality in patients with suspected blunt cardiac trauma with abnormal ECG and elevated cardiac troponin level.
427. Pericardial or cardiac injuries should be suspected if AP chest radiograph has any of the following findings—widened mediastinum, enlarged cardiomediastinal silhouette, abnormal cardiac silhouette contour, changing cardiac position after tube thoracotomy, pneumopericardium, displaced rib fractures particularly between the third and ninth ribs.
428. MRI should be considered for evaluation of symptomatic organized pancreatic or peripancreatic fluid collections, particularly when intervention is contemplated.
429. Pancreatic duct disruption should be excluded by MRI with MRCP before taking decision of any drainage procedures for necrotizing pancreatitis because drainage will most likely fail in the setting of disrupted pancreatic duct.
430. A low threshold should be maintained for screening the thoracolumbar spine with imaging in blunt trauma patients particularly in elderly patients (increased risk of spine fractures).
431. Amputation should be planned as a part of management when a part of limb is dead, deadly or dead loss.
432. A statin therapy should be continued in atherosclerotic occlusive arterial disease even if lipid profile is normal because statin may stabilize atherosclerotic plaques.
433. Minimal debridement should be considered following soft tissue trauma in face and neck region because most of the devitalized looking tissues will indeed survive due to rich vascular supply.
434. Use of vertical tracheal incision, smallest tracheostomy tube and rapid downsizing of tube must be considered for minimizing the risk of post-tracheostomy stenosis.
435. Surgeon should be alert during management of significant dogbite wounds because these wounds may require thorough assessment and surgical intervention as extensive undermined injuries may present due to large canine teeth.
436. Clenched fist injuries should be treated seriously because these wounds, though appear minor, may result in injury to the extensor tendon, joint capsule along with significant bacterial contamination from oral flora of the biting offender.
437. The decision to transport a critically ill patient of ICU for diagnostic purpose should be taken judiciously after assessing risk-benefit ratio because of potential risk of dislodgement of endotracheal tube, hemodynamic compromise during transport.
438. Subclavian site should be considered as central venous access site in patients with tracheostomy because tracheal secretions increase the chance of infection (subclavian catheters are least likely to become infected).
439. During tracheostomy, injury to the first tracheal ring should be avoided to minimize the risk of subglottic stenosis.
440. Patient's head must be flexed when the tapes of tracheostomy tube are tied otherwise it may become slack when patient changes his/her head position from extension to flexion.
441. Suction and humidification of tracheostomy tube at regular intervals should be considered to minimize the risk of aspiration and tube blockage.
442. Tracheostomy should be considered if bilateral recurrent laryngeal nerve palsy develops following total thyroidectomy.
443. Low tracheostomy, instead of endotracheal intubation should be considered to securing the airway following crush or laceration injuries to the laryngeal skeleton because severe fibrosis and loss of laryngeal function may occur following endotracheal intubation.
444. Surgeon must recognize that the patient in shock state is actively bleeding or not because in patient who is actively bleeding, the priority is to stop bleeding and in patient who is not actively bleeding, the management is to correct the shock state first.
445. For a nonfunctioning stent in malignant distal biliary obstruction, if plastic stent is present, it should be replaced by a SEMS or in case of SEMS, a plastic stent or new SEMS is to be placed within the original SEMS.

Contd...

Contd...

446.	Resectability of malignant hilar strictures should be assessed before biliary stenting because ductal decompression and imaging artifacts may affect proper assessment.
447.	If liver-directed surgery or therapy (e.g., ablation, radiofrequency embolization) is planned in colon carcinoma, hepatic MRI with extracellular or hepatobiliary gadolinium-based contrast agent should be considered for better assessment of metastatic lesions.
448.	Elective surgery should be delayed for 30 days after insertion of bare metal coronary stent and for 1 year after insertion of drug eluting stent placement (delay to decrease the risk of in-stent thrombosis). For semi-elective surgeries, surgery may be considered after 6 months.
449.	Blood glucose must be more strictly monitored during perioperative period in patients with type 1 diabetes than type 2 diabetes because these patients are more prone to become hypoglycemic during stressful condition and at more risk of developing ketoacidosis.
450.	Evaluation by a geneticist should be considered in all babies with isolated cleft palate because about half of the isolated cleft palate patients have genetic abnormalities.
451.	Assessment for sensorineural and conductive deafness by auditory brainstem responses (ABR) and tympanometry should be considered in all children with cleft lip and palate before 1 year of age.
452.	Palate should be clinically assessed in a child presenting with cleft lip.
453.	Thick split thickness skin graft (STSG) should be avoided in unhealthy wound beds, particularly in chronic ulcer because thick grafts have more metabolic demand.
454.	Thick STSG or full thickness skin graft (FTSG) should be considered for reconstruction of mechanically demanding parts, i.e., palm, sole because dermis provides the strength and viscoelastic properties of skin.
455.	Hyperthermia and hyperglycemia should be managed promptly in head injury patients because these conditions are toxic to injured neurons thereby increasing the risk of developing secondary injuries.
456.	Spina bifida occulta should be suspected if any tuft of hair, cutaneous hemangioma or sinus track is found over the lumbosacral region.
457.	Surgical closure of meningomyelocele should be considered within 24–48 hours of birth to minimize the risk of meningitis or ventriculitis.
458.	Nonsteroidal analgesics should be avoided in pregnant surgical patients due to increased risk of premature closure of ductus arteriosus.
459.	Disorder of sexual differentiation (DSD) should be ruled out in all patients with perineal hypospadias along with unilateral or bilateral undescended testes.
460.	The electrode of argon beam coagulator should be held slightly far from tissue (5–10 mm).
461.	In patients with hip prosthesis, during use of electrosurgery, the return electrode pad should be placed on the contralateral hip.
462.	If alcohol-based agents are used for antiseptic dressing, it must be ensured that the solution is not pooled near the dispersive pad and the operative field is dry before use of electrosurgery.
463.	Dose escalation (from 20 to 40 mg/day) of tamoxifen or alternate hormonal therapy should be considered in breast cancer patients with *CYP2D6* genotypes associated with reduced CYP2D6 enzyme activity.
464.	During parotidectomy for malignant parotid tumor, if gross invasion of facial nerve is not present, nerve should be preserved even peeling off the tumor from the nerve (adjuvant radiation therapy can provide adequate local control).
465.	A catheterized urine sample (not a standard midstream urinary sample) should be collected for urine examination in female patient with suspected recurrent urinary tract infection.
466.	Surgeon should carefully examine the inside of prepuce and glans to exclude carcinoma in adult phimosis patients.
467.	Surgeon must be aware during surgery for saphenopopliteal incompetence that the anatomy of the short saphenous vein is variable in popliteal fossa region.
468.	Surgeon must be aware about the existence of anterior accessory of the great saphenous vein (AAGSV) during varicose vein surgery because it is commonly mistaken for great saphenous vein.

DON'TS IN SURGERY

1. In bleeding wound, do not apply any clamp blindly (chance of nerve damage is more).
2. In contaminated wound (particularly injuries caused by road traffic accidents, explosions, high velocity penetrating injuries), don't do primary repair of the wound.
3. During management of limb injuries, if tourniquet have to applied, do not forget the time of application of tourniquet.
4. If crush injury presents several days after the incident, do not do late fasciotomy (myoglobin released from dead muscle causes glomerular deposition resulting in renal failure).
5. In skin closure, silk should not be used as suture material.
6. During skin incision, don't incise the skin obliquely (the shearing mechanism may lead to necrosis of the undercut edge).
7. Do not grasp the suture material with needle holder or hemostatic forceps (may lead to fracture of the suture material).
8. Do not use nonabsorbable suture material in the biliary tract or urinary tract (to minimize the risk of stone formation).
9. Do not use braided suture material for vascular anastomosis (to minimize risk of platelet adherence which may lead to distal embolization).
10. Do not grasp the 'shank' or 'point' of the needle by the needle-holder.
11. During resection-anastomosis, do not impinge on the mesentery by the intestinal clamps.
12. Do not give skin incision crossing skin creases or over bony prominences.
13. Do not compromise the exposure due to cosmetic ground, particularly during laparotomy.
14. Circumcision should not be done in children with hypospadias.
15. Do not do a elective surgery for 3–6 months after acute MI (to reduce the risk of perioperative reinfarction).
16. Do not place any T-tube smaller than 14 Fr after open CBD exploration.
17. In trauma setting, for establishment of airway, cricothyroidotomy should not be done in patients below age 11 years (increased risk of subglottic stenosis).
18. If a patient attends emergency with a penetrating weapon remaining in place, the weapon should not be removed in emergency, should be removed in OT with proper setup.
19. Prophylactic antibiotics should not be administered in acute burn injury (increased risk of antibiotic resistance and fungal infection).
20. When calculating burn size, first-degree burn should not be estimated.
21. Surgeon should not use electrosurgery adjacent to clip during laparoscopic cholecystectomy (conduction of thermal energy via the metallic clip may lead to delayed biliary stricture).
22. CT scan should not be initial imaging in pregnant patients presenting with acute abdominal pain.
23. Laparoscopic cholecystectomy should not be done in Child's C cirrhosis patients.
24. Routine preoperative biliary drainage should not be considered in malignant extrahepatic biliary obstruction.
25. Insertion of uncovered SEMSs should not be considered for drainage of extrahepatic biliary obstruction of unknown etiology or benign biliary strictures.
26. Forceful endoscopic dilation of an early postoperative bile duct stricture (less than 4 weeks after surgery) should be avoided.
27. PAIR technique should not be used in cystic echinococcosis of lung.
28. CL cyst (hydatid cyst) should not be treated until parasite nature is not definitely proven.
29. Biopsies should not be performed in areas with endoscopic evidence of erosive esophagitis during endoscopic surveillance for Barrett esophagus.
30. Emetic agents should not be used in immediate management of caustic injuries.
31. Esophageal dilation should not be done between 7 and 21 days after caustic injury (risk of esophageal perforation is more).
32. Lidocaine or bupivacaine combined with epinephrine should not be used for anesthesia of fingers, toes, ears, nose, or penis (risk of tissue necrosis due to epinephrine mediated vasospasm of terminal arterioles).
33. Application of iodine, povidone-iodine, hydrogen peroxide should not be used during local care of acute wound (these agents may impair wound healing).

Contd...

Contd...

34.	Attempting to neutralize acidic or alkaline material should not be done (neutralization reaction may cause further tissue damage).
35.	Stricture dilation before or immediately after stent placement in colonic obstruction, should not be done (increased risk of perforation).
36.	Colonic stenting should not be done in presence of colonic perforation.
37.	SEMS as palliative decompression (in malignant colonic obstruction) should not be considered if patient is a candidate for antiangiogenic therapy e.g., bevacizumab (more chance of perforation).
38.	Surgeon should not use hybrid cannula system (metal with plastic) in laparoscopic surgery (to avoid capacitive coupling).
39.	The last port should not be suddenly withdrawn (sudden suction effect of cannula may entrap the omentum or bowel inside the port wound).
40.	Surgeon should not burn the tissue more than required during electrosurgical monopolar coagulation (because, in coagulation current, the collagen melts and then solidifies, thereby the vessel lumen is sealed; if more burning of tissue, the melted collagen burns and sealing strength may decrease).
41.	Surgeon should better avoid division of the round ligament in open repair of inguinal hernia in women.
42.	Surgeon should not handover the scalpel to his/her assistant directly.
43.	Better to avoid 'one handed knot tied with left hand' when tying a ligature or suture in very delicate tissue.
44.	Surgeon should not attempt appendectomy in appendicular lump.
45.	Surgeon should not use monopolar electrosurgical device during neonatal circumcision (because of high risk of penile tissue loss).
46.	Surgeon should not use indwelling urinary catheter or to maintain it unless there is a specific indication (to reduce the risk of catheter-associated urinary tract infection).
47.	The clips (in laparoscopic surgery) should not be applied very close to each other (the two nearby clips nullify the dumbbell formation and both will be loose).
48.	Adrenal biopsy should not be done before biochemically excluding pheochromocytoma.
49.	Preoperative hair removal should not be done by razors.
50.	Surgeon should not rely on classic features of shock (e.g., tachycardia, hypotension) in elderly trauma patients, serum markers (e.g., base deficit, serum lactate) should be assessed for evidence of shock.
51.	A granny knot should never be used by the surgeon as it is a unsafe knot.
52.	Too tight skin suturing should not be done as it cuts through the tissue or strangulates the tissue.
53.	FAST should not be relied as the only diagnostic imaging modality to exclude intra-abdominal injury in pediatric trauma patients.
54.	Skin incisions should not be made over a previous scar. Scar should be excised (at the subdermal level) at the time of skin incision.
55.	Superior pedicles of the thyroid should not be mass ligated during thyroidectomy to avoid injury to the external branch of superior laryngeal nerve.
56.	During surgery or any procedures, gloved fingertips of the surgeon should not be projected beyond the finger.
57.	Polyfilament sutures should not be pulled roughly through the tissues because these sutures have dragging and sawing effect.
58.	Ends of the threads should not be cut too short. It should be 2–3 mm long in braided sutures and 4–5 mm long in monofilament sutures.
59.	Sutures should not be held by metal instruments because sutures are weakened by holding these instruments.
60.	Diathermy should not be activated for a prolonged period during surgical dissection.
61.	Knot should not be too tight or too loose.
62.	Balloon should not be inflated till the Foley's catheter is inserted up to its hilt.
63.	Anal speculum should not be inserted without a digital rectal examination.
64.	Ligatures should not be applied too near the cut end of a ductal structure.
65.	Excess traction should be avoided during mobilization of the splenic flexure of the colon during colonic surgery to decrease the risk of tearing of the splenic capsule (splenocolic ligament arises from the inferior pole of the spleen).

Contd...

Contd...

66. Nonessential 'out of hours' blood transfusion and overnight blood transfusion should be avoided, whenever possible.
67. Fluid infusion should not be given through a administration set which is used for transfusion of blood components.
68. Intravenous drugs should not be administered during blood transfusion through same venous access. IV drugs should be administered through another venous access or in between transfusions.
69. Platelets should not be transfused through a transfusion set already used for other blood components.
70. Prolonged pre-operative fasting should be avoided in elderly surgical patients to avoid dehydration.
71. Peripheral venous cannulation should be avoided in a limb with lymphoedema.
72. During suturing of the arteries, grasping the endothelium should be avoided.
73. During repairing of the arterial wall defect, the vessel wall should not be everted (lumen become narrowed).
74. Primary closure should not be attempted in untidy, unhealthy wounds.
75. Wounds should not be closed under tension.
76. Chest drain should not be given outside the 'triangle of safety' without USG guidance.
77. In case of accidental dislodgement or removal of chest drain, the tube should not be inserted into the previous site.
78. Chest drain should not be inserted without USG guidance if air (in suspected pneumothorax) or blood (in suspected hemothorax) or fluid (in suspected pleural effusion) cannot be aspirated during infiltration of local anesthesia.
79. Clamping of the chest drain should not be done in patients on positive pressure ventilation or noninvasive ventilation (NIV).
80. Surgical procedure should not be started just after injecting the local anesthetic. A minimum of 4–5 minutes have to be waited for onset of action.
81. Incision should not be made directly over the permanent skin marking otherwise skin tattooing may occur.
82. Hemostatic forceps should not be used on the epidermis for control of oozing from the cut edges of skin. The forceps should be used to the dermal edges.
83. Tissue glue (e.g., cyanoacrylate) should not be used for wounds where skin cannot be closely apposed.
84. In perforated appendicitis, irrigation of the intraperitoneal cavity should not be done.
85. During tendon repair, vinculum should not be injured ('vinculae' or 'vinculum' are band of connective tissue that contain tiny blood vessels).
86. During tendon repair, tendon ends should not be hold with forceps.
87. Lymph node biopsy should not be done with a cavalier attitude.
88. During lymph node biopsy, lymph nodes should not be crushed, otherwise microscopic architecture may be altered.
89. Hypotonic fluids (e.g., dextrose) should not be used as volume expander in hypovolemic shock.
90. In hypovolemic shock, vasopressor or inotropic therapy should not be initiated without adequate preload.
91. Bleeding points should not be grasped along with bunched up tissues by hemostatic forceps.
92. In reoperative surgery, diathermy dissection should not be done blindly through the scar tissue because vessels and nerves may be encased within the scar tissue.
93. In patients with severe hypovolemic shock due to hemorrhage, unnecessary investigations (e.g., CT) should not be done prior to control of hemorrhage.
94. Any healthcare worker with open and infected skin lesions should not enter the operation theater.
95. Surgeon should not use monopolar diathermy during dissection near recurrent laryngeal nerve in thyroidectomy.
96. Monopolar diathermy should not be used near the facial nerve or its branches during parotidectomy.
97. Razors should not be used for preoperative skin shaving (risk of SSI is more in comparison to clippers or depilatory cream).
98. Dissection should not be continued in the depth with continuing hemorrhage.
99. A braided suture is better avoided for vascular anastomosis (increased chance of platelet adherence leads to embolus formation).
100. Barbed sutures should not be used for fascial closures.

Contd...

Contd...

101.	Discharge should not be planned after laparoscopic surgery until patients have passed urine and adequately taking liquid and solid diets.
102.	Circumcision should not be done in infants with hypospadias.
103.	Surgeon should not do any surgery without patient's consent unless in a situation to save 'life and limb'.
104.	The informed consent for a surgery should not be taken by a junior team member who has never conducted that surgical procedure.
105.	Barium contrast study should not be done in a patient with suspected bowel perforation (barium can cause peritonitis).
106.	Capsule endoscopy should not be used in patients with known small bowel strictures.
107.	Local anesthetics with adrenaline should not be used in anatomic sites supplied by end-arteries (e.g., fingers, toes, ear, nose, and penis), patients with cardiovascular diseases or taking tricyclic antidepressants and MAO inhibitors.
108.	Surgeon should not rely on a drain if clinical findings are suggestive of anastomotic leak or intraperitoneal bleeding (blockage of abdominal drain is a common event).
109.	Drains should not be bring out through the main wound.
110.	Contaminated wound should not be closed. The wound should be left open to heal by secondary intention.
111.	Recapping needles before disposal should not be done to avoid the risk of needle-stick injuries.
112.	Surgical cricothyroidotomy should not be done in any patient below the age of 10 years.
113.	Surgeon should not use monopolar diathermy in the head-neck region in patients with cochlear implants. Bipolar diathermy should not be used within 2 cm of the implant.
114.	Surgeon should not ignore the unusual peroperative findings. He/she should either manage it accordingly or note it in the operative note for further workup.
115.	Dressing over the incision site after surgery should not be changed before 48 hours.
116.	Vigorous resuscitation with crystalloids and colloids should not be done in trauma patients with hypovolemic shock (increased risk of coagulopathy, ARDS).
117.	The distal end of the fiberoptic cable should not be placed close to the patient's skin, when the light source is on (heat generated at the end of the cable may cause burn injury).
118.	Braided suture material should not be used in potentially contaminated wound.
119.	Retention sutures for abdominal wound dehiscence should not be removed before 2 weeks.
120.	Diagnosis of abscess should not be based solely on presence of fluctuation (fluctuation is usually absent in breast abscess, perianal abscess, abscess in fingertips).
121.	During lymph node biopsy, lymph node should not be directly grasped with tissue forceps (crushing by forceps may distort the microscopic architecture of lymph node).
122.	Digital rectal examination and proctoscopy should not be done in acute anal fissure.
123.	Hemorrhoidectomy should not be considered for hemorrhoids in pregnancy or postpartum hemorrhoids (resolve spontaneously within a few weeks after delivery).
124.	Nonexpanding retroperitoneal hematoma in zone II and III should not be explored.
125.	Definitive surgical management of pancreaticoduodenal injuries should not be attempted in an institution with limited resources and expertise. Patient should be referred to a specialized center after placing a drain in the lesser sac.
126.	Do not miss the groin examination and digital rectal examination when examining a patient with acute abdomen.
127.	Surgical reduction of intussusception should not be done by pulling the proximal end. Reduction should be done by milking it in a retrograde fashion.
128.	Hernial sac of direct inguinal hernia should not be opened or excised.
129.	In sliding hernia, dissection of contents of sac from the wall of sac should not be attempted (sigmoid colon, cecum, or urinary bladder as a content forms part of the posterior wall of the sac).
130.	"Watchful waiting" policy should not be considered for asymptomatic or minimally asymptomatic femoral hernias (high risk of strangulation).

Contd...

Contd...

131. If replantation of amputated digit is planned, the amputated part should not be in direct contact with ice.
132. Blind placement of nasogastric tube should not be done in patients with suspected skull base fracture.
133. Corticosteroids should not be administered in head injury patients (associated with increased mortality).
134. Corticosteroids should not be considered for management of acute spinal cord injury (lack of evidence to support neurological improvement).
135. Neck immobilization using hard collar should not be done in trauma patients with ankylosing spondylitis or major cervical kyphosis. Neck should be immobilized in flexion by using sandbags under the occiput and either side of the head or by using halo brace.
136. Core biopsy of the thyroid swelling should not be considered due to increased risk of postbiopsy hemorrhage (due to increased vascularity of the thyroid).
137. During closure of the thyroidectomy wound, water seal closure of the strap muscles should not be done (if hemorrhage occurs during the postoperative period, the hematoma may escape into the subcutaneous tissue).
138. Adrenal biopsy should not be done until phaeochromocytoma has been biochemically excluded.
139. Intramuscular injection or IV access should not be done in the arm or forearm on the side of axillary dissection.
140. Endotracheal intubation should not be done in blunt crushing injuries of thyroid or cricoid cartilage (increased risk of fibrosis that may lead to loss of laryngeal function). A low tracheostomy should be considered.
141. In the acute stage of burn, intramuscular injections should not be given (absorption is unpredictable due to peripheral vasoconstriction).
142. Digital mammography or Digital breast tomosynthesis (DBT) should not be withheld during pregnancy (no increased risk of teratogenic effect).
143. Screening or diagnostic mammography should not be delayed due to ongoing lactation.
144. Contrast-enhanced MRI should not be considered during pregnancy due to trans-placental passage of gadolinium.
145. Continuous bladder irrigation in patients with clot retention should not be initiated until the bladder is clot free by manual irrigation and aspiration with normal saline through the 22F or 24F three-way Foley catheter.
146. Surgeon should not mobilize the testis from scrotum into the inguinal canal during hernia repair to avoid risk of testicular ischemia or torsion.
147. During hernia repair in large, complete inguinal hernia, indirect sac should not be dissected beyond the pubic tubercle to avoid the risk of ischemic orchitis.
148. The ligature should not be overtightened because it may cause weakening of the blood vessel by the cheese-wire cutting effect.
149. Forced coagulation should not be used in close proximity to important anatomical structures such as bile duct or ureter because the risk of collateral damage is higher.
150. The argon flow rate in Argon beam coagulation device should not exceed 10 L/min while operating on highly vascular organs, e.g., liver, spleen, kidneys, to minimize the risk of gas embolism.
151. Biopsy should not be done from the central crater of an ulcerated lesion because this area mostly consists of necrotic tissues.
152. Insulin administration should not be stopped for a significant length of time during perioperative period in patients with type 1 diabetes due to increased risk of acidosis.
153. Open surgical biopsy should not be done in salivary gland tumors to avoid microscopic spillage of tumor cells in surrounding tissues.
154. Blind probing of a stable wound should not be attempted in the emergency as clot may be disrupted resulting in uncontrollable hemorrhage.
155. Surgeon should not forget to examine the gynecological organs during exploratory laparotomy of a female patient with acute abdomen.
156. Surgeon should not rely on isolated readings of pulse rate and blood pressure to exclude shock in trauma patients.
157. In a trauma patient with altered consciousness, it should not be assumed that alcohol or other drugs are solely responsible for this clinical condition.

Contd...

Contd...

158.	In shotgun injuries, individual pellets should not be sought. The wound should be treated, not the weapon.
159.	During calculation of GCS score, a score of 1 should not be assigned if the component (E/V/M) is untestable.
160.	Surgeon should not use the GCS alone for monitoring coma, or to assess the severity of brain damage or predict outcome.
161.	During FNA of lymph nodes, too much local anesthetic should not be injected because the pool of anesthetic around the node makes an inadequate sample more likely.
162.	The ultrasound jelly should not be used during the aspiration part of the USG-guided FNA, or the jelly should be removed if used previously.
163.	Any additional laboratory tests specific to patients with HIV(PWH) should not be advised in PWH before any surgical procedure.
164.	Immediate reconstruction should not be considered after mastectomy for inflammatory breast cancer.
165.	Whole body bone scan should not be considered for the evaluation of distant disease in stage I and IIA breast cancer.
166.	Decision of premature debridement of muscles affected following snake bite should not be taken because signs of venom injury and muscle necrosis almost looks similar.
167.	Elective surgery should not be considered within two weeks of snake bite because coagulopathy of envenomation may persist for 2 weeks after injury.
168.	During tracheostomy in children, the head should not be over extended, otherwise, the opening may occur at the level of fifth and sixth rings.
169.	During emergency tracheostomy, no attempts should be made to control hemorrhage before establishing the airway.
170.	Surgical excision of malignant melanoma should never include the deep fascia because melanoma rarely infiltrates the deep fascia, and it acts as a barrier for local invasion to deeper structures.
171.	Spilt thickness skin graft should not be considered in aesthetically sensitive areas, e.g., eyelid, face mouth, because the shape might distort due to secondary contraction that is more prominent in STSG than FTSG.
172.	Overextension of neck should not be done during airway management in pediatric trauma patients because it may compromise the airway.
173.	Assessment of severity of hypospadias should not be done based on the location of ectopic urethral meatus only.
174.	A scratch pad should be better avoided for cleaning eschar in the tip of active electrode during use of electrosurgery because the scratch pad may cause groove on the tip that may cause further eschar formation.
175.	Chemotherapy should not be planned in breast cancer patients with pregnancy after 35 weeks of pregnancy or within 3 weeks of planned delivery to minimize the hematological complications related to chemotherapy.
176.	Overenthusiastic dissection to search for saphenopopliteal junction for ligation of short saphenous vein should not be done because the SSV may terminate amongst a plexus of thin-walled deep veins that may be injured resulting in increased risk of injury to popliteal artery and tibial nerve.

Chapter 34

Miscellaneous

(Trials, Terminologies, Classification, Criteria, Scoring, Important Facts, Most Appropriate Investigations)

IMPORTANT TRIALS IN SURGERY

ACRIN 6666 trial: A randomized control trial to study combined screening with ultrasound and mammography versus mammography alone in women at elevated risk of breast cancer.

AMAROS trial: Comparing ALND with axillary radiation in clinically node negative patients with tumors smaller than 3 cm who have a positive SLN.

APPAC trial: To compare antibiotic therapy with appendectomy in the treatment of uncomplicated acute appendicitis confirmed by computed tomography.

ARTIST trial: Capecitabine plus cisplatin versus capecitabine plus cisplatin with concurrent capecitabine radiotherapy in completely resected gastric cancer with D2 lymph node dissection.

ATLAS trial: Long-term effects of continuing adjuvant tamoxifen for 10 years versus stopping at 5 years after diagnosis of estrogen receptor-positive breast cancer.

AVOD trial: Compared intravenous fluid alone versus intravenous fluid and antibiotics in CT-confirmed uncomplicated left-sided diverticulitis.

CHINA trial: Compared the outcomes of active observation versus interval appendectomy after successful NOM of an appendix mass in children.

CLASS trial: Comparison of Laser, Surgery, and Foam sclerotherapy for treatment of varicose veins.

CLASSIC trial: Adjuvant capecitabine and oxaliplatin for gastric cancer after D2 gastrectomy.

COLOR trial: Laparoscopic versus open surgery for colon cancer.

COLOR II trial: Laparoscopic versus open surgery for rectal cancer.

COLOR III trial: Transanal TME versus laparoscopic TME for mid and low rectal cancer.

COMPETE trial: To evaluate the efficacy and safety of Peptide Receptor Radionuclide Therapy (PRRT) with 177Lu-Edotreotide compared to targeted molecular therapy with Everolimus in patients with inoperable, progressive, somatostatin receptor-positive (SSTR+), neuroendocrine tumors of gastroenteric or pancreatic origin (GEP-NET).

COOL trial: Closed or open after source control laparotomy for severe complicated intra-abdominal sepsis.

COREAN trial: Open versus laparoscopic surgery for mid or low rectal cancer after neoadjuvant chemoradiotherapy.

CRASH-2 trial: Role of tranexamic acid in the management of those with or at risk of significant bleeding after trauma.

CRISTAL trial: Effects of fluid resuscitation with colloids vs. crystalloids on mortality in critically ill patients presenting with hypovolemic shock.

CRITICS trial: Comparison between perioperative chemotherapy with preoperative chemotherapy with postoperative chemoradiotherapy in patients with resectable gastric adenocarcinoma.

CRITICS–II trial: Neoadjuvant chemotherapy followed by surgery versus neoadjuvant chemotherapy and subsequent chemoradiotherapy followed by surgery versus neo-adjuvant chemoradiotherapy followed by surgery in resectable gastric cancer.

CROSS trial: Neoadjuvant chemoradiotherapy plus surgery versus surgery alone for cancer of the esophagus or esophagogastric junction.

DIABOLO trial: Compared antibiotics versus observation in patients presenting with first episode of sigmoid diverticulitis.

ESCHAR trial: Compression therapy alone versus compression plus surgery in chronic venous ulceration.

EVRA trial: Comparison of compression therapy and early endovenous ablation versus compression therapy and deferred endovenous ablation.

HERA trial: Trastuzumab as adjuvant chemotherapy in HER2-positive early breast cancer.

IBCSG 23-01 trial: To determine necessity of ALND in patients with positive SLN.

KLASS-01 trial: Comparison between laparoscopic distal gastrectomy versus open distal gastrectomy.

KLASS-02 trial: Comparison between laparoscopic and open subtotal gastrectomy with D2 lymphadenectomy for locally advanced gastric cancer.

LOTUS trial: Randomized controlled trial comparing laparoscopic Nissen fundoplication to esomeprazole.

MAGIC trial: Perioperative chemotherapy and surgery versus surgery alone in resectable gastroesophageal cancer.

MERCURY study: Demonstrated the accuracy, feasibility, and reproducibility of magnetic resonance imaging to stage rectal cancer.

MERCURY II study: This study validated MRI low rectal plane assessment, reducing pCRM involvement, and avoiding overtreatment through selective preoperative therapy.

MINDACT trial: 70-gene signature as an aid to treatment decisions in early-stage breast cancer.

NETTER-1 trial: Comparing treatment with 177Lu-DOTA0-Tyr3-Octreotate to Octreotide LAR in patients with inoperable, progressive, somatostatin receptor-positive midgut carcinoid tumors.

NSABP B-04 trial: Compared radical mastectomy to less extensive surgery.

NSABP B-06 trial: Compared lumpectomy and ALND with or without breast irradiation with total mastectomy and ALND in tumor 4 cm or less.

NSABP B-32 trial: To determine whether SLND renders the same survival benefit and regional control that ALND does but with fewer side effects in clinically node-negative tumors.

NSABP BCPT P-1 trial: To determine whether tamoxifen administered for atleast 5 years prevented invasive breast cancer in women at increased risk.

NSABP BCP T P-2 trial: To compare tamoxifen versus raloxifene for reduction of breast cancer incidence.

PANTER trial: Randomized controlled trial comparing open necrosectomy to step-up approach in the management of infected pancreatic necrosis.

PENGUIN trial: Randomized controlled trial comparing endoscopic transgastric vs. primary necrosectomy in patients with infected necrotizing pancreatitis.

PONCHO trial: Pancreatitis of biliary origin, optimal timing of cholecystectomy.

PREVENT trial: To determine whether prophylactic placement of a polypropylene mesh decreases the incidence of parastomal hernia following permanent end-colostomy versus the traditional stoma formation without a mesh.

ProGERD study: To evaluate whether, depending on the initial presentation, non-erosive and erosive reflux disease without Barrett's esophagus will progress to more severe disease under current routine care following the resolution of the initial condition.

PROPPR trial: A pragmatic, phase 3, multisite, randomized clinical trial to determine the effectiveness and safety of transfusing patients with severe trauma and major bleeding using plasma, platelets, and red blood cells in a 1:1:1 ratio compared with a 1:1:2 ratio.

REI-EXCISE study: To evaluate the diagnostic accuracy of rapid ionization mass spectroscopy using an iKnife device for oncological margin status in breast conserving surgery.

ROLARR trial: Effect of robotic-assisted vs. conventional laparoscopic surgery on risk of conversion to open laparotomy among patients undergoing resection for rectal cancer.

TAILORx trial: Adjuvant chemotherapy guided by 21-Gene expression in hormone receptor-positive, HER2-negative, axillary node-negative breast cancer.

TOGA trial: Trastuzumab in combination with chemotherapy vs. chemotherapy alone for treatment of HER-2-positive advanced gastric or gastroesophageal junction cancer.

TOPGEAR trial: Perioperative ECF chemotherapy vs. preoperative chemoradiation for resectable gastric and esophago-gastric junction cancer.

ACOSOG ZOO11 trial: A multicenter randomized controlled trial to determine whether all patients with invasive breast cancer with positive SLN need an ALND.

IMPORTANT TERMINOLOGIES AND THEIR ABBREVIATIONS

3D-CRT : 3D Conformal Radiation Therapy
5-HT : 5-hydroxytryptamine
AAA : Abdominal Aortic Aneurysm
AACE : American Association of Clinical Endocrinologists
AAES : American Association of Endocrine Surgeons
AASLD : American Association for the Study of Liver Diseases
ABI : Ankle Brachial Index
ACC : American College of Cardiology
ACG : American College of Gastroenterology
ACR : American College of Radiology
ACS : American College of Surgeons
ADA : American Diabetes Association
ADH : Atypical Ductal Hyperplasia
ADPKD : Autosomal Dominant Polycystic Kidney Disease
AE : Alveolar Echinococcosis
AGB : Adjustable Gastric Banding
AHA : American Heart Association
AHPBA : American Hepatopancreatobiliary Association
AJCC : American Joint Committee on Cancer
ALARA : As Low As Reasonably Achievable
ALH : Atypical Lobular Hyperplasia
ALND : Axillary Lymph Node Dissection
ALPPS : Associating Liver Partition and Portal Vein Ligation for Staged Hepatectomy
AMIGO : Advanced Multimodal Image-Guided Operation suite
APA : American Pancreatic Association
APAIR : Albendazole, Percutaneous Aspiration, Injection, and Reaspiration
aPTT : Activated Partial Thromboplastin Time
ASA : American Society of Anesthesiologists
ASBO : Adhesive Small Bowel Obstruction
ASBrS : American Society of Breast Surgeons
ASCO : American Society of Clinical Oncology
ASCRS : American Society of Colon and Rectal Surgeons
ASGE : American Society for Gastrointestinal Endoscopy
ASPEN : American Society for Parenteral and Enteral Nutrition
ATA : American Thyroid Association
ATC : Acute Traumatic Coagulopathy
ATLS : Acute Trauma Life Support
AUA : American Urological Association
AVF : American Venous Forum

AWBU : Automated Whole Breast Ultrasound
BI-RADS : Breast Imaging-Reporting and Data System
BLS : British Lymphology Society
BMI : Body Mass Index
BOO : Bladder Outlet Obstruction
BPD : Biliopancreatic Diversion
BT : Bleeding Time
BTS : British Thoracic Society
BXO : Balanitis Xerotica Obliterans
CABG : Coronary Artery Bypass Grafting
CAP : College of American Pathologists
CARS : Compensatory Anti-inflammatory Response Syndrome
CBE-EMR : Complete Barrett's Eradication EMR
CCF : Congestive Cardiac Failure
CCI : Chronic Critical Illness
CDC : Centre for Disease Control and Prevention
CDH : Congenital Diaphragmatic Hernia
CE : Cystic Echinococcosis
CEDM : Contrast-enhanced Digital Mammography
CEUS : Contrast-enhanced Ultrasonography
CIKPLA : Cryptogenic Invasive *K. pneumomiae*-associated Liver Abscess
CIRCI : Critical Illness-related Corticosteroid Insufficiency
CISH : Chromogenic In Situ Hybridization
CME : Complete Mesocolic Excision
CMV : Cytomegalovirus
CNB : Core-Needle Biopsy
COX-2 : Cyclooxygenase-2
CPR : Cardiopulmonary Resuscitation
C-RADS : CT Colonography-Reporting And Data System
CRP : C Reactive Protein
CRM : Circumferential Resection Margin
CT : Clotting Time
CTA : CT Angiography
CTCAE : Common Terminology Criteria for Adverse Events
CTU : CT Urography
CTV : CT Venography
CUP : Cancers of Unknown Primary
CVP : Central Venous Pressure
DAMPs : Damage-associated Molecular Patterns

DBE : Double Balloon Enteroscopy
DCE-MRI : Dynamic Contrast Enhanced-MRI
DCIS : Ductal Carcinoma In Situ
DCR : Damage Control Resuscitation
DCS : Damage Control Surgery
DDLT : Deceased Donor Liver Transplantation
DEB-TACE : Drug-Eluting Bead-Transarterial Chemoembolization
DEXA : Dual X-ray Absorptiometry
DFS : Disease-free Survival
DIC : Disseminated Intravascular Coagulation
DPEJ : Direct Percutaneous Endoscopic Jejunostomy
DPL : Diagnostic Peritoneal Lavage
DSD : Disorders of Sexual Development
DSNB : Dynamic Sentinel Node Biopsy
DTC : Differentiated Thyroid Carcinoma
DVT : Deep Vein Thrombosis
EAES : European Association of Endoscopic Surgery
EANM : European Association of Nuclear Medicine
EASL : European Association for the Study of the Liver
EAST : Eastern Association for the Surgery of Trauma
EAU : European Association of Urology
EBV : Epstein-Barr Virus
ECCO : European Crohn's and Colitis Organization
ECF : Extracellular Fluid
ECMO : Extracorporeal Membrane Oxygenation
eFAST : Extended Focused Assessment with Sonography for Trauma
EGC : Early Gastric Cancer
EHS : European Hernia Society
EMLA : Eutectic Mixture of Local Anesthetics
EMR : Endoscopic Mucosal Resection
EMT : Epithelial–Mesenchymal Transition
ENETS : European Neuroendocrine Tumor Society
ENSAT : European Network for the Study of Adrenal Tumors
EPBD : Endoscopic Papillary Balloon Dilation
EPLBD : Endoscopic Papillary Large Balloon Dilation
EPUAP : European Pressure Ulcer Advisory Panel
ERAS : Enhanced Recovery After Surgery
ERCP : Endoscopic Retrograde Cholangiopancreatography
ERD : Erosive Reflux Disease

ERUS : Endorectal Ultrasound
ESCP : European Society of Colo-Proctology
ESD : Endoscopic Submucosal Dissection
ESE : European Society of Endocrinology
ESGAR : European Society of Gastrointestinal and Abdominal Radiology
ESGE : European Society of Gastrointestinal Endoscopy
ESMO : European Society for Medical Oncology
ESPEN : European Society for Clinical Nutrition and Metabolism
ETA : European Thyroid Association
ETGBD : Endoscopic Transpapillary Gallbladder Drainage
EUGOGO : European Group on Graves' Orbitopathy
EUS : Endoscopic Ultrasound
EUS-BD : EUS-guided Biliary Drainage
EUS-GBD : Endoscopic Ultrasound-guided Gallbladder Drainage
EUSOBI : European Society of Breast Imaging
EVTM : Endovascular Resuscitation and Trauma Management
FAST : Focused Assessment with Sonography for Trauma
FC-SEMS : Fully Covered Self-Expanding Metal Stent
FDP : Freeze-dried Plasma
FEV1 : Forced Expiratory Volume in the First Second
FFP : Fresh Frozen Plasma
FISH : Fluorescence In Situ Hybridization
FIT : Fecal immunochemical Test
FLIP : Functional Lumen Imaging Probe
FNA : Fine Needle Aspiration
FOBT : Fecal Occult Blood Testing
FUSE : Fundamental Use of Surgical Energy
GEP : Gene Expression Profiling
GRE : Glycopeptide-resistant Enterococci
GSV : Great Saphenous Vein
HAART : Highly Active Antiretroviral Therapy
HALS : Hand-assisted Laparoscopic Surgery
HBV : Hepatitis B Virus
HCV : Hepatitis C Virus
HDU : High Dependency Unit
HIDA : Hepatobiliary Iminodiacetic Acid scan
HIFU : High Intensity Focused Ultrasound
HIV : Human Immunodeficiency Virus
HPV : Human Papilloma Virus

HTLV : Human T-lymphotropic Virus
HUS : Hemolytic Uremic Syndrome
IAP : International Association of Pancreatology
IASMEN : International Association for Surgical Metabolism and Nutrition
IBTR : In-Breast Tumor Recurrence
ICG : Indocyanine Green
IDSA : Infectious Diseases Society of America
IDUS : Intraductal Ultrasonography
IGF-1 : Insulin-like Growth Factor
IGRT : Image Guided Radiation Therapy
IGT : Image Guided Therapy
IHC : Immunohistochemistry
IHD : Ischemic Heart Disease
IIONM : Intermittent Intraoperative Neural Monitoring
IL-1 : Interleukin-1
IMPT : Intensity-modulated Proton Beam Therapy
IMRT : Intensity Modulated Radiation Therapy
INR : International Normalized Ratio
IOC : Intraoperative Cholangiography
IOUS : Intraoperative Ultrasound
IPC : Intermittent Pneumatic Compression
IPMN : Intraductal Papillary Mucinous Neoplasm
IPOM : Intraperitoneal Onlay Mesh
IPSS : International Prostate Symptom Score
ISBI : International Society for Burn Injury
ISH : In Situ Hybridization
ISI : International Sensitivity Index
ISTH : International Society for Thrombosis and Hemostasis
ITP : Idiopathic Thrombocytopenic Purpura
ITU : Intensive Therapy Unit
IWGDF : International Working Group on the Diabetic Foot
KSHV : Kaposi's Sarcoma Associated Herpes Virus
LAMS : Lumen-apposing Metal Stent
LCBDE : Laparoscopic CBD Exploration
LCIS : Lobular Carcinoma In Situ
LDLT : Living Donor Liver Transplantation
LIFT : Ligation of Intersphincteric Fistula Tract
LI-RADS : Liver Imaging-Reporting and Data System
LLR : Laparoscopic Liver Resection

LMA : Laryngeal Mask Airway
LMWH : Low Molecular Weight Heparin
LPR : Laryngopharyngeal Reflux
LSC : Laparoscopic Subtotal Cholecystectomy
LSG : Laparoscopic Sleeve Gastrectomy
LUS : Laparoscopic Ultrasound
LUTS : Lower Urinary Tract Symptoms
MACE : Major Adverse Cardiovascular Events
MAFT : Minimally Invasive Anal Fistula Treatment
MBI : Molecular Breast Imaging
MDCT : Multidetector CT
MET : Metabolic Equivalent Task
MIC : Minimum Inhibitory Concentration
MMR : Mismatch Repair Gene
MODS : Multiple Organ Dysfunction Syndrome
MRA : MR Angiography
MRCP : Magnetic Resonance Cholangiopancreatography
MRE : Magnetic Resonance Elastography
MRSA : Methicillin Resistant *Staphylococcus aureus*
MRU : MR Urography
MRV : MR Venography
MSI : Microsatellite Instability
MSOF : Multiple System Organ Failure
MTC : Medullary Thyroid Carcinoma
MUSE : Medigus Ultrasonic Surgical Endostapler
NAFLD : Non-alcoholic Fatty Liver Disease
NASH : Non-alcoholic Steatohepatitis
NCCN : National Comprehensive Cancer Network
NERD : Non-erosive Reflux Disease
NGS : Next-generation Sequencing
NHTR : Nonhemolytic Transfusion Reaction
NICE : National Institute of Health and Care Excellence
NI-RADS : Neck Imaging-Reporting and Data System
NIRFC : Near-infrared Fluorescent Cholangiography
NOSES : Natural Orifice Specimen Extraction Surgery
NOTES : Natural Orifice Transluminal Endoscopic Surgery
NPUAP : National Pressure Ulcer Advisory Panel
NR-ERCP : Non-radiation ERCP
NRLN : Non-recurrent Laryngeal Nerve

NSABP : National Surgical Adjuvant Breast and Bowel Project
OGIB : Obscure Gastrointestinal Bleeding
OLT : Orthotopic Liver Transplantation
OS : Overall Survival
PACU : Postanesthetic Care Unit
PAIR : Percutaneous Aspiration, Injection, and Reaspiration
PCLD : Polycystic Liver Disease
PCR : Polymerase Chain Reaction
PCS : Postcholecystectomy Syndrome
PCSEMS : Partially Covered Self-Expandable Metal Stents
PDGF : Platelet Derived Growth Factor
PDPH : Post-dural-puncture Headache
PDT : Photodynamic Therapy
PEG : Percutaneous Endoscopic Gastrostomy
PEGJ : Jejunal Extension through a PEG
PEI : Percutaneous Ethanol Injection
PEM : Positron Emission Mammography
PET : Positron Emission Tomography
PEVAC : Percutaneous Evacuation of Cyst Content
PFS : Progression-free Survival
PICS : Persistent inflammation, Immunosuppression, and Catabolism Syndrome
PI-RADS : Prostate Imaging-Reporting and Data System
POCSL : Peroral Cholangioscopic Lithotripsy
POCUS : Point-of-care Ultrasound
POEM : Peroral Endoscopic Myotomy
PONV : Postoperative Nausea and Vomiting
PPN : Partial Parenteral Nutrition
PPPIA : Pan-Pacific Pressure Injury Alliance
PRM : Pattern Recognition Molecule
PSA : Prostate Specific Antigen
PT : Prothrombin Time
PTBD : Percutaneous Transhepatic Biliary Drainage
PTCS : Percutaneous Transhepatic Cholangioscopy
PTCSL : Percutaneous Transhepatic Cholangioscopic Lithotomy
PTFE : Polytetrafluoroethylene
PTGBD : Percutaneous Transhepatic Gallbladder Drainage
REBOA : Resuscitative Endovascular Balloon Occlusion of the Aorta
REBOVC : Resuscitative Endovascular Balloon Occlusion of the Vena Cava
RFA : Radiofrequency Ablation

RGB : Roux-en-Y Gastric Bypass
ROTEM : Rotational Thromboelastometry
RRL : Relative Radiation Level
RSI : Rapid Sequence Induction
RT : Resuscitative Thoracotomy
RT-PCR : Reverse Transcriptase Polymerase Chain Reaction
SABR : Stereotactic Ablative Radiation Therapy
SAGES : Society of American Gastrointestinal Endoscopic Surgeons
SAG-M : Saline-Adenine-Glucose Mannitol
SAMBA : Society of Ambulatory Anesthesia
SAP : Serum Amyloid Protein
SBE : Single Balloon Enteroscopy
SEMS : Self-expandable Metal Stents
SEPS : Self-expanding Plastic Stents
SILS : Single Incision Laparoscopic Surgery
SIR : Society of Interventional Radiology
SIRS : Systemic Inflammatory Response Syndrome
SLND : Sentinel Lymph Node Dissection
SNMMI : Society of Nuclear Medicine and Molecular Imaging
SNNS : Sentinel Node Navigation Surgery
SPECT : Single Photon Emission Computed Tomography
SSI : Surgical Site Infection
SSSI : Superficial Surgical Site Infection
SVS : Society for Vascular Surgery
TACE : Transarterial Chemoembolization
TACO : Transfusion-associated Circulatory Overload
TAE : Transarterial Embolization
TAP : Transversus Abdominis Plane Block
TAMIS : Transanal Minimally Invasive Surgery
TBI : Toe Brachial Index
TBI : Traumatic Brain Injury
TBSA : Total Body Surface Area
TBW : Total Body Water
TEG : Thromboelastography
TEM : Transanal Endoscopic Microsurgery
TGF-β : Transforming Growth Factor-beta
TIC : Trauma-induced Coagulopathy
TIF : Transoral Incisionless Fundoplication
TI-RADS : Thyroid Imaging-Reporting and Data System

TIVA : Total Intravenous Anesthesia
TME : Total Mesorectal Excision
TNF-α : Tumor Necrosis Factor-alpha
TOS : Thoracic Outlet Syndrome
TPN : Total Parenteral Nutrition
TRALI : Transfusion-related Acute Lung Injury
TRUS : Transrectal Ultrasound
TTP : Thrombocytopenic Purpura
TXA2 : Thromboxane A2
UGIB : Upper Gastrointestinal Bleeding
UH : Unfractionated Heparin
UOAA : United Ostomy Association of America
VAAFT : Video-assisted Anal Fistula Treatment
VAC : Vacuum Assisted Closure
VATS : Video-assisted Thoracoscopic Surgery
VBG : Vertical Banded Gastroplasty
VCE : Video Capsule Endoscopy
VEGF : Vascular Endothelial Growth Factor
vWF : von Willebrand Factor
WATS : Wide-area Transepithelial Sampling
WBCT : Whole Body CT
WHS : Wound Healing Society
WOCN : Wound Ostomy Care Nurse
WSACS : World Society of Abdominal Compartment Syndrome
WSES : World Society of Emergency Surgery

IMPORTANT CLASSIFICATIONS IN SURGERY

ASA Physical Status Classification

ASA PS classification	Definition	Adult Examples, Including, but not Limited to
ASA I	A normal healthy patient	Healthy, non-smoking, no or minimal alcohol use
ASA II	A patient with mild systemic disease	Mild diseases only without substantive functional limitations. Examples include (but not limited to): current smoker, social alcohol drinker, pregnancy, obesity (30<BMI<40), well-controlled DM/HTN, mild lung disease
ASA III	A patient with severe systemic disease	Substantive functional limitations; One or more moderate-to-severe diseases. Examples include (but not limited to): poorly controlled DM or HTN, COPD, morbid obesity (BMI ≥40), active hepatitis, alcohol dependence or abuse, implanted pacemaker, moderate reduction of ejection fraction, ESRD undergoing regularly scheduled dialysis, premature infant PCA <60 weeks, history (>3 months) of MI, CVA, TIA, or CAD/stents
ASA IV	A patient with severe systemic disease that is a constant threat to life	Examples include (but not limited to): recent (<3 months) MI, CVA, TIA, CAD/stents, ongoing cardiac ischemia or severe valve dysfunction, severe reduction of ejection fraction, sepsis, DIC, ARD or ESRD not undergoing regularly scheduled dialysis
ASA V	A moribund patient who is not expected to survive without the operation	Examples include (but not limited to): ruptured abdominal/thoracic aneurysm, massive trauma, intracranial bleed with mass effect, ischemic bowel in the face of significant cardiac pathology or multiple organ/system dysfunction
ASA VI	A declared brain-dead patient whose organs are being removed for donor purposes	

The addition of "E" denotes emergency surgery.

Bailey classification: Classification for second branchial cleft cyst.
Type I (Most superficial): Lies along the anterior surface of the sternocleidomastoid muscle, just deep to the platysma muscle;
Type II (Most common): Along the anterior surface of the sternocleidomastoid muscle, lateral to the carotid space, and posterior to the submandibular gland;
Type III: Extends medially between the bifurcation of the internal and external carotid arteries to the lateral pharyngeal wall;
Type IV: Lies in the pharyngeal mucosal space.

Baker classification (Revised): Classification of capsular contracture after prosthetic breast reconstruction.
IA: Augmented or reconstructed breast which appeared absolutely natural
IB: Soft, palpable implant on examination
II: Mildly firm reconstructed breast, implant may be visible and detectable by physical examination
III: Moderately firm reconstructed breast, implant is readily detectable
IV: Severe contracture with an unacceptable aesthetic outcome and/or significant patient symptom requiring surgical intervention.

Bismuth-Corlette classification: Details in Chapter 4 of Gallbladder and Biliary System.

Bosniak classification: A classification system for cystic lesions of the kidneys based on contrast-enhanced CT findings and categorized into—I, I, II-F, III, IV.

CEAP classification: Details in Chapter 18 of Arterial Diseases, Venous Diseases and Diseases of Lymphatics.

Cernea classification: Details in Chapter 14 of Thyroid.

Chicago Classification

This classification system is used to diagnose esophageal motility disorders based on manometric findings. This system has four major categories based on LES relaxation and motility of esophageal body: (i) Incomplete LES relaxation (achalasia or esophagogastric junction outflow obstruction); (ii) Major motility disorders (absent contractility, distal esophageal spasm, and hypercontractile or Jackhammer esophagus); (iii) Minor motility disorders (ineffective esophageal motility or fragmented peristalsis); and (iv) Normal esophageal motility.

Clavien-Dindo Classification

Classification of surgical complications.

Grade	Definition
I	• Any deviation from the normal postoperative course without the need for pharmacological treatment or surgical, endoscopic, and radiological interventions • Allowed therapeutic regimens are drugs as antiemetics, antipyretics, analgesics, diuretics, electrolytes, and physiotherapy. This grade also includes wound infections opened at bedside
II	• Requiring pharmacological treatment with drugs other than such allowed for grade I complications. • Blood transfusions and total parenteral nutrition are also included
III IIIa IIIb	• Requiring surgical, endoscopic, or radiological intervention • Intervention not under general anesthesia • Intervention under general anesthesia
IV Iva IVb	• Life-threatening complication (including CNS complications) requiring IC/ICU management • Single organ dysfunction (including dialysis) • Multiorgan dysfunction
V	Death of a patient

Suffix "d" If the patient suffers from a complication at the time of discharge, the suffix "d" (for "disability") is added to the respective grade of complication. This label indicates the need for a follow-up to fully evaluate the complication.

Couinaud classification: Details in the Chapter 5 of Liver.

DeBakey classification: Details in the Chapter 18 of Diseases of Arteries, Venous Diseases and Diseases of Lymphatics.

EHS classification: Details in the Chapter 19 of Hernia.

Fitzpatrick classification (Skin type and sunburn sensitivity):
Type I: Always burn, never tan
Type II: Always burn, sometimes tan
Type III: Sometimes burn, sometimes tan
Type IV: Sometimes burn, always tan
Type V: Never burn, sometimes tan
Type VI: Never burn, always tan

Forrest classification: Details in the Chapter 9 of Stomach and Duodenum

Gharbi classification: Details in the Chapter 5 of Liver.

Goldman classification: A widely accepted classification system for urethral injury.

Injury type	Injury description	Urethrographic appearance
I	Stretching or elongation of otherwise intact posterior urethra	Intact but stretched urethra
II	Urethral disruption above the urogenital diaphragm while the membranous segment remains intact	Contrast agent extravasation above the urogenital diaphragm only
III	Disruption of the membranous urethra, extending below the urogenital diaphragm and involving the anterior urethra	Contrast agent extravasation below the urogenital diaphragm, possibly extending to the pelvis or perineum; intact bladder neck
IV	Bladder neck injury extending into the proximal urethra	Extraperitoneal contrast agent extravasation; bladder neck disruption
Iva	Bladder base injury simulating a type IV injury	Periurethral contrast agent extravasation; bladder base disruption
V	Isolated anterior urethral injury	Contrast agent extravasation below the urogenital diaphragm, confined to the anterior urethra.

Hamburg classification: A classification system of vascular anomalies.

Hinchey classification: A classification system for perforated diverticulitis.

Hinchey classification	Modified Hinchey classification (by Sher et al.)
I Pericolic abscess or phlegmon	I Pericolic abscess
II Pelvic, intra-abdominal, or retroperitoneal abscess	IIa Distant abscess amenable to percutaneous drainage IIb Complex abscess associated with fistula
III Generalized purulent peritonitis	III Generalized purulent peritonitis
Iv Generalized fecal peritonitis	IV Fecal peritonitis

Inoue classification or Intrapapillary capillary loop (IPCL) classification: For assessment of depth of invasion using narrow band imaging and magnification.

Kajava classification: Classification of polymastia.
Class I: Consists of a complete breast including glandular tissue, nipple, and areola
Class II: Consists of only glandular tissue and nipple, without areola.
Class III: Consists of only glandular tissue and areola, without nipple.
Class IV: Consists of only glandular tissue.
Class V (pseudomamma): Consists of only nipple and areola, without glandular tissue.
Class VI (polythelia): Consists of only the nipple.
Class VII (polythelia areolaris): Consists of only the areola.
Class VIII (polythelia pilosa): Consists of only hair.

Kasai classification: Classification of biliary atresia.
Type I: Obliteration of common bile duct (patent cystic and common hepatic duct)
Type IIa: Obliteration of common hepatic duct (patent cystic and common bile duct), sometimes with a cyst at hilum
Type IIb: Obliteration of common hepatic duct, cystic and common bile duct.
Type III: Obliteration of left and right main hepatic ducts at the level of porta hepatis

Komi classification: Classification of anomalous union of the pancreaticobilio ducts (AUPBD).
Type I: Union of the ducts at a right angle to each other
Type Ia: Without dilatation or
Type Ib: With dilatation of the common channel
Type II: Union of the ducts with an acute angle between them
Type IIa: Without dilatation or
Type IIb: With dilatation of the common channel

Type III: Comprises of complex patterns of accessory pancreatic ducts, with or without intricate duct networks
Type IIIa: Is similar to the classic pancreas divisum with biliary dilatation
Type IIIb: Characterized by the absence of the Wirsung's duct
Type IIIc:
Type IIIc1: Tiny communication exists between the main duct and the accessory ducts
Type IIIc2: Comprises of a common channel made up of common and accessory ducts of equal caliber
Type IIIc3: Total or partial dilatation of the ductal system.

Kyoto classification: This classification organizes endoscopic findings related to *H. pylori* infection. The score of this classification is the sum of the scores of five endoscopic findings (atrophy, intestinal metaplasia, enlarged folds, nodularity, and diffuse redness with or without regular arrangement of collecting venules). The score ranges from 0 to 8. A score of 0 indicates no *H. pylori* infection. Score of 2 or more indicates *H. pylori* infection. Score of 4 or more might indicate gastric cancer risk.

Le-Fort classification: Classification system of midface fracture based on the direction of fractures.
Type 1 (horizontal): Transverse fracture through the maxillary sinuses, lower nasal septum, pterygoid plates
Type 2 (pyramidal): Oblique fracture crossing zygomaticomaxillary suture, inferior orbital rim, nasal bridge
Type 3 (craniofacial dissociation): Fracture above the zygomatic arch, through the lateral and medial orbital walls and nasofrontal suture.

Los Angeles classification of Esophagitis (Based on Endoscopic Assessment of Reflux Esophagitis)
Grade A: One (or more) mucosal break no longer than 5 mm that does not extend between the tops of two mucosal folds.
Grade B: One (or more) mucosal break more than 5 mm long that does not extend between the tops of two mucosal folds.
Grade C: One (or more) mucosal break that is continuous between the tops of two or more mucosal folds but which involve less than 75% of the circumference.
Grade D: One (or more) mucosal break which involves at least 75% of the esophageal circumference.

Michel's classification: This classification described the hepatic arterial anatomy and its variations, identified 10 types of anatomical variations (Type I to X).

Modified Milwaukee classification: This classification system is used to classify biliary sphincter of oddi dysfunction (SOD).

Type I: Biliary-type pain, elevated serum liver enzymes more than 1.1 times the upper limit of normal, bile duct dilation more than 9 mm.
Type II: Biliary-type pain and either elevated liver enzyme levels or dilated bile duct.
Type III: Biliary-type pain only.

Modified Johnson classification: Classification system of gastric ulcer based on anatomic location and acid secretion. Details in Chapter 9 of stomach.

Neimeier classification: Classification for gallbladder perforation

Type I	Acute free perforation into the peritoneal cavity
Type II	Subacute-localized perforation with pericholecystic abscess
Type III	Chronic perforation, with cholecystoenteric fistulas

OLGA (Operative Link for Gastritis Assessment) staging system: This staging system includes topography and extent of atrophy in gastritis.

PNM classification: Classification system for human alveolar echinococcosis. 'P' for parasitic mass (PX, P0, P1, P2, P3, P4); 'N' for involvement of neighboring organs (NX, N0, N1); 'M' for metastasis (MX, M0, M1).

Refined Hurley classification: This is the modified Hurley classification to classify the severity of hidradenitis suppurativa, subdividing stage I and II of original Hurley classification into stages A (mild), B (moderate) and C (severe), based on extent of disease and degree of inflammation.

IA: Without sinus tracts, ≤2 body areas and <5 abscesses and nodules; IB: Without sinus tracts, >2 body areas or ≥5 abscesses/nodules, fixed lesions; IC: Without sinus tracts, >2 body areas or ≥5 abscesses/nodules, migratory lesions.

IIA: With sinus tracts, no inflammation; IIB: With sinus tracts, presence of inflammation, ≤2 body areas; IIC: Presence of sinus tracts, presence of inflammation, >2 body areas.

III: ≥1% body surface area of a body site with interconnected inflammatory sinus tracts.

Regnault classification: It is the classification system of breast ptosis based on the position of nipple-areola complex relative to the inframammary crease.
Grade I: Nipple is at or up to 1 cm below the inframammary crease
Grade II: Nipple at a level 1 to 3 cm below the crease
Grade III: Nipple more than 3 cm below the crease or at the inferior pole of the breast.

Revised Atlanta classification of acute pancreatitis: Details in the Chapter 6 of Pancreatitis.
Sarin's classification: Classification of gastric varices based on location of varices as well as its relationship with esophageal varices. Details in the Chapter 9 of Stomach.
Savary-Miller classification
Siewert-Stein classification

Stanford classification: Details in the Chapter 18 of Arterial Diseases.
Strasberg classification: Details in the Chapter 4 of Gallbladder and Biliary System.

Timing of Acute Care Surgery (TACS) Classification

Timing- iTTS from diagnosis	Possible clinical scenarios	Color code	Note
Immediate surgery	Bleeding emergencies		Immediate life-saving surgical intervention, resuscitative laparotomy
Within an hour	Incarcerated hernia, perforated viscus, diffuse peritonitis, soft tissue infection accompanied with sepsis		Surgical intervention as soon as possible but only after resuscitation (within 1 to 2 hours)—administration of antibiotics upon diagnosis-no delay.
Within 6 hours	Soft tissue infection (abscess) not associated with sepsis		Administration of antibiotics upon diagnosis—no delay
Within 12 hours	Appendicitis (local peritonitis), cholecystitis (optional)		Administration of antibiotics upon diagnosis—no delay
Within 24 or 48 hours	Second-look laparostomy		Schedule in advance. Intervention should occur at day time

[iTTS: Ideal Time To Surgery]

Terblanche classification: This clinical classification is the most useful classification for assessment of long-term outcomes of surgical bile duct repair.

Grade	Result	
I	Excellent	No biliary symptoms with normal liver function
II	Good	Transitory symptoms, currently no symptoms and normal liver function
III	Fair	Clearly related symptoms requiring medical therapy and/or deterioting liver function
IV	Poor	Recurrent stricture requiring correction, or related death

Todani modification of Alonso-Lej classification: Details in the Chapter 4 of Gallbladder and Biliary System.

IMPORTANT CRITERIA

Amsterdam criteria II: Clinical criteria for diagnosis of Lynch syndrome, previously known as hereditary non-polyposis colorectal cancer (HNPCC)

There should be at least three relatives with an HNPCC-associated cancer (cancer of the colorectum, endometrium, small bowel, ureter, or renal pelvis) and:

- One should be first-degree relative to the other two;
- At least two successive generations should be affected;
- At least one should be diagnosed before age 50;
- Familial adenomatous polyposis should be excluded;
- Tumors should be verified by pathological examination.

Revised Bethesda criteria: For testing microsatellite instability (MSI) in colorectal tumors
Tumors from individuals should be tested for MSI in the following situations:

- Colorectal cancer diagnosed in a patient who is less than 50 years of age.
- Presence of synchronous, metachronous colorectal, or other Lynch syndrome-associated tumors, regardless of age.
- Colorectal cancer with a Microsatellite instability-high (MSI-H) histology (i.e., presence of tumor infiltrating lymphocytes, Crohn's-like lymphocytic reaction, mucinous/signet-ring differentiation, medullary growth pattern) diagnosed in a patient who is less than 60 years of age.
- Colorectal cancer diagnosed in one or more first-degree relatives with a Lynch syndrome-related tumor, with one of the cancers being diagnosed under the age 50 years.
- Colorectal cancer diagnosed in two or more first-degree relatives with Lynch syndrome-related tumors, regardless of age.

Choi response criteria: A tumor response criteria following targeted therapy in GIST.

Complete response: Disappearance of all target lesions

Partial response: ≥10% decrease in tumor size or ≥15% decrease in tumor attenuation at computed tomography; no new lesions.

Progressive disease: ≥10% increase in SLD of lesions; does not meet the criteria for partial response by virtue of tumor attenuation, new intramural nodules, or an increase in the size of existing intramural nodules.

Stable disease: None of the above.

The expanded Denver screening criteria: Expanded Denver criteria is used to determine indication of CT angiography to detect blunt cerebrovascular injury (BCVI) in trauma patients. CT angiography is indicated if any one or more of the criteria are present.

- Signs/symptoms of BCVI
- Arterial hemorrhage from neck/nose/mouth
- Cervical bruit in patients <50 years
- Expanding cervical hematoma
- Focal neurological deficit
- Neurological examination incongruous with head CT findings
- Stroke on secondary CT scan
- Risk factors for BCVI

(*High-energy transfer mechanism with*):

- Le Fort II or III
- Mandible fracture
- Complex skull fracture/basilar skull fracture/occipital condyle fracture
- Severe traumatic brain injury (TBI) with GCS <6

- Cervical spine fracture, subluxation or ligamentous injury at any level
- Near hanging with anoxic brain injury
- Seatbelt abrasion with significant swelling, pain or altered mental status
- TBI with thoracic injury
- Scalp degloving
- Thoracic vascular injury
- Blunt cardiac rupture
- Upper rib fracture

Milan criteria: This criterion is used for patients with hepatocellular carcinoma considered for orthotopic liver transplantation. This criterion identifies patients most likely to benefit from transplantation. *Criteria includes:* (i) Single tumor diameter less than 5 cm; (ii) Not more than three foci of tumor, each one not exceeding 3 cm; (iii) No extrahepatic involvement; and (iv) No major vessel involvement.

mRECIST criteria: Modified RECIST criteria is used for hepatocellular carcinoma.

Complete response: Disappearance of arterial phase enhancement in all target lesions.

Partial response: >30% decrease in SLD of "viable" target lesion (arterial phase enhancement)

Progressive disease: >20% increase in SLD of "viable" target lesion (arterial phase enhancement)

Stable disease: None of the above.

New Orleans criteria (NOC): Computed tomography is indicated in minor head injury with any one of the following findings. These criteria should be applied in patients who also have GCS15. **H**eadache, **E**mesis, **A**ge over 60, **D**rug or alcohol intoxication, **C**onvulsion, **T**rauma visible above the clavicles, **S**hort-term memory deficits (mnemonic 'HEAD CT').

NEXUS (National Emergency X-ray Radiography Utilization Study) criteria: This criterion is used to decide which trauma patients do not require cervical spine imaging. Criteria includes: (i) Focal neurologic deficit; (ii) Midline spinal tenderness; (iii) Altered level of consciousness; (iv) Intoxication; and (v) Distraction injury. If none of the above criteria are present, no imaging is required.

PECARN (Pediatric Emergency Care Applied Research Network) algorithm: This clinical decision tool identifies children at very low risk of clinically important traumatic brain injury (ci-TBI) and guides to take decision about CT brain.

<2-year-old
Any one of the following?
(i) GCS ≤14; (ii) Altered mental status; and (iii) Palpable skull fracture.

Then, a non-contrast CT brain (4.4% risk of ci-TBI).

One or more of the following?
(i) Non-frontal scalp hematoma; (ii) Loss of consciousness ≥5 seconds; (iii) Severe injury mechanism (pedestrian or bicyclist without helmet struck by motorized vehicle, fall >1 meter or 3 feet, head struck by high-impact object); and (iv) Abnormal activity per parents.

Then, consider a non-contrast CT brain or Observation (0.9% risk of ci-TBI).

≥2 years-18 years
Any one of the following?
(i) GCS ≤14; (ii) Altered mental status; and (iii) Signs of a basilar skull fracture.
Then, obtain a non-contrast CT brain (4.3% risk of ci-TBI).

One or more of the following?
(i) History of vomiting; (ii) Loss of consciousness; (iii) Severe injury mechanism (Pedestrian or bicyclist without helmet struck by motorized vehicle, fall >2 meter or 5 feet, head struck by high-impact object); and (iv) Severe headache
Then, consider a non-contrast CT brain or observation (0.9% risk of ci-TBI).

RECIST (Response Evaluation Criteria in Solid Tumors) Criteria
Most widely used criteria used for reporting tumor clinical response to neoadjuvant systemic therapy.

Four RECIST criteria are described:
1. Complete response (lesion not detectable)
2. Partial response (≥30% reduction in maximal lesion diameter)
3. Stable disease (<30% reduction in maximal lesion diameter)
4. Progressive disease (≥20% increase in the maximal lesion diameter)

RECIST categories are also divided into **Clinical response** (based on physical examination) and **Pathological response** (based on histological resection following surgical resection). Clinical response is denoted by "c" and Pathological response is denoted by "p".

Roizen criteria—to assess the efficacy of adequate preoperative alpha-blockade and includes:
1. No in-hospital blood pressure >160/90 mm Hg 24 hour prior to surgery
2. No orthostatic hypotension with blood pressure <80/45 mm Hg
3. No ST or T-wave changes for 1 week prior to surgery
4. No more than 5 premature ventricular contraction per minute.

Rome IV criteria: Defines Irritable bowel syndrome diagnostic criteria. Recurrent abdominal pain on average atleast 1 day/week in the last 3 months, associated with two or more of the following criteria:
1. Related to defecation
2. Associated with a change in the frequency of stool
3. Associated with a change in the form (appearance) of stool.

These criteria should be fulfilled for the last 3 months with symptom onset atleast 6 months prior to diagnosis.

Wells criteria: This scoring system stratifies patients for pulmonary embolism and provides a pre-test probability. Based on the score, physicians can decide what further testing is required (d-dimer or CT angiography). *Interpretation: 0-1: Low risk*—Pulmonary embolism rule-out criteria (PERC) can be considered as well as d-dimer; *2-6: Moderate risk*—Consider d-dimer or CT pulmonary angiography; *High risk:* d-dimer not recommended. *≤4:* Unlikely - consider d-dimer; *≥4.5:* Likely - Consider CT pulmonary angiography; >6: *High risk.*

Criteria	Score
Clinical signs and symptoms of DVT	3
An alternative diagnosis is less likely than PE	3
Heart rate more than 100	1.5
Immobilization for three or more consecutive days or surgery in the previous 4 weeks	1.5
Previous objectively diagnosed PE or DVT	1.5
Hemoptysis	1
Malignancy (on treatment, treatment in last 6 months or palliative)	1

Wells criteria for deep vein thrombosis: A scoring system for prediction of deep vein thrombosis. *-2 to 0:* Low probability; *1-2 points:* Moderate probability; *3-8 points:* High probability

Clinical characteristic	Score
Active cancer (patient either receiving treatment for cancer within the previous 6 months or currently receiving palliative treatment)	1
Paralysis, paresis, or recent cast immobilization of the lower extremities	1
Recently bedridden for ≥3 days, or major surgery within the previous 12 weeks requiring general or regional anesthesia	1
Localized tenderness along the deep venous system	1
Entire leg swelling	1
Calf swelling at least 3 cm larger than that on the asymptomatic side (measured 10 cm below tibial tuberosity)	1
Pitting edema confined to the symptomatic leg	1
Collateral superficial veins (non-varicose)	1
Previously documented deep vein thrombosis	1
Alternative diagnosis at least as likely as deep vein thrombosis	-2

IWATE criteria are used to predict the difficulty of laparoscopic liver resection from preoperative variables. The preoperative variables are tumor location (Couinaud segment), tumor size, proximity to major vessels, extent of liver resection, associated HAL/Hybrid and liver function. The grading of the operative difficulties is low, intermediate, advanced, or expert.

SCORING SYSTEMS IN SURGERY

4Ts score: It is a pretest scoring system for heparin-induced thrombocytopenia. It includes: (i) Magnitude of thrombocytopenia; (ii) Timing of platelet count fall; (iii) Thrombosis or other sequelae of HIT; and (iv) Other causes of thrombocytopenia. The score ranges between 0 to 8. Score 0–3, 4–5 and 6–8 classified as low, intermediate, and high probability of HIT, respectively.

AAST injury scoring: AAST (American Association for the Surgery of Trauma) injury scoring is the most commonly used system of grading injuries. This scoring system guides the management and aids in prognosis. Still, 32 different AAST injury scales are present.

ABC score: This score predicts need for massive transfusion in trauma patients. It includes: (i) Presence or absence of a penetrating wound; (ii) Systolic blood pressure (≥90 mm Hg/<90 mm Hg); (iii) Heart rate (<120 bpm/>120 bpm); and (iv) FAST (positive/negative). The score ranges from 0–4. Score 0–1 are less likely to require massive transfusion (>10 packed red blood cells), score 2–4 are more likely to require massive transfusion. This score has a positive predictive value of 50–55% and a negative predictive value of less than 5%. This score is better at identifying who will not need massive transfusion.

AIMS65 scoring: This scoring system is to predict in-hospital mortality from upper GI bleeding. The score includes following components: (i) Albumin <3.0 g/dL; (ii) INR >1.5; (iii) Systolic blood pressure ≤90 mm Hg; (iv) Age >65 years. If more than two components are present, risk of mortality is high.

Alvarado score: Details in the Chapter 11 of Appendix.

APACHE scoring: The APACHE (Acute Physiology and Chronic Health Evaluation) score is to evaluate critically ill patients. Original APACHE score was first used in 1981, included 34 individual variables and a chronic health evaluation.

The APACHE II scoring system was released in 1985. It is measured during the first 24 hour of ICU admission. It includes 12 physiological variables and 2 disease-related variables. The score ranges from 0 to 71 points.

The APACHE III released in 1991. The weighting of variables is more complex than the previous two versions. The APACHE IV was introduced in 2006. It includes 17 physiological variables. It is used to assess severity of illness and prognosis of ICU patients.

The APACHE II is most commonly used among all versions.

Appendicitis Inflammatory Response (AIR) Score

Findings	Score
Vomiting	1
Pain in RLQ	1
Rebound tenderness: • Light • Medium • Strong	 1 2 3
Body temperature >38.5°C	1
Polymorphonuclear leukocytes: • 70-84% • ≥85%	 1 2
WBC count: • 10.0–4.9 × 10^9/L • ≥15.0 × 10^9/L	 1 2
CRP concentration: • 10–49 g/L • ≥50 g/L	 1 2
Total score	12

Score 0–4: Low probability; *Score 5–8:* Indeterminate group; *Score 9–12:* High probability

Apfel score: This scoring system is used to predict postoperative nausea and vomiting. It includes four variables (female sex, history of motion sickness or postoperative nausea and vomiting, nonsmoker, postoperative opioid treatment is planned) and assigns one point for each. Score ranges from 0–4. If the score is 0, the probability is 10% whereas if score is 4, the probability is 78%.

Balthazar scoring: Details in the Chapter 6 of Pancreas.

Baux score: This score is for predicting mortality in burn patients. The score is calculated as: [TBSA + Age of the patient]. Score over 140 considered as being unsurvivable.

BISAP (Bedside Index for Severity in Acute Pancreatitis) score: This scoring system is used for predicting mortality and severity in acute pancreatitis. This score includes five variables: (i) Blood urea nitrogen level >25 mg/dL; (ii) Impaired mental status; (iii) Development of SIRS; (iv) Age >60 years; and (v) Presence of pleural effusion. Data should be taken from the first 24 hours of the patient admission. Score ranges from 0-5. BISAP score ≥3 seemed to be reliable to identify high-risk patients.

Boey score: This scoring system is for predicting morbidity and mortality in perforated peptic ulcer. It includes: (i) Concomitant medical illness; (ii) Preoperative shock (systolic BP <90 mm Hg); (iii) Duration of perforation >24 hours. Score ranges from 0–3 (Each factor scores 1 point if positive).

Boston Bowel Preparation Scale (BBPS): This scoring system is used for rating the bowel preparation quality during colonoscopy. A four-point scoring system depending on the degree of colon cleanliness is applied to each of the three broad regions of the colon: the right colon (including the cecum and ascending colon), the transverse colon (including the hepatic flexure and splenic flexure) and the left colon (including the descending colon, sigmoid colon and rectum). Total BBPS score ranges from 0–9.

Bristol Stool Form Scale (BSFS): BSFS was developed in the Bristol Royal Infirmary in England. Seven types of stools are described:

Type 1: Separate hard lumps, like nuts (hard to pass)
Type 2: Sausage-shaped, but lumpy
Type 3: Like a sausage but with cracks on its surface
Type 4: Like a sausage or snake, smooth, and soft
Type 5: Soft blobs with clear cut edges (passed easily)
Type 6: Fluffy pieces with ragged edges, a mushy stool
Type 7: Watery, no solid pieces, entirely liquid.

Caprini score (1991): It is a risk assessment model to determine risk of venous thromboembolism in postsurgical patients and provides validated recommendations for prophylaxis and includes 20 variables. According to the weightage of risk factor, variables are assigned different points and summation of all points constitute the score. According to the score range, risk levels are categorized into: Low risk (score 0–1); Moderate risk (score 2); High risk (score 3–40; Highest risk (5 or more).

Caprini RAM 2013 version: It includes additional risk factors include: BMI >40, Smoking, Diabetes requiring insulin, Chemotherapy, Blood transfusions, Human immunodeficiency virus infection, Length of surgery greater than 2 hours.

Child-Pugh score: Details in Chapter 5 of Liver.

CT Severity Index (CTSI): Details in Chapter 6 of Pancreas.

DeMeester score: Scoring system to categorize GERD according to severity. Details in Chapter 21 of 'Esophagus'.

Eckardt Symptom Score (ESS): It is a 4-item self-report scoring system that includes: (i) Weight loss (in kg); (ii) Chest pain; (iii) Regurgitation; and (iv) Dysphagia, for measuring achalasia symptom severity. Each item is graded on a score of 0–3, with maximum score of 12. Score ≥3 is suggestive of active achalasia.

Fournier's Gangrene Severity Index (FGSI): This scoring system is for predicting outcome in patients with Fournier gangrene. It includes following variables at admission: (i) Temperature; (ii) Heart rate; (iii) Respiration rate; (iv) Serum sodium, potassium; (v) Serum creatinine; (vi) Leukocyte count; (vii) Hematocrit; (viii) Serum bicarbonate. FGSI score >9 is sensitive and specific mortality predictor in patients with Fournier's gangrene.

Full Rockall score: This scoring system is to predict mortality from upper GI bleeding. It includes following variables: (i) Age; (ii) Pulse; (iii) Systolic blood pressure; (iv) Comorbidities; (v) Endoscopic diagnosis; and (vi) Endoscopic stigmata of hemorrhage. Score 4–5 have significantly higher mortality and score ≤2 is associated with very low chance of mortality.

General Surgery Acute Kidney Injury Risk Index: This scoring system is to stratify patients at risk of acute kidney injury related morbidity and mortality in non-cardiac surgeries. It includes nine preoperative risk factors: Age ≥56 years, Male sex, Active congestive heart failure, Ascites, Hypertension, Emergency surgery, Intraperitoneal surgery, Renal insufficiency—mild or moderate (serum creatinine value >1.2 mg/dL), Diabetes mellitus—oral or insulin therapy. Patients are stratified into classes according to presence of risk factors: Class I (0–2 risk factors), Class II (3 risk factors), Class III (4 risk factors), Class IV (5 risk factors), and Class V (6 or more risk factors).

Glasgow Blatchford bleeding score: This scoring system is for risk stratification, to predict the need for endoscopy and surgery in upper GI hemorrhage. The scoring includes: Systolic blood pressure (mm Hg), Blood urea-nitrogen (mmol/L), Hemoglobin for men (g/dL), Hemoglobin for women (g/dL), Pulse, Meleana, Syncope, Hepatic disease and Cardiac failure. Score 0–1 denotes "low risk", indicates no need for in-patient treatment and endoscopy.

Glasgow Coma Scale (GCS) [Recommended for age ≥4] Details in Chapter 16 of Trauma.

Glasgow Coma Scale (GCS): For Children (Age <4)

	Best motor	Best verbal	Best eye opening
6	Obeys		
5	Localizes	• Smiles, oriented to sound, follows objects, interacts • Crying interaction	
4	Withdraws	Consolable inappropriate	Spontaneously
3	Flexes	• Inconsistently consolable • Moaning	To speech
2	Extends	Inconsolable Restless	To pain
1	None	None	None

Glasgow Outcome Scale (GOS): This system assess outcome in patients after brain injury.

- Dead
- Persistent vegetative state
- Severe disability (Conscious but disabled)
- Moderated disability (Disabled but independent)
- Recovery

Glasgow Outcome Scale-Extended (GOS-E)

- Dead
- Vegetative state
- Low severe disability
- Upper severe disability
- Low moderate disability
- Upper moderate disability
- Low good recovery
- Upper good recovery

Gleason score: A grading system of prostate cancer based on patterns of tumor cells in prostate biopsy specimens. The score of most predominant pattern and the second predominant pattern are added. Score 6 is low grade, score 7 is intermediate grade, and score of 8–10 is high-grade cancer.

Injury Severity Score (ISS): An anatomical scoring system for trauma patients and is based on the Abbreviated Injury Scale (AIS). The ISS is calculated as the sum of the squares of the highest AIS code in each of the three most severely injured ISS body regions (Head or neck, Face, Chest, Abdominal or pelvic contents, Extremities or pelvic girdle, External). ISS score ranges from 1–75.

International Prostate Symptom Score (IPSS): This scoring system is used to measure the severity of lower urinary tract symptoms (LUTS) and is based on answers to seven questions concerning urinary symptoms (Incomplete emptying, Frequency, Intermittency, Urgency, Weak stream, Straining, Nocturia). Each question is assigned points from 0 to 5. The total score therefore ranges from 0–35. Score 0–7: mildly symptomatic; 8–19: moderately symptomatic and 20–35: severely symptomatic.

Izbicki scoring system for appendicitis: A scoring system for diagnosis of acute appendicitis, is based on 7 items (gender, leukocyte count, guarding, rebound pain, migration of pain, duration of pain, type of pain).

Izbicki pain score: A validated pain scoring system for chronic pancreatitis. It includes four questions: (i) Frequency of pain; (ii) Pain intensity (VAS score); (iii) Use of analgesics; and (iv) Disease-related inability to work. Score ranges from 0-100, where score 0 denotes no pain and sore 100 denotes excruciating pain.

Kaiser score: It is an evidence-based scoring system to distinguish benign from malignant lesions in breast MRI. It incorporates five BIRADS descriptors (spiculations, MRI enhancement curves, margins, internal enhancement patterns, edema). Score ranges from 1 (minimum) to 11 (maximum). Lesion with score >4 should be biopsied.

Karnofsky score: Karnofsky performance scale (KPS) is used to quantify performance status of a patient. It ranges from 0–100 (0, 10, 20, ...,100), where score 100 denotes normal functional status and score 0 denotes death.

Koivuranta score: This scoring system is used to predict postoperative nausea and vomiting. It includes five variables (duration of surgery >60 minutes, female sex, history of motion sickness, history of postoperative nausea and vomiting, nonsmoker) and assigns one point for each. Score ranges from 0–5.

Lansky score: Scoring system in cancer patients of less than 16 years to determine performance status. It is a parent-rated instrument. Score ranges from 10–100.

Lee index: It is a modification of the original Goldman cardiac risk index. It is used to estimate the cardiac risk in non-cardiac surgery. It includes six independent clinical determinants of major perioperative cardiac events: History of ischemic heart disease, History of cerebrovascular disease, History of congestive heart failure, Preoperative insulin treatment for diabetes mellitus, serum creatinine >2 mg/dL or 177 µmol/L, High-risk surgery. All determinants contribute 1 point. *0 point:* 3.9% risk; *1 point:* 0.9% risk; *2 points:* 7% risk; *3 points:* 11% risk; and *4–6 points:* 15% risk.

LRINEC (Laboratory Risk Indicator for Necrotizing Fasciitis): A clinical decision tool used for distinguishing necrotizing fasciitis from other soft tissue infections. It includes: (i) White blood cell count; (ii) Hemoglobin; (iii) Serum sodium; (iv) Blood glucose; (v) Serum creatinine; and (vi) C-reactive protein. Score ranges from 0–13. A score of 6 or more is suspicious for necrotizing fasciitis and score of 8 or more is strongly predictive of necrotizing fasciitis.

Manchester scoring system: A risk prediction model to assess the probability that an individual carries a BRCA mutation.

Modified Marshall scoring system: This scoring system is used to evaluate organ failure in the setting of acute pancreatitis. A score of 2 or more over a period of more than 48 hours for any one of the three organ systems (Respiratory, Renal, Cardiovascular) is defined as persistent organ failure, if it is present for less than 48 hours, is known as transient organ failure.

Oakland score: Scoring system specifically designed for lower gastrointestinal bleeding (LGIB) to classify stable bleeds (shock index <1) as major or minor. This scoring system comprises seven variables: (i) Age; (ii) Gender; (iii) Previous hospital admission with LGIB; (iv) Digital rectal examination findings; (v) Heart rate; (vi) Systolic blood pressure; and (vii) Hemoglobin. A patient with score 8 or less (minor bleed), can be discharged from the emergency department with OPD follow-up. A patient with score >8 (major bleed), is likely to benefit from hospital admission.

Ogilvie dysphagia score: *Score 0:* No dysphagia: able to eat normal diet; *Score 1:* Moderate passage: able to eat some solid foods; *Score 2:* Poor passage: able to eat semi-solid foods; *Score 3:* Very poor passage: able to swallow liquids only; and *Score 4:* No passage: unable to swallow anything.

Park's incontinence scale: I: Patients continent for solid and liquid stool and for flatus; II: Patients continent for solid and liquid stool, but incontinent for flatus (with or without urgency); III: Patients continent for solid stool, but incontinent for liquid stool or flatus; and IV: Patients incontinent for formed stool.

Pediatric Appendicitis Score (PAS): Details in the Chapter 11 of Appendix.

Pittsburgh Perforation Severity Score (PSS): A scoring system based on 10 clinical and radiological variables for decision making in patients with esophageal perforation: [Age >75 years; Pulse >100 bpm; Leukocytosis >10000 WBC/mL; Pleural effusion (on CXR, CT, or barium swallow)—Point 1 each; Fever >38.5°C; Noncontained leak (on barium swallow or CT); Respiratory compromise (respiratory rate >30, increasing oxygen requirement or need of mechanical ventilation); Time to diagnosis >24 hours—Point 2 each; Presence of cancer; Hypotension—Point 3 each]. To held decision making in esophageal perforation. Patients with score ≤2 are potential candidates for nonoperative management.

POSSUM (Physiological and Operative Severity Score for the enUmeration of Mortality and Morbidity) score: This scoring system is used for predicting 30-day risk for mortality and morbidity in postsurgical patients. It includes 18 variables: 12 physiological factors and 6 operative factors. Each variable is divided into 4 grades with an exponentially increasing score (1, 2, 4 and 8)

P-POSSUM (Portsmouth-POSSUM): The refinement of original scoring system. This system also includes 18 variables (12 physiological factors and 6 operative factors). A different formula is used to calculate mortality and morbidity. This scoring system better predicts postoperative mortality than the original one.

PULP (Peptic Ulcer Perforation) score: This scoring system is for predicting morbidity and mortality in perforated peptic ulcer. It includes: (i) Age >65 years; (ii) Comorbid active malignant disease or AIDS; (iii) Comorbid liver cirrhosis; (iv) Concomitant use of steroids; (v) Shock on admission (BP<100 mm Hg and heart rate >100 bpm); (vi) Time from perforation to admission >24 hours; (vii) Serum creatinine >130 µmol/L; (viii) ASA score 2, 3, 4, 5. Score ranges from 0–18. Score 0–7 denotes low risk (<25%) and score 8–18 denotes high risk (>25%).

quickSOFA (qSOFA) score: Patients outside the ICU are at risk of sepsis development if two or more of the following are abnormal: (i) Elevated respiratory rate ≥22 breaths per minute; (ii) Altered mental status (Glasgow coma scale <15); and (iii) Systolic blood pressure of 100 mm Hg or less.

Revised Baux score (R-Baux score): This scoring system is the modified Baux score, predicting mortality in burn patients. The score is calculated as: [TBSA + Age + (17 × R)], where R = 1, if patient has inhalation injury and R = 0, if not.

RIPASA (Raja Isteri Pengiran Anak Saleha Appendicitis) score: A scoring system for acute appendicitis. It includes 18 variables divided into 4 groups (data, signs, symptoms, and laboratory values). The maximum score is 16. Score less than 5 points—unlikely; score 5–7 points—low probability; score 7.5–11.5—high probability; and score 12 or more—diagnostic.

SAPS (Simplified Acute Physiology Score) II scoring: It estimates the mortality in ICU patients. The score includes 12 physiological variables and 3 disease-related variables. The worst physiological variables (variables with highest number of points) along with disease-related variables are counted in the first 24 hours of ICU admission. Score ranges from 0 to 163 points. Not applicable for burn points, coronary care unit points and cardiac surgery points.

SOFA (Sequential Organ Failure Assessment) score: This scoring system is a morbidity severity score and mortality estimation tool. It includes six variables, each representing a body system: (i) FIO_2/PaO_2 (Respiratory system); (ii) Platelet count (Coagulation system); (iii) Bilirubin level (Liver); (iv) Glasgow coma score (Neurological); (v) MAP/Vasopressors used (Cardiovascular); (vi) Creatinine/Urine output (Renal). Each organ system assigns a point value from 0 to 4. The worst physiological variables are collected every 24 hours during ICU admission. The SOFA score ranges from 0 to 24. SOFA score ranges 15–24 predicts >90% mortality.

TIRADS scoring: ACR TI-RADS (Thyroid Imaging Reporting and Data System) is a scoring system for thyroid nodules based on five USG features (Composition, echogenicity, shape, margin, echogenic foci), proposed by American College of Radiology. This scoring system recommends when to do FNA or USG follow-up or no FNA is required. Details of this scoring system is in Chapter 14 (Thyroid).

Tumor Regression Grade (Mandard TRG system): *TRG1:* No viable cancer cells, complete response; *TRG2:* Single cells or small group of cancer cells; *TRG3:* Residual cancer outgrown by fibrosis; *TRG4:* Significant fibrosis outgrown by cancer; and *TRG5:* No fibrosis with extensive residual cancer.

TWIST (Testicular Work-up for Ischemia and Suspected Torsion) scoring: A clinically validated scoring system based on 5 clinical variables for work-up and management of acute scrotal emergencies where testicular torsion is suspected. Details in Chapter 20 of Diseases of Testis, Scrotum, and Penis.

Vancouver Scar Scale (VSS): Most recognized burn scar assessment method. It includes four scar characteristics: (i) Vascularity; (ii) Pigmentation; (iii) Pliability; and (iv) Height. Score ranges from 0 to 13.

Visick score: The scoring system is to monitor the subjective effects of primary antireflux surgery.

Visual infusion phlebitis (VIP) score: A uniform standard scale for measuring grade and severity of infusion phlebitis.

Site observation	Score	Stage	Action
IV site appears healthy	0	No signs of phlebitis	Observe cannula
One of the following signs is evident: • Slight pain near the IV site OR • Slight redness near the IV site	1	Possibly first signs of phlebitis	Observe cannula
Two of the following are evident: • Pain at IV site • Redness	2	Early stage of phlebitis	Resite cannula
All of the following are evident: • Pain along path of cannula • Redness around site • Swelling	3	Medium stage of phlebitis	• Resite cannula • Consider treatment

All of the following are evident and extensive: • Pain along path of cannula • Redness around site • Swelling • Palpable venous cord	4	Advanced stage of phlebitis or the start of thrombophlebitis	• Resite cannula • Consider treatment
All of the following are evident and extensive: • Pain along path of cannula • Redness around site • Swelling • Palpable venous cord • Pyrexia	5	Advanced stage thrombophlebitis	• Resite cannula • Consider treatment

Watson dysphagia scale: It consists of questions about food with 9 different viscosity and solidity and patients have problems with a specific food. Score ranges from 0-45 where score 45 is the worst possible dysphagia.

Zubrod score (ECOG/WHO score): Scoring system to determine performance status in cancer patients. Score ranges from 0 to 4, with '0' being fully functional and asymptomatic, and '4' being bedridden.

IMPORTANT FACTS

1. **Sources of surgical site infection (SSI)** are patient's endogenous flora, skin colonization, and exogenous sources (operation theater, instruments, surgical team).
2. Among the connective tissues, **tendons** have the highest tensile strength.
3. **Cartilage** has minimal ability to regenerate because it has no intrinsic blood supply.
4. **Scoring systems for assessing wound infection:** (i) The ASEPSIS wound score and (ii) Southampton wound grading system.
5. **The risk of transmission of infection from a hepatitis B-positive patient to a surgeon** is much greater than the risk of transmission from a Hep B-positive surgeon to a patient.
6. **A surgeon who is hepatitis B-surface antigen positive, but e-antigen negative** can continue medical practice.
7. **Surgeons with chronic hepatitis C infection** can continue medical practice (chance of transmission of infection from surgeon to patient is extremely low).
8. **Necrosis** is a pathological process of cell death due to external factors, whereas **apoptosis** is an orderly and internally driven physiological process of cell death.
9. **Wound dehiscence** commonly develops between fifth and eighth postoperative day.
10. Decreased level of **serum potassium** is a late indicator of depletion of total body potassium. Potassium should be replaced in patients with anticipated potassium loss, even if serum potassium is below normal.
11. **Medial basilic vein** is a preferred venipuncture site. This vein is separated from the brachial artery by the bicipital aponeurosis.
12. **Hartmann's solution** is the ideal fluid in diabetic patients undergoing surgery if patients not requiring VRIII (Variable Rate Intravenous Insulin Infusion).
13. The ideal fluid in diabetic patients (requiring VRIII) undergoing surgery is **glucose 5% in saline 0.45% pre-mixed with potassium chloride**.
14. **Central venous catheterization** is technically easier in the right internal jugular vein or femoral vein due to straighter course.
15. **During cannulation of peripheral veins,** the veins become prominent in warm environment, if placed dependently or tying a tourniquet proximal to the site of cannulation.
16. **In adults, upper extremity is the preferred site** for peripheral and midline vascular catheter insertion.
17. **Routes for contamination of vascular catheter:** (i) Migration of skin flora at the catheter insertion site and then colonization at the catheter tip (most common); (ii) Direct contamination of the catheter by hand or other devices; (iii) Hematogenous seeding of organisms from other infective focus; and (iv) Contaminated infuscate.
18. **1 liter of 5% dextrose solution** provides **400 kcal energy** supplements.
19. **Gallbladder** is devoid of muscularis mucosa and submucosa layer.
20. **Crypts of Luschka** are indentations in the gallbladder mucosa that sink into muscle coat.
21. **Cantle's line** is a vertical plane (running from gallbladder fossa anteriorly to the IVC posteriorly) divides liver into right and left lobes.
22. The mucosa of the cystic duct (particularly adjacent to the gallbladder neck) have mucosal folds, known as **spiral valves of Heister**. These valves regulate the filling and emptying of the gallbladder.
23. **Sphincter of Lutkens** is the sphincter structure of cystic duct.
24. **Hepatocystic triangle** is bordered by inferior surface of liver superiorly, the cystic duct and medial border of the gallbladder laterally and medially by the common hepatic duct. This triangle is the target area for dissection during laparoscopic cholecystectomy.

25. **Cystic lymph node of Lund (also known as Node of Calot or Mascagni node):** This lymph node overlies the insertion of the cystic artery into the gallbladder wall. This lymph node acts as a anatomical landmark to identify cystic artery during cholecystectomy.
26. **The left hepatic duct** drains segment II, III and IV. The left hepatic duct is longer than the right and increased propensity for dilatation when there is distal extrahepatic biliary obstruction. **Left hepatic duct is one of the preferred site for hepaticojejunostomy.**
27. **The ducts of Luschka (Subvesical bile ducts):** Accessory small bile duct contact with the gallbladder fossa and drain into right hepatic or common hepatic duct. If this structure is not recognized during cholecystectomy, bile leak and subsequent bile accumulation (biloma) may develop.
28. In **intrahepatic gallbladder**, surgeons may face difficulty to find plane of dissection during separation of gallbladder from cystic plate during cholecystectomy. **Mesenteric pattern of gallbladder** is at risk of torsion.
29. **Caterpillar hump or Moynihan's hump** is a rare vascular anomaly where the tortuous right hepatic artery forms a U-shaped loop close to gallbladder with short cystic artery. During cholecystectomy, misidentification leads to clipping of the right hepatic artery or uncontrollable bleeding.
30. During cholecystectomy, if the **cystic duct is too short** (<2 cm), placing ligaclips or ligatures is technically difficult. If surgeon finds **wide cystic duct,** sometimes surgeon faces confusion between CBD and wide cystic duct.
31. **Characteristic features of subvesical duct are**: (i) This duct is present in 20–50% individuals; (ii) Does not drain any specific liver segment; (iii) No communication with the gallbladder; (iv) This duct joins the common hepatic duct, or the right hepatic duct; (v) May deeply embedded in the cystic plate; and (vi) During cholecystectomy, this duct may be injured and may cause bile leak.
32. **The arterial supply of the supraduodenal bile duct** is mainly axial (mostly by the 3 o'clock and 9 o'clock arteries), only 2% of the supply is nonaxial (by the branches arising from the main trunk of the hepatic artery).
33. **The plate system in liver** includes hilar plate, cystic plate, and the umbilical plate.
34. Exposure of the right intrahepatic ductal system is technically more difficult than that of the left ductal system.
35. The common hepatic artery after origin of gastroduodenal artery and right gastric artery, is known as proper hepatic artery. Middle hepatic artery comes off the left hepatic artery and supplies segment IV.
36. Weight of the liver is 1.2–1.6 kg. Gallbladder is about 10 cm long and 3–5 cm wide. The mean diameter of common hepatic duct (CHD) and common bile duct (CBD) is about 6 mm. The length of CBD is 10–15 cm. The diameter of the cystic duct is approximately 1–3 mm.
37. **The parts of sphincter of Oddi:** (i) The sphincter choledochus; (ii) The pancreatic sphincter; and (iii) The sphincter ampullae. Sphincter choledochus regulates the flow of bile and gallbladder filling. Sphincter ampullae prevents reflux of duodenal contents.
38. **Murphy sign may be absent** in diabetic and obese acute cholecystitis patients.
39. **The "rosary sign"** is a CT finding in adenomyomatosis of gallbladder. It is formed by discrete hypoattenuating intramural lesions with enhancing epithelium within. **"Pearl necklace sign"** is seen in T2-weighted MR imaging.
40. The exact **pathophysiology of pruritus** in obstructive jaundice is not known, but increased levels of bile salts and histamine in circulation are most likely responsible.
41. **Asymptomatic bile duct dilatation** may be found in older age and after cholecystectomy.
42. In USG, **acoustic shadowing** occurs when a structure attenuates sound more rapidly than surrounding tissues.
43. In USG, with positional variation, gallstones move quickly, sludge moves slowly whereas polyps are fixed.
44. Posterior acoustic shadowing is commonly absent in gallstones smaller than 3 mm.
45. **Hepatobiliary specific contrast agents for MRI** are mangafodipir trisodium, gadobenate dimeglumine, and gadoxetic acid.

46. **Causes of filling defects in cholangiogram:** (i) Calculi; (ii) Air bubbles; (iii) Blood clots; (iv) Parasites; and (v) Bile duct cancer. Calculi is the most common cause of filling defect.
47. In cholangiogram, the magnification is of the order of 40%.
48. Gallbladder perforation is more common in laparoscopic cholecystectomy than in open cholecystectomy.
49. Right hepatic vein is larger than the left and middle hepatic veins.
50. **The main portal scissura** divides the liver into right and left liver. The middle hepatic vein runs through the main hepatic scissura. The right liver is drained by the right hepatic duct and left liver is drained by left hepatic duct.
51. **Caudate lobe** is divided into right portion, left portion, and the caudate process. Caudate lobe is drained by multiple ducts that join both right and left hepatic ducts.
52. **The right hepatic duct** drains segments V, VI, VII, and VIII. **The left hepatic duct** drains segments II, III, and IV.
53. For exposure of the biliary confluence and left hepatic duct, '**lowering of the hilar plate**' at the inferior border of segment IV is necessary.
54. **Due to absence of valve in the portal venous system:** (i) High blood flow is possible at low pressure and (ii) Venous pressure measurement is feasible at any point of venous system.
55. **The portal vein** provides about 75% of the blood supply to the liver and 50–70% of the oxygen requirement. The hepatic artery provides about 25% of the blood supply to the liver.
56. The length of the portal vein is 5.5–8 cm and diameter is approximately 1 cm. Portal pressure is between 6 and 10 mm Hg. The right portal vein is larger than the left portal vein.
57. Portal vein anatomy is less variable in comparison to variation of biliary ductal system and hepatic arterial system.
58. **Hep Par-1 (Hepatocyte Paraffin 1)** is a monoclonal antibody that recognizes mitochondrial antigen of hepatocytes. This immunohistochemical marker is used to differentiate between poorly differentiated hepatocellular carcinoma and metastatic carcinoma of liver.
59. Among the coagulation factors, factor VII has the shortest half-life (about 6 hours). Deficiency of factor VII is manifested as prolonged prothrombin time (PT) or increased INR. Due to the short half-life of factor VII, patients with liver failure, vitamin-K deficiency, or oral anticoagulant toxicity initially manifest with increased PT, or INR value.
60. **Ligaments related to the liver are:** (i) The falciform ligament; (ii) Coronary ligament; (iii) Right and left triangular ligaments; (iv) The round ligament (ligamentum teres); (v) The hepatoduodenal ligament; and (vi) The ligamentum venosum.
61. **Falciform ligament** acts as an anatomical landmark for the border between left medial and left lateral sections.
62. **The round ligament (ligamentum teres)** contains the obliterated left umbilical vein. This ligament provides the landmark for identification of left portal vein and left hepatic duct.
63. **The ligamentum venosum** contains the obliterated ductus venosum. This ligamentous attachment provides the landmark for identification of left hepatic vein.
64. **The hepatoduodenal ligament** contains the bile duct, hepatic artery, and portal vein.
65. The falciform ligament, triangular ligaments, and coronary ligament are avascular. In portal hypertension, venous collaterals may develop in these ligaments.
66. The total liver volume is directly proportional to the body surface area.
67. **Urata formula** is used to estimate standard liver volume of an individual. According to this formula, LV (mL) = $706.2 \times \text{BSA}\ (\text{m}^2) + 2.4$
68. **CT or MR volumetry** is mandatory for estimation of segmental liver volume prior to major liver resections or segmental liver transplantation.

69. In most of the individuals (about 80%), middle hepatic vein joins the left hepatic vein and then the common venous channel drains into the suprahepatic IVC. The right hepatic vein drains into the IVC separately.
70. Right hepatic vein is the longest vein in the liver.
71. During liver surgery, the risk of major bleeding is more from hepatic veins than portal venous branches.
72. Most of the primary liver tumors receive the majority of their blood supply from the hepatic arterial system.
73. **The attenuation value of liver** is between 54 and 60 HU. The attenuation value of liver is more (approximately 8 HU) than the spleen (due to hepatic storage of glycogen and iron).
74. **Hypervascular benign liver lesions** are focal nodular hyperplasia, adenoma, hemangioma. **Hypervascular primary malignant liver lesions** are HCC, fibrolamellar carcinoma, peripheral cholangiocarcinoma.
75. **Hypervascular liver metastatic lesions:** Primary lesions are neuroendocrine tumors, renal cell carcinoma, melanoma, thyroid carcinoma.
76. **Hypovascular liver lesions** are most conspicuous in portal venous phase images.
77. **Adult pancreas** is approximately 15 cm in length, weight 60–100 g. The exocrine pancreas comprises about 98% of the pancreatic mass, endocrine pancreas comprises only 2% of the pancreatic mass.
78. **The duct of Wirsung** drains the head and uncinate process of pancreas, whereas the duct of Santorini drains the body and tail of the pancreas. The duct of Wirsung drains through the major duodenal papilla (ampulla of Vater). **The duct of Santorini** drains through the minor papilla 2 cm anterosuperior of the major papilla.
79. Pancreatic β-cells represent approximately 55% of islet cells, secrete insulin and amylin. Amylin is a peptide hormone that regulates plasma glucose by regulating gastric emptying and glucagon secretion. Amylin deficiency is found in patients with T1DM and T2DM.
80. Pancreatic δ-cells represent less than 10% of the islet cells, secrete somatostatin.
81. Pancreatic F-cells represent less than 5% of the islet cells, secrete pancreatic polypeptide.
82. Pancreatic €-cells represent less than 1% of islet cells, secrete human islet cells.
83. β-cells and δ-cells are distributed uniformly throughout the pancreas, whereas α-cells are in a higher proportion in body and tail of pancreas. Uncinate process has a lower proportion of α-cells.
84. **Triphasic CT protocol includes:** (i) Precontrast phase; (ii) Late arterial phase; and (iii) Portal venous phase. Four-phase CT protocol includes—All three phases of triphasic CT protocol plus 3- to 5-minute delayed phase ('late venous' or 'equilibrium' phase).
85. **'Cheatle slit'** is to make a slit in the antimesenteric border of the smaller diameter end of the bowel to increase the free edge for better apposition during end-to-end anastomosis.
86. After completion of intestinal anastomosis, the luminal patency is checked by invaginating the intestinal walls from each side through the anastomotic ring. A patent lumen is felt like a doughnut.
87. **The white line of Toldt** serves as a guide during mobilization of the ascending colon.
88. The transverse colon is the longest part (about 50 cm) of the colon. The sigmoid colon is the most muscular part of the colon.
89. **The collateral pathways of colonic arterial supply are:** (i) The marginal artery of Drummond and (ii) The arc of Riolan. The marginal artery of Drummond extends throughout the colon. The splenic flexure region is the watershed area **(Griffith point)** where collateral circulation is absent in about 50% of patients. Another watershed area is the **Sudeck point** (rectosigmoid junction) is described as the point of origin of the last sigmoid arterial branch, originating from the inferior mesenteric artery.
90. **The arc of Riolan (meandering mesenteric artery)** provides collateral pathway between the middle colic artery and proximal left colic artery.

91. Amoeboma should be suspected if a patient presents with right iliac fossa mass and history of blood-stained mucoid diarrhea (altered bowel habit is not a common presentation of right-sided colonic carcinoma).
92. Intestinal tuberculosis should be suspected in any patient who presents with weight loss, malaise, abdominal pain and features of recurrent subacute intestinal obstruction.
93. In children with intussusception, pathological lead point is not common. If present, it may be Meckel's diverticulum, enteric duplication cyst, small bowel lymphoma.
94. CT is a more reliable imaging modality than USG in obese patients with suspected appendicitis (diminished accuracy of USG in presence of subcutaneous and intra-abdominal fat).
95. USG is a reliable imaging modality to confirm presence of acute appendicitis but unreliable modality to exclude appendicitis.
96. MRI is a preferred imaging modality in children and pregnant patients with suspected appendicitis if USG is inconclusive.
97. Cosmetic outcome of circumferential incisions in breast are better than radial incisions.
98. The term 'Goiter' was derived from the Latin word 'guttur' (throat). The term 'thyroid gland' was derived from the Greek word 'thyreoeides' (shield-shaped).
99. **Heterotopic thyroid tissue** is present in about 20% of patients with thyroglossal cyst.
100. The thyroid gland is the storage site of more than 90% of the total body iodine.
101. **The type 2a variant of external branch of the superior laryngeal nerve (EB-SLN)** is at a greater risk of injury and found in about 20% of patients.
102. The EB-SLN is also termed as **"Galli-Curci Nerve"**.
103. The superior parathyroid gland commonly presents dorsal to the recurrent laryngeal nerve (RLN), whereas the inferior parathyroid glands are commonly located ventral to RLN.
104. Thyroid cancers rarely metastasize to submaxillary nodes (level I).
105. T3 is more potent (3–4 times), less tightly bound to plasma protein, much lower circulating plasma level, shorter half-life (1 day, T4: 7 days), compared to T4.
106. TSH assay is the most sensitive and specific test for diagnosis of hyperthyroidism and hypothyroidism and for adjusting the dose of T4. **Reference range of TSH:** 0.5–5 μU/mL, **Total T4:** 55–150 nmol/L, **Total T3:** 1.5–3.5 nmol/L, **Free T4:** 12–28 pmol/L, **Free T3:** 3–9 pmol/L.
107. Free T3 assay is the most useful test for confirmation of diagnosis of early hyperthyroidism.
108. In the presence of low iodide uptake, thyroid gland mainly produces T3.
109. In severely ill patients, thyroid hormone levels may be reduced without an increase in TSH level, this condition is known as **Euthyroid sick syndrome**.
110. I-123 is a pure gamma emitter, provides lower doses of radiation to the thyroid than I-131, image quality is superior, half-life is 12–14 hrs.
111. **'Galen's anastomosis'** is the anastomosis between the descending sensory fibers of the superior laryngeal nerve and the posterior branch of the recurrent laryngeal nerve.
112. Recurrent laryngeal nerve (RLN) is termed as **'recurrent'** because after branching off the vagus, it turns upwards under the subclavian artery on the right side and under the ligamentum arteriosum on the left side.
113. **Non-recurrent RLN** is a rare anomaly of the recurrent laryngeal nerve. It directly arises from the cervical vagus and is almost exclusively present on the right side. Often, the non-recurrent RLN is associated with a vascular anomaly (retro-esophageal right subclavian artery). This nerve is at higher risk of injury during thyroidectomy due to its aberrant course (along with superior thyroid pedicles or transverse course superficial or deep to inferior thyroid artery).

114. **Voice changes in thyroid disease is due to:** (i) Tumor invasion of RLN; (ii) Compression injury of nerve; and (iii) Vocal fold edema due to hormonal dysfunction.
115. **Causes of post-thyroidectomy voice change:** (i) Injury to recurrent laryngeal nerve; (ii) Injury to external branch of superior laryngeal nerve; (iii) Cervical strap muscle injury; (iv) laryngeal edema; and (v) Injury due to airway management.
116. **Risk factors for RLN injury:** (i) Recurrent goiter; (ii) Large goiter; (iii) Abnormal nerve anatomy; and (iv) Surgeon inexperience.
117. During thyroid surgery, routine identification of the recurrent laryngeal nerve is a safer approach than avoidance.
118. **Injury of the recurrent laryngeal nerve may occur in:** (i) Thyroidectomy; (ii) Parathyroidectomy; (iii) Cervical esophagectomy; and (iv) Carotid endarterectomy.
119. In preoperative assessment laryngeal assessment before thyroid surgery, a finding of vocal cord paralysis along with hoarseness is highly suggestive of RLN involvement by the thyroid disease.
120. Stretching at the ligament of Berry is the most common cause of neuropraxic injury of recurrent laryngeal nerve during thyroidectomy.
121. **Intraoperative nerve monitoring (IONM) in thyroidectomy is particularly beneficial in:** (i) Revision thyroid surgery; (ii) Total thyroidectomy; and (iii) Thyroid surgery in presence of unilateral RLN paralysis.
122. **After total thyroidectomy, expected areas of radioactive iodine uptake are:** (i) Adjacent to Berry's ligament; (ii) Superior thyroid pole; (iii) Paratracheal lobar region; and (iv) Isthmus.
123. Hemorrhage and hematoma following thyroid surgery mostly develop within the first 24 hours.
124. **The acronym DESATS** has been created to aid early identification of patients manifesting signs of potential post-thyroidectomy hematoma. **The acronym includes:** Difficulty swallowing/discomfort; Increase in early warning score (EWS) or national early warning score (NEWS); Swelling; Anxiety; Tachypnea/difficulty breathing; and stridor.
125. **'SCOOP' approach** is a systematic bedside surgical approach to open the thyroidectomy wound in patients with signs of airway compromise due to suspected hematoma. This approach includes S: skin exposure; C: cut sutures; O: open skin; O: open muscles; P: pack wound (developed by DAS, BAETS, ENT-UK).
126. Preexisting conditions (PECs) that influence outcome in trauma patients are cirrhosis, coagulopathy, COPD, ischemic heart disease, and diabetes mellitus.
127. Rib fractures, brain injury, and pelvic fracture are common injuries following trauma in geriatric population.
128. In trauma, pediatric population have increased chance of multiple injuries due to smaller body mass (greater force is transmitted per unit of body area), less body fat, closer proximity of organs.
129. **Broslow® pediatric emergency tape** is a color-coded length-based tape for appropriate fluid volume, drug doses, equipment size in pediatric emergencies.
130. The risk of hypothermia is more in pediatric patients because of surface area to body mass ratio is more compared to adults.
131. **Intraosseous infusion** is performed by bone-marrow needle. Preferred sites of intraosseous infusion are proximal tibia and distal femur.
132. **Spinal cord injury without radiographic abnormalities (SCIWORA)** is more common in children than adults.
133. Risk of upper airway obstruction is more in pediatric burn patients as their airways are smaller.
134. Hemorrhage is the most common cause of shock in trauma.
135. Tachycardia and cutaneous vasoconstriction are the early indicators of shock.
136. Tachycardia may not be present in elderly patients with hemorrhagic shock due to less response to catecholamine stimulation, use of beta-adrenergic blocker, or presence of pacemaker.

137. Pediatric surgical patients are at increased risk of fluid overload or dehydration.
138. Premature infants are extremely thermolabile because of minimal fat storage in the body and inability to shivering.
139. In patients with intubation or severe facial or eye swelling, verbal and eye responses cannot be properly elicited. In these scenarios, the score will be 1 with a modifier 'T'. *Example:* Verbal "1T". In these patients GCS ranges from 3T to 10T.
140. **Shock index** is defined as heart rate divided by systolic blood pressure. This index is also known as hemodynamic stability indicator. This index is a better indicator of shock severity than heart rate or blood pressure.
141. **Modified shock index** is defined as heart rate divided by mean arterial pressure.
142. CT scan is the best imaging modality for review if malposition of chest drain is suspected.
143. Urine output is the best marker of adequacy of fluid resuscitation.
144. In shock, global hypoperfusion is determined by measurement of serum lactate, base deficit, and mixed venous oxygen saturation.
145. **Fat fracture (post-traumatic pseudolipoma)** is caused by acute trauma, particularly in the thigh or gluteal region.
146. The risk of liver and spleen injury is higher in pediatric population because the spleen and liver are less protected by the ribs.
147. **Postconcussive syndrome** is basically the constellation of symptoms after brain injury, persisting for a prolonged period. These symptoms include headache, dizziness, confusion, difficulty with concentration, insomnia. Treatment is symptomatic and reassurance.
148. Children compensate for hypovolemic shock by increasing their heart rate.
149. Priapism develops at the moment of complete motor and sensory paraplegia.
150. The most common cause of subarachnoid hemorrhage is trauma.
151. Aneurysmal subarachnoid hemorrhage is usually associated with significant vasospasm but not in associated with traumatic subarachnoid hemorrhage.
152. **The absence of oscillation (respiratory swing)** in chest drain tube indicates any of the following: (i) The chest drain tube is blocked; (ii) The tube is no longer within the pleural cavity; and (iii) The lung is fully expanded.
153. **Omental tape technique** is used to fix the chest drain tube to the skin to prevent tube kinking and to reduce the pain due to dragging at the insertion site.
154. **Extracapsular dissection (ECD)** includes total excision of the benign parotid tumor surrounded by healthy parotid tissue without planned dissection of the main trunk of facial nerve. The recurrence rate is almost similar to superficial parotidectomy but associated with less complication rates (i.e., temporary facial nerve palsy 7% vs 25%; Frey's syndrome 0 vs 60%). ECD may be considered as a surgical choice for mobile, small benign parotid tumor located in superficial lobe without any adhesion to facial nerve.
155. During end-to-end repair of ureter, spatulation increases the circumference of the ends being anastomosed.
156. Most common cause of neck swelling in children is lymphadenopathy.
157. Jugulodigastric lymph node is the largest lymph node of all cervical lymph nodes.
158. Most of the neck masses in adults are neoplastic.
159. A nontender neck mass is most likely neoplastic.
160. Most of the malignant neck mass is due to metastasis from head and neck squamous cell carcinoma (HNSCC).
161. Cervical metastases from HPV-positive HNSCC are often mistaken for benign cyst or abscess because of cystic appearance on imaging.
162. **Normal anatomic structures commonly mistaken for a pathologic neck mass are** submandibular gland, the transverse process of C2, carotid bulb.

163. Malignant lesions in lip and oral cavity commonly metastasize to level I to III group of cervical nodes. Primary lesion in oropharynx, hypopharynx, and larynx commonly metastasize to level II to IV. Primary lesions in nasopharynx and thyroid usually metastasizes to level V.
164. **Bilateral cervical lymph node metastases** may be found in cancer of tongue base, nasopharynx, and midline oral cavity.
165. A contrast-enhanced CT or MRI for evaluation of neck mass of unknown etiology must cover from the base of the skull to the thoracic inlet.
166. MRI is preferred over CT scan in evaluation of neck metastases if primary lesion is suspected in nasopharynx or increased risk of perineural spread.
167. In patients with renal insufficiency, noncontrast MRI is a better imaging modality than noncontrast CT for assessment of neck mass (due to better soft tissue characterization of MRI).
168. If history and clinical findings of a patient with neck mass is highly suggestive of lymphoma, core needle biopsy should be considered as the first-line tissue sampling method.
169. **Causes of cystic cervical metastases:** (i) HPV-associated head-neck squamous cell carcinoma; (ii) Primary tumor in tonsil, nasopharynx, and base of tongue; and (iii) Papillary thyroid carcinoma.
170. In thyroglossal cyst, papillary cancer most commonly found, Hurthle cell, anaplastic and squamous cell carcinoma are rarely found, medullary thyroid cancer never found.
171. The most important layer to approximate during skin closure is the dermis (contains the blood supply and cellular elements needed for healing).
172. Scissors cut tissues in the sagittal plane from near to far and scalpel from far to near.
173. During surgery, the hand is most comfortable in midprone position.
174. Trainee surgeons tend to exert up to 130% more force or torque than is required by experienced one to perform the same procedure.
175. The chevron shape of the hemostatic clip ensures that the tip of the clip closes first to prevent the enclosed tubular structure from squeezing out.
176. Absorbable suture materials are degraded by hydrolysis.
177. Polyfilament sutures are always braided, rather than twisted.
178. A curved needle can be passed through the tissues with minimal trauma and with minimal force by perfect pronation and supination movements of the wrist.
179. Monofilament sutures are at greater risk of reducing strength due to improper handling than polyfilament sutures.
180. Surgical knots reduce the strength of all suture materials (about 50%).
181. The weakest part of any suture line is the knot.
182. In a suture line, the highest density of foreign body material is in the knot.
183. **Types of barbed sutures:** (i) Quill™ Knotless Tissue Closure Device; (ii) V-Loc™ unidirectional barbed suture with a fixed loop; and (iii) STRATAFIX™ Spiral- unidirectional barbed sutures with a variable loop at the end.
184. **Complete square knot** consists of two sequential throws that lie in opposite directions.
185. **A surgeon's knot** consists of a double throw followed by a single throw.
186. **Presacral veins** are prone to bleed because they are avalvular and directly communicate with the basivertebral veins.
187. **In reoperative pelvic surgery,** the chance of ureter injury is high where ureter crosses the pelvic brim or close to its insertion into the urinary bladder.
188. **In reoperative pelvic surgery**, urinary bladder may be injured during the opening of abdomen at the level of pubic symphysis.

189. Sharp dissection in the correct plane is almost bloodless. Increase in bleeding indicates that the dissection is not in a correct plane or underlying inflammatory or malignant pathology has invaded the plane.
190. Pulse oximeters cannot distinguish oxyhemoglobin from carboxyhemoglobin. Therefore, pulse oximetry is not useful to rule out CO poisoning in burn patients.
191. β-hemolytic streptococci group A in wound is a **contraindication to skin grafting**.
192. **Thickness of the skin graft** can be assessed by bleeding points on the donor surface. In a thin graft, bleeding points are closely placed whereas in a thicker graft, the bleeding points are far apart.
193. Skin grafts can be stored for up to 2 weeks in a refrigerator at 4°C into sterile gauze pad moistened with saline.
194. Most common type of congenital diaphragmatic hernia is **Bockdalek hernia**.
195. **Different skin tension lines are** Langer's line, relaxed skin tension line, and biodynamic excisional skin tension line.
196. A significant number of elderly patients with abdominal pathology present with acute onset abdominal symptoms without significant clinical findings. Proper diagnostic work-up should be done to avoid development of complications (e.g., appendicular perforation, gangrene of the gallbladder).
197. **'Honeymoon palsy'** refers to a compressive neuropathy of radial nerve due to compression of one partner's arm by another's head during overnight sleep.
198. **'English lacing'** is a method of fixing the abdominal drain where the stitch is placed through the skin and then lace it back and forth around the drain.
199. **Ureter has a characteristic vermiculating (motion resembling that of a worm) peristaltic movement. Kelly's sign** is a clinical sign to identify ureter during surgery by visible vermiculation when the ureter is pressed gently.
200. If the small intestinal wall is acutely breached, mucosa becomes everted because the area of folded mucosa is much greater than the area of submucosa and seromuscular layer. This eversion can be corrected by inverting mattress (Connell) suture during repair.
201. If fistula track is completely epithelialized, the chance of spontaneous closure is minimal.
202. Blood flow is faster in the center of the lumen of the blood vessels than the periphery.
203. Perioperative hypothermia increases the risk of infection and impairs healing.
204. **Oral hypoglycemic agents with risk of hypoglycemia during fasting:** Sulphonylurea (e.g., glibenclamide, gliclazide, glipizide)
205. **Oral hypoglycemic agents that can be continued during fasting without risk of hypoglycemia:** Metformin, DPP-IV inhibitors (e.g., sitagliptin, vildagliptin), GLP-1 analogs (e.g., exenatide, liraglutide), pioglitazone
206. **1 IU of subcutaneous rapid-acting insulin** will drop the CBG by 3 mmol/L.
207. Patients with centrally distributed fat are at increased risk of perioperative complications than those with peripherally distributed fat.
208. Calcified vessels are more difficult to control with vascular clamp.
209. Atheromatous plaques may develop in veins when they are used as arterial grafts or in arteriovenous fistulas.
210. **Zajdela technique** (also known as 'French technique' or 'fine-needle nonaspiration') is a method of FNAB where no aspiration or negative pressure are used for acquisition of the sample. Rapid down and up movement of the needle along with capillary action of the needle are utilized for acquisition of cells from the lesion.
211. Blood vessels are absent within the epidermis.
212. **Positive contrast agents** are iodinated contrast agent and barium. **Negative contrast agents** are gas (e.g., carbon dioxide).
213. **Nephrogenic systemic fibrosis**, a potentially fatal complication may develop after administration of gadolinium contrast agent for MRI in patients with severe renal insufficiency (GFR <30 mL/min).

214. In laparoscopic surgeries, electrosurgical injuries are usually recognized after 3–7 days of injury.
215. In pediatric patients, transverse supraumbilical incision is preferred over the vertical midline incision (children have wide abdomen and broad costal margin).
216. According to **Hayflick hypothesis**, normal, somatic, differentiated human cell population are permitted to undergo cell division between 40 and 60 times.
217. The growth of a human tumor can be described by the **Gompertizian curve**. In the early stage of tumor, the growth is exponential. As the tumor grows, the growth becomes slower.
218. **Norton-Simon hypothesis** states that 'chemotherapy results in a rate of regression in tumor volume that is proportional to the rate of growth for an unperturbed tumor of that size.'
219. Free air can persist for up to 5–7 days in the peritoneal cavity following abdominal surgery.
220. **Chilaiditi syndrome** is asymptomatic interposition of a loop of large intestine between the right hemidiaphragm and the liver and presented as free gas under right dome of diaphragm in X-ray.
221. **The MUST (Malnutrition Universal Screening Tool)** is a screening tool (introduced by the British Association of Parenteral and Enteral Nutrition) for screening of malnourished and at risk of undernutrition patients.
222. After postoperative paralytic ileus, peristalsis returns back first in the small intestine followed by large intestine, and then stomach.
223. **Apfel and Koivuranta scores** are two clinically validated risk scoring systems to predict postoperative nausea and vomiting (PONV).
224. **'Fragility' fracture** is a type of pathological fracture resulting from minimal trauma due to osteoporosis. Typical fragility fractures include fractures of wrist, proximal femur, vertebral fracture.
225. The normal pale-yellow color of urine is due to **urochrome**.
226. **Cornett's sign** is elicited to differentiate between abdominal wall swelling and intra-abdominal mass.
227. Elongated bilateral muscular bulge along the inguinal ligament in thin persons during straining is termed as **Malgaigne's bulge**. It is often confused with hernia during clinical examination.
228. **The short synacthen test (SST)** is the most commonly used method of assessment of adrenal insufficiency. This test includes measurement of serum cortisol before and after administration of synthetic ACTH (Tetracosactrin).
229. Ganglion cyst is also called **'Bible cyst'**.
230. **Red flag symptoms and signs of cancer:** (i) Breast lump with nipple retraction or other skin changes along with axillary lymphadenopathy—**Breast carcinoma;** (ii) Recent history of alteration of bowel habit and passage of mucus with stool—**Colorectal carcinoma**; (iii) Elderly male patient with recent onset painless hematuria—**Bladder carcinoma**; (iv) Obstructive jaundice with gallbladder lump—**Periampullary carcinoma or gallbladder carcinoma**; (v) Nonhealing ulcer over a previous burn scar—**Marjolin's ulcer (squamous cell carcinoma)**; (vi) Change in size, bleeding, itching and color changes in mole—**Melanoma**; (vii) Persistent difficulty in swallowing—**Esophageal carcinoma**; (viii) Persistent cervical lymphadenopathy—**Metastatic lymph node or lymphoproliferative disorder**; (ix) Thyroid swelling with cervical lympadenopathy—**Papillary carcinoma of thyroid**; and (x) Parotid swelling with facial nerve palsy—**Carcinoma of parotid**.
231. **TNM staging** is applicable for tumors that are **microscopically confirmed as malignant**.
232. **Hallmarks of cancer are:** (i) Self-sufficiency in growth signals; (ii) Insensitivity to growth-inhibitory signals; (iii) Evasion of apoptosis; (iv) Limitless replicative potential; (v) Angiogenic competence; (vi) Invasion and metastasis; (vii) Reprogramming of energy metabolism; and (viii) Evading immune destruction.
233. **'Stage migration'** also known as **'Will Rogers phenomenon' (Okie paradox)**: In oncology, new imaging modalities allow detection of tiny metastases. As a result, more patients are assigned into more severe metastatic disease stage from less severe single tumor stage. This 'stage migration' results in improved survival in both the less severe and more severe disease stages.

234. **Pathological diagnosis is not required in these tumors if tumor seems to be resectable in imaging findings:** (i) Carcinoma of head of pancreas; (ii) Gallbladder carcinoma; (iii) Cholangiocarcinoma; (iv) Gastrointestinal stromal tumor (GIST); and (v) Testicular tumor (imaging and tumor markers).
235. **Acute phase reactants** are classified as positive and negative. **Positive acute phase reactants** include C-reactive protein, procalcitonin, ferritin, fibrinogen. During inflammation, serum concentration of positive acute phase reactants are increased. **Negative acute phase reactants** include albumin, prealbumin, transferrin, and retinol-binding protein. Serum concentration of negative acute phase reactants is decreased during inflammation.
236. Prealbumin is a more sensitive biochemical marker of malnutrition than albumin because of its shorter half-life (2–3 days).
237. **'FAST HUG' is a checklist mnemonic for ICU patients** (by Vincent JL) that includes: **F (Feeding)**—Can the patient tolerate oral and/or enteral feeds? **A (Analgesia)**—Patient should not be in pain nor receive excessive analgesia; **S (Sedation)**—Patient should not experience discomfort but should be arousable; **T (Thromboembolic prevention)**—With chemical or medical adjuncts; **H (HOB elevated)**—Optimal 30-45°; **U (Stress Ulcers)**—H_2 antagonists or PPI; and **G (Glucose control)**—Blood sugar level and treatments.
238. **Cardinal signs of Kanavel** for diagnosis of infectious tenosynovitis are: (i) Finger is held in flexion; (ii) Fusiform swelling of the finger; and (iii) Tenderness along the tendon sheath; and (iv) Pain on passive extension of the digit.
239. **Eklund view (Implant displacement view)** is an additional mammographic view for screening of breast cancer in patients with breast implants. This includes pushing the implant against the chest wall and pulling forward of the breast tissue.
240. Among the 20,000 human genes, **less than 200 genes act as driver genes** for development of cancer.
241. Epithelial cancers are the most common type of cancer because **epithelia has the highest mitotic turnover.**
242. The stages of carcinogenesis in epithelial tumors are **"breakthrough event"**, **"expansion phase"** and **"invasion phase"**. These transformations require **at least 2 to 3 driver gene mutations**. **Order of mutations are** also important for carcinogenesis. APC mutation must have to be develop before the KRAS or BRAF mutation for malignant transformation of colonic adenoma to colorectal carcinoma.
243. Most of the mutations and epigenetic alterations found in malignant tumors are **not related to tumor itself.**
244. **Driver genes in colorectal cancer** are APC, KRAS, BRAF, PIK3CA, SMAD4, and TP53. **APC, KRAS and TP53** are commonly mutated in colorectal cancer.
245. **The lateral adherences** of epithelial cells are controlled by **E-cadherin** and **basal adherences** to the extracellular matrix are controlled by **cytokeratin.**
246. **Epithelial cell markers** are E-cadherin and cytokeratin. **Mesenchymal cell markers** are vimentin, fibronectin, and N-cadherin.
247. **Normal lymph node** is oval or reniform shaped due to central fatty hilum and peripheral thin cortex. The long axis: short axis ratio is more than 2. In a **metastatic lymph node**, the cortex gradually thickens due to deposition of malignant tumor cells near the marginal sinus.
248. **Children are at increased risk of pulmonary trauma** than adults due to increased compliance of chest wall and less muscle mass.
249. In blunt chest trauma, **proposed mechanisms for lung parenchymal injury are:** (i) The implosion effect (ii) The inertia effect and (iii) The spalling effect.
250. **The Cancer Genome Atlas (TCGA)** is a landmark cancer genomics program started in 2006. This program sequenced and molecularly characterized over 20,000 primary cancers and matched normal samples for 33 cancer types.
251. **The Cancer Microbiome Atlas (TCMA)** is a collection of curated, decontaminated microbial compositions of oropharyngeal, esophageal, gastrointestinal, and colorectal tissues. This atlas will provide valuable resource materials for studying microbiome of GI cancers.

252. **The Glue Grant Program: "Inflammation and the Host Response to Injury"** is a multicenter, multidisciplinary program by The National Institute of General Medical Sciences on 2001 in a 10-year effort to analyze the human genomic response to severe trauma and burns and the relationship of genetic expression in the context of different clinical outcomes.
253. **'Omics' technology** includes genomics (characterization and quantification of genes), epigenomics (epigenetic mechanisms), transcriptomics (expression profiling of mRNA), proteomics (characterization of proteome), and metabolomics (study of metabolites).
254. **Radiomics**, the new branch of radiology, is the extraction of high volume of meaningful data from medical images that are helpful for decision making.
255. **iKnife** is a new device to evaluate the resection margin status intraoperatively in breast cancer surgery by mass spectrometric analysis of surgical diathermy smoke.
256. **Shock-induced endotheliopathy (SHINE)** is a disease state related to acute critical illness (e.g., severe trauma) secondary to over-activation of sympathicoadrenal system characterized by damage to the endothelium, including the glycocalyx.
257. **Viscoelastic tests are:** (i) TEG (Thromboelastography) and (ii) ROTEM (Rotational Thromboelastometry). **Cartridge-based point-of-care viscoelastic tests** are ROTEM sigma and TEG 6s system.
258. In trauma patients with exsanguinating hemorrhage, **maintenance of circulation is in priority over airway management** because in presence of severe hypovolemia, positive pressure ventilation may compromise further cardiac function and precipitate cardiac arrest.
259. **Estimated blood loss** in each rib fracture: 100–200 mL, fracture tibia: 300–500 mL, fracture femur: 800–1000 mL, pelvic fracture-more than 2 liters.
260. **Deresuscitation** is aggressive and active fluid removal in patients with fluid overload using diuretics and/or ultrafiltration.
261. Core elements of **Fluid stewardship** are the **4 Ds** (drug, dose, duration, and de-escalation), the **4 questions** (when to start fluid therapy, when to stop fluid therapy, when to start and when to stop fluid removal), the **4 indications** (resuscitation, maintenance, replacement, and nutrition), the **4 fluid phases**—ROSE model (Resuscitation, Optimization, Stabilization, Evacuation).
262. In atraumatic needle, the needle is attached to the suture material by **either swaging or crimping.**
263. The **important mechanical properties of a suture material** are tensile strength, Breaking strength retention (BSR), elasticity and yield point. An ideal suture should have high tensile strength, good BSR and low-to-medium modulus of elasticity.
264. **A low-friction suture** exhibits good tissue slide and good knot run-down but less knot security.
265. **Visibility** is an important property of suture material, particularly for smaller gauge sutures. Blue-green color is the most appropriate for visibility particularly for laparoscopic surgery.
266. **Natural suture materials swell in the tissues** due to absorption of tissue fluids. This swelling increases the knot security of natural suture materials.
267. **Continuous suturing** is more waterproof and hemostatic than interrupted suturing. **Interrupted suturing** is associated with less risk of devascularization of anastomosis than continuous suturing.
268. **Interrupted suturing** is preferred over continuous suturing in esophageal and colonic anastomoses because of less risk of devascularization of anastomoses.
269. **GORE-TEX®** is a microporous, nonabsorbable monofilament made of expanded polytetrafluoroethylene (ePTFE). This suture causes the least inflammatory reaction of all biomaterials used in surgery. The microporous structure allows tissue in growth. Its easy handling property is due to its soft, flexible and compressible character. It is associated with less needle-hole leakage because the needle approximates the thread diameter.

270. During incision, **bleeding from the subcutaneous veins in the subcutaneous fat are difficult to control by electrocoagulation**. Splitting of the subcutaneous fat by distraction of the wound edges cause less bleeding in comparison to cutting the fatty layer by electrocoagulation, particularly in obese patients.
271. **In a hypersthenic patient with narrow subcostal angle**, midline incision is preferred over transverse or oblique incision for better exposure of supracolic compartment.
272. **Right subcostal nerve** is always injured in right subcostal incision and may cause neuralgic-type pain. McBurney's grid-iron incision may cause injury to the **ilioinguinal nerve,** that may be a predisposing factor for development of ipsilateral inguinal hernia due to weakness of musculoaponeurotic component of inguinal canal.
273. **Reactionary hemorrhage** is a specific bleeding complication in **laparoscopic surgery** because the vessels compressed by the pressure of pneumoperitoneum may start to bleed following desufflation.
274. **The penetrating characteristic of a needle** is determined by the sharpness of the tip and the tapering ratio. It is the ratio between the distance between the shoulder and tip and the diameter of the shaft. The needle is sharper if it has a higher taper ratio.
275. The cross-sectional shape of the body of the needle determines the **security of grip of the needle holder**. The round-bodied needle offers the least secure grip.
276. The skin cancers of the head-neck region have increased propensity to metastases to **parotid lymph nodes**.
277. Parotid gland is the main source of **stimulated salivary secretion**. Submandibular gland produces most of the saliva in **unstimulated state**.
278. Sublingual gland produces the **thickest and most viscous saliva**.
279. **Von Ebnar gland** is a type of minor salivary gland, present close to foliate and circumvallate papillae, play a role in taste perception.
280. **StoneBraker™** is a recently developed salivary pneumatic intracorporeal lithotripter that fragments stones in the parotid and/or submandibular ducts by using pneumatic force.
281. **Most of the post-parotidectomy facial palsy** are transient due to neuropraxia as a result of stretching during surgery. Most of the transient facial palsy resolves within 6 months.
282. The ½ circle needle is better for end-to-side anastomosis and the 3/8 circle is better for tissue approximation and end-to-end anastomosis.
283. The use of circular staplers undoubtedly increased the number of sphincter-saving low anterior resections without compromising the distal margin.
284. **Characteristic B-configuration of the staples** after firing of the GI-staplers is essential for inverted coaption of the edges without impairment of the vascular supply to the anastomosis.
285. **Spray coagulation using Argon beam coagulation system** is the best method of controlling surface oozing over a large area.
286. 45° laparoscopes are rarely used in abdominal laparoscopic surgery, but very useful in thoracoscopic surgery.
287. The Endocameleon® Hopkins® telescope (Storz) is a recent telescope (10 mm) that is capable of altering viewing angles (0°–90°) by adjusting knobs.
288. Humans perform precision tasks best when they look down at the task.
289. The thermal lesion after radiofrequency thermal ablation is hyperechoic and size can thus be monitored by USG.
290. The classic presentation of **'Meal-time syndrome'** in submandibular duct stone is seen only in presence of **complete duct obstruction.**
291. **Composition of salivary stone:** (a) Organic components (cellular debris, bacteria, glycoproteins, mucopolysaccharides) and (b) Inorganic components (calcium carbonates, calcium phosphates).

292. In presence of biliary obstruction and increased pressure in the bile duct, the bile becomes less lithogenic because of relative decrease in secretion of cholesterol and phospholipids in comparison to bile acid secretion. When biliary obstruction is relieved (e.g., placement of decompressive biliary stent), the bile becomes more lithogenic due to relative increase in secretion of cholesterol and phospholipids.

293. Clinical cholangitis and bacteremia never develop unless biliary obstruction causes an increase of intraductal pressure. The chill and rigor of cholangitis is due to systemic bacteremia.

294. The CT value of bile duct stones depends on the amount of calcium phosphate or calcium carbonate in the stones.

295. The physiologic derangements caused by obstructive jaundice (e.g., functions of Kupffer cell, lymphocytes, neutrophil) take several weeks to reverse even after biliary decompression by endoscopic or percutaneous stenting.

296. The amount of damage following penetrating trauma depends more on the speed of the object rather than its weight.

297. Analysis of multiple microscopic sections is essential for confirmation of diagnosis of mucinous carcinoma (colloid carcinoma) because cancer cells may not be evident in all sections due to mucinous component.

298. **Air transport of trauma patients** may develop some unique complications—expansion of gas in the body cavities (in pneumothorax patients) or within the equipment (e.g., endotracheal cuff balloons).

299. Penetrating injury to the '**cardiac box'** may be indicative of injury to the heart. This box is bordered by the clavicles superiorly, costal margins inferiorly, and laterally midclavicular line.

300. **'The Deadly Dozen'** are the major thoracic injuries that are classified into the **Lethal six** (airway obstruction, tension pneumothorax, cardiac tamponade, open pneumothorax, massive hemothorax, and flail chest) and the **Hidden six** (thoracic aortic disruption, tracheobronchial disruption, myocardial contusion, diaphragmatic tear, esophageal injury, and pulmonary contusion).

301. **Circumcision at puberty or at adult life** do not have any protective role in carcinoma penis.

302. In carcinoma penis, corporal bodies are rarely involved as **Buck's fascia** act as a natural barrier.

303. **Partial transection of artery** often causes more significant hemorrhage than complete transection because in **complete transection**, the retraction of intima and media prevents exsanguinating hemorrhage.

304. Palpable pulse or detection of pulse wave in Doppler imaging **does not exclude vascular injury** because pulse wave may propagate through soft clots or an intimal flap.

305. **Kernohan notch** is the impression of transtentorial brain herniation on the contralateral brainstem.

306. **Grading of concussion:** Grade 1 (no loss of consciousness; confusion without amnesia); Grade 2 (no loss of consciousness; confusion with amnesia); Grade 3 (Loss of consciousness).

307. Sealed peptic perforation of stomach or duodenum is also termed as **'forme fruste' of acute free perforation.**

308. **Forme froste choledochal cyst** is a type of choledochal cyst that has minimal or no dilatation of extrahepatic bile duct and is associated with pancreaticobiliary malunion.

309. Postoperative depression is also termed as **'postoperative blues'**, is a common manifestation after any major surgical procedure.

310. Airbags do not provide protection from side-impact events and in accidents where the vehicle rolls over.

311. **"Talk and die syndrome"** represents a group of patients with potentially salvageable primary traumatic head injury who develops rapid deterioration of conscious level into coma and death.

312. **Reverse triage** is the process of refocusing the hospital resources on critically ill patients in the scenario of mass casualty event or disaster by identifying and discharging the patients who have a relatively low risk of complications.

313. The **CBRNE** (Chemical, Biological, Radiological, Nuclear, High-yield explosives) injuries are special type of injuries associated with war, terrorist attacks, and industrial accidents.

314. While calculating GCS score in trauma patients, **the best eye-opening response (E) cannot be assessed** in patients with bilateral complete third nerve palsies or bilateral orbital hematomas. In these patients, the best eye-opening response should be recorded as 'C' for closed eyes.
315. **The best verbal-response cannot be assessed in patients** who are dysphasic or artificially ventilated via tracheostomy tube or endotracheal tube. In these patients, the best verbal response should be recorded as 'D' for dysphasia or 'T' for tube.
316. **The best motor response cannot be assessed in patients** with complete paralysis of the limbs or because of sedatives or muscle relaxant drugs, the best motor response should be recorded as 'P' for paralysis.
317. **Glasgow coma score** (total score, e.g., 3–15) is applicable when all three components are testable. **Glasgow coma scale** (component score, e.g., E1 VNT M3) is applicable when any of the three components are not testable.
318. **True sebaceous cysts** develop in a rare condition known as steatocystoma multiplex.
319. **The Human papilloma virus (HPV) causing skin warts** is not oncogenic.
320. **Thickened hyalinized collagen** (keloidal collagen) is the hallmark of keloid.
321. **Reporting categories of core biopsy of breast lesions:** B1 (normal tissue); B2 (benign lesion); B3 (lesion of uncertain malignant potential); B4 (suspicious); B5 (malignant)—B5a-carcinoma in situ, B5b-invasive carcinoma, B5c-not possible to say whether carcinoma in situ or invasive carcinoma.
322. Potential immunohistochemistry markers for unknown primary cancers (to determine most likely cell lineage)—**Pankeratin (AE1/AE3, CAM 5.2)**—Carcinoma; **CK5/6, p63/p40**—Squamous cell carcinoma; **S100, SOX10**—melanoma and sarcoma.
323. **Anticipatory nausea and vomiting (ANV),** also known as conditioned, learned, or psychological nausea and vomiting develops in approximately 20% of patients before any cycle of chemotherapy.
324. **Maternofetal transmission of cancer** is rare, but reported in metastatic melanoma, lung cancer and certain hematologic malignancies.
325. HIV Medicine Association of the Infectious Diseases Society of America, International Anal Neoplasia Society, and the Association of Coloproctology of Great Britain and Ireland **recommend routine anal Pap test in people with HIV (PWH).**
326. Overall health status (e.g., organ dysfunction, nutritional state) are **more reliable predictors of surgical outcome than CD4+ T-cell count or viral load in patients with HIV**.
327. **Superficially invasive squamous cell carcinoma (SISCCA)** is defined as anal cancer that has been completely excised, with less than or equal to 3 mm basement membrane invasion and maximal horizontal spread of less than or equal to 7 mm. This histological type is commonly found incidentally following excision of a potentially benign lesion such as hemorrhoids, anal skin tag, or condyloma.
328. **Additional treatment strategies for people living with HIV (PLWH) who have anal cancer:** (a) Normal tissue-sparing radiation techniques; (b) Consideration of non-malignant causes for lymphadenopathy; and (c) More frequent surveillance anoscopy.
329. The presence of jaundice in gallbladder cancer patients carries poor prognosis.
330. MRI is the preferred imaging modality for evaluating masses within the gallbladder and demonstrating bile duct involvement.
331. **ER-low-positive breast cancers** are eligible for endocrine treatment but their biologic behavior is more similar to ER-negative cancers.
332. **RAHI (Retroauricular hairline incision) approach** initially developed for benign upper neck lesions for better cosmetic outcomes than traditional cervical incisions.
333. **'Rusty pipe syndrome':** Unilateral or bilateral bloody nipple discharge may be present during pregnancy or early lactation due to proliferative epithelial changes and increased vascularity of the breast. This condition is usually self-limited.

334. **Breast-implant associated anaplastic large cell lymphoma (BIA-ALCL)** is a disease of breast implant capsule and not of the breast tissue itself. Most of the BIA-ALCL are associated with textured implants.
335. **"Linguini" or "wavy-line" sign** in MRI without IV contrast is the most specific sign of intracapsular implant rupture.
336. **Silicone adenitis** may develop in the axillary lymph nodes following silicone implant rupture.
337. **DBT-ductography** (a technique combining digital breast tomosynthesis and ductography) is a promising tool for pathologic nipple discharge.
338. **Most of the recurrences in the reconstructed breast** are found in the skin and subcutaneous tissues.
339. **Targeted axillary dissection (TAD)** after neoadjuvant therapy in node-positive breast cancer is a new approach that includes clipping of the biopsy-proven metastatic nodes before neoadjuvant chemotherapy followed by excision of marked lymph node ("clipped node") and sentinel lymph nodes after neoadjuvant therapy.
340. Luminal subtype of breast cancers has a propensity to develop bone metastasis first, HER2-enriched cancers to liver and lung metastases, and basal-type cancers to liver and brain metastases.
341. American Board of Internal Medicine, European Society for Medical Oncology (ESMO), and Spanish Society of Medical Oncology (SEOM) discourage the use of imaging in asymptomatic patients with newly diagnosed early stage breast cancer.
342. Functional imaging studies of breast include: (i) Contrast-enhanced digital mammography (CEDM); (ii) Molecular breast imaging (MBI); (iii) FDG-PET breast dedicated; (iv) MRI breast; and (v) Abbreviated breast MRI (AB-MRI).
343. **Cisgender** terminology is used to describe any individual whose gender identity matches the sex assigned at birth. **Transgender** terminology is used for any individual whose gender identity differs from the sex assigned at birth.
344. A transfeminine is one who was assigned male at birth but identifies with the female side of the gender spectrum. A transmasculine is one who was assigned female at birth but identifies with the male side of the gender spectrum.
345. Gender-affirming breast surgeries, also known as "top surgery" includes reduction mammoplasty or mastectomy in transgender men and breast augmentation in transgender women.
346. **'Commotio cordis'** is fatal ventricular arrhythmia following blunt chest injury. It is an uncommon injury, but an important cause of sudden death in young players.
347. **Pancreatic duct disruption** is a complication particularly of necrotizing pancreatitis. This complication is better assessed by MRI with MRCP than CT. This complication should be excluded before planning for continuing conservative management or any drainage procedure because in the presence of duct disruption, these measures most likely fail.
348. Sport hernia (athletic pubalgia) is not a true hernia.
349. **Water-soluble contrast challenge** is a new protocol for predicting the success of conservative management of small bowel obstruction. This protocol includes oral or enteric tube administration of 100 mL of hyperosmolar iodinated contrast agent (diatrizoate meglumine or diatrizoate sodium diluted in 50 mL of water) followed by radiograph at 8 hours and 24 hours. Surgery is rarely required if contrast reaches the colon by 24 hours.
350. In February 2018, FDA has approved two blood-based biomarkers, ubiquitin C-terminal hydrolase L-1 (UCH-L1) and glial fibrillary acidic protein (GFAP) for determining the necessity of head CT in patients with mild TBI.
351. **The NeuroImaging Radiological Interpretation System (NIRIS)** is a recently developed CT scoring system which offers better prediction of management in TBI patients (who need prolonged admission/neurological intervention) as well as mortality. **NIRIS 0:** may be discharged; **NIRIS1:** hospital admission/follow-up imaging required; **NIRIS 2:** advanced care/critical care required; **NIRIS 3:** neurointervention or neurosurgery required; **NIRIS 4:** high risk of death.

352. **'Vibration white finger'** is the Raynaud's phenomenon of occupational origin following the use of vibrating tools.
353. **Superficial femoral artery** is the most commonly affected artery in chronic occlusive arterial disease.
354. **Sunset foot sign or dependent rubor** is found in critical limb ischemia. The leg becomes pallor on elevation to 45° and then reactive hyperemia on lowering of the leg.
355. **'Corkscrew collaterals'** is a characteristic arteriographic finding in Buerger's disease.
356. **Second branchial cleft fistula** passes through the bifurcation of carotid artery, whereas **third branchial cleft fistula** passes posterior to the carotid bifurcation.
357. **Based on the risk of nephrogenic systemic fibrosis (NSF), gadolinium-based contrast agents are classified into three groups:** (i) Class I- maximum risk of NSF; (ii) Class II- very low risk of NSF; and (iii) Class III- limited data.
358. An isolated cleft palate cannot be diagnosed by **antenatal ultrasound**. Cleft lip can be detected by antenatal USG scan after 18 weeks.
359. **Thin split thickness skin grafts have a better chance of engraftment** in comparison to thick STSG because they contain mostly epidermis (epidermis has less metabolic demand) whereas thick STSG contain more dermis (dermis has more metabolic demand).
360. **Primary contraction** is more significant in full thickness skin graft (FTSG) than STSG. **Secondary contraction** is more prominent in STSG than FTSG.
361. **Meshing of the STSG** significantly alters the aesthetics of the graft.
362. **Measures to minimize pain during injection of local anesthetics:** (i) Distracting conversation with the patient during injection; (ii) Stretching the area of injection; (iii) Use of smaller diameter needle; (iv) Skin piercing at an angle of 90° (traversing of minimum nerve endings); (v) Insertion of needle in a quick short manner; (vi) During injection, tapping of the adjacent skin with a finger (Gate control); and (vii) Injection of small volume pulses, not continuously.
363. **The second trimester is the safest period for surgery in pregnant surgical patients** because organogenesis has occurred and no risk of anesthetic induced malformation or spontaneous abortion.
364. Severe hypospadias associated with unilateral or bilateral undescended testes is associated with increased risk of **disorder of sexual differentiation (DSD)** than severe hypospadias with normally descended testes.
365. **Traditional monopolar electrosurgical devices** become less functioning in **liquid environment** because current is dispersed through liquid.
366. **Electrocautery** uses direct current whereas **electrosurgery** uses alternate current.
367. **Argon beam coagulator** is operated at a higher power setting than monopolar electrosurgery in coagulation mode.
368. For clinical use of Laser, **chromophore** is required to absorb the laser energy. In the human body, **melanin, hemoglobin and water are the available chromophores.**
369. The age-related increase in cancer risk is not applicable to childhood cancers.
370. **Climacteric** is the period of starting the decline in ovarian activity until after the end of ovarian function. This period includes peri-menopausal, menopausal, and post-menopausal state.
371. In female breast cancer, incidence rate increases rapidly with increasing age and then decline around climacteric. This point of inflection in incidence is termed '**Clemmesen's hook**'.
372. **'Breast tissue age'** is a better marker of risk for breast carcinoma in female breast cancer than chronological age.
373. **Obesity related increased risk of cancers**—endometrial cancer (strongest association), esophageal adenocarcinoma, carcinoma of gastric cardia, hepatocellular carcinoma, renal cell carcinoma, multiple myeloma, gallbladder carcinoma, and pancreatic carcinoma.

374. **Mammary analog secretory carcinoma** is a newly described salivary gland carcinoma that have *NTRK* gene fusion.
375. **Androgen receptor** is commonly absent in malignant salivary gland tumors except in salivary duct carcinoma and adenocarcinoma NOS.
376. **HER2 overexpression** may be found in **mucoepidermoid carcinoma of salivary gland** but not found in adenoid cystic carcinoma.
377. **Chronic dental disease** may be the risk factor for **cancers** in some specific sites of oral cavity, e.g., in the **lateral tongue, alveolar ridge, buccal mucosa.**
378. **The anterior accessory of the great saphenous vein (AAGSV)** accompanies the GSV, superficial to the GSV and not surrounded by saphenous fascial sheath. It is one of the causes of postoperative recurrence because it is often mistaken for GSV.
379. The great saphenous vein is the **most common site for venesection** and the **most commonly used conduit** for coronary artery bypass grafting.
380. Superficial veins of the lower limb lie superficial to the deep fascia but deep to the saphenous fascia.
381. Venous cut down in great saphenous vein is commonly performed at the ankle because of the predictable and superficial location of the vein.

MOST APPROPRIATE INVESTIGATIONS

1. Bowel ischemia or infarction is suspected: Contrast-enhanced CT
2. Hollow viscus perforation is suspected: Chest X-ray in erect posture
3. Assessment of spinal trauma: CT scan
4. Suspected head injury: Noncontrast CT scan (NCCT)
5. Bowel obstruction is suspected: Contrast-enhanced CT abdomen
6. Diverticulitis is suspected: Contrast-enhanced CT abdomen
7. Suspected acute cholecystitis: USG abdomen
8. Acute renal colic: Noncontrast CT KUB
9. Suspected abdominal aortic aneurysm rupture: CT angiography
10. Metastatic lung deposit: CT chest
11. Suspected intra-abdominal neoplasm: CT abdomen with IV contrast
12. Suspected abdominal wall mass: MRI abdomen without or with IV contrast
13. Acute onset flank pain (suspicion of urolithiasis) in pregnant patient: Color Doppler US of kidney and bladder
14. Acute onset scrotal pain, without trauma, without antecedent mass: Duplex Doppler US of scrotum
15. Suspected acute pancreatitis, initial presentation with typical symptoms and signs, significantly elevated amylase and lipase: USG abdomen.
16. Suspected acute pancreatitis, initial presentation and serum amylase, lipase values equivocal, other diagnostic possibilities (e.g., bowel ischemia, bowel perforation): CT abdomen and pelvis with IV contrast.
17. Acute pancreatitis, critically ill, development of SIRS, severe clinical scores, more than 48–72 hours after onset of symptoms: CT abdomen and pelvis with IV contrast.
18. Suspected necrotizing pancreatitis: CT abdomen and pelvis with IV contrast.
19. Male younger than 25 years with indeterminate palpable breast mass: USG breast.
20. Male 25 years or older with indeterminate palpable breast mass: Diagnostic mammography or diagnostic digital breast tomosynthesis (DBT).
21. Male of any age with palpable breast mass suspicious for breast cancer: Diagnostic mammography or diagnostic DBT.
22. Female younger than 30 years with clinically significant noncyclical mastalgia: USG breast.
23. Female of 30–39 years with clinically significant noncyclical mastalgia: Diagnostic mammography or diagnostic DBT.
24. Female 40 years or older with clinically significant noncyclical mastalgia: Diagnostic mammography or diagnostic DBT.
25. Subacute or chronic traumatic brain injury with new neurologic deficit: MRI head without IV contrast.
26. Suspected CSF rhinorrhea: CT maxillofacial without IV contrast.
27. Suspected CSF otorrhea: CT temporal bone without IV contrast.
28. Suspected cephalocele following trauma: MRI head without IV contrast.
29. In patients with suspected sclerosing cholangitis or biliary stricture: MRCP.
30. For characterization of indeterminate focal liver lesions of any size: MRI without and with contrast.
31. Suspected acute mesenteric ischemia: CTA abdomen and pelvis with IV contrast.
32. Suspected chronic mesenteric ischemia: CTA abdomen and pelvis with IV contrast or MRA abdomen with pelvis without and with IV contrast.

33. Known breast cancer, axillary evaluation: USG of axilla.
34. To determine response after completion of neoadjuvant chemotherapy for breast cancer: MRI of breast.
35. After completion of neoadjuvant therapy, axillary evaluation: USG of axilla.
36. Penetrating neck injury with clinical soft injury signs: CTA neck with IV contrast.
37. Penetrating neck injury, normal or equivocal CTA, suspected aerodigestive tract injury: Panendoscopy (laryngoscopy, bronchoscopy, and esophagoscopy).
38. Suspected appendicitis: CT abdomen and pelvis with IV contrast.
39. Suspected appendicitis in pregnancy: USG abdomen or MRI abdomen and pelvis without IV contrast.
40. Suspected lower extremity deep vein thrombosis: Duplex Doppler USG of lower extremity.
41. Suspected choledocholithiasis: MRCP.
42. Suspected hemopericardium following chest trauma: USG of the pericardium.
43. Diffuse axonal injury (DAI) is suspected: MRI of brain.
44. Sphincter of Oddi dysfunction: Sphincter of Oddi manometry.
45. For diagnosis of non-obstetric abdominal pain in pregnancy: USG or MRI without IV gadolinium.
46. Suspected emphysematous cholecystitis: CT abdomen.
47. Suspected gangrenous cholecystitis: CT abdomen.
48. Hydatid cyst of liver: USG abdomen.
49. Hydatid cyst of lung: CT scan of thorax
50. Hydatid cyst of brain: CT brain.
51. For delineation of anatomy and location of paraesophageal hernia: Barium esophagram.
52. Screening for Barrett's esophagus: Conventional endoscopy.
53. Suspected esophageal perforation: Contrast-enhanced CT or CT esophagography.
54. Suspected necrotizing fasciitis: MRI.
55. Patient with obscure gastrointestinal bleeding: Small-bowel video capsule endoscopy.
56. For evaluation of pancreatic cyst: Gadolinium-enhanced MRI with MRCP.

Index

A

Abdomen 49, 331
anterior 613, 614
computed tomography scan of 52, 84, 90, 112, 115, 124, 126, 226, 236, 238, 253, 272, 298, 304, 316, 318, 339, 360, 373
examination of 101, 157, 158, 237, 290, 373, 615, 751
plain X-ray of 298, 304
secondary survey of 581
straight X-ray of 52, 316, 372, 751
ultrasonography of 52, 80, 388, 684
X-ray of 112, 114, 253
Abdominal closure, techniques of 646
Abdominal compartment syndrome 645
management of 170
Abdominal esophagus 774
perforation, management of 787
Abdominal procedures 395
advantages of 395
disadvantages of 395
Abdominal tenderness 253, 339
degree of 679
Abdominal wall 218, 220
compliance 645
defects 891
congenital 220
elevation of 933
hernia 730
injuries 617
Abdominal wound, penetrating 614
Abdominoperineal excision 426
types of 426
Abdominoperineal resection 426, 429
Aberrant obturator artery 729
Aberrant tissue 303
Ablation 135, 140
Abscess 120, 380
acute pilonidal 417
amebic liver 102, 111, 119, 120
anorectal 401
breast 446
central 440
cold 741
complex 826
deeper 401
drainage of 332, 401, 878
intersphincteric 402
ischiorectal 402
submucosal 402
supralevator 402
formation 113
interloop 229
intra-abdominal 228, 295
intraperitoneal 228, 229
liver 101, 112, 113, 129, 144, 157
lung 114
multiple 113, 229
pelvic 230
perianal 401
peri-areolar 440
perinephric 878
peripheral 440
pilonidal 417, 443
pyogenic 157
recurrent subareolar 441
renal 879
retroperitoneal 228, 233
septic epidural 114
simple 826
splenic 211
subareolar 453
superficial 401
visceral 228
Absorbable mesh 629
Abstinence 183
Acceleration injury 582
Accessory spleen 209
location of 209
Accidental intermediate host 123
Acetic acid injection 140
Achalasia 778, 794
dilator 780
manometric subtypes of 779
Achilles reflex 491
Acid
base balance, disorders of 16
neutralizing 247
production 564
Acidic substances, injury patterns of 789
Acidosis 644
metabolic 27, 643
respiratory 28, 943
Acinetobacter 38
Acne inversa 825
Acoustic shadowing 1071
Actinomyces israelii 852
Actinomycosis 404, 853
Activated partial thromboplastin time 32
Acute care surgery classification 1059
Acute cholangitis
development of 74
management of 47, 75
Acute cholecystitis 45-47, 120, 157, 201
characteristic of 45
complications of 48
diagnostic criteria for 45
severity grading for 46
Acute lung injury, transfusion-related 37, 39
Acute nonimmune-mediated reactions 36, 37
Acute pancreatitis
classification of 164
grading of severity of 168
phases of 164
score 1065
Adalimumab 310, 311, 825
Addison's disease 493, 511
Adductor reflex 742
Adenocarcinoma 88, 89, 93, 264, 323, 324, 340, 357, 426, 794, 808, 897, 899
affects 794
esophageal 795
histologic appearance of 357
mucinous 265, 357
papillary 89, 265
risk factors for 794
tubular 265
Adenoma 88, 111
carcinoma
ex pleomorphic 808
sequence 356
lactating 446
microscopic features of 546
multiple 135
pleomorphic 803, 807
synchronous 423
toxic 492, 504
tubular 351
tubulovillous 351
villous 351
Adenomyomatosis 53
Adenosine diphosphate receptor antagonists 32
Adenosis, sclerosing 443
Adhesions 294, 295
classification of 296
peritoneal 295
Adhesive small bowel obstruction 301
Adiposis dolorosa 823
Adjuvant bisphosphonate therapy 479

Adjuvant endocrine therapy 478
- selection of 479

Adjuvant systemic therapy 478, 837
Adnexa, diseases of 816
Adrenal artery
- inferior 544
- middle 544
- superior 544

Adrenal crisis 554
Adrenal Cushing's syndrome 548
- surgery for 551

Adrenal gland
- diseases of 544
- microscopic features of 545

Adrenal hyperplasia, congenital 757
Adrenal insufficiency, acute 554
Adrenal mass 558
Adrenal medulla, diseases of 555
Adrenal surgery, approaches of 559
Adrenal vein drains 544
Adrenalectomy 547
- laparoscopic 547, 560

Adrenocorticotropic hormone
- deficiency 447
- stimulation test 553

Adrenogenital syndrome 552
Advanced endoscopic imaging
- modalities 267, 272
- techniques 267

Advanced laparoscopic cholecystectomy technique 47
Aerodigestive tract injury 581
Afferent loop syndrome 288
Aflatoxin 136
Agenesis, bilateral renal 861
Agitation 577
Agranulocytosis 500
- management of 500

Air plethysmography 696
Airway 598
- injury
  - major 609
  - management of 596
- maintenance 577
- management 576, 652
- obstruction 591, 603
  - signs of 577
- surgical 591

Alanine transferase, increased level of 114
Albendazole therapy 159
Albumin, serum 345
Albuterol 22
Alcohol
- active 143
- consumption 177
- use 794

Alfuzosin 902
Alimentary tract, physiological narrowing of 791
Alkali administration 27
Alkaline
- reflux gastritis 288
- substances 789

Alkalosis
- metabolic 27
- respiratory 28

Allergic reaction 36
Allgrove disease 778
Allis tissue forceps 1000
Alloimmunization 37
Alonso-Lej classification 79, 1059
Alpha1-antitrypsin deficiency 685
Alpha-adrenergic blockers 556, 902, 907
Alpha-blockers 902
Alpha-fetoprotein 924
Alpha-methydopa 234
Alpha-methyltyrosine 556
Altemeier procedure 396
Alvarado score 378, 379
Alveolar echinococcosis 123
Amastia 438
Amazia 438
Ambulatory reflux monitoring 775, 776
Amenorrhea 496
American Association for Surgery of Trauma
- duodenal injury scale 619
- grading of renal injuries 634
- liver trauma grading 627
- pancreatic injury scale 621
- splenic trauma grading 630

Aminoglycosides 21, 25
Amiodarone 489, 492
Amnesia 988
Amniotic fluid 221
Amphotericin 21, 25
Amputation 678, 709
Amyand's hernia 749
Amylase 163
- serum 166

Anabolic androgenic steroid therapy 135
Anal canal 402, 430
- anatomical 430
- cancer 430, 1084
  - nonmetastatic 431
- diseases of 390
- invasive carcinomas of 430
- palpation of 404
- surgical 430

Anal crypts 401
Anal cushions 409
- blood supply of 409
- prolapse of 409

Anal fissure 398
- acute 399
- chronic 399
- management of low-pressure 399

Anal fistula
- complex 403
- simple 403

Anal intraepithelial neoplasia, treatment of 431
Anal stenosis, causes of 414
Anal subepithelial muscles, rupture of 409
Anal transitional zone 430
Analgesia 655, 988, 1080
- epidural 987

Analgesic
- abuse 897
- nonopiod 988

Anaphylactic reaction 37
Anaplastic carcinoma 513, 523
- treatment of 524

Anastomotic biliary stricture 78
Androgen 908
- ablation 910
  - methods of 910
- deficiency 447
- receptor 808, 1087
- therapy 449

Anemia 291, 308, 373
- pernicious 493, 511

Anesthesia 981
- epidural 987
- general 722
- induction of 990
- local 983
- maintenance of 991
- neuroaxial 985
- regional 722
- spinal 986
- types of 983

Aneurysm 681
- aortic 683
- distal 211
- proximal 211
- size 684
- true 682
- types of 681

Angiectasia bleeding, management of 370
Angina, intestinal 680
Angiodysplasia 259
Angioembolization 370, 630
- indications of 256
- role of 628, 630

Angiogenesis 6
Angiography 627
Angiomyolipoma 882
Angioplasty, percutaneous transluminal 678
Angiosarcoma 701, 838
- forms of 838

Animal bites 641
Anion gap 27
Anisocoria 585
Anisocytosis 214
Ankaferd blood stopper 258, 371

Ankle
brachial index 676, 704, 708
flare 694
Ankylosing spondylitis 234
Anoderm 430
Anomalous biliopancreatic duct junction, presence of 79
Anorectal abscess 401
drainage tract, epithelialization of 403
horseshoe type 402
occult 401
types of 401
Anorectal disorders, treatment of 420
Anorectal lesions 308
management of 313
Anorectal manometry 394
Anorectal ring 430
Anorectal sepsis, complex 401
Anorectal suppurative process 403
Anorexia 137, 281, 324
Anterior compartment group 965
Anterior cord syndrome 599
Anterior cranial fossa fracture 584
signs of 580
Anterior flail segment 602
Anterior spinal artery 598
injury of 599
Anterior urethra 639, 640, 910
penetrating injuries of 640
straddle injuries of 640
Antiandrogens 910
Antibiotics 33, 85, 116, 380, 907
oral 158
prophylaxis 156, 215, 722
selection of 116
therapy 117
parenteral 117
Antibody
antimitochondrial 86
synthesis of 208
Anticholinergic 346, 902
agents 902
Anticoagulant drugs 33
Anticonvulsants 590
judicious use of 590
Anti-inflammatory property 697
Anti-integrin therapy 310
Antimicrobial
prophylaxis 992
topical 657
Antiplatelet therapy 677
Antireflux surgery 778
indications of 777
Anti-saccharomyces cerevisiae antibodies 309
Antithyroid drugs 489, 490, 500, 509
side effects of 500
Antitubercular therapy 316
Anti-tumor necrosis factor therapy 346
Antral sparing 281
Anus
cancer of 430
tumors of 430
visual inspection of 412
Anxiety 311
Aorta 611
abdominal 672
descending thoracic 611
infrarenal 683
Aortic dissection 686
diagnosis of 687
proximal 687
Aortitis, inflammatory 686
Aortobifemoral bypass 678
Aortoiliac occlusive disease 678
Ape-hand deformity 952
Aperture, abnormal 747
Apfel score 1065, 1079
Apocrine gland bearing 825
Aponeurosis 740
Apoptosis 1070
Appendage
testicular 766
torsion 760
Appendectomy 380, 381
different laparoscopic approaches of 380
drain after 382
laparoscopic 383, 384
open 381
Appendiceal mass 386
Appendicectomy 387
Appendicitis
acute 232, 376-380, 385
complicated 378, 379
inflammatory response score 379, 1064
Izbicki scoring system for 1066
subhepatic acute 46
Appendicular lumen, obstruction of 376
Appendicular stump closure, methods of 384
Appendix 374
cannulation of 387
different positions of 377
epididymis 760
neoplasm of 387
testis 760
torsion of 760
Apple-core lesion 795
Appropriate repair technique, selection of 689
Aqueous glutaraldehyde solution 938
Argon beam coagulation system 629, 1082
Aromatase inhibitors 478
Arterial diseases 665
Arterial injury
hard signs of 632
soft signs of 632
Arterial occlusion, chronic mesenteric 680
Arterial occlusive disease 676
Arterial tumor contact 195
Artery 632
occlusion
large 844
small 844
partial transection of 1083
renal 633
Arthritis, septic 114
Arthropathy 308
Artificial bowel sphincter 420
Arytenoid cartilage resection 951
Ascaris lumbricoides 44, 84, 302
Ascites 409
refractory 152
Ashkenazi Jewish heritage 454
Aspergillus 162
flavus 136
parasiticus 136
Aspiration
percutaneous 122
pneumonia 326
test 933
therapeutic 915
Aspirin 32, 677
low-dose 692
Ataxia-telengiectasia 265
Atelectasis 114
Athelia 438
Atherectomy 678
Atheroma
development, stages of 668
pathophysiology of 668
Atherosclerosis 667, 682
Atherosclerotic plaques 669
complications of 669
Atlanta classification, revised 1059
Atracurium 988
Atresia
biliary 78
congenital 294
esophageal 501
intestinal 221, 327
Atrial fibrillation 496, 670
Atrial myxoma 670
Atrial septal defect 490
Atrophic gastritis, multifocal 262
Atrophie blanche 694
Atrophy 675
Atypia 443, 453
Augment residual reservoir function 426
Autogenous vein bypass graft 678
Autoimmune
diseases 493, 511, 831
disorders 210, 234, 701
Autoimmunity, role of 85
Autologous fat 951
Autologous reconstruction method 472

Autologous vein graft 596
Axilla 825, 951
  examination of 484
  management of 475
Axillary dissection 475
  complications of 475
Axillary line, anterior 57
Axillary lymph node
  dissection, indications of 475
  level of 475
Axillary reverse mapping 476
Axillo breast approach, bilateral 528
Axillobifemoral bypass 678
Axillo-bilateral breast approach 528
Axonotmesis 948, 949
Azathioprine 310

B

Babbitt's theory 79
Babcock tissue forceps 1001
Babesiosis 38
Bacilis fragilis 48
Backwash ileitis 87
Bacteria
  anerobic 254
  opsonization of 208
  pyogenic 702
Bailey classification 1055
Bail-out procedure 58
Baker classification 1055
Balanitis xerotica obliterans 917
Ball of Wool' sign 127
Balloon
  angioplasty 680
  dilation 260, 779
  embolectomy 671
  enteroscopy 324
    simple 326
  guided endoscopy 326
  tamponade 151
Balthazar original grading
    system 169, 1065
Band ligation 370
Barbed sutures, types of 1077
Barbiturates 988
Bard Parker handle 997
Barium 785, 791
  enema 344
  enteroclysis 324
  esophagogram 781, 795
  study 316, 795
  swallow 787, 795
Barrett's epithelium 792
Barrett's esophagus 241, 264, 792-794
  diagnosis of 793
  management of 793
  nondysplastic 793
  risk factors for 792
  surveillance of 793
Barrett's technique 129
Barrter's syndrome 27
Bartholin's duct 803
Basal adherences 1080
Basal cell
  carcinoma 829
  nevus syndrome 830
Bascom's technique 419
Bascom's theory 417
Basophilic stippling 214
Bassini repair, modified 724
Baux score 1065
  revised 1068
Bazin's ulcer 852
B-cell lymphoma, diffuse large 280
Beck's triad 610
Beckwith-Wiedemann syndrome 220, 222
Beger procedure 184, 187
  Berne modification of 184
Behavior, aggressive 561
Behçet's disease 690
Bell-Clapper deformity 759
Benign colonic obstruction 340
  causes of 340
Bent inner tube sign 335
Benzodiazepines 988
Berg's level 475
Berry aneurysm 682
Best eye-opening response 1084
Best motor response 588
Best possible score 588
Beta-blockers 234, 556
Beta-cell function, impaired 181
Bethesda criteria, revised 1060
Bethesda system 507
Bevacizumab therapy 364
Bevan technique 727
Bezoars 283
Bible cyst 1079
Bicarbonate synthesis 27
Bilayer mesh repair 725
Bile duct 80
  carcinoma of 80
  cyst 111
  dilatation, asymptomatic 1071
  epithelium of 92
  injury 61
    classification of 61
  intrahepatic 85
  obstruction 181
  stone, secondary 66
Bile reflux gastritis 263
Bile stone, primary 66
Bilhemia, causes of 77
Biliary atresia 78
  classification of 1057
Biliary enteric bypass 73, 85, 199
  methods of 199
Biliary obstruction, malignant 111
Biliary pancreatitis 170
  management of 170
  mild 51, 170
Biliary stenting 95, 199
  approaches of 96
  complications of 97
Biliary stones, irretrievable 97
Biliary stricture 78, 83, 129
  diagnosis of 78
  management of 78, 184
  nonanastomotic 78
Biliary symptoms, history of 52
Biliary system
  anomalous anatomy of 99
  cholangiographic evaluation of 65
  endoscopic therapeutic
      approaches of 98
  pathologies of 43
Biliary tract 77, 111
  exploration, different option of 51
  pathology of 115
Biliary tree 77
Bilio-enteric fistula, types of 52
Bilirubin, significant elevation of serum 46
Bimodal age distribution 305
Biochemical tests 556
Biologic mesh 749
Biomarkers, serum 138, 379
Biopsy 90, 138, 278, 309, 344, 431, 441, 449,
    886, 895
  endoscopic 266
  excision 459, 460, 836
  preoperative 236
  proven axillary metastases 475
  stereotactic 462
  techniques 459, 462
  transperitoneal 94
  treatment of 431
Bipolar electrosurgery 939, 940
Bird Beak sign 337
Bisegmentectomy 142
Bismuth quadruple therapy 248
Bismuth-Corlette
  classification 1055
  staging system, modified 93
Bisphosphonates 24, 241
Black pigment stone 43, 43
Bladder 897
  augmentation 892
  calculi 892
  cancer 896
    schistosoma associated 895
  exstrophy of 891
  injury 638, 726
    uncomplicated extraperitoneal 638
  lesions 897
  neck contracture 903
  outlet obstruction 892

pain 860
psoas hitch 637
trauma, internal iatrogenic 638
tumor 896
types of 896
washings 898
Blair incision, modified 811
Bland transarterial embolization 144
Blast injuries 614
Blatchford score 256
Bleeding 97, 322, 326
causes of perioperative 58
gastric ulcer, emergency surgery of 259
gastrointestinal 320, 369
major 692
management of 9, 277, 364
painless 412
peptic ulcer 255, 256, 281
nonoperative management of 256
rectal 412, 422
risk factors for 255
sources of internal 578
time 32
vessel 629
proximal control of 689
Bleomycin 690, 972
Blind
clamping 578
loop syndrome 319
Blisters 656
deroofing of 656
management of 656
Blood 639
components 36
flow, stasis of 690
gas analysis 915
group antigen-binding adhesin 242
loss, estimated 1081
pressure 547
product resuscitation 38
stained nipple discharge 450
transfusion
complications of 36
massive 38
vessels 537
Bloody nipple discharge 449, 453
Bloody stool, pathophysiology of 304
Bloom syndrome 265
Blue dot sign 760
Blue dye 476, 477
Blue light cystoscopy 898
Blue nevus 827, 828
Blue toe syndrome 670
Blumgart staging system 93
Blunt cardiac injury 603, 610
Blunt esophageal rupture 603
Blunt liver trauma 627
Blunt scrotal injury 643
Blunt trauma 217, 611, 613, 615, 622, 643, 784
abdomen 617
management of 614
mechanisms of 572
Boari bladder flap 637
Bochdalek hernia 749, 1078
Boerhaave syndrome 281, 784
Boey score 254, 1065
Bolus obstruction, causes of 302
Bone
disease 537
metastasis 458
pain 24
Bony structures, examination of 592
Borrmann's classification system 266
Bosniak classification 1055
Boston bowel preparation scale 1065
Botulinum toxin 399, 779
injection 813
Bowel injury 617, 726
Bowel preparation, preoperative 992
Bowen's disease 829, 917
Bowenoid papulosis 917
Brachial plexus 951
Brain
computed tomography scan of 584
contusion 584
injury, secondary 582
metastasis 458
tumors 353
Branchial cyst 970
types of 970
Branchial sinus 971
Breast 436, 690
abscess 446
drainage of 440
lactational 439
nonlactational 440
treatment of 439
approach, endoscopic 528
biopsy
excisional 461
stereotactic 463
cancer 145, 454, 464, 468, 476, 483
axillary 482
early 467, 469
inflammatory 483
invasive 464
ipsilateral 469
major 482
molecular subtypes of 467
positive 1084
screening 464, 465
syndrome, hereditary 265, 454
carcinoma 446, 448, 449, 451, 453, 454, 468, 485, 1079
management of 482
spread of 458
suggestive of 458
conserving therapy 480
advantages of 469
cyst 446
density category 466
development of 438
diagnostic magnetic resonance imaging of 466
disease 438
fibrocystic 449
examination 484
normal 451
hypertrophy, juvenile 444
imaging-reporting and data system 466
irradiation, whole 481
lesions
core biopsy of 1084
histologic classification of benign 443
nonpalpable 461, 462
palpable 459
pain 451
chart, maintenance of 452
reconstruction 471
types of 471
screening of 465
tissue age 1086
tuberculosis of 442
ultrasonography of 441, 442, 484
ultrasound of 451
Breath sounds 605
abnormal 577
Breathing 578, 653
Bristol stool form scale 1065
Broad-spectrum antibiotics 116, 299
Bromocriptine 452
Bronchitis, chronic 309
Bronchodilators 21
Bronchoscopy 796
Bronchus 350
Brooke ileostomy 348
Broslow pediatric emergency tape 1075
Brown pigment stones 43, 84
pathogenesis of 44
Brown-Séquard syndrome 599
Bruit 675
Brush cytology 795
Brushite stone 867, 888
Buccal mucosa 1087
Buck's fascia 766, 917, 1083
Budd-Chiari syndrome 134, 148, 154
causes of 148
Budesonide 346
multimatrix 346
Buerger's disease 679, 690, 844
Buffalo hump 704
Bupivacaine 985, 986
Burn 649
care of 662
chemical 662

contact 651
deep dermal 657
depth of 653
electric 660
estimation of percentage of 653
flame 651
injury 241
management of 652
mechanisms of 651
treatment of 654
late complications of 662
scar 659
wound
cleansing of 656
surgical management of 658
zone of 654
Bypass grafting 680

C

Cajal interstitial cells 278
Calcification
eggshell' pattern of 683
metastatic 537
Calcitonin 535
estimation of serum 551
Calcium 23
bilirubinate stones 77
carbonate apatite stones 868
channel blockers 557
topical 399
dobesilate 413, 697
gluconate, intravenous 26
high serum 537
homeostasis 535
ionized 39
oxalate stone 867, 870, 888
phosphate stone 867
formation 867
serum 23
Calculi, secondary 892
Calorie requirements, calculation of 659
Calot's triangle
dissection of 50, 60
exposure of 60
Calprotectin 345
Cambridge classification 182
Cameron ulcer 259, 774
Cancer 9
anal canal 430, 1084
breast 467
colon 354, 364
colorectal 145, 146, 412, 1080
development of 757
esophageal 259
esophagogastric junction 794
gallbladder 89
gastric 241, 259, 268, 273, 289
gastroesophageal junction 264
genome atlas 1080
hallmarks of 1079
invasive breast 464
likelihood of 466
maternofetal transmission of 1084
metastatic 796
nonmelanoma skin 833
pancreatic 689
perianal 430
predisposition 350, 353
syndromes, hereditary 265, 794
rectal 421, 423
signs of 1079
small cell 93
surveillance 354
symptoms of 1079
synchronous 361
testicular 922
thyroid 513, 523
urothelial 888, 897
Candida albicans 787
Cannula, different sizes of 1017
Cantle's line 1070
Cantrell pentalogy 220
Capecitabine 92
Caprini score 692, 1065
Capsule, incomplete 807
Carbimazole 500
dosage of 500
Carbohydrate 659, 992
Carbuncle 825, 879
Carcinoembryonic antigen
estimation 360
role of 423
Carcinogenesis, late 348
Carcinoid syndrome, symptoms of 324
Carcinoma 90, 512, 766
adenoid cystic 807, 808
adenosquamous 357
anal 430
anaplastic 513, 523
basal cell 829
bile duct 80
bladder 1079
breast 446, 448, 449, 451, 453, 454, 468, 485, 1079
colon 311, 356
colorectal 348, 1079
embryonal 923
esophageal 794, 1079
fibrolamellar hepatocellular 137
follicular 512, 513, 515, 518-520
gallbladder 91, 102, 141, 1079
hepatocellular 136, 141
inflammatory 439
intramucosal 796
liver 447
medullary 357, 513
thyroid 520
mixed 265
mucoepidermoid 807, 808
neuroendocrine 357
pancreatic 181, 191
papillary 513, 514, 1079
penis 917
periampullary 1079
prostate 907
rectal 422
rectum 311, 425
renal cell 145, 882
scrotum 766
small cell 357, 897, 899
spindle cell 357
squamous cell 93, 357, 430, 701, 794, 818, 831, 895, 897, 899, 1079
thyroid 513, 514, 523
types of 829
verrucous 833
Card-board rigidity 253
Cardiac arrest management 576
Cardiac emboli 670
sources of 670
Cardiac failure, congestive 152, 496, 697
Cardiac injury
inadvertent 612
penetrating 610
Cardiac malformations 490
Cardiac monitor 941
Cardiac tamponade 603
Cardiac valves 537
Cardiff breast clinic 452
Cardiopulmonary arrest 576
Cardiopulmonary disease, severe 143
Cardiorespiratory disease 339
Cardiovascular dysfunction 46
Caroli's disease 77, 80, 83
Carotid
artery, internal 595
body tumor 971
subclavian bypass 676
Cartilage 1070
based point-of-care viscoelastic tests 1081
color of 433
Caruncle, inflammation of 497
Caseation necrosis 315
Catecholamine excess, documentation of 556
Caterpillar hump 1071
Catheter drainage 122
Catheterization 638, 892
Cattell-Braasch maneuver 633
Cauda equina syndrome 599, 600
Caudate lobe 1072
Caustic injury 788, 790
complications of 789
histopathologic phases of 789
severity of 788

Cavernosal tissue, excessive debridement of 642
Cavernospongious shunt 916
Cavity
abdominal 932
pelvic 613
peritoneal 227, 717, 746
Cecal bascule 337
Cecal volvulus 337
types of 337
Cecum 362
dilation 339
Ceftriaxone 156
Celiac angiography, venous phase 212
Celiac axis 195
Celiac disease 87, 309, 323, 324
Celiac plexus nerve block 183
Cellular component 669
Cellulitis 826
Cellulose, oxidized regenerated 34
Centchroman 452
Central cord syndrome 599, 600
Central nervous system disease 990
Central vascular ligation 361
Central venous catheterization 1070
Cephalosporin 33
Cerebral concussion 582
Cernea classification 527, 1056
Certolizumab pegol 310, 311
Cervical anastomosis 797
advantages of 797
Cervical collar 851
Cervical esophagus 784
perforation, management of 786
Cervical incision 797
Cervical lymph node metastases 968
bilateral 1077
Cervical pap test 431
Cervical spinal injury 598
Cervical spine 581
motion, respiratory swing of 577
secondary survey of 581
Cetrimide solution 128
Cetuximab 281
Chagas disease 38
Charcot's triad 75
Cheatle slit 1073
Chemical
promoting platelet aggregation 32
sterilization, different methods of 938
Chemoembolization, transarterial 145
Chemoradiotherapy, concurrent 431
Chemosis 497
Chemotherapy 122, 128, 226, 280, 445, 690, 924
adjuvant 478, 479
systemic 479
antitubercular 967
neoadjuvant 92, 481
principles of 131
regimens 479
systemic adjuvant 479
Chest
computed tomography scan of 360, 373
drain 607, 608
indications of 607
insertion, techniques of 608
tube, tip of 609
pain, pleuritic 451
secondary survey of 581
tube 609
X-ray 114, 253, 449, 604, 608
Chicago classification 1056
Chief cell 534
Chilaiditi syndrome 1079
Child-Pugh scoring 139
Chimney Sweeper's cancer 766, 831
Chlamydia
pneumoniae infection 682
trachomatis 761
Chlorpromazine 450
Choanal atresia 501
Cholangiocarcinoma 86, 87, 92
distal 94, 103
extrahepatic 93
hepatocellular 137
intrahepatic 93, 94, 95
metastatic extrahepatic 95
mimic extrahepatic 94
molecular profiling of 93
resectable hilar 95
Cholangiogram 1072
Cholangiohepatitis, oriental 83
Cholangitis 66, 75, 87, 94, 97, 170
acute 74
concomitant primary sclerosing 309
management of 85
recurrent 80
bacterial 83, 84
pyogenic 83
sclerosing 234, 511
secondary sclerosing 86
Cholecystectomy 44, 48, 53, 54, 56, 58, 67, 78, 92, 102, 106
complications of 58
delayed 102
early 102
extended 106
laparoscopic 50, 56, 57, 103
prophylactic 56
Cholecystitis 97
acute 45-47, 120, 157, 201
acalculous 54
emphysematous 48
chronic 49
calculous 102
gangrenous 48
Cholecystoenteric fistula 48
Cholecystojejunostomy 199
Cholecystoses 53
Cholecystostomy, percutaneous 48, 54
Choledochal cyst 77, 79, 80
classification of 79
Choledochoduodenostomy 73
complications of 73
Choledochojejunostomy 199
Choledocholithiasis 66, 86, 103
predictors for 67
Choledocholithotomy 72
Choledochoscope 69
Cholelithiasis 80, 308
Cholera, pancreatic 565
Cholestasis 179, 500
Cholesterol 667, 677
esters 53
polyp 53
precursors 53
pseudopolyp 88
stones 43, 77
pathogenesis of 44
Cholesterolosis 53
polyp 53
Cholestyramine 285
Chondrocalcinosis 537
Choriocarcinoma 923
Chromaffin cells 545
Chromoendoscopy, virtual 267
Chromophobe renal cell cancer 884
Chromophore 1086
Chronic calculous cholecystitis 102
gold standard treatment of 50
Chronic hepatitis 102
C infection 1070
Chronic idiopathic inflammatory disease 305
Chronic pancreatitis 177-182, 212
classification of 177
stages of 179
Chronic subdural hematoma 587
pathophysiology of 587
Chvostek's sign 23, 543
Chylocele 765
Chylomicron, presence of 707
Chylothorax 707
Chylous ascites 707, 926
Chylous pleural effusion 707
Chyluria 707
Cilostazol 677, 709
Cimetidine 448
Circumcision 767
clamps 767
complications of 767
indications of 767
methods of neonatal 767
radical 919

Circumferential resection margin 361, 423
Cirrhosis 50, 87, 136, 149, 241
  alcoholic 447
  compensated 149
  decompensated 137, 149
  nonalcoholic 447
  secondary biliary 80
Cisplatin 21, 25, 92
Clamping, duration of 629
Clarithromycin triple therapy 248
Classical surgical method 767
Claudication
  distance 674
  intermittent 674
Claus model 455
Clavien-Dindo classification 1056
Claw hand deformity 952
Clear cell 534
Cleft
  fistula, second branchial 1086
  lift technique 419
  lip 976, 978, 979
    classification of 978
    repair, principles of 979
  palate 976, 980
Clemmesen's hook 1086
Clindamycin 825
Clinical activity score 497
Clinical scoring system 378
Clips
  migration, complications of 58
  types of 937
Clonorchis sinensis 44, 84, 93
Clopidogrel 677
Cloquet's hernia 728, 749
Closed loop obstruction 296
Clostridium
  difficile colitis 343
  perfringens 48
Clot
  formation time 33
  initiation 33
  lysis of 33
  strength 33
Clothesline injury 596
Clotting time 32
Coagulation 30
  infrared 414
  waveform 940
  zone of 654
Coagulopathy 39, 643, 644
Coated vicryl plus 1013
Cock's peculiar tumor 818
Coffee bean sign 335, 337
Coils, migration of 762
Cold
  nodule 506
  sensitivity test 821
  snare polypectomy 352
Colectomy
  laparoscopic 364
  minimally invasive approaches of 364
  total abdominal 348
  types of 362, 363
Colitides, infectious 343
Colitis
  amebic 351
  fulminant 311, 342
  ischemic 351
  mild 342
  severe 311, 342
Collagen
  types of 6, 8
  vascular disease 7
Collar stud abscess 967
Colles' fascia 766
Colloid 29
  goiter 504
  role of 655
Colon
  adenocarcinoma of 340
  ascending 362
  cancer 354, 364
    management of 361
    resectable 361
    spread of 358
    surgery 421
    types of 354
  cut-off sign 165
  diverticular disease of 330
  injuries 623
  interposition 796
  ischemia, features suggestive of 339
  metastatic tumor of 340
  regional lymph nodes of 358
Colonic arterial supply, collateral pathways of 1073
Colonic obstruction 340
  benign 340
  malignant 340
Colonography, computed tomography scan of 373
Colonoscopy 94, 309, 316, 360, 373, 394, 422, 423
  guided biopsy 373
  surveillance 348
Colorectal anastomosis 336
Colorectal cancer 145, 146, 412, 1080
  hereditary nonpolyposis 354
  management of 429
  molecular pathways of 355
  synchronous 423
Colostomy 420
Comet tail 88
Common bile duct, tangential injury of 62
Common hepatic duct 100
Commotio cordis 1085
Compartmental syndromes 645
Complete esophageal obstruction, clinical signs of 791
Complete mesocolic excision 361
Complete rectal prolapse 392-394
  differential diagnosis of 393
Complete square knot 1077
Complex esophageal stricture 787
Component separation technique 739
Compound nevus 827
Compound volvulus 338
Compression
  garment 706
  stockings, types of 697
  therapy 697, 701
Computed tomography
  abdominal 617, 627
  angiography 676, 680
  contrast-enhanced 335
  scoring system 167
Concussion, grading of 1083
Concussive 614
Confocal laser endomicroscopy 267, 272
Congenital umbilical hernia 730, 731
  spontaneous closure of 732
Conjunctival calcification 537
Conjunctival redness 497
Conn's syndrome 546
Connective tissue disorders 713, 830
Consciousness, level of 579, 588
Conservative surgery, complications of 129
Constipation, chronic 409, 750
Contact thermal therapy 370
Contamination 11
Continuous closed postoperative lavage approach 172
Continuous fascial traction 646
Contusions 587
  pulmonary 578, 603
Conventional abdominoperineal excision 426, 427, 428
Conventional white light endoscopy 267
Cooper's ligament 718, 719, 725
  repair 725
Cord
  compression 598
  hemisection of 599
  hydrocele of 763
  injury, mechanisms of 598
Core-cut biopsy 441, 459
Core-needle biopsy 236, 450, 459,, 460
Corkscrew collaterals 1086
Corneal calcification 537
Cornett's sign 1079
Corona
  mortis 718, 719
  phlebectatica 694
Coronal sulcus 642
Coronary ligament 109

Corporal ligation, deep 642
Corpus spongiosum 910
Correa cascade 268
Corrosive stricture 794
Cortex 545
Corticospinal tract 599
Corticosteroids 241
  intralesional 9, 14
  maintenance therapy 552
  systemic 346
Cortisol 554
Costochondritis 451
Cough 113
  chronic 722, 750
Couinaud classification 1056
Cowden syndrome 265, 454
Cranial vault, fracture of 584
Craniofacial dysjunction 593
Craniotomy flap, large 586
C-reactive protein 345
Cremasteric reflex 759, 760
Cretinism 490
  myxoedematous 490
  neurological 490
Cricothyroidotomy, open 578
Crisis, hypercalcemic 537
Crohn's colitis 343
  surgical options for 311
Crohn's disease 241, 263, 302, 305, 308-313, 315, 323, 324, 327, 351, 408
  cardinal symptoms of 308
  characteristic features of 307
  granulomas of 315
  oral lesions in 309
  perianal fistulizing 404
Cryoablation 140, 144
Cryoprecipitate 35
Cryptoglandular theory 401
Cryptorchid testis 756
  possible sites of 754
Cryptorchidism 755, 759
  acquired 754
  congenital 754
  recurrent 755
Cryptosporidium 162
Crystalloid 29
Crystals, appearance of 870
Cullen sign 165
Curlicue ureter sign 743
Curling's ulcer 241
Cushing's disease 548
Cushing's syndrome 548, 550
  adrenal 548
  diagnostic of 550
  iatrogenic 549
  pituitary 548, 551
Cushing's ulcer 241
Cutting Seton technique 407
Cyanoacrylate glue 258
Cyanosis 577
Cyclophosphamide 897
Cyclosporine 25
Cystadenoma, serous 190
Cystectomy
  partial 128
  radical 899
Cystic artery 42
Cystic cervical metastases, causes of 1077
Cystic duct 1071
  insertion, variations of 100
Cystic echinococcosis 123
  surgical options for 129
Cystic fibrosis 180, 241
  gene 162
Cystic lesions 189, 190, 818
  mucin-producing 190
Cystine 888
  stone 868, 870
Cystobiliary communication 125, 128
  intraoperative management of 129
Cystocele 394
Cystoduodenostomy 174, 175, 203
Cystogastrostomy 174, 175, 203
Cystography, computed tomography scan of 638
Cystojejunostomy 174, 175
Cystolithotripsy
  percutaneous 893
  transurethral 893
Cystoscopy 889, 898
Cysts 81-83, 111, 124, 125, 128, 159, 183, 212, 443
  apocrine 446
  bile duct 111
  bone 537
  branchial 970
  breast 446
  characteristic features of 863
  choledochal 77, 79, 80
  chylolymphatic 231
  complex 446
  complicated 446
  congenital 111
  daughter 124
  dermoid 231, 818
  duplication 303
  enterogenous 231
  epidermal 818
  epididymal 766
  extrusion of 129
  fluid analysis reveals 189
  gastrostomy, open 172
  hydatid 111, 123, 124, 126, 238
  management of 446
  mesenteric 231, 238
  multiple 863
    hepatic 152
    sebaceous 818
  nonparasitic 210
  ovarian 238
  parasitic 210
  sebaceous 448, 766, 818
  second branchial 970
  secondary infection of 173
  simple 132, 446, 863
  spontaneous rupture of 80
  true sebaceous 1084
  urachal 224
  vitelline 223
Cytohistologic diagnosis 78
Cytokeratin 1080
Cytology 907
Cytomegalovirus 38, 339, 343
Cytotoxin-associated antigen 242
Czerny retractor 1006
  uses of 1006

D

Damage control
  approach 689
  laparotomy, principles of 643
  surgery 622, 637, 643
Danazol 452
  therapy 449
Dance sign 304
Dartos fascia 766
Daseler's quadrilateral area 921
Daughter cysts 124
  endogenous 124
  multiple 126
De Garengeot hernia 749
De Quervain's thyroiditis 508, 509
Dead-end host 123
Death
  crown of 719
  early 573
  immediate 573
  late 573
Deaver retractor 1006
  uses of 1006
Debakey classification 1056
Debridement 701
Deceleration injury 582
Decompression 152, 254, 299
  biliary 84
  delayed 646
  immediate 645
  invasive 170
  prophylactic 646
Deep vein thrombosis 690
  outcomes of 691
  pathophysiology of 690
  prophylaxis, types of 692
  Wells criteria for 1062
Defecography 394
Degloving injuries 640

Dehydroemetine 122
Dehydroepiandrosterone 447
Delaire technique 979
Delorme procedure 396
DeMeester score 776, 1065
Dengue 38
Dental
  abnormalities 980
  disease, chronic 1087
Depressed fracture 584
  treatment of 584
Depression 311, 704
  respiratory 655
Dercum's disease 823
Dermal nevus 827
Dermoid cyst 231, 818
  congenital 818, 819
  implantation 819
  sequestration 818
Dermopathy 494
Desarda technique 723
Desflurane 989
Desiccation 939
Desjardin's choledocholithotomy forceps 1008
Detachable loops, application of 258
Devascularization procedure 153
Device-assisted enteroscopy 326
  types of 326
Dexamethasone suppression tests 550
Dextrose solution 22
Diabetes mellitus 7, 87, 135, 136, 181, 377, 511, 667, 671, 682, 701, 844
  control of 677
  management of 709
  pancreatogenic 181
Diabetic foot 846
  ulcer 846
    assessment of 847
Diabetic gastroparesis 283
Diagnostic flexible fiberoptic upper gastrointestinal endoscopy 785
Diagnostic mammography 450
  indications of 466
Diagnostic peritoneal lavage 615, 616
Diaphragm, traumatic defects of 283
Diarrhea 496
  postvagotomy 285
Diarrheal episode 393
Diastasis recti 225
  classification system for 225
Diathermy, unipolar 812
Diet
  high-fiber 332
  low iodine 516
  modification of 287
Dietary habits 323
  modification of 367
Dietary modification 420
Diethylenetriaminepentaacetic acid 865
Dieulafoy's lesion 259, 282
Different minimal access techniques 931
Different scar scale 8
Different suturing techniques 1015
Diffuse axonal injury 582, 587
DiGeorge's syndrome 23
Digital breast tomosynthesis 451
Digital chromoendoscopy 272
Digital rectal examination 393, 399, 412, 422, 431, 751
Digoxin 447
Dilated pancreatic duct 190
Diltiazem 399, 448
Diosmin 697
Direct pancreatic function test 182
Direct vision internal urethrotomy 911
Disability 579, 653
Distal perfusion, assessment of 656
Distal rectal stump, washout of 626
Distal splenorenal shunt 154
Distal transverse colon 363
Distal ureteral stone 888
Distant metastasis 445, 458
Distress, respiratory 113
Diuresis 24
Diuretics
  loop 21
  therapy 19
Diversion 626
Diverticula 319, 330
  acquired 319
  duodenal 319
  esophageal 781
  jejunal 318
  jejunoileal 318
  long 320
Diverticular bleeding, management of 370
Diverticular disease, symptomatic uncomplicated 330
Diverticulectomy 319, 322, 782, 783
Diverticulitis 321, 322, 412
  clinical presentation of 331
  complicated 330, 331
  reduce risk of 332
  uncomplicated 330, 331
Diverticulosis 330
Diverticulum
  epiphrenic 782
  incidental 322
  inversion 319
  mid-esophageal 783, 784
  short 322
Doom, triangle of 719
Doppler ultrasound 676
Dorsal column 599
Dorsalis pedis pulse, absence of 675
DOTATOC scan 562
Double closed loop obstruction 338
Double hook retractor 1006
Double-balloon enteroscopy 326
Doughnut sign 304
Doxazosin 556, 902
Doxorubicin 226, 690
Doxycycline 33, 765, 825
Drainage 401, 402, 440, 626, 878
  biliary 85, 102
  laparoscopic 174
  procedures 250
Draining seton 407, 408
Drugs 450, 489
  antineoplastic 7
  cytoprotective 247
  sympathomimetic 915
Dryness 704
Duct
  distal part of 223
  ectasia 441, 443, 449, 453
  involution 453
  obstruction 177
  parotid 594
Ductal abnormalities 176
Ductal adenocarcinoma 192
Ductal carcinoma
  in situ
    nuclear grading of 457
    treatment of 469
  invasive 457
Ductal epithelial cells 192
Ductal hypertension 51, 180
Ductogram 451
Ductography 441, 442, 450, 451
  contraindications of 451
Ductoscopy 450
  advantages of 451
Dunphy sign 377
Duodenal C loop, widening of 620
Duodenal diverticula 319
  intraluminal 319
  types of 319
Duodenal resection 319
Duodenal sweep 791
Duodenal ulcer
  clinical presentation of 244
  pathophysiology of 243
  surgery for intractable 248
Duodenum 52, 241, 564, 565
  kocherization of 73
  preserving pancreatic head resection 184
Duplex scan 676
Dutasteride 902
Duval's procedure 184, 185
Dyselectrolytemia 339
  correction of 260, 372
Dyskinesia, biliary 55
Dyslipidemia 135

Dyspepsia 324
Dysphagia 347, 779, 798
Dysplasia 348, 793
 degree of 793
 fibromuscular 685
 high-grade 311, 793, 796
 low-grade 311, 793
Dyspnea 523
Dysthyroid optic neuropathy 502

E

Ear lobule 808
Early dumping syndrome 287
E-cadherin 1080
Eccentric breast mass 449
Ecchymosis, bilateral periorbital 580
Echinococcus tapeworms found 123
Echocardiography, transesophageal 672
Eckardt symptom score 779, 1065
Ectocyst 124
Ectodermal dysplasia complex 438
Ectopia vesicae 891
Ectopic adrenocorticotropic hormone syndrome 549, 551, 552
Ectopic parathyroid, sites of 534
Ectopic testis 754
 possible sites of 754
Ectopic ureter, termination of 862
Eczema 694
Edema
 cerebral 582
 peripheral 281
Edematous foreskin, manual compression of 768
Efferent loop obstruction 288
Ehler-Danlos syndrome 330, 685, 686, 713
Ejaculatory dysfunction 902, 926
Eklund view 1080
Elastic stockings 692, 709
Elastography, rotational 39
Elective open splenectomy 213
Elective sigmoid colectomy 332
 principles of 332
Electric burn 660
 injury, severity of 660
 management of 661
Electrocautery 940, 1086
Electrocoagulation 1082
 unipolar 370
Electrode monitoring system 941
Electrolyte 589
 abnormalities 25
 balance, disorders of 16
 imbalance 20, 37
  correction of 299
Electroporation, irreversible 140, 145
Electrosurgery 940
 complications of 941
 safety precautions for 941
 unipolar 939, 940
Electrosurgical tissue effects 939
Electrosurgical unit, waveforms of 940
Elephantiasis neuromatosa 824
Elston-Ellis modification 457
Emboli 670
Embolic occlusion 671
 acute 671
Embolism 683, 844
 pulmonary 690
Embolization 135, 627
 angiographic 281
 retrograde 762
Emergency surgical intervention 335, 338
Emetine 122
Empyema gallbladder 49
En bloc
 hepatic resection 92, 106
 splenectomy 196
Encephalitis 804
Endarterectomy 678
 aortoenteric 678
Endoanal advancement flap 407, 408
Endocarditis 112
Endoclot 258, 371
Endocrine
 disorders 24
 therapy 445, 469
Endometriosis 295
Endoneurial tube 948
Endoneurium 823
Endophthalmitis 114
Endoscope
 classification system for 937
 sterilization of 937
Endoscopic ablation, techniques of 796
Endoscopic approach 68, 85, 87
Endoscopic balloon dilation 340
Endoscopic clip application 258
Endoscopic drainage, complications of 173
Endoscopic eradication therapy 793
Endoscopic hemostasis therapy 370
Endoscopic management 184, 256, 258, 889, 911
Endoscopic mucosal resection 259, 276, 352
 complications of 267
 techniques of 267
Endoscopic pancreatic function test 182
Endoscopic pilonidal sinus treatment 418
Endoscopic procedures 784
Endoscopic resection 793
 techniques of 796
Endoscopic retrograde
 cholangiopancreatography 194
  complications of 68
 pancreatography 182
Endoscopic scoring systems 309
Endoscopic severity score 345
Endoscopic submucosal dissection 259
 advantages of 267
Endoscopic therapy 796
Endoscopic transluminal necrosectomy 171, 172
Endoscopic transmural drainage 172, 173
Endoscopic transpapillary drainage 75, 172, 173
Endoscopic treatment 785, 889
Endoscopic ultrasonography 166, 194, 267, 272, 795, 796
Endoscopic ultrasound 200, 309, 562, 564
 guided angiotherapy 258
Endoscopically placed duodenal stent 199
Endoscopic-assisted linea alba reconstruction 225, 732
 plus mesh augmentation 225
Endoscopy 280, 774, 779, 789, 792
 emergent 792
 endoluminal 931
 flexible 792
 high-resolution 795
 intraoperative 595
 nonurgent 792
 submucosal 781
 third-space 781
Endosymbiont Wolbachia 765
Endothelial cell migration 6
Endothelial damage 690
Endothelial injury 668
Endotheliopathy, shock-induced 1081
Endotracheal cuff balloons 1083
Endovascular aortic aneurysm repair 684, 685
Endovascular therapy 678
 types of 678
Endovenous thermal ablation 698
 complications of 698
 contraindications of 698
Enema
 contrast 304, 335
 reduction, contraindications of 304
Energy devices 34
Enhanced recovery after surgery pathway 992
Enteral nutrition 170, 327
 total 659
Enteral tube feeding 170
Enterocele 394, 721
 partial 749
Enteroclysis 325
Enterocolitis, necrotizing 327
Enterolithotomy 53
Enteroplasty
 serial transverse 327, 329
 tapering 327, 329

Enteroscopy, intraoperative 326
Enuresis 861
Enzymes, pancreatic 180
Epidermal growth factor receptor ligand 281
Epidermis 831
Epididymis 760
Epididymitis, acute 759, 761
Epididymo-orchitis, acute 759
Epidural analgesia 987
  indications of 987
Epidural anesthesia 987
  indications of 987
Epigastric fullness 291
Epigastric hernia 714, 732, 733
  repair, principles of 733
Epigastric port 57
Epigastric vessels, inferior 718
Epilepsy 582, 820
Epinephrine 258, 985
  injection therapy 370
Epineurium 823, 948
Episcleritis 308
Epithelia 1080
Epithelial cell markers 1080
Epithelialization 6, 403
Erectile dysfunction 675
Erysipelas 826
Erythema nodosum 308
Erythrocyte sedimentation rate 345
Erythrocytosis 137
Escharotomy 656
  complications of 656
  principles of 656
Escherichia coli 116, 761
Esophageal adenocarcinoma 795
  development of 792
Esophageal caustic injuries
  classification of 789
  management of 790
Esophageal dilation, complications of 788
Esophageal disorders 794
Esophageal food bolus impaction 792
Esophageal impedance measurement 775
Esophageal injury 611, 784
  management of 596
Esophageal perforation 603, 784, 785
  causes of 784
  spontaneous 784
Esophageal reconstruction 790
Esophageal spasm, diffuse 781
Esophageal stents 788, 798
Esophageal stoma, construction of 786
Esophageal stricture 790
  acquired causes of 787
  simple 787
Esophageal transection 155
Esophageal tumors, classification of 795
Esophageal varices 281
Esophagectomy 780
  principles of 796
  transhiatal 797
  transthoracic 796
Esophagitis, Los Angeles classification of 1058
Esophagogastric devascularization procedures 155
Esophagogastric junction 276
Esophagogastrostomy 277
Esophagoscopy 787
Esophagram, contrast 789
Esophagus 791
  abdominal 774
  caustic injury of 788
  cervical 784
  diseases of 771
  location of 797
  proximal 241
  sigmoid 780
  stricture of 787
Estrogen 447, 449, 690, 908
Ethanol 146, 258
Ethanolamine 258
Ethilon 1014
Ethylene oxide sterilization 938
Etomidate 988
European Group of Graves' Orbitopathy classification of severity of ophthalmopathy 497
European Hernia Society
  classification 1056
  groin hernia classification system 720
  parastomal hernia classification 745
  primary abdominal wall hernia classification 731
Euthyroid 491
  hyperthyroxinemia 500
  sick syndrome 1074
Evening primrose oil 452
Exercise rehabilitation 677
Exocrine pancreas 181
  diseases of 181
Exomphalos 220
Exophthalmometer 499
Exophthalmos 497
Extensor tendons, injury of 959
External beam radiation therapy 140
External iatrogenic bladder
  injury, signs of 638
  trauma 638
Extracellular matrix 669
Extracorporeal shock wave lithotripsy 871
Extracorporeal therapy 19
Extraesophageal symptoms 775
Extrahepatic bile duct 85
  injury 618
Extrahepatic biliary system 40
Extrahepatic cholangiocarcinoma 93
  diagnosis of 94
Extrahepatic portal vein obstruction 147, 148
Extraintestinal manifestations 308, 347, 353
  presence of 353
Extralevator abdominoperineal excision 426, 428
Extraperitoneal bladder injury, mechanisms of 638
Extraperitoneal fat, protrusion of 728
Extraperitoneal rectal injury, management of 626
Extremities
  acute arterial occlusion of 669
  chronic occlusive disease of 674
Eye
  opening 588
  protrusion of 497
  signs 498
Eyed needle, sterilization of 1004
Eyeless needle, sterilization of 1004
Eyelid
  erythema 497
  swelling 497

F

Face, soft tissues of 592
Facial nerve 811, 951
  identification of 811
  injury 594, 813
    risk of 813
  intraoperative transection of 813, 951
Falciform ligament 109, 1072
Fan sign 968
Fascia lata, minced autologous 951
Fascial defect 237
Fascicles 948
Fasciitis, necrotizing 708, 1067
Fasciocutaneous flaps 767
Fat 58
  fracture 1076
  necrosis 447, 448
    mammographic features of 447
    scrotal 759, 766
Fatty liver disease, nonalcoholic 136
Fatty streak 668
Febrile nonhemolytic transfusion reaction 37
Fecal calprotectin 309, 345
Fecal incontinence 420
  risk factors for 406
Feeding, oral 170
Femoral artery aneurysm 685
Femoral canal 728
  boundaries of 728
Femoral hernia 714, 720, 725, 728, 749
  repair, uncomplicated 729
  variants of 728

Femoral ring 713
  rigidity of 728
Femoral vein 729
Femur 690
Fibrin 258
  glue 408
  polymerization 33
  sealants 35
Fibrinogen concentrate 36
Fibroadenoma 443, 446, 453
  excision of 443
  operated specimen of 443
  percutaneous excision of 444
Fibroblasts, mitogenic factor for 6
Fibromatosis
  aggressive 226
  colli 972
Fibromyalgia 451
Fibroplasia 6
Fibrosis 192
  mediastinal 234, 511
  retroperitoneal 87, 234
Fibrous tissue 58
Field triage decision scheme 574
Filarial dance sign 765
Filariasis 705
Finasteride 902
Fine tremor 496
Fine-needle aspiration 117, 459, 491
  biopsy 459, 515
  cytology 431, 441, 459, 484
Fingers
  papillary carcinoma of 23
  thoracostomy 605
Finney pyloroplasty 250
First variceal hemorrhage, prevention of 156, 284
Fissure
  acute 398, 399
  anal 398
  chronic 398
  multiple 398
Fistula 308, 441, 841, 853
  aortoenteric 259
  biliary 33, 129
    enteric 77
  closure 53
  complex 405
  enteroatmospheric 368
  external 853
    pancreatic 173
  extrasphincteric 403
  internal 853
  management of 333
  mucous 366
  multiple urethrocutaneous 404
  parotid 813
  perianal 311
  plug 408
  postoperative pancreatic 198
  repair 53
  simple 405
  suprasphincteric 403
  tract 405
    course of 971
  transperitoneal 403
Fistula-in-ano 401, 403
  classification of 403
  management of 408
  recurrent 308, 404, 405
Fistulectomy 406
Fistulography 64
Fistulotomy 406, 408
Fitzpatrick classification 1056
Fixation
  methods, types of 593
  tapes 851
Flail
  chest 578, 602, 603
  segment, lateral 602
Flap based procedures 418, 419
Flat epithelial atypia 443
Flavonoids 413
Fleischer's syndrome 438
Flexor tendon
  injury of 960
  sheath infection 958
Florid ductal hyperplasia 443
Fludrocortisone 554
Fluid 589
  balance 19
    disorders of 16
  calculation of 655
  collection
    abdominal 645
    acute peripancreatic 164
  input-output 19
  intake 870
  management 601
    perioperative 992
  overload, consequences of 19
  respiratory swing of 609
  resuscitation 170, 254, 299, 304, 339, 372, 654, 655, 663, 681, 751
    aggressive 578
    principles of 654
  stewardship 1081
  therapy 991
  types of 655
Fluoroquinolones 761
Fluorouracil 241
Foam
  cells die 668
  sclerotherapy 698
Focal nodular hyperplasia 111, 134
  cut section of 135
Foley self-retaining catheter 1009
Follicle excision, midline 418
Follicular
  adenoma 512
  cells 512
  neoplasm 519
  occlusion tetrad 416
Fondaparinux 692
Fontaine classification 674
Fontaine sign 971
Food bolus impaction 791
Foot
  care 677
  deformities, assessment of 848
  ulcer, prevention of 849
Formaldehyde 938
Forrest classification 256, 1056
Fossa 60
  ischioanal 402
  lateralis 719
  medialis 719
  peritoneal 746
  vesicalis 719
Fothergill's sign 226
Four-layer bandage 701
Fournier's gangrene 766, 767, 826
  severity index 766, 826, 1065
Foveolar hyperplasia 281
Fowler-Stephens orchidopexy 758
Fox's sign 165
Fracture
  depressed 584
  immobilization 576
  mandible 593
  maxilla 593
  nasal bone 594
  nondepressed 584
  pyramidal 593
  severe depressed 584
  sternal 603
  vertebral 597
Fragility fracture 1079
Frank necrosis 697
Frantz tumor 190
Free flap 472
  advantages of 474
  disadvantages of 474
Free-swimming bifid-tailed cercaria 894
Fresh-frozen plasma 35
Frey procedure 184, 187, 188
  Hamburg modification of 184, 187
Frey syndrome 813
Frimann-Dahl sign 335
Frontotemporoparietal flap 586
Fruchaud myopectineal orifice 717
Frusemide 26
Frykman-Goldberg procedure 396
Fulguration 939
Full Rockall score 1065
Full-template inguinal lymph node dissection 921

Functional lumen imaging probe 779
Fundoplication
laparoscopic 777
partial 777, 783
Furosemide 447
Fusiform 682

G

G6PD deficiency 210
Gadolinium contrast 523
Gail model 455, 464
Galactocele 446
Galactography 441, 450
Galactorrhea 449
causes of 450
Galen's anastomosis 1074
Gallbladder 40, 42, 49, 76, 80, 88, 89, 350, 618, 1070
acute inflammation of 54
anomalous anatomy of 99
arterial supply of 100
defect, focal 48
disorder, functional 55
dissection of 60
inflammation of 52
intrahepatic 1071
lymphatics drain 42
malignancy, risk factors for 88
mesenteric pattern of 1071
mucocele of 49
palpable 94
pathology of 43, 115
perforation 48
classification of 1058
polyp 87, 88
Galli-Curci nerve 1074
Gallstone 43, 54, 77, 162, 289, 302
disease 49
spectrum of 44
ileus 52, 77
impaction, sites of 52
multiple 49
pancreatitis 66, 167
Ganglion 819
after excision of 819
true 819
Gangrene 675
atherosclerotic 707
Gangrenous sigmoid colon, resection of 335
Gardner's syndrome 353, 354, 818
Gastrectomy 273
distal 273, 276, 277, 291
partial 283
proximal 273, 276, 277
pylorus-preserving 276, 277
sleeve 283
subtotal 280, 281
total 273, 276, 277, 281
types of 273, 276
Gastric 353
antral vascular ectasia 259
antrum 274
atony, postvagotomy 285
cancer 241, 259, 268, 273, 289
distal 264
early 267
guideline of 795
hereditary diffuse 265, 266, 454
unresectable 277
conduit 796
emptying 285
delayed 198
gastrointestinal stromal tumor 279
resection of 280
intubation 580
lymphoma 280
metaplasia 241
mucosa, heterotopic 241
outlet obstruction 172, 199, 260, 291, 790
causes of 261
functional 285
malignant causes of 261
palliation of 198
polyps 353
resection 273
rugal folds, massive 281
ulcer 243, 244, 283
benign 245
clinical presentation of 244
malignant 245
pathophysiology of 243
surgery for intractable 251
varices
isolated 284
types of 284
volvulus 282, 283
acute 283
Gastrinoma 563, 564
triangle 563
Gastritis 241, 262, 263
acute 46, 101, 201
assessment staging system 1058
atrophic 262
autoimmune 262
classification of 262
eosinophilic 263
erosive 263
granulomatous 263
hypertrophic lymphocytic 281
lymphocytic 263
nonatrophic 262
Gastrocolic ligament 209
Gastroduodenal artery 256
Gastroesophageal junction 275, 773
Gastroesophageal reflux disease 775
Gastroesophageal varices 284
Gastrograffin 785, 791
Gastrohepatic ligament 106
Gastrointestinal anastomosis staplers 432
Gastrointestinal bleeding 320, 369
causes of 369
lower 369, 370
overt 369
upper 369
Gastrointestinal endoscopy, lower 344
Gastrointestinal linear stapler 432
Gastrointestinal loss 21, 25
Gastrointestinal stromal tumor 259, 278, 324
Gastrointestinal superficial neoplastic lesions 267
Gastrojejunostomy 250
laparoscopic 199
stoma 241
Gastropexy 283
Gastroschisis 221, 327
Gastrostomy, fundoantral 283
Gaze evoked orbital pain 497
Gelatin foam 34
Gelfoam 34
Gemcitabine 92
General anesthesia 722
complications of 991
effects of 987
indications of 991
General surgery 296
acute kidney injury risk index 1065
Genetic
disorders 867
factors 493, 908
mutations 523
risk model 455
testing 353
Genital defects 891
Genitofemoral nerve 718, 727
Genitofemoral reflex arc 759
Genitourinary function 425
Genitourinary injuries 634
Germ cell tumor
extragonadal 923
neoplasia in situ 922
Germinative membrane 124
Germline mutation 353, 886
Gharbi classification 127, 1056
Giant cell 447
arteritis 686
Giant fibroadenoma 444, 453
Giant hemangioma 134
Gigantomastia 453
Gland injury 594
Glandular hyperplasia 899
Glansectomy 919
Glasgow Blatchford bleeding score 1066

Glasgow coma
 scale 588
 score 1084
Glasgow criteria, modified 167
Glaucoma 820
Gleason score 908, 1066
Glibenclamide 1078
Gliclazide 1078
Glioblastoma multiforme 353
Glipizide 1078
Glomus tumor 821
Glossitis 309
Glucagonoma 561, 565
Glucocorticoids 24, 235
 replacement 554
Glucose control 1080
Glue grant program 1081
Gluteal cleft 416, 417
Glycemic control, perioperative 993
Glycogen storage disease 135
Goiter
 diffuse nontoxic 504
 multinodular 505
 substernal 505
 toxic multinodular 492, 503
Gold standard treatment 50, 211
Goldman classification 1056
Gompertizian curve 1079
Gonads, bilateral nonpalpable 757
Gonorrhea, low risk of 761
Gonorrheal acute epididymitis, risk of 761
Goodsall's rule 405
Goose neck deformity 316
Gorlin syndrome 818
Gout 701
Gracilis muscle flap 426
Graciloplasty, dynamic 420
Graft versus host disease, transfusion-associated 38
Graham's omental patch repair 290
Graham's omentopexy 254, 255
 modified 254
Granulomas 315
 caseating 315
 characteristic features of 315
 confluent 315
 pyogenic 821
 umbilical 224
Granulomatous diseases 315
Graves' disease 492, 493, 500, 502
Graves' ophthalmopathy 497
 management of 502
Graves' orbitopathy 497
Grayhack shunt 916
Great saphenous vein 1087
Great vessel injury 611
Greenish discharge 449
Grey Turner's sign 165
Groin 722
 anatomy of 717
 hernia 717
  management, international guidelines for 726
  Nyhus classification of 719
 pain 726
Gross hematuria 638, 858
Growth
 factors 7
  role of 7
 failure 308
Grynfeltt-Lesshaft
 hernia 741, 749
 triangle 740
Gunshot
 injuries, high-energy 614
 wound 611, 613, 614
Gustatory sweating 813
Gynecomastia 447, 448
 differential diagnosis of 448
 grading of 448
 neonatal 447
 pathological 447
 physiological 447
 refeeding 448
 senile 447
 types of 447

H

Hadfield's operation, modified 442
Haemophilus influenzae B vaccine 215
Haggitt's criteria 352
Hair debris 416
Hairy cell leukemia 210
Hairy mole 828
Halo sign 580
Halothane 989
Hamartoma, cystic dilation of 133
Hamburg classification 1057
Hamoudi tumor 190
Hand
 assisted laparoscopic colectomy 364
 infections 957
 instruments 936
  classification system for 937
  sterilization of 938
 surgery of 954
Hanging drop test 933
Hanley technique 402
 modified 402
Hannington-Kiff sign 742
Hannover classification 61, 62
Harmonic scalpel 942
Hartley–Dunhill procedure 501
Hartmann's procedure 335, 336
Hartmann's solution 1070
Hashimoto thyroiditis 489, 493, 509, 511
Hasson's technique 50, 934
Hayflick hypothesis 1079
Head injury 241, 582, 586
 classification of 588
 types of 582
Healed venous ulcer 696
Hearing loss 804
Heart
 disease, ischemic 989
 failure, congestive 339
Heartburn 775
Heat
 intolerance 496
 probe 370
 sink effect 143
Heineke-Mikulicz pyloroplasty 250
Heinz bodies 208, 214
Heister spiral valves 1070
Helicobacter pylori
 infection 241
 role of 241
 stool antigen test 246
 virulence factors of 242
Heller myotomy
 modified 780
 original 780
Hemangioma 111, 134, 808
 hepatic 134
Hematocele 765
Hematogenous spread 358, 835, 925
Hematological disorders 915
Hematological dysfunction 46
Hematoma 741
 acute subdural 586
 duodenal 619
 epidural 585
 evacuation of 586
 extradural 585
 intracerebral 587
 intracranial 582
 need surgical evacuation of 585
 rectus sheath 225
 retroperitoneal 233
 scrotal 759
 spontaneous retroperitoneal 233
 subdural 586
Hematopoiesis
 extramedullary 208
 splenic 208
Hematuria 639, 858, 887, 893
 causes of 859
 microscopic 858
 painless 858
Hemicolectomy 362, 387
Hemidiaphragm 114
Hemiscrotum, contralateral 759
Hemobilia 77
 causes of 77
Hemochromatosis, hereditary 136, 180
Hemodialysis 22, 24
Hemoglobin level 345

Hemoglobinuria, paroxysmal nocturnal 148
Hemolysis 152
Hemolytic transfusion reaction 37, 39
Hemophilus influenzae 804
Hemorrhage 30, 34, 135, 198, 903
- acute variceal 156
- control of 578, 688
- external 578
- intracystic 133
- prevention of recurrent 156
- reactionary 1082
- retroperitoneal 234, 762
- risk of 904
- stigmata of 256
- types of 34

Hemorrhagic disorders 33
- acquired 33
- congenital 33

Hemorrhoidectomy 414
- closed 415
- complications of 414
- indications of 414
- open 415
- types of 414

Hemorrhoidopexy, stapled 416
Hemorrhoids 409
- fourth degree 411
- secondary 409
- symptomatic 412
- third-degree 434
- thrombosed external 416
- types of 411

Hemospray 32, 258, 371
Hemostasis 30, 214
- instruments used for 998
- methods of 34

Hemostatic agents, topical 34, 629
Hemostatic topical powder 370, 371
Hemothorax 603, 607
- massive 578, 603, 607

Henoch-Schönlein purpura 303
Heparin
- low dose unfractionated 692
- therapy 32
- unfractionated 33

Hepatectomy 77
- partial 141

Hepatic artery route 112, 113
Hepatic disease 7
Hepatic duct 42, 1071, 1072
Hepatic dysfunction 46
Hepatic function, assessment of 139
Hepatic resection, extended 92
Hepatic vein 544
Hepaticojejunostomy 199, 1071
Hepatitis 500
- acute viral 101, 120, 157
- B infection 136
  - detection of 139
- C infection 136
  - detection of 139
- chronic 102

Hepatobiliary disease 308, 990
Hepatobiliary iminodiacetic acid 55
Hepatocystic triangle 1070
Hepatocyte paraffin 1072
Hepatoduodenal ligament 1072
Hepatolithiasis 77, 80, 93
- secondary 77

Hepatomegaly 125
Hepatopulmonary syndrome 152
Hermaphroditism, true 447
Hernia 711, 713, 749, 756
- abdominal wall 730
- amyand's 749
- asymptomatic sliding 774
- bilateral 720
- bochdalek 749, 1078
- Cloquet's 728, 749
- composition of 713
- congenital umbilical 730, 731
- contents of 743
- De Garengeot 749
- defect 733
  - clear delineation of 734
  - length of 737
  - multiple hepatic 737
  - width of 737
- development of 713, 742
- direct inguinal 720, 721, 727
- epigastric 714, 732, 733
- external 713
- femoral 714, 720, 725, 728, 749
- giant paraesophageal 773
- groin 717
- Hesselbach's 728, 749
- hiatal 773, 774
- incarcerated 716, 759
- incisional 715, 734
  - abdominal wall 730
- indirect inguinal 721
- inguinal 294, 714, 720, 721
- inguinofemoral 744
- internal 713, 746
- interparietal 744
- interstitial 744
- irreducible 716, 721
- ischiorectal 743
- Laugier's 728, 749
- lesser sac 747
- Littre 749
- lumbar 715, 740
- Maydl's 749
- medium-sized 732, 733
- Morgagni 749
- obstructed 295, 716
- obturator 715, 741, 742
- occult femoral 728
- open incisional 737
- orifice, types of 746
- Pantaloon 749
- paraduodenal 747
- paraesophageal 283, 773
- parastomal 745
- paraumbilical 731
- pericecal 746
- perineal 716, 743
- Petersen 749
- Petit 741, 749
- posterior perineal 743
- primary abdominal wall 730, 731
- primary acquired 741, 743
- properitoneal 744
- pudendal 743
- recurrent 719
  - incisional 736
  - inguinal 722
- repair 721, 741
  - laparoscopic 726, 738
  - open femoral 728
  - open groin 717
  - principles of 722
- retroanastomotic 747
- Richter's 728, 749
- Romberg 749
- sac
  - course of 742
  - treatment of 723
- saddle bag 749
- sciatic 716, 741, 743
- Serafini's 728, 749
- sigmoid mesocolon-related 747
- sliding 723
- small
  - epigastric 733
  - umbilical 732
- spigelian 715, 740, 749
- strangulated 716, 722
- superficial 744
- superior lumbar 741
- symptomatic inguinal 722
- transmesenteric 747
- trocar site 748
- types of 713, 721
- umbilical 222, 714, 730, 732
- ureteric sciatic 743
- Velpeau's 728, 749
- ventral 730

Hernia-en-glissade 727
Hernioplasty 722
Herpes zoster 451
Hesselbach's hernia 728, 749
Hiatal hernia 773, 774
- sliding 773
- types of 773

Hibernomas 823
Hidradenitis suppurativa 443, 767

High tie technique 425
High-anion gap metabolic acidosis 27
Hilar cholangiocarcinoma 92-94, 141
  classification of 93
Hilar plate, lowering of 1072
Hildreth's test 821
Hill-Baker procedure 249
Hinchey classification 1057
  modified 1057
Hinge injury 597
Hirschsprung's disease 778
Hirsute 417
Histoplasmosis 315
Hoarse voice 577
Holding tissues, instruments used for 1000
Hole sign 48
Holy plane 424, 425
Homan's sign 690
Homboid flap 419
Homocystinuria 690
Honeycomb appearance 159
Honeymoon palsy 1078
Hook retractor, uses of 1006
Hopkins rod lens system 935
Hormone 535
  replacement therapy 554
Horseshoe kidney 862
Hostile abdomen 684
Hot nodule 506
Hot snare polypectomy 352
Howell-Jolly bodies 208, 214
Howship-Romberg sign 742
Human bites 641
Human cadaveric allograft 658
Human chorionic gonadotropin 924
Human immunodeficiency virus cholangiopathy 86
Human leukocyte antigen haplotype 85
Human papilloma virus 1084
Hurley staging system 825
Hurthle cell
  carcinoma 515, 520
  tumor, benign 520
Hutchinson's lentigo 828
Hutchinson's sign 835
Hyaline cartilage 8
Hybrid parastomal endoscopic re-do technique 746
Hydatid cyst 111, 123, 124, 126, 238
  risk of 123
Hydatid disease, polycystic 123
Hydatid thrill 125
Hydralazine 234
Hydration 24
Hydrocarbons, organic 831
Hydrocele 756, 762, 763, 765
  congenital 762, 769
  fluid 763
  primary 765
  secondary 763, 765
Hydrocelectomy 765
Hydrocortisone 554
Hydrofluoric acid burn 662
Hydrogen
  ion
    gastrointestinal loss of 27
    renal loss of 27
  peroxide 128, 405
Hydronephrosis 864
  bilateral 864
  causes of 864, 865
  severe 235
  unilateral 864
Hydropneumothorax 604
Hydrothorax, hepatic 152
Hydroxyurea 701
Hygroma, cystic 820, 972
Hyperactivity 496
Hyperaldosteronism 546
Hyperamylasemia, persistent 620
Hypercalcemia 24, 137, 162
  asymptomatic 24
  familial hypocalciuric 24
  mild 24
  moderate 24
Hypercholesterolemia 137, 667
Hypercoagulability 148
Hypercoagulable states 148
Hypercortisolism 548
Hyperemia, zone of 654
Hyperextension injury 597
Hypergastrinemia, causes of 564
Hyperglycemia 550
Hyperhomocysteinemia 667
Hyperkalemia 22, 37
Hyperkeratosis 704
Hypermagnesemia 26
  mild asymptomatic 26
Hypermetabolism 659
Hypernatremia 20
Hyperparathyroidism 241, 537
  primary 24, 536-538, 542
  secondary 23, 541
  tertiary 24, 542
Hyperpigmentation, mucocutaneous 350
Hyperplasia
  atypical
    ductal 443
    lobular 443
  benign prostatic 899
  epithelial 453
  prostatic 722
  stromal 899
Hyperreflexia 496
Hypersplenism 212
Hypertension 546, 550, 667
  control of 677
  intra-abdominal 645
  intracranial 590
  intraoperative 557
  management of 709
  pathophysiology of 547
  secondary 546
  segmental portal 179
  sinistral 150
  systemic 686
  venous 693
Hyperthyroidism 24, 492
  overt 500
  subclinical 500
Hypertonic saline 128
Hypertriglyceridemia 162, 667
Hypertrophy
  adolescent 453
  congenital 353
Hyperuricosuria 866
Hyperventilation 589
Hypoalbuminemia 281
Hypocalcemia 23, 37
  acute 23
  chronic 23
Hypochondrium 90, 101, 125
Hypodense lesion 146
Hypoechoic lesion 115
Hypoglossal nerve 803
Hypoglycemia 137, 563
  prevention of 563
  risk of 1078
Hypokalemia 21, 546, 547
  causes of 21
  pathophysiology of 547
  severe 21
Hypomagnesemia 23, 25
  asymptomatic 25
  mild 25
  severe 25
  symptomatic 25
Hyponatremia 20
  true 20
Hypoparathyroidism 23, 542
  clinical presentation of 543
  treatment of 543
Hypoperfusion, systemic causes of distal 656
Hypoplasia, pulmonary 220
Hypospadias 913, 917
  classic triad of 913
  distal 914
  middle 913
  pelvic 913
  perineal 913
  proximal 914
Hyposplenism, causes of 212
Hypotension 590
  permissive 578
  systemic 605
Hypothermia 579, 643, 644
  intraoperative 992

Hypothyroid 491
Hypothyroidism 283, 489, 509
- adult 491
- causes of 489
- clinical 491
- congenital 490
- secondary 491
- subclinical 491
- transient 490

Hypotrophy, testicular 761
Hypovolemia 19, 578, 590, 656
- mild 19

I

Iatrogenic bladder injury 638
- management of 638

Iatrogenic trauma 636
- risk factors for 636

Ibandronate 24
Idiopathic thrombocytopenic purpura 210
Ifosfamide 21
Ileal diverticula 318
Ileal pouch, types of 347
Ileocecal region 315
Ileorectal anastomosis 348, 354
Ileosigmoid knotting 338
- characteristic features of 338

Ileostomy 314
- continent 348
- loop 366, 429

Ileum 317
Ileus
- paralytic 926
- postoperative 993

Iliac vessels 636, 718, 719
Iliofemoral bypass 678
Ilioinguinal nerve 1082
- pragmatic resection of 727

Iliopubic tract 717, 719
- repair 725

Imamura-Doppman procedure 562
Imatinib 226
- mesylate, uses of 280

Immobilization 24, 690
- position of 957
- splint 851

Immune hemolytic reaction, acute 36
Immune system 660
Immune-mediated diseases 87, 309
Immunochromatographic tests 246
Immunology 278
Immunomodulation, transfusion-associated 37
Impaired incretin secretion 181
Impetigo 825, 826
Implant displacement view 1080
Incarcerated rectal prolapse, management of 394
Incidentaloma 514
- adrenal 558
- management of 559

Incisional hernia 715, 734
- classification 736
- concomitant 745
- development of 735
- mesh repair of 751
- repair 737

Incisions 440, 525, 956
- abdominal 797
- subcostal 213
- types of 735

Incontinence 348
Indirect inguinal hernia 721
- types of 727

Indirect pancreatic function test 182
Infections 7, 64, 148, 172, 439, 582, 831, 958
- active 329
- adenovirus 303
- bacterial 38, 44, 162
- clinical evidence of 701
- fungal 162, 704
- hematogenous 875
- local 11
- parasitic 162
- stone 868
- systemic 11
- viral 38, 136

Infectious diseases 38
Inferior lumbar triangle 740
- boundaries of 740

Inferior thyroid vessels
- dissection of 526
- ligament 526

Infertility 756
Inflammation 259, 497
- chronic 908
- local 180
  - signs of 45
- systemic signs of 45

Inflammatory bowel disease 87
- chronic immune-mediated 341

Infliximab 310, 311, 408
Inflow occlusion 629
Inframesocolic space 227
Ingestion, accidental foreign body 791
Ingrowth 97
Inguinal area, bilateral palpation of 918
Inguinal canal 744
Inguinal floor
- reconstruction of 724
- strengthening of 724

Inguinal hernia 294, 714, 720, 721
- bilateral 722
- congenital 720
- indirect 721
- large 727
- repair, laparoscopic 718
- sliding 727
- strangulated 727, 741

Inguinal lymph node 431
- bilateral 921
- dissection 705
- unilateral 921

Inguinal ring, deep 713
Inguinodynia 727
Inhalation
- agents 557, 989
- injury 652
  - treatment of 654

Injection therapy 258
Injury
- abdominal 613
  - wall 617
- arterial 632
- bony 591
- colonic 623
- complete 599
- diaphragmatic 611
- duodenal 618, 619
- electrical 661
- esophageal 611, 784
- examination of 592
- head 241, 582, 586
- high velocity 583
- impact 582, 583
- incomplete 599
- inhalation 652
- intraperitoneal 625
- management of 620-622
- mechanical 582
- mechanisms of 582, 597
- midfacial 591
- minor 62
- pancreatic 620
- patterns 572, 789
- penetrating 582, 583, 633, 640, 951
- posterior urethral 639
- rectal 625
- repair of 612
- retroperitoneal 632
- scrotal 643
- severity score 1066
- small 622
- splenic 217, 617, 629
- strangulation 641
- testicular 643
- types of 572, 582, 591
- ureteral 636, 926
- urethral 639

Inoue classification 1057
Insufflator, important indicators of 934
Insulation failure 941
Insulin resistance 135
Insulinoma 562, 563
- localization of 562

Interferon, low-dose 226
Internal hernia 713, 746
- common type of 747
- types of 746

Internal rectal prolapse 394
- operations for 396

International Prostate Symptom Score 901, 1066
Intersphincteric fistula 403
- tract, ligation of 408

Interstitial thermal therapy, large 140, 144
Intestinal adaptation, phases of 327
Intestinal obstruction 294, 308, 321, 322
- acute 372
- management of 312

Intestinal transplantation, isolated 329
Intestine 292
- color of 300
- large 341, 353
- segment of 300
- weakest part of 318

Intestinopathy 152
Intra-abdominal pressure
- actual 934
- monitoring of 644

Intracavernosal injection 915, 917
Intracellular shift 21, 25
Intracranial hypertension 590
- management of 590

Intracranial pressure monitoring 590
Intraductal papillary mucinous neoplasms 189, 190, 192
Intralesional corticosteroid 9, 14
- injection 9

Intramesosigmoid type 747
Intramuscular route 655
In-transit metastases, treatment of 837
Intraosseous infusion 1075
Intrapapillary capillary loop classification 1057
Intraperitoneal bladder injury 638
- mechanisms of 638

Intrathecal space 985
Intravenous loop diuretics 26
Intubation, elective 577
Intussusception 232, 294, 303, 304, 392
- ileocecal 321
- retrograde 303
- types of 303

Invasive breast cancer 464
- treatment of 469

Iodine
- contrast agent 516
- deficiency 489
  - maternal 490

Ipilimumab 886
Iron
- metabolism 208
- overload 38

Irradiation 447
- pelvic 897

Irrigation fluid 903
Ischemia 759
- acute limb 670
- bowel 298
- cerebral 582
- colonic 335
- critical limb 674
- nonocclusive mesenteric 681

Ischemic priapism 915
- causes of 915
- management of 915

Ischioanal abdominoperineal excision 426
Islet autotransplantation 184, 188
Islet cell tumor 563
Isoflurane 989
Ivor Lewis esophagectomy 797
Iwate criteria 1063
Izbicki pain score 180, 1066
Izbicki procedure 184, 187

J

Jaboulay gastroduodenostomy 250
Japan Research Group for Study of Hepatolithiasis 77
Japanese Endoscopic Society 267
Japanese Gastric Cancer Association 270
Jaundice 66, 137, 172
- obstructive 33, 66, 103, 137, 198, 199
- painless 94
  - progressive 94
- palliation of 92

Jejunum 52, 317
Jod-Basedow phenomenon 503
Johnson classification, modified 243, 1058
Joint movement
- early 957
- range of 704

Junctional nevus 827
Junostomy 203
Juvenile polyposis syndrome 265, 350, 354
- clinical diagnosis of 350

K

Kaiser score 1067
Kajava classification 1057
Kallmann syndrome 447
Kanavel cardinal signs 1080
Kangari cancer 831
Kaposi sarcoma 837
Karnofsky score 1067
Karydaki's procedure 418
Karydaki's theory 417
Karydakis flap 419
Kasabach-Merritt syndrome 134
Kasai classification 1057
Katayama fever 895
Kausch-Whipple procedure 184, 186
Kelly's sign 1078
Keloid 8, 659
- formation 8
- over deltoid region 8
- scar 662

Keratinocytes 831
Keratosis
- actinic 828
- senile 828
- solar 828

Kernohan notch 1083
Ketamine 988
Ketoconazole 447
Key muscles, monitoring of 598
Keyhole repair, laparoscopic 746
Ki-67 index 561
Kidneys 634, 863
- cancer syndromes, hereditary 882
- characteristic features of 863
- congenital malformations of 861
- disease, polycystic 863
- infections of 875
- simple cyst of 863
- supernumerary 861
- tuberculosis of 879
- tumors 881

Killian's triangle 782
Klatskin tumor 92
Klebsiella pneumoniae 113, 116
Klinefelter's syndrome 447
Klippel-Trenaunay-Weber syndrome 134, 820
Kocher's hemostatic forceps 999
Kock pouch 348
- complications of 348

Koivuranta score 1067, 1079
Komi classification 1057
Kugel technique 724
Kulchitsky cells 387
Kyoto classification 1058

L

Laceration, deeper 631
Lacrimal apparatus injury 594
Lactate dehydrogenase 924
Lactobezoars 284
Landzert fossa 747
Lanes tissue forceps 1001
Langenbeck retractor 1006
- uses of 1006

Langerhans islets 561
Lanreotide 563
Lansky score 1067
Laparoendoscopic approach 726, 728
Laparoscope, angle of 935

Laparoscopic cholecystectomy 50, 56, 57, 103
  basic steps of 59
  indications of 56
  principles of 50
Laparoscopic colectomy 364
  approaches of 364
Laparoscopic instruments
  classification system for 937
  dimension of 937
  sterilization of 937
Laparoscopic mesh
  rectopexy 396
  repair techniques 746
Laparoscopic omental patch technique 254
Laparoscopic repair techniques 737, 738
Laparoscopic splenectomy 213, 214, 631
  indications of 213
Laparoscopic ventral hernia repair 738
  contraindications of 738
Laparoscopy 931
  complications of 943
  diagnostic 194, 378, 617
  staging 272, 291
Laparotomy 238, 615, 751, 797
  anterolateral 797
  exploratory 290, 751
  indications of 614
Lapatinib 480
Laryngeal nerve, recurrent 527, 951, 1075
Laser therapy 919
Late dumping syndrome 288
Lateral internal sphincterotomy 400
Lateral sphincterotomy
  complications of 400
  contraindications of 400
Latex agglutination test 246
Latissimus dorsi flap 473
Laugier's hernia 728, 749
Lauren classification system 265
Lax hydrocele 765
Leather bottle stomach 266
Lee index 1067
Lee-Huang point 933
Le-Fort classification 593, 1058
Leg ulcer, causes of nonvenous 701
Legionella 162
Lentigo 827
Leprosy 315
Leptomeningeal angiomatosis 820
Leptospira 162
Lesions
  benign pigmented 827
  excision of primary 837
  malignant 829
  nonproliferative 443
  proliferative 443
  sclerosing 453
  tubercular 880
Lesser sciatic foramen 743
Less-open sublay operation 732
Leukemia 831, 868
  acute myeloid 210
  prolymphocytic 210
Leukocytes 5
Leukocytosis 114, 157, 372
Levofloxacin 248
Levothyroxine 490, 516
Leydig cell
  hypoplasia of 756
  tumor 447, 923
Lichtenstein repair 724, 725
Lidocaine 985, 986
Lieberkühn crypts 387
Li-Fraumeni syndrome 265, 445, 454
Ligament 317, 1072
  inguinal 717
Ligamentum
  teres 109, 1072
  venosum 1072
Lilly's procedure 80
Limb
  body wall defect syndrome 221
  hypertrophy 820
  infusion, isolated 837
  perfusion, isolated 837
  volume, assessment of 704
Limberg flap 419
  modified 419
Linea alba 713
  fatty hernia of 733
  weakened decussating fibers of 733
Linear ulceration, deep 309
Linezolid 33
Lingual nerve 809, 810
Linitis plastica 266
Linoleic acid 452
Linolenic acid 452
Lip swelling 309
Lipid 669
  emulsion therapy 985
Lipid-laden macrophages 447
Lipoblastomas 823
Lipodermatosclerosis 694, 696
Lipoma 448, 741, 822, 823
  aborescens 823
  operated specimen of 822
  subcutaneous 822
  uncommon varieties of 823
Lithium 489
Lithotomy position 426
Littoral cell angioma 212
Littre hernia 749
Liver 35, 123, 126, 863
  abscess 101, 112, 113, 129, 144, 157
    favor of 157
    polymicrobial 113
    pyogenic 111, 117, 118, 120
  adenomatosis 135
  anatomy 110
  attenuation value of 1073
  biopsy 77, 86, 135
  cells 119
  cirrhosis of 241
  cysts, fenestration of remnant 133
  disease 33, 107
    end-stage 139
    polycystic 111, 133
    radiation-induced 144
  dullness, obliterated 253
  failure 144
  fluke infections 93
  function
    compromised 733
    test 67, 449
  hydatid cyst of 124
  imaging reporting and data system 138
  lesions
    hypervascular 1073
    hypovascular 1073
    malignant 1073
  metastases 145, 429
    colorectal 145, 358
    management of 361
    metachronous 358
  resection 142
    complications of 141
    indications of 118, 141
    segmental 85
  right lobe of 159
  segmental anatomy of 110
  shadow, enlargement of 114
  simple cyst of 132
  transplantation 78, 133, 135, 143, 153
  trauma 627, 628
    penetrating 628
  tumors, parenchymal 94
  volume 143
Living donor transplantation 143
Llyod-Davies position 426
Lobectomy 129
  plus isthmusectomy 515
    disadvantages of 515
Lobular carcinoma in situ 443, 456
Lobules 119
Local anesthetic
  systemic toxicity, treatment of 985
  toxicity of 985
Local excision, approaches of 424
Local infection 11
  classic signs of 11
Lockwood's infra-inguinal approach 729
Locoregional therapy 140, 143
Long-acting somatostatin analog 287
Longitudinal intestinal lengthening and tailoring procedure 327, 329

Longmire 196
Loop sigmoid colostomy 429
Lothessein's transinguinal approach 728
Love's test 821
Low anterior resection syndrome 424-426
Low Maruyama index surgery 271
Low molecular weight heparin 33, 692
Low spinal cord reflexes, assessment of 598
Low tie technique 425
Low velocity injuries 583
Low-birth-weight 222
Lower leg
  anterior aspects of 494
  lateral aspects of 494
Lower limb
  examination of 14, 709
  lymphedema 705
Lower midline syndrome 220
Lower rectum, adenocarcinoma of 426
Lower urinary tract symptoms 900
  causes of 900
Low-friction suture 1081
Lumbar hernia 715, 740
  acquired 741
  classification of 741
  congenital 741
  inferior 741
Lumbar triangle 740
  inferior 740
Lumen apposing metal stent 173
  uses of 173
Lumpectomy 445, 469
Lund's node 42
Lund-Browder chart 653
Lung 129, 690
  metastasis 458
    management of 361
  parenchymal injury 1080
Lupus 830
Luschka crypts 1070
Luschka ducts 1071
Lymph node 106, 269, 475, 796
  apical 358
  cystic 1071
  dissection 273, 837
    extent of 273
    quality of 926
    therapeutic 523
  enlarged pelvic 921
  epicolic 358
  inguinal 431
  intermediate 358
  metastasis 836
  metastatic 515, 1079, 1080
  normal 1080
  paracolic 358
  parotid 1082
  primary neoplasm of 969
  principal 358
  regional 920
Lymph scrotum 765
Lymphadenectomy 92, 106, 196
  pelvic 921
  radical inguinal 236
  standard 196
Lymphadenitis
  acute 232, 702
  nonspecific 967
  tuberculous 967
Lymphadenopathy 966
  axillary 449
  mesenteric 303
Lymphangiography 705
Lymphangioma 707, 808, 820
  cystic variety of 972
Lymphangiomatosis, superficial scrotal 765
Lymphangiosarcoma 704, 707, 838
Lymphangitis, acute 702
Lymphatic
  abnormality, congenital 707
  acute inflammation of 702
  diseases 665
  drainage
    manual 706
    simple 706
  filariasis, urological complications of 765
  spread 358, 835
  system, diseases of 702
  tumors of 707
Lymphedema 702
  assessment of 704
  chronic 838
  classification of 703
  congenita 704
  filarial 703
  postradiation 767
  praecox 703, 704
  primary 703, 704
  tarda 704
  upper limb 705, 706
Lymphocele, symptomatic 926
Lymphoma 88, 93, 303, 324, 831
  primary gastrointestinal 280
Lymphoproliferative disorder 1079
Lymphoscintigraphy 705
Lynch syndrome 265, 354, 361
  diagnosis of 354

M

Macrocysts 453
Macrophages 668
Madden-Auchincloss mastectomy 471
Mafenide acetate 657
Magnesium
  ammonium phosphate 868
  foods rich in 25
  serum 21, 26
Magnetic resonance venography 690
Magnetic sphincter augmentation 778
Main bile duct, strictures of 62
Malabsorption 180
Malaise 137, 324
Malaria 38
Malformations
  arteriovenous 281, 821
  congenital 490, 861
  penile 756
  venous 820
Malgaigne's bulge 1079
Malignancy 162, 234, 327, 329, 690
  hypercalcemia of 24
  increased risk of 348
  intra-abdominal 886
  risk factors for 88
Malignant tumor 812, 881
  high-grade 807
  low-grade 807
Mallampati classification 990
Mallory–Weiss tear 259
Malnutrition 7, 447
  universal screening tool 1079
Mammary analog secretory carcinoma 1087
Mammary duct fistula 453
Mammary ductoscopy 451
Mammography 441, 442, 451, 464, 465
  diagnostic 450
  screening 464
  types of 464
Mammotome 462
Manchester scoring system 1067
Mandible, fracture of 592
Mannitol 589, 590
Manometry 774
  esophageal 775, 776, 781
  high-resolution 776, 779
Marfan syndrome 222, 330, 685, 686, 713
Marfanoid habitus 567
Marjolin's ulcer 662, 701, 831, 839, 1079
Marshall scoring system, modified 1067
Maruyama index 271
Mascagni's lymph node 42
Mass, palpable 125
Massive transfusion
  complications of 39
  protocol 38, 578
Mast cells 5
Mastalgia 451-453
  cyclical 451, 453
  non-cyclical 451
  non-focal 451
Mastectomy
  indications of 470

partial 445
radical inguinal 471
simple 471
total 445
types of 470
Mastitis
lactational 439
periductal 441, 453
recurrent periductal 441
treatment of 439
Mastocytosis, systemic 241
Mastoid process 807
Matrix metalloproteinases 6
Mattox maneuver 633
Maxillofacial injuries, treatment of 591
Maydl's hernia 749
Mayo's endoscopic subscore 345
Mayo's scissors 1007
uses of 1007
McBurney's point 377
McCune-Albright syndrome 135
McEvedy's high approach 729
McGill pain questionnaire 180
McIndoe scissors, uses of 1007
McMahon classification 61, 62
McVay repair 725
Mealtime syndrome 805, 1082
Meandering mesenteric artery 1073
Mechanical obstruction 340
suggestive of 339
Mechanical small bowel obstruction, different types of 301
Meckel's diverticulum 221, 224, 241, 303, 320-322
neoplasm of 321
surgical management of symptomatic 323
Meckel's scintigraphy 322
Meconium ileus 294
Medial basilic vein 1070
Medialization thyroplasty 951
Median nerve 952
injury 952, 959
Median umbilical fold 718
Mediastinum 923
Medical therapy 343
Medium-chain-triglyceride rich diet 707
Medulla 545
Medullary thyroid carcinoma 520
distinctive features of 520
inherited forms of 520
types of 520
Medulloblastoma 353
Meek micrografting technique 658
Megacolon, toxic 343
Meggitt-Wagner wound classification 848
Melanocytes 833
Melanoma 833, 834, 1079
classification of 833
cutaneous 833
malignant 836
mucosal 833
noncutaneous 833
Menetrier's disease 281
Meningeal artery, middle 585
Meningitis 114, 804
Meningococcal vaccine, revaccination of 215
Menstruation, cyclical changes of 453
Mesalamine 346
multimatrix preparation 346
Mesenchymal cell markers 1080
Mesenteric arterial
embolism 327
occlusion, acute 679
Mesenteric artery, superior 680
Mesenteric lymph nodes, self-limiting inflammation of 232
Mesenteric venous occlusion 681
Mesentery 218
Mesh 748
fixation methods 749
infection 726
mediated techniques 646
migration of 726
placement, techniques of 738
rectopexy 395
repair 722-724, 729, 733, 751
Meshed split-thickness skin graft 643, 767
Mesoappendix dissection, techniques of 384
Mesosigmoidoplasty 335, 336
Metabolic acidosis 27, 643
types of 27
Metabolic alkalosis 27
biological effects of 27
hypochloremic 261
Metabolic disorders 136, 915
Metabolic syndrome 135
Metabolism, inherited errors of 136
Metacestodes 123
Metaiodobenzylguanidine scanning 556
Metallic bougie 1010
Metastasis 88, 836
peritoneal 358
secondary 897
sites of 358
synchronous 358
Metastatic breast carcinoma, primary management of 482
Metastatic disease 146, 884, 895
high-volume 146
treatment of 910
Methimazole 500
dosage of 500
embryopathy, syndrome of 501
Methotrexate 226, 235, 310, 701
Methysergide 234
Metoclopramide 450
Metronidazole 122
Metzenbaum scissors 1007
use of 1007
Michel's classification 1058
Microabscess 113
Microcarcinoma 514
Microdochectomy 442
Microfibrillar collagen 34
Microfilaria, detection of 765
Microhamartoma, biliary 133
Microlithiasis
occult 162
testicular 923
Micronized purified flavonoid fraction 697
Microporous polysaccharide spheres 34
Microsatellite instability testing 272, 360
Microwave ablation 140
Middle cranial fossa fracture 584
signs of 580
Midgut volvulus 294
Midstream urine sample, microscopic analysis of 858
Migratory necrolytic erythema 565
Mikulicz's procedure 336
Milan criteria 1061
Mild lower limb, management of 706
Milk stasis 439
Millard rotation 979
Milwaukee classification, modified 1058
Mineral deficiency 7
Mineralocorticoid
replacement 554
therapy 554
Minimal mesenteric dissection 329
Minimally invasive
colectomy 361, 364
esophagectomy 796, 797
Ivor Lewis esophagectomy 797
McKeown esophagectomy 797
retroperitoneal necrosectomy 171, 172
surgery 929, 938, 943
advantages of 942
disadvantages of 942
extracavitary 931
Minimum alveolar concentration 989
Minocycline 825
Minor depressed fractures 584
Minor salivary gland 803, 806
tumors 806
Mirizzi syndrome 46, 76
management of 76
types of 76
Mismatch repair 272, 360
Mitotic index 561
Mitotic rate 279, 836
Mohs surgery 831, 919
Molecular classification 135
Mondor's disease 451, 443
penile 443

Monocytes 668
Monomicrobial cryptogenic invasive liver abscess 114
Monopolar electrosurgery 941
Montreal classification system 342
Morgagni hernia 749
Mosquito hemostatic forceps 999
Motility disorder 261
Motor neuropathy 846
Motor-vehicle accidents, types of 572
Moynihan's cholecystectomy forceps 1007
Moynihan's hump 1071
Moynihan's modification 45
Mucinous adenocarcinoma 265, 357
  prognosis of 357
Mucocele 806
Mucogingivitis 309
Mucoid discharge 412
Mucopolysaccharidoses 222
Mucosa
  colonic 353
  jejunal 241
Mucosal prolapse 392-394
  differential diagnosis of 393
Mucus retention cyst 806
Mule spinner's cancer 766
Mulliken technique 979
Multidimensional scale 180
Multifocal idiopathic fibrosclerosis, components of 511
Multigene assay 477, 479
Multi-layer inelastic lymphoedema bandaging 706
Multinodular goiter 505
  histology of 505
Multiple array needle electrode 144
Multiple endocrine neoplasia 561, 566, 567
  syndromes 566
Multiple organ dysfunction 681
Mumps orchitis 759
Mumps virus 804
Murphy's percussion test 45
Murphy's sign 45, 101, 1071
  elicitation of 45
  sonographic 45
Muscle 803
  flap 786
  invasive urothelial blader cancer 898
  wasting 496
Musculoskeletal system, secondary survey of 581
Mutations 360, 834
Mycoplasma 162
Mycotic aneurysm 682
Myelofibrosis 148
  idiopathic 210
Myeloproliferative disorders, primary 148
Myocardial infarction 339
Myocardial rupture 603
Myochosis coli 330
Myopathy 550
  proximal 496
Myopectineal orifice 717
Myotomy 779
  esophagogastric 783
  surgical 780
    cricopharyngeal 782
Myxedema, pretibial 494

N

Naffziger test 499
Narrowed-spectrum endoscopy 267
Nasal cannula 851
Nasogastric
  decompression 290, 372
  drainage 170
  intubation 993
  tube 254, 851
Nasotracheal intubation 591
Natalizumab 310
Natatory ligament 958
Nausea
  anticipatory 1084
  postoperative 992
Nealon classification 176
Near-infrared fluorescent cholangiography 58
Neck 575, 822
  computed tomography scan of 524
  dissection 968, 969
    classification of 968
    complications of 969
    extended 969
  exploration
    bilateral 538, 540, 541
    principles of 595
  incision 797
  injuries 594
    penetrating 594
  lymphatic levels of 964
  mass, malignant 966
  swelling 962, 966
    congenital 966
    cystic 966
    midline 966
    neoplastic 966
  X-ray of 524
Necrosectomy, open 172
Necrosis
  cystic medial 686
  pancreatic 171
  transmural 790
  zone of 654
Necrotic tissue 12
Necrotizing pancreatitis 164, 171
  management of 171
Necrotizing soft tissue infection 826
  severe type of 766
Needle
  cricothyroidotomy 578
  holder, grip of 1082
  thoracocentesis 605
Negative pressure wound therapy 12, 646
Neimeier classification 1058
Neoadjuvant systemic therapy 467, 481
  advantages of 481
  indications of 481
Neoplasia 756
Neoplasms 295, 321
  malignant 323
  mucinous cystic 189, 190, 192
  retroperitoneal 235
  solid pseudopapillary 190
Neoplastic lesion 259, 295, 809
Nephrectomy 635, 874
  palliative 886
  partial 635, 874
Nephrocalcinosis 537
Nephrogenic systemic fibrosis 1078
  risk of 1086
Nephrolithiasis 308, 537
Nephrolithotomy 874
  percutaneous 873, 888
Nephron-sparing surgery 886
Nephroscope 873
Nephrostomy tube 874
Nephroureterectomy, radical inguinal 886, 889, 890
Nerve
  anatomy of 948
  block 984
  entrapment 726
  fiber 948
  grafting 951
  hypertrophy, pancreatic 180
  injury 946, 959
    classification of 948
    major 596
    management of 950
  monitoring, intraoperative 1075
  repair, principles of 950
  tension free primary anastomosis of 951
  transfer 951
Nervousness 496
Neural crest cells 971
Neurectomy 727
Neurilemmomas 808
Neuroendocrine tumor 387, 561
  high grade 357
  pancreatic 190, 561
Neurofibroma 808, 823
Neurofibromatosis 561
  multiple hepatic 823, 824

Neuroimaging radiological interpretation system 1085
Neurologic deficit, severe 580
Neurologic disorders 915
Neurological system, secondary survey of 581
Neurolytic therapy 183
Neuromas, mucosal 567
Neuromodulation, sacral 420
Neuromuscular blockade 991
  reversal of 988
Neuron 948
Neuropathy
  autonomic 846
  peripheral 847
  severe peripheral 697
Neuropraxia 948, 949
Neurotmesis 948, 949
New Orleans criteria 1061
New pulp score 254
Nicotine consumption 177
Niemeier classification 48
Nifedipine 399
Nigro regime 431
Nipple
  cracked 439
  discharge 449, 450
    assessment of 449
    causes of 449
    cytologic examination of 450
    pathologic 449
  eversion 453
  Paget's disease of 483
  retraction 441, 449, 453
    causes of 441
Nissen fundoplication, laparoscopic 777
Nitroglycerine, topical 399
Nitrous oxide 989
Nivolumab 886
Nocturia 860
  causes of 860
Nodular thyroid disease, benign 523
Nodule, management of 507
Nonabsorbable suture 222, 237
Non-anion gap metabolic acidosis 27
Noncirrhotic portal fibrosis 147
Noncolorectal metastases 145
Nonfistulizing lesions 308
Nonhealing bruise 704
Nonimmune hemolytic reactions 37
Noninvasive tests 246
Nonischemic priapism 915
  management of 916
Non-mesh mediated techniques 646
Non-muscle invasive urothelial bladder cancer 898
Non-neuroendocrine metastases 145
Nonocclusive mesenteric insufficiency 681
Nonoperative management 299, 380, 614, 627, 628
  trial of 254
Nonresectional operative procedures 337
Nonseminoma 925
Non-staghorn calculi 871
Non-steroidal anti-inflammatory drugs
  role of 242
  topical application of 452
Nonsteroidal aromatase inhibitors 478
Nontoxic multinodular goiter 505
Non-transecting anastomotic urethroplasty 912
Non-variceal upper gastrointestina bleeding, management of 258
Northern exposure sign 335
Norton-Simon hypothesis 1079
Nottingham modification 457
Nuck
  hernia canal 763, 749
  hydrocele of canal of 763
Nuclear polymorphism 457
Numbness 675
Nutcracker esophagus 781
Nutrition 850
  parenteral 170
Nutritional supplement, composition of 659
Nylon 1014

O

Oakland score 1067
Obesity 135, 136
Obliteration, total failure of 224
Obraztsova's sign 377
Obstipation 297
Obstruction 295, 302
  causes of 376
  colonic 340
  duodenal 181
  four cardinal features of 297
  intestinal 294, 308, 321, 322
  level of 297
  management of 277, 333, 365
  pathophysiology of 295
  strangulation 296
  types of 334
Obturator
  canal 742
  foramen 742
  membrane 742
  nerve 742
  sign 377
Occlusion, causes of 667
Ochsner-Mahorner test 695
Octreoscan 562
Octreotide 287, 563
Oddi sphincter 42, 77, 177, 1071
Off-midline excisional procedure 418
Ogilvie dysphagia score system 787, 1067
Ogilvie syndrome 339
Okuda staging 140
Oligomenorrhea 496
Olsalazine 346
Omental graft 232
  uses of 232
Omental tape technique 1076
Omentoplasty 129
Omentum 629, 631
  functions of 232
Omics' technology 1081
Omphalocele 220
Omphalomesenteric duct
  anomalies 223, 320
  vestigial remnant of 320
Oncocytoma 881
Oncogenes 513
Oophoritis 804
Oozler's operation 283
Open abdomen
  classification 646
  complications of 646
Open adrenalectomy
  approaches of 558
  different approaches of 560
Open cholecystectomy
  basic steps of 60
  scar 8
Open colectomy 364
  conventional 364
Open dressing 657
Open mesh repair techniques 746
Open prostatectomy 904
  approaches of 904
  indications of 904
Open repair techniques 737
Open splenectomy 213
  indications of 213
Operative management, principles of 300, 628
Ophthalmopathy
  mild 502
  sight-threatening 502
Opioid 436
  analgesics 655, 988
Opisthorchis viverrini 93
Optical fibers 935
Optimal tumor response 481
Oral hypoglycemic agents 1078
Oral pancreatic enzyme supplementation 183
Orbit, computed tomography scan of 500
Orbital pain, spontaneous 497
Orbitopathy 497
Orchidectomy 760
Orchidopexy 757
  benefits of 757

complications of 758
laparoscopic 758
Orchiectomy
bilateral
simple 760
subcapsular 760
indications of 760
partial 924
radical inguinal 760, 923, 924
transcrotal 924
unilateral simple 760
Orchiopexy, standard 758
Orchitis 447, 804
ischemic 726
Organ
failure 168
sparing approaches 918
support 645
Ormeloxifene 452
Ormond disease 234
Orotracheal intubation 577
Orthodontic management 980
Orthophthalaldehyde 938
Orthotopic liver transplantation 83
Oscillation, absence of 1076
Osler-Weber-Rendu syndrome 134
Ossification, heterotopic 662
Osteitis fibrosa cystica 537
Osteogenesis imperfecta 713
Osteoma 353, 818
Osteomyelitis 112, 114
Osteonecrosis 308
Osteopenia 87, 537
Osteoporosis 87, 181, 537
Ostomy 367
types of 366
Ovarian cancer syndrome, hereditary 265, 454
Ovarian cyst 238
torsion of 232
Overnight dexamethasone suppression test 550
Overwhelming post-splenectomy infection 214, 215
prevention of 215
Oxaliplatin 92
Oxygen saturation probe 851
Oxyphil 534
Oxyphilic cell carcinoma 520
Oxyuris vermicularis 376

P

Pacemaker 941
Paget's disease 483
penoscrotal 767
Pain 157, 180, 412, 670, 859, 893
abdominal 94, 113, 125, 163, 172, 180, 281, 297, 338, 339, 681
acute-onset severe unilateral scrotal 770
assessment of 180
bilateral aching 451
biliary 451
chronic postoperative inguinal 727
extramammary 451
groin 726
intractable abdominal 184
management of 9, 183, 199
prostatic 860
renal 859
scrotal 770
site of 859
triangle of 719
ureteral 859
urethral 860
Palatal ulcerations 309
Palliative therapy 204, 798
Pallor 670
Palm, rule of 653
Palmer's point 932
Palpitations 496
Pamidronate 24
Pancreas 196, 690
adult 1073
annular 162
benign cystic neoplasm of 189
carcinoma of head of 94, 103
cystic neoplasm of 176
diseases of 160
distal 564
divisum 177
endocrine 532
head of 564
neuroendocrine tumors of 561
premalignant tumors of 192
pseudocyst of 176
tail of 192, 209
Pancreatectomy 188, 189
distal 196, 621
total 184, 188
Pancreatic body 195
Pancreatic cancer 689
screening 191
Pancreatic duct 564
disruption 1085
Pancreatic endocrine
neoplasm 562
tumors 145
Pancreatic exocrine insufficiency 180
causes of 180
Pancreatic head 195
Pancreatic islet D cell 565
Pancreatic protocol computed tomography abdomen 193
Pancreatic pseudocyst 164
drainage, laparoscopic 172
Pancreatic resection 174, 180
Pancreatic stone, management of 184
Pancreatic stricture, management of 184
Pancreatic tissue 166
nonviable 166
Pancreaticoduodenectomy 196, 204, 622
complications of 198
pylorus-preserving 186
Pancreaticogastrostomy, techniques of 197
Pancreatico-pleural fistula 181
Pancreatitis 80, 97, 326, 804
acute 46, 101, 163-166, 201, 372, 1059
biliary 51
on chronic 166
biliary 51, 170
chronic 177-182, 212
critical acute 168
interstitial edematous 164
mild 169
acute 168
moderate 169
acute 168
non-gallstone 167
severe 169
acute 168, 177
biliary 51
Pancreatoduodenectomy 189
partial 184, 186
Pancreatogram 182
Pancuronium 988
Pantaloon hernia 749
Pap test 1084
Papillary apocrine change 443
Papilloma 821
intraductal 443, 449
Papillotomy, endoscopic 72
Paradoxical movement 602
Paraesophageal hernia 283, 773
asymptomatic 774
surgical repair of 774
Paragangliomas 555
extra-adrenal 971
Paralysis 670
Paramyxovirus 804
Paraneoplastic syndrome 137, 884
Paraphimosis 768
Parasite 84
infestations 44
Parastomal hernia 745
classification of 745
repair, methods of 745
Paratesticular abnormalities 756
Parathyroid 532
agenesis 23
diseases of 535
exploration 566
hormone 535
sonographer 539
surgery 538
surgical anatomy of 534

Parathyroidectomy 538
- indications of 538
- subtotal 541, 542
- total 541

Parenchyma, renal 633
Parenchymal injury, pulmonary 609
Parenteral nutrition 170
- indications of 170

Paresthesia 23, 670, 675
Paris classification 267
Park's incontinence scale 1067
Parkinson's disease 339
Parkland formula, modified 655
Paronychia
- acute 957
- chronic 957

Parotid
- carcinoma of 1079
- dissection of 812
- gland 803, 804, 807, 808
  - duct of 803
  - lower part of 808
  - superficial lobe of 807
  - tumors, majority of 806

Parotidectomy 812
- complications of 812
- incisions for 811
- partial superficial 812
- superficial 811
- total 807

Partial splenectomy 213, 631
- contraindications of 213
- indications of 213

Partington and Rochelle modification 184, 185
Passaro's triangle 563
Patent urachus 224, 891
Patey-Dyson mastectomy 471
Pathognomonic keratin-plugged punctum 818
Pathology
- behind syndrome 288
- inflammatory 61

Pazopanib 886
Pearl Necklace sign 1071
Peau D'orange appearance 458
Pediatric appendicitis score 379, 1067
Pedicled flap
- advantages of 474
- disadvantages of 474

Pelvic examination 422, 431
Pelvic floor
- defects 891
- hernia, types of 743
- rehabilitation 420

Pelvic fracture 633, 639, 640
- clinical findings suggestive of 581
- urethral injury 640

Pelvic radiotherapy, postoperative 705
Pelvic surgery
- abdominal 692
- reoperative 1077

Pelvic wall, hernia of 741
Pelvis
- computed tomography scan of 298, 360, 373
- contrast-enhanced computed tomography scan of 90, 236
- magnetic resonance imaging of 309
- renal 350
- secondary survey of 581

Pembrolizumab 796
Penectomy
- partial 918, 919
- total 918-920

Penetrating injury 582, 583, 633, 640, 951
- management of 614

Penile curvature, correction of 913
Penile fracture
- causes of 642

Penile injury 640
- different types of 640

Penile intraepithelial neoplasia 917
Penis
- carcinoma of 917
- diseases of 752
- fracture of 642

Peptic perforation 201, 751
Peptic ulcer
- clinical presentation of 244
- complications of 245
- disease 102, 241, 259
- perforation score 1067
- recurrent 248
- refractory 248
- sites of 241

Percutaneous catheter drainage 117, 158, 171
Percutaneous drainage 172, 173, 229
- complications of 173

Percutaneous ethanol injection 140, 143
Percutaneous nephrolithotomy 873, 888
- complications of 874
- contraindications of 873

Percutaneous transhepatic
- cholangioscopic lithotomy 77
- gallbladder drainage 47, 102

Perforation 253, 316, 335, 339
- abdominal 784, 785
- duodenal 97, 619
- sites of 784
- tubercular 316

Perianal abscess 401
- drainage of 402

Perianal cancer 430
- treatment of 431

Perianal fistulizing disease, management of 311
Perianal hidradenitis suppurativa 825
Perianal region
- inspection of 404
- palpation of 404

Pericardial tamponade 610
Pericarditis 309
Pericyst 124
Pericystectomy 128, 129
Periductal mastitis 441, 453
- pathophysiology of 441
- suggestive of 458

Perinatal care 220
Perineal dissection 427
Perineal hernia 716, 743
- anterior 743
- secondary acquired 743
- types of 743

Perineal procedures 395
- advantages of 395
- disadvantages of 395
- indications of 395

Perineal reconstruction, indications of 426
Perineal wound 426
- reconstruction options for 426

Perineum, inspection of 393, 404
Perineurium 948
Perinuclear antineutrophil cytoplasmic antibodies 344
Perioral region, papillary carcinoma of 23
Peripheral artery disease 674
Peripheral nerve
- lesion 846
- trunk 948

Peristalsis 300
Peritoneal cavity 227, 717, 746
- spaces of 227

Peritoneal fluid, cytologic testing of 272
Peritoneal irrigation, intraoperative 382
Peritoneal ligament 746
Peritoneal mesothelioma, malignant 230
Peritoneal neoplasm, primary malignant 230
Peritoneal tissues, protection of 128
Peritoneum 218, 227, 358, 581
Peritonitis, signs of 254
Perivascular epithelioid cells 882
Periwound skin protectants 10
Peroral cholangioscopic lithotripsy 77
Peroral endoscopic myotomy 780
Perthe's test, modified 696
Pertuzumab 480
Petersen hernia 749
Petit hernia 741, 749
Peutz-Jeghers
- polyps 350
- syndrome 265, 323, 324, 350, 354, 454

Peyer's patch 314
hypertrophied 303
Peyronie's disease 234, 916
Phallus 757
Pharmacologic therapy 420
Phenol application 418
Phenothiazines 447
Phenotypic classification 310
Phenoxybenzamine 556
Phenylephrine 915
Phenytoin 447
Pheochromocytoma 522, 555, 556, 559
bilateral 558
extra-adrenal sites of 555
intraoperative management of 557
syndrome associated 555
Phimosis 767, 917
complications of 767
pathologic 767
physiologic 767
Phlebotonics act 413
Phlebotropic drugs, use of 710
Phlegmasia
alba dolens 691
cerulean dolens 691
Phlegmon 380
Phyllodes tumor 444, 445, 485
Phytobezoars 283, 302
special type of 283
Pigment stone, intrahepatic 83
Pigmentation, mucocutaneous 350
Pigtail catheter drainage 112
Pilonidal disease 416
chronic 418
spectrum of 416
Pilonidal sinus 416
unusual sites of 416
video-assisted ablation of 418
Pilosebaceous follicles 818
Ping pong fracture 584
Piperacillin 33
Pittsburgh perforation severity score 785, 1067
Planned open cholecystectomy, indications of 56
Plaque, growth of 667
Plasma metanephrines evaluation 556
Plastic stent
composition of 96
diameter of 96
Platelet 208
concentrates 35
dysfunction 32
Platinum based chemotherapy 899
Platysma 968
Pleural effusion 165
Pleuritis 46
Plexiform neurofibromatosis 824
Plica circulares 317
Plication technique 764
Plug-and-patch
repair 725
technique 724
Plummer disease 503
Plummer-Vinson syndrome 794
Pluripotent 320
Pneumatic compression, intermittent 692, 707
Pneumatic dilation 780
Pneumobilia 77
causes of 77
Pneumococcal vaccine, revaccination of 215
Pneumonia 46, 112
Pneumoperitoneum
physiology of 932
significant 254
Pneumothorax 578, 603
open 578, 603, 606
simple 603, 604
PNM classification 1058
Poikilocytosis 214
Poikilothermy 670
Pointing finger 952
Point-of-care
testing 39
ultrasound 378
Poland syndrome 438
Polidocanol 258, 698
Poliglecaprone 1013
Polyarteritis nodosa 234, 685, 701
Polycystic kidney disease
autosomal dominant 863
autosomal recessive 863
Polycythemia vera 241, 701
Polydioxanone 1013
Polyester fiber suture 1014
Polyglactic 910 1013
Polyglycolic suture 1013
Polymastia 438
Polypectomy 351
Polyphosphazene-coated polymethylmethacrylate microspheres 144
Polypoidal lesion 88
Polyposis
colonic 818
familial adenomatous 265, 324, 353
syndrome 423
autosomal dominant 353
juvenile 265, 350, 354
Polypropylene 724, 1014
Polyps
adenomatous 351, 353
colonic 353
colorectal 349
duodenal 353
extracolonic 353
extraintestinal sites of 350
hamartomatous 323, 349
hyperplastic 281, 349
inflammatory 351
intestinal 303
juvenile 281, 349
multiple
adenomatous 353
hepatic 352
pedunculated 352
periampullary 353
synchronous 423
true 88
Polythelia 438
Polytrauma 652
Polyvinyl alcohol articles 145
Pond fracture 584
Popliteal artery aneurysm 685
recognition of 685
Porcine derived collagen agents 34
Porphyria cutanea tarda 136
Port placement, principles of 935
Porta hepatis 106
Portal cavernoma 148
Portal hypertension 87, 144, 147, 148, 150, 212, 409
causes of 147
clinically significant 139
Portal hypertensive gastropathy 152
Portal scissura 1072
Portal vein 142, 148, 188, 1072
bifurcation 110
branches of 77
Portal venopathy, obliterative 134
Portal venous
flow 113
route 112, 113
system 1072
Portocaval shunt
end-to-side 154
side-to-side 154
Portosystemic collaterals, decompression of 152
Port-wine stain 820
Positive overnight dexamethasone suppression test 550
Positive pressure ventilation 578
Postablation whole body iodine scan 516
Postanesthesia care unit 991
Postauricular sequestration dermoid cyst 818
Postburn pruritus, management of 659
Postconcussive syndrome 1076
Postembolization syndrome 144
Post-endoscopic retrograde cholangiopancreatography pancreatitis 162
Posterior mesh rectopexy 395-397
Posterior wall defect 719

Postgastrectomy syndromes 286
Postoperative pain management 993
Post-parotidectomy facial palsy 1082
Postpolypectomy bleeding, management of 370
Post-splenectomy blood picture 214
Post-thyroidectomy voice change, causes of 1075
Post-transfusion purpura 38
Post-traumatic seizure 590
  risk factors for 590
Postvagotomy syndromes 285
Postvoid residual urine 902
Potassium
  chloride 241, 1070
  foods rich in 22
  serum 1070
  supplementation 21
Pouchitis 348
Poupart's ligament 744
Povidone-iodine solute 128
Prader orchidometer 761
Prague classification 793
Prazosin 556
Preanesthetic medication 992
Pregabalin 183
Pregnancy 148, 385, 409, 490, 686
  epithelial hyperplasia of 453
Prehn's sign 761
Prentiss maneuver, modified 758
Preperitoneal mesh placement 740
Preperitoneal space 726
  landmarks 718
Presacral drain 626
Presacral veins 1077
Pressure
  flow urodynamic studies 902
  necrosis 844
  offloading 848
  ulcer 849
    development 849
    medical device-related 851
Priapism 915
  history of 915
  ischemic 915
  management of 916
Primary duct stone, management of 74
Primary sclerosing cholangitis 85, 93, 308
  complications of 87
Primary thyroid malignancy 512
  pathogenesis of 513
Primary tumor 559
  treatment of 918
Primary ureteroureterostomy over ureteral stent 637
Pringle maneuver 629
Probenecid 868
Proctectomy 408
Proctitis 348
Proctoscopy 399, 405, 412, 431
Profibrinolytic action 697
Prokinetics 170
Prolactinoma 450
Prolapse 409, 412
Prolene 1014
  hernia system 723
Prone jack-knife position 426
Prophylactic bilateral central neck dissection 522
Prophylaxis 691
  against thromboembolism 992
  potential candidates of 691
Propofol 988
Propylthiouracil 500
  dosage of 500
Prostaglandin 242, 913
Prostate
  cancer grading system 908
  carcinoma 907
  cryosurgical ablation of 909
  holmium laser resection of 904
  photoselective vaporization of 904
  specific antigen 901, 909
  transurethral holmium laser
    ablation of 904
    enucleation of 904
  transurethral
    incision of 904
    resection of 903
Prostatectomy
  radical 909, 910
  retropubic 905
  transvesical 906
Prostatitis 907
  types of 907
Prosthesis
  penile 917
  testicular 760
Prosthetic valve 670
Protein 659
  C deficiency 148
  losing hypertrophic gastropathy 281
  S deficiency 148
Prothrombin complex concentrate 36, 39
Proton pump inhibitor therapy, trial of 775
Protoscolicidal agents 128
Protoscolicide 128
Pruritus 94
  pathophysiology of 1071
Pseudoachalasia 779
Pseudoaneurysm 682
  arterial 181
Pseudocyst 166, 172, 174, 176, 179, 181, 184, 190
  causes of 172
  characteristic features of 181
  management of 172, 184
  pancreatic 164
  treatment of 172
Pseudogynecomastia 448
Pseudohematuria 858
Pseudo-hernia 741
Pseudohypernatremia, causes of 20
Pseudohypokalemia, causes of 21
Pseudohyponatremia 20
  causes of 20
Pseudohypoparathyroidism 543
Pseudokidney sign 304
Pseudolipoma, post-traumatic 1076
Pseudolithiasis, biliary 43
Pseudomonas aeruginosa 116
Pseudomyxoma peritonei 230
Pseudo-obstruction, acute colonic 339, 340
Pseudopolyp 88, 351
Pseudopseudohypoparathyroidism 543
Psoas sign 377
Psoriasis 309
Psychiatric illness 614
Puberty 447
Puestow-Gillesby procedure 184-186
Pulp space infection 957
Pulsation, arterial 675
Pulselessness 670
Pulsion diverticulum 782
Punch biopsy 836
Pupil size, assessment of 589
Pure uric acid stones 868
Push and pull technique 326
Push enteroscopy 325
Pyelolithotomy 874
Pyelonephritis 888
  acute 875
  chronic 877
  reflux-associated 877
Pyloric exclusion procedure 619
Pyloric stenosis, congenital hypertrophic 261
Pyloroplasty 250
Pylorus, circular muscles of 261
Pyocele 765
Pyoderma gangrenosum 308
Pyonephrosis 879, 888
Pyriform sinus fistula 508

Q

Quackel shunt 916
Quantitative disease activity score 345
Quartz-rod lenses 935
Queyrat erythroplasia 829, 917
Quick sequential organ failure assessment score 1068
Quinolones 33

R

Radial margins 361
Radial nerve 952
  injury 952, 959

Radial scar 443
Radiation 513
  boost dose of 481
  enteritis 327
  pneumonitis 144
  therapy 140, 234, 524
    adjuvant 480, 830, 837
    intensity modulated 140
Radical neck dissection 968
  modified 516, 969
Radical prostatectomy 909, 910
  approaches of 910
  complications of 910
Radioactive iodine
  therapy 489, 516, 519
  treatment 522
Radioembolization, transarterial 144
Radiofrequency
  ablation 140, 143, 146, 258, 698
  electrosurgery 938
Radio-guided occult lesion localization 461
Radioisotope 476, 477
Radiological signs 316
Radionuclide thyroid scan 500, 506
Radiopaque stones 868
Radiotherapy 226, 280, 295, 909
Raised intracranial pressure 582
Raloxifene 478
Rampley's swab holding forceps 996
Ramstedt pyloromyotomy 261
Ramucirumab 796
Randall's plaque 866
Ranitidine 448, 450
Rank and Wakefield classification 3
Ranson criteria 167
  modified 167
Ranula 803, 806
  simple 806
  treatment of 809
Rapunzel syndrome 283
Raynaud's disease 844
Reanastomosis 155
Rebleeding
  prevention of 284
  risk of 256
Reconstruction
  complications of 474
  implant-based 472, 474
  methods after gastrectomy 277
  techniques of 724
Rectal cancer 421, 423
  asymptomatic 146
  obstructing 429
  protocol 423
  spread of 421
  surgery 421
Rectal injury 625
  intraperitoneal 625
Rectal mobilization, posterior 395, 396
Rectal prolapse 392, 412
  external 394
  internal 394
  mucosal 393
  surgical procedures for 395
  types of 392
Rectal tube placement 170
Rectocele 394
Rectopexy 395
  complications of 396
Rectosigmoid growth, large 409
Rectum 241, 348, 751
  diseases of 390
  intussusception of 392
  length of 421
  lower third of 421, 424
  mid part of 421, 424
  upper third of 421, 424
Rectus abdominis muscles, diastasis of 225
Recurrent laryngeal nerve 527, 951, 1075
  injury 527
    mechanisms of 528
    risk factors for 527
    symptoms of 527
Red pulp 208
Reductase inhibitors 902
Refined Hurley classification 1059
Reflux
  duodenal 51
  esophagitis 1058
  testing, methods of 776
Refractory stricture 788
Regnault classification 1059
Regorafenib 280
Regurgitation 601, 775, 779
Relieving worm bolus obstruction, operative technique of 302
Renal agenesis, unilateral 861
Renal artery 633
  aneurysm 685
Renal calculi, types of 867
Renal cell cancer
  metastatic 886
  papillary 884
Renal disease 537, 989
  chronic 7
Renal dysfunction 46
Renal excretion 26
Renal failure, chronic 241
Renal injury 634
  delayed complications of 634
  early complications of 634
  suggestive of 634
Renal pelvis 350
  urothelial tumors of 888
Renal preservation techniques 634
Renal stone 537, 866
  open surgery for 874
Renal system 660
Renal transplant recipients 897
Renal vasculature, anomalies of 862
Renorrhaphy 635
Resectable mid bile duct tumors 95
Resection
  extent of 362, 363
  principles of 141
  types of 189, 273
Respiratory acidosis 28, 943
  acute 28
  chronic 28
Respiratory alkalosis 28
  acute 28
  chronic 28
Respiratory dysfunction 46
Respiratory swing 609, 1076
Response evaluation criteria in solid tumors criteria 481, 1062
  modified 1061
Resuscitation
  endovascular 627
  goals 169
  neonatal 220, 222
Retained antrum syndrome 289
Retention cyst, types of 818
Retinal pigmented epithelium 353
  congenital hypertrophy of 353
Retractors 1005
  sterilization of 1006
Retroauricular hairline incision 1084
Retrocaval ureter 864
Retro-orbital fibrosis 511
Retroperitoneal fibrosis 87, 234
  idiopathic 234, 511
Retroperitoneal lymph node dissection 926
  complications of 926
Retroperitoneum 218, 746, 923, 925
  midline 633
  pelvic 633
Reynold's pentad 75
Rheumatoid arthritis 87, 234, 309, 493, 701
Rhomboid flap 419
Rib 602
  fracture 602
    multiple hepatic 602
    types of 602
  upper 602
Richter's hernia 728, 749
Riedel's thyroiditis 87, 234, 511
Ringer's lactate 169, 576, 578, 655
Ripstein and McMahan procedure, modified 396
Rives' technique 724
Rivinus ducts 803
Robotic colectomy 364
Rodent ulcer 829
Rogers score 692

Roizen criteria 557, 1062
Rokitansky-Aschoff sinuses 53
Romberg hernia 749
Ropivacaine 986
Rosary sign 1071
Rosemont classification 183
Rotavirus infection 303
Round ligament 109, 1072
Roux stasis syndrome 289
Roux syndrome 289
Roux-en-Y
- choledochojejunostomy 87
- gastric bypass 87, 283
- gastrojejunostomy 303
- hepaticojejunostomy 65, 77
- pancreaticojejunostomy 621
- reconstruction 198

Rovsing sign 377
Rubber band ligation 413
Rummel tourniquet 629
Ruptured aneurysm, management of 684
Rusty pipe syndrome 1084
Rutherford classification 674
Rutkow-Robbins repair 725
Ryle's tube 260, 1016
- catheterization 751

S

Sac
- dissection of 729
- ligation of 723
- narrowness of 728
- opening of 723

Saint's triad 331
Salicylates 868
Saline
- irrigation 260
- normal 578

Salivary gland
- diseases of 801, 803
- lymphomas 808
- major 803, 806
- pathology, surgical procedures for 809
- tumor 806, 807
  - majority of 806

Salivary neoplasm, benign 807
Salivary stone, composition of 805, 1082
Salivary tumor, malignant 807
Salmonella 162, 343
- typhi 314

Sandwich technique 746
Sandy batches 895
Santorini duct 1073
Sapheno-femoral junction 709
- incompetent 694

Sapheno-popliteal junction 709
Sarcoidosis 87, 315
Sarcoma 93
Sarfeh's portocaval shunt 154
Sarin's classification 284, 1059
Satellite lesions 835
Saturday night palsy 952, 953
Scald 651
Scalp
- aplasia cutis of 501
- defects, reconstruction of 232
- ear-nipple syndrome 438
- injury 583

Scalpel, safe handling of 997
Scar
- abnormal 9
- contracture 662
- hypertrophic 8, 659, 662
- hypertrophied 8

Scarff-Bloom-Richardson grading system 457
Scarpa's fascia 766
Schistosoma haematobium infection 895
Schistosomiasis 315, 404, 894
- hepatic 894
- urinary 894

Sciatic hernia 716, 741, 743
- types of 743

Scleritis 308
Scleroderma 685, 830
Sclerosant 152, 258, 414
- therapy 258

Sclerosing cholangitis, primary 85, 93, 308
Sclerosis 453
- multiple 309
- systemic 87
- tuberous 561, 882
- variceal 152

Sclerotherapy 414, 820
- antegrade 762
- complications of 698, 762
- mechanisms of action of 698
- retrograde 762
- types of 698

Scoop approach 1075
Screening tests 32
Scrotal diseases 766
Scrotal edema, idiopathic 759, 766
Scrotal skin, characteristic features of 767
Scrotectomy 767
- indications of 767

Scrotum 643, 756, 766
- acute 759, 760
- carcinoma of 766
- diseases of 752
- filarial 767

Seatbelt
- injury 572
- sign 622
- syndrome 622

Sebaceous horn 818
Seddon's classification 948
Sedentary lifestyle 667
Segmental nomenclature, Couinaud system of 109
Segmentectomy 142
Selective estrogen
- down regulators 478
- receptor modulators 478

Selective neck dissection 969
Self-expanding metal stenting 364
Self-retaining retractor 1006
- uses of 1006

Semen analysis, abnormal 761
Seminoma 922, 925, 926
- cut section of 922
- mediastinal 923

Sengstaken-Blakemore tube application 281
Sensation, loss of 847
Sensory
- function 598
- loss 952
- neuropathy 846

Sentinel loop sign 165
Sentinel lymph node 461
- biopsy 469, 475, 476, 836
  - incisions for 477
  - indications of 475
  - techniques of 476

Sentinel piles 398
Sepsis 152, 348
- control of 368
- management of 659
- pelvic 348
- presence of 254
- transfusion related 37
- uncontrolled 152

Sequential organ failure assessment score 1068
Serafini's hernia 728, 749
Serial pneumatic dilation 780
Serological tests 246, 895
Seropurulent discharge, active 404
Serrated polyposis syndrome 354
Sertoli cell tumor 447
Serum lipase 166
- activity 166
- level 166

Serum tumor markers 924
- measurement of 923

Sessile polyp, resection of 352
Seton, types of 407
Sevoflurane 989
Sexually transmitted infections 761
Shamblin classification 971
- modified 971

Shave biopsy 836
Shearing injury 597
Shigella 343

Shock
  hypovolemic 297
  index 1076
    modified 1076
  obstructive 605
  septic 254
  wave break stones 872
  wave lithotripsy
    complications of 872
    contraindications of 872
Shoeshine maneuver 777
Short bowel syndrome 327
  etiologies of 328
Short gastric vessels
  division of 213
  ligation of 213
Short synacthen test 1079
Shouldice
  repair 724
  technique 722
Shunts, proximal 916
Sialadenitis 166, 804
  acute bacterial 804
  autoimmune 804
  sclerosing 234
  viral 804
Sialocele 813
Sialolithiasis 803, 805
Sickle cell
  anemia 701
  disease 210, 915, 916
Sigmoid
  colectomy 332, 333
  colon 363
    endoscopic fixation of 336
    resection of 336
  diverticulitis, classic presentation of 331
  end colostomy 429
  resection 397
  volvulus 334, 336
    X-ray signs in 335
Sigmoidopexy 336
Sigmoidoplasty
  extraperitoneal 335
  intraperitoneal 335
Sigmoidoscopy 353
Signet ring cell
  adenocarcinoma 357
  carcinoma 265
Silastic stent 95
Silent thyroiditis 508, 509
Silodosin 902
Silver sulfadiazine 657
Simple clinical colitis activity index 345
Sinus 841, 852
  persistence of 853
  tachycardia 496
  tract 416
Sister Mary Joseph nodule 838
Sistrunk's operation 973
Sjögren syndrome 804
Skeletal defects 891
Skin
  assessment 850
  breakdown 697
  cancer, common 829
  care of 659
  closure 526
    techniques of 1015, 1016
  cystic lesions of 818
  diseases of 816
  graft 658, 1078
    full-thickness 658
    thickness of 1078
  hyperpigmentation of 550
  incision 933
  infection 824, 826
  manifestations 308
  metastases 838
  perianal 402, 430
  preparation 992
  sparing mastectomy 471
  stapler 1016
  substitutes, permanent 658
  temperature 675
  tension lines 1078
Skip lesions 305
Skull
  bone 537
    fracture 582
  fracture 583, 584
  osteoma of 353
Sluggish peristaltic sound 253
Small bore chest drains 609
Small bowel
  bleeding 369, 370
  endoscopy 325
  imaging 309
  injury 622
  obstruction 294, 298
  polypectomy 350
  volvulus 298
Small capsular laceration 631
Small intestinal obstruction 294, 298
  causes of 294
Small intestine 323
  acquired diverticula of 319
  lipoma of 323
  neoplasm of 323
  polyposis of 350
  true diverticulum of 320
Smoking 7, 667
  cessation of 332, 502, 679
Smooth muscle
  antibodies 86
  cells 668
  recruitment 668
Snip open vesicle 656
Snodgrass modification 914
Snowflake sign 127
Sodium morrhuate 258
Soft tissue
  infection 826
    non-necrotizing 826
  injuries 591
  necrosis 739
Solid mass lesion 923
Solid organ injury 617
Solitary adrenal mass, finding of 547
Solitary thyroid nodule 506
Somatostatin receptor scintigraphy 562, 564
Somatostatinoma 561, 565
Sorafenib 226
Spades sign, ace of 335
Spatulation 636
Speculum, rectal 1011
Speech difficulty 980
Spencer Well's hemostatic forceps 998
Sperm banking 924
Spermatic cord 923
Spermatocele 766
Spherocytosis, hereditary 210
Sphincter sacrificing procedures 406
Sphincter, external 403
Sphincteroplasty 420
  transduodenal 74
Sphincterotomy 68, 77, 400
  calibrated 400
  chemical 399
  closed 400
  endoscopic 68, 99, 259
  lateral internal 400
  open 400
Spigelian fascia 740
Spilled gallstones, complications of 58
Spinal artery, anterior 598
Spinal cord
  injury 339, 581
    incomplete 599
    neurological classification of 598
    types of 599
  lesion 846
Spinal immobilization 598
Spinal injury 597
  evaluation of 600
  management of 598, 600
Spine
  immobilization 575
  examination of 598
  fracture of 690
Spinothalamic tract, damage of 599
Spiral intestinal lengthening and tailoring 327, 329
Spironolactone 447, 547
Spleen 205, 208, 863

abscess of 210
accessory 209
central area of 631
cysts of 212
functions of 208
peliosis of 212
preservation of 629
thalassemic 210
tumors of 212
Splenectomy 209-211, 213, 631
common indications of 210
complications of 214
elective 215
emergency 215
iatrogenic 210
incidental 210, 211
indications of 210
laparoscopic 213, 214, 631
minimally invasive approaches of 213
partial 213, 631
staging 210
Splenic artery
aneurysm 210, 211, 685
distribution of 207
ligation of 214
Splenic autologous transplantation 631
Splenic flexure 363
Splenic pedicle, ligation of 214
Splenic vein thrombosis 181, 210
Splenomegaly
massive 210, 212
mild 212
moderate 212
Splenoplexy 209
Splenorenal shunt, proximal 154
Splenosis 209
Split-thickness skin graft 640
donor sites for 658
Split-wall sign 335
Sporadic gastrinoma 563
Sporadic hamartomatous polyp 349
characteristic features of 349
Sporadic medullary thyroid carcinoma 520
surgery for 522
Squamous cell carcinoma 93, 357, 430, 701, 794, 818, 831, 895, 897, 899, 1079
invasive 430
risk factors for 794
superficially invasive 1084
Stab wound 611, 613, 614
Stafne's bone cavity 804
Stafne's bone cyst 804
Staghorn calculus 868, 871
Standard anesthetic protocol 992
Stanford classification 1059
Staphylococcal infection 824
Staphylococcus 766, 824
aureus 116, 804, 825
Staplers, types of 432
Starch microspheres 145
Stasis 44
zone of 654
Statin therapy 709
Steatorrhea 180
Stemmer's sign 704
Stenosis 62, 294
pulmonary 490
Stensen's duct 803
Stent
complications of 798
dysfunction 97
migration 97, 152
occlusion 97
types of 798
Stereotactic body radiation therapy 140
Sterile 763
Sterilization 996
Sternotomy wound 8
Steroidal aromatase inhibitors 478
Steroids 7
anabolic 447
Stewart-Treves syndrome 838
Stewart-Way classification 61, 63
Stierlin sign 316
Stiffness 957
Stigmata, high-risk 189
Stoma 366, 367, 426, 624
Stomach 280
adenocarcinoma of 264
diseases of 239
gastrointestinal stromal tumor of 264
injuries 618
malignant neoplasms of 264
proximal 275
regional lymph nodes of 270
Stone
biliary 68
extraction 68
instruments used for 68
formation 80, 84, 867
intrahepatic 77, 111, 113
peripheral, presence of 77
radiolucent 868
removal of 873
types of 43
Stool antigen test 246
Straddle
fracture 640
injuries 640
Strangulation
features of 297
increased risk of 742
obstruction 296
pathophysiology of 296
Strasberg classification 61, 1059
Strawberry
gallbladder 53
nevus 820
Streptococcus milleri 116
Stress 311
ulcer 1080
prophylaxis 655
Stretta procedure 778
Stricture formation 84
Stricturoplasty 312
indications of 312
types of 312
Stridor 577
String sign 316
String technique 641
Stroke 339
Stromal development 453
Struvite calculi 870
Struvite stones 868
formation 868
Stump appendicitis 385
Sturge-Weber syndrome 820
Stuttering priapism 915
management of 916
Subarachnoid space 985
Subclavian arterial occlusion, management of 676
Subclavian steal syndrome 676
Subclavian subclavian bypass 676
Subcostal nerve 1082
Subcutaneous onlay laparoscopic approach 732
Subcutaneous rapid acting insulin 1078
Subfascial endoscopic perforator ligation 700
Subhyoid 973
Sublingual gland 803
ducts of 803
excision of 809
neoplastic lesion of 809
tumor 806
Submandibular duct 809
Submandibular gland 803, 805
excision of 810
Submandibular stone, surgical management of 805
Substance abuse 143
Subvesical duct 1071
Succinylcholine 988
Sugarbaker technique, laparoscopic modified 746
Sulfasalazine 346
Sulfur granules 852
Sump syndrome 73
Sunburn sensitivity 1056
Sunderland's classification 948
Sunitinib 280, 489, 886
Superficial dermal burn 657
Superficial epidermal burn 657

Superficial femoral artery 1086
Superficial inguinal dissection 920
Superior laryngeal nerve 1074
injury, external branch of 527
Superior lumbar triangle 740
boundaries of 740
Superior thyroid vessels
dissection of 526
ligation of 526
Supraduodenal bile duct 1071
Suprahyoid 973
Supramesocolic space 227
Surgery 294, 449, 501
abdominal 295
general 296
indications of 256, 281, 822
laparoscopic 1082
radical 128
types of 184, 273
Surgical abdominal decompression 645
Surgical drainage
approaches of 118
indications of 118
Surgical energy, fundamental use of 942
Surgical gut 1012
Surgical management 87, 399, 563, 601, 870
principles of 222, 786
Surgical site infection, sources of 1070
Surgical wound, classification of 4
Suture
material
length of 735
properties of 1011
rectopexy, posterior 395-397
repair 222, 237, 729, 733, 737
selection, principles of 1012
Swelling 722, 763, 768, 957
appears 237
cystic 223
labial 639
nonneoplastic 819
oral mucosal 309
pseudocystic 819
scrotal 766
testicular 726, 760
transilluminant scrotal 762
unilocular 819
Swimmer's itch 895
Swollen leg 694
Sydney system 262
Synovial sheath 958
Synthetic monofilament suture 612
Syphilis 682
Systemic inflammatory response syndrome 167
Systemic lupus erythematosus 234, 701
Systemic therapy 140, 524

T

Tachyarrhythmia 557
Takayasu's arteritis 686
Takihara orchidometer 761
Talk and die syndrome 1083
Tamoxifen 226, 452, 469, 478
therapy 449
Tamsulosin 902
Tangential excision 658
Tanner's operation 283
Taper cut needle 1005
TAPP repair 726
Taylor procedure 249
Tear, longitudinal 398
Teduglutide 327
Teeth, supernumerary 353
Telangiectasia, hereditary hemorrhagic 134
Telangiectatic hepatocellular adenoma 135
Telescope 935
length of 935
Temporary abdominal closure, techniques of 646
Temporary plastic biliary stent 74
Tenderness, abdominal 253, 339
Tendon 1070
injury 959
sheaths 958
pneumothorax 578, 603, 605
Teratoma 923
cut section of 923
cystic 238
types of 923
Terazosin 556, 902
Terblanche classification 1059
Terminal ileum, intubation of 309
Testicular failure, secondary 447
Testicular prosthesis 760
placement of 924
Testicular tenderness, generalized 759
Testicular tumor 765, 925
classification of 922
Testicular volume 761
measurement of 761
Testicular workup 759
Testis 755, 761, 766, 770, 923
appendix 760
atrophic 756
bilateral nonpalpable 757
cryptorchid 756
diseases of 752
ectopic 754
examination of 756
germ cell tumors of 447
hard 760
high lie of 759
intra-abdominal 756
retractile 755
rupture of 643
salvaging 643
sparing surgery 924
strictures of 447
torsion of 756
undescended 754, 757
vanishing 755, 756
Testosterone 449
Tetanus prophylaxis 655
Tetany 543
Tetracaine 986
Tetracyclines, oral mucosal 825
Thalassemia 210, 701
major 210
Theophylline 447
Therapeutic central neck dissection 516
Therapeutic flexible endoscopy, timing of 792
Thermal ablation 140
mechanisms of action of 698
Thermal therapy
contact method of 258
noncontact 258, 370
Thiazide diuretics 21, 25
Thickened hyalinized collagen 1084
Thiersch procedure 396
Thiersch-Duplay technique 914
Thiopurines 310, 346
Thomas sign 192
Thoracic anastomosis, advantages of 797
Thoracic damage control
surgery 612
basic principles of 612
techniques 612
Thoracic duct injury 596
Thoracic esophagus
perforation, management of 786
upper 797
Thoracic injury, life-threatening 603
Thoracic perforation 784, 785
Thoracic trauma 602
Thoracoabdomen 613
Thoracoabdominal staplers 432
Thoracoscopy 931
Thoracotomy 607, 797
anterolateral 797
Thrombin 258
Thromboangiitis obliterans 679
Thrombocytopenia 33
Thromboelastometry 39
rotational 33
Thromboembolic prevention 1080
Thrombolytic therapy 673
Thrombophlebitis 762
migrans 689
superficial 689
Thromboprophylaxis 692
Thrombosis 670, 683

Thrombotic thrombocytopenic purpura 210
Thyroglobulin 514
 estimation, postoperative 516
Thyroglossal cyst 973
Thyroglossal duct, part of 973
Thyroid 524
 acropachy 496
 associated orbitopathy 497
 cancer 513, 523
 carcinoma 513, 514, 523
  papillary 514
  radiation-induced 513
 cytopathology 507
 disease 1075
 disorders of 487, 489
 failure, primary 491
 gland 508
  dysgenesis 490
 hormone 490, 516
  factitious ingestion of 492
  replacement, postoperative 516
 imaging reporting and data system scoring 1068
 malignancy
  primary 512
  secondary 512
 malignant neoplasms of 512
 neoplasm 512
  benign 512
 nodule 506
  functions of 517
  sonographic pattern of 506
  types of 506
 papillary carcinoma of 1079
 scan 973
 scintigraphy 517
 stimulating antibodies, elevated 500
 storm 502
 surgery 527, 528
  complications of 526
 swelling 505
  diffuse 523
  large 523
 tissue, heterotopic 1074
 vein, middle 525
Thyroidectomy 502, 516, 527, 528, 1075
 basic steps of 525
 completion 515, 519
 near-total 523
 prophylactic total 522
 subtotal 501
Thyroiditis 492, 508
 acute 508
 autoimmune 234, 509
 chronic lymphocytic 509
 invasive fibrous 511
 painless 492
 postpartum 509
 subacute 492, 508
  granulomatous 508
  lymphocytic 508, 509
 suppurative 508
Thyrotoxic phase, treatment of 509
Thyrotoxicosis 492, 497, 500
 causes of 492
 signs of 500
 symptoms of 500
Tibia 690
Tibial occlusive disease 678
Tidy wound 3
Tietze syndrome 451
Tillaux's sign 231
Tillaux's triad 231
Tissue
 adhesives 35
  topical 1015
 based reconstruction 474
 injury, deep 851
 repair, primary 722-724
 resistance 660
 retrieval, best option for 90
 sealants 258
 transfer procedure 911
 type 433
T-lymphocytes 5
Tobacco use 794
Tocolytics 21
Toe-brachial index 704
Toes, papillary carcinoma of 23
Tofacitinib 346
Tongue, lateral 1087
Toremifine 226
Torsion, increased risk of 209
Total abdominal colectomy 348
 complications of 348
Total leukocyte count 67
Total mesorectal excision 421, 424
 advantages of 424
 principles of 424
Total pericystectomy
 closed 128
 open 128
Total proctocolectomy 348
 complications of 347, 348
Total thyroidectomy 501, 515, 516, 519, 522, 1075
 advantages of 515
Tourniquet use 578
Towel clip 996
Toxicity, systemic 984
Toxoplasma 162
Trabucco technique 723
Tracheobronchial injuries 603, 609
Tracheostomy 523
 tube 851, 1016
Traction injury 951
Tranexamic acid 39
 pre-emptive use of 578
Transanal colonoscopic decompression tube placement 340
Transanal endoscopic microsurgery 424
Transanal minimally invasive surgery 424
Transanal total mesorectal excision 428
Transcystic common bile duct exploration 69, 70
Transforming growth factor alpha, role of 281
Transfusion reaction
 acute adverse 36
 delayed 36
Transgender 1085
Transient responders 627, 632
Transinguinal preperitoneal repair 724
Transitional cell 897
 carcinoma 888
 papilloma 896
Transjugular intrahepatic portosystemic shunt 152
Transmural inflammation 305
Transnasal ultrathin endoscope 795
Transoral incisionless fundoplication 778
Transoral ultrathin endoscope 795
Transosseous wiring 593
Transperitoneal approach 558, 684
Transplantation, intestinal 327, 329
Transrectus preperitoneal approach 724
Transurethral microwave thermotherapy 904
Transversalis fascia 718
 failure of 717
Transverse colon
 mid part of 362
 right part of 362
Transversus abdominis 737, 739
Trastuzumab 480, 796
Trauma 447, 570, 572
 abdominal 613
 deaths 573
 management system 573, 627
 maxillofacial 590
 penetrating 611, 613
 penile 915
 pulmonary 1080
 quality improvement program 38
 renal 634
 splenic 210, 630
 ureteral 636, 637
Traumatic aortic disruption 603
Traumatic brain injury 582, 589
 mild 588
 moderate 588
 severe 588
Traumatic diaphragmatic injury 603
Treitz ligament 317
Trendelenburg's operation 699, 710
Trendelenburg's test 694
Trephine stoma 429

Trichobezoars 283, 302
Triglyceride level 707
Triphasic waveform 676
Triple-A syndrome 778
Tris-acyl gelatin microspheres 144
Troisier's sign 968
Trophozoites enter periportal sinusoids 119
Trousseau's sign 23, 543
Trousseau's syndrome 689
Troxerutin 697
Truncal vagotomy 249
T-tube 72, 74, 1009
  placement 71
    complications of 72
  refashioning of 72
  tract 98
Tube thoracostomy 604, 605, 707
Tuberculosis 315, 404, 442, 682, 853, 879
  abdominal 315
  ileocecal 316
  intestinal 315, 316
  visceral 315
Tubularization technique 914
Tubule formation 457
Tumors 134, 274, 275, 362, 363, 421, 423, 481, 926
  adrenal cortical 447
  assessment of 422, 431
  benign 111, 821, 881
    epithelial 807
    nonepithelial 807
  biopsy 884
  bleeding 271
  carcinoid 145, 324
  colorectal 356
  common benign 808
  debulking 340
  desmoid 226, 353, 818
  functional 971
  growth, different patterns of 897
  localization of 564
  location of 424, 425
  macroscopic appearance of 267
  malignant 812, 881
  metastatic 141, 324, 340, 881
  nonepithelial 808
  parotid 806
  perianal 430
  primary 559
  recurrent aggressive 226
  regression grade 1068
  resection of 972
  second primary 387
  size 279
  solid 195
  spread of 835, 884
  sternomastoid 972
  submandibular 806
  suppressor genes 135, 513
  testicular 765, 925
  universal 822
  unresectable 277
  urothelial 888
Tunica vaginalis, hydrocele of 763
Turcot's syndrome 353354,
Turner's syndrome 438
Twist scoring system 760
Tylosis 794
Typhoid
  enteritis 314
  ulcers 314
Tyrer-Cuzick model 455
Tyrosine kinase
  inhibitor 48, 226, 489
  therapy 280

U

Ugahary technique 724
Ulcer 251, 252, 259, 701, 841, 843, 846
  actinomycotic 852
  anastomotic 259
  arterial 844
  decubitus 849
  deep 844
  depth 848
  dressing, basic principles of 852
  ischemic 844
  marginal 289
  neuropathic 846
  refractory 248
  traumatic 844
  tubercular 316, 852, 854, 880
  types of 844
  venous 845
Ulcerative colitis 341, 344, 348, 351, 361, 373
  acute severe 346
  chronic refractory 347
  distinguishing features of 307
  endoscopic index 345
  initial presentation of 342
  severity of 342
  surgical options for 347
Ulcerative proctitis, mildly active 346
Ulnar bursa 958
  infections of 958
Ulnar nerve 952
  injury 959
Ulnar-mammary syndrome 438
Ultra-short bowel syndrome 329
Ultrasonography 52, 80, 304, 388, 450
  abdominal 331
  endoscopic 166, 194, 267, 272, 795, 796
  testicular 449
  transabdominal 163, 182
Ultrasound
  classification 127
  contrast-enhanced 190
  endoanal 431
  endoscopic 200, 309, 562, 564
Umbilical hernia 222, 714, 730, 732
  acquired 731, 732
  anatomical classification of 730
  congenital 730, 731
  infantile 222, 237
  large 732, 733
  repair
    incisions for 730
    surgical principles of 732
  sac 730
  types of 731
Umbilical port 57
Umbilical sinus 223
Umbilical vein 188
Umbilicus 733
Umbrella sign, inverted 316
Unconsciousness 988
Unilateral neck exploration 538, 539
Upper extremities, arterial occlusive disease of 676
Upper gastrointestinal
  bleeding 369
    endoscopic management of 258
  contrast series 319
  endoscopy 94, 245, 272, 344, 775
Urachus
  distal part of 224
  proximal part of 224
Urata formula 143, 1072
Urea breath test 246
Urease 242
  producing bacteria 866
Ureter 350
  congenital malformations of 861
  duplication of 862
  mobilization of 636
  omental wrapping of 235
  postcaval 864
  urothelial tumors of 888
Ureteral calculi 887
Ureteral catheter 888
Ureteral drainage 235
Ureteral injury 636, 926
  repair of 636
Ureteral reimplantation 637
Ureteral stone, proximal 888
Ureteral trauma 636, 637
  iatrogenic 636
Ureterocele 864
Ureterolysis, surgical 235
Ureteroscopy, flexible 889
Urethra
  anterior 639, 640, 910
  bulbar 640

dimension of 1010
penile 640
posterior 639, 640, 910
Urethral catheterization 1010
complications of 1010
contraindications of 1010
major 1010
Urethral dilation 911
Urethral injury 639
causes of 639
clinical presentation suggestive of 639
iatrogenic causes of 639
staging of 640
Urethral stents 911
Urethral stricture 910
etiologies of 910
sites of 910
Urethroplasty 911, 914
anastomotic 912
complications of 912
Urethrorrhagia 639
Uric acid 868
stone 868, 870
formation 868
Urinalysis 901
Urinary bladder 350, 894, 899
Urinary catecholamines 551
Urinary catheter 290, 993, 1009
Urinary cytology 889
Urinary incontinence 910
Urinary retention 639
Urinary stone
classification of 869
recurrence of 875
Urinary stream, interruption of 893
Urinary tract infection, symptoms of 893
Urine 870
culture 907
examination 878, 881
microscopic examination of 895
pH, low 868
Urochrome 1079
Urodynamic study 394
Uroflowmetry 902
Urogenital remnant cyst 231
Urography, intravenous 865
Urology 856
Ustekinumab 310
Uveitis 308

V

Vacuum-assisted biopsy 462
Vacuum-assisted closure
system, components of 13
therapy 12, 13
Vagal transection, incomplete 285
Vaginal hydrocele, primary 763
Vaginal introitus 639
Vaginal laceration 639
Vagotomy 249
highly selective 249
selective 249, 250, 285
supradiaphragmatic 249
Vague abdominal pain 324
Valentino syndrome 380
Valsalva maneuver 733, 761
Valve
anomalies, congenital 686
dysfunction of 348
prolapse 348
Vancomycin 33
Vancouver scar scale 1068
Vandetanib 489
Variceal hemorrhage
management of 156
treatment of 284
uncontrollable 152
Varicella zoster virus 339
Varicocele 761
bilateral palpable 761
clinical grading of 761
repair
complications of 762
inguinal approach of 762
Varicose vein 693, 696, 709, 820
Vas deferens 718
Vas rectae penetrate circular muscle 330
Vascular catheter, contamination of 1070
Vascular clamp 629
use of 596
Vascular disease, aneurysmal 681
Vascular injuries 688, 726, 960
management of 595, 633
Vascular lesion 259
Vascular thrombosis 409
Vascular trauma 688
consequences of 688
Vasoactive intestinal peptide-secreting tumor 565
Vasoconstriction 32
Vasoconstrictors, withdrawal of 681
Vasopressor support 681
Vater ampulla 319
Vecuronium 988
Vedolizumab 310, 346
Vein
compressibility, lack of 690
graft, cryopreserved 678
peripheral 1070
Velpeau's hernia 728, 749
Vena cava filter, inferior 692
Venous leg ulcer 701
management of 701
workup of 701
Venous system, duplex scanning of 696
Venous thrombosis 327
Ventilation 578
adequate 578
mask 851
Ventral mesh rectopexy 395-397
Ventricle 610
Ventricular mural thrombus 670
Ventricular septal defect 490
Venulitis 690
Verapamil 447
Veress needle 50
insertion angle of 933
placement of 933
Vertical compression 597
Vertical rectus abdominis muscle flap 426
Vessels 718
Vibration white finger 1086
Vicryl mesh 631
Video capsule endoscopy 325
Video-assisted anal fistula treatment 408
Video-assisted retroperitoneal debridement 171
Villous atrophy, congenital 327
Vinblastine 226, 690
Virchow's node 968
Virchow's triad 690
Virilizing signs 550
Viscera, herniated 220, 221
Visceral artery aneurysm 685
Viscoelastic tests 1081
Viscous saliva 1082
Visick score 1068
Vismodegib 830
Visual infusion phlebitis score 1068
Vitamin 7
A 7
B_{12}
deficiency anemia 319
level, monitoring of 277
C 659
D 908
K
deficiency 32, 33
parenteral 33
low serum level of lipid soluble 181
Vitelline duct 320
cell lining of 320
Vitellointestinal duct anomalies 223
Vitiligo 511
Vocal cord
assessment of 515
injection technique 951
medialization, open 951
Voice therapy 951
Voltage electrical injuries 652
Volvulus
development of 337
double 338
mesenteroaxial 282
organoaxial 282
secondary 283

Vomiting 297, 1084
postoperative 992
von Ebnar gland 1082
von Hippel Lindau syndrome 134, 561
von Meyenburg complexes 133
von Recklinghausen's disease 236, 823
V-Y advancement flap 419

W

Waldeyer's fossa 747
Wallace's rule of nines 653
Walled-off necrosis 164, 166, 171, 176
Wandering spleen 209, 283
Wantz technique 724
Warfarin therapy 32
Warm nodule 506
Warren shunt 154
Warthin's tumor 808
Water-Lily sign 127
Water-soluble contrast enema 339
Watertight mucosa-to-mucosa anastomosis 636
Watson dysphagia scale 1069
WDHA syndrome 565
Weakness
acquired 713
congenital 713
Webspace infection 958
Wegener's granulomatosis 234
Weight loss 94, 281, 308, 332, 779
Wells procedure
modified 396
original 396
Wermer's syndrome 566
Whipple procedure 196
Whipple triad 562
Whirl sign 335, 337
White light
cystoscopy 898
endoscopy 793
White pulp 208
Will Rogers phenomenon 1079
Wilms' tumor 886
Wilson's disease 136
Windsock sign 319
Winslow hernia foramen 629, 747
Wire-guided localization 461, 462
Wireless video capsule endoscopy 324
Wirsung duct 1073
Wolff-Chaikoff effect 503
Worms, bag of 761
Wound 3, 10, 12
acute 3
assessment 10
bed preparation 10
biopsy 701
care 657
local 848
chronic 3
classification of 3
colonized 12
contraction 6
debridement 11
methods of 11
dehiscence 1070
dressing 12, 657
advantages of 657
edges, marsupialization of 406
exudate 10
types of 10
formation, mechanisms of 9
healing 1, 3, 7
abnormal 8
phases of 5
types of 4
hypoxia 7
hypoxic 7
infection 11, 1070
stages of 11
malignant 9
management 10, 661
open 4
perineal 426
repair 6
Wrist, dorsum of 819

X

Xanthine stone 868
Xanthinuria, hereditary 868
Xenograft 658
Xeroderma pigmentosum 265, 829, 830
Xiphoid 733
X-marks-the-spot sign 335
X-ray, abdominal 283

Y

Yersinia 38
Yolk sac tumor 923

Z

Zajdela technique 1078
Zarger endoscopic classification 790
Zenker diverticulum 782
Zig-zag pattern 329
Zinc deficiency 659
Zipper injuries 641
Zoledronic acid 24
Zollinger-Ellison syndrome 180, 241, 248
Z-plasty 419
Zubrod score 1069
Zuska disease 441